KINN'S

THE Administrative
Medical
Assistant
An Applied Learning Approach

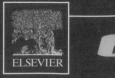

KINN'S

THE Administrative
Medical
Assistant

An Applied Learning Approach

SIXTH EDITION

Alexandra Patricia Young, BBA, RMA, CMA

Adjunct Instructor
Everest College, Arlington Midcities Campus
Arlington, Texas
Professional Writer
Grand Prairie, Texas

With over 270 illustrations

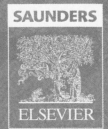

SAUNDERS

ELSEVIER

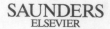

SAUNDERS
ELSEVIER

11830 Westline Industrial Drive
St. Louis, Missouri 63146

Executive Editor: Susan Cole
Developmental Editor: Celeste Clingan
Publishing Services Manager: Patricia Tannian
Project Manager: Sarah Wunderly
Senior Book Designer: Julia Dummitt

Printed in United States of America

Last digit is the print number: 9 8 7 6 5 4 3 2

DEDICATION

To my dad, J.W. Crumley, my grandmother, Lucille Saxton,
and to all of the healthcare professionals who cared for them during their illnesses.
Thank you for your dedication to medicine and to your patients.
To all medical assisting students who seek to improve their lives by helping others.

Alexandra Patricia Young, BBA, RMA, CMA

PREFACE

Medical assisting as a profession has changed dramatically since *The Administrative Medical Assistant* was first published in 1982. This updated sixth edition continues to represent a long-standing commitment to quality medical assisting education with its engaging, straightforward writing style and demonstrated positive outcomes. Hundreds of instructors in classrooms all across the country have used this text to teach thousands of students over the years. Many of these students have gone on to teach students of their own with this very same trusted resource. To continue the use and growth of this text and its features, the sixth edition has undergone a massive revision in an effort to offer the most comprehensive, up-to-date, and innovative approach to teaching this subject today. I appreciate the opportunity to explore the exciting field of medical assisting with you!

DISTINCTIVE FEATURES OF OUR APPROACH

This textbook has endured throughout the years because it has been able to keep pace with an ever-changing profession while producing students who are well trained and qualified to enter medical practices across the country. This dependability is why the market continues to rely on this text edition after edition. Underlying this dependability is a foundation of pedagogical features that has stood the test of time and that has been expanded and improved upon yet again in this new edition. Such features include the following:

- An easy-to-read, highly interactive writing style that engages students through practical applications of medical assistant competencies.
- An emphasis on skill development with procedural steps outlining each skill, supported by rationales that provide meaning to each step.
- A pedagogical framework based on the use of learning objectives, vocabulary terms, and supportive student supplements.
- A package of supportive materials to accommodate a wide variety of student learning types and instructor teaching styles.

NEW FEATURES IN THIS EDITION

The medical field is an ever-changing one, with constant advances in diagnostic procedures and treatment protocols.

Accrediting agencies, including the Committee on Accreditation of Allied Health Programs (CAAHEP) and the Accrediting Bureau of Health Education Schools (ABHES), place demands on faculty and medical assistant programs to maintain accreditation standards. The influence of current risk management practices and the potential of electronic technology as a resource for student and patient education have both complicated and expanded the opportunities available to medical assistant professionals.

To build on the long-established strengths of the Kinn textbook, the sixth edition expands and supplements the techniques used so successfully in past editions. The combined talents and backgrounds of the primary author and contributor have resulted in a text that adheres to the Kinn tradition while meeting the needs of a new generation of medical assistant educators and students. The result is an innovative text that comprehensively meets the educational and accreditation needs of all types of medical assistant programs while effectively training tomorrow's medical assisting professionals.

This edition of *Kinn's The Administrative Medical Assistant* incorporates a unique approach that is reflected in the subtitle: An Applied Learning Approach. It is believed that learning takes place only when students are engaged and when the learning requires something from them in response to information that is being imparted to them.

This "applied" theme is set up-front in the first chapter, which introduces students to the concepts of critical thinking and the impact of individual learning styles on student success. This in turn transitions into time management and problem-solving skills, as well as effective study skills and test-taking strategies. The text develops from there true to the original Kinn textbook, and is rounded out by the last chapter that helps students focus on preparing for and nurturing their career as a medical assistant.

This pedagogical theme and other new enhancements can be found throughout the book and its supplements in the following features:

- Each chapter opens with a Scenario related to the chapter's focus. This introduces students to a medical assistant and a situation, with questions to consider, that provide a way for students to directly apply concepts they are learning. These features challenge them to think about how they would behave and the decisions they would make in certain situations.

- Each chapter also opens with national curriculum competency tables that outline current competencies for CAAHEP and ABHES, two primary accrediting associations. Furthermore, within the chapters specific CAAHEP and ABHES competencies are identified within the Procedures to ensure that students attain the necessary requirements to achieve employment in the medical assisting profession.
- Throughout the chapter, Critical Thinking Applications are designed to allow the student to use a concept that has just been learned in the context of the overall chapter scenario. These exercises help students look at the big picture and consider various angles, or approaches, to the challenges in which they will eventually find themselves in the medical office. These exercises provide a wonderful opportunity for discussion and further reflection.
- Chapters end with a Summary of Scenario that identifies concepts for student focus, as well as a discussion, where relevant, of patient education as it relates to the chapter focus and concepts within the chapter. The answers to Scenario questions provide relevant information that the student may encounter as a professional in the field.
- Well-developed Learning Objectives emphasize the cognitive and performance objectives addressed in the chapter, and are summarized at the end of each chapter for student review of learning.
- The artwork throughout provides a more attractive textbook for student use. Many photographs better support the revised content and are relevant to the actual medical office. Many photographs were replaced with new images that show more updated equipment and better illustrate key procedural steps.
- Chapter 8 on computers has been revised and thoroughly updated to include timely information to reflect the more sophisticated computer systems found in today's busy medical practice. It provides easy-to-understand details about subjects such as the elements of microprocessors, an "inside-the-computer" section, file formats, Internet connectivity, networking basics, computer security, and ergonomics. The medical records management and health information chapters also include an in-depth discussion of computer-based medical records.
- More than any previous edition, customer service is stressed throughout the chapters. As patients become more involved in their healthcare, medical assistants must realize that the healthcare field is a service industry and that patients should be treated more like customers.
- New to this edition, the Office Environment and Daily Operations chapter provides information about procedures for managing an office, expenses involved in the operation of a medical office, proper waste management, and basic safety and security.
- Also new to this edition, the Privacy in the Physician's Office chapter explains how the HIPAA Privacy Rule benefits the healthcare industry and the patient, discusses rights of patients under the Privacy Rule, and what is expected of healthcare providers.
- New compliance regulations in medical billing and coding have lent a far greater emphasis on reimbursement than ever

before. The billing and coding unit has been expanded and updated and includes the following: basics of diagnostic coding, basics of procedural coding, basics of health insurance, and the health insurance claim form. Chapter 20 includes an introduction to and directions for using the new CMS 1500 (08/05 version) that will be required in April of 2007.
- The Connections heading at the end of each chapter integrates text content with accompanying ancillaries and Internet sites. These provide students and instructors with a means to enhance their understanding of chapter concepts as well as to stay current on medical news, trends, and industry developments.

EVOLVE

Stay current with trends, developments, and news in the medical field, as well as access additional chapter supplemental features, advice on your externship, interviewing techniques, and more through EVOLVE, the website that is provided complimentary to this textbook. This exciting website is an interactive learning environment that adds an incredibly powerful set of instructional resources to your classroom experience. EVOLVE works in coordination with Kinn's *The Administrative Medical Assistant: An Applied Learning Approach,* Sixth Edition, by providing Internet-based course content and Internet web links to reinforce and expand your learning experience.

In addition to the Evolve Learning Resources available to students, there is an entire suite of tools available to instructors that allows for communication between instructors and students, including discussion boards, e-mail, chat rooms, and more.

To access this comprehensive online resource, simply go to the EVOLVE Home Page at http://evolve.elsevier.com and enter your user name and password provided to you from your instructor. If your instructor has not set up a Course Management System, you can still access all the learning resources available free with this textbook by going to http://evolve.elsevier.com/Kinn/admin/.

EXTENSIVE SUPPLEMENTAL RESOURCES

The diversity of students, instructors, programs, institutions, and teaching environments using this textbook required that we develop an integrated, comprehensive, and flexible package of supplements to support Kinn's *The Administrative Medical Assistant: An Applied Learning Approach,* Sixth Edition. Each of these innovative supplements is designed to enhance the teaching and learning experience, with the outcome of producing students well equipped to pass any certification examination, and who will go on to experience successful professional careers in medical assisting. These supplements and their unique features include the following.

Student Software Program

The free CD-ROM that comes with your textbook includes three programs designed for you to apply the key content and skills you've learned throughout the textbook. The Medical

Assisting Competency Challenge provides realistic scenarios, with you making the decisions and getting feedback on each decision you make, plus a skill-building section that lets you practice both administrative and clinical competencies. All forms used throughout are included for reference in a format suitable for printing. The Anatomy and Physiology animations will help you strengthen your knowledge of the body and medical terminology. The Altapoint demo is derived from a real medical office software program and lets you practice front office skills on the computer.

Study Guide

This practical tool takes the "applied learning approach" to a whole new level, giving you the opportunity to apply the knowledge and skills you are learning in the textbook. Some of the outstanding features of this study guide include:

- Procedure checklists that serve as a valuable tool for checking your competency, as well as a tool for your instructor to gauge your skill level and proficiency for each skill in the textbook.
- A multitude of exercises to reinforce key content throughout the textbook, including vocabulary exercises that help you recall and apply medical terms.
- Coding applications, documentation scenarios, and telephone screening examples provide you with the opportunity to apply administrative concepts to clinical situations.
- Chapter quizzes at the end of each chapter exercise set allow you to further test your knowledge.
- Study tips for all medical assisting students, as well as a section on study tips specifically designed for ESL (English-as-a-Second-Language) students, written by an ESL consultant.
- A glossary of English-Spanish terms, based on the text glossary, gives students an excellent resource for working with patients who speak English as a second language. This glossary is likewise extremely helpful for those medical assisting students who themselves speak English as a second language.

Instructor's Resource Manual

This complete instructor teaching tool includes extensive curriculum materials in both print and electronic formats. Beginning and veteran instructors alike will be able to easily prepare their lectures, presentations, labs, and assessments with an extensive course syllabus, multiple course outlines, chapter Internet addresses, and ready-made tests for each chapter. Answer keys for all text and Student Study Guide questions are also included. In addition, special tips for instructors with ESL (English-as-a-Second-Language) students have been provided, written by an ESL consultant.

Test Bank

Our test bank provides an accurate and exhaustive source of test items for a wide variety of examination styles. It contains more than 1,000 questions, and is available in both printed and electronic format so you can easily prepare your quizzes and exams, tailored to your classroom format.

PowerPoint Presentation Slides

The instructor CD-ROM includes a PowerPoint viewer and a set of over 600 PowerPoint slides. The slides include a summary of key chapter material, and can easily be customized to support your lectures and enhance your classroom presentation. All slides have been formatted to reflect the text design, and include many images from the text. These slides can also be easily formatted within the PowerPoint program for student note taking or as overhead transparencies.

TEACH Lesson Plan Manual

The TEACH Lesson Plan Manual includes a print version of the lesson plan manual as well as a CD containing all TEACH resources. Assets are also available via the Evolve website. The TEACH Lesson Plan Manual provides instructors with customizable lesson plans and lecture outlines based on learning objectives. With these valuable resources, instructors will save valuable preparation time and create a learning environment that fully engages students in classroom preparation. The lesson plans are linked to each chapter and are divided into 50-minute units in a three-column format. Instructors will also have lecture outlines in PowerPoint with talking points, thought-provoking questions, and unique ideas for lectures. The **Instructor's Electronic Resource** on CD contains a test bank in ExamView with over 500 questions and PowerPoint slides.

KINN'S ADMINISTRATIVE MEDICAL ASSISTING ONLINE

Today's educational environment has the potential to be more interactive than ever before. The more resources available to facilitate learning, and the more varied those resources are, the greater the chances are for material to be comprehended and retained.

Kinn's Administrative Medical Assisting Online has been developed with this creative approach to education in mind. Offering a multidimensional experience that is not possible in a traditional classroom setting, these unique and innovative new products are complete courses that simulate the externship experience by creating a virtual medical practice where students have an opportunity to learn by doing.

Lessons draw on the text for reading assignments, then provide an opportunity for you to apply text content by entering the simulated environment, complete with an office manager who acts as your supervisor/mentor through the courses, other office personnel, physicians, and realistic patient cases. This environment is an exciting way for you to discover what it is like to work in the field of medical assisting before you ever enter your externship.

A wide range of visual, auditory, and interactive elements create this exciting environment and work together to amplify key learning objectives from the textbook, giving you the opportunity to practice key skills first by being guided through a practice of each skill, then by trying to perform that skill in a realistic application exercise. This combination of guided practice and application of skills gives you the confidence to perform these skills with competence in your classroom or on the job.

Providing a myriad of learning opportunities, Kinn's Administrative Medical Assisting Online accommodates diverse learning styles and circumstances through the use of a sophisticated learning management system that lets your instructor tailor the program's content either to support a traditional classroom learning experience or as a true distance education course. You log on through the Evolve portal to complete lessons, take quizzes and exams online, participate in threaded discussions, post assignments to your instructor, or chat with your instructor or fellow classmates, all from any location that has an Internet connection.

Alexandra Patricia Young

SPECIAL FEATURES

A **Scenario** at the beginning of each chapter is presented so that the student can think about a real-world situation when reading the chapter content.

Scenario questions provide a way for students to directly apply concepts they are learning and think about decisions they would make in certain situations.

Learning Objectives emphasize the cognitive and performance objectives presented in the chapter.

National Accreditation and Competencies and Content tables outline current competencies for CAAHEP and ABHES.

The Medical Assisting Profession
3

SCENARIO

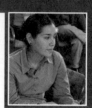

Sandra Rameriz is a single mother who has decided on medical assisting as a career. She has always been interested in the medical field and wants a job that will allow her to spend evenings and weekends with her 3-year-old son, Roberto. The idea of working in a physician's office appeals to her, and she has applied to a school that is close to her apartment and day care provider. She plans to attend day classes and work part-time after school until it is time to pick up her son.

Sandra is very excited about her new career and has set several goals for her training. First, she hopes to attain perfect attendance, and second, she would like to graduate with honors. She has budgeted her study time and plans to ask her instructors during the first 2 weeks of school for suggestions about how she can better prepare for classes and examinations. Sandra will find medical assisting to be a rewarding career and respected profession.

While studying this chapter, think about the following questions:

- What obstacles might prevent Sandra from attending all of her classes, and how can she prepare in advance to overcome them?
- How can Sandra begin to explore the type of physician offices in which she would enjoy being employed after graduation?

- What goals might Sandra have at the commencement of her training? At the end of training?
- How can Sandra make the most of her time attending school to become a medical assistant?

LEARNING OBJECTIVES

1. Define, spell, and pronounce the terms listed in the vocabulary.
2. Briefly discuss the history of medical assisting as a profession.
3. Differentiate between administrative and clinical medical assisting duties.
4. Discuss the versatility of a career in medical assisting.
5. Explain the reasons that hiring an individual who has no formal training is often more expensive than hiring a professional medical assistant.
6. Identify several considerations to keep in mind when choosing a position as a medical assistant other than financial compensation.
7. Discuss the aspects of the medical assistant's performance on a successful externship.
8. List three unacceptable behaviors on the externship site.
9. Explain why continuing education is so important to the medical assistant.
10. Discuss the difference between a CMA and an RMA.

National Accreditation Competencies and Content

ABHES COMPETENCIES	ABHES COMPETENCIES
Professionalism	**Communication**
1.a. Project a positive attitude	2.p. Professional components
1.b. Maintain confidentiality at all times	2.q. Allied health professions and credentialing
1.c. Be a "team player"	
1.d. Be cognizant of ethical boundaries	**Legal Concepts**
1.e. Exhibit initiative	5.f. Maintain licenses and accreditation
1.f. Adapt to change	
1.g. Evidence a responsible attitude	
1.h. Be courteous and diplomatic	
1.i. Conduct work within scope of education, training, and ability	

Each chapter contains **Vocabulary** with definitions.

Critical Thinking Application boxes are linked to the Scenario and prompt students to apply what they have learned at the end of major sections.

Illustrated step-by-step Procedures show how to perform and document administrative and clinical procedures encountered in the health-care setting.

Vocabulary page (UNIT ONE, page 36)

36   UNIT ONE   INTRODUCTION TO MEDICAL ASSISTING

VOCABULARY

allied health fields Occupational disciplines in which professionals involved with the delivery of healthcare or related services assist physicians with the diagnosis, treatment, and care of patients in many different specialty areas.

benefits Services or payments provided under a health plan, employee plan, or some other agreement, including programs such as health insurance, pensions, retirement planning, and many other options that may be offered to employees of a company or organization.

certification (ser-tuh-fuh-ka'-shun) The attesting of something as being true, as represented, or as meeting a standard; the result of having been tested, usually by a third party, and awarded a certificate based on proven knowledge.

continuing education units (CEUs) Credits for courses, classes, or seminars related to an individual's profession, designed to promote education and to keep the professional up to date on current procedures and trends in his or her field; CEUs are often required for licensing.

cross-training Training in more than one area so that a multitude of duties may be performed by one person or so that substitutions of personnel may be made in an emergency or at other necessary times.

externship or internship A training program that is part of a course of study of an educational institution and is taken in the actual business setting of that field of study; the terms are often interchanged in reference to medical assistant training.

intangibles (in-tan'-juh-buls) Qualities that are incapable of being perceived, especially by touch, or incapable of being precisely identified or realized by the mind.

invasive Involving entry into the living body as by incision or insertion of an instrument.

perks Extra advantages or benefits from working in a specific job that may or may not be commonplace in that particular profession; a shortened form of *perquisites*.

phlebotomy (fli-bah'-tuh-me) The invasive procedure used to obtain a blood specimen for testing, experimentation, or diagnosis of disease.

profit sharing Offer of a part of a company's profits to employees or other designated individuals or groups.

stock options Offers of stocks for purchase to a certain group of individuals or certain groups, such as employees of a for-profit hospital.

versatile (vur'-suh-til) Embracing a variety of subjects, fields or skills; having a wide range of abilities.

According to the U.S. Department of Labor's *Outlook Handbook,* medical assisting is pr one of the fastest growing occupations i States over the 2004-2014 period. Much of this result of the increase in the number of group prac and other facilities that need a high number of su nel. This makes the flexible medical assistant wh both clinical and administrative duties particularl the physician.

A career as a medical assistant is challengin job satisfaction, opportunities for service, financi possibilities for advancement. Men and women c successful as medical assistants. Individuals co medical assisting discipline must be dedicated an and must have a strong desire to become caregive are people who have the ability to put the needs first and have a sincere concern for those who ar

---

Clinical page (UNIT SIX, page 626)

626   UNIT SIX   FUNDAMENTALS OF CLINICAL MEDICAL ASSISTING

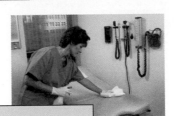

and recording vital signs. During the examination, the physician may expect the medical assistant to do the following:

- Hand instruments and equipment as requested and provide supplies as needed.
- Alter the position of a gooseneck lamp to better illuminate the area being examined, and turn lights off and on during specific phases of the examination.
- Position and drape the patient during the different phases of the examination.
- Assist in collecting and properly labeling specimens such as urine, Pap smear samplings, and throat cultures.
- Conduct follow-up diagnostic procedures as ordered including an **electrocardiogram** (ECG), eye or ear screening, urinalysis, and phlebotomy.
- Schedule postexamination diagnostic procedures such as a mammogram, x-ray examination, or **colonoscopy**.

CRITICAL THINKING APPLICATION

Felicia's first patient for the day is Harry Garcia, a 51-year-old truck driver who is scheduled for a complete physical examination. Mr. Garcia's insurance has changed since his last visit. The physician ordered an ECG to be performed and a complete blood panel to be drawn before the physical. What does Felicia need to complete before Dr. Kosto sees the patient?

Supplies and Instruments Needed for the Physical Examination

The instruments typically used during the physical examination are displayed in Figure 31-2. They enable the physician to see, feel, inspect, and listen to parts of the body. All equipment must be in good working order, properly disinfected, and readily available for the physician's use during the examination. The instruments most frequently used for the physical examination are described in the following paragraphs. Physical examinations are typically conducted from the head to the feet; the instruments are listed in the order in which the physician would typically request them.

Ophthalmoscope. An ophthalmoscope is used to inspect the inner structures of the eye. It has a stainless-steel handle containing batteries, onto which a head is attached. The head is equipped with a light and magnifying lenses and an opening through which the eye is viewed. Examination rooms are usually equipped with wall-mounted electrical units for the ophthalmoscope and otoscope, a dispenser for disposable speculums, and a wall-mounted sphygmomanometer (Figure 31-3).

Tongue Depressor. A tongue depressor is a flat, wooden blade used to hold down the tongue when examining the throat (Figure 31-4).

Otoscope. An otoscope is used to examine the external auditory canal and tympanic membrane. It has a stainless-steel handle containing batteries or is part of a wall-mounted electrical unit (see Figure 31-3). The head of the otoscope contains a light that is focused through a magnifying lens and should be covered with disposable ear speculum. The light may also be used to illuminate the nasal passages and throat.

Procedure page (UNIT EIGHT, page 896)

896   UNIT EIGHT   ASSISTING WITH MEDICAL SPECIALTIES

PROCEDURE 41-4

Prepare Patient for and Assist with Routine and Specialty Examinations: Obtain Pediatric Vital Signs and Vision Screening

CAAHEP COMPETENCIES: 3.b.(4)(b), 3.b.(4)(e)
ABHES COMPETENCIES: 4.d, 4.h

GOAL: To accurately obtain vital signs for and assess vision of a pediatric patient.

EQUIPMENT and SUPPLIES

- Digital or tympanic thermometer
- Pediatric blood pressure cuff
- Wristwatch with sweep second hand
- Weight scale with height bar
- Stethoscope
- Snellen E eye chart and oculator
- Pen
- Patient's chart

PROCEDURAL STEPS

1. Gather equipment.
   PURPOSE: Efficiency.
2. Wash your hands.
   PURPOSE: Infection control.
3. Explain the procedure to the parent, and if you want the parent to help by holding the child, explain the technique you want him or her to employ.
   PURPOSE: Explanations ahead of time save time and enhance cooperation.
4. Help the child stand in the center of the scale, and weigh the child. Ask the child to turn around, and obtain the child's height. Record your findings.
5. Obtain tympanic or axillary temperature using the procedure explained in Chapter 30 (Figure 1).
6. Record the temperature. Indicate the method used: A = axillary, T = tympanic.
   PURPOSE: A procedure is not done until it is recorded in the patient's record.
7. Place the stethoscope on the child's chest at the midpoint between the sternum and the left nipple. Listen for the apical beat (Figure 2).

8. Count the apical beat for 1 full minute.
9. Record the apical pulse. Be sure to place an Ap before the rate to indicate that this is an apical pulse reading.
   PURPOSE: A procedure is not done until it is recorded on the patient's record.
10. Place your flat hand on the child's chest, and count the respirations for 1 full minute.
11. Record the respiration rate.
    PURPOSE: A procedure is not done until it is recorded on the patient's record.
12. Check to be sure that you have the correct-size blood pressure cuff, then proceed with taking the blood pressure. Follow procedure in Chapter 30 (Figure 3).
13. Record the blood pressure.
    PURPOSE: A procedure is not done until it is recorded in the patient's record.
14. If vision screening is to be done, familiarize the child with the E chart by asking him to make an E point the same way as your

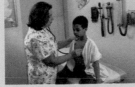

FIGURE 2

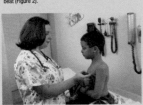

FIGURE 1

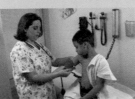

FIGURE 3

Continued

n table.

on according to office policy. In to make a copy of the patient's atient first enters the office or y changes in insurance infor-een to the office regularly. urine and blood if they have ysician. t, weight, body mass index

tigation into the reason for the patient the examination nswer patient questions about y fears. e needs to empty the bladder cause a full bladder may inter-s well as be uncomfortable for

prepare for the examination. clothing should be removed, on the gown (open either to pending on the type of exam-ape to ensure patient privacy.

ence of events, explain what is maintain patient privacy and

he chart, completing all forms

n the designated area for the rt holder on the examination that no identifiable patient rding to the Health Insurance bility Act (HIPAA), patient ted at all times. he medical assistant should ician complete the physical and efficiently as possible. room so all equipment and d working order and prepared d information and measuring

- Reinforce the instructions the physician gave the patient.
- Be sure you are comfortable performing a procedure.
- If you have any concerns about a procedure, discuss them with the physician privately before proceeding.
- Do not perform a procedure if you are uncomfortable; get someone to help you.

Always remember: You are the assistant, and this is the physician's patient. The physician is ultimately responsible for every aspect of the patient's care. If you feel uncertain or unsure of any order that the physician has written for a patient, you must get it clarified before you proceed. Always stay within the legal and ethical guidelines of the medical assisting profession in your state.

SUMMARY OF SCENARIO

Kaiwan is becoming more and more comfortable in his position as an orthopedic medical assistant at the sports medicine clinic. His enthusiasm is contagious. Patients consistently comment on his positive, upbeat manner. Kaiwan is motivated to learn new things and methods for better assisting the physicians with routine procedures. He always seeks answers to questions that occur with new patients. He has gained a great deal of confidence and now remembers to always check the paraffin bath temperature before starting a treatment. One of the most enjoyable aspects of his job continues to be assisting Dr. Alexander with treating the team members. Kaiwan has attended two sports medicine continuing education seminars with Dr. Alexander. He is now thinking about continuing his education part-time to become an athletic trainer while continuing to work at the clinic. Kaiwan recognizes the importance of continuing education in maintaining orthopedic skills.

At the end of the chapter, the Summary of Scenario provides students with relevant information that they may encounter as a professional in the field.

SUMMARY of LEARNING OBJECTIVES

1. Define, spell, and pronounce the terms listed in the vocabulary.
   * Spelling and pronouncing medical terms correctly adds credibility to the medical assistant. Knowing the definition of these terms promotes confidence in communication with patients and co-workers.
2. Describe the principal structures of the musculoskeletal system and their functions.
   * The main structures of the musculoskeletal system include the skeletal muscles, which provide movement; tendons, which connect muscles to bones; bones, which provide support, protection, mineral storage, and blood cell development; and ligaments, which connect bone to bone.
3. Differentiate among tendons, bursae, and ligaments.
   * Tendons are the tough bands that connect muscles to bones; ligaments provide support by connecting bone to bone and preventing a joint from moving beyond its normal ROM. Bursae prevent friction between different tissues in the musculoskeletal system.
4. Summarize the major muscular disorders.
   * Fibromyalgia is a condition of unknown origin that causes widespread connective tissue and muscular pain with sleep disorders and extreme fatigue. Myasthenia gravis is an autoimmune disorder that affects the use of ACh at the neuromuscular junction, resulting in muscular weakness, especially in the face and eyes. A sprain is the tearing of ligaments and a strain is the overstretching or tearing of a muscle or tendon.
5. Identify and describe the common types of fractures.
   * The common types of fractures are explained in Table 42-3.

6. Explain the difference between osteomalacia and osteoporosis.
   * Osteomalacia is the softening of bone because of a problem with the metabolism or absorption of vitamin D, calcium, and phosphorus; in children the condition is called *rickets*. Osteoporosis is a decrease in bone density caused by many factors including lack of dietary calcium earlier in life; it leads to brittle bones that easily fracture.
7. Classify typical spinal column disorders.
   * Spinal column disorders are related to the shape of the spine; scoliosis is a lateral deviation, lordosis or swayback is a pronounced curve of the lower back, kyphosis is a pronounced cervical curve or hunchback.
8. Differentiate among the various joint disorders.
   * Joint disorders include dislocations when the two bones of the joint are no longer approximated; gout, which is a form of arthritis caused by a collection of uric acid crystals most commonly in the synovial membrane of the great toe; SLE, which is a widespread autoimmune disorder that can affect any organ system in the body; Lyme disease, a form of infectious arthritis that is caused by ba... and that can result in exten... if left untreated; OA, caused... cartilage of synovial joints; R... causes crippling pain and d... and bursitis, which are infla... tissue that are typically caus...
9. Summarize the medical assista... procedures.
   * The medical assistant is res...

Summary of Learning Objectives reviews important points of the chapter's focus, reinforcing content students must master.

SUMMARY of LEARNING OBJECTIVES
Continued

rapid, weak, and thready pulse; tachypnea; and altered levels of consciousness. If the process is not reversed, the central nervous system becomes depressed and acute renal failure may occur.
10. Summarize the characteristics of common vascular disorders.
   * Varicose veins are dilated, tortuous, superficial veins in the legs that develop because the valves do not completely close, allowing blood to flow backward, thus causing the vein to distend from the increased pressure. Phlebitis is an inflammation of the veins most commonly seen in the lower legs. DVT is a thrombus with inflammatory changes that has attached to the deep venous system of the lower legs and has caused a partial or complete obstruction of the vessel. If a thrombus becomes dislodged and begins to circulate through the general circulation, it is then called an embolus. Arteriosclerosis is a general term for the thickening and loss

of elasticity of arterial walls; it can occur in arteries throughout the body and cause systemic ischemia and necrosis over time. Atherosclerosis is a form of arteriosclerosis in which the formation of an atheroma occurs. An aneurysm is a ballooning or dilation of the wall of a vessel caused by weakening of the vessel wall. Peripheral arterial disease affects the vessels outside of the heart, especially the legs and feet, in which circulation is decreased and ischemia can occur.
11. Outline typical cardiovascular diagnostic procedures.
   * Cardiovascular diagnostic procedures include Doppler studies of the patency of blood vessels; angiography to show arterial pathways; echocardiography to assess the structure and movement of the parts of the heart, especially the valves; and cardiac catheterization to show the heart chambers, valves,

CONNECTIONS

 Study Guide Connection: Go to Chapter 46 Study Guide. Read the Case Study and Workplace Applications and complete the assignments. Do online research for answers to the questions in the Internet Activities associated with assisting in cardiology.

 CD Connection: Go to the Medical Assisting Competency Challenge CD and do the training activities under Diagnostic Testing. For a better understanding of the function of the heart, view the animation for normal cardiopulmonary physiology.

evolve **Evolve Connection:** For more information related to assisting in cardiology, go to evolve.elsevier.com/kinn and visit related weblinks for Chapter 46. Click on the Medical Assisting Exam Review and do the practice questions to sharpen your test-taking skills.

Connections information at the end of the chapter presents ancillary products and resources that are available to assist students' comprehension of concepts and to enhance their learning experience

REVIEWERS

I am deeply grateful to the numerous people who have shared their comments and suggestions on this edition. Reviewing a book or supplement takes an incredible amount of energy and attention, and I am glad so many of my colleagues were able to take time out of their busy schedule to help ensure the validity and appropriateness of content in this edition. The reviewers provided me with additional viewpoints and opinions that combine to make this text an incredible learning tool.

I wish to thank the following editorial reviewing team:

Michelle Buchman RN, BSN, BC
Nursing Director, St. John's Marian Center
Owner/Manager Educational Support Services, LLC
Springfield, Missouri

Amy DeVore, BA, CMA
Instructor
Butler County Community College
Butler, Pennsylvania

Monica D. Flowers, CMIS, CHI
Administrative Medical Assisting and Medical Office Specialist
Instructor
Arlington Career Institute
Grand Prairie, Texas

Deborah Holmes, RN, CMA-C
Former Medical Assisting Program Chair
Iowa Western Community College
Council Bluffs, Iowa

Maureen Messier, CMA, RMA, AS, BA
Instructor, Medical Assisting/General Education
Branford Hall Career Institute
Southington, Connecticut

Andrea Potteiger, CPC, CMAA, CBCS, CHI, NR-CAHA, NR-CMA, NR-CPT, NR-CEKG
Lead Healthcare Instructor
New Horizons
Harrisburg, Pennsylvania

Donna M. Schenkel, BA
Coding Instructor
Southeast Technical Institute
Sioux Falls, South Dakota

Janet Sesser, RMA(AMT), CMA, BSEd Admin
Director of Education for Allied Health
High-Tech Institute, Inc.
Phoenix, Arizona

Lynn Slack, CMA
Medical Programs Director
ICM School of Business and Medical Careers
Pittsburgh, Pennsylvania

CONTRIBUTOR TO THIS EDITION

The preceding section demonstrates the amount of feedback and developmental input that went into shaping the sixth edition of this book. Because the medical assisting curriculum is so broad in scope, no individual can be an expert in all areas. I therefore extend a special acknowledgment to the following person who brought their expertise to bear by contributing one or more chapters to this edition:

Carline A. Dalglcish, MA, BS, CMA
Owner/Director
COUGAR-Ed.net LLC Department of Medicine
Arlington, Texas

AUTHOR ACKNOWLEDGMENTS

I consider it a privilege to be one of the authors of this incredible textbook. I appreciate the dedication and tireless work performed by the editorial, design, and production team that partnered with us on *Kinn's The Administrative Medical Assistant: An Applied Learning Approach*, Sixth Edition. This textbook has led countless medical assistants into a career that has allowed them to express compassion, caring, and dedication to health and wellness.

Years before I became associated with the writing of this textbook, I used it to teach my own students. Thousands of medical assistants today owe a great debt to Mary Kinn, the original author, for her innovation and dedication to the medical assisting field. I personally appreciate her vision, her past input, and her contributions that brought the text from its first edition through many subsequent editions. As we publish this tenth edition, our appreciation for Mary Kinn is heartfelt and sincere.

Susan Cole, Executive Editor, is a dedicated, sharp editor with a keen insight into the allied health profession and her professionalism is absolutely second to none. She listened to ideas, provided insight, encouragement, and endless support to me as I revised the book, determined to make the text even better than the last edition. I especially want to thank Susan for her support and her ability to help me refocus during the difficult months that my family faced while I was writing this revision.

Celeste Clingan, Developmental Editor, assisted every step of the way and her wonderful attitude made the writing process much easier. Celeste was always open to new ideas and concepts, and was complimentary to us as a writing team when those ideas worked. I know that this is a project that she will be proud of, because she did a gigantic amount of work, kept us organized, and remained supportive throughout the entire process.

I sincerely appreciate the work and contributions of Sarah Wunderly, Senior Project Manager. She was consistently cooperative and helpful during the production stages of this process. A warm thank-you goes to each one of her team members who worked on the Kinn project.

During the revision of this edition, I experienced several devastating losses and challenging times. Three individuals who inspired me and were crucial parts of my life passed away, and my son was diagnosed with a curable cancer. These events brought me into contact with the healthcare professionals that I write about in this text. As I experienced life on the other side of the thermometer, so to speak, I was reminded of the reasons that I entered the healthcare profession long ago in 1981. The dedication of the professionals who cared for my family was heartwarming and encouraging. The healthcare profession is the most rewarding career field available, and my hope is that more and more individuals choose allied health careers in the future.

And last, my family deserves so many thanks, because they allowed me to work on this textbook when they would rather have had my time to themselves. My children, Jimmie, Jonathan, Jessica, and Stacey, inspire me daily. My mother, Patricia Crumley, has been supportive ever since she held up flash cards in the wee hours of the morning while I was learning medical terminology during my own school years. Thanks also go to my sisters, Alisha Crumley and Karry Chapman, for endless encouragement and support. And last of all, tremendous thanks to my fiancé, Bentley Charles Adams. You are my rock, the man that I can always depend on, the man to whom I can release all of my concerns and know that they will be handled with care. Thank you for your belief in me and my abilities as a writer. I look forward to the rocking chairs on the front porch of our home in years to come.

Alexandra Patricia Young, BBA, RMA, CMA

CONTENTS

List of Procedures

Becoming a Successful Student

SCENARIO

Shawna Long is a newly admitted student in a medical assistant program at your school. Shawna is anxious about starting classes and very concerned that she may not be a successful student. She had trouble with some of her classes in high school and must continue to work part time while taking medical assistant classes. Based on what you discover about the learning process in this chapter, see if you can help Shawna take steps toward success.

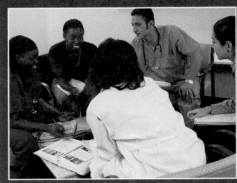

While studying this chapter, think about the following questions:

- Why is it important for Shawna to understand how she learns best?
- Time management is an important part of being a successful student as well as a successful medical assistant. What are some strategies Shawna can implement to help her manage her time as effectively as possible?
- Shawna will face many problems and conflicts while working through the MA program. How can she develop workable strategies for dealing with these issues?
- Studying may be a challenge for Shawna. What skills can she use to help her learn new material and prepare for examinations?

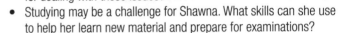

LEARNING OBJECTIVES

1. Define and spell the terms listed in the vocabulary.
2. Assess the importance of developing professional behaviors as a member of the allied health team.
3. Evaluate the concept of critical thinking and how it affects your actions.
4. Examine your learning preferences.
5. Interpret how your learning style affects your success as a student.
6. Apply time-management strategies to make the most of your learning opportunities.
7. Use problem-solving techniques to manage conflict and barriers to your success.
8. Integrate effective study skills into your daily activities.
9. Design test-taking strategies that help you take charge of your success.
10. Incorporate critical thinking and reflection to make mental connections as material is learned.

VOCABULARY

critical thinking The constant practice of considering all aspects of a situation when deciding what to believe or what to do.

empathy (em′-puh-the) Sensitivity to the individual needs and reactions of patients.

learning style The way that an individual perceives and processes information to learn new material.

perceiving (pur-sev′-ing) How an individual looks at information and sees it as real.

processing (pro′-ses-ing) How an individual internalizes new information and makes it his or her own.

professional behaviors Those actions that identify the medical assistant as a member of a healthcare profession, including being dependable, performing respectful patient care, exercising initiative, demonstrating a positive attitude, and using teamwork.

reflection (re-flek′-shun) The process of considering new information and internalizing it to create new ways of examining information.

You have taken the first step toward becoming a successful student by choosing your profession and field of study. The medical assistant profession is both challenging and rewarding. Becoming a medical assistant opens the doors to a wide variety of opportunities in both administrative and clinical practice at ambulatory or institutional healthcare settings. Medical assistants are important members of the healthcare team, and as a healthcare professional you will be expected to practice certain **professional behaviors** (Figure 1-1). These professional behaviors, which are discussed in depth in Chapter 4, include demonstrating dependability, respectful patient care, **empathy,** initiative, a positive attitude, and teamwork. In order to become a successful medical assistant you must first become a successful student. This chapter helps you discover the way that you learn best and provides multiple strategies to assist you in your journey toward success.

WHO YOU ARE AS A LEARNER: HOW DO YOU LEARN BEST?

Think about what you do when you are faced with something new to learn. How do you go about understanding and learning the new material? Over time you have developed a method for **perceiving** and **processing** information. This pattern of behavior is called your **learning style.** Many different ways of examining learning styles exist, but most professionals agree that the success of students depends more on whether they can "make sense" of the information than on whether or not they are "smart." Education that is based on attention to individual learning styles is sensitive to the different ways that students learn and approaches new material with a wide variety of methods so that all students have the opportunity to learn. Determining your individual learning style and understanding

how it applies to your ability to learn new material are the first steps toward becoming a successful student (Figure 1-2).

Learning Style Inventory

For you to learn new material, two things must happen. First you must perceive the information. This is the method you have developed over time that helps you examine the material and recognize it as real. Then you must process the information. Processing the information is how you internalize it and make it your own. By investigating various learning styles, you can figure out how to combine different methods of perceiving and processing information. In his book *Becoming a Master Student*, David Ellis discusses these different methods of information perception, processing, and learning.

Information perception involves how you go about examining new material and making it real. Learners perceive new material in two ways. Some people are concrete perceivers who learn information through direct experience by doing, acting, sensing, or feeling. Concrete learners prefer to learn things that have a personal meaning or things that they feel are relevant. Other learners are abstract perceivers who take in information through analysis, observation, and **reflection.** Abstract learners like to think things through. They analyze the new material and build theories to help understand it. They prefer structured learning situations and use a step-by-step approach to problem solving.

Information processing is how you internalize the new information and make it your own. There also are two different methods for processing material. Active processors prefer to jump in and start doing things immediately. They make sense of the new material by immediately using it. They look for practical ways to apply the new material and typically do not mind taking

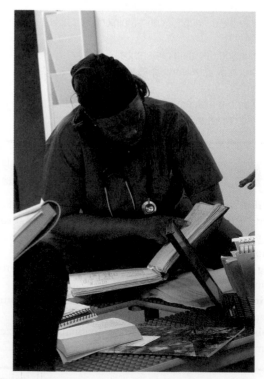

FIGURE 1-2 Student learning.

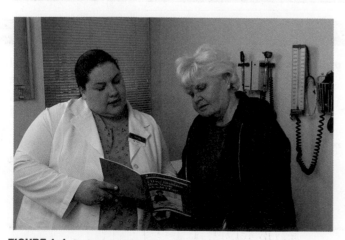

FIGURE 1-1 Professional interaction with patient.

risks to get the desired results. They learn best with practice and hands-on activities. Reflective processors, however, have to think about the information before they can internalize it. They prefer to observe and consider what is going on. The only way they can make sense of new material is to spend time thinking and learning a great deal about it before acting.

CRITICAL THINKING APPLICATION

- Consider the two ways to perceive new material. Are you a concrete perceiver who ties the information to a personal experience, or do you prefer abstract perception in which you like to analyze or reflect on the meaning of the material? Choose which one you think most accurately describes your method of investigating new information.
- Then think about the way you process learning. Are you an active processor who is always looking for the practical application of what you learn, or are you a reflective processor who has to think about new material before internalizing it?
- After completing this activity write down the combination of your perceiving and processing learning styles and share it with your instructor.

Using Your Learning Profile to Be a Successful Student: Where Do I Go from Here?

No one falls completely into one or the other of these categories. However, by being aware of how we generally prefer first to perceive information and then to process it, we can be more sensitive to our learning style and can approach new learning situations with a plan for learning the material in a way that best suits our learning preferences. Your preferred perceiving and processing learning profile will fall into one of the following stages in the Learning Style Inventory created by David Kolb of Case Western Reserve University.

Learners in Stage 1 have a concrete reflective style. These students want to know the purpose of the information and have a personal connection to the content. They like to consider a situation from many different points of view, observe others, and plan before taking action. Their strengths are in understanding people, brainstorming, and recognizing and creatively solving problems. If you fall into this stage, you enjoy small group activities and learn well in study groups.

Stage 2 learners have an abstract reflective style. These students are eager to learn just for the sheer pleasure of learning rather than because the material relates to their personal lives. They like to learn lots of facts and arrange new material in a logical and clear manner. Stage 2 learners plan studying and like to create ways of thinking about the material but do not always make the connection with the practical application of the material. If you are a Stage 2 learner, you prefer organized, logical presentations of material and therefore enjoy lectures and generally dislike group work. You also need time to process and think about the new material before applying it.

Learners in Stage 3 have an abstract active style. Learners with this combination of learning style want to experiment and test the information that they are learning. If you are a Stage 3

learner, you want to know how techniques or ideas work, and you also want to practice what you are learning. Your strengths are in problem solving and decision making, but you may lack focus and may be hasty when making decisions. You learn best with hands-on practice by doing experiments, projects, and laboratory activities. You also enjoy working alone or in small groups (Figure 1-3).

Stage 4 is made up of concrete active learners. These students are concerned about how they can use what they learn to make a difference in their lives. If you fall into this stage, you like to relate new material to other areas of your life. You have leadership capabilities, can create on your feet, and are usually vocal in a group, but you may have difficulty completing your work on time. Stage 4 learners enjoy teaching others and working in groups and learn best when they can apply the new information to real-world problems (Figure 1-4).

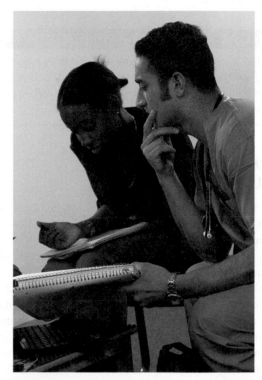

FIGURE 1-3 Learning in a small group.

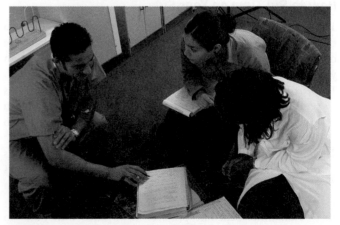

FIGURE 1-4 Teaching and working with others.

To get the most out of knowing your learning profile, you need to apply this knowledge to how you approach learning. Each of the learning stages has pluses and minuses. When faced with a learning situation that does not match your learning preference, see how you can adapt your individual learning to make the best of the information. For example, if you are bored by lectures, look for an opportunity to apply the information being presented to a real problem you are facing in the classroom or at home. If you are an abstract perceiver, take time outside of class to think about new information so that you are ready to process it into your learning system. If you benefit from learning in a group, make the effort to organize review sessions and study groups. If you learn best by teaching others, offer to assist your peers with their learning. By taking the time now to investigate your preferred method of learning, you will perceive and process information more effectively throughout your school career.

CRITICAL THINKING APPLICATION

Take a few minutes to reflect on a time when you really enjoyed learning about something new. How was the material presented, and what did you do to "make it your own"? What do you need to do to become a more effective learner?

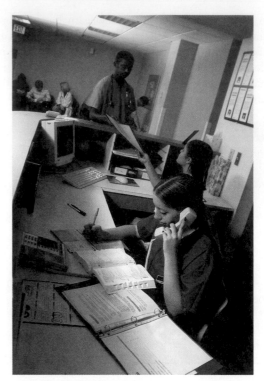

FIGURE 1-5 Time management in a busy medical practice.

TIME MANAGEMENT: PUTTING TIME ON YOUR SIDE

One of the most complicated tasks for a professional medical assistant is to effectively manage time. No other workplace can compete with the distractions and demands of a busy healthcare setting. Do you think that you practice effective time-management skills? Do you believe that you are in control of your time, or do you think that other people or situations control it? How frequently do you say that you just do not have enough time to do what you are supposed to do, let alone those things you would like to do? Time management gives you the opportunity to spend time in the way you choose. Effective time management is also crucial to your success as a student and as a future healthcare professional (Figure 1-5).

How to Put Time on Your Side

The following time-management skills are designed to help you effectively deal with the demands on your time. Highlight the ones that you think will be most useful in helping you deal with your situation.

1. *Determine your purpose.* What do you want to accomplish this semester, in this course, or in this unit of study? What do you want to achieve as a student? What is one thing you can do to help achieve your goals?
2. *Identify your main concern.* Besides school, what other demands do you have on your time? Based on the learning goals you have established, what do you need to do to accomplish your goals?
   - Plan time: Schedule projects in advance with notes to yourself on deadlines.

   - Use down time: Take your work with you everywhere you go. Do small bits at every opportunity.
   - Guard time: Avoid distractions (e.g., television, music) that will interfere with your concentration. Notice how others abuse your time. Learn to say no to outside demands on your time.
   - Discover time: Steal time from other activities in your schedule.
   - Assign time: Ask for help when you need it from friends and family.
3. *Be organized.* What materials (e.g., books, research, supplies) do you need to have an effective study session? What preparation is needed to make the most of your time?
   - Record time: Use a day planner or calendar to write down due dates for assignments and tests. If a paper or project is due on a specific date, write yourself a reminder in your day planner to start the project on a specific date so you are sure to have it done when it is due.
   - Optimal time: Take advantage of the time of day when you study and learn the best. Schedule study time during your peak performance time—which means if you are an early riser make time for homework first thing in the day, or at night if you are a night owl. Plan on dedicating at least some of your optimal time to your school work.
4. *Stop procrastinating.* If you avoid working on your goals, you may not achieve them. Examine the following suggestions as ways to break the procrastination cycle.
   - Make the work meaningful: What is important about the work you are putting off and what are the benefits of getting it done? Reflect on your long-range goals. Is it important to do a good job on the work so you

can earn an acceptable grade, do well in the course, complete the medical assisting program, and ultimately find employment?

- Plan work deadlines: Break assignments into achievable sections that can be completed in the time slots available. Schedule those work sections in your day planner to prevent forgetting deadlines for assignments.
- Ask for help: Let your support system know you have work to get done. Ask them for encouragement to stay on track. If you have school-age children you can set an excellent example by planning "family" homework sessions. You can get some of your work done while role modeling learning behaviors for your children. Let your partner know when due dates are looming or tests are scheduled. Ask for help in meeting day-to-day demands so you can study or prepare for school.
- Prioritize: If you keep avoiding a certain task, reevaluate its priority. If it is really worth worrying about, get started now, not later. Don't waste time worrying about how you are going to get things done. Spend that time actually working on the projects that worry you the most.
- Reward yourself: Create a reward that is meaningful and something you will work for. If you want to spend time with your family or friends on the weekend, develop a plan and stick to it so you can share that special time as a reward.

5. *Remember you.* It is very easy to become overwhelmed with responsibilities both in school and at home. Part of successful time management includes setting aside time to do things you enjoy. You have chosen a profession that can be very demanding. Now is the time to remember that you have to take care of yourself as well as meet your professional and personal responsibilities. So remember to plan some time for yourself as well (Figure 1-6).

CRITICAL THINKING APPLICATION

How do you spend your time? Over 3 days this week write down the amount of time you spend on each activity. How much television do you watch? How much time do you spend talking on the phone? How about driving time, visiting time, work time, time for family and friends, and so on? At the end of the 3-day period, add up the various categories of time. Do you recognize any time you might be wasting? Can you implement any of the suggested time-management strategies to make more time available?

PROBLEM SOLVING AND CONFLICT MANAGEMENT

As a future member of the healthcare team, you will frequently face problems and conflict. Although we usually look at these situations as negative factors in our lives, problem solving and conflict management actually give us the opportunity to positively affect a potentially negative situation. Learning how to manage problems can be very useful for your practice as a medical assistant, as well as for your success as a student.

The first step in reaching an equitable solution to a problem or conflict situation is to identify the central issue. How many times have you known that you were upset about something but were not really sure why? You cannot solve a problem or resolve a negative situation unless you are sure what is at the root of your feelings. You need to understand the problem and gather as much information about the situation as possible before you decide to act. One way of doing this is to ask yourself these questions:

- When does the situation occur and under what circumstances?
- How does it make you feel?
- Is there someone else involved?
- What interferes with making a decision or resolving the conflict?

Once you understand the situation and how you feel about it, you need to decide if it is worth the effort to resolve it. Prioritize your involvement. Sometimes situations and problems may arise that you are unable to resolve or that you may decide are not important enough for you to act on. For example, if one of your co-workers refuses to take out the garbage when it is his or her turn, does that really bother you? If it does, then you need to deal with the issue. However, if the individual helps out in other ways then perhaps the garbage isn't worth the effort to resolve the conflict.

After you have gathered the details about the problem or conflict and you have decided it is important enough to act on, it is time to determine possible solutions. One way to do this is to ask for advice or brainstorm ideas with individuals you respect. Sometimes another person can give you special insight into the problem that you were unable to see on your own. After brainstorming for possible solutions, you should then get feedback regarding the workability of the suggested solutions. An alternative to brainstorming possible solutions to the problem is to list on a piece of paper the pros and cons of possible solutions. Simply looking at a list of the positive and negative aspects of the solution may clarify how you should solve the problem. Before deciding on a particular solution, make sure you critically analyze the consequences of each proposed solution: Which one best meets your needs and has the potential for providing an outcome you can live with?

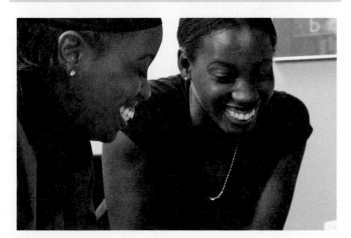

FIGURE 1-6 Making time for you.

Finally you are ready to implement the chosen solution. However, your work is not over yet. You need to evaluate the outcome of your decision and see if it truly did meet your needs. If not, it may be time to review other possible solutions and try another approach.

Conflict management requires some additional consideration. If you are in conflict with a peer, instructor, or co-worker, it is important to follow certain guidelines. You should attempt to solve the conflict in a private place at a prescheduled time. This ensures that the person will meet with you and that neither one has to worry about others overhearing the conversation. At the meeting clearly state your feelings about the conflict and how you would like it resolved. Then try to come to an agreeable solution. The best way to deal with conflict situations is through open, honest, assertive communication. However, just as with problem solving, it is important to follow up on the decided course of action to see if it effectively dealt with the source of the conflict (Figure 1-7).

CRITICAL THINKING APPLICATION

Think about a serious problem you are currently facing. Use the brainstorming and/or pros-and-cons method for creating solutions to the problem. Implement your chosen solution, and follow up on its effectiveness. Did the problem-solving process help you manage the situation more effectively?

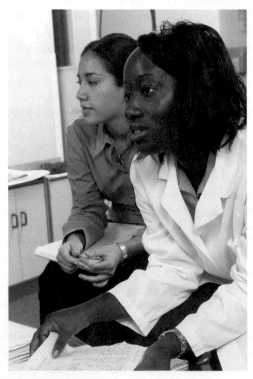

FIGURE 1-7 Dealing with conflict.

STUDY SKILLS: TRICKS TO BECOMING A SUCCESSFUL STUDENT

So far in this chapter we have looked at the influence of individual learning styles and time management on learning success. Now we will investigate some ideas that are useful in learning new material. These study skills include memory techniques, active learning, brain tricks, reading methods, and note-taking strategies.

Several techniques can help you store and remember information. The first of these involves organizing information into recognizable groups so the brain can easily find it. You can organize information by getting the big picture first before trying to learn the details. One way to implement this strategy is to skim a reading assignment before actually reading and taking notes on the material, thus getting a general impression of what you need to learn before tackling the details. Depending on your learning style, it may also help to find a way of making the new information meaningful. Think about your educational goals and how the new material will help you achieve those goals. Another way of remembering material is to create an association with something you already know. By grouping new material with already stored material, your brain will remember it much easier.

A useful study skill for some learners is to be physically active while learning. Some students learn best if they walk or talk out loud while studying. Besides encouraging learning, moving and talking while studying relieve boredom and keep you awake. Another way to be actively involved in learning is to use pictures or diagrams to represent the material you are studying. Some people are visual learners, and creating pictures of the material is the easiest method for them to retain the information. Other students find that rewriting notes or making lists of information helps them retain the material. Writing also helps those students who need to "do" something in order to learn.

Studying will go much more smoothly if you work *with* your brain rather than *against* it. If you tend to get anxious and worried while studying, you may be acting as your own worst enemy. One way of dealing with a topic that you find anxiety producing is to overlearn it. If material is overlearned, you are much less likely to experience test anxiety. Another method for remembering material is to quickly review it after class. This minireview will help the new information become part of your long-term memory system. Many students find creating songs, dances, or word associations an effective way to learn and remember new material. Putting details into a familiar song and moving to it can help trick the brain into remembering the information. This is especially helpful when trying to learn anatomy and physiology. Another excellent way of learning information is to actually teach it to someone else. Teaching requires you to have a good understanding of the material as well as the ability to describe it for others. It can be an effective reinforcer of complicated material (Figure 1-8).

A great deal of the learning process is expected to take place from assigned readings. You can use several methods to make reading assignments more meaningful. If you find a reading assignment challenging or difficult to understand, the first step

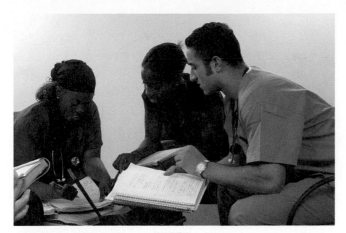

FIGURE 1-8 Effective study skills.

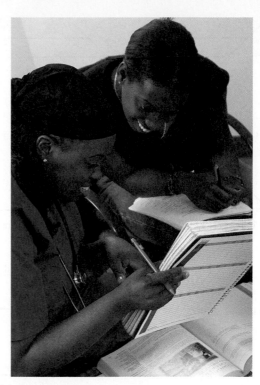

FIGURE 1-9 Sharing notes.

is to take the time to read it again. Sometimes the first time through the material is not enough to gain understanding. As you read, highlight important words or thoughts and stop periodically to summarize the material. If you get bored while reading, use your body—walk or talk your way through the assignment. Take the time to look up words or terms you do not understand, or ask your instructor or tutor for help. Outlining the material can help you create a brief overview of what you need to learn. And finally, the best way to determine if you learned anything from your reading is to try to explain it to someone else. If that is effective, you know you acquired the knowledge needed from the reading assignment.

Many students find effective note taking a challenge. The big question is, "How much of what the instructor says do I actually need to write down?" The first step in effective note taking is to come to class prepared. The more familiar you are with the material, the easier it will be to determine the important parts of the instructor's lecture. Pay attention to the instructor, and look for clues about what he or she thinks is important. Ask questions about the material if you do not understand it rather than writing down information that makes no sense to you. Think critically about what you hear before you write it down so you can start to build relationships among the things you want or need to know.

When it comes to actual note taking, some strategies can make the process of recording notes an active learning tool. Organize the information as much as possible while you are writing, in either an outline or paragraph format. Use only one side of the paper for easier reading and leave blank spaces where needed to fill in details later. Use key words to help you remember the material, and create pictures or diagrams to help visualize it. If permitted, use tape recorders when appropriate and make sure you have either handouts or notes that cover material written on the board, in an overhead, or in a PowerPoint presentation. Another helpful tool is to develop your own system of abbreviations to help simplify the writing load.

The most effective way to use your notes is to review them shortly after class. This is the time to add details, clarify information, or make notes about asking the instructor for explanations during the next class. You could even exchange

notes with students you trust to compare information (Figure 1-9). Some students find it beneficial to type or rewrite their notes. This can give you an opportunity to learn the material as you are transcribing it. As you are reviewing your notes you can also draw mind maps of the information or diagram outlines to help you better understand and remember the material.

Creating mind maps is a way of representing the main idea of the topic and supporting important details with a figure or picture. Healthcare textbooks are made up of complicated concepts with multiple main ideas, each with its own important details. Mind maps are a way of consolidating complex details and organizing them into a format that is easier to remember. The spider map example in Figure 1-10 presents a method for including several main ideas with details in one study guide. The fishbone map in Figure 1-11 can be used to learn complicated causes of disease. The chain-of-events map in Figure 1-12 displays the cause and effect of events such as infection control or the history of medicine. The cycle map in Figure 1-13 shows the connection between factors, such as with the chain of infection. Creating your own mind maps is a way of making the information more meaningful and easier for you to understand.

Although many techniques can help you study, perhaps the most important one is your attitude toward learning. Some students fall into the "I can't possibly learn this material" trap. That type of attitude only leads to self-defeat. The way to solve barriers is to first recognize that they exist. Once you know your weak spots, use the suggested study skills to improve in those areas. Do not be afraid to ask questions or to seek out help if you do not understand the material. Employ as many different strategies as necessary to become a successful student.

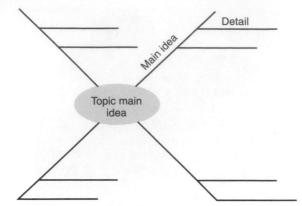

FIGURE 1-10 Spider map displays multiple main ideas with supporting details.

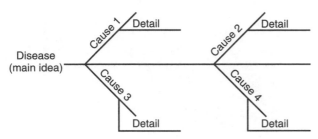

FIGURE 1-11 Fishbone map used to describe causes of disease.

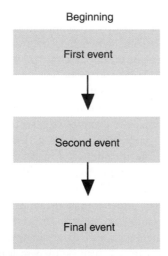

FIGURE 1-12 Chain-of-events map displays the cause and effect of events.

CRITICAL THINKING APPLICATION

Write down at least two barriers to your learning. Review the study skill suggestions discussed, and choose four you want to try out. Use them over the next week to help you when learning new material. Reflect on whether the chosen study skills helped you learn the material better.

TEST-TAKING STRATEGIES: TAKING CHARGE OF YOUR SUCCESS

What happens when you do not know the answer to the first question on a test? What if you do not know the next one? Are you able to go on without panicking? Many people find taking

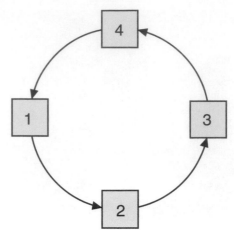

FIGURE 1-13 Cycle map shows how one action leads to another.

tests the most challenging part of being successful students. Multiple approaches are available that you can employ to take charge of your success and improve your ability to take tests. These include such strategies as adequate preparation, controlling negative thoughts during test time, and understanding how to manage various types of questions.

The first step is to go into a test adequately prepared. Use the time-management skills already outlined in this chapter to get prepared for the big day. Recognize and employ your preferred learning style to overlearn the material and increase your confidence. Use memory tools like flash cards, checklists, and mind maps to help visualize the material. Form a study group if you are the type of learner who benefits from studying in groups (Figure 1-14). Schedule and plan study time, and reward yourself for your hard work. It is also important to go into the test rested and relaxed, so eat, exercise to relieve stress, and sleep before the test so that you are as alert as possible.

Before you start the test make sure you read directions carefully and, if possible, begin with the easiest or shortest questions to build your confidence. Be aware of the amount of time allotted for the examination, and pace yourself accordingly. As you go through the test, look for clues to answers in other questions. During test time remember to use positive self-talk at the first indication of panic. Repeatedly remind yourself that you are well prepared, relax, and think about the material before you get worried. You need to stop negative thoughts as soon as they arise, and instead visualize yourself being successful. Use slow deep breathing to relax and, if helpful, close your eyes for a minute and visualize a relaxing place before you go on with the test. You may find it helpful to wear a thick rubber band on your wrist and to snap it as soon as you start to think negatively. This will provide a physical reaction to interfere with the power of your negative thoughts and serve as a reminder of what you should be concentrating on.

Some strategies can be employed when answering certain types of questions. With multiple choice questions, try to identify key words or clues in each question. Read the question carefully and answer it in your head before you review the provided answers. If you are not absolutely sure of the answer, make an educated guess or follow your instincts in choosing an

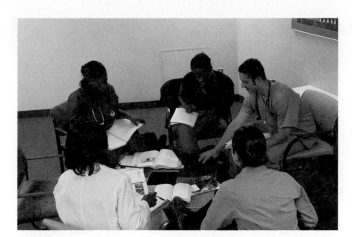

FIGURE 1-14 Study group.

answer. "True-or-false" questions give you a "50/50" chance of being correct. Remember that if any part of the question is not true, then the statement is false. Again, check the statements for key words that will help indicate the direction of the answer. Look for qualifying terms (e.g., "always," "never," "sometimes") that are key to understanding the meaning of the true-or-false statement.

CRITICAL THINKING APPLICATION

Think about a time you experienced test anxiety. Write down the details about the situation and how you felt. Choose four test-taking strategies that you think would be beneficial in handling similar situations in the future.

BECOMING A CRITICAL THINKER: MAKING MENTAL CONNECTIONS

The ability to process information and arrive at reasonable conclusions is crucial to all healthcare workers. The process of **critical thinking** involves sorting out conflicting information, weighing the knowledge you possess about that information, ignoring or letting go of personal biases, and deciding on a reasonable belief or action. Critical thinking is actually an active search for the truth. Critical thinking could be described as thorough thinking because it requires learners to be open-minded to all possibilities. Successful students are thorough thinkers because they must determine the facts about the topic being learned and come to logical conclusions about the material. Critical thinkers are also inquisitive learners who are constantly in the process of analyzing and sorting out conflicting information to reach conclusions. A crucial step in critical thinking is evaluating the results of your learning. Reflection is key to critical thinking. "How did I learn what I learned?" and "What does it mean in my life?" are questions that must be consistently asked in order to continue to learn. Becoming a successful student and ultimately a successful member of the allied health team requires the possession of critical thinking skills. Both the material presented in this chapter and the critical thinking application exercises are designed to encourage you along this lifelong learning path of critical thinking.

SUMMARY OF SCENARIO

One of the things Shawna can do to improve her learning is to determine her individual learning style. By understanding how she typically perceives and processes new information she can plan the best methods for learning the material. In addition to understanding who she is as a learner, Shawna needs to practice successful time-management skills to keep up with school and work responsibilities. Effective problem solving and developing study skills that work for her are also key to her success as a student.

SUMMARY of LEARNING OBJECTIVES

1. Define, spell, and pronounce the terms listed in the vocabulary.
   - Spelling and pronouncing medical terms correctly adds credibility to the medical assistant. Knowing the definitions of these terms promotes confidence in communication with patients and co-workers.
2. Assess the importance of developing professional behaviors as a member of the allied health team.
   - Medical assistants play a vital role in the healthcare team and are expected to display such professional behaviors as being dependable, practicing respectful patient care, having empathy,

showing initiative, having a positive attitude, and using teamwork.
3. Evaluate the concept of critical thinking and how it affects your actions.
   - Incorporate critical thinking and reflection to make mental connections as material is learned. Critical thinkers can evaluate conflicting information and make a decision to act based on their knowledge and willingness to be open-minded to all possibilities.
4. Examine your learning preferences.

Continued

SUMMARY of LEARNING OBJECTIVES
Continued

- Learning preferences are the ways that you like to learn and that have proven successful in the past.

5. Interpret how your learning style affects your success as a student.
   - Learning styles are determined by your individual method of perceiving or examining new material and the way that you process it or make it your own. People are either concrete or abstract perceivers and either active or reflective processors.

6. Apply time-management strategies to make the most of your learning opportunities.
   - Effective time-management strategies such as setting goals, prioritizing, getting organized, and avoiding procrastination will make you a more successful student as well as an effective medical assistant.

7. Use problem-solving techniques to manage conflict and barriers to your success.
   - Problem-solving and conflict-management techniques are key to your success. First, identify the central issue and how you feel about it; then consider possible solutions and their potential results, implement the chosen solution, and analyze the results.

8. Integrate effective study skills into your daily activities.
   - Study skills such as memory techniques, active learning, brain tricks, effective reading methods, note-taking strategies, and mind maps all help students to be more successful.

9. Design test-taking strategies that help you take charge of your success.
   - Test-taking strategies include preparing adequately for the examination, controlling negative thoughts during the examination, and understanding how to deal with different types of questions.

10. Incorporate critical thinking and reflection to make mental connections as material is learned.
    - Critical thinking can be described as thorough thinking because it considers all sides of the information without bias. Reflection is the process of thinking about or reviewing information before acting.

CONNECTIONS

 Study Guide Connection: Go to Chapter 1 Study Guide. Read the Case Study and Workplace Applications and complete the assignments. Do online research for answers to the questions in the Internet Activities associated with becoming a successful student.

 CD Connection: Go to the Medical Assisting Competency Challenge CD and review the content of the training activities. These will be referred to throughout the textbook to enhance your learning experience.

 Evolve Connection: For more information related to becoming a successful student, go to http://evolve.elsevier.com/kinn/admin and visit related weblinks for Chapter 1. Click on the Medical Assisting Exam Review and do the practice questions to sharpen your test-taking skills.

The Healthcare Industry

SCENARIO

Carlos Santos, CMA, is a medical assisting instructor with 10 years' experience in the clinical area. He worked for a group of family practitioners and for an allergist during his career as a medical assistant before becoming an instructor. Mr. Santos believes that it is very important to give his students an overview of the healthcare industry early in their training. He knows that it is exciting to show them the history and progress of medicine and introduce them to the current types of facilities available for patient care on both a national and a local level. This helps the student to understand where he or she fits into the whole picture as a medical assistant. Often Mr. Santos assigns the students a short report on one person who contributed to the progress of medicine. He finds that this is a good way to encourage the students to use the Internet and conduct research right from the start of their training; the students get a chance to grow more comfortable speaking in front of a group. The knowledge that the students will gain about the different areas of patient care will be useful once they graduate and begin working in a healthcare facility. All of these skills will make Mr. Santos's students more versatile and valuable to their eventual employers.

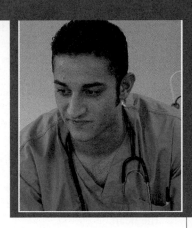

While studying this chapter, think about the following questions:

- Why is continuing medical research so important to the healthcare industry?
- How can the individual medical assistant contribute to the progress of medicine in today's world?
- What is the value in gaining an overview of the entire healthcare industry as one begins a career in medical assisting?

LEARNING OBJECTIVES

1. Define, spell, and pronounce the terms listed in the vocabulary.
2. Identify the ancient cultures that contributed a major portion of our medical terminology.
3. Explain the history of medicine and how it has affected today's medical industry.
4. Distinguish between and describe the two medical symbols in general use today.
5. Explain why a medical education at Johns Hopkins was considered superior, even in its early years.
6. List several medical pioneers, and discuss the importance of their contributions to the medical profession.
7. Explain the roles of the world healthcare organizations.
8. Discuss the various types of ambulatory care.
9. Distinguish among different types of doctors and medical practices.
10. Identify the medical specialties recognized by the American Board of Medical Specialties.
11. Discuss various healthcare occupations and the role these professionals play in the healthcare industry.

National Accreditation Competencies and Content

ABHES COMPETENCIES

Communication
2.g. Use appropriate medical terminology
2.q. Allied health professions and credentialing

Legal Concepts
5.f. Maintain licenses and accreditation

accreditation (u-kre-duh-ta'-shun) The process through which an organization is recognized for adherence to a group of standards that meet or exceed expectations of the accrediting agency.

advent A coming into being or use.

allopathic (al-o-pa'-thik) A word used to contrast homeopathic medicine with mainstream medicine; describes medicine supposedly characterized by an effort to counteract the symptoms of a disease by administration of treatments that produce effects that are opposite to the symptoms.

alternative medicine A variety of therapeutic or preventative health care practices that are alternatives to mainstream medicine, such as chiropractic, homeopathy, naturopathy, and herbal medicine.

ambulatory (am'-bu-la-to-re) Able to walk about and not be bedridden.

amenities Things that contribute to comfort, enjoyment, or convenience.

cardiac arrhythmias (kar'-de-ak ah-rith'-me-ahs) Irregular heartbeats resulting from a malfunction of the electrical system of the heart.

case management The process of assessing and planning patient care, including referral and follow-up, to ensure continuity of care and quality management.

chiropractic (ki'-ruh-prak-tik) A medical discipline that focuses on the nervous system and involves manual adjustment of the vertebral column to affect the nervous system to treat various disorders and to promote patient wellness.

cited Quoted by way of example, authority, or proof or mentioned formally in commendation or praise.

contamination (kun-ta-mu-na'-shun) A process by which something is made impure, unclean, or unfit for use by the introduction of unwholesome or undesirable elements.

credentialing (kri-den'-shuh-ling) The act of extending professional or medical privileges to an individual; the process of verifying and evaluating that person's credentials.

dissection (di-sek'-shun) Separation into pieces and exposure of parts for scientific examination.

encounter Any contact between a healthcare provider and a patient that results in treatment or evaluation of the patient's condition; not limited to in-person contact.

fermentation (fur-men-ta'-shun) An enzymatically controlled transformation of an organic compound.

holistic (ho-lis'-tik) Related to or concerned with all of the systems of the body, rather than breaking it down into parts.

homeopathy (ho-me-uh'-puh-the) A type of alternative medicine that attempts to stimulate the body to recover itself; a system of therapy based on the concept that disease can be treated with minute doses of drugs thought capable of producing the same symptoms in healthy people as the disease itself.

hospice (hos'-pus) A concept of care that involves health professionals and volunteers who provide medical, psychologic, and spiritual support to terminally ill patients and their loved ones.

indicators An important point or group of statistic values that, when evaluated, indicate the quality of care provided in a healthcare facility.

indicted (in-di'-ted) Charged with a crime by the finding or presentment of a jury according to due process of law.

indigent (in'-di-junt) Totally lacking in something of need.

innate Existing in, belonging to, or determined by factors present in an individual since birth.

innocuous (i'-nuh-kyu-wus) Having no effect, adverse or otherwise; harmless.

mysticism The experience of seeming to have direct communication with God or ultimate reality.

naturopathy (na-chu-ra'-puh-the) An alternative to conventional medicine in which holistic methods are used, as well as herbs and natural supplements, with the belief that the body will heal itself. Naturopathic physicians can currently be licensed in 15 states, Puerto Rico, and the Virgin Islands.

osteopathic (us-te-uh-pa'-thik) A type of medicine based on the theory that disturbances in the musculoskeletal system affect other bodily parts, causing many disorders that can be corrected by various manipulative techniques in conjunction with conventional medical, surgical, pharmacologic, and other therapeutic procedures.

pandemic (pan-de'-mik) A condition in which the majority of the people in a country, a number of countries, or a geographic area are affected.

peer review organization A group of medical reviewers contracted by the Centers for Medicare and Medicaid Services to ensure quality control and medical necessity of services provided by a facility.

philanthropist (fu-lan'-thruh-pist) An individual who makes an active effort to promote human welfare.

putrefaction (pyu-truh-fak'-shun) Decomposition of animal matter that results in a foul smell.

robotics Technology dealing with the design, construction, and operation of robots in automation.

staff privileges Allowance of a healthcare professional to practice within a specific facility.

standards Item or indicator used as a measure of quality or compliance with a statutory or accrediting body's policies and regulations.

subluxations (suh-blek-sa'-shuns) Slight misalignments of the vertebrae or a partial dislocation.

telemedicine The use of telecommunications in the practice of medicine, in which great distances can exist among healthcare professionals, colleagues, patients, and students.

teleradiology The use of telecommunications devices to enhance and improve the results of radiologic procedures.

treatises (truh-te'-ses) Systematic expositions or arguments

List continues on next page

List continued from previous page

in writing including a methodic discussion of the facts and principles involved and the conclusions reached.
triage (tre′-azh) The sorting of and allocation of treatment to patients according to a system of priorities designed to maximize the number of survivors and treat the sickest patients first.

The growth of today's healthcare industry seems unstoppable. Thanks to modern technologic advances, medicine speeds forward faster than ever in its quest to improve the health of humankind. Modern advances, such as **telemedicine,** are experiencing significant growth, and the images produced with **teleradiology** have vastly improved in their resolution. **Robotics** is assisting healthcare professionals in surgery and even delivers drugs to hospital floors using laser sensors. Education in medicine has grown exponentially: computers, the Internet, and video have enabled an instructor in New York to communicate with a student in Los Angeles. The key to this technology lies within the development and widespread use of elaborate information systems that have revolutionized the way that medicine is practiced today. Technology is advancing at an astounding rate of speed; the healthcare environment of the future is barely imaginable. This chapter looks back at the history of medicine, gazes at its present, and glances toward its future.

THE HISTORY OF MEDICINE

Medical Language and Mythology

Today's medical professional uses words with origins stemming from the romance and fantasy of classical and ancient languages. The study of anatomy reaches back to the dawn of recorded history. Today's modern terms are often similar to their original versions. Some terms are inaccurate when translated literally, because the ancients did not fully understand body functions. The word *artery*, for example, which comes from the Greek word *arteria*, literally means "a windpipe." The early Greeks believed that the arteries carried air, not blood. Greek and Roman mythology have contributed a major portion of our medical terminology, but we have also borrowed liberally from Arabic, Anglo-Saxon, and Germanic sources. Several terms originate from the Bible.

The human head rests on the first cervical vertebra, which is called the *atlas*. Atlas was the famous Greek Titan who was condemned by Zeus to bear the heavens on his shoulders. Achilles was held by the heel as his mother dipped him into the river Styx, so that he would become invulnerable. However, his heel was not immersed, and he later died from a wound in that area. "Achilles heel" is a common expression used today to show a point of weakness. Aphrodite, the Greek goddess of love and beauty, is the source of the name for drugs used to enhance sexual arousal, called *aphrodisiacs*. The equivalent Roman goddess of love, Venus, is associated with lustful desires.

A portion of the female anatomy, the mons *veneris* (mons pubis), and *venereal* diseases were named after her.

Aesculapius, the son of Apollo, was revered as the god of medicine. The early Greeks worshiped the healing powers of Aesculapius and built temples in his honor where patients were treated by trained priests. His daughters were Hygeia, goddess of health, and Panacea, goddess of all healing and restorer of health. Our modern word "hygiene" has its origin in Hygeia, and the modern meaning for panacea is "a remedy for all ills and difficulties." The staff of Aesculapius is a common medical icon. It depicts a serpent encircling a staff and signifies the art of healing. The staff of Aesculapius has been adopted by the American Medical Association as the symbol of medicine. The mythologic staff belonging to Hermes, the messenger of the gods, is the caduceus, which was thought to have magical powers. The caduceus is a staff encircled by two serpents with wings at the top. This icon is the medical insignia of the U.S. Army Medical Corps and is often misused as a symbol of the medical profession (Figure 2-1).

Medicine in Ancient Times

Although religious and mythologic beliefs were the basis of care for the sick in ancient times, evidence suggests the use of drugs, surgery, and other treatments based on theories about the body from as early as 5000 BC. In the well-developed societies of the Egyptians, Babylonians, and Assyrians, certain men acted as physicians and used the little knowledge they had to try to treat illness and injury.

Moses presented rules of health to the Hebrews at approximately 1205 BC. He was the first advocate of preventive medicine and is considered the first public health officer. Moses knew that some animal diseases could be passed to humans and that **contamination** existed, so a religious law was developed

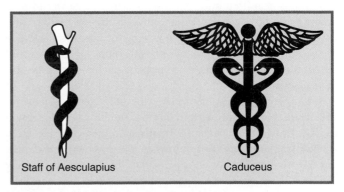

Staff of Aesculapius   Caduceus

FIGURE 2-1 Staff of Aesculapius and the caduceus.

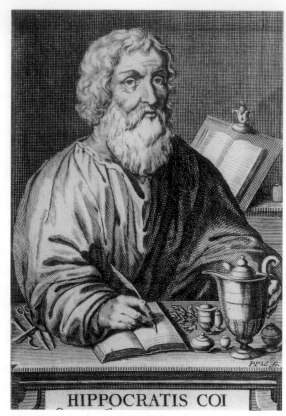

FIGURE 2-2 Hippocrates is known as the Father of Medicine. (Courtesy National Library of Medicine.)

forbidding humans to eat or drink from dirty dishes. The people of that era believed that doing so would defile their bodies and they would lose their souls.

Hippocrates, known as the Father of Medicine, is the most famous of the ancient Greek physicians (Figure 2-2). He was born in 450 BC on the island of Cos in Greece. He is best remembered for the Hippocratic Oath, which has been administered to physicians for more than 2000 years. Hippocrates is credited with taking **mysticism** out of medicine and giving it a scientific basis. During this period of history, most believed that illness was caused by demon possession; for the illness to be cured, the demon had to be removed from the body. Hippocrates' clinical descriptions of diseases and his volumes on epidemics, fevers, epilepsy, fractures, and instruments were studied for centuries. He believed that the body had the capacity to heal itself and that the physician's role was to help nature. Very little was known about anatomy, physiology, and pathology, and there was no knowledge of chemistry. Despite these limitations, many of the classifications of diseases and descriptions of symptoms that Hippocrates developed are still in use today.

Galen was a Greek physician who migrated to Rome in 162 AD and became known as the Prince of Physicians. He is said to have written more than 500 **treatises** on medicine. He wrote an excellent summary on anatomy as it was known at the time, but his work was faulty and inaccurate because it was largely based on the **dissection** of apes and swine. He is considered the Father of Experimental Physiology and the first experimental neurologist. He was the first to describe the cranial nerves and the sympathetic nervous system, and he performed the first experimental section of the spinal cord, producing hemiplegia. Galen also produced aphonia by cutting the recurrent laryngeal nerve, and he gave the first valid explanation of the mechanism of respiration. Galen was also a champion of medical ethics: he felt that physicians "must learn to despise money," and that if a physician was interested in profit, he was not serious in his devotion to the art of medicine. Galen's beliefs about monetary profit from medicine parallel the views of many modern healthcare professionals, who understand the nature of the healthcare crisis the world faces today. Although much of what he believed about the body was incorrect, Galen's teachings remained intact until human dissections began and physicians were able to visualize exactly what was inside the human body.

Because both Hippocrates and Galen were highly respected, the authority of their observations went unquestioned. This had a negative effect on the progress of science throughout the Dark Ages and well into the sixteenth century. Their theories and descriptions were considered immutable principles, so few physicians were innovative and curious enough to challenge them. Those who did experiment in medicine were scorned by their colleagues, and physicians continued to use methods that were at best ineffectual or **innocuous** and at worst harmful to the patient. However, the establishment of universities led to a study of theories of disease rather than observation of the sick.

Early Development of Medical Education

Medical knowledge developed slowly, and distribution of such knowledge was poor. Before the printing press was invented in the mid-fifteenth century, very little exchange of scientific knowledge and ideas occurred; scientists were not well informed about the investigations of other scientists. The printing press allowed books to be distributed faster and over a widespread area. Another development important to science occurred in the seventeenth century, when European academies or societies were established, consisting of small groups of men who met to discuss subjects of mutual interest. The academies provided freedom of expression that, with the stimulus of exchanging ideas, contributed significantly to the development of scientific thought. One of the earliest of the academies was the Royal Society of London, formed in 1662. The development of communications during this era was important, and these societies contributed to the exchange of information.

Our world became more complex over the centuries, which prompted a greater need for regulation. The passage of the Medical Act of 1858 in Great Britain was considered one of the most important events in British medicine. The act established a statutory body, the General Medical Council, which controlled admission to the medical register and had regulatory power over medical education and examinations.

In the United States, medical education was greatly influenced by the Johns Hopkins University Medical School in Baltimore, Maryland, established in the early 1890s. The school admitted only college graduates with a year's training in the natural sciences. The clinical education at Johns Hopkins was superior because the school partnered with Johns Hopkins Hospital, which had been created expressly for teaching and research by members of the medical faculty. The first four professors at Johns Hopkins were Sir William Osler (Professor of Medicine), William H. Welch (Chief of Pathology), Howard A. Kelley (Chief of Gynecology and Obstetrics), and William D. Halsted (Chief of Surgery). Together these four men transformed the organization and curriculum of clinical teaching and made Johns Hopkins the most famous medical school in the world at that time.

The earliest medical school **accreditation** resulted from a report published by Abraham Flexner. He received a grant from the Carnegie Foundation Commission to study the quality of medical colleges in the United States and Canada. His report, called the Flexner Report, resulted in the closure of many low-ranking schools and the upgrading of others. These events legitimized medical education and opened new doors for many individuals to the world of medicine.

CRITICAL THINKING APPLICATION

■ Mr. Santos asks his class to identify which of the individuals involved in early medicine have had the most impact on modern healthcare. Whom would you choose, and why?

■ The students point out that early research was often viewed in a negative manner. How does research affect us now, and how is it viewed by the public?

Early Medical Pioneers

Andreas Vesalius (1514-1564) was a Belgian anatomist known as the Father of Modern Anatomy (Figure 2-3). At the age of 29 he published his great *De Corporis Humani Fabrica*, in which he described the structure of the human body. This work marked a turning point by breaking with past traditional beliefs in Galen's theories. Vesalius introduced many new anatomic terms, but because of his radical approach, he was subjected to persecution from his colleagues, teachers, and pupils. Despite his great

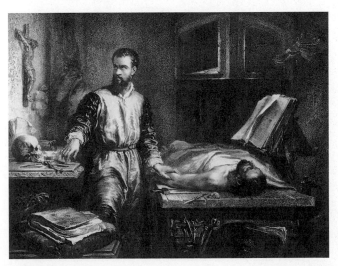

FIGURE 2-3 Andreas Vesalius is known as the Father of Modern Anatomy. (Courtesy National Library of Medicine.)

contributions to the science of anatomy, his name is not used to identify any significant anatomic structures.

Other important advances and discoveries took place throughout the world. Gabriele Fallopius (1523-1562), an Italian student of Vesalius, was also an accurate dissector. He described and named many parts of the human anatomy. He named the fallopian tubes after himself and also named the vagina and placenta. In 1628 William Harvey (1578-1657) announced his discovery that the heart acts as a muscular pump, forcing and propelling the blood throughout the body. He revealed that the blood's motion is a continuous cycle, basing his conclusion on his experimental vivisection, ligation, and perfusion as well as brilliant reasoning. Harvey's writings were recognized in Germany before the English permitted their publication at home. Modern England now considers Harvey to be its medical Shakespeare.

The unseen world of microorganisms was first revealed by Anton van Leeuwenhoek (1632-1723), a Dutch linen draper and haberdasher. Haberdashers made their living dealing in men's clothing and accessories, but it was Leeuwenhoek's hobby of grinding lenses that eventually led to his amazing discovery of the magnification process. He ground more than 400 lenses during his lifetime, some of which were no larger than a pinhead. In the grinding process, Leeuwenhoek learned how to use a simple biconvex lens to magnify the minute world of organisms and structures, never before seen. Leeuwenhoek was the first to ever observe bacteria and protozoa through a lens, and his accurate interpretations of what he saw led to the sciences of bacteriology and protozoology.

Marcello Malpighi (1628-1694) was born near Bologna, Italy, and attended the University of Bologna, where he earned a doctorate in both medicine and philosophy. He pioneered the use of the microscope in the study of plants and animals. Microscopic anatomy became a prerequisite for advances in physiology, embryology, and practical medicine. In 1661 he described the pulmonary and capillary network connecting the smallest arteries with the smallest veins. This was one of the most important discoveries in the history of science, and it validated Harvey's work. Malpighi is commonly regarded as the first histologist.

Medical Advances in the Eighteenth and Nineteenth Centuries

English scientist John Hunter (1728-1793) is known as the Founder of Scientific Surgery. An army surgeon, he became an expert on gunshot wounds and experimented with tissue transfer. His surgical procedures were soundly based on pathologic evidence. He was the first to classify teeth in a scientific manner and introduced artificial feeding by means of a flexible tube passed into the stomach. He provided a classic description of the syphilitic chancre, which is sometimes called a Hunterian chancre. During his studies of venereal diseases, he inoculated himself with what he thought was gonorrhea, but instead he acquired syphilis. His results in this study actually caused confusion in the medical community because he mistakenly thought that gonorrhea was a symptom of syphilis. This misconception was not corrected until the beginning of the twentieth century. His collection of anatomic and animal specimens formed the basis for the museum of the Royal College of Surgeons. After Hunter's death he was buried in St. Martin. His remains were later moved, however, to Westminster Abbey as a gesture of honor. A tablet was placed over his grave by the Royal College of Surgeons to "record their admiration of his genius as a gifted interpreter of the Divine Power and Wisdom at work in the laws of Organic Life and their grateful veneration for his services to mankind as the Founder of Scientific Surgery." Today in Australia the John Hunter Hospital serves more than 600 inpatients and 1000 outpatients per day.

Edward Jenner (1749-1823) was a student of John Hunter and a country physician from Dorsetshire, England. He is considered one of the immortals of preventive medicine for his development of the smallpox vaccine. While Jenner was serving as an apprentice, he assisted in treating a dairymaid. Smallpox was mentioned, and she commented, "I cannot take that disease, for I have had cowpox." Smallpox at that time was a deadly **pandemic.** Jenner observed that those who had contracted cowpox never contracted smallpox. Later, as a practicing physician, Jenner continued investigating the relationship between cowpox and smallpox almost obsessively, but the medical society members grew bored with his obsession and threatened to expel him from their ranks. On May 14, 1796 Dr. Jenner took purulent matter from a pustule on the hand of Sarah Nelmes, a dairymaid, and inserted it through two small superficial incisions into the arm of James Phipps, a healthy 8-year-old boy. This was the first vaccination. On July 1 a virulent dose of smallpox matter was given to the boy in the same arm. Phipps' vaccination kept him safe from the dreaded disease, and Jenner's method of vaccination spread throughout the world. The results of his experiments were published in 1798. He called this method of protection *vaccination,* from the Latin word *vacca,* which means "cow," and at that time, cowpox was called *vaccinia.* Today smallpox has been eradicated throughout the world as a result of a planned program of global vaccination.

Austrian physician Leopold Auenbrugger (1722-1809) developed the use of percussion in diagnosis. He became physician-in-chief to the Hospital of the Holy Trinity at Vienna in 1751, where he tested his discovery. Although scorned and ignored by his contemporaries, his techniques later made him famous and are still used today during physical examinations. René Laennec (1781-1826) was a French physician who developed the stethoscope in 1819. At first he used only a cylinder of rolled paper in his hands; later he used a wooden device because of its sound-conducting properties. With today's sophisticated stethoscopes physicians are able to hear sounds in the body, including a fetus inside the mother. Laennec's book, *Treatise on Mediate Auscultation and Diseases of the Chest,* was readily accepted and translated into many languages. It is said to be the most important treatise on diseases of the thoracic organs ever written.

Several men of the early 1800s are remembered for their fight against puerperal fever and their concern for women's health. Puerperal fever, an infectious disease that can be contracted during childbirth, was also called *puerperal sepsis* or *childbed fever.* The term *puerperal,* denoting a woman in childbed, originates from the Latin *puer,* "a child," and *pario,* "to bring forth." The word *puerperium* now designates the period from delivery to the time the uterus returns to normal size (approximately 42 days after childbirth).

The best known of these men was the Hungarian physician Ignaz Philipp Semmelweis (1818-1865); history has called him the Savior of Mothers. His fight against puerperal fever is a sad story of hardships. His theories were resisted by many professionals, including his instructors. Semmelweis noted that the fever often attacked women who were delivered by medical students coming straight from the autopsy or dissecting rooms. Semmelweis directed that in his wards the students were to wash and disinfect their hands before going to examine the women and deliver the children. This process brought about a marked reduction of cases of puerperal fever on his ward, but he still faced unrelenting opposition. As his theories were proved correct, Semmelweis felt an incredible guilt that the doctors themselves had caused so many deaths. He died at the age of 47—ironically, from the very disease he had fought. He was infected with puerperal fever from a cut on his finger during an autopsy. His grave had hardly been closed when scientists began to understand the causes of this disease, largely as a result of the investigations of two great scientists, Louis Pasteur and Joseph Lister.

Pasteur (1822-1895) was a Frenchman who did brilliant work as a chemist, but it was his studies in bacteriology that made him one of the most famous men in medical history (Figure 2-4). He was bestowed the title of Father of Bacteriology and has also been honored as the Father of Preventive Medicine. He gave unselfishly of his time outside his profession to help others solve problems. Pasteur's adventures included studying

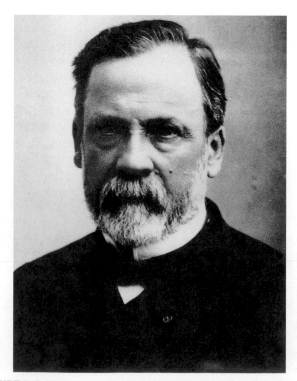

FIGURE 2-4 Louis Pasteur was a brilliant chemist who made numerous contributions to medicine. (Courtesy National Library of Medicine.)

the difficulties in the **fermentation** of wine. He averted disaster in France's critical winemaking industry by a process he developed, now called *pasteurization.* This achievement alone would have made him an immortal among the French. Through a process of supplying enough heat to destroy microorganisms, wine was prevented from turning to vinegar. The French people called on Pasteur again to help the ailing silkworm industry. He devoted years to the conquest of diseases that infected the silkworm. His efforts were impeded when he was stricken with hemiplegia, but after a long, difficult recovery, he was able to continue with a stiff hand and a limp.

Convinced that the infinite world of bacteria held the key to the secrets of contagious diseases, Pasteur left chemistry again to continue studying his theory. Many renowned scientists denied the germ theory of disease and devoted themselves to degrading Pasteur's theories and experiments. In the midst of this controversy he became involved in the prevention of anthrax, which threatened the health of cattle and sheep. Pasteur was eventually honored for his work with many other diseases, such as rabies, chicken cholera, and swine erysipelas. He devoted the last 7 years of his life to the Pasteur Institute, which was founded as a clinic for rabies treatment, a research center for infectious disease, and a teaching center. The Pasteur Institute still exists today. He died in 1895, with his family at his bedside. It is said that his last words were, "There is still a great deal to do."

Joseph Lister (1827-1912) revolutionized surgery through the application of Pasteur's discoveries. He understood the similarity between infections in postsurgical wounds and the processes of **putrefaction.** Pasteur proved that these processes were caused by microorganisms. Before this time, surgeons accepted that infections in surgical wounds were inevitable. Lister reasoned that microorganisms must be the cause of infection and should be kept out of wounds. His colleagues were indifferent to his theories, because most believed infections were God-given and natural. Lister disagreed, and he developed antiseptic methods by using carbolic acid for sterilization. By spraying the rooms with a fine mist of the acid, soaking the instruments in carbolic solutions, and washing his hands in a similar solution, he was able to prove his theories. He is honored as the Father of Sterile Surgery. Pasteur and Lister met after years of great mutual admiration. The meeting was filled with emotion, and it was written in *Pathfinders in Medicine* that "a new star should have appeared in the heavens to commemorate the event." Medicine truly owes a deep gratitude to these two pioneers for the knowledge they imparted to the art.

Robert Koch (1843-1910) is a familiar name to all bacteriologists because of his famous Koch's Postulates—his theory of rules that must be followed before an organism can be accepted as the causative agent in a given disease. Koch was a German physician who earned great honors in bacteriology and public health. He introduced many of the tools used in the laboratory, such as the culture-plate method for isolation of bacteria. He discovered the cause of cholera and demonstrated its transmission by food and water. This discovery completely transformed health departments and proved the importance of bacteriology in everyday life. Koch's greatest disappointment was his failure to find a cure for tuberculosis, but in his attempt he isolated tuberculin, the substance produced by tubercle bacteria. Its use as a diagnostic aid was of immense value to medicine. In 1885 the University of Berlin created the Chair of Hygiene and Bacteriology in honor of Robert Koch. He became a Nobel Laureate in 1905.

One of Koch's students was a German physician named Paul Ehrlich (1854-1915). He pioneered the fields of bacteriology, immunology, and especially chemotherapy. Chemotherapy is the process of treating diseases by injecting chemicals into the body to destroy microorganisms, and this was a new science in Koch's day. Ehrlich was only 28 when he wrote his first paper on typhoid, but his greatest gift to humanity was called his "magic bullet," or formula 606, which was designed to fight syphilis. With the organism identified by scientists Bordet and Wasserman, Ehrlich set out to find a chemical that would destroy the organism but not harm the host, specifically, the human body. The six hundred–sixth drug that Ehrlich tried finally brought about healing. He called it *salvarsan* because he believed that it offered mankind salvation from the disease. This endeavor also marked the beginning of the practice of injecting chemicals into the body to destroy a specific organism. In 1908 Ehrlich shared the Nobel Prize with Eli Metchnikoff, who is remembered for his theory of phagocytosis and immunology.

Crawford Williamson Long (1815-1878) was the first to employ ether as an anesthetic agent. Early in 1842 a group of students would have a social gathering after chemistry lectures and inhale ether, a chemical commonly found in chemistry labs, as a form of amusement. Ether, an intoxicant similar to nitrous oxide, functions as a soporific or sleep-inducing agent. However, at one of these "ether frolics," as they were called, Dr. Long also observed that people under the influence of ether did not seem to feel pain. After considerable thought, he decided to use ether for a surgical operation. In March 1842 he removed a tumor from the neck of James M. Venable after placing him under the influence of ether. Dr. Horace Wells was a dentist who reported using nitrous oxide as an anesthetic in 1844. Another dentist, Dr. William T.G. Morton, reported using ether in 1846 when he extracted a tooth from a patient, and he also used the gas at Massachusetts General Hospital for a surgical procedure.

Surgeons are grateful to Wilhelm Konrad Roentgen (1845-1923), a professor of physics at the University of Wurzburg, Germany. Roentgen discovered the x-ray in 1895 while experimenting with electrical currents passed through sealed glass tubes. He was awarded the Nobel Prize in Physics in 1901. Although he called it an *x-ray,* history has honored him by calling it the *roentgen ray.* Marie and Pierre Curie discovered radium in 1898, and they were awarded the 1902 Nobel Prize in Physics for their work on radioactivity. Unfortunately, Pierre was killed 3 years later while crossing a street in a rainstorm. Marie was awarded his teaching position at the Sorbonne, a medical university in France; no woman had taught at the school in its 650-year history. In 1911 she was awarded the Nobel Prize for her discoveries of radium and polonium, the first person to receive the award twice. She died in 1934 from pernicious anemia, which was believed to have been caused by her overexposure to radiation and years of overwork.

Nineteenth Century Women in Medicine

Many other women made great contributions to medicine in the early nineteenth century. Florence Nightingale (1820-1910) is known as the founder of nursing and is fondly called the Lady with the Lamp (Figure 2-5). She was of noble birth, and somewhat late in life she sought nursing training in both England and Europe. By the dawn of the Crimean War in 1854, she had established a fine reputation for her work in hospital organization. She was invited by the British Secretary of War to visit the Crimea to help correct the terrible conditions that existed in caring for the wounded. She created the Women's Nursing Service in Scutari and Balaklava. The physicians treated her and the other 38 nurses poorly until a crisis brought thousands of wounded and sick soldiers to the army hospitals. The bravery and competence of the nurses helped the doctors realize their value to the medical profession. In 1860 she founded the Nightingale School and Home for Nurses in London, which marked the beginning of professional nursing education.

Clara Barton (1821-1912), an American, began her nursing career early in life. When she was 11 years of age her brother fell from the roof of their barn, and Clara nursed him back to health over a 2-year period. She later was a battlefield nurse and **philanthropist** whose work during the Civil War led her to recognize that very poor records were kept in Washington to aid in the search for missing men who were wounded or killed in combat. Her efforts to remedy this led to the formation of the Bureau of Records. Her organization and recruitment of supplies for the wounded led to her eventual involvement with the Red Cross in the Franco-Prussian War. In 1881 she organized a Red Cross Committee in Washington, the original formation of the American Red Cross. She served as its first president from 1881 to 1904. Her retirement came at the age of 82, just after personally leading dangerous expeditions to help victims of fires, hurricanes, and floods. The American Red Cross remains a vital organization to this day.

Elizabeth Blackwell (1821-1910) was the first woman in the United States to receive the Doctor of Medicine degree from a medical school (Figure 2-6). Blackwell's family immigrated to New York from England in 1832. She began her medical education by reading medical books and later obtained private instruction. Medical schools in New York and Pennsylvania initially refused her applications for formal study, but finally in 1847 she was accepted at the Geneva Medical College in New York. Ten years later, she established the New York Infirmary for Indigent Women and Children, the first hospital staffed entirely by women. In 1869 Blackwell returned to her native England and became a professor of gynecology at the London School of Medicine for Women, of which she was a founder.

Lillian Wald (1867-1940), a social worker and nurse, made great contributions to medical care when she founded the Henry Street Settlement in New York City. Wald operated a visiting nurse service from this establishment. When one of her nurses was assigned to the city's public schools in 1902, the New York City Municipal Board of Health established the world's first public school nursing system.

Margaret Sanger (1883-1966) was born in Corning, New York, and trained as a nurse at the White Plains Hospital. She became the American leader of the birth control movement. While working among the poor in New York City, she came to understand the public's need for information about contraception. She left nursing to devote herself to that objective. In 1873 the federal Comstock law declared it illegal to import or distribute any device, medicine, or information designed to prevent conception or induce abortion, or to mention in print the names of sexually transmitted diseases. Nurses and physicians were legally prohibited from providing this information to their patients. In 1914 Sanger was **indicted** for circulating the magazine *The Woman Rebel*, in which she attacked the legislative

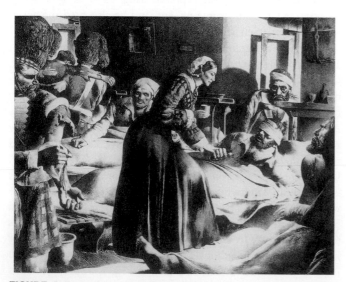

FIGURE 2-5 Considered the founder of nursing, Florence Nightingale is also known as the Lady with the Lamp. (Courtesy National Library of Medicine.)

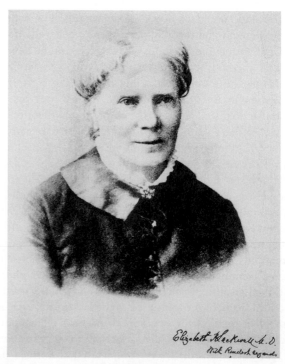

FIGURE 2-6 Elizabeth Blackwell was the first woman to receive a degree as a medical doctor in the United States. (Courtesy National Library of Medicine.)

restrictions of the Comstock law. The case was dismissed 2 years later. In the same year she established the first American birth control clinic; this led to her arrest, conviction, and time in the county jail. She continued her work, and after World War II, she successfully advocated research into hormonal contraception, because of the newfound concern about population growth. This research ultimately led to development of the birth control pill. When the Planned Parenthood Federation of America was formed in 1941, she was named honorary chairperson.

CRITICAL THINKING APPLICATION

Mr. Santos asks his students to tell him which of these early pioneers they would most like to have worked with. Whom would you choose, and why? What difficulties did they face as they worked?

MEDICAL MILESTONES

In recognition of the achievements of scientists of the past, Sir Isaac Newton spoke of our ability to discover and innovate in the medical field. He humbly said, "If I have seen a little further than others, it is because I have stood on the shoulders of giants." Great strides in medicine accompanied the twentieth century, and technology began to advance rapidly. Medical leaders continued their contributions, and knowledge, treatment, and research grew by leaps and bounds.

Walter Reed was a U.S. Army pathologist and bacteriologist who proved that yellow fever was transmitted by the bite of a mosquito. Persons with diabetes should be grateful to Sir Frederick Grant Banting, a Canadian physician who isolated insulin for treatment, along with Charles Herbert Best, a Canadian physiologist. In 1928 Sir Alexander Fleming discovered penicillin accidentally while researching influenza and working with staphylococcal bacteria. He found a substance in mold that prevented growth of bacteria even when the substance was diluted 800 times.

Cardiologist Helen Taussig and surgeon Alfred Blalock explored the health issues of children born with cyanosis resulting from a malformed heart. Dr. Taussig collaborated with Dr. Blalock to develop a lifesaving operation for these children, called "blue babies." History often omits the contributions of Vivien Thomas, an African-American who was Dr. Blalock's surgical research technician at Johns Hopkins Hospital. Thomas was a former carpenter who constructed several of the medical instruments used in the Blalock-Taussig procedure. Thomas actually created the blue-baby condition in dogs, on which he regularly practiced the surgical procedure. When Dr. Blalock and Dr. Taussig performed the first blue-baby operation at Johns Hopkins University, Thomas stood over Blalock's shoulder and advised him during the procedure, since Thomas had done the surgery several more times than Blalock. This happened at a time when African-Americans were not allowed on the main floors of the hospital, much less in the surgical suite. This surgery became known as the Blalock-Taussig procedure, and although the first blue-baby operation prolonged the patient's life by only 2 months, subsequent operations were successful

and children were able to leave the hospital with hope of a healthy life.

Jonas Edward Salk and Albert Sabin almost eradicated poliomyelitis, once the killer and crippler of thousands in the United States. Salk's injectable vaccine was developed in 1952, and after wide-scale testing in 1954 it was distributed nationally, greatly reducing the incidence of the disease. Sabin's live-virus vaccine, in a form that could be swallowed, became available less than a decade later. Werner Forssmann, a German surgeon, originated a cardiac technique called *catheterization* that is used in the diagnosis and treatment of heart disease. Christiaan Barnard, a South African surgeon, performed the first human-heart transplant in 1967. Dr. Elisabeth Kübler-Ross, a Swiss-born psychiatrist who died in 2004, was shocked at the treatment of terminally ill patients at her hospital in New York. She wrote the best-selling book *On Death and Dying*, which helped professionals and laypersons alike to understand the stages of grief.

CRITICAL THINKING APPLICATION

- During class discussion Mr. Santos points out that the leaders in the healthcare industry had specific goals for their careers and achieved worldwide recognition for their contributions. What individuals have made contributions to medicine in recent years?
- How can the individual medical assistant make a contribution to medicine?

MODERN MEDICINE

Many modern physicians are making important discoveries and contributions to the field of medicine. Dr. David Ho is considered by many to be one of the most brilliant minds today helping to piece together the puzzle of the human immunodeficiency virus (HIV). Ho is the scientific director and chief executive officer (CEO) of the Aaron Diamond AIDS Research Center in New York City and is also a professor at Rockefeller University. He was born in Taiwan in 1952, and his family immigrated to the United States when he was 12 years of age. He eventually entered college to study physics—medicine was actually his second choice—but once he discovered molecular biology and the concept of gene splicing, he decided to become a researcher. He still does calculations in Chinese. Ho was named *Time* magazine's "Man of the Year" in 1996 for his work in the battle against HIV and acquired immunodeficiency syndrome (AIDS).

Dr. Eve Slater served as the Assistant Secretary for Health at the U.S. Department of Health and Human Services (DHHS). Dr. Slater was former Secretary Tommy G. Thompson's primary advisor on matters regarding issues concerning the nation's public health and oversaw DHHS's U.S. Public Health Service (PHS). Before she joined DHHS, Dr. Slater served as a senior vice president of Merck Research Laboratories' external policy, and also as Vice President of Corporate Public Affairs. Dr. Slater was the first woman to hold this rank. During her time with Merck, she spearheaded the approval of major medicines used to treat the HIV infection, osteoporosis, cardiovascular disease, arthritis, chickenpox, and many others. In 1976, Dr. Slater became the first woman appointed chief resident in medicine at Massachusetts General Hospital. She served as an assistant professor at Harvard Medical School and directed laboratory research funded by the National Institutes of Health (NIH) and the American Heart Association. Currently, Dr. Slater is a board member of several prestigious medical organizations, including Theravance, Inc. and VaxGen, the company co-founded by Dr. Don Francis, who led the fight against AIDS when the disease was first discovered.

Dr. C. Everett Koop was graduated from Cornell University as a medical doctor in 1941 and spent most of his career as a pediatric surgeon. During his terms as the U.S. Surgeon General, he became a proponent of tobacco awareness, insisting that tobacco advertisements must be less attractive to the youth of today. Dr. Koop is a professor at Dartmouth Medical School. He founded the Koop Institute, an organization whose mission is to "promote the health and well-being of all people." Dr. Koop has been honored with many awards, including 41 honorary doctorates.

Dr. Marcia Angell is the former editor-in-chief of the *New England Journal of Medicine* (NEJM), one of the most prestigious medical publications in the United States. Her career with NEJM began in 1979, and her excellent articles spanned a variety of subjects, from the pharmaceutical companies' profit margins to the effects of socioeconomic status on Americans seeking healthcare services. Angell was named one of the 25 most influential Americans in 1997 by Time magazine. She has written and contributed to several books, including *Science on Trial: The Clash of Medical Evidence and the Law in the Breast Implant Case*. Angell is a board-certified pathologist and currently serves as senior lecturer in the Department of Social Medicine at Harvard Medical School.

As the director of the National Institute of Allergy and Infectious Diseases at the NIH, Dr. Anthony Fauci leads research efforts on immune–mediated disorders. His scientific leadership has resulted in major advances in several diseases, such as polyarteritis nodosa and Wegener's granulomatosis. Many of his studies now relate to HIV and the body's response to the AIDS virus, and ways to improve HIV treatment and prevention, including HIV vaccine development. Out of more than one million scientists who published during the period between 1981 and 1994, Dr. Fauci was the fifth most **cited.** He received his MD from Cornell University Medical College, and his career with the NIH has spanned more than 30 years.

Dr. Antonia Novello was the first woman, and the first Hispanic, to be honored with the post of Surgeon General. She served at the NIH and was the honorary chairperson of the National Youth Summit for Mothers Against Drunk Driving (MADD). Novello played a key role in writing the warning labels on cigarette packages. She supported and promoted the National Organ Transplant Act of 1984 and has contributed to the efforts of the United Nations Children's Fund (UNICEF). Novello was a clinical professor at Georgetown University Hospital and in 1994 was inducted into the National Women's Hall of Fame. She currently serves as New York State's health commissioner.

THE NATIONAL VIEW OF HEALTHCARE

World Health Organization

The World Health Organization (WHO), founded in 1948, is a specialized agency of the United Nations. The organization promotes cooperation among nations in their efforts to control and eliminate diseases worldwide. The purposes of WHO are as follows:

- To give worldwide guidance in the field of health
- To set global standards for health
- To cooperate with governments in strengthening national health programs
- To develop and transfer appropriate health technology, information, and standards

One of the greatest accomplishments of this agency was the eradication of smallpox. Other diseases, such as polio and leprosy, are on the verge of eradication. The agency also created and maintains the International Classification of Diseases (ICD) coding system. ICD-9 is used today to identify diseases and conditions using a specific code number. The original purpose of this system was to track worldwide morbidity and mortality statistics. WHO is committed to research and delivery of needed drugs and medical supplies to various areas of the world. In addition, WHO promotes the sharing of health information, and WHO officials meet with the leaders of the worldwide health industry to discuss various ethical and moral implications that face today's healthcare professionals.

U.S. Department of Health and Human Services

The Department of Health and Human Services (HHS) is the principal U.S. agency for providing essential human services and protecting the health of all Americans, especially those who are unable to help themselves. HHS is made up of more than 300 programs involved in the following:

- Medical and social science research
- Immunization services
- Financial assistance for low-income families
- Child support enforcement services
- Improvement of infant and maternal health
- Child and elder abuse prevention services
- Assistance programs for elderly Americans

HHS also oversees the Medicare and Medicaid programs. Medicare is the nation's largest health insurer, and HHS processes more than one billion claims every year. It is the largest grant-making agency in the federal government, providing more than 60,000 grants annually. With a budget of more than $581 billion and more than 67,000 employees, HHS works side by side with local and state governments in its effort to serve the healthcare needs of the public.

U.S. Army Medical Research Institute of Infectious Diseases

The primary focus of the U.S. Army Medical Research Institute of Infectious Diseases (USAMRIID) is protecting military service members, but the Institute conducts key research programs in national defense and infectious diseases that benefit

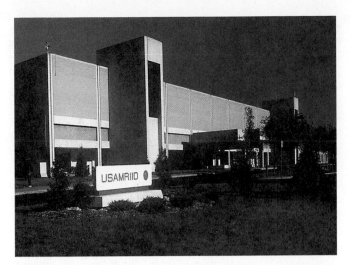

FIGURE 2-7 U.S. Army Medical Research Institute of Infectious Diseases in Fort Detrick, Maryland. (Courtesy USAMRIID, Ft. Detrick, Md.)

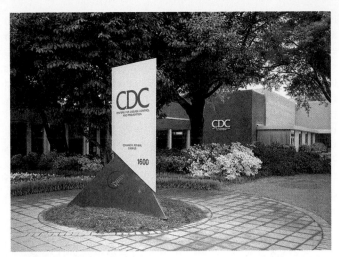

FIGURE 2-8 The headquarters of the Centers for Disease Control and Prevention (CDC) are located in Atlanta, Georgia. (Courtesy Centers for Disease Control and Prevention, Atlanta, Ga.)

everyone (Figure 2-7). USAMRIID, located at Fort Detrick in Maryland, works extensively with the Centers for Disease Control and Prevention (CDC) and WHO. USAMRIID also controls an internationally known reference laboratory with state-of-the-art facilities. This laboratory is instrumental in identifying biologic threats and the diseases those threats produce. USAMRIID is the only laboratory facility operated by the Department of Defense that is equipped to study biosafety level IV viruses and pathogens.

Four biosafety levels are commonly accepted among laboratory professionals. Biosafety level I consists of well-known agents that have a minimal or low biohazard potential to laboratory personnel and to the environment as a whole. At this level the laboratory is not necessarily separated from the regular areas of the facility. Examples of level I pathogens include *Pneumococcus* and *Salmonella*. In the biosafety level II section of the laboratory, substances with a moderate biohazard potential are studied. At levels I and II laboratory personnel have specific training in handling pathogens, and specialized equipment is used to avoid splashes and splatters. Pathogens classified as biosafety level II are hepatitis, the Lyme disease virus, and influenza virus.

Personnel working in biosafety level III have very specific training in working with the potentially deadly pathogens found at this level. All procedures performed on level III pathogens have a high biohazard risk and are done inside protective safety cabinets. Laboratory personnel are required to wear heavy personal protective equipment. Special regulations concerning exhaust air and ventilation are strictly followed, and access to the laboratory is limited when work is in progress. Human immunodeficiency virus (HIV), anthrax, and typhus are some of the pathogens classified as biosafety level III. Biosafety level IV is applied to the most deadly pathogens, which often produce incurable diseases. The biohazard risk of transmission of these agents is extreme and includes the risk of airborne transmission. Laboratory personnel are highly trained in the manipulation and handling of these dangerous pathogens. Laboratory access is strictly controlled in this section. Some of the pathogens

studied at biosafety level IV include Ebola virus, Lassa virus, and hantavirus.

Centers for Disease Control and Prevention

The headquarters for the CDC are located in Atlanta, Georgia, (Figure 2-8). The CDC is the principal U.S. federal agency concerned with the health and safety of people throughout the world and is a part of HHS. It is a clearinghouse for information and statistics associated with healthcare. Several divisions within the CDC focus on specific health-related issues, such as the National Center for HIV, STD, and TB Prevention; the Public Health Practice Program Office; the National Center on Birth Defects and Developmental Disabilities; and the National Center for Health Statistics. Branch offices are located throughout the United States and in several foreign countries. The CDC has over 9000 employees who are dedicated to public health. Extensive publications and information services provide healthcare professionals all over the world with the information needed to care for patients.

The agency conducts research into the origin and occurrence of diseases and develops methods for their control and prevention. In addition, it develops immunization services and aids in the training of healthcare workers. In recent years the CDC has been intricately involved in the battle against HIV, which in its advanced form is the acquired immunodeficiency syndrome (AIDS). The agency has developed guidelines emphasizing that universal blood and body fluid precautions be used in all situations in which the risk of contamination by body fluids exists. These recommended precautions are the basis for the laws enforced by the Occupational Safety and Health Administration (OSHA) regarding blood-borne pathogens.

National Institutes of Health

The National Institutes of Health (NIH) began as a one-room laboratory in the marine hospital on New York's Staten Island in 1887. Its first major contribution to medicine was the isolation of the bacterium that causes cholera. Tuberculosis was the number one cause of death at that time. There were few drugs that could alleviate or cure diseases, and there were no vaccines, except for smallpox vaccine. There were no antibiotics, and even aspirin was not yet available. Doctors could diagnose some conditions but fell short on treatments. In 1891 the laboratory moved from Staten Island to Washington, DC. In 1930 the laboratory became the NIH, an agency of HHS. The mission of the NIH is to uncover new knowledge that will lead to better health for everyone. As a part of the public health service, it seeks to improve the health of the American people, supports and conducts biomedical research into the causes and prevention of diseases, and uses a modern communications system to furnish biomedical information to the healthcare professions.

The NIH moved from Washington, DC, to Bethesda, Maryland, in 1938 and today occupies more than 60 buildings covering 30 acres. It consists of 27 different Institutes and Centers and the National Library of Medicine. Thousands of research projects are underway in NIH laboratories and clinics at any given time. The NIH also provides support to other research projects conducted at universities, medical schools, and hospitals.

HEALTH INDUSTRY COUNCILS

Health industry councils are organizations that seek to organize and unify all of the entities providing healthcare in a certain region or community. These organizations keep statistical records about the medical trends in the area and are an important factor in drawing new businesses related to the medical field to the area that they represent. These councils are designed to function as developmental groups that promote the industry in their area and work together for the good of all those involved in healthcare. The organizations represented within the council may fiercely compete in the area market, but they work together to promote the healthcare industry in the region where they are located. The councils usually are made up of task forces and committees that study communications concepts, home health, managed care, membership and development, new business promotion, and design and construction. They are an excellent source of medical information and trends in medicine locally, statewide, and nationally. These councils are valuable assets to any region that wishes to remain on the cutting edge of healthcare.

TYPES OF HEALTHCARE FACILITIES

Hospitals

Several different types of hospitals exist. They are classified according to the type of care and services that they provide to patients, as well as by type of ownership. Acute-care hospitals offer intensive care units and emergency or trauma departments and are equipped to handle the most severely ill or injured patients. Subacute-care hospitals offer patient care for those who do not require extensive services but still need hospital super-

vision and treatment. Specialty hospitals, such as a psychiatric hospital, offer specific services. Teaching hospitals provide a learning environment and often have research departments as well. These hospitals are usually affiliated with medical schools, and interns or residents provide care supervised by licensed physician instructors. Community hospitals provide care in rural areas or in specific areas within a metropolis. Regional hospitals are usually acute-care facilities and serve a large area that may not offer intensive care in its local communities.

Private hospitals are run by a corporation or other organization and are usually designed to produce a profit for the owners or stockholders. Nonprofit hospitals exist to serve the community in which they are located and are normally run by a board of directors. The term *nonprofit* is sometimes misleading, because a difference exists between "profit" and "making money." A nonprofit hospital or organization may make money in a campaign or fund-raiser, but all of the money is returned to the organization. Nonprofit hospitals and organizations must follow strict guidelines in the area of finance and must account to the government how much money is brought in and for what purposes it is used. Sometimes the term *county hospital* is used to designate the hospital to which **indigent** patients are taken. These hospitals provide emergency care to those who cannot pay for medical expenses. Today, however, many people without insurance go to the emergency department (ER) for routine illnesses. This is one reason that ERs are busy and full. If patients have no other options, the ER physicians become primary care providers. This is a major cause of the long waiting times experienced in hospital ERs. Managed care has eased this problem somewhat by refusing to cover visits to the ER that are not true emergencies. **Triage** procedures are used to determine which patients have the most severe conditions and should be seen first.

Hospitals have various departments that are organized to provide efficient patient care. The admissions department gathers information and enters it into a computer for use by the rest of the hospital staff. Nursing service supervises all of the nursing care given to the patients and is involved in **case management.** The laboratory provides diagnostic testing on blood, body fluids, and tissues, and the radiology or nuclear medicine department offers diagnostic imaging and x-ray services. The respiratory services department offers a broad spectrum of diagnostic tests and various treatments. Most hospitals also have a physical medicine and rehabilitation department, which offers both physical and occupational therapy. The dietary department employs professionals who carefully plan menus to meet the needs of each patient served. Most modern hospitals have a surgery department, and many offer day surgery services that allow patients to have a procedure performed and go home the same day, if they recover as expected. The medical records department is responsible for the patient records related to every **encounter** that takes place in the facility. Social services works with patients to ensure continuity of care, patient education, and social intervention, all of which assist patients with emotional, economic, and social concerns.

The hospital administrators manage the hospital on a day-to-day basis, and human resource responsibilities are usually a part of the administration department. Almost every hospital has a board of directors to assist the administrators in governing the hospital, and usually a medical staff committee, led by the hospital's chief of staff, assists in the management of the facility and the **credentialing** process for the physicians that have **staff privileges.** Credentialing involves determining whether a practitioner should be allowed to practice medicine in a facility, based on his or her education, license, past performance, and other qualifications.

The National Practitioner Data Bank also gathers information that helps healthcare facilities identify physicians who are incompetent. It provides information about physicians who have had licensure problems, made malpractice settlements, had clinical privileges revoked or restricted, or had action taken against them by a professional society. This process is incredibly important, because if an incompetent physician is allowed to have staff privileges at a hospital, patients could be harmed and the facility could be held liable for the physician's actions and named as a codefendant in medical professional liability cases. Physicians' backgrounds should be carefully scrutinized by the credentialing committee and staff to avoid this threat of liability. Various types of **peer review organizations** (PROs) are also critical to good healthcare facility management.

Accreditation is considered the highest form of recognition for the quality of care that a facility or organization provides. Not only does it indicate to the public that the facility is concerned with offering high-quality care, it also provides professional liability insurance benefits and plays a role in regulatory agency relicensure and certification efforts. Hospitals and other healthcare facilities are often accredited by the Joint Commission on Accreditation of Healthcare Organizations (JCAHO), an organization that is concerned with the quality of care given in healthcare facilities. **Standards** or **indicators** have been developed that help to determine when patients are receiving high-quality care. The term *quality* refers to much more than whether the patient liked the food served or had to wait to have a procedure or test performed. Categories of compliance include the following:

- Assessment and care of patients
- Use of medication
- Plant, technology, and safety management
- Orientation, education, and training of staff
- Medical staff qualifications
- Patient rights

Ratings from 1 to 5 are given to the facility on its performance in specific areas. A "1" rating means that the facility is in full compliance with that standard, and the other ratings indicate different levels of noncompliance. HHS also regulates healthcare facilities, as does OSHA.

CRITICAL THINKING APPLICATION

- Mr. Santos has assigned his students to groups and asked them to investigate local hospitals. What types of hospitals are found in your local area, and what services do they provide? How might a hospital board decide what services are offered to the community?
- How might Mr. Santos' students find out whether a physician has staff privileges at a certain hospital?

Ambulatory Care

Many other types of healthcare facilities operate in the industry today. **Ambulatory** care centers include a wide range of facilities that offer healthcare services to patients who are able to walk around and are not bedridden. Physicians' offices, group practices, and multispecialty group practices are common types of ambulatory care facilities. Group practices may be of a single specialty, such as pediatrics, or may be multispecialty. A multispecialty practice might consist of an internal medicine specialist, an oncologist, a family practitioner, and an endocrinologist. Usually the physicians within the practice refer to each other when indicated. This is not only more convenient for the patients, but also more profitable for the physicians.

Occupational health centers are concerned with helping patients return to work and productive activity. Often, physical therapy is used in conjunction with rehabilitation services that assist the patient in regaining as much of the previous level of ability as possible. Also, freestanding rehabilitation centers can assist patients with a wide range of services. Pain management centers help patients deal with discomfort that is associated with their condition. Sleep centers diagnose and treat people who have sleep problems. Difficulty in sleeping is a symptom, like pain, and the cause of the disturbance must be found so that proper treatment can be provided. Freestanding urgent or emergency care centers provide patients with an alternative to hospital ERs. They are less expensive, have a shorter waiting time, and are conveniently located in many areas. Most have flexible hours, many are open well into the evening hours, and walk-in appointments are usually accepted.

Surgery has become more convenient because of the number of ambulatory surgical centers that exist today. Day surgery performed in hospitals has continued to provide patients with alternatives to overnight hospital care after surgery. Many insurance companies now prefer day surgery because it is more cost effective. Not many years ago, however, the only alternative to inpatient surgery was the same hospital's day-surgery department. Today more and more freestanding surgical centers are available. Patients can be treated with laser surgery, radial keratotomy, and cataract removal during the day and recover at home that same evening. Plastic surgeons are becoming very innovative in the physical structure of their offices and the types of surgery they offer on an outpatient basis. Many plastic surgeons offer breast augmentation and reduction and even abdominoplasty ("tummy tuck") and liposuction in the office setting. It was not long ago that having abdominoplasty meant staying for several days in the hospital. The new trend is becoming more accepted, partially as a result of the new "office-based surgery" accreditation offered by the Ambulatory Care Accreditation Program of the JCAHO.

Dialysis centers offer services to patients with severe kidney disorders, and many of the larger cities across the country have cancer centers for patients who need treatment by oncologists. Many other types of ambulatory care facilities exist, including centers that provide magnetic resonance imaging (MRI), student health clinics, dental clinics, endoscopy centers, community health centers, mobile health services, podiatric care centers, and women's health centers.

Geriatric and long-term patients have more options today for ambulatory care than ever before. In the past, nursing homes were the only alternative to keeping elderly patients in their own homes. These nursing homes provided care for residents who needed more than just assistance with day-to-day activities. Now there are many attractive options to traditional nursing homes or skilled nursing facilities. One of the most popular is assisted living. Most assisted living facilities provide 24-hour supervision of their residents, most meals, and a broad range of services, from the very basic, such as transportation to physician office visits and errand-running, to the extravagant, such as shopping trips and day-long outings. Most also provide exercise programs, social services, laundry and linen services, and housekeeping. The cost ranges from approximately $1000 to $3000 per month, depending on the location and the **amenities** desired by the resident. There are many new assisted-living facilities specifically designed for Alzheimer's or other memory-care patients.

Independent retirement communities offer residents the opportunity to come and go as they please. Many have a resort-like design, catering to the desire of retirees to enjoy their golden years. Usually the communities consist of apartments or duplex units, and some even offer small cottages. Activities are planned to enhance the social life of the residents, and some communities offer libraries with computer access, restaurant-style dining, beauty salons, and even gardens to grow food. The units usually have special emergency call bells and other protective devices for safety.

Other Healthcare Facilities

Several other types of healthcare facilities deserve attention in the broad overview of the healthcare industry. Diagnostic laboratories offer testing services for patients referred by their physicians. Since the enactment of the Clinical Laboratory Improvement Act (CLIA) in 1967 and its amendment in 1988, many physician offices have stopped providing laboratory tests that were performed inside their offices. These types of labs are called physician office laboratories (POLs). CLIA was enacted to ensure high-quality laboratory testing. The regulations set forth by both OSHA and CLIA rules often made it more cost effective to have the patient go to an outside laboratory to have tests done. The medical assistant should note that OSHA is an organization and division of the U.S. Department of Labor that enforces many laws related to workplace safety. CLIA is a law, not an agency. However, both influence safety and quality testing.

Home health agencies were tremendously successful in the late 1980s to the mid 1990s, but cuts in Medicare funding have caused them to suffer severe losses in recent years. This concept of care is very popular. Unfortunately, the influx of too many home health agencies and the subsequent drop in payments made to them have resulted in fewer home healthcare providers over the past several years. In addition, many hospitals began offering home healthcare, which added to the already heavy competition that smaller firms faced. Home healthcare offers its patients home care, therapy services, administration and assistance with medications, and other services so that the patient can remain at home yet still obtain the care that is needed.

Medical suppliers are retail operations that offer all types of medical devices and products. Diabetic patients can purchase glucose monitoring machines. Special hospital beds can be ordered for those who need them. All types of durable medical equipment (DME), such as bedpans, crutches, bathing assistance devices, wheelchairs, and walkers, are available, often without a physician's prescription. Most medical suppliers serve both the public and the profession.

Hospice centers play an important role in the acceptance of terminal illnesses. These facilities are designed to care for the patient with a terminal disease and provide support to family members. The goal of hospice is to provide peace, comfort, and dignity while controlling pain and promoting the best possible quality of life for the patient. Most patients involved in hospice care have a life expectancy of less than 6 months.

MEDICAL PRACTICES

Three general types of business structures exist in medical practices today: the sole proprietorship, the partnership, and the corporation. Sole proprietorships dominated medical practice until the last quarter of the twentieth century. These practices are on the decline as a result of the **advent** of managed care and its favor of the multispecialty group practice.

Sole Proprietorship

A sole proprietor is an individual who holds exclusive right and title to all aspects of the medical practice. The sole proprietor may employ other physicians to participate in the practice. The employed physician is entitled to employee benefits; however, the owner is not considered an employee and is not so entitled. In addition, the owner would be potentially liable for all of the acts of his or her professional employees and staff members. Although practicing alone has many advantages, including flexibility and independence, it also has heavy disadvantages. The drawbacks include having total responsibility for covering the practice 24 hours a day, 7 days a week. In an unincorporated solo practice, the business dies when the owner leaves it, unless it is sold to someone else. Many modern physicians do not see sole proprietorship as an avenue for a decent income as a doctor, because managed care companies often offer participation to group practices over the single-practice physician, enabling them to provide more options to the patients. Some doctors organize associate practices. In this case, physicians share office space, and often equipment and employees, but they operate their practices as sole proprietorships. Agreements such as these should always be in writing to avoid misunderstandings and legal concerns.

Partnership

When two or more physicians elect to associate in the practice of medicine, they may enter into a partnership agreement. This agreement specifies all of the rights, obligations, and responsibilities of each partner. They have more potential for profit as a partnership than they would in practice as sole proprietors, because various expenses are shared and resources are pooled. Each physician has more freedom, because the doctors rotate an "on-call" schedule so that each has some time away from the office and patients. However, one disadvantage of the partnership is the liability of each for the actions and conduct of all the others. In a partnership arrangement, the partners often pool employees, equipment, insurance, facilities, and even profits, and these resources are divided according to the specifications of the partnership agreement or contract.

A group practice is a body of at least three licensed physicians who engage in full-time practice in a formally organized and legally recognized entity. A group practice may take the form of a partnership, or it may be formed as a corporation. The group may share income and expenses, equipment, records, and personnel and may combine patient care and business management. The group practice may be an association of the same specialty or may be a multispecialty organization. Usually a group practice will take the form of a partnership or a corporation.

Corporation

A corporation may be defined as an artificial entity having a legal and business status that is independent of its shareholders or employees. Corporations are regulated by statutes of the state in which the incorporation takes place. In most cases the physician shareholders are employees of the corporation. Even one physician in a solo practice can incorporate the practice. All employees of the corporation receive income and tax advantages. Corporations are usually able to offer better benefit packages, which may include pension and profit-sharing plans, medical expense reimbursement, life insurance, disability income insurance, and many other benefits. Some offer cafeteria plans, which the employees can customize according to their specific needs, including benefits such as child care reimbursement and tuition reimbursement. Most benefits are tax deductible to both the employer and employee, and some plans offer pretax benefit packages as well. Professional employees of a corporation are liable for only their own acts, although it is always a good idea for any professional in the medical field to carry his or her own malpractice insurance. Another advantage of the corporate entity is the continuous life of the corporation. It does not dissolve with a change in shareholders.

HEALTHCARE PROFESSIONALS

Title of "Doctor"

Doctors of Medicine

Medical doctors (MDs) are considered to be **allopathic** physicians and are the most widely recognized type of physician. They diagnose illness and disease and prescribe treatment for their patients. MDs are allowed to write prescriptions and perform surgeries. They offer advice on nutrition and preventive medicine. To become an MD usually requires 4 years of undergraduate training (premed) and 4 years of medical school. Some extraordinary students are allowed entry after 3 years of undergraduate studies, but competition for entry into medical school is intense, so grades and other experience in healthcare are strongly considered. Premed students study biology, physics, organic and inorganic chemistry, mathematics, English, humanities, and social sciences. There are approximately 125 allopathic medical schools in the United States. After medical school the student faces 3 to 8 years of internship and residency programs. An intern is a medical student still in training at medical school but treating patients under the supervision of licensed doctors. A residency is a graduate medical education program, often in a specialty, and is usually a paid "on-the-job training" hospital position. Often MDs specialize in a certain field, such as cardiology or pediatrics. These doctors usually invest 3 to 6 years of training in the specialty after medical school and can obtain board certification in one or more of 24 different specialty areas recognized by the American Board of Medical Specialties (Table 2-1). An MD must have a state license to practice, and continuing education is required to maintain the license. Graduates of foreign medical schools can usually obtain a license in the United States after passing an examination and completing a residency program in this country.

Doctors of Osteopathy

Osteopathic physicians (Doctors of Osteopathy [DOs]) complete requirements similar to those of MDs to graduate and practice medicine. Osteopaths use medicine and surgery, as well as osteopathic manipulative therapy (OMT), in treating their patients. Andrew Taylor Still is considered the originator of osteopathic medicine, which he began in 1874. He believed in a more **holistic** approach to medicine, and although he was an MD, he founded the American School of Osteopathy in Kirksville, Missouri. The school was originally chartered to offer an MD degree but later focused more on the osteopathic approach. DOs stress preventive medicine and holistic patient care, as well as a special focus on the musculoskeletal system and OMT. Osteopathic medicine also promotes the **innate** ability of the body to heal itself, and many osteopaths tend to take a more conservative approach to using medications and surgical procedures than allopathic physicians. Many DOs practice **homeopathy,** believing in the body's ability to heal itself. Premed students moving toward osteopathic medicine also study biology, physics, organic and inorganic chemistry, mathematics, English, humanities, and social sciences. They also usually complete 4 years of undergraduate studies, then begin 4 years of medical studies at a school for osteopathic medicine. Most DOs participate in a 12-month rotating internship in the various specialty areas before entering a residency program lasting from 2 to 6 years, and they are eligible for board certification through either the American Board of Medical Specialists or the American Osteopathic Association. Approximately one in 20 physicians in the United States is a DO. DOs participate

TABLE 2-1 Types of Medical Specialties Recognized by the American Board of Medical Specialties

MEDICAL SPECIALTY	TITLE OF PRACTITIONER	DESCRIPTION OF SPECIALTY
Allergy and Immunology	Allergist, Immunologist	An allergist/immunologist is trained to evaluate disorders and diseases of the immune system. These include conditions such as adverse reactions to drugs and foods, anaphylaxis, problems related to autoimmune diseases, asthma, and insect stings.
Anesthesiology	Anesthesiologist	An anesthesiologist provides pain relief and management during surgical procedures and for patients with long-standing conditions accompanied by pain, such as cancer patients. Anesthesiologists also provide critical care and resuscitation for patients during cardiac or respiratory emergencies.
Colon and Rectal Surgery	Colon and Rectal Surgeon	This type of surgeon diagnoses and treats conditions affecting the intestines, rectum, and anal area, as well as organs that can cause intestinal disease. They often treat cancers that appear in these areas, as well as disorders such as hemorrhoids and fissures.
Dermatology	Dermatologist	The dermatologist works with adult and pediatric patients in treating disorders and diseases of the skin, hair, nails, and related tissues. Dermatologists are specially trained to manage conditions such as skin cancers, cosmetic disorders of the skin, scars, allergies, and other disorders, both malignant and benign.
Emergency Medicine	Emergency Physician	An emergency physician is an expert in triage and in treating patients to prevent death or serious disability. This physician gives immediate care to stabilize the patient, then refers to the appropriate professional for further care. These physicians are usually found in hospital emergency rooms or freestanding emergency centers.
Family Practice	Family Practitioner	The family practitioner offers care to the whole family, from newborns to elderly adults, and is familiar with a wide range of disorders and diseases. Preventive care is of primary concern. This is one of the more common specialties that physicians choose.
General Surgery	Surgeon	Surgery is the correction of deformities, defects, diseases, or injured parts of the body by means of operative treatment. A surgeon must be familiar with the various specialties to effectively treat patients. General surgery includes all of the aspects of surgery other than those separated into a subgroup specialty.
Internal Medicine	Internist	Internists are concerned with comprehensive care, often diagnosing and treating those with chronic, long-term conditions. They also offer treatment for common illnesses and preventative care. Internists must have a broad understanding of the body and its ailments in order to diagnose and provide treatment to the patient.
Medical Genetics	Geneticist	A geneticist is a physician trained to diagnose and treat patients who have conditions related to genetically linked diseases and may provide special genetic counseling when indicated. Often associated with research projects, this physician may participate in screening programs for defects and abnormalities, sometimes before the birth of an infant.
Neurological Surgery	Neurological Surgeon	The neurological surgeon offers nonoperative and operative care for patients with conditions of the central, autonomic, and peripheral nervous systems, including the supporting structures and vascular supplies of related organs.
Neurology, Psychiatry	Neurologist, Psychiatrist	The neurologist diagnoses and treats disorders of the brain, spinal cord, nerves, and the blood vessels that support those organs. Generally, the neurologist manages infectious, metabolic, degenerative, and systemic involvement of the nervous system. A psychiatrist is a physician whose specialty is the diagnosis and treatment of persons with mental, emotional, or behavioral disorders. The psychiatrist is qualified to conduct psychotherapy and to prescribe medications when necessary.
Nuclear Medicine	Nuclear Medicine Specialist	This specialist uses radioactive substances for the diagnosis and treatment of disease. Radiation and imaging instruments are used to detect diseases often before the affected organ is shown to be abnormal by other methods. The nuclear medicine specialist is aware of the effects of radiation on various structures, as well as the fundamentals of the principles of radiation and physics.

Continued

TABLE 2-1 Types of Medical Specialties Recognized by the American Board of Medical Specialties—*cont'd*		
MEDICAL SPECIALTY	**TITLE OF PRACTITIONER**	**DESCRIPTION OF SPECIALTY**
Obstetrics and Gynecology	Obstetrician and Gynecologist	Obstetricians provide care to women of childbearing age and monitor the progress of the developing child. They deliver the baby, and care for the mother for approximately 6 weeks after birth. Gynecologists are concerned with the diagnosis and treatment of the female reproductive system.
Ophthalmology	Ophthalmologist	Ophthalmologists diagnose, treat, and provide comprehensive care to the eye and its supporting structures. These physicians also offer vision services, including corrective lenses. Screening tests are promoted as a measure of preventative care.
Otolaryngology	Otolaryngologist	These physicians treat diseases and conditions that affect the ear, nose, throat, and structures related to the head and neck. Problems that affect the voice and hearing are also referred to this specialist.
Pathology	Pathologist	Pathologists study the causes of diseases that affect the body and determine what may have caused the death of a patient. These physicians study tissues and cells, body fluids, and actual organs to assist in diagnosing the patient's ailments. Pathologists often perform autopsies.
Pediatrics	Pediatrician	Pediatricians promote preventative medicine and treat diseases that affect children and adolescents. They monitor the child's growth and development and provide a wide range of health services to keep their patients healthy.
Physical Medicine and Rehabilitation	Physiatrist	Physicians of this specialty assist patients who have physical disabilities. This may include those with musculoskeletal disorders or who are suffering from pain as a result of injury or trauma. Their primary goal is to restore the patient to the state of health the patient had before the injury or trauma as nearly as possible through rehabilitation.
Plastic Surgery	Plastic Surgeon	The plastic surgeon works with patients who have had some type of injury or condition that has left them with a physical defect. The surgeon performs reconstructive procedures, using grafts, flaps, and tissue transfer and replanting. These surgeons also perform cosmetic enhancements and procedures that are elective in nature.
Preventative Medicine	Preventative Medicine Specialist	Preventative Medicine is concerned with preventing the occurrence of both mental and physical illness and disability. Analysis of present health services and planning for future medical needs are part of this specialty. Preventative medicine consists of several components, including biostatistics, environmental studies, occupational studies, and clinical preventive medicine activities.
Radiology	Radiologist	Radiology is a specialty in which x-rays are used for diagnosis and treatment of disease. A diagnostic radiologist specializes in using x-rays, ultrasound, nuclear medicine, computed tomography, and magnetic resonance imaging for detection of abnormalities throughout the body.
Thoracic Surgery	Thoracic Surgeon	This surgical specialty is concerned with the operative treatment of the chest and chest wall, lungs, and respiratory passages. Specialists in this field are involved with heart surgery, including both valvular and coronary heart surgery.
Urology	Urologist	Urology is a medical specialty concerned with the treatment of diseases and disorders of the urinary tract. They diagnose and manage problems with the genitourinary system and practice endoscopic and percutaneous procedures related to these structures.

in continuing education programs to renew their licenses annually.

Doctors of Chiropractic

Chiropractors (Doctors of Chiropractic [DCs]) are typically thought of as "bone doctors" but actually focus on the nervous system to help patients live healthier lives. The nervous system is the master system of the body, controlling and coordinating all the other systems. Information from the environment, both internal and external, moves through the spinal cord to get to the brain, and in the same manner, information from the brain moves through the spinal cord to reach the body in a two-way flow of communication. The intention of the **chiropractic** adjustment is to remove any disruptions or distortions of this energy flow that may be caused by slight misalignments that chiropractors call **subluxations.** Chiropractors are trained to locate these subluxations and remove them, using touch as well as x-ray films, thereby restoring the normal flow of nerve energy so that the entire body functions in an optimal fashion. They believe that the same innate inner intelligence that grows the body from a single cell into a complex human being can also heal the body if it is free of disturbance to the nervous system. The philosophy is that health, not merely absence of symptoms, comes from within the body, not from the outside. Chiropractic colleges require undergraduate studies in biology, organic and inorganic chemistry, physics, English, and the humanities, and then 3 to 4 years are spent studying chiropractic. Each state offers licensing. Some chiropractors devote their practices to a specific specialty, but more often they practice general chiropractic. Continuing education is required for relicensure. Chiropractic is one of the most common fields of **alternative medicine.**

CRITICAL THINKING APPLICATION

- Mr. Santos challenges his new medical assisting students to interview several types of doctors at some point during their studies. The class discusses the different philosophies of medicine among allopathic, osteopathic, and chiropractic physicians. Discuss with your class the similarities and differences of these three aspects of medicine.
- Most of Mr. Santos' students have visited one or more of these types of doctors. What experiences have you had with medical doctors (MDs), osteopaths (DOs), or chiropractors?

Dentists

The two basic types of dentists in the United States are Doctors of Dental Medicine (DMD) and Doctors of Dental Surgery (DDS). Dentists treat and prevent problems dealing with the teeth and gums and the tissue surrounding them. They can perform oral surgery and write prescriptions for antibiotics and analgesics. Some specialist dentists perform straightening, called *orthodontics,* and some perform root canal therapy, called *endodontics.* Dental school usually lasts 4 years after completion of undergraduate studies, and state licensing is required.

Optometrists

The optometrist (OD) is trained and licensed to examine the eyes to test visual acuity and to treat vision defects by prescribing correctional lenses and other optical aids. A program of exercise may be planned for the patient's eyes. Optometrists study at accredited schools for optometry for 4 years after completing undergraduate studies in the sciences, mathematics, and English. They must be licensed in the state in which they practice. Optometrists should not be confused with ophthalmologists, who are licensed MDs.

Podiatrists

Podiatrists, or Doctors of Podiatric Medicine (DPM), are educated in caring for the feet, including surgical treatment. Normal persons spend an extraordinary amount of time on their feet, resulting in wear and tear and chronic pain. Podiatrists are trained to find pressure points and weight-distribution

problems. These doctors train for 4 years at accredited colleges after undergraduate studies in the sciences.

Other Doctorates

Other individuals may be called "doctor" based on the degree they have earned in their field. For instance, a person with a PhD has a doctoral degree in philosophy, may be addressed as "doctor," and might work as a professor at a university or in a field related to his or her discipline. A PsyD is a Doctor of Psychology, and an EdD is a Doctor of Educational Psychology. Doctors who practice **naturopathy,** called naturopathic physicians, use only natural means to help the body to heal. These medical professionals are licensed in 15 states.

Licensed Medical Professionals

Many types of licensed medical professionals assist the physician in diagnosing and treating the patient (Table 2-2). Some of the professionals that the medical assistant will commonly encounter are listed in this section. Medical assistants are usually certified professionals and are discussed in detail in Chapter 3.

Physician Assistants

Physician assistants (PAs) provide direct patient care services under the supervision of licensed physicians. They are trained to diagnose and treat patients as directed by the physician, and in 46 states and the District of Columbia they are allowed to write prescriptions. These professionals take patient histories, order and interpret tests, perform physical examinations, and even make diagnosis decisions. They can be found in physician offices, in hospitals, on military bases, and in other healthcare facilities.

Nurse Practitioners

Nurse practitioners (NPs) provide basic patient care services, including diagnosis and prescribing for common illnesses. These professionals must have advanced academic training beyond the RN degree and also have vast clinical experience. Usually the focus of nurse practitioners is on preventive care and disease prevention, and an NP is allowed to practice independently or as a part of a team of healthcare professionals.

Nurse Anesthetists

Nurse anesthetists are registered nurses (RNs) who administer anesthetics to patients during care by surgeons, physicians, dentists, or other qualified health professionals. They practice in many different settings, including offices, traditional hospitals, labor and delivery units, ophthalmology offices, plastic surgery offices, and many others. This practice is quite advanced, and they are compensated well for their skills. Nurse anesthetists can be found in both metropolitan and rural communities.

Registered Nurses

The RN has many career options available. Many nurses work in an administrative capacity within hospitals or other types of healthcare facilities as managers. They also provide direct patient care, where they are vital in assessing the patient and providing a care plan. Usually nurses find a specialty area that

TABLE 2-2 Allied Health Careers from the Health Professions Career and Education Directory

OCCUPATION	CREDENTIAL	BRIEF JOB DESCRIPTION
Anesthesiologist Assistant	AA	Functions as a specialty physician assistant under the direction of a licensed and qualified anesthesiologist; assists in developing and implementing the anesthesia care plan
Art Therapist	ATR	Uses drawings and other art or media forms to assess, treat, and rehabilitate patients with mental, emotional, physical, and/or developmental disorders
Athletic Trainer	ATC	Provides a variety of services, including injury prevention, assessment, immediate care, treatment, and rehabilitation after physical injury or trauma
Audiologist	CCC-A	Identifies individuals with symptoms of hearing loss and other auditory, balance, and related neural problems; assesses the nature of those problems and helps individuals manage them
Blindness and Visual Impairment Professions	LVT, O&M, VRT	Helps people learn to use their vision more efficiently, both with and without optical devices; provides training and offers recommendations to help patients function more successfully in their environments
Blood Bank Technology, Specialist in	SBB	Performs routine and specialized tests in blood center and transfusion services, using methods that conform to the accepted standards in the blood bank industry
Clinical Laboratory Science or Medical Technologist	MT, MLT	Performs tests in conjunction with pathologists to diagnose the causes and nature of disease; develops data on blood, tissues, and fluids of the human body using a variety of methodologies
Counseling-Related Occupations	LPC, LMHC	Deals with human development concerns through support, therapeutic approaches, consultation, evaluation, teaching, and research; practices the art of helping people to grow
Cytotechnologist	CT	Works with pathologists to evaluate cellular material from all body sites primarily using the microscope; looks for normal and abnormal cytologic changes, including malignancies
Dance Therapist	DTR, ADTR	Uses the psychotherapeutic properties of movement as a process that furthers the emotional, cognitive, social, and physical integration of the patient as a tool for healing
Dental Assistant, Dental Hygienist, Dental Laboratory Technician	CDA, RDH, CDT	Performs a wide range of tasks from assisting the dentist to instructing patients as to how they can prevent oral disease and maintain oral health
Diagnostic Cardiovascular Sonographer or Technologist	RDCS, RVT	Performs diagnostic examinations and therapeutic interventions of the heart and/or blood vessels at the request of a physician using invasive and/or noninvasive techniques.
Dietetic Technician, Dietician	DTR	Integrates and applies the principles derived from the sciences of food, nutrition, biochemistry, physiology, food management, and behavior to achieve and maintain health status
Electroneurodiagnostic Technology	REEG-T	Records and studies electrical activity in the brain and nervous system; obtains interpretable recordings of patients' nervous system function
Emergency Medical Technician, Paramedic	EMT, Paramedic	Provides medical care to people who have suffered from an injury or illness outside the hospital setting, most often in an emergency; provides basic and/or advanced life support
Genetic Counselor	IGC	Provides genetic services to individuals and families seeking information about the occurrence or risk of a genetic condition or birth defect
Health Information Management	RHIA, RHIT	Provides expert assistance in the systems and processes of health information management, including planning, engineering, administration, application, and policy making
Kinesiotherapist	RKT	Provides rehabilitation exercise and education designed to reverse or minimize debilitation and enhance the functional capacity of medically stable patients
Massage Therapist	MT	Applies manual techniques and may apply adjunctive techniques with the intention of positively affecting the health and well-being of the client
Medical Assistant	CMA, RMA	Functions as a member of the health care delivery team and performs both administrative and clinical procedures and duties; multiskilled health professional

Continued

TABLE 2-2 Allied Health Careers from the Health Professions Career and Education Directory—*cont'd*

OCCUPATION	CREDENTIAL	BRIEF JOB DESCRIPTION
Medical Illustrator	MI	Specializes in the visual display and communication of scientific information; creates visuals and designs communications to teach medical professionals as well as the public
Music Therapist	MT-BC	Uses music within a therapeutic relationship to address physical, emotional, cognitive, and social needs of individuals of all ages; assesses strengths and needs of clients
Nuclear Medicine Technologist	RT	Uses the nuclear properties of radioactive and stable nuclides to make diagnostic evaluations of the anatomic or physiologic conditions of the body and provide therapy with unsealed radioactive sources
Occupational Therapist	OTR	Uses purposeful activity and interventions to achieve functional outcomes to maximize the independence and the maintenance of health for those limited by physical injury or illness
Ophthalmic Laboratory Technician, Medical Technician or Technologist	COT, COMT	Collects data and performs clinical evaluations; performs tests and protocols required by ophthalmologists; assists the physician in treating the patient
Orthoptist	CO	Performs a series of diagnostic tests and measurements on patients with visual disorders; helps design a treatment plan to correct the disorders of vision, eye movements, and alignment
Orthotist and Prosthetist	RTO, RTP, RTPO	Designs and fits devices (orthoses) to provide care to patients who have disabling conditions of the limbs and spine and/or partial or total absence of a limb
Perfusionist	CCP	Operates extracorporeal circulation and autotransfusion equipment during any medical situation in which the patient's respiratory or circulatory function must be supported or temporarily replaced
Pharmacy Technician	CPhT	Assists pharmacists with duties that do not require the expertise or judgment of a licensed pharmacist
Physical Therapist	PT	Helps to improve patient strength and mobility, relieve pain, prevent or limit permanent physical disabilities; takes a personal, direct approach to meeting individual health goals
Physician Assistant	PA	Practices medicine with the direction and responsible supervision of a licensed doctor of medicine or osteopathy; makes clinical decisions and provides a range of services
Radiation Therapist, Radiographer	RRT	Delivers prescribed dosages of radiation to patients for therapeutic purposes; provides appropriate patient care and maintains accurate records of treatment provided
Rehabilitation Counselor	CRC	Determines and coordinates services to assist people with disabilities in moving from psychologic and economic dependence to independence
Respiratory Therapist, Respiratory Therapy Technician	RRT, CRT, RPFT, CPFT	Evaluates, treats, and manages patients of all ages with respiratory illnesses and other cardiopulmonary disorders; advanced RTs exercise considerable independent judgment
Surgical Assistant	CSA	Provides aid in exposure, hemostasis, closure, and other intraoperative technical functions that help the surgeon carry out a safe operation with optimal results for the patient
Surgical Technologist	ST, CST	Assists in preparing patients for surgery and maintaining the sterile field within the surgical suite, making certain that all members of the surgical team adhere to sterile technique
Therapeutic Recreation Specialist	CTRS	Uses treatment, education, and recreation services to help people with illnesses, disabilities, and other conditions develop and use their leisure in ways that enhance their health

they enjoy and practice within that area, although they may also "float" to different departments within the hospital. Some function as home health nurses, visiting patients and providing home care. Some work in nursing homes or in public health, and others serve in physicians' offices.

Licensed Practical and Vocational Nurses

Licensed practical nurses (LPNs) and licensed vocational nurses (LVNs) offer bedside care, assisting with the actual day-to-day personal care required by inpatients. They assess patients, chart their progress, and administer medications and intravenous fluids where allowed by law. They often work in hospitals or skilled nursing facilities and are also found in physicians' offices. They sometimes supervise nursing assistants and may also provide patient education services.

Medical Technologists

Medical technologists (MTs) perform diagnostic testing on blood, body fluids, and other types of specimens to assist the physician in arriving at a diagnosis. These professionals work with bacteria and viruses and use their technical skills combined with their knowledge of disease to perform their duties. They can make quality-control decisions and can act independently within their profession. Hospitals, teaching universities, research organizations, and laboratories employ most of the medical technologists. Usually they have a Bachelor of Science (BS) degree in addition to certification or a license.

Medical Laboratory Technicians

Medical laboratory technicians (MLTs) perform most of the same test procedures that the medical technologist performs; the difference between the two is that MLTs do not work independently. They are usually supervised by an MT and have at least an associate's degree and a certification or license. MLTs work in the same types of facilities as MTs.

Physical Therapists

Physical therapists (PTs) assist patients in regaining their mobility and improving their strength and range of motion, which may have been impaired by an accident or injury or as a result of disease. After assessing the patient, the PT devises a treatment plan in conjunction with the patient's physician. The goal of the PT is to improve how the patient functions at work and at home.

Respiratory Therapists

Most respiratory therapists (RTs) work in the hospital environment. All types of patients receive respiratory care, including newborns and geriatric patients. RTs commonly use oxygen therapy to assist with breathing, and they also perform diagnostic tests that measure lung capacity.

Occupational Therapists

Occupational therapists (OTs) work with patients who have developed conditions that disable them developmentally, emotionally, mentally, or physically. OTs assist in helping the individual to compensate for loss of function. The goal of OTs is to bring their patients to a level of living healthy, productive lives.

Diagnostic Cardiac Sonographers

Diagnostic cardiac sonographers or technologists (DCSs or VTs) assist in the diagnosis and treatment of cardiac and vascular diseases and disorders. They perform noninvasive tests, including echocardiographs and electrocardiographs. Often ultrasonography is used by the cardiovascular technician to assist the physician in discovering the malfunction of the heart and its structures.

Diagnostic Medical Sonographers

Diagnostic medical sonographers (DMSs) assist physicians in the diagnosis of various disorders by means of ultrasound waves, which produce images of the internal structures of the body. These professionals are often called *sonographers*. Ultrasonography is used to assist the physician in many ways, including the monitoring of fetal development.

Radiology Technicians

Radiology technicians (RTs) use various machines to help the physician diagnose and treat certain diseases. These machines may include x-ray equipment, ultrasonographic machines, and MRI scanners. RTs explain procedures to patients and know correct positioning techniques, so that the images recorded are accurate and helpful for the diagnosing physician.

Paramedics

Paramedics are specially trained to provide emergency care to patients in life-threatening situations. Paramedics are highly efficient and well versed in the functions of the body. They perform advanced skills and, with more experience, are able to supervise or direct the operations of an emergency care ambulance facility.

Emergency Medical Technicians

Emergency medical technicians (EMTs) progress through several levels of training, each providing more-advanced skills. Their medical education encompasses managing respiratory, cardiac, and trauma cases and often emergency childbirth. Specialties within the EMT field also exist in certain states, such as EMT Cardiac, which includes training in **cardiac arrhythmias,** and EMT Shock Trauma, which includes starting intravenous fluids and administration of medication.

Registered Dietitians

Registered dietitians (RDs) have thorough training in nutrition and the different types of diets that patients are placed on to improve or maintain their condition. They use the advice of the physician and information about the patient to design healthy diets during hospital stays and even help to plan menus for home use. They also provide education for the patient about the diet and alternatives that will help in choosing attractive foods.

CLOSING COMMENTS

The healthcare industry is certainly one of the most exciting career fields to enter in today's world. The constant change and development of new technology and theories make medicine an attractive option for career choices. The needs of medicine extend far beyond the boundaries of the United States, and collaborative efforts among countries promote a faster move forward with new discoveries and hope for those affected by disease. Headlines grace newspapers and computer screens daily, detailing stories of human cloning, designer babies, genetic discoveries, and computer capabilities that amaze us all. Medications are being developed that bring us to the brink of eliminating certain diseases. The mapping of the human genome may lead to incredible breakthroughs in the study of colon, breast, and ovarian cancers, cystic fibrosis, neurologic degeneration, sickle cell anemia, and countless other conditions. There has never been a more thrilling time to become a part of the world of medicine and make a contribution as a healthcare professional.

SUMMARY OF SCENARIO

Mr. Santos is an effective instructor, and one who is concerned about providing interesting material for his students. He wishes to instill a strong respect in the students for the people who played a role in early medical advances. His classroom discussions will help the students to think about what it was like to present new ideas to the public and often be ridiculed.

While teaching them about the history of medicine and the state of healthcare today, he also provides opportunities for the students to work together in discussion groups and present information to the class. He encourages Internet research, a valuable skill that will help the medical assisting student in many areas of training. By allowing the students to speak in front of the class while giving reports on the medical forefathers, Mr. Santos teaches the students to be more at ease when speaking in public and when articulating instructions and details to patients and co-workers. All of these skills make a well-rounded medical assistant who will become a great asset to the facility in which he or she is employed.

Mr. Santos explains that continuing medical research is critical to the healthcare industry because new and more-effective drugs and treatments are necessary and because many diseases and conditions do not as yet have a cure. Medical research constantly looks for better ways to make patients well and continually strives to find cures for diseases that medicine has not yet conquered. Medical assistants may work for physicians who are involved in research projects, and this may afford them the opportunity to contribute to medical research.

By providing his students with an overview of the healthcare industry, Mr. Santos helps them to become more familiar with the professionals whom they encounter in various medical facilities and to have a better awareness of their duties and responsibilities.

SUMMARY of LEARNING OBJECTIVES

1. Define, spell, and pronounce the terms listed in the vocabulary.
   - Spelling and pronouncing medical terms correctly adds credibility to the medical assistant. Knowing the definition of these terms promotes confidence in communication with patients and co-workers.
2. Identify the ancient cultures that contributed a major portion of our medical terminology.
   - Greek and Roman mythology contributed the major portion of the medical terms we use today. Terms have also been borrowed from Anglo-Saxon, German, Arabic, and other sources, including the Bible.
3. Explain the history of medicine and how it has affected today's medical industry.
   - The history of medicine clearly influences medical practice today, because yesterday's discoveries are today's medications and treatments. Research is an ongoing necessity in the medical field. As technology becomes more and more sophisticated, medical advancements follow.
4. Distinguish between and describe the two medical symbols in general use today.
   - The American Medical Association adopted the staff of Aesculapius as the symbol of medicine. The symbol is a staff encircled by a serpent. The caduceus is often mistakenly used to represent medicine but is actually the medical insignia of the U.S. Army Medical Corps. This icon is a staff encircled by two serpents, bearing wings at the top.
5. Explain why a medical education at Johns Hopkins was considered superior, even in its early years.
   - Johns Hopkins University Medical School has been recognized as a leader in healthcare education for over a century. The university was one of the first institutions to partner with a hospital for training purposes, resulting in its superior medical education. Johns Hopkins contained a research department as well, where faculty members investigated new methods and treatments for patients. Combining the medical education with readily available patients brought the discovery of illness and disease into a new light for early medical students. Today Johns Hopkins is a multibillion-dollar organization, incorporating three acute-care hospitals and other entities in an integrated healthcare system.

Continued

SUMMARY of LEARNING OBJECTIVES
Continued

6. List several medical pioneers, and discuss the importance of their contributions to the medical profession.
   - Numerous early pioneers made tremendous contributions to the medical field. Constant growth and research have pressed the medical profession forward, and with the assistance of technology the growth speeds along today faster than ever.

7. Explain the roles of the world healthcare organizations.
   - World healthcare organizations provide information, medication, and personnel to attempt to eradicate diseases and treat those diseases for which no cure exists. Many of these organizations operate with restricted funding and rely often on volunteer donations and volunteer workers to operate. These agencies often work together in an effort to effectively solve problems of epidemics and learn more about diseases. All of the national healthcare organizations are a vital part of the medical industry today.

8. Discuss the various types of ambulatory care.
   - Physicians' offices, group practices, and multispecialty group practices are a few types of ambulatory care. This division of medicine also includes occupational health centers, dialysis centers, rehabilitation clinics, and sleep centers. Patients who are ambulatory are able to move from place to place, usually on their own or with the assistance of a wheelchair or walker.

9. Distinguish among different types of doctors and medical practices.
   - Three main provider portals of entry into the healthcare system exist today; they are medical doctors, osteopathic physicians, and chiropractic physicians. These different disciplines have some similar training, but osteopathic physicians usually use a holistic approach, and chiropractors concentrate many of their efforts on the alignment of the spine in an effort to promote a healing of the body. Most physicians work in a sole proprietorship, a group practice, or a healthcare corporation.

10. Identify the medical specialties recognized by the American Board of Medical Specialties.
    - Numerous specialties focus on particular areas of the practice of medicine. The American Board of Medical Specialties recognizes over 20 specialty groups that support various organizations designed to promote that particular branch of medicine. Although other specialties and subspecialties of medicine exist, the most common and most generally recognized are those associated with the American Board of Medical Specialties.

11. Discuss various healthcare occupations and the role these professionals play in the healthcare industry.
    - The American Medical Association recognizes more than 60 allied healthcare occupations. These allied health professionals contribute to the field of medicine, each playing a specific role in the healthcare industry.

CONNECTIONS

Study Guide Connection: Go to Chapter 2 Study Guide. Read the Case Study and Workplace Applications and complete the assignments. Do online research for answers to the questions in the Internet Activities associated with the healthcare industry.

CD Connection: Go to the Medical Assisting Competency Challenge CD and review the content of the training activities. These will be referred to throughout the textbook to enhance your learning experience.

Evolve Connection: For more information related to the healthcare industry, go to http://evolve.elsevier.com/kinn/ admin and visit related weblinks for Chapter 2. Click on the Medical Assisting Exam Review and do the practice questions to sharpen your test-taking skills.

The Medical Assisting Profession

3

SCENARIO

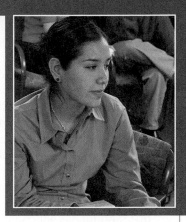

Sandra Rameriz is a single mother who has decided on medical assisting as a career. She has always been interested in the medical field and wants a job that will allow her to spend evenings and weekends with her 3-year-old son, Roberto. The idea of working in a physician's office appeals to her, and she has applied to a school that is close to her apartment and day care provider. She plans to attend day classes and work part-time after school until it is time to pick up her son.

Sandra is very excited about her new career and has set several goals for her training. First, she hopes to attain perfect attendance, and second, she would like to graduate with honors. She has budgeted her study time and plans to ask her instructors during the first 2 weeks of school for suggestions about how she can better prepare for classes and examinations. Sandra will find medical assisting to be a rewarding career and respected profession.

While studying this chapter, think about the following questions:

- What obstacles might prevent Sandra from attending all of her classes, and how can she prepare in advance to overcome them?
- How can Sandra begin to explore the type of physician offices in which she would enjoy being employed after graduation?

- What goals might Sandra have at the commencement of her training? At the end of training?
- How can Sandra make the most of her time attending school to become a medical assistant?

LEARNING OBJECTIVES

1. Define, spell, and pronounce the terms listed in the vocabulary.
2. Briefly discuss the history of medical assisting as a profession.
3. Differentiate between administrative and clinical medical assisting duties.
4. Discuss the versatility of a career in medical assisting.
5. Explain the reasons that hiring an individual who has no formal training is often more expensive than hiring a professional medical assistant.
6. Identify several considerations to keep in mind when choosing a position as a medical assistant other than financial compensation.
7. Discuss the aspects of the medical assistant's performance on a successful externship.
8. List three unacceptable behaviors on the externship site.
9. Explain why continuing education is so important to the medical assistant.
10. Discuss the difference between a CMA and an RMA.

National Accreditation Competencies and Content

ABHES COMPETENCIES	ABHES COMPETENCIES
Professionalism	**Communication**
1.a. Project a positive attitude	2.p. Professional components
1.b. Maintain confidentiality at all times	2.q. Allied health professions and credentialing
1.c. Be a "team player"	
1.d. Be cognizant of ethical boundaries	**Legal Concepts**
1.e. Exhibit initiative	5.f. Maintain licenses and accreditation
1.f. Adapt to change	
1.g. Evidence a responsible attitude	
1.h. Be courteous and diplomatic	
1.i. Conduct work within scope of education, training, and ability	

VOCABULARY

allied health fields Occupational disciplines in which professionals involved with the delivery of healthcare or related services assist physicians with the diagnosis, treatment, and care of patients in many different specialty areas.

benefits Services or payments provided under a health plan, employee plan, or some other agreement, including programs such as health insurance, pensions, retirement planning, and many other options that may be offered to employees of a company or organization.

certification (ser-tuh-fuh-ka′-shun) The attesting of something as being true, as represented, or as meeting a standard; the result of having been tested, usually by a third party, and awarded a certificate based on proven knowledge.

continuing education units (CEUs) Credits for courses, classes, or seminars related to an individual's profession, designed to promote education and to keep the professional up to date on current procedures and trends in his or her field; CEUs are often required for licensing.

cross-training Training in more than one area so that a multitude of duties may be performed by one person or so that substitutions of personnel may be made in an emergency or at other necessary times.

externship or internship A training program that is part of a course of study of an educational institution and is taken in the actual business setting of that field of study; the terms are often interchanged in reference to medical assistant training.

intangibles (in-tan′-juh-buls) Qualities that are incapable of being perceived, especially by touch, or incapable of being precisely identified or realized by the mind.

invasive Involving entry into the living body as by incision or insertion of an instrument.

perks Extra advantages or benefits from working in a specific job that may or may not be commonplace in that particular profession; a shortened form of *perquisites*.

phlebotomy (fli-bah′-tuh-me) The invasive procedure used to obtain a blood specimen for testing, experimentation, or diagnosis of disease.

profit sharing Offer of a part of a company's profits to employees or other designated individuals or groups.

stock options Offers of stocks for purchase to a certain group of individuals or certain groups, such as employees of a for-profit hospital.

versatile (vur′-suh-til) Embracing a variety of subjects, fields or skills; having a wide range of abilities.

According to the U.S. Department of Labor's *Occupational Outlook Handbook,* medical assisting is projected to be one of the fastest growing occupations in the United States over the 2004-2014 period. Much of this growth is a result of the increase in the number of group practices, clinics, and other facilities that need a high number of support personnel. This makes the flexible medical assistant who can handle both clinical and administrative duties particularly valuable to the physician.

A career as a medical assistant is challenging and offers job satisfaction, opportunities for service, financial reward, and possibilities for advancement. Men and women can be equally successful as medical assistants. Individuals considering the medical assisting discipline must be dedicated and committed and must have a strong desire to become caregivers. Caregivers are people who have the ability to put the needs of the patient first and have a sincere concern for those who are not at their best. A caregiver must feel an obligation to assist the patient in whatever way possible and have patience with those who, at times, are more difficult. This strong inner desire is one of the most important qualities of the successful professional medical assistant. Through development of this "caregiving" mentality, many personal rewards will follow, as will a long and beneficial career.

THE HISTORY OF MEDICAL ASSISTING

The first medical assistant was probably a neighbor of a physician who was called on to help when an extra pair of hands was needed.

As time passed and the practice of medicine became more organized and more complicated, some physicians hired nurses to help in their office practices. Gradually, record keeping, data reporting, and an increasing number of business details became important to physicians, and they realized a need for an assistant with both administrative and clinical training. Nurses were likely to have training only in clinical skills, so many physicians began training them or other individuals to assist with all of the office duties. Community and junior colleges began offering training programs that focused on both administrative and clinical skills in the late 1940s. Medical assistant organizations at the local and state level began developing around 1950, and soon after, certifying examinations became available. Today medical assisting is one of the most respected **allied health fields** in the industry, and training is readily available through community colleges, junior colleges, and private educational institutions throughout the United States.

THE SCOPE OF PRACTICE OF A MEDICAL ASSISTANT

Versatile is an excellent descriptive term for today's medical assistant. The duties that medical assistants perform vary not only from office to office, but even within the same clinic. Medical assistants perform routine duties within the offices of many types of health professionals, including physicians, chiropractors, podiatrists, and others. Individuals with medical assisting training can accomplish many jobs in the hospital environment, and some are employed by freestanding emergency centers or surgery centers. Opportunities for medical assistants are growing because of the constant change within the medical profession and the surge of **cross-training**, which means that one individual is trained to do a variety of duties. Medical assistants work under the direct supervision of a physician in the office and perform tasks delegated by the doctor or supervisor.

The American Association of Medical Assistants (AAMA) once defined the scope of practice as the "performance of delegated clinical and administrative duties within the supervising physician's scope of practice consistent with the medical assistant's education, training, and experience." This definition remains accurate today. The duties performed by the medical assistant do not constitute the practice of medicine.

The two major categories of duties that medical assistants perform are administrative tasks and clinical tasks (Figure 3-1). On the administrative end of the spectrum, medical assistants greet patients who arrive in the office or clinic and obtain basic registration information. They may enter information into a computer and assemble the patient's medical record. They are trained to do office accounting, which may be done electronically or manually. The medical assistant is trained in filing procedures and in proper techniques for adding information to the medical record. A basic knowledge of procedure and diagnosis coding is important to today's medical assistant, and some medical assistants concentrate strictly on the billing and coding career option. They are able to complete insurance claim forms and determine insurance coverage and limitations for the patient. Medical assistants answer telephones, schedule appointments, update medical records, and handle all types of correspondence. Often the medical assistant schedules outpatient procedures and hospital admissions and may coordinate consultations with physicians. Those who enjoy the administrative side of the profession often enter into office management positions.

The clinical duties that medical assistants perform are just as broad as the administrative duties. These professionals prepare patients and the equipment needed before examinations and assist the physician during patients' office visits. They assist with or perform basic testing procedures and are usually proficient in **phlebotomy.** Medical assistants are trained in first aid skills and cardiopulmonary resuscitation. They collect and prepare laboratory specimens and know how to adhere to U.S. Occupational and Health Administration (OSHA) and Clinical Laboratory Improvement Amendment (CLIA) regulations. Often medical assistants working in the clinical area are responsible for inventorying and ordering supplies. If directed by a physician and allowed by the state, they may administer various types of medications and perform x-ray examinations. Medical assistants also perform electrocardiograms and prepare patients for x-ray evaluations. They assist in minor surgical procedures, prepare sterile trays, and perform autoclave sterilization procedures for instruments. Other clinical duties involve taking medical histories from patients, patient teaching, and obtaining and recording vital signs. Medical assistants who enjoy the clinical side of the profession may become office managers or may supervise other medical assistants.

Duties and restrictions related to medical assisting vary from state to state, but in most of the United States the medical assistant performs as an agent of the physician and is under the physician's supervision. This means that the medical assistant performs actions that he or she is told to perform by the physician and that the physician is responsible for those actions. The command may be related to the medical assistant from the physician verbally, through a supervisor, or by way of the office policy and procedure manual. *Respondeat superior* is a Latin term meaning "let the master answer." Physicians are responsible not only for their own actions, but for the actions of employees performing within the scope of their employment.

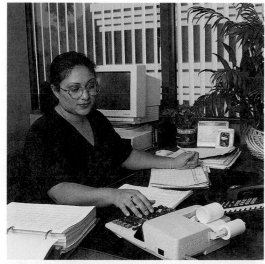

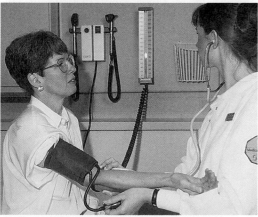

FIGURE 3-1 The responsibilities of a medical assistant include both administrative and clinical duties. (Bottom photo from Chester GA: *Modern medical assisting,* Philadelphia, 1998, Saunders.)

CRITICAL THINKING APPLICATION

- Sandra is not sure whether she will enjoy administrative or clinical assisting more. How can she begin to explore both avenues during her classroom training? During her externship or internship?
- How could Sandra explore the medical specialties and determine what areas might be of interest to her as a potential job site?

A CAREER IN MEDICAL ASSISTING

Trained medical assistants are equipped with a flexible, adaptable career in which they experience the rewards of helping other people (Figure 3-2). The skills acquired by the medical assistant are valuable, and employment is readily available anywhere in the world that medicine is practiced. Many medical assistants pursue their careers far beyond the usual retirement age, because physicians realize the value of the experienced, mature employee. This career attracts the nontraditional student who may be older than the average postsecondary student by a decade or more. Although many older students feel intimidated by the classroom, they normally have excellent experiences in school and reach the top of the class. Medical assisting is more than suitable for the student just exiting high school. Many individuals plan to work as medical assistants to earn a viable income while pursuing further academic studies.

The practice of medicine has changed dramatically in the past several decades. Increasing costs have created a trend away from hospital-based treatment and toward the delivery of care in physicians' offices and in outpatient ambulatory clinics. Although physicians have employed medical assistants in their practices for many years, computerization and technologic advances have created more opportunities for formally trained medical assistants, and their responsibilities have similarly increased. Clearly defined educational requirements have been established, and these requirements have resulted in improvement of the quality and accessibility of medical assistant training. These requirements have resulted in creating a healthy respect for medical assistants, who are considered an integral part of today's allied health field.

Employment for medical assistants is abundant. In the United States in 2004 approximately 387,000 jobs were held

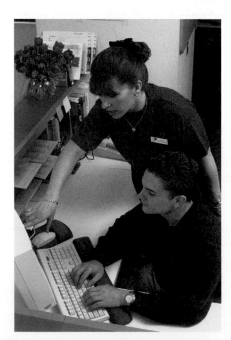

FIGURE 3-2 Medical assisting is a career with many benefits and perks, not to mention the internal rewards of assisting patients in need.

by medical assistants; approximately 60% of those were in physicians' offices, and approximately 15% were in hospitals. Career opportunities abound in public health facilities, hospitals, laboratories, medical schools, research centers, voluntary health agencies, and medical firms of all kinds. Jobs may also be available with federal agencies such as the Department of Veterans Affairs, the U.S. Public Health Service, and armed forces clinics or hospitals.

Most medical assistants derive a high degree of satisfaction from their work. Job turnover among medical assistants is surprisingly low; some begin working with a physician when the practice is opened and stay until the physician's retirement. In the past, physicians would often hire any individual to perform office and clinical duties, but these people were often untrained and unprofessional. Therefore they could be paid a minimum amount for their work. Most physicians have learned that hiring an untrained person to work in the medical office is usually more expensive in the long run. Untrained assistants often make errors that are costly to the practice, and these assistants require much more supervision. Formal training and **certification** are valuable not only to the medical assistant, but to the physician-employer.

Medical assistants are compensated in various ways, some by hourly wages and some by salary. The earnings vary from place to place. Overall, medical assistants can expect a healthy return on their investment in training, experience, and skills. Most physicians realize that a good medical assistant is worth a higher-than-average wage, and a medical assistant with formal training is almost always compensated on a higher scale than one with no training. The *Occupational Outlook Handbook,* a Department of Labor publication, reports statistics on the average salaries for many different career fields, including medical assisting. This information can be accessed at www.bls.gov/oco. More information on salaries may be obtained by monitoring the local classified advertisements and by checking online job information on sites such as Yahoo! Careers. It is important to determine a realistic entering salary. Often graduates in many fields expect to make a much higher salary than is reasonable right after graduation, with little or no experience in the medical field.

The medical field offers good **benefits** to employees. Usually, the larger the organization, the better the benefits and **perks.** Most employers offer a health insurance plan or managed care plan to their employees. Often a life insurance program is included, and dental insurance is always a valuable benefit. Some companies have **profit sharing** plans and **stock options.** Some organizations give their employees access to credit unions, and many have discount options to local businesses, such as uniform shops. Remember that benefits and perks should be considered when contemplating a job opportunity. Many medical assistants may choose to work for less money if the benefits and the opportunities for advancement are good. Consider driving time, holidays, paid parking, sick days, vacation days, and facilities when choosing a job. Do the co-workers seem to enjoy one another's company and get along? Is the physician friendly or more "aloof and cold"? All of these should be weighed carefully before making the final decision as to which position to accept. It is a truism that "money is a byproduct of services rendered." Nowhere is this more accurate than in the medical field. When the patients are served well, the medical assistant becomes more and more valuable to the employer and is compensated accordingly.

CRITICAL THINKING APPLICATION

- Sandra knows that she needs certain benefits as a single mother. What might she need to look for in a potential job after her graduation?
- What are some ways that Sandra can compare positions and opportunities?
- What types of websites might help Sandra in learning about opportunities in her geographic location?

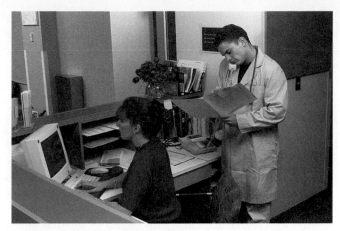

FIGURE 3-3 Medical assistants must have a professional appearance and demeanor in the medical office environment.

PROFESSIONAL APPEARANCE

A well-groomed medical assistant in appropriate attire has a positive psychologic effect on patients. The essentials of a professional appearance are good health, good grooming, and suitable dress.

Good health requires getting adequate sleep, eating balanced meals, and exercising enough to keep fit. Medical assistants can set a good example by following a sensible and healthy lifestyle that includes regular checkups of their own physical condition, both medical and dental. A radiantly healthy office staff promotes the best possible public relations image for the physician.

Good grooming is little more than attention to the details of personal appearance. Personal cleanliness, which includes taking a daily bath or shower, using deodorant, and practicing good oral hygiene, is vital. The use of perfume or aftershave cologne should be avoided or limited, because patients and co-workers may be allergic to some scents. A female medical assistant's makeup should be conservative and moderately applied. Heavy or exaggerated makeup is out of place in the professional office; subtle eye and lip makeup is best for the physician's office. Clear or muted shades of nail polish are best, and long nails are not only inappropriate but can be dangerous to the patient and the medical assistant. Nails must be kept clean and at a very conservative length. Both male and female assistants should be sure that their hair is shiny clean, neatly styled, and off the collar.

The medical assistant usually wears a uniform or lab coat, which not only presents a professional appearance but also identifies the assistant as a member of the healthcare team (Figure 3-3). Fashionable styling makes it possible for the medical assistant's uniform to be both practical and attractive. Women may choose to wear pantsuits, which are available in white or a variety of colors; a two-piece dress uniform in white or a color; an attractively styled traditional white uniform; or a scrub set. Scrubs have become increasingly popular and much more attractive over the past decade. They are now often made of pretty fabrics in rich colors and patterns and are much better suited for the professional office than the old green or blue scrubs worn in the surgical suites of hospitals. Men

may also wear the newer scrubs or may choose white slacks with a white or colored shirt, jacket, or pullover top. If it is acceptable in the facility, a lab coat may be worn over street clothes, but it is important that the lab coat be buttoned when **invasive** procedures are performed. Uniforms should be laundered daily, because medical assistants are exposed to ill patients throughout their workday. Shoes should be appropriate for a uniform, spotless, and comfortable. Many attractive styles that resemble running or tennis shoes are available at uniform shops, specially conditioned for the medical professional who is on his or her feet the majority of the day. White shoes must be kept white by daily cleansing and touchups. Remember that if laced shoes are worn, the laces also need cleaning.

In some facilities the physician prefers that the staff not wear uniforms. Some psychiatrists and some pediatricians, for example, believe that the clinical appearance of a uniform may affect patients adversely. However, today's uniforms reflect so many styles and patterns that the right one for the particular office should be readily available. Some of the fabrics depict cartoon characters or drawings that will appeal to children yet still function as a durable uniform. A medical assistant who does not wear a uniform should follow the dictates of good taste and should be conservative in choosing a professional wardrobe. Jeans are rarely acceptable in the medical facility, unless the office is extremely casual or it is a special day.

The garments worn while on duty must be comfortable, allow easy movement, and still look fresh at the end of a busy day. Whatever uniform style the assistant chooses, it should be personally becoming and worn over appropriate undergarments. The lines, colors, and ornamentation of the undergarments should not be seen through the uniform; therefore it is best to wear a neutral color without a pattern. Thongs and high-cut underwear should be avoided. When a uniform is worn, jewelry should be limited to an engagement ring, wedding band, and professional pin. No more than two earrings per ear lobe should be worn, and the clothing or hairstyle should always cover tattoos. Facial and tongue piercings are unacceptable in the medical arena and must be removed during working hours. A name badge will help patients identify each staff person by name.

Be sure that the dress code that is required in the office setting is clearly understood. Adherence to that code is a demonstration of responsibility and the willingness to cooperate with office rules. Compliance with office regulations will be a factor in office promotion decisions.

EDUCATION AND TRAINING

Ideally, a medical assistant should have both administrative and clinical skills, although he or she may have a personal preference for one over the other. The physician's staff must be able to handle all responsibilities of the office except those requiring the services of the physician or another licensed professional. In an office with several assistants, each should be able and willing to substitute in an emergency for any of the others and should be cross-trained on the basics of the others' duties. Teamwork is a very important part of any occupation, and even more so in the medical environment.

Certain knowledge and skills are expected of a trained medical assistant. The skills mentioned within this chapter are not all-inclusive but suggest what may be expected on entry into employment as a professional medical assistant.

Classroom Training

Formal training is essential for today's medical assistant. Many community colleges, junior colleges, and private career institutions offer courses in medical assisting. After satisfactory completion of the program, the student usually receives a certificate or diploma. Private career institutions offer training that usually takes 7 to 10 months to complete and offer enrollment as often as monthly. Students who attend community colleges, junior colleges, and some private career institutions to study medical assisting may complete the educational requirements to obtain an associate degree in medical assisting. Courses at the community college level usually take 1 to 2 years to complete and offer enrollment from every few weeks to two or three times per year.

Currently the trend is toward offering the medical assisting program in modules, so that the student receives some clinical training, some administrative training, and some theory in each module taken. Some classes are taught in traditional classrooms, and the clinical aspect is usually taught in a laboratory at the school. Much of the equipment that the medical assistant will use in practice is found in the laboratory, such as an autoclave, medical instruments and trays, and specimen-collection equipment. Medical assisting training usually involves the study of medical terminology, anatomy and physiology, aseptic technique, clinical procedures, medical law and ethics, principals of pharmacology, insurance billing and coding, receptionist and telephone technique, patient communication, human relations, management duties, and receptionist duties, among other subjects.

Instructors are important allies as the medical assisting student pursues his or her education, and the relationship between instructor and student should be one of mutual respect (Figure 3-4). Students must realize that instructors have a strong desire to share their knowledge and that they want each student

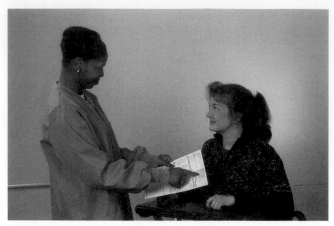

FIGURE 3-4 Get to know instructors and ask their advice on study habits and test preparation. Instructors are valuable references when the medical assistant begins the job search.

to succeed. Individual schools have certain rules and regulations that must be enforced, many of them a result of state or federal regulation or legislation. The guidelines that students must follow are not designed to hinder the education, but rather to make certain that the school graduates competent medical assistants. Complete assignments accurately, turn them in on time, and take pride in all of the work done for class. School days should be missed only when absolutely necessary. Develop good habits in school, and they will become valuable assets to future employers.

CRITICAL THINKING APPLICATION

- How can Sandra develop a positive, nurturing relationship with her instructors?
- What should she do if she has difficulty in the classroom or if her grades begin to fall?
- How can Sandra study effectively and prepare for examinations?

Externships and Internships

Most medical assisting training programs require an **externship** or **internship** before the student graduates. For the purposes of this text, the terms are interchangeable and have the same meaning. This on-the-job training allows students to put the skills they have learned in the classroom setting to use with real patients and staff members. In the majority of cases, externships and internships are unpaid positions that are a part of the medical assistant training program, not a separate entity. Most accreditation organizations do not allow student externs or interns to be paid.

The physician, probably more than any other employer, expects employees to carry out their duties independently, with little or no direct supervision. Someone at the externship site will be designated as the student's supervisor. The medical assisting student should consult frequently with the externship supervisor to determine what is expected of the student and what progress is being made (Figure 3-5).

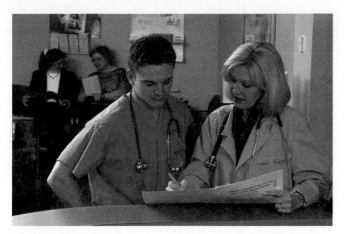

FIGURE 3-5 The externship or internship provides practical experience in the skills learned in the classroom. It is usually listed first on the resume once the medical assistant graduate prepares a resume, so it is vital to perform well and make a good impression.

Benefits of Externship

- The school has a line of communication to the community and is better able to assess the needs and expectations of the public for which it is training prospective employees.
- The externship agency benefits from the new ideas and methods that the trainee may introduce. If the facility is looking for additional help, this is an ideal way to evaluate the performance of a trainee without involvement in the hiring process.
- The trainee benefits most of all by exposure to practical experience in a variety of settings. This experience in the real world removes a great deal of the anxiety that might otherwise be present in a first employment situation.

The student must be open to constructive criticism and a willing learner. Techniques may be learned on the externship that were not included in the classroom training, or optional methods may be taught for various procedures. The medical assistant should never argue with the staff at the clinical site that a method taught by the school is the only correct way. Often several methods are available to obtain the same result. The medical assisting student should treat the externship experience as if it were a probationary period on an actual job. Remember, the externship is often the first medical reference that the student will be able to list on the resume.

Several general rules must be remembered on the externship site. First, the medical assistant will have to gain the trust of the employees there. This is done by eagerly performing the duties assigned in a timely manner and performing those duties to the best of the student's ability. If any questions arise at any time, the student should ask the externship supervisor instead of assuming or performing the duties the wrong way.

It is often helpful to read the job description of the medical assistant in the facility so that the student will understand what is expected of him or her. The student medical assistant must show responsibility and dependability. There should never be a time that the student is not busy while at the externship site. If all assigned duties are completed, the extern should offer to assist others in their duties or ask for additional responsibilities. Counters always need cleaning, and filing always needs to be done. The student who does these duties without being told shows initiative and a strong work ethic. In addition, all of the rules for professional appearance apply to the site and should be meticulously followed, because the medical assisting student will be working with actual patients.

The medical assistant may find it necessary to educate the patient about the definition of what a medical assistant is and does. Often, patients assume that those assisting in the offices are nurses, but medical assistants should never represent themselves in this manner. When making introductions or assisting with patients, one should state, "I am Sandra Rameriz, Dr. Patrick's medical assistant extern," or "I am Sandra, a medical assistant intern here in Dr. Patrick's office." These words accurately portray the duties performed and help the patient to know who is caring for him or her in the physician's office.

Externs need to know a few other rules. A medical assisting student must never attempt to form a romantic relationship with patients or co-workers on the externship site. Patient confidentiality must be respected at all times, and anything that the student discovers about a patient must not be revealed or discussed under any circumstances. The student must not use any of the drug samples at the office unless specifically given permission by the physician. The student should never go to the drug storage area alone without permission or unless directed by the supervisor or physician. Externs should be extremely careful if asked to handle petty cash in the office. No student wants to be accused of any impropriety while performing their externship hours. Students must never ask the physician to treat them or any members of their family or friends. If the physician offers this as a benefit, it is acceptable, but one must not assume the physician is available for and willing to give free treatment. An extern must not ask the physician to provide prescriptions; for liability reasons, most physicians will not prescribe medications for people who are not their patients.

The externing student should bring **intangibles** to the physician's office not found in any job description. Courtesy toward others and a capacity for teamwork, a positive attitude, enthusiasm, initiative, and dedication are important personal attributes for the professional medical assistant. After becoming comfortably acquainted with what is expected on the externship, the student should concentrate on developing his or her skills and learning as much as possible during this short period. An extern becomes a valuable team player by assisting others and being reliable. By performing at peak level, the student gains the respect and trust of those on the externship site, and these people can become an excellent reference to use in beginning the search for that first paid position. Remember, the professional services of a medical assistant are extremely personal. Therefore the manner in which these services are performed can affect the health and welfare of a patient in either a positive or a negative way. When medical assisting students do their best to be sure that all contact with patients is positive in nature, they win the praise of patients, supervisors, and co-workers alike.

Continuing Education

Education does not end with the completion of formal training. The amount of medical knowledge gained in a given year is astounding. The practicing medical assistant must keep current with the rapid changes within the profession. Most physicians appreciate the medical assistant who asks questions about unfamiliar conditions and procedures and are willing to teach students about the function of the body and treatments that benefit the patient. Much can be learned by reading or reviewing the medical literature that arrives in the daily mail or articles that appear in newspapers, magazines, and medically related newsletters.

Continuing education classes are available to enhance the knowledge of the professional medical assistant. **Continuing education units (CEUs)** may be required to maintain the medical assistant's certification. These credits can be obtained through many sources, including the AAMA, the American Medical Technologists (AMT), and various other agencies and educational institutions. Professional seminars and workshops often offer CEUs. Notices of continuing education classes are sent in bulk to medical facilities and physicians' offices, so the staff should watch for courses that pertain to their particular job duties and take advantage of them as available.

PROFESSIONAL ORGANIZATIONS

By joining a professional organization and taking part in the activities it offers, a medical assistant can grow personally and professionally, keeping abreast of current trends. Participation in a recognized professional organization shows that the employee takes the career seriously and wants to be an asset to the employer. National organizations, state chapters of these organizations, and local groups meet to promote the profession of medical assisting. The organizations offer many benefits to members. Some offer health, disability, and malpractice insurance programs. Some offer credit card options and discount programs that are exclusive to their membership. All extend an opportunity for continuing education and learning beyond the classroom. Some schools that offer medical assistant training form local or school-based chapters of professional organizations. Both the AAMA and AMT offer discounted student memberships.

American Association of Medical Assistants and Certified Medical Assistants

AAMA was formally organized in 1955 as a federation of several state associations that had been functioning independently. Today the AAMA has 51 state societies (including Washington, DC) and more than 375 local chapters. The organization, whose national headquarters are located in Chicago, Illinois, was the driving force behind establishing a national certification program for medical assistants. AAMA has also been instrumental in the accreditation of medical assisting training programs in community colleges and private career institutes and in setting the minimum standards for entry-level medical assistants. At meetings held on national, state, and local levels, medical assistants can participate in workshops, learn about all types of advancement in the field, hear prominent speakers, and network with other medical assistants from other parts of the country. AAMA publishes a bimonthly journal called *CMA Today*, which includes articles with tests that may be submitted for CEU credit.

Since 1963 the AAMA has administered the certified medical assistant (CMA) examination. Those who pass the examination are awarded the CMA credential (Figure 3-6). Examinations are given in January, June, and October of each year at more than 200 centers throughout the United States. Certification is available to graduates of medical assisting programs accredited by the Commission on Accreditation of Allied Health Education Programs (CAAHEP) or by the Accrediting Bureau of Health Education Schools (ABHES). Recertification is required every 5 years and can be accomplished through CEUs or reexamination. More information is available at www.aama-ntl.org. CAAHEP competencies for medical assistants are located at the back of

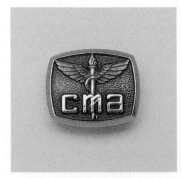

FIGURE 3-6 This pin is worn by the certified medical assistant. (Courtesy American Association of Medical Assistants, Chicago, Ill.)

this text. These competencies detail the administrative, clinical, and transdisciplinary skills required of the competent medical assistant graduate.

American Medical Technologists and Registered Medical Assistants

In the early 1970s the AMT, a national certifying body for laboratory professionals, began offering a certifying examination for medical assistants. This led to the formation of the registered medical assistant (RMA) program within the AMT organization in 1976. AMT offers this national certification to medical assistants who meet established standards and pass the examination (Figure 3-7). Several other certification examinations are offered by AMT that may be of interest to medical assistants. The certified office laboratory technician (COLT) examination is available to those who have completed certain educational and work experience requirements. Most medical assistants who work in the clinical area and have at least 6 months' experience will qualify to take the examination. Medical assistants may also qualify to take the phlebotomy technician certification examination (RPT) offered by AMT after meeting specific work-related requirements. The Certified Medical Administrative Specialist (CMAS) examination is offered to those who have graduated from an accredited administrative program or who have 5 years' experience in the field. RMAs with 2 years' administrative exprience may also take the examination.

AMT also provides societal benefits, including publications such as *AMT Events*, a quarterly magazine with useful information and articles relating to the professions served by the organization. AMT also offers national, state, and local meetings to enhance the knowledge and networking opportunities of its members. CEU credits are available to assist in increasing a medical assistant's level of competence and are a requirement for those who first became certified (or will recertify) after January 1, 2006.

The national headquarters for AMT are located in Park Ridge, Illinois. More information about the RMA examination is available on the website www.amt1.com. The ABHES competencies for medical assistants are located at the back of this text. These competencies detail the administrative, clinical, and general skills required of the medical assistant graduate.

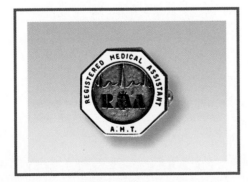

FIGURE 3-7 This pin is worn by the registered medical assistant. (Courtesy RMA/American Medical Technologists, Park Ridge, Ill.)

National Healthcareer Association

Some schools also offer certification through the National Healthcareer Association. These include the Certified Medical Administrative Assistant (CMAA), the Certified Clinical Medical Assistant (CCMA), as well as the Certified Billing and Coding Specialist (CBCS) and Certified Medical Transcriptionist (CMT). The costs for these certification examinations range from approximately $100 to $150. The National Healthcareer Association's website can be found at www.nhanow.com.

Taking Certification Examinations

Both the CMA and RMA certifications are national credentials. The CMA credential is offered by the AAMA, and the RMA credential is offered by the AMT. Because medical assistants are not required to be licensed, both of these examinations are voluntary. A medical assistant may practice in the United States without either certification, but most employers today require at least one certification. Both organizations have committees that develop the examinations, and they are both based on the roles that medical assistants fulfill in the workplace.

Students should take the examination soon after graduation; the intricate knowledge gained in school will be easier to recall the sooner it is taken. In addition, the fee for the CMA examination will increase 1 year after the graduation date. Although the graduate is not guaranteed more wages with certification or registration, most employers are willing to pay more for a graduate who has been through formal training and the certification or registration procedure.

The CMA examination covers three general categories, including administrative, clinical, and transdisciplinary competencies. The examination is scored by tallying correct responses, so making a guess will not count against the student. The minimum score to obtain the CMA credential is currently 425, and students are allowed 4 hours to complete the examination. AAMA offers two practice tests on its website that cover both anatomy and physiology and medical terminology review. AAMA requires either continuing education credits or reexamination to continue using the CMA credential.

The RMA examination can be scheduled nearly every day of the year other than Sundays and holidays at over 200 testing centers throughout the United States, its territories, and Canada. Applicants for the RMA examination must be graduates of a medical assisting course accredited by ABHES or by CAAHEP, or they must meet requirements related to their experience. The RMA examination covers administrative skills, clinical skills, and general skills and contains over 200 questions. Examinees are allowed 3 hours to take the paper-based test, and $2\frac{1}{2}$ hours to take the computer-based test. The scoring is based on a scale with a minimum passing score of 70. Practice examinations are available on the AMT website.

The AMT has recently mandated a point system to prove compliance with continuing education requirements. RMAs, CMASs, and COLTs are required to earn 30 points, and RPTs are required to earn 20 points. Points can be earned through continuing education, employer evaluations, professional and formal education, and various other methods.

Medical Assistant's Creed

I believe in the principles and purposes of the profession of medical assisting.

I endeavor to be more effective.

I aspire to render greater service.

I protect the confidence entrusted to me.

I am dedicated to the care and well-being of all patients.

I am loyal to my physician-employer.

I am true to the ethics of my profession.

I am strengthened by compassion, courage, and faith.

The Difference Between CMAs and RMAs

Two major differences between these two credentials are the examination consultant organizations and the cost. The CMA examination fee for the 2006 testing year is $95 for recent CAAHEP or ABHES graduates. The annual membership fees vary from state to state and are substantially lower if one joins while still a student. Student membership costs range from $20 to approximately $35 but must be applied for before graduating. Nonmembers must pay $170 to take the CMA examination. Annual dues thereafter are between $67 and $97, depending on the state association joined. The RMA examination cost is $90, which includes the first year's dues. Annual dues thereafter are currently $48. See Table 3-1 for a detailed comparison of the CMA and RMA.

CRITICAL THINKING APPLICATION

- Why is it important for Sandra to obtain one of the medical assisting certifications after graduation?
- How might certification help her career as a medical assistant?
- When and where can the tests be taken in your area?

CLOSING COMMENTS

This chapter has presented the advantages of becoming a trained medical assistant and some of the many career opportunities available. The necessary skills that must be developed and the general knowledge that must be acquired to function effectively have been presented. However, skills and knowledge alone do not ensure success. Personality traits and professional appearance are also critical. Professional societies and continuing education are vital to the professional medical assistant. The individual who accepts this career must be willing to accept the responsibilities inherent in its standards. The importance of gaining a national certification cannot be stressed enough. Whatever the career goals of the medical assistant, the ideas expressed in this chapter will be useful to all.

Medical assisting has grown into one of the most respected professions in the allied health field. When asked about the field, one should share the role a medical assistant plays in the office and the training involved. Others may be interested in a career change or have a desire to enter the medical field. A medical assistant should always be an exceptional ambassador for the profession.

TABLE 3-1 Differences between the Certified Medical Assistant and the Registered Medical Assistant

	CERTIFIED MEDICAL ASSISTANT (CMA)	REGISTERED MEDICAL ASSISTANT (RMA)
Credential awarded by	American Association of Medical Assistants (AAMA)	American Medical Technologists (AMT)
Address of certification or registration organization	American Association of Medical Assistants 20 N. Wacker Drive, Suite 1575 Chicago, IL 60606-2903 800-228-2262	American Medical Technologists 10700 West Higgins Road, Ste 150 Rosemont, IL 60018 800-275-1268
Organization website	www.aama-ntl.org	www.amt1.com
Mailing address for certification applications	AAMA Certification 7999 Eagle Way Chicago, IL 60678-1079	RMA Certification/AMT 10700 West Higgins Road, Ste 150 Rosemont, IL 60018
Requirement for certification or registration	Federal licensing is not required; certification or registration is optional in most states.	Federal licensing is not required; certification or registration is optional in most states.
Qualifications to take examination	Applicants must fall into one of three categories to qualify to take the CMA examination: • Category One: Graduating student or recent graduate of a CAAHEP-accredited medical assisting program • Category Two: Nonrecent graduate of a CAAHEP-accredited medical assisting program • Category Three: Graduating student or graduate of an ABHES-accredited medical assisting program	Good moral character and at least 18 years old High school graduate or acceptable equivalent Must be a graduate of, or scheduled to graduate from: • a medical assistant program accredited by either ABHES or CAAHEP • a medical assistant program in a postsecondary school that is accredited by a regional or national organization, is recognized by the U.S. Department of Education, and includes a minimum of 720 clock hours including externship • a formal medical services training of the U.S. Armed Forces Must have 5 years of work experience unless graduated from the medical assisting program within the last 3 years
Examination approval organization	National Board of Medical Examiners (NBME) www.nbme.org	National Commission for Certifying Agencies www.noca.org/ncca/ncca.htm
Cost of examination	AAMA members pay $95 (can be a student member, which costs $25-$35, depending on the state)	$90 (membership in AMT not required)
Length of time required to take examination	4 hours	3 hours
Content of examination	Three sections of 100 questions each, covering general or transdisciplinary skills, clinical skills, and administrative skills	More than 200 questions, covering general subject areas, clinical areas, and administrative areas
Testing sites	Over 200 centers throughout the United States, assigned when approved to take examination	Over 200 centers throughout the United States; list of sites available at www.pearsonvue.com/amt
Where to obtain practice test	www.aama-ntl.org/becomeCMA/exam_outline.aspx	www.amt1.com/site/epage/15340_315.htm
Testing dates	The application date for the January examination is October 1 of the previous year. The application date for the June examination is March 1 of the same year. The application date for the October examination is July 1 of the same year.	Testing dates are ongoing and are arranged at PearsonVue Centers throughout the United States.

SUMMARY OF SCENARIO

Sandra has chosen to embark on an exciting career and will find her work very rewarding. She knows that she will be proud of her efforts and looks forward to becoming a respected member of the healthcare team in a physician's office. She has set goals for her class work and attendance and is determined to meet them. Obstacles usually arise whenever one embarks on a new project, and Sandra must plan for the days that she or her child may be ill or her transportation fails. Having a backup plan in advance will help her to overcome these minor setbacks.

Many opportunities exist for the medical assistant in both administrative and clinical positions, and as Sandra progresses through her training she will find areas that appeal to her more than others. All are vitally important so that she will be a versatile medical assistant, able to perform front- and back-office duties. Exposure to various duties will be provided during the externship, and these experiences will help her to determine where she might enjoy working once she graduates. It is important that Sandra glean as much experience and knowledge as possible while in school so that she will have more options after her training.

Sandra should develop a good relationship with her instructors and go to them when she has questions or concerns. These professionals are anxious to share their knowledge and experiences with students to best prepare them for the work environment. If Sandra's grades ever drop or she is struggling, Sandra should seek the advice of the instructor to determine how to improve her performance. The externship is also critically important, because it is usually the first medical reference a new graduate will have. Any difficulties at the externship site should be brought to the attention of the externship supervisor or an instructor at her school. Learning to set goals will help her to achieve more throughout her education, and this is a habit she should carry into her career.

With so many benefits available at different facilities in the medical field, Sandra will need to carefully weigh what she needs for herself and her son before taking any position. She should look at all of her options and choose the best one after careful evaluation. Her time in school should be spent getting to know her instructors and understanding their expectations, studying hard, learning to budget time and money, and discovering as much as possible about her new career. This will result in her satisfaction with her job and new career.

SUMMARY of LEARNING OBJECTIVES

1. Define, spell, and pronounce the terms listed in the vocabulary.
   - Spelling and pronouncing medical terms correctly adds credibility to the medical assistant. Knowing the definition of these terms promotes confidence in communication with patients and co-workers.
2. Briefly discuss the history of medical assisting as a profession.
   - The first medical assistants were probably neighbors and friends of the physician. The field has grown into one of the most respected and versatile professions in allied health.
3. Differentiate between administrative and clinical medical assisting duties.
   - Administrative duties are those that involve running the office, such as scheduling appointments and filing insurance. Administrative medical assistants usually spend most of the day in the front office of the facility. Clinical duties include more patient contact and assisting the physician in the back office. Often, new graduates move toward one or the other divisions, but they should always be ready and willing to adapt to new duties or fill in at other areas when necessary.
4. Discuss the versatility of a career in medical assisting.
   - Medical assistants are versatile enough to work in many different settings. Most often they are found in physician offices, but they also work in hospitals, insurance companies, clinics, laboratories, and many other facilities. The combination of administrative and clinical training makes the medical assistant quite valuable to the employer.

5. Explain the reasons that hiring an individual who has no formal training is often more expensive than hiring a professional medical assistant.
   - Medical assistants who have been formally trained certainly deserve a fair wage, comparable to the national average for a person in whatever position they hold. When supervisors or employers attempt to find "bargain help" at a cheaper rate, often they do not hire the high-quality employee who is so necessary in the physician's office. Because medical assistants help care for the patient, they should be compensated well so that the retention of the office staff will be continuous and stable. This can only help the physician care for patients in a more effective manner and gives the patients a sense of familiarity and security as well.
6. Identify several considerations to keep in mind when choosing a position as a medical assistant other than financial compensation.
   - The medical assistant should consider many factors other than the salary when choosing a position. Location, perks, benefits, and the atmosphere of the office are all important. Many assistants are interested in growth within the organization and welcome those opportunities. Working for a friendly, caring physician and/or supervisor is invaluable. Sometimes, taking a lesser position in a well-known and reputable facility is temporarily worth a lower wage because of future opportunities. Consider all aspects of a position before accepting a job offer.

Continued

SUMMARY of LEARNING OBJECTIVES
Continued

7. Discuss the aspects of the medical assistant's performance on a successful externship.
   - The medical assisting externship offers the student an opportunity to put the skills learned in the classroom to good use. If completed successfully, this is an excellent reference for the resume. The student should perform at the optimal level and never hesitate to complete duties assigned. Offer to go above and beyond to secure the support of the externship site as the job search begins.

8. List three unacceptable behaviors on the externship site.
   - An externing medical assistant should never attempt to form relationships with patients outside the office or view the chart for personal information. Do not ask the physician to treat family members, and do not take medications without explicit permission from the physician or supervisor. Be very careful when handling cash and drugs in the office. The student should make every effort to never be late to the externship site unless a severe emergency occurs.

9. Explain why continuing education is so important to the medical assistant.
   - Continuing education is important to medical assistants so that the latest trends and information are readily available and accessible. Take advantage of local seminars and continuing education classes. Often the employer will agree to pay for classes or seminars that the medical assistant takes if they relate to his or her employment at the facility. Some will provide tuition reimbursement for college expenses, often even if the college courses are not related to the position the employee holds at the facility.

10. Discuss the difference between a CMA and an RMA.
    - The main difference between the CMA and RMA credentials is the agency that provides each certification. The CMA credential is awarded by the AAMA, and the RMA is awarded by the AMT. Both are nationally recognized certifications.

CONNECTIONS

Study Guide Connection: Go to Chapter 3 Study Guide. Read the Case Study and Workplace Applications and complete the assignments. Do online research for answers to the questions in the Internet Activities associated with the medical assisting profession.

 CD Connection: Go to the Medical Assisting Competency Challenge CD and review the content of the training activities. These will be referred to throughout the textbook to enhance your learning experience.

 Evolve Connection: For more information related to the medical assisting profession, go to http://evolve.elsevier.com/kinn/admin and visit related weblinks for Chapter 3. Click on the Medical Assisting Exam Review and do the practice questions to sharpen your test-taking skills.

Professional Behavior in the Workplace

4

SCENARIO

Karen Yon has wanted to work in the medical field for most of her adult life. She studied very hard in high school and graduated with honors. She volunteered in a local hospital, then after working for 3 years in restaurants as a server, she enrolled in medical assistant classes. After her externship, she was asked to continue as a regular employee at a family practice in her area.

Karen strives to do all of her duties professionally and compassionately in the physician's office. She maintains a professional image to patients and co-workers. However, it was difficult to learn how to be professional at all times and show compassion to patients through only the classroom experience. These are important aspects of her job, and she was able to gain valuable experience in these areas on her externship. Because this is her first job in the medical field, she wants to make a good impression on her employer and be a team player.

Throughout most of Karen's training as a medical assistant, her grandmother was confined to a rehabilitation center after a stroke. Although she has progressed well with treatment, Karen is the only relative who lives close to the rehabilitation center, and her family depends on her to check on her grandmother from time to time. Karen enjoys spending time at the center reading to her grandmother, because they are close. Still, Karen realizes that the stroke has caused permanent damage, and her grandmother's health seems to be on the decline.

While studying this chapter, think about the following questions:

- How do professional medical assistants put aside personal issues and devote themselves to the patients in the office?
- How can Karen meet her familial and work obligations equally well?
- What steps should Karen take to ensure that both her family and her supervisors understand her obligations to the other?
- How can Karen exhibit professional behavior and compassion for patients on a daily basis at the physician's office?

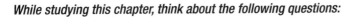

LEARNING OBJECTIVES

1. Define, spell, and pronounce the terms listed in the vocabulary.
2. Explain the meaning of the word professionalism.
3. Discuss several of the characteristics of professionalism.
4. Explain why confidentiality is so important in the medical profession.
5. Discuss the role of the medical assistant's attitude in caring for patients.
6. List some examples of office politics.

7. Identify specific ways that teamwork can be promoted in the physician's office.
8. Discuss the meaning of insubordination and why it is grounds for dismissal.
9. Identify several categories of prioritizing tasks and their meaning.
10. Talk about goal setting and how this helps in achieving career success.

National Accreditation Competencies and Content

ABHES COMPETENCIES

Professionalism

1.a. Project a positive attitude
1.b. Maintain confidentiality at all times
1.c. Be a "team player"
1.d. Be cognizant of ethical boundaries
1.e. Exhibit initiative
1.f. Adapt to change
1.g. Evidence a responsible attitude
1.h. Be courteous and diplomatic
1.i. Conduct work within scope of education, training, and ability

Communication

2.p. Professional components

Legal Concepts

5.e. Maintain liability coverage

VOCABULARY

characteristics Distinguishing traits, qualities, or properties.

commensurate (ku-men′su-rut) Corresponding in size, amount, extent, or degree; equal in measure.

competent Having adequate or requisite capabilities.

connotation (kah-nuh-ta′-shun) An implication; something suggested by a word or thing.

credibility The quality or power of inspiring belief.

demeanor (di-me′-nur) Behavior toward others; outward manner.

detrimental (de-truh-men′-til) Obviously harmful or damaging.

discretion (dis-kre′-shun) The quality of being discrete; having or showing good judgment or conduct, especially in speech.

disseminated (di-se′-muh-na-ted) To disburse; to spread around.

initiative To cause or facilitate the beginning of; to initiate something into happening.

insubordination (in-suh′-bor-din-a-shun) Disobedience to authority.

morale (mo-ral′) The mental and emotional condition, enthusiasm, loyalty, or confidence of an individual or group with regard to the function or tasks at hand.

optimistic Inclined to put the most favorable construction on actions and events or to anticipate the best possible outcome.

persona (pur-so′-nuh) An individual's social facade or front that reflects the role in life the individual is playing; the personality that a person projects in public.

procrastination (pruh-kras-tuh-na′-shun) Intentionally putting off doing something that should be done.

professionalism The conduct or qualities characterized by or conforming to the technical or ethical standards of a profession; exhibiting a courteous, conscientious, and generally businesslike manner in the workplace.

reproach An expression of rebuke or disapproval; a cause or occasion of blame, discredit, or disgrace.

What is professional behavior? We tend to hold medical personnel to a higher standard of **professionalism** than those in most other career fields. The medical assistant who works to improve his or her professional approach in the workplace will be an asset to the employer and will be promoted to positions of more responsibility quickly within the healthcare industry.

THE MEANING OF PROFESSIONALISM

Professionalism is defined as exhibiting a courteous, conscientious, and generally businesslike manner in the workplace. It is characterized by or conforms to the technical or ethical

standards of a certain profession. Conducting oneself in a professional manner is essential for successful medical assistants. The attitude of those in the medical profession is generally more conservative than in other career fields. Patients expect professional behavior and will base much of their trust and confidence in those who exhibit this type of **demeanor** in the physician's office (Figure 4-1).

CHARACTERISTICS OF PROFESSIONALISM

Many **characteristics** make up the professional posture required of medical assistants. Student medical assistants should begin developing these characteristics while in school; these qualities

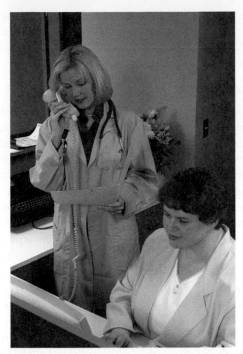

FIGURE 4-1 The professional medical assistant is an asset to the physician's office.

will not magically appear when the student begins working with actual patients. Although we might think that we would always behave appropriately during an externship or in a job setting, the habits developed in school will carry over into these experiences. If the behavior is unacceptable, it will be **detrimental** to the medical assistant's professional career. If the medical assistant wishes to advance and receive wage increases, promotions, and the trust of the employer, the following characteristics must be a part of his or her **persona.**

CRITICAL THINKING APPLICATION

- How can students practice professional behavior while still in the classroom situation?
- When students are practicing clinical skills, how can they demonstrate proficiency in professional behavior?

Loyalty

Loyalty is a faithfulness or allegiance to a cause, ideal, custom, institution, or product. Loyalty to an employer means that the employee is appreciative of the opportunity provided through the job and supports the company by giving the best effort possible. Many individuals today are interested only in what the employer can provide them. However, this is an immature approach to take toward a job. When a person is employed by a company, use of skills is exchanged for different types of compensation. Each benefits the other. Often we forget that experience alone is a great benefit from working. Loyalty to the employer is important, and the employee should feel a sense of loyalty from the company as well.

CRITICAL THINKING APPLICATION

- How can Karen demonstrate loyalty to her employer?
- What are some ways that her employer can reciprocate Karen's loyalty?

Dependability

One of the most valuable traits of a successful medical assistant is dependability. Be on time and make every attempt to be at work every day. When staff members arrive late, the schedule for the entire day can be delayed (Figure 4-2). A medical assistant must follow through when the physician or supervisor gives an order. That person will count on the medical assistant to remember and complete all assigned duties. Supervisors should be confident that once given a task to do, the medical assistant will carry it out accurately and in a timely manner.

Courtesy

Show courtesy to the patients and co-workers in the physician's office. Kind words and compassion go far in building trust between the medical assistant and patients (Figure 4-3). All

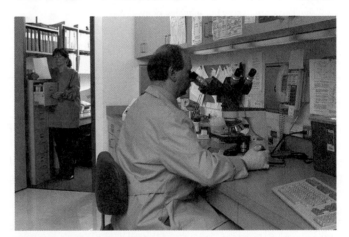

FIGURE 4-2 The physician will depend on the medical assistant to be at work on time and on each scheduled day. Absent or tardy employees cause scheduling difficulties and can greatly inconvenience the patients and remaining staff.

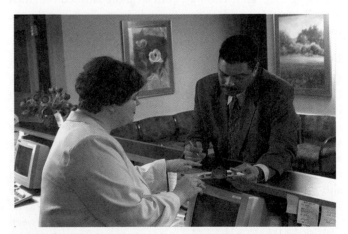

FIGURE 4-3 Taking a few moments to explain forms and bills to a patient is a courteous way to avoid misunderstandings and promote goodwill.

visitors and staff members in the office should be shown kindness and consideration. The fact that a medical assistant is having a bad day is no excuse for inflicting his or her anger or irritation on patients. Always demonstrate a good attitude and offer patients and visitors a sincere smile.

Initiative

Employee lack of **initiative** is one of the more common complaints from supervisors. Taking initiative means that the medical assistant looks for the opportunity to be of help, assisting others as the workload demands. Instead of waiting to be told to perform a task, the **competent** medical assistant looks for jobs that need to be completed; never remain idle. Some task can always be done in the medical office. Filing needs to be done on a continual basis. Inventories, supply ordering, or restocking can be performed when there is extra time. Cleaning countertops and straightening areas as work is done will help to keep the facility tidy. The medical assistant should also keep an eye on the reception area, since it may need attention several times during the day.

CRITICAL THINKING APPLICATION

- How can Karen show her initiative on the job?
- What types of duties can she perform when she has finished her workload for the day and there is still time left before leaving the office?

Flexibility

A medical assistant must be able to adapt to a wide variety of situations. An emergency could occur in the office, and the staff must be flexible enough to adjust the schedule and care for all patients. Being flexible also means that staff members are willing to assist one another in the performance of their duties. No one in the physician's office should ever say, "That's not my job." The patients must come first, and every staff member must be willing to lend a hand where needed. Some medical assistants trade or rotate their duties. If one assistant does not particularly enjoy doing a certain task, perhaps another assistant would be willing to trade tasks. This way, both are more satisfied with their jobs. Being able to adapt quickly and cheerfully will make the medical assistant a valuable asset to the office.

Credibility

Credibility is the perceived competence or character of a person. It leads to the belief that a person can be trusted. Because trust is a vital component of the physician-patient relationship, the credibility of the physician and those who assist in the office should be strong. The information provided to patients must be accurate. Patients expect that the physician and medical assistant will instruct them in a manner that will enhance their health and provide positive results. One must take care in giving any advice to patients, because they view the medical assistant as an agent of the physician. Patients may not distinguish between the medical assistant's comments and the physician's orders. Remember that giving anything that could be construed as

medical advice is outside the scope of the duties of the medical assistant. To avoid charges of practicing medicine without a license, a medical assistant must be sure to suggest only what the physician has authorized.

Confidentiality

The importance of confidentiality cannot be stressed enough in the medical environment. Patients are entitled to privacy where their health is concerned, and they should be confident that medical professionals use information only to care for them. Never reveal any information about any patient to anyone without specific permission to do so. Always verify that the person seeking information has the right to see it and that the patient has signed a consent form. Casual conversations in hallways, elevators, and break rooms between staff members can be overheard by a family member or friend of the patient. These are a few places in the facility where confidentiality is often breached.

The rules regarding confidentiality extend beyond the medical office. While at home, medical assistants should not discuss details about patients with their families and friends. Those outside the medical profession do not understand how vital it is to keep information confidential and may pass along damaging facts to others. Medical assistants must make it a rule never to discuss a patient with anyone unless information must be shared for patient care and treatment. The Health Insurance Portability and Accountability Act (HIPAA) was created in part to assure patient confidentiality. HIPAA will be discussed more in later chapters.

Attitude

Possibly the most important asset a medical assistant brings to the office is a good attitude. A good attitude involves courtesy and kindness to others, refraining from jumping to conclusions, giving the other person the benefit of the doubt, and being **optimistic.** This trait alone can influence promotions, terminations, and the entire atmosphere of the office (Figure 4-4). Individuals are able to control their attitudes with practice. It takes skill to react calmly to people who are very upset, rather than to respond in kind, especially if being harassed or accused. Speaking in an even tone and perhaps a little softer than normal will force the listener to lower his or her voice to hear. Offer to help resolve the problem and attempt to move to a private room out of the hearing range of other patients to talk. Always display a good attitude with co-workers and be willing to assist them with their duties, especially on hectic days.

OBSTRUCTIONS TO PROFESSIONALISM

It is not always easy to be a professional. Sometimes patients, co-workers, and supervisors try our patience, and it can be hard to maintain a professional attitude in these cases. Some of the obstructions to professional behavior are discussed in this section.

Personal Problems and "Baggage"

Everyone has a life outside of the workplace, and sometimes we face challenges and difficult times that are hard to put aside.

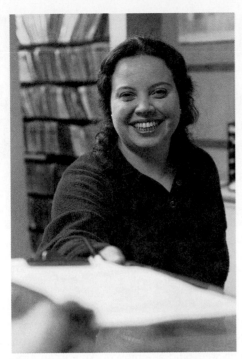

FIGURE 4-4 A good attitude goes a long way in patient and staff relationships.

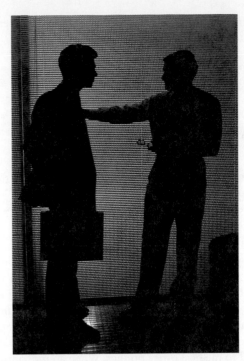

FIGURE 4-5 Gossip and rumors have no place in the medical profession. Avoid employees who participate in this type of activity.

During working hours our thoughts should be on the job at hand, especially when we are dealing with patients. However, there may be situations in our lives that are so critical or distracting that we find ourselves thinking of them constantly. This personal baggage can interfere with our ability to properly perform job duties.

When a situation intrudes on thoughts at work, it is often best to take the time to talk with a supervisor. It is not always necessary to share the intimate details, but a quick explanation that some difficulties are occurring outside of work will help the supervisor to understand any changes in habit or attitude. However, some supervisors are uncaring and are concerned only with satisfactory job performance. The medical assistant will have to use some **discretion** when discussing private affairs with the supervisor.

Never transfer personal problems and baggage to the patient. A professional medical assistant does not share personal information or problems with anyone at the medical facility, especially patients. The workday should be centered around patient care, so never allow personal business to impinge on time that should be spent assisting patients and the physician.

CRITICAL THINKING APPLICATION

It is often hard to keep from thinking about a problem while you are working. How can Karen do this if she is concerned about a grandmother who is critically ill?

Rumors and the "Grapevine"

A rumor by definition is talk or widely **disseminated** opinion with no discernible source, or a statement that is not known to be true. The definition alone suggests that spreading rumors should be avoided. Most people enjoy working in an environment in which employees cooperate and get along with each other, but rumors can cause problems with employee **morale** and are often great exaggerations or manipulations of the truth. By promoting the grapevine, rumors are passed along and become more and more outrageous with each retelling. A medical assistant should refuse to participate in the office rumor mill and should attempt to be cordial and friendly to everyone at work (Figure 4-5). Supervisors regard those who spread or discuss rumors as unprofessional and untrustworthy. Avoid passing along work-related rumors to patients, family, and friends.

Personal Phone Calls and Business

It is wise to avoid receiving unnecessary phone calls to the office from friends and family. The office phone should be considered a business line and must be used as such, except in emergencies. Using personal cell phones during working hours is not acceptable. Use breaks and lunch hours to take care of business on the phone. Never take a personal call or respond to text messages on a cell phone while working with a patient. If a phone must be carried, place it on the vibrator setting, and always step into a hall or break area if a call absolutely must be taken. This should only happen in rare cases. Visitors should not frequent the office, especially not in the area where the medical assistant is working. If someone must come to the office, always offer the reception area as a waiting room. Visitors should never be allowed to enter patient areas.

Checking personal email should also be avoided in the workplace. Any type of personal business, such as studying, looking up information on the Internet for personal use, or balancing a personal checkbook, should be done at home and not in the office setting. All of these actions distract the medical assistant from the job at hand; the focus should be on serving the patients in the office at all times.

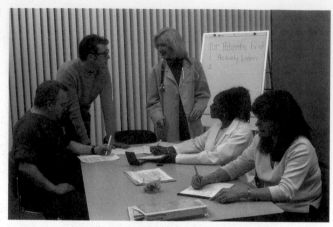

FIGURE 4-6 Teamwork is a vital part of the medical profession. All staff members must work together to care for the patient and perform required duties in the physician's office.

> **CRITICAL THINKING** APPLICATION
>
> ■ Karen has a friend who works in a video store close to her office. Her friend has begun the habit of stopping in daily during her lunch hour to chat with Karen. How can Karen politely discourage her friend from doing this?
>
> ■ Karen feels the need to check on her grandmother's condition as often as possible during the days she is ill. How might she accomplish this in a professional way?

Office Politics

Most people associate office politics with some underhanded scheme or plans to move upward in the company in whatever way possible, whether the methods used are ethical or not. The tendency is to give the word politics a negative **connotation.** *Politics* can be defined as the art or science of influencing and guiding government or some other organization. The same can be applied to medical office politics. When an individual wishes to move upward in an organization, he or she may use a positive strategy. Many people develop a specific plan regarding how they will advance and in what time period they will accomplish their goals. Medical assistants who wish to advance should be productive workers, accept responsibility, be dependable, and always conduct themselves in a professional manner. Using underhanded techniques and instigating trouble is not an effective method of career advancement.

Procrastination

Procrastination is often a symptom of the fear of failure. Some people procrastinate because this gives them an excuse for failure. Others procrastinate because they are perfectionists and feel that only they can complete a project the right way. Procrastination is the surest way to see that goals remain unfulfilled. The best way to stop this habit is to *do* something. Divide projects into small steps, and complete one at a time. When a project is divided into small segments, it is much less overwhelming. The stronger the motivation, the easier it is to fight the urge to procrastinate.

PROFESSIONAL ATTRIBUTES

Teamwork

If managers were asked what the most important attributes would be for medical professionals, teamwork would be high on the list (Figure 4-6). Staff members must work together for the good of the patients. They must be willing to perform duties outside the formal job description if they are needed in other areas of the office. Many supervisors frown on employees who state, "That's not in my job description." Any order that is given by a supervisor becomes mandatory, and an individual who refuses to perform such a task can have his or her employment terminated for **insubordination.** A medical assistant should

perform the duty and later discuss with the supervisor any valid reasons that it should have been assigned to someone else.

Although we would all enjoy working in an office in which everyone gets along and likes every other employee, this does not always happen. Personal feelings must be set aside at work, and all employees must cooperate with others to get the job done efficiently. If a medical assistant has an issue with another employee, the first move would be to discuss it privately with the other person. Then, if the situation does not improve, perhaps a supervisor should be involved for further discussions.

Time Management

We have often heard the expression "work smart." This means that we are to use our time efficiently and concentrate on the duties that are most important first. To do this we must first prioritize our duties and arrange our schedules to ensure that these duties can be performed. The first way to improve time management is to plan the tasks that need to be done that day. Taking 10 minutes to write down the tasks for the day will help to ensure that they are done. Then it is important to stay on schedule throughout the day, unless emergencies disrupt the schedule. Even then, when office days are well planned, allowances can be made for emergencies, even if they happen often, and the majority of the tasks can still be completed. The key to managing time is prioritizing.

Prioritizing

Prioritizing is simply deciding which tasks are most important. Many people make a "to do" list for the day's activities, but the secret to success is prioritizing those activities into categories that give order to the tasks.

Most tasks can be prioritized into three general categories: those that must be done that day, those that *should* be done that day, and those that could be done if time permits. Once you have a general list of tasks, review the list and further prioritize it, using a code such as M for must, S for should, and C for could (or this might be further simplified by using the letters A, B, and C). Once the tasks are divided into these categories, they can be further classified within each section. For instance, if there are six A category duties, meaning they must be done that day, these six can be numbered in the order they should be performed. The same process is completed with the B and C categories, and then as the tasks are completed, they are checked off for that day. Other categories can be added to customize the list. For example, an H category can be used for duties to perform at home, P could represent phone calls that need to be made, and E could represent errands to run. Customizing the categories will make the list more user-friendly.

Setting Goals

Those who succeed in life are planners and goal-setters. The first step in becoming a proficient goal-setter is to take the time to really think about what is to be accomplished throughout one's lifetime. These goals must be written down and reviewed often. Goals should be set for all areas in a person's life, including personal growth, career, home life, family, spiritual needs, and any others that apply to the individual. The goals should not be unreasonable. They should be measurable and specific, with written steps detailing how they will be reached. Determination and persistence in reaching the goals will help to make them happen, along with a healthy dose of hard work. The goals should be reviewed often and progress evaluated; then goals can be reset as necessary.

Remember to celebrate accomplishments and move past any goals that are missed, evaluating and restating the goals if necessary. Charles Kettering, an inventor who is most well known for his invention of the automobile self-starter, once said, "The only time you can't afford to fail is the last time you try." Never quit trying to improve and experience personal growth.

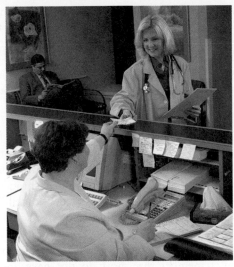

FIGURE 4-7 Knowing which employee to call when help is needed promotes goodwill among employees and often gets a task done more efficiently.

CRITICAL THINKING APPLICATION

- What are some goals that Karen might set related to her behavior on the job?
- List several goals for the new medical assistant to work toward during his or her first year in the field.

KNOWING THE FACILITY AND ITS EMPLOYEES

A much-circulated story tells of a college professor who used to end a critical test with the question, "What is the name of the woman who cleans our wing of the building?" This would perplex most students, but the question makes a good point. A professional medical assistant should attempt to get to know the people who work in the facility and should have a good idea of who handles which duties (Figure 4-7). When patients have specific problems with which they need help, they can be referred to the person who knows the most about that particular issue. It is wise to express appreciation to others whenever possible. Say "thank you" often or "I appreciate your help" when working with others. This will make co-workers more likely to assist at other times when their help is needed.

DOCUMENTATION

From the standpoint of professional behavior, documentation skills are vital to medical assistants. Charting accurately with legible, neat handwriting can make a difference in the perception of professionalism in the medical office. Be complete in any narrative regarding patients. Be sure to state facts, not opinions, and never use sarcastic remarks when charting. Phone messages must be documented carefully as well, and handled in a professional manner. Never use sarcasm when reporting messages to the physician or anyone else in the office. Use conservative speech and proper wording in all situations in the medical facility.

Note Taking

Whenever office meetings or seminars are held, be prepared by having a pad and pencil ready for note taking. A medical assistant should never be without paper and pen so that accurate information from the meeting can be jotted down for future reference. It is wise to keep a notebook or file on office meetings to refer to in case clarification of an order or a point is needed. Another good idea is to keep a small spiral notebook in a pocket with a pen, so that if an order is given in passing by the physician, the medical assistant will have a place to jot it down until he or she has access to the patient's chart. This avoids giving incorrect dosages of medication or forgetting to order a laboratory test, as well as many other errors that could be made by relying on memory.

WORK ETHICS

Work ethics can involve a whole range of activities, from individual acts to the philosophy of the entire facility. A person who has good work ethics is one who arrives on time, who is rarely absent, whose work output is **commensurate** with the pay received, and who uses his or her best abilities. Work ethics also involves other situations. If another employee is seen taking drugs from the supply cabinet or money from the cash box, the act should certainly be reported. However, if the guilty employee is also a close friend of the person who witnesses the act, an ethical dilemma is present. Ways to solve ethical problems are discussed in Chapter 6. A medical assistant must always act in such a way that his or her actions are above **reproach.**

INTERPERSONAL SKILLS

Interpersonal skills are paramount in working with patients and other health professionals. A medical assistant should work hard to perfect his or her communication techniques. Often the success of a business is directly related to the ability of its employees to communicate effectively. Interpersonal skills are discussed in detail in Chapter 5.

When speaking to patients and providing them with information, remember that most do not have any medical background and do not understand many of the phrases used by the medical community. A medical assistant must be patient and explain in a courteous manner any aspect of the instructions or details that the patient does not understand. When educating the patient, the medical assistant should have a professional attitude of concern and helpfulness. Assure the patient that medical assistants and the rest of the staff in the facility are bound by rules of patient confidentiality if the patient seems concerned about revealing pertinent information.

CLOSING COMMENTS

Patients expect and deserve professional behavior from those who work in medical facilities. Always show compassion, caring, and consideration for a person who comes to the office, whether a patient, visitor, or co-worker. By displaying these traits, the medical assistant will earn the respect of co-workers and become indispensable to the physician-employer. Behaving in a professional manner in the medical office will help to gain the patient's trust. Trust is one of the most important factors in avoiding cases of medical professional liability. Treating patients with care and not subjecting them to poor attitudes and unnecessary information will keep the patient-physician relationship a strong one, conducive to the health and recovery of the patient.

SUMMARY OF SCENARIO

Karen is happy to be employed in a family practice in which providing quality patient care is paramount. She is learning to be careful of what she says and to remain focused on the patient instead of any difficulties she may be having. Karen knows that it is her responsibility to be a team player and to assist the other staff members as much as possible. She maintains a good attitude, even when personal issues could distract her from her duties. Karen gets a strong sense of pride in being a part of the medical profession. She insists on a neat appearance and arrives on time for each scheduled workday. She always asks others if they need help when she has any extra time throughout the day. Karen looks forward to a long relationship with her employer. The rewards she feels as a member of the health team are second to none.

Although Karen is concerned about her grandmother's health, those concerns must be minimally invasive on her work duties and her attitude toward her patients and co-workers. By making an appointment to speak with her supervisor and explaining the situation with her grandmother, Karen takes a proactive role in assuring that the supervisor understands the pressures Karen is facing. Most supervisors will be sympathetic and understanding when issues outside the practice affect employees; however, this should not happen on a regular basis. By encouraging Karen to call and check on her grandmother periodically, the supervisor helps Karen to feel more confident and less distracted during the day. By finding her supervisor a supportive ally, Karen can relax and carry out her duties professionally and competently throughout the workday. Karen puts the patients first, and this is a fine example of both professionalism and patient compassion.

SUMMARY of LEARNING OBJECTIVES

1. Define, spell, and pronounce the terms listed in the vocabulary.
   - Spelling and pronouncing medical terms correctly adds credibility to the medical assistant. Knowing the definition of these terms promotes confidence in communication with patients and co-workers.
2. Explain the meaning of the word professionalism.
   - Professionalism is the characteristic of being or conforming to the technical or ethical standards of a profession. It involves exhibiting courtesy, being conscientious, and conducting oneself in a businesslike manner at the workplace. Professionalism is vitally important in the medical profession.
3. Discuss several of the characteristics of professionalism.
   - Some of the characteristics of professionalism include loyalty, dependability, courtesy, initiative, flexibility, credibility, confidentiality, and a good attitude.
4. Explain why confidentiality is so important in the medical profession.

Continued

SUMMARY of LEARNING OBJECTIVES
Continued

- Confidentiality is vitally important in the medical profession. Patients depend on medical personnel to keep their health information confidential and private. Breach of patient confidentiality is one reason that an employee could be immediately terminated from his or her position and can result in litigation between the patient and the physician-employer.

5. Discuss the role of the medical assistant's attitude in caring for patients.
   - Because most patients are not at their best when visiting the physician's office, the attitude of the staff plays an important role in patients' attitudes while in the office. Medical assistants need patience when working with those who are ill. A smile or a reassuring pat on the back will go a long way and be encouraging.

6. List some examples of office politics.
   - Office politics can be negative or positive. A person who uses others to be promoted in the company or takes credit for a team effort may be using office politics in a negative way; a person who strategically plans advancement through outstanding performance, dependability, and teamwork uses office politics in a positive manner. Knowing when to speak and when to listen will help the medical assistant to play the game of politics well in the medical facility.

7. Identify specific ways that teamwork can be promoted in the physician's office.
   - Teamwork makes any job easier to complete. By helping those who may be overwhelmed with duties, the medical assistant may find willing co-workers who will help when the situation is reversed in the future. If two assistants both have duties they dislike, they might trade the duties and both be satisfied. Everyone must work together for the good of the facility and the patients it serves.

8. Discuss the meaning of insubordination and why it is grounds for dismissal.
   - Insubordination can be used as grounds for immediate dismissal. Insubordination is being disobedient to any type of authority figure, usually the supervisor. When given a task to complete, the medical assistant should carry out the order unless it is unlawful or unethical. If the medical assistant does not carry out an order, the patient's life may be at risk. If the medical assistant feels that the duty should have been performed by someone else or there was some reason it should not have been performed, the supervisor should be consulted. Discuss the issue and attempt to reach an agreement about the appropriateness of performing the task in the future.

9. Identify several categories of prioritizing tasks and their meaning.
   - Prioritizing tasks can help the medical assistant to accomplish more tasks. Prioritizing can be used for work, home, and extracurricular activities. Tasks can be identified as those that must, should, or could be done that day. Then within each of these categories the tasks can be numbered in the order in which they should be completed.

10. Talk about goal setting and how this helps in achieving career success.
    - Goals should be written down and reviewed often to check progress. Taking small steps toward goals will help ensure that they are eventually reached. Individuals should set goals in each area of their lives, breaking the tasks down into manageable parts. Goals should not be unreasonable or unattainable but should provide the opportunity for small successes along the way to reaching the ultimate goal.

CONNECTIONS

Study Guide Connection: Go to Chapter 4 Study Guide. Read the Case Study and Workplace Applications and complete the assignments. Do online research for answers to the questions in the Internet Activities associated with professional behavior in the workplace.

CD Connection: Go to the Medical Assisting Competency Challenge CD and do the training activities under Communication.

Evolve Connection: For more information related to professional behavior in the workplace, go to http://evolve.elsevier.com/kinn/admin and visit related weblinks for Chapter 4. Click on the Medical Assisting Exam Review and do the practice questions to sharpen your test-taking skills.

Interpersonal Skills and Human Behavior

5

SCENARIO

Many types of patients seek medical attention and care in the physician's office. Each has different needs and different concerns, even if the diagnoses are similar. Communication and interpersonal skills are vitally important in meeting these needs and providing optimal care to the patient. However, the patient is not the only individual to consider. Family members are often instrumental in the health and well-being of the patient.

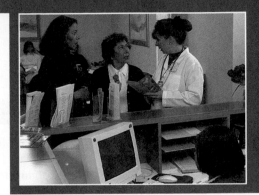

Lucille Cloyd is an 83-year-old patient who has been diagnosed with pancreatic cancer and is seeing Dr. Neill for treatment. Her daughter, Sarah Smithson, helps to care for her; she is very close to her mother emotionally. Sarah is also Dr. Neill's patient. Although Sarah does not wish to see her mother in pain, she suffers with the knowledge that life will be very different without her. Mrs. Cloyd is widowed and visits the physician once a month in addition to receiving hospice services. She is a good-humored woman who feels she has led a fruitful life, yet she has moments of depression. She has been living with Sarah and her family for 2 months and enjoys interacting with her two grandchildren and the family's pets.

The medical assistant must consider not only Mrs. Cloyd, but also her extended family. Compassion and sensitivity will be necessary to care for this patient, as well as excellent listening skills. A good knowledge of human relations will help the medical assistant make Mrs. Cloyd's medical care as pleasant as possible under the circumstances.

While studying this chapter, think about the following questions:

- How can the medical assistant treat patients as individuals during a busy workday?
- How does the medical assistant effectively communicate with a patient's family members?
- How will developing good listening skills make the medical assistant more effective?
- How do friends and family members play a role in the health of the patient?

LEARNING OBJECTIVES

1. Define, spell, and pronounce the terms listed in the vocabulary.
2. Explain why first impressions are critically important.
3. Differentiate between verbal and nonverbal communication.
4. Explain the different levels of spatial separation.
5. Discuss the value of touch in the communication process.
6. Describe the elements of the transactional communication model.
7. Explain some of the barriers to effective communication.
8. List and explain the levels of Maslow's hierarchy of needs.
9. Discuss defense mechanisms, and be able to recognize commonly used defense mechanisms.
10. Describe the value of listening.
11. List several ways to deal with conflict.
12. Explain the stages that patients go through when facing death.
13. Discuss why physical and emotional needs affect our daily performance at work.

National Accreditation Competencies and Content

CAAHEP COMPETENCIES

General

3.c.(1)(b). Recognize and respond to verbal communications
3.c.(1)(c). Recognize and respond to nonverbal communications

ABHES COMPETENCIES

Communication

2.a. Be attentive, listen, and learn
2.b. Be impartial and show empathy when dealing with patients
2.c. Adapt what is said to the recipient's level of comprehension
2.d. Serve as liaison between physician and others
2.h. Receive, organize, prioritize, and transmit information expediently
2.i. Recognize and respond to verbal and nonverbal communication
2.k. Principles of verbal and nonverbal communication
2.l. Recognition and response to verbal and nonverbal communication

Instruction

7.b. Instruct patients with special needs

VOCABULARY

adage (a′-dij) A saying, often in metaphoric form, that embodies a common observation.

aggressive Forceful or intended to dominate; hostile, injurious, or destructive, especially when referring to a behavior caused by frustration.

ambiguous (am-bi′-gu-wus) Capable of being understood in two or more possible senses or ways; unclear.

animate To fill with life; to give spirit and support to expressions.

battery An offensive touching or use of force on a person without his or her consent.

caustic (kos′-tik) Marked by sarcasm.

channels Means of communication or expression; courses or directions of thought.

comfort zone A place in the mind where an individual feels safe and confident.

congruent (kun-gru′-unt) Being in agreement, harmony, or correspondence; conforming to the circumstances or requirements of a situation.

decodes Converts, as in a message, into intelligible form; recognizes and interprets.

defense mechanisms Psychologic methods of dealing with stressful situations that are encountered in day-to-day living.

encodes Converts from one system of communication to another; converts a message into code.

encroachments Actions that advance beyond the usual or proper limits.

enunciate (e-nun′-se-at) To utter articulate sounds; the act of being very distinct in speech.

external noise Sounds or factors outside the brain that interfere with the communication process.

externalization The attribution of an event or occurrence to causes outside the self.

feedback The transmission of evaluative or corrective information to the original or controlling source about an action, event, or process.

grief Reaction to an unfortunate outcome; a deep distress caused by bereavement, a loss, or a perceived loss.

internal noise Factors inside the brain that interfere with the communication process.

language barrier Any type of interference that inhibits the communication process and is related to languages spoken by the people attempting to communicate.

litigious (luh-ti′-jus) Prone to engage in lawsuits.

malediction (ma-luh-dik′-shun) Speaking evil or the calling of a curse.

media Term applied to agencies of mass communication, such as newspapers, magazines, and telecommunications.

paraphrasing To express an idea in different wording in an effort to enhance communication and clarify meaning.

perception Capacity for comprehension; an awareness of the elements of the environment.

physiologic noise Physiologic interferences with the communication process.

pitch Highness or lowness of a sound; the relative level, intensity, or extent of some quality or state.

proxemics (prok-se′-miks) The study of the nature, degree, and effect of the spatial separation individuals naturally maintain.

sarcasm A sharp and often satirical response or ironic utterance designed to cut or give pain.

stereotype Something conforming to a fixed or general pattern; a standardized mental picture that is held in common by many and represents an oversimplified opinion, prejudiced attitude, or uncritical judgment.

stressors Stimuli that cause stress.

subtle Difficult to understand or perceive; having or marked by keen insight and ability to penetrate deeply and thoroughly.

thanatology (tha-nuh-tah′-luh-je) The study of the phenomena of death and of psychologic methods of coping with death.

vehemently (ve′-uh-ment-le) In a manner marked by forceful energy; intensely emotionally.

volatile (vah′-luh-til) Easily aroused; tending to erupt in violence.

The interpersonal skills developed by the medical assistant help to set the tone of a medical office. Interpersonal skills include the communications process and how we relate to one another during that process. Human relations can be defined as the study of the problems that arise from organizational and interpersonal contact. The two entities intersect each other, and the successful medical assistant will work to enhance these attributes on a continual basis. Patients who visit the healthcare facility may not be at their best, and the way in which the medical assistant reacts to and interacts with them can make an incredible difference in their **perception** of the office, the physician, and the medical staff. These interactions may also affect the patient's treatment and recovery.

FIRST IMPRESSIONS

Our elders have stressed all of our lives that first impressions are lasting ones, and this old **adage** is still true! The opinions formed in the early moments of meeting someone remain in our thoughts long after the first words are spoken. The first impression involves much more than just physical appearance or dress; it includes attitude and compassion, and the all-important smile (Figure 5-1).

One of the primary objectives of the professional medical assistant is to care for and about the people that are being served. Patients are the reason for the existence of the facility, and they should be offered the best customer service available. They must be warmly welcomed, and it is important to call patients by their names. People enjoy hearing their names, and it gives a patient confidence that the medical staff members know for whom they are caring.

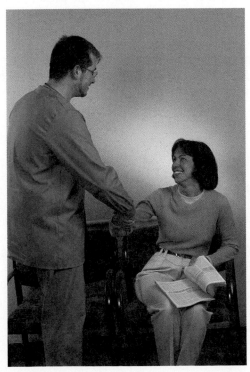

FIGURE 5-1 First impressions are critical in gaining the patient's trust.

Think for a moment about how it feels to be a new patient who is entering the unknown territory of the physician's office. Staff members of the facility are in familiar surroundings and already have some information about the new patient. However, the patient knows nothing about the staff members. One way to break that barrier is to have all staff members wear name badges, with letters large enough to be read at a distance of 3 feet. Include the staff position if several divisions of responsibility exist, for example, "medical assistant," "insurance biller," and "office manager." When the patient approaches, even when wearing a name badge, make introductions and smile. Smiles should show both facially and in the voice and eyes. Genuinely welcome the patient to the office. This small effort will help put the patient at ease in the office environment.

Some physicians make brief notes in the chart about the personal life of the patient. When the patient arrives for an appointment, the physician can ask about his or her recent trip abroad or new grandchild. This tells the patient that the doctor and the office staff see him or her as more than just an illness or a chart number. It gives the impression that they truly care, and that impression should be an accurate one. Once an impression is formed in the patient's mind, it is very difficult to change, so make the first impressions of your office positive ones.

COMMUNICATION PATHS

Verbal Communication

Messages are conveyed by the use of language, which may be written, spoken, or communicated in another way. Verbal communication depends on words and sounds. The **pitch** of the voice is a part of verbal communication. The voice lifts at the end of a question. It drops at the end of a statement. Usually when a speaker intends to continue a statement, the voice will hold the same pitch, the head will remain straight, and the eyes and hands will be unchanged. This is not an appropriate time to interrupt. If the message is interrupted, the train of thought may not be completed. Tone of voice and choice of words also affect messages.

The medical assistant should speak clearly and **enunciate** words properly. Speak loudly enough that the patients are able to hear clearly, and pay particular attention to those who wear some type of hearing assistance device. It is wise to note this information on the patient's chart to jog the memory when a patient with a hearing problem visits the office. Never assume that just because a patient is elderly, he or she has a hearing problem. When talking with patients, be sure to use the volume of speech to an advantage. Always speak at a clearly audible level, but at times it will be necessary to increase or decrease the volume of speech. When a patient is upset, for instance, it often helps to lower the volume of speech, because the patient tends to get quieter to hear the person speaking.

Eye contact is critical. Look at the person being spoken to, and do not forget a genuine smile. Many people feel that a person who speaks and cannot look another in the eyes is being deceptive. It can also mean that the speaker is very shy and has little self-confidence. Use gestures where appropriate to liven speech and **animate** the conversation.

Medical assistants must become aware of how they express themselves and how they affect the feelings of others. The tone of voice is vitally important. There is no place for **sarcasm** or **caustic** remarks. For example, saying "I hope you can manage to be on time for your next appointment" to a patient is needless and rude. The medical assistant must be conservative when speaking and not be too familiar. The patient expects professionalism and has the right to demand this in the healthcare setting. Never make an inappropriate remark and follow with "I was just kidding." This has no place in a medical facility or in any type of interpersonal communication. Take special care not to hurt anyone's feelings with words and phrases. Be very careful about what is said, especially to patients (Procedure 5-1).

Remember that patients are in the facility to be treated or cared for by the physician and staff. They are usually concerned about their illness and may have great apprehensions and fears about the future. It is completely out of place for the medical assistant to talk about his or her personal life and challenges with the patients. Allow the patient to speak, and listen instead of offering personal information. Often patients will casually mention things to the medical assistant that might influence their care. The saying that we are given "one mouth and two ears" stresses which should get more use!

Nonverbal Communication

Both verbal and nonverbal communications are important in the art of expression, and both are needed to succeed in the communication exchange. Nonverbal communications are messages conveyed without the use of words. They are transmitted by body language, gestures, and mannerisms that may or may not be in agreement with the words a person speaks. Body language is partly instinctive, partly taught, and partly imitative. It involves eye contact, facial expression, hand gestures, grooming, dress, space, tone of voice, posture, touch,

and much more. We are often unaware of our own nonverbal signals and consciously recognize only a small number of the signals sent by others. Our ability to help others increases as we hone our own skills in interpreting nonverbal communication. Nonverbal communication is almost always more accurate than verbal communication and tends to convey our true feelings and beliefs (Procedure 5-2).

Appearance is an integral part of nonverbal communication. It influences the way others view us and can present a conflicting message, or even a totally incorrect message. When we see someone who dresses or grooms in a way that is very different from our own style, we tend to assume that the personalities are also very different. This is not always true. Although we should not judge people by the way they dress, it is difficult not to form opinions based on what is seen. Visible piercings and tattoos are often looked on unfavorably in the medical profession, as are brightly painted long nails. Although these do not signify that the wearer is not professional, many patients, especially older patients, look on these trends unfavorably. For this reason alone, the medical assistant who is less conservative may be diminishing the chance for certain jobs and advancements. It is healthy to express oneself, yet in the medical profession, conservative appearance is preferred to avoid blocks in communications.

The successful medical assistant expresses self-esteem and confidence by stance, vocabulary, facial expression, and a caring attitude. The experience of speaking to someone who does not make eye contact helps one to realize the importance of greeting the patient with the eyes as well as the voice and body language. Facial expressions often convey our true feelings and are not masked by the words we use. Our eyes often tell the truth when our words are misleading or false. It is important to have an open body stance when dealing with patients. Crossed arms and legs hint that one is "closed" to the person being spoken to, and this may be construed as disinterest or disbelief.

PROCEDURE 5-1

Recognize and Respond to Verbal Communications

CAAHEP COMPETENCY: 3.c(1)(b)
ABHES COMPETENCY: 2.I

GOAL: *To be able to recognize verbal communication and respond to it in a professional manner.*

EQUIPMENT and SUPPLIES

- Cards with various patient scenarios

PROCEDURAL STEPS

1. Select a classmate as a partner for this procedure.
   PURPOSE: To practice communications with a partner whose responses will not be predictable.
2. Taking turns, draw a card and role-play the scenario described on it. Make certain that the partner understands the role on the card.
   PURPOSE: To send a clearly communicated message.

3. Allow your partner to respond to the sent message.
   PURPOSE: To make certain that your partner understood your message and allow him or her to communicate a response.
4. Restate your partner's response.
   PURPOSE: To assure understanding of the partner's message.
5. Clarify any issues that are unclear.
   PURPOSE: To make certain that the meaning of each message sent is understood.
6. Refrain from using slang or other unprofessional wording.
   PURPOSE: To maintain professional communication.
7. Continue to communicate back and forth, and be sure that each partner communicates accurately.

PROCEDURE 5-2

Recognize and Respond to Nonverbal Communications

CAAHEP COMPETENCY: 3.c(1)(c)
ABHES COMPETENCY: 2.I

GOAL: *To be able to recognize nonverbal communication and respond to it in a professional way.*

EQUIPMENT and SUPPLIES

- Cards with various statements that can be communicated in a nonverbal way

PROCEDURAL STEPS

1. Select a classmate as a partner for this procedure.
   PURPOSE: To practice nonverbal communications with a partner whose responses will not be predictable.

2. Taking turns, draw a card and communicate the thought on the card to your partner.
3. Determine if the receiver understood the message correctly.
   PURPOSE: To send a nonverbal message that is understood by the receiver.
4. Continue to communicate back and forth and be sure that each message sent is conveyed to the receiver accurately.

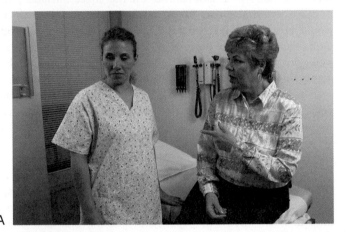 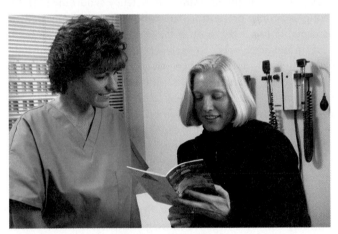

A   B

FIGURE 5-2 A, Pointing is often an accusatory gesture and causes discomfort. **B,** A bright smile helps to put the patient at ease and relax.

Nonverbal and verbal communications are dependent on each other (Figure 5-2). They must be in harmony to convey an accurate message that can be easily interpreted by the receiver. If the two are not **congruent,** the nonverbal is usually dominant and expresses the true message.

The need for personal space is demonstrated by how patients in the reception area will choose a seat. **Proxemics** is defined as the study of the nature, degree, and effect of the spatial separation individuals naturally maintain and how this separation relates to cultural and environmental factors. Seldom will a person sit in a seating space adjoining that of a stranger if there is another option. Although the need for space varies with the individual culture, some might even remain standing to satisfy the need for personal space. Public space is usually accepted as a distance of 12 to 25 feet, and social space is usually considered to be 4 to 12 feet. Personal space ranges from 1½ to 4 feet, and intimate contact includes physical touching to approximately 1½ feet. The medical assistant can often tell when he or she has invaded someone's personal space, because the person will tend to back up a step or two. If this happens, take a small step back and respect the boundaries that are being set. The more familiar and comfortable patients are with the medical assistant, the closer the space they will allow.

Touch is a powerful communicator. The soft acceptance of someone's hand in yours, to the good-natured pat on the back, to the harsh slap on the face all relay different messages that need no words to accurately express. In the medical profession, as in any business, touch can be comforting or can promote a sexual harassment suit. Individuals who have experienced sexual abuse or other traumatic experiences may not want to be touched at all. Unfortunately, one must be extremely careful when using this effective communication tool. In today's **litigious** society, any nonconsensual touching may be considered **battery,** and touch should be used with great discretion and cautious care.

The medical assistant should not be afraid to touch the patient appropriately, for example, using a pat on the back or a squeeze of the hand (Figure 5-3). Some patients are receptive to a brief sideways hug, whereas others would take this as an intrusion into their personal space. Certainly patients with

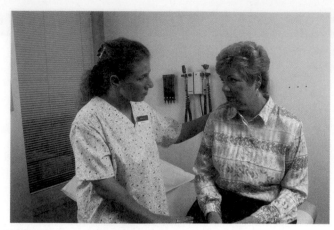

FIGURE 5-3 Touching the patient communicates care and compassion.

serious illnesses appreciate touch as an expression of empathy. Never be afraid to touch sick patients, especially those with diseases such as acquired immunodeficiency syndrome (AIDS), as long as proper precautions are followed where indicated. It is acceptable to ask a person if he or she minds being hugged. These individuals need to feel acceptance, and the attitude of the medical staff members they encounter will directly influence their adherence to keeping their appointments with the physician. If they do not feel accepted and cared for, they will not return to the physician's office. A gentle touch and a smile do wonders for showing care and concern.

Posture can signal depression, excitement, anger, or even an appeal for help. When the physician sits at the front of the chair and leans forward, he or she is giving the message of caring and interest. Positioning is important as well. Sitting behind a desk promotes an air of authority. Standing or sitting across a room may convey a negative message of denying involvement or reluctance to talk. Sitting side by side with a patient will help to initiate trust and promote open conversation. The medical assistant should practice good postural techniques as a part of projecting a positive image and for personal health reasons.

CRITICAL THINKING APPLICATION

- How might touch be an important communication tool with Mrs. Cloyd?
- How can Sarah be affected by using touch?
- Could laughter affect either of these women as they deal with death?

THE PROCESS OF COMMUNICATION

Anyone who works within the realm of public service should develop good communication skills. It is important to be able to interact with others and put them at ease, so that their comfort level increases and they develop trust. To communicate well, we must first have a general understanding of the process of communication. Once a message is sent, it cannot be retrieved and restated or expressed in a different way. Especially

in the medical profession, communication must be clear and concise, and the message we intend to send must match what the receiver understands.

Although many different scientific models of communication exist, the one that best fits most types of communication is the transactional communication model. Before understanding how this model works, one must understand the elements we use to communicate.

Usually when two people interact, both people act as senders and as receivers. The sender is the person who sends a message through a variety of different **channels.** Channels can be spoken words, written messages, and body language. The sender **encodes** the message, which simply means that he or she chooses a specific way of expression using words and other channels. The receiver **decodes** the message according to his or her understanding of what is being communicated. However, sometimes the receiver incorrectly understands the message. This often is a result of noise, which is anything that interferes with the message being sent. It can be literal noise, such as a radio or a jackhammer on the street outside. This is called **external noise.** Or it can be **internal noise,** which would include the receiver's own thoughts or prejudices and opinions. **Physiologic noise** interferes with communication as well. This includes any biologic factor that would preclude the communicator from sending or receiving accurate messages, such as not feeling well or being overly tired. **Feedback** can be given through verbal expressions or body language, such as a simple nod of understanding. The perception of the receiver is very important and is discussed later in this chapter.

The transactional communication model (Figure 5-4) depicts "communicators" instead of one sender and one receiver. If two people are communicating, both are sending and receiving messages and both are encoding and decoding what is being offered. Even when two people are speaking one at a time, messages are continually sent with words, body language, facial expressions, and gestures. Various channels of communication are used, and both communicators offer feedback, even if it is done subconsciously. Noise may or may not be present, but even the best communicators experience some type of noise, even if that is only thinking of what to say next.

Listening

Listening is just as important to good communication as the spoken word. Hearing is the process, function, or power of perceiving sound, whereas *listening* is defined as paying attention to sound or hearing something with thoughtful attention. People need to know that the medical assistant is listening. This is actually true in all interpersonal relationships, including husband-wife, parent-child, supervisor-employee, and doctor-patient interactions. When listening to someone who is attempting to communicate, the first rule is to look at the speaker and pay attention. Sometimes it is important not to respond immediately, but to remain silent and offer an understanding and reassuring nod.

Sometimes it is hard to listen. We may not be able to listen effectively because we are distracted by our own thoughts. Perhaps the situations occurring in our own lives make the

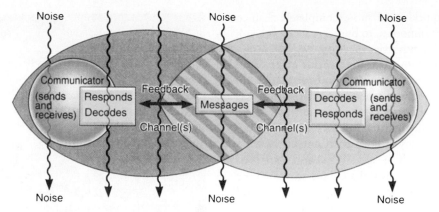

FIGURE 5-4 The transactional communication model. (From Adler RB, Towne N: *Looking out, looking in: interpersonal communication*, San Antonio, 1996, Harcourt Brace.)

conversation we are hearing seem meaningless and unimportant. Or so many messages may be attacking at once that we are unable to focus on any specific one to hear what is being communicated. At other times, such as in anger, we are so rapidly preparing our response that we cannot hear what is being said. We may simply be too tired to listen, or we may have prejudged the speaker and decided that there is no need to listen. However, while working with patients the medical assistant must be diligent in not only hearing the words being spoken, but also listening to them and to what the patient is attempting to communicate.

Active listening is the skill whereby **paraphrasing** and clarifying what the speaker has said take place. Paraphrasing is listening to what the sender is communicating, analyzing the words, and restating them to confirm that the receiver has understood the message as the sender intended it. This process clarifies the speaker's thoughts and helps to indicate that there is a common understanding of the message between both people. When communicating in this way, the receiver should reword what the sender has said and then ask a clarifying question. Consider the following example:

Patient: I have not been feeling well lately.

MA: You say you have not been feeling well. What exactly is the trouble?

This type of communicating may seem awkward at first, because most of us believe that listening involves lack of speech. Active listening means that the speaker's words are heard, and a restatement is used to verify that the message was understood correctly. This statement gives the speaker the opportunity to correct any misconceptions or misunderstandings. Consider the following example:

Patient: My back hurts.

MA: Where does it hurt?

Patient: In the middle.

MA: Can you point to exactly where it hurts?

Patient: Yes, right here. (points)

MA: Is it a sharp or dull pain?

Patient: Very sharp.

MA: How often does it occur?

Patient: Several times a day.

MA: Can you tell me on an average day how many times it bothers you?

Patient: About six times.

MA: How long does it last?

Patient: About 10 or 15 minutes.

MA: How long has this been a concern?

Patient: For about 2 weeks.

MA: So you have had a sharp pain in this part of your back, about six times a day lasting for up to 15 minutes for 2 weeks? Is that correct?

Patient: Yes.

It would have been easier if the patient had said, "I have had a sharp pain in my back that lasts up to 15 minutes, and it happens about six times a day." This example shows how the medical assistant can continue clarifying until the answer is specific enough, which is critical when obtaining information from the patient.

It is also best to ask "open" questions, as opposed to "closed" questions. An open question requires more than a "yes" or "no" answer. It forces the patient to provide more detail and expand on his or her thoughts. A closed question can be answered with "yes" or "no" and compels the medical assistant to spend more time obtaining the answers needed to accurately document the patient's needs.

CRITICAL THINKING APPLICATION

- How can the medical assistant be sure that Mrs. Cloyd understands how she is to take her medication?
- Often older patients do not appreciate instructions being given to their caregiver instead of directly to them. How can the medical assistant place the primary focus on communicating with Mrs. Cloyd, yet make sure that Sarah understands the instructions and care at the same time?

Often when a person or patient is talking with the medical assistant, he or she is looking for a specific type of response. Some patients want advice, some want sympathy, and others are looking for reassurance. Many patients will open up to the medical assistant more quickly and more completely than to the physician. Because it is important to build good rapport with patients, this can be a very positive aspect of the relationship the medical assistant has with the patient. However, the medical assistant should never agree to withhold information from the physician under any circumstances. If the patient asks that the assistant not reveal something to the physician, the medical assistant should politely explain that he or she has an ethical obligation to report any and all pertinent information to the physician, especially if it affects medical care. For example, if the patient asks the medical assistant not to tell the physician that the patient has been smoking against medical advice, the assistant could be jeopardizing the patient's care if the information is not reported.

This does not mean that specific details must always be aired. If, for example, the patient reveals that stress levels have been high because she has filed a sexual harassment suit against her boss, the medical assistant could report to the physician that the patient is having some legal problems that have resulted in additional stress at work. Never agree to lie to the physician! The patient must understand that if the physician questions any information given by the patient, it must be revealed so that the physician is assured that the care being provided is the right care. It is also critical to note that the physician may have worked with the patient for a long period and may have a better understanding of the patient's needs than the medical assistant. One patient may be able to handle a high degree of stress, and another may crumble at the first sign of stress. A good physician knows his or her patients and keeps accurate, complete records that will help with decision making in these situations.

If ever in doubt about telling the physician something a patient has said, the best solution is to tell. Remember, medical professionals are legally bound to confidentiality, and the patient may need to be reminded of this. Encourage him or her to talk to the physician and communicate all of his or her concerns, no matter how insignificant they may seem. Never display a judgmental attitude or express negativity about the patient's activities, thoughts, or behavior. Offer to be with the patient, if he or she desires, as the patient discusses difficult issues with the physician, or to make arrangements for a special counseling session with the physician if this is indicated. Some patients are hesitant to initiate conversation with the physician because they feel they are taking too much of his or her time. The medical assistant can help to ensure that critical issues receive the doctor's attention.

WARNINGS AGAINST ADVISING A PATIENT

The medical assistant must be extremely careful when making suggestions or comments to a patient, in order to avoid legal accusations of practicing medicine without a license. Often a patient will ask for an opinion as to which course of action to take. Medical assistants are not qualified to give any type of advice to a patient. Strict laws in most states prohibit anyone other than a licensed physician from offering medical advice. Even if the patient asks what the medical assistant would do if presented with the same options, the assistant cannot encourage

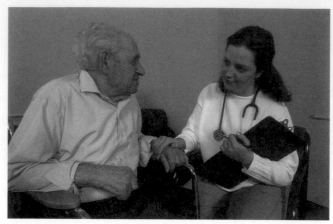

FIGURE 5-5 Careful listening and asking questions will help the patient express thoughts and feelings.

the patient to choose one option over another. The assistant can offer a listening ear, though, and help the patient process his or her own thoughts. This can be done in much the same way as using active listening techniques (Figure 5-5). When a patient expresses a concern, the medical assistant should restate the concern, then ask a clarifying question. For example:

> Patient: I don't know if I should take the chemotherapy treatments the doctor suggested.
>
> MA: You seem worried about the treatments. What are you concerned about specifically?

Patients must come to their own decisions about treatments and options that they have when faced with a medical decision. The medical assistant is often looked on not only as an authority figure, but also as an extension of the physician. Patients may mistakenly think that the medical assistant has the same opinion as the physician. It is important that all communication with the patient be professional and accurate. Always attempt to get the patient to openly discuss all of his or her concerns and fears with the physician.

The medical assistant should never agree to withhold any information from the physician, because even a small piece of information could completely change the plan of treatment. When giving instructions to patients, it is always best to have them in writing and keep a copy for the patient's chart so that a written record of what was communicated to the patient is available. Use excellent documentation technique when adding information to the patient's chart. Remember that all of the patients in the facility deserve to be treated with respect and compassion. Help the physician to establish trust with the patient. An open, trusting relationship with the patient will help to avoid legal issues in the future.

CRITICAL THINKING APPLICATION

- How should the medical assistant handle Sarah's questions about the various aspects of her mother's treatments?
- How does her mother's decision not to have chemotherapy treatments affect Sarah? What barriers to communication between them might be present?

OBSERVING CAREFULLY

In the fast-paced world of medicine, sometimes nonverbal signals sent by patients that play a critical role in their care are missed. If the patient hesitates when speaking, it may be an indication that he or she has more to say. As mentioned previously, the inability to look a person directly in the eyes sometimes, but not always, indicates deception. The medical assistant must pay close attention to what is seen as well as what is heard when communicating with the patient. Look into the patient's eyes, and watch intently for signs of trouble.

When a patient cries, the medical assistant should always question what is causing the tears. Some patients may refuse to discuss the issue or insist that nothing is wrong, but tears are always a sign of some emotion, whether it is anger, frustration, fear, pain, or some other concern. It is unwise to allow patients who are obviously emotionally upset to leave the office without reasonable assurance that they are going to be safe. The medical assistant might wish to suggest that a friend come to the office and escort the patient home. On rare occasions, it is better to be firm with the patient and insist on help getting home if he or she is in a **volatile** state. This action may save the patient from being hurt or hurting someone else. Careful observation of the patient as a whole is worth the time investment and may even save the patient's life.

DEFENSE MECHANISMS

Anxiety or stress causes the human body to react in many different ways. Some people handle **stressors** more easily than others. Most people use **defense mechanisms** when they feel pressured or attacked in some way. These are often subconscious reactions designed for emotional protection; they help us to deal with whatever difficult event has triggered such a response. Often people may not even realize that they are using these mechanisms and may **vehemently** deny that they do so. Many types of defense mechanisms exist, and the medical assistant should be familiar with them to better communicate with patients and others they come into contact with in the course of their duties.

Verbal Aggression

When a person verbally attacks another without addressing the original complaint, or disregards it, he or she is being verbally **aggressive** (Figure 5-6). Such people may attack, or they may change the subject. Some individuals get very angry at any suggestion of wrongdoing. They lash out, usually quite loudly, and attack back quickly in hopes of diminishing their role in any wrongdoing.

"When are you going to clean the drug sample closet?"
"Who are you to ask me that? You haven't finished your duties today, either!"

Sarcasm

This word has its origin in the Greek *sarkasmos,* which means "to tear flesh" or "to bite the lips in rage." This is quite an accurate definition of the nature of sarcasm. It is a biting edge added to

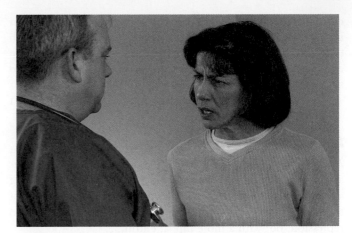

FIGURE 5-6 Remain calm even if a patient becomes verbally aggressive, and attempt to calm him or her by listening and expressing empathy whenever possible.

words that a person states with the intent to cause pain or anger. Sarcasm is hostile and cruel in most cases, and some individuals use it constantly, thinking that it is quite witty. On the contrary, it often makes bitter enemies of its victims.

"Of course it's a nice dress, if you like tents."

Rationalization

Rationalizing is attributing actions to rational and credible motives without analyzing underlying methods. When people rationalize their behavior, they are offering excuses for what has been done or said and trying to convince others that the behavior was completely justified.

"He only hits me because he is stressed at work."

Compensation

A person who compensates makes up for one behavior by stressing another. Compensation is a psychologic mechanism through which feelings of inferiority, frustration, or failure in one area are counterbalanced by achievement in another. Compensation is not always a negative response, but it is often used as an excuse for not accomplishing what should be accomplished.

"I know I gained 5 pounds, Dr. George, but I exercised three times last week."

Regression

Regression is the reversion to an earlier mental or behavioral level. Some people regress to a childlike state or period or exhibit qualities inherent to an earlier time in life. This can include making excuses for not doing a certain thing, saying that it cannot be done, instead of the truth, which is that the person does not want to do it. Replacing the word "can't" with "won't" is a good gauge of using regression.

"I'd like to get better grades, but I can't find time to study."

Repression

The process whereby unwanted desires or impulses are excluded from the consciousness and left to operate in the unconscious is called *repression.* Blocking a problem out of the mind, or changing the subject when it is mentioned, are both types of repression. The repressed urges or desires may seethe beneath the surface, absorbing energy, and force the continual repression of the desires, which takes more and more concentration to do successfully.

"I should phone my brother since we fought, but I just can't deal with that now."

Apathy

Apathy is a lack of feeling, emotion, interest, or concern. It is an indifference to what is happening or a pretense of not caring about a situation. Usually, apathy is not a true reflection of the inner feeling. It is a defense mechanism that is similar to repression, but with a more flippant attitude.

"I don't care what grade I got on the test, because I am not going to pass the class anyway."

Displacement

Displacement is the redirection of an emotion or impulse from its original object, such as an idea or person, to another object. When challenged or attacked by one person or event, displacement is used to channel negative feelings to some other area, which gives a false sense of control over issues that may not be controllable. The venting of hostile feelings is directed somewhere other than where it should be directed, but usually this is a result of a lack of confidence in addressing the true issues at hand.

"I have enough problems at work and don't need to come home to a nagging wife!"

Denial

Denial is a psychologic defense mechanism in which confrontation with a personal problem or with reality is avoided by denying the existence of the problem or reality. This is where the common expression, "He's in denial" originates. For whatever reason, the individual is unable to cope with the stress of a situation and completely pushes it or any person or thing representing it away.

"My husband can't have cancer. He is completely healthy."

Physical Avoidance

Some events are so painful for people that they completely avoid any representation of the event. This could be a person, a place, an object, or just about anything that serves as a reminder of the event that induces the negative feelings. If the problem is a person, that person may be avoided forever. If it is a place, such as a home that a couple lived in before one of them died, the other person may physically move. In some cases, such as physical abuse, the avoidance may be necessary, but it can also be quite unhealthy and may need to be explored further through therapy.

"I will never go to that restaurant again, because that is where my ex-husband told me he wanted a divorce."

Projection

Projection as a defense mechanism is the attribution of one's own ideas, feelings, or attitudes to other people or to objects.

This especially includes the **externalization** of blame, guilt, or responsibility as a defense against anxiety. Some people project their feelings about a certain thing onto others, who may not be affected by the negative connotations the first person feels. Projection is a way to avoid dealing with the root issues of a problem.

"Everyone else is always late, so why am I getting reprimanded for it?"

DEALING WITH CONFLICT

Conflict is defined as the struggle resulting from incompatible or opposing needs, drives, wishes, or external or internal demands. We deal with conflict in our lives in some capacity almost daily. Knowing how to recognize the signs of conflict and what patterns people use to deal with conflict will be of great benefit to the medical assistant. This will enable the professional to be understanding and empathetic to patients, co-workers, supervisors, and others in the day-to-day work environment.

Conflict is not always negative; sometimes it is beneficial to relationships. It can be constructive and allow people to learn more about each other. This may promote a stronger understanding and deeper levels of intimacy. Unless both parties are aware that a problem exists between them, no conflict exists. The conflict begins when both realize there is a problem that needs resolution. People handle conflict in different ways. Some avoid it at all costs, and on the other end of the spectrum, some seem to thrive on conflict.

In order to understand the thought processes of others and how best to respond to them, as well as discerning how others respond, it is helpful to define some of the many types of conflict. Of itself, assertion is not conflict; assertion is stating or declaring positively, often forcefully or aggressively. Being assertive or aggressive can be very productive. Assertive people often receive job promotions and reach the goals they set for their lives. Too much aggression can make a person seem pushy, so it should be controlled and used at the appropriate times. Remember, there is a difference between assertion and aggression, which will be discussed in the following paragraphs.

Nonassertion is the inability to express needs and thoughts or the refusal to express them. Some avoid conflict and some accommodate by putting others' desires before their own. Sometimes nonassertion is justifiable. Anyone who has been involved in a long-term relationship realizes that there will be occasions when the other person's needs must come first. Many have learned the truth of the old saying, "Choose your battles wisely."

CRITICAL THINKING APPLICATION

- Why might Mrs. Cloyd and Sarah experience conflict at this stage in their lives?
- How might each deal better with disagreements, especially regarding Mrs. Cloyd's decisions about her medical care?

Aggression is defined in several ways. It can be a hostile, injurious, or destructive behavior or outlook, especially when caused by frustration. It is also the practice of making attacks or **encroachments,** especially if the acts are unprovoked. In the realm of psychologic studies, there are different types of aggression. Direct aggression occurs when a person directly attacks another, whether by criticism, **malediction,** ridiculing, or other methods. This behavior causes the victim to feel embarrassment, shame, anger, or a range of other emotions. *Passive aggression* is a familiar term, but many may not know its definition. A passive-aggressive person expresses himself or herself in an obscure, **ambiguous** way. People who experience passive aggression may have feelings of rage, inadequacy, or resentment that they cannot articulate in a direct manner. Unfortunately, this behavior usually will not provide the results that are needed or expected.

The Crazymakers: Passive-Aggressive Communications

In the book *Looking Out, Looking In: Interpersonal Communication* by Ronald B. Adler and Neil Towne, the concept of "Crazymakers" is discussed and credited to George Bach. Bach was a psychologist who developed the theory of creative aggression; he nicknamed this passive-aggressive behavior *crazymaking*. He said that two types of aggression exist: clean fighting and dirty fighting. Crazymaking was his name for dirty fighting, which is a detrimental behavior for all involved. The term *partner* is loosely used to indicate the opposite side or victim of the crazymaker.

Following are brief descriptions of the characteristic types of passive-aggressive persons described by Bach.

The Avoider

Avoiders refuse to fight. When a conflict arises, they leave, fall asleep, pretend to be busy at work, or keep from facing the problem in some other way. This behavior makes it difficult for the partner to express feelings of anger and hurt, because the avoider will not fight back.

The Pseudoaccommodator

Pseudoaccommodators refuse to face up to a conflict either by giving in or pretending nothing is wrong. This drives the partner crazy, because the partner definitely feels there is a problem, and causes feelings of guilt and resentment toward the accommodator for bringing the situation up for discussion in the first place.

The Guiltmaker

Instead of saying straight out that they don't want or don't approve of something, guiltmakers try to make their partners feel responsible for causing pain. A guiltmaker's favorite line is, "It's OK, don't worry about me...," followed by a long sigh.

The Subject Changer

Really an avoider, the subject changer escapes facing up to aggression by shifting the conversation whenever it approaches an area of conflict. Because of their tactics, subject changers and their partners never have the chance to explore their problems and do something about them.

The Distracter

Rather than come out and express their feelings about an object of dissatisfaction, distracters attack other parts of their partners' lives. Thus they never have to share what is really on their minds and can avoid dealing with painful parts of their relationships.

The Mind Reader

Instead of allowing their partners to express feelings honestly, mind readers go into character analysis, explaining what the other person really means or what is wrong with the other person. By behaving this way, mind readers refuse to handle their own feelings and leave no room for their partners to express themselves.

The Trapper

Trappers play an especially dirty trick by setting up a desired behavior for their partners; then, when the behavior is manifested, they attack the very thing they requested. An example of this technique is for the trapper to say, "Let's be totally honest with each other," then attack the partner's words of honesty.

The Crisis Tickler

Crisis ticklers bring what is bothering them almost to the surface but never quite express their true feelings. Instead of admitting concern about the finances, they innocently ask, "Gee, how much did that cost?" dropping a rather obvious hint but never really dealing with the crisis.

The Gunnysacker

Gunnysackers do not respond immediately when angry. Instead, they put their resentment into a gunnysack, which after a while begins to bulge with both large and small gripes. Then, when the sack is about to burst, the gunnysacker pours out all the pent-up aggressions on the overwhelmed and unsuspecting partner.

The Trivial Tyrannizer

Instead of honestly sharing their resentments, trivial tyrannizers do things they know will bother their partners—leaving dirty dishes in the sink, clipping fingernails in bed, belching out loud, turning up the television too loud, and so on.

The Beltliner

Everyone has a psychologic "beltline," and below it are subjects too sensitive to be approached without damaging the relationship. Beltlines may have to do with physical characteristics, intelligence, past behavior, or deeply ingrained personality traits a person is trying to overcome. In an attempt to "get even" or hurt their partners, beltliners will use intimate knowledge to hit below the belt, where they know it will hurt.

The Joker

Because they are afraid to face conflicts squarely, jokers kid around when their partners want to be serious, thus blocking the expression of important feelings.

The Blamer

Blamers are more interested in finding fault than in resolving a conflict. Needless to say, they usually do not blame themselves. Blaming behavior almost never resolves a conflict and is an almost sure-fire way to make receivers defensive.

The Contract Tyrannizer

Contract tyrannizers will not allow their relationships to change from the way they once were. Whatever the agreements the partners had for roles and responsibilities at one time, they will remain unchanged.

The Kitchen Sink Fighter

Kitchen sink fighters are so named because in an argument they bring up things that are totally off the subject—as in everything, including the kitchen sink. Perhaps it is the way the other person behaved last New Year's Eve, or bad breath, or the unbalanced checkbook; any past imperfection is fair game for picking a fight.

The Withholder

Instead of expressing their anger honestly and directly, withholders punish their partners by holding something back—courtesy, affection, good cooking, humor, sex. Such withholding is likely to build up even greater resentments in the relationship.

The Benedict Arnold

Benedict Arnolds get back at their partners by sabotage, by failing to defend them from attackers, and even by encouraging ridicule or disregard from outside the relationship.

BARRIERS TO COMMUNICATION

Physical Impairment

Patients may have physical troubles that impair their ability to communicate effectively. This could be a vision or hearing problem, or one of many other conditions that makes communicating a bit more difficult than usual. The medical assistant should use more descriptive language when speaking with the patient who has a visual disturbance. This helps the patient to "see" what is being discussed. The person with diminished hearing may be very sensitive and in denial of the condition. Be certain that you have his or her attention and that you are face to face with the person while speaking. People who are hearing impaired are often very dependent on lip reading for comprehension. Being elderly is not an impairment at all. Many older patients are physically fit and mentally sharp and do not expect special treatment. Never increase the volume of your speech in an assumption that an older patient is hard of hearing. Some physicians make a note in the patient's medical record that indicates the patient has a hearing problem or other impairment, similar to notations about patient allergies. With such notations in an easily noticeable place, everybody that handles the record will know about the impairment and take proper measures to adapt.

CRITICAL THINKING APPLICATION

- What must be considered when communicating verbally with Mrs. Cloyd? With Sarah?
- How can the medical assistant show compassion to a terminally ill patient during her appointment when the office is extremely busy?

Language

With non–English-speaking patients the medical assistant may need to use gestures and more body language to convey messages. In such cases, be alert to the possibility of misunderstandings. Confirm that the message being sent is the message that the listener received by asking for feedback. Ask the listener to repeat the message, and if family members are present, be sure they have a good understanding of what is being communicated as well.

It is always helpful to have a bilingual staff member so that there is less chance of miscommunication with those who speak a different language (Figure 5-7). Many regions offer bilingual classes for medical professionals to assist them with basic communications with their patients. The medical assistant will find it well worth the time and financial investment to investigate such classes, because bilingual employees are quite valuable to the physician and may be able to command a higher salary.

Prejudice

Personal and social bias, or prejudice, brings about discrimination. *Discrimination* is a word that is used to describe unfair

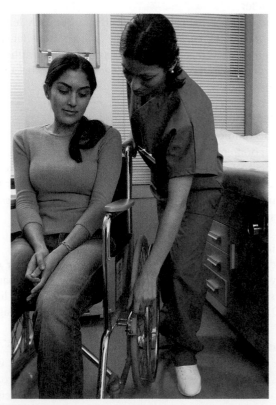

FIGURE 5-7 Bilingual staff members are valuable in ensuring accurate communications with patients who speak a different language.

treatment of a person because of race, gender, religious affiliation, or handicap, or for any other reason. Discrimination is unethical, morally and socially wrong, and in many situations illegal. It also prevents us from communicating effectively.

Some discrimination is very **subtle;** it is not expressed openly or in a blatant manner. Subtle discrimination is based on a person's appearance, values, lifestyle, or some other personal factor. Examples include discrimination against those who are obese, divorced individuals, homosexuals, welfare recipients, or those with sexually transmitted diseases. Sometimes we are not aware that our words or actions reflect subtle discrimination against others.

Personal prejudices must be recognized before one can change them. Medical professionals are exposed to a wide variety of persons who need excellent medical care. The professional cannot allow personal prejudice to affect the care of any individual. Everyone has the right to be honored as a human being and treated respectfully. This enforces the Golden Rule: treating others as you would wish to be treated. Realize the worth of each individual person, and allow that attitude to reflect in all of the actions taken with a patient.

Stereotyping

Stereotyping is defined as the application of a standardized mental picture that is held in common by members of a group and that represents an oversimplified opinion, prejudiced attitude, or uncritical judgment. It is unfair to **stereotype** anyone or categorize him or her based on preconceived, often incorrect, assumptions. Although sometimes there is a degree of truth to the assumption based on stereotypic categories, people should not be judged before there has been an opportunity to get to know them as individuals. The medical assistant should push preconceived notions aside and look at the individual when forming and building a relationship. In the medical profession, stereotypic categories should not be considered when caring for patients and developing good rapport with them.

Perception

Perhaps one of the most important issues to consider when discussing barriers to communication is the concept of perception. Perception means the capacity for comprehension, or the discernment of what is being communicated, according to the message receiver's point of reference. When we discussed the transactional communication model earlier in the chapter, it was obvious that because of different types of noise and channels, there would be times that the message sent would be distorted; the receiver would not always get the message that the sender meant to send. The receiver's perceptions could completely alter the message, no matter how clearly it was sent. If the receiver believes that all attorneys are corrupt, he or she will probably be unable to get past this perception when speaking with one and therefore may not be able to trust any attorney.

Often our perceptions stem from some experience that happened in the past with a certain group of people. This perception goes unresolved or has affected us so strongly that we group all people from that walk of life into a negative category. This is an unfair way to deal with people; everyone

should be viewed as an individual, not as a part of a stereotypic group. Remember, perception is an individual's point of view, right or wrong. The issue of interpretation also plays a role—the determination of what is meant by a certain message. There must be an attempt to understand both points of view and a willingness to discuss them calmly, even when discussing subjects that cause anger. Most people do not truly enjoy conflict. Have a healthy respect for others' opinions. The differences among individuals are part of what makes each of us unique.

COMMUNICATION DURING DIFFICULT TIMES

Communication is not an art that comes easily to everyone. It is often difficult to express feelings in an honest and open way. When a crisis occurs, it is much harder to communicate effectively and we sometimes say things that we do not mean. The medical assistant must develop communication skills that can be used in times of trouble. There must be an understanding of why a patient or co-worker is unable to communicate.

Patience is important, too, because people are not always at their best when they are concerned about their condition or that of a loved one. Always remain calm when dealing with a person who is experiencing a traumatic event or has any depressive condition. Remember that he or she may be reacting to many emotions—fear, anger, doubt, inadequacy, or many others. The key is to listen and determine the best way to help the patient out of any immediate danger and help him or her establish some type of support system.

Anger

One of the most difficult times to communicate is when we are angry. Anger is a normal emotion that all of us feel at one time or another. Usually the expression of anger is a healthy thing. Some people bottle up their emotions and do not express what they truly feel inside. If this is done repeatedly, at some point the anger will erupt, possibly over a tiny event or at an inappropriate time. Others explode over every little situation, and people who do this need anger management skills and training.

Anger, like most emotions, can cause physiologic changes. When a person feels anger, the blood pressure rises and the heart rate increases. Many things can trigger anger, from a simple traffic backup to a real or perceived betrayal, the diagnosis of a disease, or the death of a close relative. "Road rage" is one example of anger out of control and is a serious problem on our public highways today. Unexpressed anger can cause or contribute to all types of health problems, including depression and hypertension.

The medical assistant can help to calm an angry patient by speaking calmly and refusing to return the emotion. If the volume is gradually lowered with every sentence spoken, the angry person will have to lower the volume as well to hear what the assistant is saying. Suggest that the person breathe deeply and stop talking for a few minutes. Remember that the anger that is being expressed is usually not directed intentionally toward the medical assistant. Be a good listener and allow the person to speak as long as it is not abusive speech. Using logic with the angry individual may also help. Some will use words such as "never" and "always"; for example, "My wife never balances the checkbook!" or "You always make me wait for my appointment!" These statements are broad generalizations and usually untrue. Using a logical approach and maintaining a calm attitude will help the angry individual.

Address the root of the problem, and be willing to admit if the physician's office has made a mistake or contributed to a problem. Do not be afraid to say, "I'm sorry, we made an error." Arguing will never solve the situation and will only increase the intensity of the patient's feelings. Four words that will often disarm an angry person are "Let me help you." There will be times in the career of a medical professional that a patient, a co-worker, or even the physician will lash out, even though the medical assistant is not the cause of the anger. Realize that this is a part of being human, and be as caring and kind as possible. If the anger becomes abusive, either refer the situation to a supervisor or, if that is not possible, tell the patient that you can no longer discuss the situation and offer to schedule an appointment so that the matter can be discussed at a later time. By then, the patient will probably have calmed down and will be able to discuss the situation rationally.

Shock

When an event or a circumstance arises that is especially painful, an individual may experience emotional shock. This may happen when a person has just been told that a family member has been killed in an automobile accident or some other catastrophe has taken place. Many different types of shock occur, but in this chapter, the emotional aspect is discussed. Often the person cannot think or move, and other coping reactions may take place. One person may scream in agony, whereas another may calmly sit down and begin to talk about a completely unrelated subject. The person who appears calm is probably more at risk, because in addition to shock, he or she may be experiencing a denial process. We never really know in advance how we will react to events that are traumatic. Also, our reactions may differ from time to time. What else is happening in a person's life will determine how he or she will be able to cope with a traumatic event.

Never leave a person in emotional shock alone. If the healthcare professional cannot stay close by, arrangements should be made for someone to stay near, especially during the early stages, if at all possible. Because the thought processes the person is experiencing may not be under control, he or she could be a danger to himself or herself or others. People who are in shock have a strong need to get away from the situation they have found themselves in. They may try to literally run away, or they may speed off in a car, which compounds the situation. The event does not have to be a life-threatening one, but the patient may perceive it as such. For instance, a teenager who becomes pregnant may not be able to focus on anything except her perception that her life is ruined. As with anger, listening is a good disarming tool for dealing with a person in emotional shock.

The medical assistant should watch for several signs of emotional shock, including hyperactivity, disruptions in

breathing patterns, a blank staring, sudden hysterics, and shaking. Humans have an innate sense of threat or danger, and this sense may initiate what psychologists call the "fight or flight" syndrome. When a person feels a threat of some kind, the hormone adrenaline is released in the body quickly, and this hormone promotes an increased heart rate and blood pressure. The oxygen level in the body increases, which prepares the muscles to help the body flee. Awareness is increased, as are energy and performance. The individual either runs, avoiding the danger, which is the "flight" aspect, or stays to "fight," facing the stressors or threat. With either choice, the body must have this increased energy level and awareness to deal with the situation. When the immediate period of shock abates, the individual may feel a debilitating, drained sensation as the hormonal levels return to normal.

CRITICAL THINKING APPLICATION

- Is it possible that Sarah might experience shock months after her mother's death?
- How can the medical assistant help Sarah to deal with these emotions?

Death and Dying

Years ago patients who were considered terminally ill were placed in hospital wards and left to their demise. The medical community did not focus on understanding the fears and concerns of the dying, and very few measures that preserved their dignity were offered to them. However, in 1969 a ground-breaking book, *On Death and Dying*, was published by Dr. Elisabeth Kübler-Ross, who studied **thanatology.** Kübler-Ross (Figure 5-8), a Swiss psychiatrist, realized that terminally ill patients were somewhat ignored, even by medical professionals, and she spent many hours interviewing these patients, discovering their fears and concerns. Kübler-Ross listened to them and realized that there were certain stages that patients passed through as they dealt with their impending death. She held seminars during which she interviewed dying patients as medical students listened. When the book was published, she was recognized internationally as an authority on the subject of death. She wrote more than 20 books about the process of dying. In *Life Lessons*, she shares many of the truths she learned from the dying to encourage us to live. Dr. Kübler-Ross died in August 2004.

Kübler-Ross believed that the process of dealing with death or loss has five specific stages. These stages include denial, bargaining, anger, depression, and acceptance. She believed that all people go through each stage in the grieving process, but they may not go through the stages in the same order. A stage could take days to work through or several months. Although she related these stages to dying patients, they are not exclusively limited to those who are dying. Anyone experiencing **grief** may progress through these five stages, and having a good understanding of them will help the medical assistant to better care for the patient.

Denial is the first stage, during which the patient or grieving person denies the issue that is causing the grief and thinks,

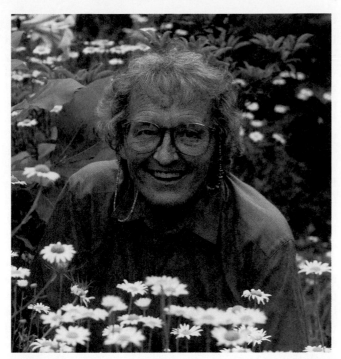

FIGURE 5-8 Dr. Elisabeth Kübler-Ross is the author of more than 20 books, many of which deal with the subject of death and dying, and is considered an international authority on the stages of grief. Dr. Kübler-Ross died in 2004. (Photograph copyright Kenneth Ross, 1985.)

"No, not me." The person is shocked and rejects the facts. The denial is a defense mechanism that helps the individual to deal with the news. The second stage is anger, when the dying patient begins to ask, "Why me?" The anger is often directed at others, and that may include the people in the family taking care of the patient, or it may include healthcare workers who cannot present a cure. In the third stage the patient begins to bargain in an attempt to postpone death or eliminate it altogether. This bargaining is usually with God, and the patient may pray to see a child marry or to witness some other upcoming event. The event is not the true hope of the patient, but life itself is. These patients say, "Yes, me, but…" in the attempt to postpone death. The fourth stage is depression, and during this stage patients realize that they are going to die and may feel regret for the goals they did not accomplish or for not taking better care of themselves. These patients say, "Yes, it's me…" and they must be allowed this period of grieving. However, family and friends should watch the patient carefully for signs of deep depression. The final stage of grief is acceptance, during which the patient is able to say, "Yes, me, and I'm ready." The reality of the impending death or distressing situation is accepted, and although the patient may continue to experience some depression, he or she is better equipped to deal with the arrangements that have to be made and may even demonstrate good humor during this time.

Patients who are dying must be treated with dignity and respect. This does not mean that they are unable to laugh and enjoy the life they are still living. Gentle touch and kind words will help patients to know the medical assistant cares for them. It is important to be careful with words and phrases around dying patients, but be natural in your conversations with them and do not be afraid to laugh. Never suggest to such patients that you "know how they feel." This phrase belittles their situation, and we never really know how another person feels. Asking questions is a good method of communication when you are not sure what to say. Use questions such as, "How do you feel about that?" or "What does your family think about your plans to discontinue treatment?" Then listen to the patient and make eye contact with him or her as you listen. You may also ask, "How can I help you?" as opposed to "Is there anything I can do?" There will be a natural tendency for the patient to say "No" to the second question. However, if you ask specifically how to help, they may open up and allow you or the office staff to be of help. They may simply need suggestions about who could cut their grass or how to contact Meals on Wheels. Hospice services provide terminally ill patients and their families with care and support, often from the point of diagnosis to bereavement. Many have found hospice services invaluable in the process of coping with a loved one close to death. The medical office should have listings of community resources to assist in these types of situations.

CRITICAL THINKING APPLICATION

- Often people put off writing a will. Could this be procrastination or a fear of death?
- When is it important to have a will?
- How can the medical assistant help Sarah to deal with her mother's impending death?
- What stage of grief might Mrs. Cloyd currently be experiencing? What stage might Sarah be experiencing?

MULTICULTURAL ISSUES

Cultural differences influence the way we deal with those from various parts of the world. We often become isolated in our thinking and incorrectly assume that people all over the world think and do things the same way that we do. However, there are vast differences in cultures from country to country, and even from areas within the same country. In the United States we see a difference between northerners and southerners. The speech of people in New York is significantly different from that of people in south Texas, and the dialect changes again from Texas to the West Coast. We picture Texans with cowboy boots and hats, but that is not how most Texans dress. Some of us still associate Alaska with Eskimos and igloos. Perhaps this stems from the books we read in elementary school, but cultures today are much more widely mixed in the United States, and because many people immigrate to our country for various reasons and opportunities, it is wise to learn a bit more about the cultures and the variety of people who inhabit the world.

We sometimes stereotype people of other cultures and think that we understand what they are like and how they live. Often, some type of **media** has influenced our thinking. There is much to learn from other cultures, and sharing is a way to gain an understanding of the experiences in other places. This helps us to be more well-rounded individuals and to enjoy and appreciate our own cultural differences. Remember that those people who have come to the United States from other countries have to deal with their ideas of both their own homeland and this country as well. There may be significant misconceptions, so in the medical facility, patience will be necessary as explanations are provided. Take extra time and care with patients of other cultures, without assuming they know or understand local culture. Also understand that culture is something that is passed from generation to generation, so many of the ideas people hold dear have been handed down for centuries.

Some people who enter a new country go through a period of what is called "culture shock"—a state of being in unfamiliar surroundings and being away from the things that were present in everyday life in the homeland. Street signs are different; in some cases, people drive on the opposite side of the street. Affected people quickly realize that their "normal" ways of doing things no longer work, and they must make some type of adaptation to survive. This adaptation may mean changing the habits and customs of a lifetime. This can be a very exciting prospect for some, but a very frightening prospect for others. Simple processes, such as enrolling in school, become extremely difficult tasks. Patience is a critical tool to help others adjust to the American way of life.

Examples of Cultural Traditions

- A husband speaks for his wife. The wife does not speak to the physician.
- The palm of the hand, facing down, is used to beckon someone. The hand motion signaling one to come or follow, performed with the back of the hand toward the patient, is used only when calling an animal. An open hand is used to point, rather than one finger.
- A female's clothing is not removed without the presence of another female family member.
- Emotional crying and sobbing denote femininity.
- Going to the doctor is a sign of weakness.
- The female medical assistant never touches the male patient.
- Acquaintances are not permitted to stand within 3 feet of the patient; only immediate family members are permitted to stand within this space.
- The Chinese do not like to be touched by people they do not know.
- The Laotian's "yes" response may not mean "yes," because it is considered rude to say "no" to others or to cause conflict.
- A native of Cambodia, as well as a Laotian, will not look into the eyes of the person being addressed because long eye contact means disrespect and is impolite.
- Cambodians do not like to have their blood drawn because they believe it will weaken them.
- Afghans and Mexicans have a concept of time that is less precise than in the United States.
- Vietnamese consider the head to be a sacred part of the body and are offended by being touched on the head or shoulders. Only the elderly may touch the head of a child without giving offense.

Communicating with People of Other Cultures

People from other cultures want to be treated just as you would like to be treated if you were visiting another country; they wish to be respected and treated fairly. Much can be learned about the background of others, and much can be shared about the culture we know, too. Cultural differences are responsible for many misunderstandings. We must make an attempt to understand people of other walks of life.

When speaking with those from a foreign country, there may be a **language barrier.** Even if the person knows some English, there will be words and phrases that do not make sense in the way that we use them in the United States. A period of time must pass during which the words are heard frequently before they will take on meaning to a person who is unfamiliar with them. It is important to speak a little more slowly than usual to a person whose primary language is not English—not to insinuate they are less intelligent but to give them a chance to absorb the words and mentally translate them into their own language, then prepare a response. There is no need to increase the volume of speech; people from other cultures are not hard of hearing. They merely need a little more time to process the words that are said.

Medical assistants should have an awareness of the nonverbal messages being sent by the persons who are interacting. In our society a simple up-and-down nod of the head means "yes" and a side-to-side shake means "no." However, in Bulgaria and some other countries, these signals have the opposite meaning. It is important to be sensitive to and aware of the beliefs of the many cultures that will be represented in the patient population. If you work in a practice that predominantly serves a distinct ethnic group, discuss possible cultural differences with the physician and with influential people within the cultural group. Learning to understand cultural differences helps you to gain the confidence and respect of patients.

EMOTIONAL AND PHYSICAL NEEDS

Human beings have certain emotional and physical needs that must be met for us to live balanced lives and a healthy existence. Many of us take these needs for granted until they become an absolute necessity; then our focus becomes directed toward meeting them. Few in the United States have faced hunger as those in some Third World countries have, and when hunger is our need, it suddenly becomes our prime concern. This section provides some insight into the needs we have as humans and their role in the total health of the body, mind, and spirit.

Maslow's Hierarchy of Needs

Psychologist Abraham Maslow created what he called the hierarchy of needs (Figure 5-9). A hierarchy is defined as "things arranged in order, rank, or a graded series." Maslow believed that our human needs can be categorized into five levels and that the needs on each level must be satisfied before we can move to the next level. These levels are often depicted as a triangle, with the most basic needs at the bottom and the highest potential for growth as a human being at the top.

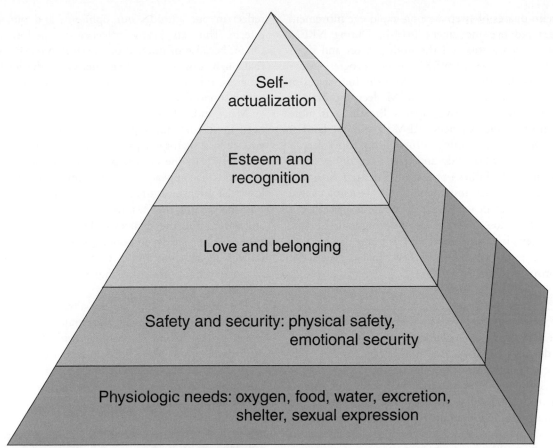

FIGURE 5-9 Maslow's hierarchy of needs. (From Adler RB, Towne N: *Looking out, looking in: interpersonal communication,* San Antonio, 1996, Harcourt Brace.)

The needs we have as humans, at the most basic level, are those that involve our physical well-being. These include food, rest, sleep, water, air, and sex. The second level includes issues related to our safety. We need to feel safe and secure in our homes and our environments, as well as the places where we work. The third level involves our social needs for love, a sense of belonging, and interaction with others. The fourth level relates to our self-esteem. We have an inner need to feel good about ourselves and to know that others view us in a positive manner. The last level is the self-actualization stage, in which we maximize our potential. In this level, we attempt to be at our best and to live our lives to the fullest extent possible.

Approval, Acceptance, and Achievement

Three specific needs that we have, apart from Maslow's hierarchy of needs, are critical to our happiness. These three needs are approval, acceptance, and achievement. Although most would agree that we do not need everyone's approval at all times, there exist specific people whose approval we do seek. Children usually wish to please their parents, even when the child is an adult. We seek to please our supervisors, and even our own children. However, this need to please can be taken too far. Various books address personalities called *pleasers,* who often place their own needs second to the needs of those they feel they must please in order to feel of worth.

We have a healthier self-esteem if we feel accepted by others. This resembles the sense of belonging discussed earlier but is a bit more extensive in nature. A feeling of acceptance includes the belief that our actions, words, dress, mannerisms, and other personality traits are acceptable to others we wish to impress.

Last, we have an inner need for achievement. Most humans want to do something great and contribute to their world in some way. A great thing to one person may be winning an Olympic race, but to another it may be reading to an elderly grandmother at a nursing home. We all enjoy praise for a job well done, or for losing weight, or for passing a difficult examination. It is beneficial to all when legitimate praise is shared freely and appreciated. This is especially true in our close relationships but is just as important in the workplace. It is much easier to work for a supervisor who praises for work well done than for one who never offers a pat on the back.

A Good Night's Sleep

Many of us do not realize the value of our sleep time. Sleep is one of the most important physical needs that we have and is the one most often sacrificed during busy, stressful periods of life. This is called *sleep deprivation.* Human beings need approximately 8 hours of sleep each night, although many can function for a period of time with less sleep. Eventually this lack of sleep will take a physical and emotional toll on the body.

The two main phases of sleep are non–rapid eye movement (NREM) and rapid eye movement (REM). During NREM sleep the eyes are fairly still and the body relaxes and slows down. There are four stages of NREM, which progress into a deeper sleep. After the body moves through the four stages of NREM, it enters REM sleep. During REM sleep the brain is highly active and the eyes move rapidly. Breathing is more irregular, and most people experience REM sleep in the last few hours of the sleep cycle. Dreaming occurs during REM sleep.

Many professionals who study and treat sleep disturbances agree that if an individual does not reach REM sleep, he or she will have provided physical rest for the body but not mental rest. This rest is critical in stress management, and because it occurs at the end of most sleep cycles, or during its last hours, those who cut their sleep time short may not enter REM sleep often. Thus they do not get the mental rest that is needed for them to perform at optimal levels.

Healthy Nutrition

We have been taught since we were children that good nutrition is vital to healthy bodies. Our bodies are machines whose performance depends on good health. We care for the body with a balance of good nutrition, activity, and health care. A balanced diet is essential to ensure that the organs and systems within us function at optimal levels. When the body is not receiving the nutrients and vitamins that it needs, various parts may malfunction, and this can lead to conditions or diseases or a worsening of the problems already present.

In today's diet-conscious society, some people attempt to lose weight by eating less food or cutting out meals altogether. This is a dangerous practice. Losing weight quickly through fad diets and "miracle" supplements is usually a guarantee that the weight will eventually return.

One should always begin weight loss programs under the advice and care of a physician. Do not skip meals in an effort to lose weight, and do choose foods from the four basic food groups. Avoid unhealthy snacks and sodas, and drink at least 8 to 10 glasses of water every day. Exercise regularly and take walks to provide cardiovascular benefits to the body. If you take good care of your body, the chances are increased that it will function properly for a longer period of time, resulting in a longer, healthier lifetime to enjoy to the fullest.

CRITICAL THINKING APPLICATION

- Could Sarah's sleep and nutrition habits affect her ability to care for her mother?
- How might these affect Sarah's personal stress levels, and how can she ensure that she is caring for herself, when her thoughts are primarily on her mother?

Positive Relationships

As mentioned earlier in this chapter, all of us need to feel approval, acceptance, and achievement. This is a vital component within our relationships as well. When we are involved in a relationship that is not going well, it will naturally reflect in our attitude, our opinions, and our sense of self-esteem. This can greatly influence our performance at work. Often, because of infatuation, we find ourselves in a situation that might not be a positive one. Once the relationship is in progress, it is sometimes hard to end it and find a connection with a supportive, caring individual.

Many individuals really have not determined what they need from a relationship. It is helpful to make a list of what you are looking for in a partner and commit not to compromise with regard to the critical points on the list. The sparks and fireworks that appear in the beginning of a relationship may lose their intensity as time goes on, and a firm foundational base must be present after the newness wears off. Choose carefully and wisely, and the chances of becoming involved in healthy relationships greatly increase. In addition, more and more individuals are choosing to remain single and are enjoying life to the fullest. Certainly this choice is better than being a part of a destructive partnership.

Harmful relationships are not always just between partners. Often we experience stress and strain with relatives, friends, and co-workers. Sometimes contact with the person causing the discontent cannot be avoided, at least for a period of time. In these cases we must learn coping techniques for dealing with the difficult relationship. Open, honest communication is of paramount importance.

CRITICAL THINKING APPLICATION

- Often survivors feel a sense of "unfinished business" with a person who has died, and have a more difficult time bringing closure to the relationship. How might Sarah spend high-quality time with her mother and come to terms with her death in a positive way?
- Is there anything that should not be discussed with a terminally ill patient?

Healthy Self-Esteem

Self-esteem is a confidence and satisfaction in oneself. To have high self-esteem, an individual must also be self-aware, and that takes some honesty. It means taking a look at your strengths and your weaknesses and knowing what you have to offer as a person. To feel well and accomplish goals in life, you must develop positive attitudes and positive responses to the pressures in life. It can sometimes be difficult to keep a positive attitude when others are being negative. Some people believe that if they inflict their bad feelings on others, they will feel better about themselves. It is important to remember, though, that no one can make you feel a certain way; it is a choice that you make. Blaming others for one's situation in life or negative emotions is self-defeating.

We are able to control two things in life—our attitude and our actions. Even when faced with a potentially volatile situation, our attitude and reactions are decisions that we make. These decisions should be made with careful thought, even if the reaction must be a swift one. Think before speaking. Pause a moment if needed, before reacting. Take a time out. Choose your battles wisely. All of these suggestions will help you to react in a more positive, constructive way when faced with a difficult situation.

Improving Yourself

No matter how great the training or how many opportunities are placed in front of a person, fear and doubt can sabotage efforts to improve the self-image, confidence, and potential of an individual. Almost every failure or mistake experienced can be traced to fear or doubt; either we are afraid to take a specific action or we doubt our own abilities. Blaming the circumstances around us is no excuse for a poor performance. It is also important to remember that small, daily decisions make a huge impact on our lives, sometimes even more than what we consider critical life decisions. For example, a student decides not to study for 30 minutes daily for an upcoming major examination, then fails it. This small decision to do something other than study results in failing an examination, which may force course repetition and delay the graduation date.

Self-esteem will improve if a person is able to adapt to situations well. To be human is to be a changing, growing, imperfect, but amazing living creation. Adapting means being flexible and open to the actions of others. Although we should have empathy for others, we cannot allow others to ruin our day or lower our confidence level. Inventor-philanthropist Charles Kettering once said, "The only time you can't afford to fail is the last time you try." Our failures often teach us much more than our successes. The important thing is to get up, evaluate why the failure occurred, then move forward armed with the new knowledge gained from mistakes.

Procrastination is often a symptom of the fear of failure and the fear of success. Many people procrastinate because they feel it will give them an excuse for their failure. They say, "There is no way I could pass that test—I only had 2 days to study!" Others are perfectionists and put off doing a job or delegating because they feel no one can do it as well as they can. The best way to stop procrastinating is to do something! Divide projects into small steps and complete one at a time. This makes tasks much less overwhelming.

The self-improvement process is ongoing. Periodically stop and evaluate where you stand in relation to the goals you have set for your life. Set goals—short- and long-term goals—for all of the areas of life, including career, relationships, and personal growth. Write the goals down; make them specific and measurable. Be sure that the goals are reasonable. Start with smaller, short-term goals and work toward long-term goals. Be persistent and never give up. Post a list of them on the refrigerator, and note progress. Do not count on having a whole lifetime to pursue goals; instead, move toward them consistently and enthusiastically.

Comfort Zones

We all have comfort zones. When faced with new ideas or changes, many of us tend to be a bit unsure of ourselves. Think back to the first day at school, the first day on a new job, the first time going to a fancy restaurant, a first date—these events often make us feel a bit uncomfortable. New experiences may be outside of our **comfort zone.** Psychologists often speak about a comfort zone, which is a place in the mind where we feel safe and comfortable, where we can perform comfortably and confidently. Most goals, however, require movement outside the comfort zone to reach them. Striving to reach a goal means trying new things, and this can be quite stressful. Because we do not want to become so stressed that we give up on our goals, we should take slow, small steps that are challenging, then move to the next step. Procrastination is a failure concept, but it can be overcome through dedication and consistent planning. Remember, too, that patients are usually outside of their comfort zones while visiting the physician's office. Do everything possible to make them feel at home and comfortable.

CLOSING COMMENTS

Interpersonal skills are critically important to the successful medical assistant. Communication will be a part of all interactions throughout the day, and the better developed these skills are, the better the medical assistant will be able to serve the patients in the facility. Every attempt should be made to enhance the interpersonal and human relations skills that the medical assistant currently has and to strive to better these skills continually. This will ensure that effective communication will be a part of the relationship with patients as well as others with whom the medical assistant interacts.

SUMMARY OF SCENARIO

Mrs. Cloyd and her daughter are facing a difficult time. Death is inevitable for everyone, but when a loved one is diagnosed with a terminal illness, it is particularly distressing. Both of these women need compassion and caring from the medical team. They will need to feel as if they are being heard and that their opinions are important. Some of their needs are similar, but they have differing needs as well. A gentle touch and laughter will brighten their day, and these expressions are critical to a person experiencing the stress of a devastating illness.

The medical assistant must ensure that Mrs. Cloyd understands her medications and treatments. The office should assist her and her daughter in finding community resources for which she might be eligible. Be sure to instruct Mrs. Cloyd primarily, and make certain that Sarah also understands any directions her mother should follow. Sarah will need compassion as she deals with her mother's illness and impending death. Because she is also a patient of the clinic, she should be given care and attention and may have emotional needs or periods of great stress also. Even on the busiest of days, these two women deserve warmth from the staff and should be made as comfortable as possible as they seek medical care.

Although the medical office is always a busy place, the medical assistant can take a moment to individualize the care that they provide to patients. Looking into the patients' eyes and genuinely asking how they have been getting along demonstrates interest in them. Call patients by their name and ask about their families. These techniques allow the medical assistant to develop rapport, which will result in a more pleasant office visit for the patient.

Often, the patient will be accompanied by a relative or friend, and the medical assistant may find it necessary to interact with these individuals. Remember that all information about the patient must be kept in strict confidence. Friends and family play a role in the overall health of the patient. When relations are strained, patients may feel depressed and stressed. This can affect their health in a negative way. The patient with strong family support will often heal faster and have a better outlook toward their health issues.

Listening is a skill that must be practiced and refined. The patient needs to know that the medical assistant is focusing attention on him or her, hearing their concerns and paraphrasing to make certain that the patient is understood correctly. Listening is one of the most important skills that the medical assistant can develop.

SUMMARY of LEARNING OBJECTIVES

1. Define, spell, and pronounce the terms listed in the vocabulary.
   - Spelling and pronouncing medical terms correctly adds credibility to the medical assistant. Knowing the definition of these terms promotes confidence in communication with patients and co-workers.
2. Explain why first impressions are critically important.
   - First impressions are critical in the medical profession. Dress, attitude, and appearance all influence the credibility of the medical assistant. The medical assistant should always treat patients and visitors to the office as individuals who deserve the best in customer service.
3. Differentiate between verbal and nonverbal communication.
   - Verbal communication depends on words and sound, whereas nonverbal communication consists of messages that are conveyed to another without the use of words. Body language, eye contact, facial expressions, and hand gestures are some of the many ways we use body language. Sometimes our body language conflicts with verbal communication, and a mixed signal is sent to the receiver. Often we are unaware of nonverbal signals and notice only a small number of the signals that other people send.
4. Explain the different levels of spatial separation.
   - Spatial separation can be defined as the space of comfort between individuals. Public space is usually considered to be 12 to 25 feet, whereas social space is approximately 4 to 12 feet. Personal space is the range of $1\frac{1}{2}$ to 4 feet, and intimate space would include touching up to approximately $1\frac{1}{2}$ feet.
5. Discuss the value of touch in the communication process.
   - Touch is important in the process of communication because it projects an air of care and compassion to the receiver. The medical assistant should never be afraid to touch patients, as long as precautions are taken with those who are contagious. Touching the patient shows empathy and often can be more eloquent than the spoken word.
6. Describe the elements of the transactional communication model.
   - The transactional communication model includes a sender and a receiver who both offer messages to each other using various channels. The sender encodes a message, then the receiver decodes it, to the best of his or her ability. Often some type of noise interferes as well, such as internal, external, and physiologic noise. Perception is important when communicating because messages are sometimes easily misinterpreted.
7. Explain some of the barriers to effective communication.
   - Some of the barriers to communication include physical impairment, language differences, prejudice, stereotyping, and perception. Barriers may also be present during difficult times, such as when a crisis occurs, when a person is angry or

Continued

SUMMARY of LEARNING OBJECTIVES

Continued

in shock, or when a patient or family member is experiencing an impending death or illness or has experienced a serious accident.

8. List and explain the levels of Maslow's hierarchy of needs.
   - Maslow's hierarchy of needs includes five levels, beginning with our most basic needs, such as food, rest, sleep, water, and anything that involves our physical well-being. The second level is related to safety issues, and the third, our social needs, such as love and interaction with others. The fourth level deals with our self-esteem, and the fifth is self-actualization, where our potential is maximized.

9. Discuss defense mechanisms, and be able to recognize commonly used defense mechanisms.
   - Defense mechanisms are psychologic methods of dealing with stressful situations and include sarcasm, denial, repression, compensation, and several others. Often these mechanisms are our only way of dealing with circumstances that are difficult to cope with.

10. Describe the value of listening.
    - Listening is one of the most important skills the medical assistant can possess. Listening involves not only silence, but active feedback as well. Open-ended questions help the medical assistant to restate what the patient is saying, to be sure that the patient is understood clearly.

11. List several ways to deal with conflict.
    - Everyone experiences conflict in daily living, so it is necessary to develop skills in dealing with conflict in as positive a way as possible. Conflict is not always negative and can be quite

beneficial to relationships. Knowing the different types of conflict, as well as how people attempt to process conflict, will help the medical assistant to recognize patterns and respond appropriately. Some individuals deal with conflict by being aggressive, assertive, or nonassertive. There are also many passive-aggressive methods of dealing with conflict, such as avoidance, changing the subject, distraction, blaming, and several others.

12. Explain the stages that patients go through when facing death.
    - Elisabeth Kübler-Ross suggests that there are five stages to the process of grief: denial, bargaining, anger, depression, and acceptance. She believes that all stages are experienced while grieving, but not necessarily in the same order. The medical assistant can better care for the patient and the patient's loved ones when a good understanding of the grieving process is present.

13. Discuss why physical and emotional needs affect our daily performance at work.
    - Everyone needs physical and emotional rest to function throughout the day. A good night's sleep, consisting of at least 8 hours, regular exercise, and healthy nutrition will help to keep the medical assistant fit for duty. When these needs are not being met, work performance may suffer and the medical assistant may not be able to give proper attention and care to the patients. Exhaustion will affect the ability to perform, as will pressing concerns that linger in the mind. Make every effort to clear all negative thoughts and completely focus on the patients.

CONNECTIONS

 Study Guide Connection: Go to Chapter 5 Study Guide. Read the Case Study and Workplace Applications and complete the assignments. Do online research for answers to the questions in the Internet Activities associated with interpersonal skills and human behavior.

 CD Connection: Go to the Medical Assisting Competency Challenge CD and do the training activities under Communication.

 Evolve Connection: For more information related to interpersonal skills and human behavior, go to http://evolve. elsevier.com/kinn/admin and visit related weblinks for Chapter 5. Click on the Medical Assisting Exam Review and do the practice questions to sharpen your test-taking skills.

Medicine and Ethics

6

SCENARIO

Monica Johnson has been employed for 6 months as a medical assistant in a family practice. She works as the clinical medical assistant for Dr. Richard Wray. One of Dr. Wray's patients, Anna Walsh, recently adopted a baby after 8 years of trying to conceive a child. The baby, Delaney Gracelia, was born to a single mother, Susan, who participated in an open adoption in which she and the Walshes met and got to know each other during her pregnancy. Susan dated the baby's father for about 6 months before discovering that she was pregnant, and they are no longer dating. Susan wanted to make a good decision for the baby and decided to place her for adoption.

Dr. Wray performed some genetic testing on Delaney, and the adoptive parents were involved throughout the pregnancy, even meeting Delaney's birth mother for physician appointments from time to time. Monica observed both Susan and the Walshes and saw many benefits from the arrangement, noticing that everyone was primarily concerned with Delaney and her happiness and well-being. However, there were periods that were difficult, as well, for both sides. This prompted Monica to give some thought to her own feelings and ideas about many different ethical situations and issues and how she would react in the face of having to make ethical decisions.

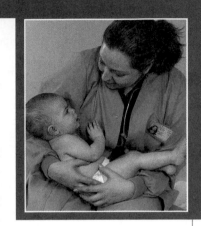

While studying this chapter, think about the following questions:

- What difficulties do patients who are placing their babies for adoption face?
- What difficulties do adoptive parents face when participating in an open adoption?
- How can the medical assistant be supportive of both the adoptive parents and the birth mother?
- Should the medical assistant discuss personal beliefs about ethical situations with patients?

LEARNING OBJECTIVES

1. Define, spell, and pronounce the terms listed in the vocabulary.
2. Explain rights and duties as related to ethics.
3. List and define the four types of ethical problems.
4. Discuss the process used for making an ethical decision.
5. Detail the impact that the CEJA has on the ethical decisions made by healthcare professionals.
6. Describe the way unique identifiers help HIV-positive patients to avoid some discrimination.
7. Note some of the concerns regarding ethics that surround genetic information.
8. Explain why confidentiality is an ethical issue.
9. Discuss several of the CEJA opinions and how they might differ from the views of the class as a whole.

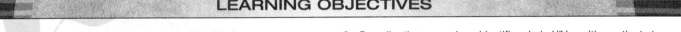

National Accreditation Competencies and Content	
CAAHEP COMPETENCIES	**ABHES COMPETENCIES**
General	**Professionalism**
3.c.(2)(b). Perform within legal and ethical boundaries	1.d. Be cognizant of ethical boundaries

VOCABULARY

advocate (ad'-vuh-kat) One who pleads the cause of another; one who defends or maintains a cause or proposal.

allocating (a'-luh-ka-ting) Apportioning for a specific purpose or to particular persons or things.

annotations (a-nuh-ta'-shun) Notes added by way of comment or explanation.

beneficence (buh-ne'-fuh-sens) The act of doing or producing good, especially performing acts of charity or kindness.

clinical trials Research studies that test how well new medical treatments or other interventions work in the subjects, usually human beings.

disparities (di-spar'-uh-tes) Marked differences or distinctions.

disposition (dis-puh-zi'-shun) The tendency of something or someone to act in a certain manner under given circumstances.

duty Obligatory tasks, conduct, service, or functions that arise from one's position, as in life or in a group.

euthanasia (yu-thuh-na'-zhe-uh) The act or practice of killing or permitting the death of hopelessly sick or injured individuals in a relatively painless way for reasons of mercy.

fidelity (fuh-de'-luh-te) Faithfulness to something to which one is bound by pledge or duty.

gametes (ga'-mets) Mature male or female germ cells, usually possessing a haploid chromosome set and capable of initiating formation of a new diploid individual; a sex cell, whether sperm or ovum.

genome (jeh'-nom) The genetic material of an organism.

idealism The practice of forming ideas or living under the influence of ideas.

impaired Being in a less-than-perfect or less-than-whole condition; includes having handicaps or functional defects and being under the influence of drugs, alcohol, and/or controlled substances.

infertile Not fertile or productive; not capable of reproducing.

introspection (in-truh-spek'-shun) An inward, reflective examination of one's own thoughts and feelings.

nonmaleficence (non-mal-fe'-zens) Refraining from the act of harming or committing evil.

opinions Formal expressions of judgment or advice by an expert; formal expressions of the legal reasons and principles on which a legal decision is based.

philosopher A person who seeks wisdom or enlightenment; an expounder of a theory in a certain area of experience.

postmortem Done, collected, or occurring after death.

procurement (pro-kuhr'-ment) To get possession of, to obtain by particular care and effort.

public domain The realm embracing property rights that belong to the community at large, are unprotected by copyright or patent, and are subject to use or appropriation by anyone.

ramifications (ra-muh-fuh-ka'-shuns) Consequences produced by a cause or following from a set of conditions.

reparations (re-puh-ra'-shuns) Amends, acts of atonement, or satisfaction given as a result of a wrong or injury.

sociologic Oriented or directed toward social needs and problems.

surrogate (suhr'-uh-gat) A substitute; to put in place of another.

unique identifiers Codes used instead of names to protect the confidentiality of the patient in a method of anonymous HIV testing.

veracity (vuh-ra'-suh-te) A devotion to or conformity with the truth.

---

*E*thics is defined as the thoughts, judgments, and actions on issues that have implications of moral right and wrong. The concept of ethics concerns itself with the philosophies underlying ideal relationships between human beings, as well as the promotion of the highest good for humanity as a whole. Various beliefs exist about what is and is not ethical in everyday life and in the medical profession. The decisions that people make based on ethical beliefs can quite possibly alter the course of human existence.

A medical assistant not only must have a strong knowledge base about ethical issues that might be faced throughout the profession, but also must come to terms with some of the deeply rooted value systems that have been a part of his or her life since youth. The trials and tribulations we have experienced, as well as the joys, will all influence our thought patterns when we are faced with an opportunity to make a good ethical decision.

HISTORY OF ETHICS IN MEDICINE

From earliest recorded history, humans have pondered ethics—the judgment of right and wrong. Ethics should not be confused with etiquette. *Etiquette* refers to courtesy, customs, and manners, whereas ethics explores the moral right or wrong of an issue. It is not surprising that for centuries the field of medicine has set for itself a rigid standard of ethical conduct toward patients and professional colleagues.

The earliest written code of ethical conduct for medical practice was conceived in approximately 2250 BC by the Babylonians and was called the *Code of Hammurabi*. It elaborated on the conduct expected of a physician and even set the fees that a physician could charge. The Code was quite lengthy and detailed, which is the probable reason it did not survive the ages. In approximately 400 BC Hippocrates, the Greek physician known as the Father of Medicine, developed a brief statement

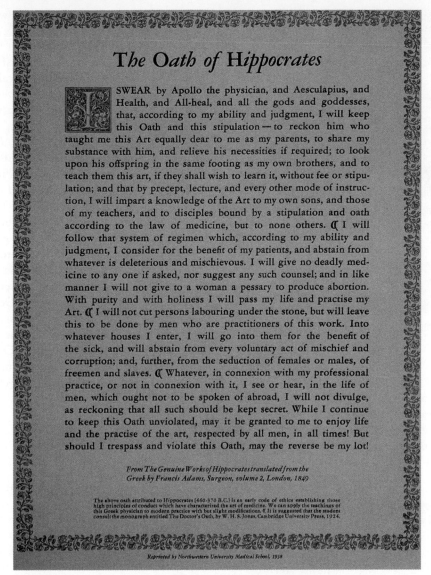

The Oath of Hippocrates

I SWEAR by Apollo the physician, and Aesculapius, and Health, and All-heal, and all the gods and goddesses, that, according to my ability and judgment, I will keep this Oath and this stipulation — to reckon him who taught me this Art equally dear to me as my parents, to share my substance with him, and relieve his necessities if required; to look upon his offspring in the same footing as my own brothers, and to teach them this art, if they shall wish to learn it, without fee or stipulation; and that by precept, lecture, and every other mode of instruction, I will impart a knowledge of the Art to my own sons, and those of my teachers, and to disciples bound by a stipulation and oath according to the law of medicine, but to none others. ❨ I will follow that system of regimen which, according to my ability and judgment, I consider for the benefit of my patients, and abstain from whatever is deleterious and mischievous. I will give no deadly medicine to any one if asked, nor suggest any such counsel; and in like manner I will not give to a woman a pessary to produce abortion. With purity and with holiness I will pass my life and practise my Art. ❨ I will not cut persons labouring under the stone, but will leave this to be done by men who are practitioners of this work. Into whatever houses I enter, I will go into them for the benefit of the sick, and will abstain from every voluntary act of mischief and corruption; and, further, from the seduction of females or males, of freemen and slaves. ❨ Whatever, in connexion with my professional practice, or not in connexion with it, I see or hear, in the life of men, which ought not to be spoken of abroad, I will not divulge, as reckoning that all such should be kept secret. While I continue to keep this Oath unviolated, may it be granted to me to enjoy life and the practise of the art, respected by all men, in all times! But should I trespass and violate this Oath, may the reverse be my lot!

*From The Genuine Works of Hippocrates translated from the
Greek by Francis Adams, Surgeon, volume 2, London, 1849*

The above oath attributed to Hippocrates [460-370 B.C.] is an early code of ethics establishing those high principles of conduct which have characterized the art of medicine. We can apply the teachings of this Greek physician to modern practice with but slight modifications. ❨ It is suggested that the student consult the monograph entitled The Doctor's Oath, by W. H. S. Jones, Cambridge University Press, 1924.

Reprinted by Northwestern University Medical School, 1938

FIGURE 6-1 The Oath of Hippocrates. (Courtesy National Library of Medicine.)

of principles that remains an inspiration to the physicians of today. The Oath of Hippocrates has been administered to many medical graduates (Figure 6-1). The most significant contribution to medical ethics after the time of Hippocrates was that of Thomas Percival. Percival was a physician, **philosopher,** and writer from Manchester, England. In 1803 he published his Code of Medical Ethics. Percival was very interested in **sociologic** matters and took a great interest in the study of ethical concepts as related to the medical profession.

In 1846, as the American Medical Association (AMA) was being organized in New York City, medical education and medical ethics were already considered important aspects of the profession. At the first annual AMA meeting in 1847, a Code of Ethics was formulated and adopted. It specifically acknowledged Percival's code as its foundation, and this document became a part of the fundamental standards of the AMA and its component parts. Even today sections of the AMA Code of Ethics stem from Percival's writings.

WHO DECIDES WHAT IS ETHICAL?

When we weigh the question of who decides what is ethical, the answer is evident: you do. Every day medical professionals face the task of making ethical decisions. Although many different groups of people meet to discuss the ethics of a procedure or decision from the local level to national and worldwide levels, fundamentally, each individual decides what is ethical and what is not for him or her and the individuals these decisions will affect. As with any important choice, one must consider the short- and long-term effects and consequences. Although it is a completely acceptable practice to depend on groups and committees to guide ethical decisions, the responsibility for making these decisions ultimately rests with the individual (Figure 6-2).

Organizations that study ethical dilemmas may decide that a concept such as abortion is an ethical medical practice. But if an individual does not find abortion to be an acceptable

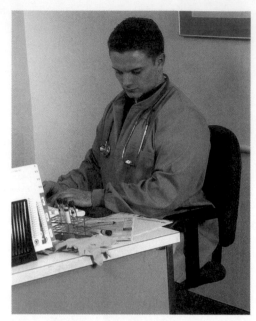

FIGURE 6-2 Medical assistants may find themselves making ethical decisions on a daily basis.

practice for religious or other reasons, abortion is not ethical for that individual. A great freedom that Americans often take for granted is that we can exercise free will in decisions related to individual conscience in this country, that we can choose from a variety of options—but we must exercise this responsibility carefully.

CRITICAL THINKING APPLICATION

- Monica knows that she has deep-rooted thoughts and ideas about many ethical matters. However, she has never really thought about where she formed her ideas. Where do we get most of our opinions on ethical or moral issues?
- What is the difference between an opinion's being personal and its being someone else's?

THE ROLE OF THE AMERICAN MEDICAL ASSOCIATION AND THE COUNCIL ON ETHICAL AND JUDICIAL AFFAIRS WITH REGARD TO ETHICS

The AMA serves physicians as a national organization providing various types of information and support. One of the most important facets of the AMA is its Council on Ethical and Judicial Affairs (CEJA). The CEJA consists of nine active members of the AMA, including one resident physician member and one medical student member, and is responsible for interpreting the *AMA Principles of Medical Ethics* as adopted by the House of Delegates of the AMA. The AMA's Code of Ethics has four components:

- Principles of medical ethics
- The fundamental elements of the patient-physician relationship

- Current opinions of the CEJA with **annotations**
- Reports of the CEJA

The *Code of Medical Ethics: Current Opinions with Annotations* is a publication that contains the first three components, with discussion of more than 135 ethical issues encountered in medicine. A separate publication, *Reports of the Council on Ethical and Judicial Affairs,* discusses the rationale of the Council's **opinions** (Figure 6-3).

The *AMA Principles of Medical Ethics* has been revised several times to follow current trends in medicine, but there has never been a change in the moral intent or overall **idealism** of the statements. In 1957 the *AMA Principles of Medical Ethics* was condensed to a preamble and 10 sections. In 1980 the principles were reduced to seven sections to clarify and update the language, eliminate reference to gender, and seek a proper and reasonable balance between professional standards and contemporary legal standards in our changing society. The most recently adopted changes, presented at the 2001 Annual Meeting of the AMA House of Delegates, reflect wording consistent with today's privacy issues and stress the importance of informed consent in deoxyribonucleic acid (DNA) database information in genomic research. Opinions are issued on a variety of subjects at the annual and interim meetings, and often older opinions are updated or changed based on current societal trends.

MAKING ETHICAL DECISIONS

Before discussing the opinions of AMA's CEJA, it is best to understand a few of the elements of ethics, the different types of ethical problems, and how a good ethical decision is made. Then, as some of the opinions are presented in this text, students can begin to evaluate their own positions regarding each issue. This section will enable the medical assistant to recognize the type of ethical problems that might arise in the physician's office and will provide a pattern to follow when making an ethical decision.

Elements of Ethics

Ruth Purtilo, in her book *Ethical Dimensions in the Health Professions,* presents three general elements of ethics: duties, rights, and character traits. A **duty** is an obligation that a person has or perceives himself or herself to have. A daughter may feel the obligation to care for her elderly parents, or a husband who has hurt his spouse may feel an obligation to somehow make up for his act.

Purtilo mentions several types of duties that relate to the medical profession. **Nonmaleficence** refers to refraining from harming the self or another person. **Beneficence** refers to bringing about good. **Fidelity** is the concept of promise-keeping, and **veracity** refers to the duty of telling the truth. Justice, in relation to medical ethics, deals with the fair distribution of benefits and burdens among individuals or groups in society having legitimate claims on those benefits. When a person has wronged another, he or she has a duty to make **reparations,** or right the wrong. Last, a person should feel grateful after being

FUNDAMENTAL ELEMENTS OF THE PATIENT-PHYSICIAN RELATIONSHIP

From ancient times, physicians have recognized that the health and well-being of patients depend on a collaborative effort between physician and patient. Patients share with physicians the responsibility for their own healthcare. The patient-physician relationship is of greatest benefit to patients when they bring medical problems to the attention of their physicians in a timely fashion, provide information about their medical condition to the best of their ability, and work with their physicians in a mutually respectful alliance. Physicians can best contribute to this alliance by serving as their patients' advocates and by fostering these rights:

1. The patient has the right to receive information from physicians and to discuss the benefits, risks, and costs of appropriate treatment alternatives. Patients should receive guidance from their physicians as to the optimal course of action. Patients are also entitled to obtain copies or summaries of their medical records, to have their questions answered, to be advised of potential conflicts of interest that their physicians might have, and to receive independent professional opinions.
2. The patient has the right to make decisions regarding the healthcare that is recommended by his or her physician. Accordingly, patients may accept or refuse any recommended medical treatment.
3. The patient has the right to courtesy, respect, dignity, responsiveness, and timely attention to his or her needs.
4. The patient has the right to confidentiality. The physician should not reveal confidential communications or information without the consent of the patient, unless provided for by law or by the need to protect the welfare of the individual or the public interest.
5. The patient has the right to continuity of healthcare. The physician has an obligation to cooperate in the coordination of medically indicated care with other healthcare providers treating the patient. The physician may not discontinue treatment of a patient as long as further treatment is medically indicated, without giving the patient reasonable assistance and sufficient opportunity to make alternative arrangements for care.
6. The patient has a basic right to have available adequate healthcare. Physicians, along with the rest of society, should continue to work toward this goal. Fulfillment of this right is dependent on society providing resources so that no patient is deprived of necessary care because of an inability to pay for the care. Physicians should continue their traditional assumption of a part of the responsibility for the medical care of those who cannot afford essential healthcare. Physicians should advocate for patients in dealing with third parties when appropriate.

FIGURE 6-3 Fundamental elements of the patient-physician relationship. (From Report of the Council on Ethical and Judicial Affairs of the American Medical Association. Originally adopted June 1990; last updated August 2001. Report 26, 1990. Available at: www.ama-assn.org/ama/pub/category/8313.html. Accessed June 26, 2006.)

the beneficiary of someone else's goodness. This is also a type of duty.

Rights are defined as claims that a person or group makes on society, a group, or an individual. The Bill of Rights appended to the U.S. Constitution guarantees certain liberties that we enjoy as American citizens. However, some individuals think that they have rights that are really privileges. For instance, Americans do not have the "right" to healthcare services. Individuals may "expect" to be cared for when sick, but this is not a right that is guaranteed to anyone in America. Some countries provide medical care to all their citizens, but the United States is not one of those countries. A right applies to all people within a group, without prejudice. One of the most intense ethical arguments faced today is the right-to-life concept. If our Constitution states that we all have the right to life, liberty, and the pursuit of happiness, how can abortion be considered ethical? Or if an individual is trying to end his or her suffering from a terminal illness, could the "pursuit of happiness" be interpreted to include seeking a physician's help in committing suicide? These are the types of ethical questions that arise in the healthcare field.

Character traits are defined in Purtilo's book as a **disposition** to act in a certain way. A person who feels honesty is an important character trait can usually be trusted to speak the truth. One who feels that it is acceptable to take small items from work for use at home may not be able to resist an opportunity to take something more valuable. Character traits will certainly not always provide an indication of how a person will react in all situations. No human being is perfect, and we are sometimes unpredictable. Stress can also interfere with our normal reactions, and other factors, such as depression or anger, influence how we act as well. The phrase that someone is acting "out of character" usually means that he or she is deviating from his or her normal behavior patterns.

With an understanding of these basic elements of ethics, we have a good foundation that will help us to look more objectively at ethical problems and solve them to the best of our ability.

Types of Ethical Problems

Purtilo presents four basic types of ethical problems (Figure 6-4). They are:

- Ethical distress
- Dilemmas of justice
- Ethical dilemmas
- Locus of authority issues

Ethical distress is the type of problem faced when a certain course of action is indicated, but some type of hindrance or

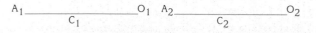

WHAT SHOULD BE DONE?

1. **Ethical Distress**
   I know which course of action I (the "agent") should take for the patient's benefit, but there is a structural barrier to my being able to do it.

   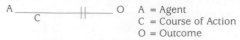

   A ———— ‖ ———— O   A = Agent
      C   C = Course of Action
                        O = Outcome

2. **Ethical Dilemma**
   There are two (or more) courses of action, each of which is right (or wrong). No matter which one I (the "agent") choose, something of value will be compromised.

   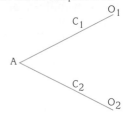

3. **Distributive Justice**
   There are benefits to be distributed among several potential beneficiaries. Not everyone can receive a full measure of the benefit. On what basis should the distribution be made?

   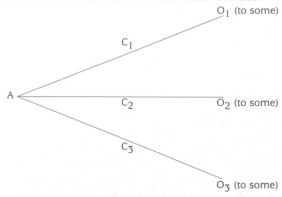

   WHO SHOULD DO IT?

4. **Locus of Authority**
   There are 2 (or more) agents or "authorities" in this situation. Each believes he or she knows what outcome will benefit the patient the most, but only one authority will prevail.

   A_1 ———————— O_1 A_2 ———————— O_2
          C_1 C_2

FIGURE 6-4 Summary of types of ethical problems. (From Purtilo R: *Ethical dimensions in the health professions*, ed 4, Philadelphia, 2005, Saunders.)

barrier prevents that action. A professional knows the right thing to do but for some reason cannot do it.

An ethical dilemma is a situation in which an individual is faced with two or more choices that are acceptable and correct, but doing one precludes doing another. A choice must be made, and something of value may be lost if a second choice is eliminated. This could be viewed as the proverbial "being caught between a rock and a hard place," whereby a choice must be made that has more of an effect than what may be seen on the surface.

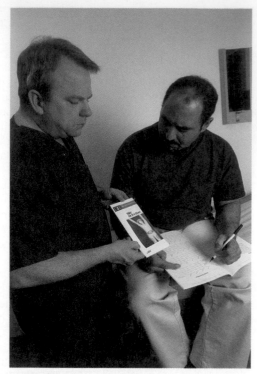

FIGURE 6-5 One of the duties of a medical assistant is to ensure that the patient understands the instructions given. Only when the patient fully understands the choices available can he or she make sound decisions.

The third type of ethical problem is the dilemma of justice. This problem focuses on the fair distribution of benefits to those who are entitled to them. Choices must be made regarding who receives these benefits and in what portion. A few examples of the dilemma of justice would include organ donations and distribution of scarce or costly medications.

In locus of authority issues, two or more authority figures have their own ideas about how a situation should be handled, but only one of those authorities will prevail. If one physician feels a patient should have surgery and another does not, how does the patient decide (Figure 6-5)?

Recognizing the type of ethical problem is not always easy. Sometimes a medical professional is faced with an issue that is a mixture of one or more types of ethical problems. When possible, it is wise to take some time in weighing the right course of action to take before making an important decision. Unfortunately, this is not always possible in the fast pace of the medical profession. Some decisions must be made in a split second, so it is wise to have a thorough grasp of ethical decision-making before the need arises.

The Ethical Decision-Making Process

In her book Purtilo presents a five-step process for ethical decision making. The steps include:
- Gathering relevant information
- Identifying the type of ethical problem
- Determining the ethics approach to use
- Exploring the practical alternatives
- Completing the action

To gather information a medical professional should ask questions, review charts, talk to the patient and other professionals, and search for other data so that the full view of the situation is available for scrutiny. Once the information is gathered, the medical professional must decide which ethical problem or problems are being presented. In determining the ethical approach to use, we must consider duties, rights, and character traits of all the individuals involved with this issue, paying close attention to the **ramifications** of all possible decisions. All of the alternatives must be considered and evaluated, and then an action should be taken (Procedure 6-1).

Although it is best to have time to give these areas some thought, this may not always be possible. It is a good practice for those entering the medical profession to take stock of what their core beliefs are. Scan the newspapers and search professional journals for ethical situations, think about the facts, then decide how you would react to each one. This is excellent preparation for the day that you will be faced with making a quick ethical decision.

CRITICAL THINKING APPLICATION

- What are the ramifications of an open adoption such as Delaney's? What problems might occur during the first year of her life?
- How might these problems be avoided?
- What are the positive aspects of the adoption?

CURRENT OPINIONS OF THE COUNCIL ON ETHICAL AND JUDICIAL AFFAIRS AND MEDICINE'S ETHICAL ISSUES

Now, armed with a basic knowledge about the types of ethical problems and the process used to solve them, we will take a look at some of the Council opinions. Remember, physicians and other medical professionals are not bound to abide by the CEJA opinions. They have the freedom to make their own decisions, but many of the medical professionals in our country tend to agree with the decisions made by the committee.

Abortion

In 1973 the U.S. Supreme Court heard the case of *Roe v. Wade*. Norma McCorvey (using the name Jane Roe) petitioned the court for permission to have an elective abortion when at age 21 she found herself pregnant with her third child. The class action suit she filed against Henry Wade, then the District Attorney in Dallas, Texas, eventually was appealed to the United States Supreme Court. Although she won her case, it was too late for her to have an abortion, and her child was born and placed for adoption. McCorvey went public with her true identity in the early 1980s and later became a staunch opponent of abortion and has spent many years promoting the overturn of *Roe v. Wade* (Figure 6-6).

Since the ruling was handed down in 1973, abortion has been one of the most volatile issues in medical ethics. According to

---

PROCEDURE 6-1

Perform Within Ethical Boundaries

CAAHEP COMPETENCIES: 3.c(2)(b)
ABHES COMPETENCIES: 1.d

GOAL: *To enable the medical assistant to perform in an ethical manner in all situations.*

EQUIPMENT and SUPPLIES

- Copy of the AAMA Code of Ethics
- Copy of the Medical Assistant Creed
- Copy of the Oath of Hippocrates

PROCEDURAL STEPS

1. Become familiar with the AAMA Code of Ethics and the Medical Assistant Creed.
   PURPOSE: To understand the purpose of medical assisting and the ethical boundaries that surround the profession.
2. Study the Oath of Hippocrates.
   PURPOSE: To gain knowledge of the roots of ethical behavior.
3. Consider the ethical problem at hand.
4. Gather relevant information about the problem.
   PURPOSE: To make certain that all of the facts are considered when solving the problem.

5. Identify the type of ethical problem.
   PURPOSE: By accumulating information about the problem and determining the type of ethical problem, the medical assistant will be better able to solve the problem.
6. Determine the ethical approach to use.
   PURPOSE: Knowing the type of problem helps the medical assistant to determine which ethical approach to use to solve the issue.
7. Explore practical alternatives.
   PURPOSE: Considering all practical alternatives helps the medical assistant to make the best ethical decisions.
8. Make the best ethical decision.
   PURPOSE: By gathering information, identifying the problem and the best ethical approach to use, and considering all practical alternatives, the medical assistant can arrive at a sound ethical decision.

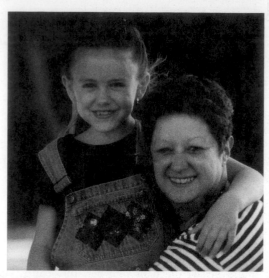

FIGURE 6-6 Norma McCorvey was "Jane Roe" in *Roe v. Wade*, the Supreme Court decision that legalized abortion. More than 20 years later, she became one of the pro-life movement's biggest advocates and has worked to get *Roe v. Wade* overturned.

the *AMA Principles of Medical Ethics,* the AMA does not prohibit a physician from performing an abortion in accordance with good medical practice and under circumstances that do not violate the law. In recent years laws have been passed in some states requiring mandatory parental notification of a minor's intent to have an abortion. In some cases this means that the minor must have parental consent, and in others, parents only must be notified of their daughter's intent to have an abortion. Some states also require a 24-hour or more waiting period after the notification has been made. However, CEJA states that the patient, even if an adolescent, should ultimately be in control of the decision as to whether parents should be involved in the abortion decision.

The AMA strongly encourages physicians to persuade the minor toward seeking counseling with someone she trusts, such as a school counselor, teacher, or relative, if the minor's parent is not to be involved in the abortion decision. However, the AMA agrees that the physician should not feel compelled to require minors to involve the parent in the decision. Medical professionals must be aware of the laws in their respective states that deal with the mandatory notification requirements and should contact the medical societies in their region to determine what constitutes proper notification.

Case to Discuss

Should a woman who has been raped and become pregnant seek an abortion?

Abuse

The AMA requires that a physician be familiar with the signs of physical, psychologic, and sexual abuse of spouses, children, mentally incompetent persons, and the elderly. Discovery of abuse creates a difficult situation for a medical professional. The patient may be the object of abuse but may deny its existence because of fear of further attacks. The law requires that abuse

be reported, and if the physician does not report abuse, ethical standards have been breached. In addition, the abuse may continue. Any medical assistant who suspects abuse must report this information to the physician first, who must determine whether the incident is reportable by law and take action. If action is not taken, the medical assistant is responsible for making a report to the proper authority in the city or state.

Case to Discuss

What harm can come to a patient's family if the medical professionals are incorrect about their assessment of abuse?

Allocation of Health Resources

Sometimes society must decide who will receive care when serving all who need care is not possible. Decisions must be made fairly and should be weighed carefully. The criteria to consider when **allocating** health resources include urgency of need, likelihood of benefit, duration of benefit, amount of resources required for successful treatment, and potential for change in quality of life. Nonmedical criteria, such as ability to pay, social worth of the individual, age, obstacles to treatment, and the patient's contribution to the illness, should not be considered. The physician who is treating the patient must remain the **advocate** of the patient and should not be involved in making allocation decisions for that patient. Procedures for such allocations are determined in an objective manner by the institutions involved in the patient care.

Case to Discuss

If the chief executive officer (CEO) of American Airlines, the winner of last year's Academy Award for Best Actor, and a drug-abusing mother of three all were equally ill and needed a liver transplant, which should receive the organ, and on what would you base the decision?

Artificial Insemination

Any individual or couple considering artificial insemination must be thoroughly counseled and endure lengthy screening procedures for communicable and genetic diseases that the donor and/or recipient may have. Informed consent must be provided, and further regulations are based on the marital status of the people involved. If the recipient is married to the donor, the resultant child will have all of the rights of a child naturally conceived. If the donor is anonymous, the husband must sign consent if he is to become the legal father of the resultant child. If the donor and recipient are not married, the recipient is considered the sole parent, unless both parties agree to recognize a right to paternity. It is not considered unethical to provide artificial insemination to a single woman or a woman who is a part of a homosexual couple. It is usually considered unethical to offer compensation to donors other than reimbursement of actual expenses and/or compensation for the donor's time.

Physicians should keep permanent records regarding donors so that:

- Individuals who test positive for communicable diseases can be excluded from the donor pool

- The number of pregnancies resulting from a single donor source can be limited
- Donors can be notified about screenings that demonstrate the presence of a communicable disease
- Donors can be notified about a disease or disorder found in a child born through artificial insemination that may have been transmitted by the donor

Much discussion is ongoing about the use of extra embryos that are harvested for reproductive purposes. The control and use of these **gametes** should logically be left to the man and woman who produced them, but the AMA agrees that both must give their consent regarding how they are used. In vitro fertilization is considered an ethical procedure.

Case to Discuss

A man fertilized eggs that were frozen for later use, but he died without having made provision for the use of those eggs after his death. Should the man's wife be able to use those eggs after her marriage to a second man?

Stem Cell Research

Many organizations feel that using human embryos for stem cell research destroys the most vulnerable of beings, and laws are designed to protect them. Others want to explore the possibility of developing cures from this research for diseases such as Alzheimer's disease, diabetes, Parkinson's disease, and heart disease. Stem cell research continues to be an area of disagreement because of the controversy regarding the point at which life begins. Those who believe that life begins at conception usually oppose stem cell research, because it involves experimentation and testing on a "viable human being." Many physicians believe that their commitment is first to "living persons" as opposed to embryos, and therefore support stem cell research. One of the strongest proponents of stem cell research was actor Christopher Reeve, who played Superman in several movies and was later paralyzed in an equestrian accident (Figure 6-7).

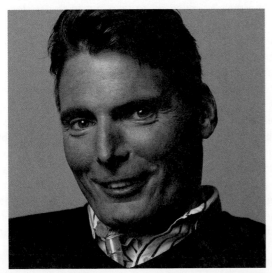

FIGURE 6-7 Christopher Reeve played the role of Superman in movies but was more admired for his untiring efforts toward medical research after the equestrian accident that left him paralyzed. Reeve died in 2004. (Courtesy Corbis.)

Case to Discuss

A medical student is recruited to work with a physician who is researching paralysis. Once the project is underway, the student discovers that the physician is using embryos that have been questionably obtained in the experimentation. What should the medical assistant do?

Surrogate Motherhood

Surrogate motherhood introduces many different ethical, legal, and social problems to the individuals involved. However, this could be the only opportunity for **infertile** couples to have a child. The benefits of surrogacy must be heavily weighed against the possible risks and psychologic problems that might arise. The AMA feels that the birth mother must be given a period of time during which she can reverse her decision to give up the child she has delivered and void the contract. However, in cases of gestational surrogacy, the legality and ethical implications are more complicated. In gestational surrogacy the child is not genetically linked to the birth mother. Usually the couple engaging the surrogate mother would be the genetic parents of the resultant child. One must also consider what will happen if the child were to be born with a deformity or handicap. This is a contract that should never be entered into without strong forethought and counseling.

Case to Discuss

What is a fair length of time to give a surrogate mother to petition to void a surrogacy contract?

Human Cloning

The AMA agrees that physicians should not at this time participate in human cloning, or somatic cell nuclear transfer, because of the numerous legal and moral issues that must be explored. Most agree that our current ethical and moral standards would interpret that a "cloned human" be granted the same rights as "normal humans," much in the same way as an adopted child is accepted legally and socially as part of a family. The AMA does not feel there has been nearly enough research into the long-term effects of cloning and therefore does not advocate the practice today.

Case to Discuss

If a couple loses a child through death but it were possible to clone the child, what concerns would be present for the family?

Genetic Counseling

Genetic counseling is also an area in which the AMA recommends caution. Through genetic counseling, parents of tomorrow may be able to choose eye color, talents, and intellect levels for their children (Figure 6-8). There are already humans who were conceived as "designer babies" in the world today. In 1980 the Repository for Germinal Choice (more commonly known as the "Genius Sperm Bank") was founded. Although it was not established to create a perfect "master race," it did attempt to produce leaders and creators. As with cloning, the AMA

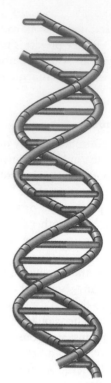

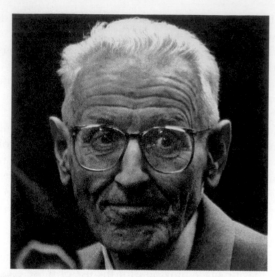

FIGURE 6-9 Dr. Jack Kevorkian, after being acquitted for numerous assisted suicides, was convicted in 1999 of second-degree murder and delivery of a controlled substance in the death of Thomas Youk, 52, who had amyotrophic lateral sclerosis (ALS or Lou Gehrig's disease). (© AFB/CORBIS.)

FIGURE 6-8 DNA, known as the "blueprint of the body," contains all the genes and chromosomes that make each human a unique creation, unlike any other human. (From Chester GA: *Modern medical assisting*, Philadelphia, 1998, Saunders.)

recommends that much more research be done before instituting genetic counseling on a global scale.

Case to Discuss

What could happen if parents were to "design" a baby, but it arrived flawed in some way or did not meet their expectations?

CRITICAL THINKING APPLICATION

- How might the genetic testing done in Delaney's case have caused an ethical dilemma?
- Discuss whether genetic testing can be counted on to predict disease.
- How many in your class would have genetic testing done on their own child before birth?

Physician-Assisted Suicide

The AMA believes that physician-assisted suicide interferes with the fundamental purpose of being a physician—being a healer. The CEJA advocates that physicians aggressively provide care and alternatives in treatment for those who are near the end of life but not promote or provide the means with which the patient could end his or her own life. This includes not only assisting the patient to inject chemicals that will induce death, but also prescribing drugs and information about lethal doses or administering a lethal dose of a drug to a patient to promote death (Figure 6-9). This is sometimes called **euthanasia,** or mercy-killing.

Case to Discuss

If a parent mentioned in passing that he or she would want the right to commit suicide in the event of a terminal illness, would you support that decision if the situation did in fact arise?

Surrogate Decision Making

According to CEJA, physicians should encourage patients to document their preferences regarding advance directives through a living will or durable power of attorney. However, many patients do not have any type of documentation of their wishes available when tragedy strikes. In these cases a surrogate may be asked to make decisions for the patient with regard to his or her medical treatment. Even when such provisions have been made, the documents are sometimes unavailable in an emergency, so patients should discuss treatment options in advance with those who may be called on to be a surrogate decision maker. If patients cannot make medical decisions for themselves and documented advance directives are unavailable or nonexistent, absent any state regulation to the contrary the physician should approach the patient's family, domestic partner, or a close friend as the surrogate decision maker. There may be cases in which family members disagree about the decisions that are necessary for the health and well-being of the patient. In these instances the physician should work to resolve the conflict through mediation or should consult the facility's ethics committee. The ultimate goal of the physician is to act in the best interests of the patient, and in the absence of any other basis for interpreting how a patient would wish to proceed with treatment, the physician should make the decision that would, in the physician's professional opinion, most benefit the patient.

Case to Discuss

A physician recommends that a patient be taken off life support. The patient lives with his homosexual partner and has not had contact with his parents in more than 10 years. Both the partner and the parents discuss the situation with the physician. The partner does not wish to remove life support, stating that the patient would want to have every opportunity to live. The parents insist that they know what is best for their son and demand that he be taken off life support. Who should prevail?

Withholding or Withdrawing Life-Prolonging Treatment

A physician is committed to saving life and relieving suffering. Sometimes these two goals are incompatible, and a choice between them must be made. If possible the patient should decide what treatment is given. Often the patient makes his or her wishes known to a responsible relative or other representative, in case the patient becomes incapacitated. Some patients wish to have a "do not resuscitate" (DNR) or "no code" order added to their charts. Usually such an order is desired so that no heroic measures are taken in a situation in which a patient would be unable or incompetent to make a decision. In any case, the decision to withdraw life support should be made before any mention of organ donation is made by the medical professionals tending the patient. In the best situation the patient has formally completed advance directives. Two types of advance directives are usually used in the United States. These documents are written instructions for healthcare and usually are in the form of a living will or a durable power of attorney. This documentation is strongly recommended by the AMA.

Patients are urged to create a living will. This is a document that states the wishes of the patient in case of terminal illness or an accident after which the patient cannot express his or her wishes. A durable power of attorney is a legal document that allows the patient to appoint someone who is trusted to make medical decisions for the patient in the event that the patient cannot make those decisions. This person is sometimes called a *patient advocate* or *healthcare proxy*. Federal law requires that patients be given information about advance directives by all facilities that participate in the Medicare and Medicaid programs.

Case to Discuss
How would a medical assistant handle the family of a patient who asks for advice about withdrawing life-prolonging treatment? To whom should the medical assistant defer the question?

Quality of Life

Physicians must sometimes participate in or advise on decisions affecting the fate of a person whose prognosis is poor, such as a deformed newborn or a person of advanced age with many physical problems. The first thought may be the burden that the patient's care will place on the family or society. However, the AMA insists that the physician's primary consideration be what is best for the patient.

Case to Discuss
A mentally ill single woman who is institutionalized becomes pregnant and refuses to give up her maternal rights so that the child can be adopted. Even if she were to reconsider, what complications result if the child is born deaf and has a severe liver disorder? Should the child be fed and cared for by the hospital staff?

Clinical Trials and Investigation

Without **clinical trials** and investigation, no new drugs or procedures would be developed. However, all such investigation must follow a competently designed systematic program with due concern for the welfare, safety, and comfort of patients. The physician-patient relationship does exist in clinical investigation, and when treatment of the patient is involved, voluntary written consent must be obtained from the patient or the patient's legally authorized representative. Additional restrictions apply to minors or mentally incompetent adults. Physicians must show the same concern for the welfare and safety of the person involved in the clinical trials as they would if the person were a private patient.

Case to Discuss
If your brother were homosexual and wanted to participate in clinical trials for a vaccination against human immunodeficiency virus (HIV), would you support his decision?

Cost of Healthcare Services

Concern for the quality of patient care should be the physician's first consideration. However, the physician should be conscious of costs and should not provide or prescribe unnecessary services. Access to an adequate level of healthcare for all members of our society is now a moral expectation, but certainly not a right. Cost must be considered when providing these services, as well as the degree of benefit to the patient, the duration of the benefit, and the number of people who will benefit.

Case to Discuss
Should an 87-year-old patient with cardiovascular disease and stomach cancer undergo expensive breast reconstruction surgery?

Organ Donation

Organ donation is not only considered ethical by the AMA, it is encouraged. However, it is considered unethical to participate in proceedings in which the donor receives payment, except reimbursement of expenses directly incurred in the removal of the donated organ. The rights of both the patient and the donor must be equally protected. In cases in which the donor has lost his or her life, the death must be certified by a physician other than the recipient's physician.

Because the need for donated organs is so extreme, protocols have been established by healthcare facilities to determine when it is proper to harvest organs. Organ **procurement** may occur immediately after a person has died, or it may happen after a patient has been kept alive artificially for a period of time. Hospitals also have specific guidelines for donation of organs from living donors, such as a kidney donation. When donations are made from one living person to another, both patients must have an advocate team that includes a physician, so that the interests and well-being of each patient are addressed. Payment to a living donor other than legitimate expenses incurred in connection with removal of the organ is also considered unethical.

Blood donations are probably the most common form of organ donation. Some religions do not believe in transfusing blood, and cases in which such beliefs come to bear must be dealt with carefully. If the patient is a minor and the parents refuse the child a blood transfusion, or any other medical care, some states would hold the parents liable for danger to or abuse of a child. However, the court system is reluctant to fight the parents over their religious beliefs and would intervene only in extreme circumstances.

CEJA has recommended that two proposals related to organ donation be considered; these are aimed at increasing organ donations and would change the approach to consent for deceased donations. The two proposed models include the mandated choice model and the presumed consent model. The mandated choice model would require individuals to express their preferences regarding organ donation at the time of performing some state-regulated task, such as renewal of a driver's license. This method would be ethically appropriate only if the individual's choice was made in accordance with the principles of informed consent. The presumed consent model would mean that deceased individuals were presumed to be organ donors unless they indicated their refusal to donate. It is unknown at this time whether the implementation of such models would affect the number of organs transplanted in a positive way, but CEJA encourages physicians to support policies that would increase the number of organ donors in the United States.

Case to Discuss

A woman dies with a living will that states that she wishes her organs to be donated. Her mother, still living, disagrees with the decision and does not want her daughter's organs donated. What should health professionals do in this situation?

CRITICAL THINKING APPLICATION

- Monica has often thought about being an organ donor. She is very much in favor of organ donation because of her interest in the medical field. Her parents are very opposed to this because of their religious beliefs. How can Monica deal with this conflict within her family?
- If Monica dies before her parents do, how can she ensure that her wishes are carried out?

Capital Punishment

The CEJA does not consider participation in the act of capital punishment by a physician to be ethical. The physician may certify the death of the person but should not administer a lethal injection or induce death in any way. This conflicts with the physician's role as a healer, much in the same manner as physician-assisted suicide does.

Case to Discuss

A very emotional patient, the parent of a child who was raped and killed, has been given the opportunity to attend the execution of the murderer. During a visit to her family physician, she expresses concerns about being able to cope with the memory of her daughter during the execution and asks you if you would attend in the same situation. How do you handle this situation?

ETHICAL ISSUES SURROUNDING HIV

Being HIV positive creates a whole new world of ethical concerns for patients as well as those who support and care for them. When the HIV crisis first came to public attention, many variables about the virus were unknown and this created a wealth of misinformation. Those infected with the virus were often forced to leave their homes and lost their jobs, were shunned in society, and faced rejection seemingly everywhere they turned, all because of fear of the illness (Figure 6-10).

Today clinical trials are underway for vaccinations against HIV, but clinical trials need volunteers for testing. Because vaccinations are often made of an attenuated or weakened strain of a virus, serious concerns exist about who will receive the vaccination. Researchers have considered testing the vaccination in several Third World countries that have a high number of prostitutes and a thriving sex industry. These people, with no intentions of changing their lifestyle no matter the risks, may see vaccination trials as their chance of not contracting HIV. However, the situation raises the question of the ethics of not submitting our own citizens to testing instead of those from disadvantaged countries.

Because of the discrimination practiced even today against people who are infected with HIV, problems occur with testing in some states that report the names of HIV-positive patients to various health departments and agencies. Although the stated intention is to ensure that these patients receive care, the accompanying effect is the risk of discriminatory practices. Some states use code systems called **unique identifiers** to assist in helping maintain the confidentiality of those getting tested for HIV. However, other states insist by statute that the names

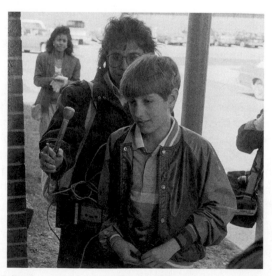

FIGURE 6-10 After a long court battle, Ryan White won the right to attend public school, despite his HIV status. (© Bettmann/CORBIS.)

be reported. Some states require mandatory HIV testing for prisoners and those who have committed sex crimes. Insurance is a difficult issue when a person is infected with HIV, and some policies can be cancelled if HIV infection is discovered. This may prompt providers who want to treat patients infected with HIV to delay reporting the infection as long as possible, using other diagnoses regarding symptoms as opposed to the underlying cause of the patient's problems. Many details are involved when HIV is a factor, even the reporting of HIV-positive status on the **postmortem** report. All of these ethical issues are difficult to resolve, and great care should be taken when making decisions surrounding a patient who is HIV positive.

ETHICS AND THE HUMAN GENOME

The mapping of the human **genome** has been in the news for several years. The genome project formally began in 1990 with the goals of identifying all of the 20,000 to 25,000 genes present in the human body, determining the sequences of the three billion chemical base pairs that make up human DNA, and finding ways to catalog this information in databases to make it readily available to those who need it. The project was completed in 2003, but the data discovered during the 13 years of the project will be studied for years to come.

Highlights of the project included the completion of the sequence mapping of chromosome 19, which is the most "gene-rich" of all of the human chromosomes. Chromosome 13 sequence mapping provided information about the genes that carry breast cancer type 2, as well as information about bipolar disorder and schizophrenia. The medical potential of the analysis of information provided by the Human Genome Project is mind boggling and will surely provoke advances in various medical fields and new technology and procedures.

Access to genetic information prompts many concerns and presents ethical, legal, and moral questions. Most of the major healthcare agencies and organizations in the United States and worldwide will be involved in the decisions made about this type of information, including the Centers for Disease Control and Prevention (CDC), National Institutes of Health (NIH), Department of Health and Human Services (DHHS), Food and Drug Administration (FDA), Centers for Medicare and Medicaid Services (CMS), and many others. Experts will be needed to educate Congress, federal agencies, and state and local governments, because laws must be passed regarding the use of genetic information. The rapid pace of science surpasses the ability of lawmakers to keep up, so the challenge ahead with regulation of the use of genetic information is a mammoth one.

The mapping of the human genome and the information provided have raised concerns about privacy and confidentiality issues. Who actually owns genetic information, and who will be allowed to control it? Logically, it would seem that the patient owns his or her own genetic information, but if that is so, then the patient should be able to control access to it. Also, decisions must be made regarding the fair use of genetic information. Employers, schools, courts, insurance companies, adoption agencies, and the military are just a few examples of organizations that could potentially misuse genetic information and discriminate against those whom they may wish to target for inclusion or exclusion. Reproductive issues arise, as well, along with questions about the reliability of genetic testing.

Patients will have to be counseled thoroughly about the risks and limitations of genetic technology. The answers to many questions are uncertain. Should a parent be allowed to test a minor child for adult-onset diseases? Should testing be performed for diseases that have no cure? All of these issues need resolution before the use of genetic information is widespread.

OTHER ETHICAL ISSUES

Interprofessional Relationships

If a medical assistant recognizes or suspects an error in a physician's orders, he or she has an ethical obligation to report this to the physician. Questioning a possible error is necessary, even if it means risking the displeasure of the physician or supervisor. It could save a life or prevent a lawsuit if an error has been made.

Physicians often refer a patient to another physician for diagnosis and treatment when it is necessary. A physician should make these referrals only when confident that the patient will receive competent treatment. It is considered unethical to offer a financial incentive or other valuable consideration to patients in exchange for recruitment of other patients.

Unless the state imposes legal restrictions, a physician in private practice is free to choose whom he or she will treat. Although private practitioners may refuse certain patients, they must treat those who have already been accepted in the practice or face possible charges of neglect. This does not include referring a patient to another physician for a condition that is not within the scope of the original physician's practice.

A sports medicine physician must keep in mind that the professional responsibility at a sporting event is to protect the health and safety of the participants, with personal judgments being governed only by medical considerations. Players should not be allowed to play and risk injury to ensure winning games.

In years past it was considered unethical for a physician to have any type of romantic relationship with nurses or assistants in the office or hospital. Although this is not as stringent a rule today, it is wise to not fraternize with co-workers, especially subordinates, at the workplace.

Confidentiality and Patient Privacy

Confidentiality is one of the cardinal rules of the medical profession. It is completely unethical and unacceptable to divulge any information about a patient to any other person not directly related to the patient's care. The places where confidentiality is often breached include elevators, hallways, waiting or reception areas, break rooms, and lunch rooms. One never knows whose relative is standing behind the medical assistant, listening to conversations that would be inappropriate for those not personally involved in the patient's care to hear. Breach of patient confidentiality is grounds for immediate termination from a healthcare facility or physician's office.

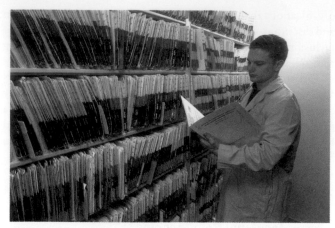

FIGURE 6-11 Confidentiality issues apply to all information about the patient, including what is charted and what is spoken between the patient and the medical assistant.

Confidentiality restrictions apply to information in patient records and charts, as well as what the medical assistant is told by the patient or patient's family (Figure 6-11). Never investigate a patient record strictly for curiosity. All information in the record must be kept in confidence. If records are computer based, accessing records of patients who do not fall directly under the medical assistant's realm of duty is also considered unethical. Never share information about patients with anyone outside the medical facility or office, including your own immediate family.

The prime objective of the medical profession is to render service to humanity, and this must be a medical assistant's first concern as well. The importance of respecting the confidentiality of information learned from or about patients in the course of employment cannot be overemphasized. It is unethical to reveal patient confidences to anyone, and this includes family, spouse, best friends, and other medical assistants. A medical assistant must never mention the names of patients outside the place of employment, because sometimes the doctor's specialty reveals the patient's reason for consultation. Confidential papers, case histories, and even the appointment book should be kept out of sight of curious eyes. In addition, outside observers should be present during the patient encounters with the physician only with the patient's explicit permission. Outside observers may include a friend who drove the patient to the physician's office or a medical student or intern who is observing in the clinic. It is advisable to document this permission in the patient's chart.

Never discuss one patient's case with another patient. If curious patients ask questions about others, simply explain that medical assistants are obligated to keep all patient information confidential. This can be done in a tactful and kind manner. Patients who ask questions of a medical nature about their own case should be referred to the physician for information and instructions, unless the physician has authorized the medical assistant to provide this information. When minors request confidential services, physicians should encourage them to include their parents. However, if the minor does not wish to involve them and the law does not require otherwise, physicians

should allow competent minors to consent to medical care and should not notify the parents without the minor patient's consent.

Remember that the Health Insurance Portability and Accountability Act (HIPAA) provides strict regulations for patient confidentiality and disclosure of private health information. Make certain that the physician's office is abiding by its own privacy policy and that all patients have been given the opportunity to review that policy. A document stating that the patient has read and understands the privacy policy or that he or she has refused to sign should be a part of the patient's medical record.

Patients may not always understand the ethical standards to which physicians and medical assistants adhere. They may ask questions about their own health or the health of a fellow patient. Medical assistants must educate patients regarding the issues of confidentiality in such a way that the patients are not offended, explaining that all patients deserve to have their medical and personal information kept private. Now more than ever the obligation of the medical assistant to keep information private is not only an ethical responsibility but also a legal responsibility. All patients should understand they are entitled to confidential treatment of their records and that the facility is dedicated to that principle.

CRITICAL THINKING APPLICATION

- Susan, Delaney's birth mother, comes to the office for a checkup 6 weeks after the baby was born. Susan looks a little sad, and when Monica questions her, she asks how Delaney is doing. What should Monica tell her?
- How can the office protect itself from issues involving confidentiality in this unusual adoption scenario?

Advertising

The only restrictions on advertising by physicians are those that specifically protect the public from deceptive practices. Standards regarding advertising and publicity have been liberalized over the years, but any advertisement or publicity must be true and not misleading. Testimonials of patients, for instance, should not be used in advertising, because they are difficult to verify or measure by objective standards. Statements regarding the quality of medial services are highly subjective and difficult to verify.

Communications with the Media

Although information regarding some patients such as celebrities and politicians may be considered news, the physician cannot discuss any patient's condition with the press without authorization from the patient or the patient's legal representative. The physician may release only authorized information or that which is public knowledge. Certain kinds of news are a part of public records. This is known as news in the **public domain** and includes births, deaths, accident reports, and police cases.

A medical assistant must be aware that only the physician is authorized to release information, and under no circumstances should the medical assistant violate the confidential nature of the physician-patient relationship. It is unethical even to certify or verify that the patient is under the physician's care without the patient's permission. Policy must be in place for every medical office regarding how media inquiries should be handled and to whom they should be referred. Never voluntarily speak to the press without authorization from the physician. Communications with the media fall within the HIPAA guidelines. Do not release a patient's health information without written permission.

Physician Obligations in Disaster Preparedness and Response

Physicians are ethically obligated to provide urgent medical care during disasters. Because extensive physician involvement is required during national, state, regional, and local disasters, physicians are expected to contribute both their time and their skills to assist in such emergencies. Examples of instances when the physician would be obligated to act include natural disasters, epidemics, and terrorist attacks.

Malevolent Use of Biomedical Research

Because biomedical research may produce information that has potential for both harmful and beneficial applications, the physician must assess the possible ramifications of participation in such research before engaging in projects. One of the most harmful uses of biomedical research involves biologic weapons. Physicians are expected to hold public trust as sacred and consider the welfare of society as a whole as well as the welfare of individual patients.

Racial and Ethnic Healthcare Disparities

Patients are entitled to the same quality of care regardless of their race or ethnic background. CEJA demands that physicians strive to eliminate biased behavior toward patients. Discrimination toward any patient or patient group cannot be tolerated. In addition, physicians must take into account any language barriers that might hinder effective treatment of the patient. Every effort must be made to make certain that the patient understands the physician and that the physician understands the patient. Physicians should also participate in efforts to encourage diversity in the profession.

Diagnostic Imaging on Request

Patients may request diagnostic imaging services for reasons such as determination of a baby's sex. Physicians should perform diagnostic imaging only when they believe that the benefits of the imaging service outweigh the risks involved.

Computers

The expanding uses of computer technology permit the accumulation of an unlimited amount of medical information. With the use of computers in the physician's office and the employment of computer service organizations, confidentiality becomes even more difficult to maintain. In general, all

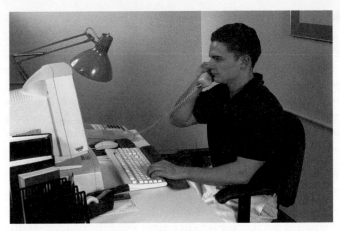

FIGURE 6-12 With the advent of advanced computer technology, a medical assistant must be particularly careful about using information about patients on the computer.

information must be entered and accessed only by authorized personnel, and a tracking system should be used to identify which employees access information. Breaches in computer policies should be considered a breach of patient confidentiality, and the consequences should be stringent enough to deter employees from accessing information to which they are not entitled (Figure 6-12). Information from the computer should be disseminated only to those who have a legitimate reason for needing the information.

Fees and Charges

Charging or collecting an illegal or excessive fee is unethical. The medical assistant is responsible for keeping informed about current billing regulations and to see that they are conscientiously followed.

Requesting that payment be made at the time of treatment is entirely appropriate and very common in today's medical offices. Often, managed care patients are asked to remit their co-payment before seeing the physician on the day of the visit. If the patient is notified in advance, adding interest or other reasonable charges to delinquent accounts is also considered ethical. Most offices use a patient information booklet that provides a written reference of all policies and that is given to new patients on their first visit. A reasonable charge may be made for the cost of duplicating patient records.

Fee Splitting and Contingent Fees

If a physician accepts payment from another physician solely for the referral of a patient, both are guilty of an unethical practice called *fee splitting*. This practice, whether with another physician, a clinic, a laboratory, or a drug company, is unethical.

Although attorneys often accept a case on a contingent fee basis, it is unethical for a physician to engage in this practice. The fee in this case is contingent on a successful outcome, but a physician should never set his or her fee on the successful outcome of medical treatment. A physician's fee must always be based on the value of service provided to the patient.

Insurance Forms

Although physicians' offices in times past would willingly file the claim on all insurance policies for their patients, some have changed their policies to a payment up-front system and give patients the information needed to file the claim themselves. Many offices will still file at least one insurance claim for established patients but may charge for multiple or complex insurance filing. This practice is entirely ethical if in conformity with local custom.

Waiver of Insurance Copayments

Physicians may opt to write off or waive copayments to facilitate patient access to medical care. If access to care is directly threatened because the patient cannot make the copayment, the physician may forgive the payment. However, routine waiver of copayments may violate the policies of some insurers, both public and private. Physicians should ensure that their policies on copayments are consistent with applicable law and within legal boundaries of their contracts with insurers.

Professional Courtesy

Professional courtesy is defined as the provision of medical care to physician colleagues or their families and staff free of charge or at a reduced fee. This is a long-standing tradition but certainly not an ethical requirement. Physicians make the decision as to who will receive professional courtesy in their offices, and this should be written into the office policy manual. In some cases, extending professional courtesy is contrary to insurance and/or managed care contracts. In addition, some physicians have stopped offering professional courtesy because of the rising costs of healthcare and shrinking reimbursements.

Appointment Charges

It is ethical for a physician to charge for a missed appointment or one that was not cancelled within a stated time if the patient has been fully advised in advance that such a charge may be made. Discretion should be used in applying such charges, however, since the patient may have encountered an emergency. Often, adding a missed appointment charge to the bill of a patient who never cancels in advance will prompt a call in the future when the appointment cannot be kept.

Prescribing Drugs and Devices

The physician should not be influenced in the prescribing of drugs, devices, or appliances by a direct or indirect financial interest in the supplier. A physician may own or operate a pharmacy but generally may not ethically refer his or her patients to that pharmacy. Patients should enjoy the same freedom of choice in deciding who will fill their prescriptions as they do in choosing a physician.

Professional and Contractual Relationships

Physicians often enter into contractual relationships, which may be as simple as monthly pest control services for the office. However, contracts can be quite complicated and contain numerous provisions, necessitating the assistance of an attorney. Physicians should negotiate the wording of contracts such that there is no question of financial incentives for the physician that would in any way compromise professional judgment or integrity.

Health Facility Ownership by a Physician

A physician may ethically own or have a financial interest in a for-profit or other health care facility, such as a freestanding clinic or health club. However, before admitting or referring a patient to that facility, the physician has an ethical obligation to reveal such ownership to the patient. In general, physicians should not refer patients to a health facility that is outside their office practice and at which they do not directly provide care or services.

Ghost Surgery

The substitution of another surgeon without the patient's consent is called *ghost surgery*. The patient has a right to choose his or her own physician or surgeon. Ghost surgery may happen when the patient has already received anesthesia and has no idea that a substitution has been made. To make a substitution without consulting the patient is deceitful and unethical.

Discipline within Medicine

A physician should expose incompetent, corrupt, dishonest, or unethical conduct on the part of members of the profession without fear of loss of favor. A physician may be subject to civil or criminal liability, including loss of license to practice medicine, for violation of government laws. Expulsion from membership is the maximum penalty that may be imposed by a medical society for violation of ethical standards.

Physician Health and Wellness

Physicians are responsible to maintain their own good health and be well enough to treat their patients. When the physician is not well, both physically and mentally, his or her health can interfere with the ability to provide good care to patients and engage in the safe execution of professional medical activities and decision making. When a physician is not in such good health, he or she is said to be **impaired.**

CEJA recommends that all physicians have their own personal doctor who will use uncompromised objectivity in caring for the physician's health. Healthcare providers are expected to intervene promptly when the health or wellness of a colleague appears to have become compromised. CEJA suggests types of intervention such as the offer of encouragement as well as referrals to physician health programs or other programs that will restore and maintain the physician's health and wellness.

A physician who knows that he or she has an infectious disease should not engage in any activity that creates an identified risk of transmission to the patient. Simple colds and other minor illnesses will arise occasionally, but illnesses that would cause a significant risk to the patient should not be given a chance to cause infection.

Substance Abuse

It is unethical for a physician to practice medicine while under the influence of a controlled substance, alcohol, or other chemical agents that could impair the ability to properly care for the patient or perform procedures. Healthcare providers who are aware of other providers with substance abuse problems must take action to ensure patient safety, which may include reporting the physician to the appropriate authority in the city or state in which he or she practices medicine.

Unethical Conduct by Members of the Health Profession

In rare instances a medical assistant is faced with a situation in which the physician-employer's conduct appears to violate established ethical standards. Before making any judgments, the medical assistant must be absolutely sure of all the information and circumstances. If unethical conduct occurs, the medical assistant must then make his or her own decision about continued employment in the facility and whether the unethical behavior should be reported to a law enforcement agency, the local medical society, or the hospital where the physician has been granted privileges. Would it be wise to remain in the office under the circumstances? Would it be better to seek other employment? Would remaining adversely affect future opportunities for employment with another physician?

These decisions are difficult, especially if the relationship and employment conditions have been favorable and congenial. An ethical medical assistant will not wish to participate in known substandard or unlawful practices, especially those that might be harmful to patients. In addition, the medical assistant must never make inaccurate reports regarding unethical behavior and should realize that some states can prosecute individuals who file a false report. Be absolutely certain of the facts before making such accusations against any health professional.

CLOSING COMMENTS

Medical assistants have an ethical obligation to keep abreast of current developments that affect the practice of medicine and care of the patients. Membership in a professional organization provides access to continuing education for maintaining knowledge and skills pertaining to the performance of medical assisting.

The study of ethics requires much thought and honest appraisal of what the medical assistant believes. Sometimes **introspection** of this type is difficult. Often our beliefs are a result of our environment, upbringing, and other factors that have influenced our thinking and actions from the time we were small children to our current age. It is important that our belief system be one that we have created personally, not just a set of beliefs accepted from another source. Medical assistants should take a serious look at the thoughts and concepts that make up their own concepts of ethics. It is important to approach ethical decisions calmly, logically, and without haste.

SUMMARY OF SCENARIO

Pregnancy is usually a joyous time, but Monica has learned that even such an anticipated event can bring ethical issues to light. She has realized that there are two or more sides to every situation and that she must be open and willing to look at all sides when making an ethical decision.

Medical assisting is a rewarding career, but sometimes the decisions that face medical professionals are quite difficult. Monica must learn to be nonjudgmental and not to inflict her opinions on her patients. They must make their own decisions regarding their health and emotional well-being, and the medical assistant should not influence their thinking unfairly.

Monica will continue to evaluate her own ideas and beliefs throughout her career as a medical assistant. Periodic self-evaluation is good for everyone, and she will grow emotionally from the experiences that patients bring about where ethical issues are concerned.

Patients who place their babies for adoption often feel the same type of grief experienced on the death of a loved one. Sometimes this loss does not register with the patient for many years after the event. Adoptive parents face many fears as well, such as the concern that the adoptive mother will change her mind about the proceedings and want the child back. Some families find the adjustment to having an adopted child in the family a difficult one. Siblings may be less than accepting of the new child, and later in life other children may tease the adopted child. However, adoption is most often a positive event in the life of a family.

The medical assistant should be supportive to both adoptive parents and birth mothers. Personal beliefs should be set aside as the patient and others involved make the best decisions they are able to make for their own lives.

SUMMARY of LEARNING OBJECTIVES

1. Define, spell, and pronounce the terms listed in the vocabulary.
   - Spelling and pronouncing medical terms correctly adds credibility to the medical assistant. Knowing the definition of these terms promotes confidence in communication with patients and co-workers.

2. Explain rights and duties as related to ethics.
   - Ethics are judgments of right and wrong or actions on issues that have implications of a moral right and wrong. Etiquette deals with courtesy, customs, and manners. A duty is an obligation that a person has or perceives himself or herself to have. Rights are claims that are made by a person or group on society, a group, or an individual. Although these terms have different definitions, the concepts are interrelated, and often all are involved in ethical questions.

3. List and define the four types of ethical problems.
   - Ethical distress is caused when a problem has an obvious solution but some type of barrier hinders the action that needs to be taken. An ethical dilemma is a situation that has two or more solutions, but if one is chosen, something of value is lost in not choosing the other. A dilemma of justice involves allocation of benefits and how they are to be fairly distributed. Two or more authority figures, each with his or her idea of how to handle a certain situation, are the center of the locus of authority ethical problem. Only one of the authority figures can prevail. Often an ethical problem has several aspects and more than one type of problem is presented.

4. Discuss the process used for making an ethical decision.
   - Making an ethical decision is easier when the situation is approached logically and considered using a five-step process. First, one gathers relevant information; then the type of problem is identified. After determining the ethical approach to use, one should explore alternatives. Finally, all that is left is to complete the action and make the decision.

5. Detail the impact that the CEJA has on the ethical decisions made by healthcare professionals.
   - Although healthcare professionals do not have to abide by the opinions of the CEJA, the Council's opinions are highly regarded, and many professionals practice in accordance with these opinions. Often providers will abide by the opinions to avoid controversy, but many still openly oppose the decisions of the CEJA.

6. Describe the way unique identifiers help HIV-positive patients to avoid some discrimination.
   - Unique identifiers maintain the confidentiality of patients who are tested for HIV. Some individuals might hesitate to be tested if they were concerned that their names would be reported to various agencies. Using the unique identifiers, patients may have much more confidence that the chances of discrimination resulting from HIV status are lessened.

7. Note some of the concerns regarding ethics that surround genetic information.
   - Many ethical concerns exist regarding genetic testing. Many patients are concerned about how the information gained will be used and who will have access to the information. Questions arise regarding the ownership of the information. When negative information is found, other ethical problems arise that will need to be addressed. Knowledge of a person's genetic blueprint could lead to discrimination. Countless issues must be examined before the use of genetic information becomes widespread.

8. Explain why confidentiality is an ethical issue.
   - Confidentiality is of major importance in the medical profession. The patient's privacy should be of prime concern to a medical assistant. It is a serious enough issue that a breach of patient confidentiality is sufficient reason for immediate termination of an employee. Because it is such a critical aspect of patient care, it is considered highly unethical to reveal any information about a patient to anyone else. All medical assistants are required and expected to uphold the confidentiality of the information with which they come into contact.

9. Discuss several of the CEJA opinions and how they might differ from the views of the class as a whole.
   - The opinions put forth by CEJA are just one group of opinions. Class members may share very differing views based on culture, past experience, or serious consideration of the issues. Each individual is entitled to have an opinion, and these opinions should be discussed and shared calmly and respectfully.

CONNECTIONS

 Study Guide Connection: Go to Chapter 6 Study Guide. Read the Case Study and Workplace Applications and complete the assignments. Do online research for answers to the questions in the Internet Activities associated with medicine and ethics.

 CD Connection: Go to the Medical Assisting Competency Challenge CD and do the training activities under Legal Concepts.

evolve **Evolve Connection:** For more information related to medicine and ethics, go to http://evolve.elsevier.com/kinn/admin and visit related weblinks for Chapter 6. Click on the Medical Assisting Exam Review and do the practice questions to sharpen your test-taking skills.

Medicine and Law

7

SCENARIO

Barbara Johnson is the new office manager for two neurologists in an urban area. Recently she was subpoenaed to appear in court with medical records to testify about a patient. This particular patient was referred to one of the physicians in the clinic, Dr. Rebecca Patrick. Dr. Patrick saw the patient several years ago, and the patient has brought a medical professional liability case against a surgeon in another city. Barbara is considered the custodian of medical records and will take them to court and answer questions about the information contained within them.

One of Barbara's first priorities at her new job is to make certain that the office is operating in compliance with the legal regulations that affect the facility. She is knowledgeable about OSHA requirements, and because her father was an attorney, she is very familiar with legal issues.

Two of the employees Barbara supervises, Samantha and Lynda, are newly graduated from medical assisting school and are anxious to learn more about the statutes and laws that affect the physicians' office. Barbara is more than happy to share what she has learned with them. She is excited about her new job and eager to be a great success.

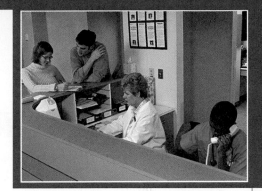

While studying this chapter, think about the following questions:

- How can the medical assistant help to comply with legal regulations in the medical office?
- How can new graduates learn about the laws that affect them in their state?
- What are some ways that medical professional liability suits can be avoided?
- What should the medical assistant do if the employer is not in compliance with legal regulations?

LEARNING OBJECTIVES

1. Define, spell, and pronounce the terms listed in the vocabulary.
2. Distinguish among an act, a statute, and an ordinance.
3. Know the two types of law.
4. Explain the three basic categories of criminal law.
5. Distinguish which type of civil law deals with medical professional liability.
6. Explain the four essential elements needed for a valid contract.
7. Distinguish between interrogatories and depositions.
8. List three things to remember when testifying in court.
9. Discuss the advantages of arbitration.
10. Differentiate among malfeasance, misfeasance, and nonfeasance.
11. Explain the "four D's" of negligence.
12. Define the types of damages.
13. Explain the importance of informed consent.
14. List several legal disclosures the physician must make.
15. Explain the importance of the Health Insurance Portability and Accountability Act.
16. Distinguish between OSHA and CLIA, explaining which of the two is an actual agency.
17. Discuss the three ways in which a physician can obtain a license to practice medicine.
18. Discuss the ways that a physician might lose a license to practice medicine.

National Accreditation Competencies and Content

CAAHEP COMPETENCIES

General
3.c.(2)(a). Identify and respond to issues of confidentiality
3.c.(2)(b). Perform within legal and ethical boundaries
3.c.(2)(d). Document accurately
3.c.(2)(e). Demonstrate knowledge of federal and state health care legislation and regulations

ABHES COMPETENCIES

Legal Concepts
5.a. Determine needs for documentation and reporting
5.b. Document accurately
5.c. Use appropriate guidelines when releasing records or information
5.d. Follow established policy in initiating or terminating medical treatment
5.e. Dispose of controlled substances in compliance with government regulations
5.f. Maintain licenses and accreditation
5.g. Monitor legislation related to current healthcare issues and practices

Office Management
6.e. Maintain liability coverage

VOCABULARY

abandonment To withdraw protection or support; in medicine, to discontinue medical care without proper notice after accepting a patient.

act The formal action of a legislative body; a decision or determination of a sovereign state, a legislative council, or a court of justice.

allegation (a-li-ga'-shun) A statement by a party to a legal action of what the party undertakes to prove; an assertion made without proof.

appeal A legal proceeding by which a case is brought before a higher court for review of the decision of a lower court.

appellate (uh-pe'-lut) Having the power to review the judgment of another tribunal or body of jurisdiction, such as an appellate court.

arbitration (ar-buh-tra'-shun) The hearing and determination of a cause in controversy by a person or persons either chosen by the parties involved or appointed under statutory authority.

arbitrator (ar-buh-tra'-ter) A neutral person chosen to settle differences between two parties in a controversy.

assault An intentional, unlawful attempt of bodily injury to another by force.

assent To agree to something, especially after thoughtful consideration.

bailiff An officer of some U.S. courts usually serving as a messenger or usher, who keeps order at the request of the judge.

battery A willful and unlawful use of force or violence on the person of another.

Code of Federal Regulations (CFR) A coded delineation of the rules and regulations published in the *Federal Register* by the various departments and agencies of the federal government. The CFR is divided into 50 titles that represent broad subject areas, and then chapters that provide specific detail.

concurrently Occurring at the same time.

contributory negligence Statutes in some states that may prevent a party from recovering some damages if he or she contributed in any way to the injury or condition.

damages Loss or harm resulting from injury to person, property, or reputation; compensation in money imposed by law for losses or injuries.

decedent (di-se'-dent) A legal term for a deceased person.

defendant A person required to make answer in a legal action or suit; in criminal cases, the person accused of a crime.

docket A formal record of judicial proceedings; a list of legal cases to be tried.

due process A fundamental constitutional guarantee that all legal proceedings will be fair; that one will be given notice of the proceedings and given an opportunity to be heard before the government acts to take away life, liberty, or property; a constitutional guarantee that a law will not be unreasonable or arbitrary.

emancipated minor A person under legal age who is self-supporting and living apart from parents or guardian; a mature minor considered by the courts to possess a sufficient understanding of self-care and responsibility.

expert witnesses People who provide testimony to a court as experts in certain fields or subjects to verify facts presented by one or both sides in a lawsuit, often compensated and used to refute or disprove the claims of one party.

felony A major crime, such as murder, rape, or burglary; punishable by a more stringent sentence than that given for a misdemeanor.

fine A sum imposed as punishment for an offense; a forfeiture or penalty paid to an injured party or the government in a civil or criminal action.

guardian ad litem Legal representative for a minor.

implied consent Presumed consent, such as when a patient offers an arm for a phlebotomy procedure.

informed consent A consent, usually written, which states understanding of what treatment is to be undertaken and of the risks involved, why it should be done, and alternative methods of treatment available (including no treatment) and their attendant risks.

List continues on next page

List continued from previous page

infractions (in-frak'-shuns) Breaking the law; minor offenses against the rules, usually punishable by fines.

judicial (ju-di'-shuhl) Of or relating to a judgment, the function of judging, the administration of justice, or the judiciary.

jurisdiction (jur-uhs-dik'-shun) A power constitutionally conferred on a judge or magistrate to decide cases according to law and to carry sentence into execution; jurisdiction is original when it is conferred on the court in the first instance, called *original jurisdiction;* or it is appellate when an appeal is given from the judgment of another court.

jurisprudence (jur-uhs-proo'-dens) The science or philosophy of law; a system or body of law or the course of court decisions.

law A binding custom or practice of a community; a rule of conduct or action prescribed or formally recognized as binding or enforceable by a controlling authority.

liable (li'-uh-buhl) Obligated according to law or equity; responsible for an act or circumstance.

libel A written defamatory statement or representation that conveys an unjustly unfavorable impression.

litigious (luh-ti'-juhs) Prone to engage in lawsuits.

manifestation (ma-nuh-fuh-sta'-shun) Something that is easily understood or recognized by the mind.

misdemeanor (mis-duh-me'-nuhr) A minor crime, as opposed to a felony, punishable by fine or imprisonment in a city or county jail rather than in a penitentiary.

municipal (myu-ni'-suh-puhl) **courts** Courts that sit in some cities and larger towns and that usually have civil and criminal jurisdiction over cases arising within the municipality.

negligence (ne'-gli-jents) Failure to exercise the care that a prudent person usually exercises; implies inattention to one's duty or business; implies want of due or necessary diligence or care.

ordinance (or'-di-nens) Authoritative decree or direction; law set forth by a governmental authority–specifically, municipal regulation.

other potentially infectious materials (OPIM) Substances or materials other than blood that have the potential to carry infectious pathogens, such as body fluid, urine, semen, and others.

paraphrased Restated; applies to restatement of text, passage, or work to convey the meaning in another form.

perjured testimony The voluntary violation of an oath or vow either by swearing to what is untrue or by omission to do what has been promised under oath; false testimony.

physician office laboratories (POLs) Laboratories owned by a private physician or corporation, such as the laboratory inside a physician's office or a freestanding laboratory.

plaintiff The person or group bringing a case or legal action to court.

precedence (pre-sed'-ens) To surpass in rank, dignity, or importance; to be, go, or come ahead or in front of.

precedents (pre'-suh-dens) A person or thing that serves as a model; something done or said that may serve as an example or rule to authorize or justify a subsequent act of the same kind.

preponderance of the evidence Evidence that is of greater weight or more convincing than the evidence offered in opposition to it; evidence that as a whole shows that the fact sought to be proven is more probable than not.

prudent Marked by wisdom or judiciousness; shrewd in the management of practical affairs.

quackery The pretense of curing disease.

reasonable doubt Doubt based on reason and arising from evidence or lack of evidence; it is not doubt that is imagined or conjured up, but doubt that would cause reasonable persons to hesitate before acting.

recourse A turning to something or someone for help or protection.

relevant Having significant and demonstrable bearing on the matter at hand.

respondent (ri-spahn'-dunt) The person required to make answer in a civil legal action or suit; similar to a defendant in a criminal trial.

slander Oral defamation; a harmful, false statement made about another person.

statutes (sta'-choots) Laws enacted by the legislative branch of a government.

stipulate To specify as a condition or requirement of an agreement or offer; to make an agreement or covenant to do or forbear from doing something.

subpoena (suh-pe'-nuh) A writ or document commanding a person to appear in court under a penalty for failure to appear.

subpoena duces tecum A legally binding request to appear in court and provide records or documents that pertain to a particular case.

testimony A solemn declaration usually made orally by a witness under oath in response to interrogation by a lawyer or authorized public official.

Uniform Commercial Code (UCC) A unified set of rules covering many business transactions; it has been adopted in all 50 states, the District of Columbia, and most U.S. territories. It regulates the fields of sales of goods; commercial paper, such as checks; secured transactions in personal property; and particular aspects of banking, letters of credit, warehouse receipts, bills of lading, and investment securities.

verdict The finding or decision of a jury on a matter submitted to it in trial.

Law is a fascinating subject. When law is applied to medicine, it can provoke interesting case studies and complex decisions. In today's **litigious** society, medical assistants, as well as physicians and other staff members, must take steps to protect themselves from lawsuits. Legal issues underlie many aspects of the provision of healthcare in a physician's office. Although the wording of **statutes** and regulations is often long and complicated, medical assistants must stay abreast of the rules governing medical facilities and do everything possible to remain in compliance with the standards and regulations for all organizations that oversee the medical industry.

Generally, the law holds that every person is **liable** for the consequences of his or her own **negligence** when another person is injured as a result. In some situations this liability also extends to the employer. Physicians may be held responsible for the mistakes of those who work in their healthcare facility, and sometimes they must pay **damages** for the negligent acts of their employees.

Under the doctrine of respondeat superior, physicians are legally responsible for the acts of their employees when the employees are acting within the scope of their duties or employment. Physicians are also responsible for the acts of assistants who are not their own employees if the assistant commits acts of negligence in the presence of the physician while under the physician's immediate supervision. *Respondeat superior* is a Latin term meaning "let the master answer." When physicians practice as partners, they are liable not only for their own acts and those of their partners, but also for the negligent acts of any agent or employee of the partnership. A medical assistant acting within the scope of the employment contract is considered an agent of the employer.

Medical assistants who are guilty of negligence are liable for their own actions, but the injured party generally sues the physician, because the chance of collecting damages is greater. However, even an assistant who has no money can still be liable for any negligent action. This fact illustrates the continuing importance of exercising extreme care in performing all duties in the professional office.

JURISPRUDENCE AND THE CLASSIFICATIONS OF LAW

Jurisprudence, the science and philosophy of law, comes from the Latin words *juris*, which means "law, right, equity, or justice," and *prudentia*, which means "skill or good judgment."

Law is a custom or practice of a community. It is a rule of conduct or action prescribed or formally recognized as binding or enforceable by a controlling authority. Law is the system by which society gives order to our lives. The U.S. Constitution is the supreme law of the land, which takes **precedence** over federal statutes, court opinions, and state constitutions. However, within the states the state constitution is the supreme law within the boundaries of that state, unless it conflicts with the U.S. Constitution. States cannot pass laws that conflict with the U.S. Constitution, nor can local governments pass laws that conflict with the state constitution.

A law enacted at the federal level, which must be passed by Congress, is called an **act.** Statutes are laws that have been enacted by state legislatures. Local governments create and enact **ordinances.** Much of our law is based on previous **judicial** and jury decisions, which are called **precedents.** Often judges and juries follow precedents when making a decision on a case before them. The two basic categories of jurisprudence are criminal law and civil law.

Criminal Law

Criminal law governs violations of the law that are punishable as offenses against the state or the government. Such offenses involve the welfare and safety of the public as a whole rather than of one individual. Criminal offenses are classified into three basic categories: misdemeanors, felonies, and treason. In order to ensure fair treatment under the law, all physicians are entitled to **due process,** which guarantees that the accused will have an opportunity to defend himself or herself against any charges brought in opposition.

Misdemeanors

A minor crime, as opposed to a **felony,** is called a **misdemeanor.** Such a crime is punishable by **fine** or imprisonment in a city or county jail rather than in a penitentiary. Misdemeanors vary from state to state and are often divided into subgroups or classes, such as class A, class B, or class C misdemeanors. In most states the subgroups are divided from most serious offenses to lesser offenses. Some states have created a subcategory of misdemeanors for **infractions,** which are often called *violations*. Infractions are minor offenses, such as traffic tickets, which are punishable only by a fine.

Felonies

A felony is a major crime, such as murder, rape, or burglary, and is punishable by a more stringent sentence than that given for a misdemeanor. Federal law and most state statutes classify felonies as crimes punishable by imprisonment for more than 1 year, whereas misdemeanors are punishable by imprisonment for 1 year or less. Usually a convicted felon cannot vote, hold public office, or possess a firearm. Felonies are often divided into subgroups or degrees, such as first degree, second degree, and third degree. The first-degree offense is normally the most serious.

Treason

Treason, the most serious crime, is the offense of attempting to overthrow the government. High treason constitutes a serious threat to the stability or continuity of the government, such as an attempt to kill the president. The President of the United States has the right to declare an action against the United States to be an act of war, as opposed to an act of treason, which is considered a crime. For instance, although the terrorist attacks of September 11, 2001, were certainly a threat against the United States, they were declared acts of war.

Civil Law

Civil law is concerned with acts that are not criminal in nature but involve relationships of individuals with other individuals, organizations, or government agencies. Many types of civil law address numerous issues. The three that most directly affect the medical profession include tort law, contract law, and administrative law.

Tort Law

Tort law provides a remedy for a person or group that has suffered harm from the wrongful acts of others. Four elements must be established in every tort action. First, the **plaintiff** must establish that the **respondent** or **defendant** was under a legal duty to act in a particular fashion. Second, the plaintiff must demonstrate that the defendant breached this duty by failing to conform his or her behavior accordingly. Third, the plaintiff must prove that the breach of the legal duty proximately caused some injury or damage. Fourth, the plaintiff must prove damages, the injury or loss suffered. Medical professional liability, or medical malpractice, falls into the category of tort law. **Libel** and **slander** are common complaints that fall into the category of tort law.

Contract Law

A contract is an agreement creating an obligation. Contract law touches our lives in many ways practically every day, but we usually do not give much thought to its influences. If a person parks a car in a parking garage for a monthly fee and signs a contract for a year, then begins parking elsewhere and refuses to pay the fee, the person may be liable for the fees for the duration of the entire contract. If damage occurs to the person's vehicle while it is parked in the garage, the garage may be responsible for reimbursement, if the contract does not **stipulate** otherwise. A contract does not have to be formalized in writing to be binding on the parties involved. Oral contracts are also valid in many states in most situations. The **Uniform Commercial Code** is a long, elaborate act that attempts to harmonize the law of sales and other commercial transactions in all 50 states. This code directly affects contract law.

Administrative Law

Administrative law involves regulations set forth by governmental agencies. For example, the Internal Revenue Service (IRS) has thousands of regulations and codes, and the typical American does not understand all of them, which may result in errors when filing taxes. The laws that allow the IRS to collect taxes and pursue restitution are administrative laws. Other agencies that are involved with administrative law include the Social Security Administration (SSA), Citizenship and Immigration Services (USCIS), and the Centers for Medicare and Medicaid Services (CMS).

ANATOMY OF A MEDICAL PROFESSIONAL LIABILITY LAWSUIT

A medical liability case often stems from a breach of trust or miscommunication between the physician and the patient. These cases fall into the category of tort law. Even when the physician has made an error, often the level of trust between the physician and patient will determine whether a lawsuit

will be pursued. First, the physician-patient relationship must be formed. Before discussing this relationship, it is important to understand what is necessary for a contract to be valid and enforceable.

What Constitutes a Valid Contract?

A valid legal contract has four essential elements. First, there must be **manifestation** of **assent** or a "meeting of the minds." This element is proven by an "offer" and the "acceptance" of that offer. The parties to the contract must understand and agree on the intent of the contract. Second, the contract must involve legal subject matter. An obligation that requires an illegal action, such as a gambling contract, is not an enforceable contract. Third, both parties must have the legal capacity to enter into a contract. This means that each party must be an adult of sound mind or an **emancipated minor.** Fourth, some type of consideration must be present. Consideration is an exchange of something of value, for example, money for the physician's time.

CRITICAL THINKING APPLICATION

Barbara works for Dr. Rebecca Patrick, who saw the patient bringing the lawsuit against the surgeon as a referral patient. Does Dr. Patrick have a contract with the patient, based on a physician-patient relationship? Why or why not?

The physician-patient relationship is generally held by courts to be a contractual relationship that is the result of three steps:
- The physician invites an offer by establishing availability.
- The patient accepts the invitation and makes an offer by arriving for or requesting treatment.
- The physician accepts the offer by accepting the patient and undertaking treatment. The physician may explicitly accept the patient's offer or implicitly accept the offer by exercising their independent medical judgment on behalf of the patient.

Before accepting a patient, the physician is under no obligation, and no contract exists. However, once the physician has accepted the patient, an implied contract does exist (Figure 7-1). This implied contract assumes that the physician will

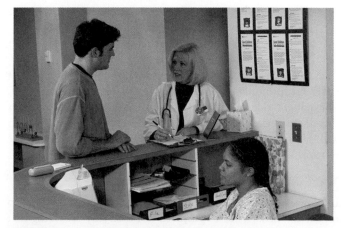

FIGURE 7-1 The physician-patient relationship is built on a strong foundation of trust, but it is also a contractual relationship.

treat the patient using reasonable care and that the physician possesses a degree of knowledge, skill, and judgment that might be expected of any other physician in the same locality and under similar circumstances. It is extremely important that no express promise of a cure be made by anyone in the office, including the physician, because this would become a part of the contract.

The patient's responsibility in this agreement includes the liability of payment for services and a willingness to follow the advice of the physician. Most physician-patient contracts are implied contracts. Although many forms may be completed by the patient before he or she is accepted by the physician, they do not in most cases constitute a formal contract for each specific visit to the physician.

CRITICAL THINKING APPLICATION

- If the patient does not pay for the services rendered by the physician, does this negate the physician-patient contract?
- How might Barbara, Samantha, and Lynda ensure that patients understand that they are expected to follow the advice of the physician?

After the physician-patient relationship has been established, the physician is obligated to attend the patient as long as attention is required, unless the physician or patient terminates the contract. When a physician terminates the contract, the patient must be given notice of the physician's intentions so that the patient has sufficient time to secure another physician. The physician may write a letter of withdrawal from medical care of the patient, and it should be delivered by certified mail, return receipt requested. A copy of the letter and the return receipt should be attached to the patient's chart and permanently retained. Reasonable time should be allowed for the patient to secure other medical care.

To protect the physician against a lawsuit for **abandonment,** the details of the circumstances under which the physician is withdrawing from the case should be included in the patient's medical chart. The letter of withdrawal does not have to specify a reason for withdrawal unless the physician so chooses, but it should state the following:

- That professional care is being discontinued
- That the physician will provide copies of the patient's records to another physician on request
- That the patient should seek the attention of another physician as soon as possible

A patient who wishes to terminate the physician-patient relationship simply no longer seeks the physician for treatment. The patient does not have to inform the office; however, if this is done, the office manager or physician should follow up with a letter confirming notice that the patient has ended the relationship.

The Statute of Frauds

In 1677 a statute was adopted in England that was designed to reduce the occurrence of **perjured testimony** by providing that certain contracts could not be enforced if they depended on the **testimony** of witnesses alone and were not evidenced in writing.

The provisions of this English statute have been closely followed by statutes adopted in all 50 states in the United States.

The promise to pay the debts of another person is an example of a contract that usually must be made in writing. If a third party who is not otherwise legally responsible for a patient's medical bills agrees to pay them, the agreement cannot be enforced unless it is in writing. If a physician were to enter into an agreement to perform a series of treatments for a given sum, and this series covered a time span of more than 1 year, the contract would have to be in writing to be enforceable.

Preliminaries of Litigation

Once a patient has decided to file a lawsuit against a physician, the first step is usually to find an attorney who will accept the case. This may be a frustration to many patients: attorneys may not wish to initiate litigation against a physician. Like physicians, attorneys do not have to accept cases they do not wish to pursue; this often occurs because the attorney does not see enough of a financial benefit from the time it would take to work on the case. Although this sounds a bit harsh, the attorney runs a business, as does a physician, and must make good business decisions as to how his or her time is spent and invested.

CRITICAL THINKING APPLICATION

- For what reasons might a physician not wish to accept a patient?
- Must the physician treat every patient who attempts to make an appointment?
- How might Barbara tactfully explain that the physician will not accept the patient into treatment?

Lawsuits are filed in a variety of different courts, and different states have different types of courts at various levels. The state judiciary has several branches. At the local level are usually **municipal courts.** These are courts in a city or town that usually deal with ordinance violations. Municipal judges may issue search and arrest warrants. Some states also have justice of the peace courts, which have **jurisdiction** over many misdemeanors and some civil matters, as well as concurrent jurisdiction over some matters along with the municipal courts. The judges that preside over justice of the peace courts may also issue search warrants and arrest warrants. They often function as small claims courts, with which the medical assistant may have contact in cases of patients who do not pay their bills. Both municipal and justice of the peace courts are local trial courts with limited jurisdiction.

County courts are higher than municipal and justice of the peace courts. These courts handle misdemeanors and civil matters up to a certain monetary limit. District courts have unlimited jurisdiction in criminal and civil matters. They are the highest state courts, other than **appellate** courts. When one party of a lawsuit is dissatisfied with a lower court's decision, it has the right to **appeal** to a higher court for review and possible reversal of the decision. Most states have an appellate court for both criminal and civil matters. The U.S. District Court handles federal matters of both a criminal and a civil nature. States

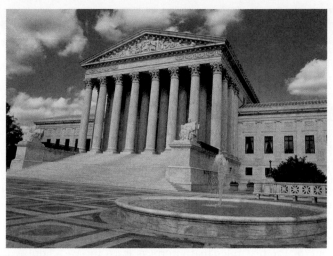

FIGURE 7-2 The U.S. Supreme Court. The Supreme Court decides cases that involve interpretation of the Constitution of the United States.

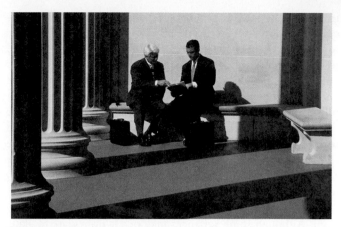

FIGURE 7-3 Preparation is of primary importance to the physician facing a medical professional liability case. A competent and experienced attorney is necessary to provide an adequate defense and present the physician's views to the court. Always be completely honest with the representing attorney.

also have Supreme Courts that handle a limited number of appellate cases.

The U.S. Supreme Court has authority given by Article III, Section One of the Constitution to ensure equal justice under the law (Figure 7-2). The Supreme Court interprets and guards the Constitution. The Court's one Chief Justice and eight Associate Justices are appointed by the President and confirmed by the Congress. The current Chief Justice of the Supreme Court is the Honorable John G. Roberts, Jr., who was appointed by President George W. Bush and confirmed by the U.S. Senate in 2005. The other Justices include Justice John Paul Stevens, Justice Antonin Scalia, Justice Anthony M. Kennedy, Justice David H. Souter, Justice Clarence Thomas, Justice Ruth Bader Ginsburg, Justice Stephen G. Breyer, and Justice Samuel Anthony Alito, Jr. Justice Sandra Day O'Connor, the first woman appointed to be a Supreme Court Justice, retired in 2005. Approximately 8000 cases are on the **docket** per term, which runs from the first Monday in October to the first Monday of October in the next year. Only 80 to 90 cases are chosen each year for full oral argument in front of the Justices.

CRITICAL THINKING APPLICATION

Samantha and Lynda are curious as to how Supreme Court decisions affect the individual physician's office. What Supreme Court decisions have affected the medical profession?

Preparing for Court

Medical professional liability suits are far from rare, and every physician faces the probability of being sued at least once during his or her career. When a suit is filed, preparation for court should start expeditiously. A medical assistant may be involved in preparing materials for court and scheduling or participating in depositions. The best advice for a medical assistant in this position is to remember to tell the truth. Attorneys will help to prepare the defense of the physician and the staff, but everyone should be truthful in the answers that are

given to the court to avoid losing his or her credibility in the trial and to avoid charges of perjury. Be especially careful to present a true and complete statement to the representing attorney. Unless he or she knows the whole truth, an appropriate defense cannot be prepared (Figure 7-3).

Interrogatories

Before the trial, the physician may be requested to complete an interrogatory, which is a list of questions from each party to the other in the lawsuit. Answers to the interrogatory must be provided within a specified time, and the answers are considered to be given under oath. Only the parties named in the lawsuit may be questioned through interrogatories.

Depositions

A deposition is testimony taken from a party or witness to the litigation and is not limited to the parties named in the lawsuit. A witness who is not a party to the lawsuit may be summoned by **subpoena** for the deposition. The deposition is usually taken in an attorney's office in the presence of a court reporter and is taken under oath. The person giving the deposition is called the *deponent*. The transcribed deposition, once finished, is sent to the deponent for review, and the deponent is at liberty to request any necessary changes or corrections in the document.

CRITICAL THINKING APPLICATION

■ Samantha and Lynda are anxious to hear about Barbara's experiences in testifying in court. She mentions that attorneys often advise witnesses to "answer the question, then be quiet." What might be meant by this advice?

■ Discuss the phrase, "the truth, the whole truth, and nothing but the truth."

Subpoenas

A subpoena is a document issued by a court requiring a person to be in court at a specific time and place to testify as a witness in a lawsuit, either in a court proceeding or in a deposition. A **subpoena duces tecum** is a legally binding request to provide records or documents to appear in court and is usually issued to the person considered the custodian of the records. This may be the medical assistant or office manager. A fee may be demanded for the time spent in compiling the records and for photocopying charges, but this fee must be requested at the time the subpoena duces tecum is served, or it is considered to be waived. Physician approval must be obtained to release or copy any patient records. Original records should never be released under any circumstances. Release only the information requested in the subpoena.

Before responding to a subpoena, make certain that it is valid. Although some variances may occur from state to state, some general rules can be used to judge the validity of a subpoena:

- A subpoena issued in one state court is generally not valid in another state. Always verify the state in which the subpoena was issued.
- A subpoena issued by a federal court in one state is generally not valid in another state unless a federal statute authorizes nationwide service of process.
- Any duly authorized law officer may execute a valid subpoena anywhere in the same state. The officer will notify the issuing court once the subpoena has been served.
- Generally, the person or entity who is issued a subpoena has 21 days to respond to the subpoena, but this time period can differ from place to place.
- A subpoena duces tecum should be filed no less than 15 days before a trial. One served less than 15 days before a trial should not be honored.

Read the subpoena carefully to determine exactly what records are being requested. The physician should always be notified of subpoenas served to the medical facility. Never copy records required in a subpoena without bringing the matter to the attention of the physician and/or office manager. It is also advisable to keep a log of subpoenas served to the office, what records were involved, and the disposition of the request, including when the records were presented to the court.

Discovery

Discovery is the pretrial disclosure of pertinent facts or documents by one or both parties to a legal action or proceeding. Many states have extensive discovery statutes that require each side to reveal to the other the facts that they "discover" while investigating the case. Discovery is also considered the process of uncovering facts in a lawsuit before the court proceedings.

Presentation of evidence may be by testimony. A witness is called who has some information about an aspect of the case and is asked questions by one or both attorneys. The witness will not know about every part of the case, but something that the person knows will be **relevant** to the case.

Another type of evidence may be documentary evidence. This is any type of evidence brought before the court by document or display. It could be a patient's chart, or a letter, a laboratory result, or a photograph. All of these are usually entered into evidence and numbered for easy reference.

CRITICAL THINKING APPLICATION

Samantha wonders what she should do if she ever finds negative information during a medical professional malpractice case that might harm her employer's defense. What advice would you offer? Would it be considered an obligation or a choice to report the employer of wrongdoing?

Preparing Witnesses and Testifying

Attorneys will prepare witnesses who may be called to testify during the court proceedings. They will review the questions that will be asked and potential questions that the opposite side may present. The attorney will help the witness to clarify the answers that he or she gives so that they are sharp and succinct. One of the first rules that attorneys learn in law school is to never ask a question to which they do not already know the answer.

Witnesses should be certain that they know the exact location of the courthouse and to which floor and courtroom they are to report. They should always be on time for a court appearance, because the judge and jury may frown on those appearing late. That frown may also include a fine or confinement in jail for contempt of court! When called to testify, it is critical that the witness dress conservatively and in a manner that shows respect for the court. Normal business attire should be adequate, but if any doubt is present, consult the attorney.

If any documents are to be referenced while testifying, the witness should review the documents before the court appearance if possible, so that the needed information will be easy to locate and discuss. The witness should speak clearly and at a volume audible to the attorneys and parties to the suit, the judge, the jury, and the court reporter. The witness should always answer each question aloud, because the court reporter must record those answers and cannot specify that the witness "nodded yes" as a response to a question.

If a question is confusing, the witness should ask the attorney to restate or repeat it. Attorneys may ask the witness to speak up, but this should not be intimidating to the witness. If the witness does not know the answer to a question or does not recall, that should be stated clearly and confidently. Above all, the parties involved are expected to tell the truth and must be seen as credible witnesses (Figure 7-4). Lying under oath constitutes perjury, which carries stiff penalties. Listening is as important as speaking, so the witness should be sure to listen to the question, and answer it, elaborating only if the attorney asks for more details.

If an attorney lodges an objection to a question, the witness should be silent until the judge rules on the objection. The objection may be sustained or overruled. Sustaining the objection means that the judge agrees with the objection and will not allow the question stated in that manner. If the judge allows the question, he or she will overrule the objection. Then the witness will be allowed to answer. The witness should never display a combative or hostile attitude and should not make sarcastic remarks while testifying in court. This is the fastest way to show disrespect for the judge, the jurors, and the court itself. No

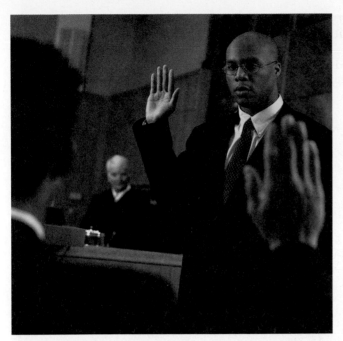

FIGURE 7-4 Witnesses must be credible and tell the truth on the stand in court to avoid charges of perjury.

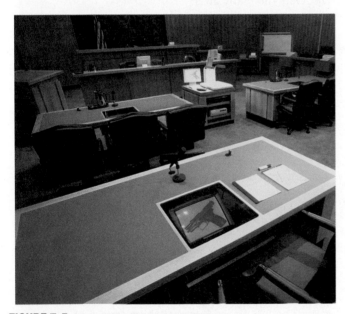

FIGURE 7-5 The inside of a typical U.S. courtroom.

matter the circumstances, the court is no place to express discontent. The witness should be professional at all times and restrain inappropriate comments and belligerent behavior. Using "yes, sir" and "no, ma'am" is appropriate in the courtroom. Always address the judge as "Your Honor."

Inside the Courtroom

Today's courtrooms are a far cry from the ones depicted on television shows representing the old west. Modern courtrooms are equipped with computer and video equipment, and elaborate security systems often monitor those who enter the building (Figure 7-5). The advent of Court TV has changed the way Americans see the justice system. By simply turning on our televisions, we can watch justice at work.

It is beneficial to know the role of each person in a court of law. The person or body bringing the lawsuit to court is referred to by different terms, depending on what type of case is to be presented. In a criminal court, the government brings the case and is represented by a prosecutor. Legal documents will read, for example, "The State of Texas v. Robert Smith" in criminal cases. In this case, the fictitious Robert Smith is the defendant. In civil court, the person or group bringing the case to court is called the *plaintiff* (or *complainant* in some court systems), and the opposite party is called the *defendant* or *respondent*. A judge will preside over the case, providing instructions concerning the law to the jury, if a jury is present. If no jury is present, the judge decides the case. This is called a "bench trial." A witness is a person who gives testimony, knowing some pertinent information about the case (Figure 7-6). Often a court reporter takes notes of the proceedings, and a **bailiff** may be present, who assists in keeping order. All of these individuals should be treated with respect and courtesy.

Burden of Proof

In a criminal case the burden of proof is on the prosecution, which must prove guilt beyond any **reasonable doubt.** Reasonable doubt is defined as the level of certainty a juror must have to find a defendant guilty of a crime. It is real doubt, based on reason and common sense after careful and impartial consideration of all the evidence, or lack of evidence, in a case.

Civil cases must be proven by a **preponderance of the evidence.** This means that there must be a greater weight of evidence that points to the defendant or respondent as being responsible for the act involved in the case.

To understand the difference between reasonable doubt and preponderance of the evidence, think of the scales of justice (Figure 7-7). For a case to be proven beyond a reasonable doubt, the scales should tip heavily toward either guilt or innocence. However, for a case to be proven by preponderance of the evidence, the scales need only tip slightly one way or the other.

To illustrate the difference in the burden of proof in criminal and civil cases, consider "The People of the State of California v. Orenthal James Simpson." In O.J. Simpson's criminal trial, although there was much circumstantial evidence, there was also enough doubt that the scales could not tip heavily toward a **verdict** of guilty, and Mr. Simpson was acquitted. But in the civil trial brought by family members of Nicole Brown Simpson and Ron Goldman after the criminal trial had ended, there was just enough evidence to tip the scales in favor of the families' claim that Mr. Simpson was somehow responsible for the deaths of the two victims. This is the equivalent of a preponderance of the evidence.

CRITICAL THINKING APPLICATION

A discussion of the burden of proof prompts Barbara, Samantha, and Lynda to discuss the case of O.J. Simpson. Discuss whether reasonable doubt existed in his criminal trial.

HUMOR IN THE COURTROOM

Mary Louise Gilman has very possibly heard it all. As the editor of the *National Shorthand Reporter*, she collected enough courtroom bloopers to fill two books: "*Humor in the Court*" and "*More Humor in the Court.*" Here are a few examples!

Q: Were you acquainted with the deceased?
A: *Yes, Sir.*
Q: Before or after he died?

Q: What happened then?
A: *He told me, he says, "I have to kill you because you can identify me."*
Q: Did he kill you?
A: *No.*

Q: When he went, had you gone and had she, if she wanted to and were able, for the time being excluding all the restraints on her not to go, gone also, would he have brought you, meaning you and she, with him to the station?
A: *Objection. That question should be taken out and shot.*

Q: And lastly, Gary, all your responses must be oral. O.K.? What school do you go to?
A: *Oral.*
Q: How old are you?
A: *Oral.*

Q: ...and what did he do then?
A: *He came home, and next morning he was dead.*
Q: So when he woke up the next morning he was dead?

Q: ...any suggestions as to what prevented this from being a murder trial instead of an attempted murder trial?
A: *The victim lived.*

Q: What is your date of birth?
A: *July fifteenth.*
Q: What year?
A: *Every year.*

Q: This myasthenia gravis–does it affect your memory at all?
A: *Yes.*
Q: And in what ways does it affect your memory?
A: *I forget.*
Q: Can you give me an example of something you've forgotten?

Q: What was the first thing your husband said to you when he woke that morning?
A: *He said, "Where am I, Cathy?"*
Q: And why did that upset you?
A: *My name is Susan.*

Q: She had three children, correct?
A: *Yes.*
Q: How many were boys?
A: *None.*
Q: Were there any girls?

Q: Doctor, before you performed the autopsy, did you check for a pulse?
A: *No.*
Q: Did you check for a blood pressure?
A: *No.*
Q: Did you check for breathing?
A: *No.*
Q: So, then it is possible that the patient was alive when you began the autopsy?
A: *No.*
Q: How can you be sure, Doctor?
A: *Because his brain was sitting on my desk in a jar.*
Q: But could the patient have still been alive nevertheless?
A: *Yes, it is possible that he could have been alive and practicing law somewhere.*

FIGURE 7-6 Humor in the courtroom. (From Gilman M, editor: *More humor in the court*, Vienna, Va, 1985, National Shorthand Reporters Association.)

Outcome of the Case

Once both sides have presented their case to the judge or jury, they are usually given the opportunity to present a final summation of their case. After this is done, the jury retires to consider the verdict. This can take minutes, hours, days, or weeks. After the jury reaches a decision, the judge may enter it as a final verdict or may disregard it if the evidence does not support the jury's decision. The judge may also revise the verdict to comply with statutes, such as statutory limits on the amount of punitive damages. The final decision of the trial court is reflected in the judgment, signed by the judge.

Either side normally has the right to appeal the decision to a higher court. However, not all appellate courts are required to hear all cases. For instance, the U.S. Supreme Court chooses the cases that it hears each year, and it is restricted to cases that involve interpretation of the Constitution and how that interpretation affects the people it governs.

In criminal cases when a person is found guilty of the crime with which he or she is charged, a sentencing date will be set, usually a few weeks to a few months after the verdict is announced, at which time the punishment will be announced.

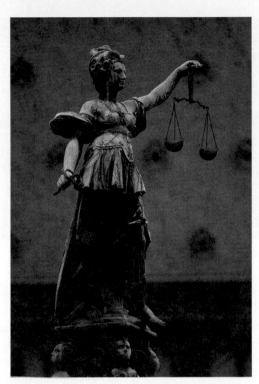

FIGURE 7-7 "Lady Justice." Justitia was the Roman goddess of justice and is the figure depicted in statues across the world, often holding both scales and a sword. Her scales imply the weighing of justice, and the blindfold represents the impartiality of justice.

ARBITRATION

Arbitration is an alternative to trial that uses a third party who has been selected because of the party's familiarity with or knowledge of the law or the issues involved to hear evidence and make a decision. Arbitration is common in modern business life. It is recognized by statute in the majority of the states and is usually available to the medical profession, affording an alternative method for resolving legal disputes between physician and patient. Many physicians and attorneys see arbitration as one way to solve the crisis of litigation in this country. Court battles can take years and can be extremely expensive, and much of the money will revert to the attorneys involved in the case instead of the victors of the lawsuit.

In arbitration the patient and the physician agree to submit the dispute to an **arbitrator** in an informal hearing. The arbitrator will render a legally binding decision based on very specific rules of arbitration. Arbitration applies essentially the same rights and the same measure of damages as a court. It is fair, less expensive, faster, and more confidential than court litigation.

The staff of each medical office should know whether arbitration statutes exist in the state where the office conducts business. The state medical board or local medical society should be able to provide this information. An arbitration agreement is a contract and is subject to the judgment of the courts only as to the fairness of the agreement. The agreement is precisely worded by an attorney and should not be **paraphrased** when explaining it to a patient. Signing the agreement is a voluntary

act by the patient, who has a grace period in which to revoke the agreement if he or she later decides against it. Likewise, a physician always has the option to decide not to care for a patient but must formally notify a patient if the decision is made to no longer render care.

If a physician elects to implement an arbitration agreement procedure with patients, every member of the physician's staff should know the details of the agreement, how and when the patient should sign up, and how to answer the patient's questions. The way that the program is presented to the patient and the willingness with which the office personnel answer the patient's questions will play a large part in whether courts will uphold the arbitration agreement as being fair and legal.

Both the patient and the physician have the opportunity to agree on who will arbitrate the case, so that it does not favor one side over the other. By prior agreement the arbitrator (or arbitrators) may be appointed by or from the American Arbitration Association, which is a neutral, private, nonprofit association dedicated to the advancement of out-of-court remedies. Its panels of arbitrators are made up of persons from business, the professions, and public interest groups.

MEDICAL PROFESSIONAL LIABILITY AND NEGLIGENCE

When injury results to a patient as a result of a physician's negligence, the patient may initiate a malpractice lawsuit to recover financial damages. However, experience has shown that the incidence of malpractice claims is directly related to the personal relationship and trust that exist between the physician and the patient. A deterioration of the physician-patient relationship is a common reason for the patient's decision to sue the physician for malpractice, even in situations in which no real injury has been sustained by the patient.

Medical professional liability, commonly called *medical malpractice,* is governed by the law of torts. The term *medical professional liability* encompasses all possible civil liability that can be incurred during the delivery of medical care. Medical professional liability is much more easily prevented than defended.

To understand medical malpractice, one must first understand the term *negligence.* Negligence, in general, implies inattention to one's duty or business, or the implication of a lack of necessary diligence or care. In medicine, negligence is defined as the performance of an act that a reasonable and **prudent** physician would not do or the failure to do an act that a reasonable and prudent physician would do. This, of course, also applies to any other healthcare professional. The standard of prudent care and conduct is not defined by law but would be left to the determination of a judge or jury, usually with the help of **expert witnesses** (Figure 7-8). Expert witnesses are members of the profession involved—in this case, medicine. To be considered an expert witness, a person usually belongs to a certifying or qualifying organization against which the qualities of the defendant may be compared.

Professional negligence in medicine falls into one of three general classifications:

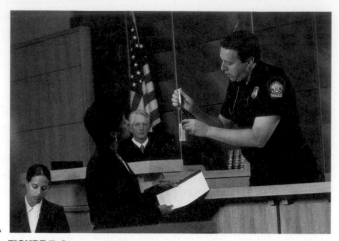
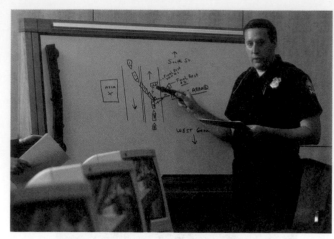

FIGURE 7-8 Expert witnesses help attorneys to prove or disprove the case in question by drawing on their experience with a given subject.

- Malfeasance: The performance of an act that is wholly wrongful and unlawful
- Misfeasance: The improper performance of a lawful act
- Nonfeasance: The failure to perform an act that should have been performed

A physician who performs an operation carelessly or fails to render care that should have been given may be found to have been negligent. Although a medical assistant acts as an agent of the physician in carrying out the majority of his or her duties, it is possible for the medical assistant to perform an act that can result in litigation.

For instance, if the medical assistant gives a patient the wrong medication or the wrong dose of medication, both the physician and the medical assistant can be held liable for the error. Some states limit the scope of practice of medical assistants where medications are involved; however, if medical assistants are performing within the realm of duties for which they have received training and the physician is accepting responsibility for the actions of those in the medical office, they are usually allowed to dispense and administer medications unless prohibited by state law. The medical assistant should always perform within the legal boundaries of his or her state (Procedure 7-1).

CRITICAL THINKING APPLICATION

Lynda is curious as to whether a physician is guilty of medical professional liability if he or she makes a mistake in diagnosing a patient. When might this be considered malpractice, and when might it not be considered malpractice?

What if the patient makes his or her condition worse? Is the physician then fully responsible? **Contributory negligence** exists when the patient contributes to his or her own condition and can lessen the damages that can be collected or even prevent them from being collected altogether.

The Four D's of Negligence

Negligence is not presumed; it must be proven. The Committee on Medicolegal Problems of the American Medical Association

(AMA) has determined that patients must present evidence of four elements before negligence has been proven. These elements have become known as the "four D's of negligence":

- Duty: Duty exists when the physician-patient relationship has been established. The patient has sought the assistance of the physician, and the physician has knowingly undertaken to provide the needed medical service.
- Dereliction: Dereliction, or failure to perform a duty, is the second element required. There must be proof that the physician somehow neglected the duty to the patient.
- Direct cause: There must be proof that the harm to the patient was directly caused by the physician's actions or failure to act and that the harm would not otherwise have occurred.
- Damages: The patient must prove that a loss or harm has resulted from the actions of the physician.

If all four of these elements exist, then the patient may obtain a judgment against the physician in a medical professional liability case.

Types of Damages

Several types of damages are commonly seen in tort cases. They are nominal, punitive, compensatory, general, and special damages.

Nominal damages are small awards that are token compensations for the invasion of a legal right in which no actual injury was suffered. For instance, if an unauthorized medical facility employee accesses a patient's medical record and is discovered but has not revealed any of the information in the record, the patient has not actually been harmed but may be awarded nominal damages in a lawsuit for the invasion of the patient's privacy.

Punitive damages are designed to punish the party who committed the wrong in such a way so as to deter the repetition of the act and are sometimes called *exemplary damages*. These damages were historically set so that the amounts would discourage intentional wrongdoings, misconduct, and outrageous behaviors. The amount of damages awarded would coincide in some percentage with the wealth of the defendant. Today there is much discussion of tort reform, which would place a cap on

PROCEDURE 7-1

Perform Within Legal Boundaries

<u>CAAHEP COMPETENCY:</u> 3.c.(2)(b)
<u>ABHES COMPETENCY:</u> 5.g

GOAL: *To perform duties within legal boundaries in the state where employed as a medical assistant.*

EQUIPMENT and SUPPLIES

- Computer
- Access to text of various laws and regulations affecting the practice

PROCEDURAL STEPS

1. Become familiar with the laws that affect medical practices in your state.
   <u>PURPOSE:</u> To understand which laws apply to the employer's facility.
2. Read the laws and regulations thoroughly.
   <u>PURPOSE:</u> To understand the concept and intent of the laws and regulations.
3. Obtain additional training on compliance with the laws and regulations, if necessary.
   <u>PURPOSE:</u> To make certain that all actions and procedures in the office are in compliance with applicable, current laws.
4. Read journals and any information available about the laws.

<u>PURPOSE:</u> To remain current in compliance activities.
5. Stay aware of licensure issues that affect the physician, including:
   - Licensure
   - Registration
   - Certification
   - Suspension
   - Revocation
   <u>PURPOSE:</u> To ensure that the physician is always practicing legally.
6. Know the scope of practice for a medical assistant.
   <u>PURPOSE:</u> To ensure that the medical assistant is always practicing legally.
7. Make certain that information is available on current laws and regulations at all times.
8. Perform all activities in accordance with applicable laws and regulations.
   <u>PURPOSE:</u> To insure compliance with applicable laws and regulations.

---

the amount of money that could be collected during personal injury litigation, including medical malpractice cases. Some have suggested a specific monetary figure, such as $500,000, as a limit on punitive damages, and others have suggested that plaintiffs be allowed to collect only up to three times the amount of compensatory damages.

CRITICAL THINKING APPLICATION

Samantha and Lynda disagree as to whether punitive damages should be awarded in medical professional liability cases. Samantha feels that nothing will compensate for certain losses, but Lynda feels that monetary compensation is reasonable when a loss has been suffered. Discuss both sides of the issue.

Compensatory damages are designed to compensate for any actual damages that are caused by the negligent person. They are intended to make the injured person "whole." Of course, nothing can substitute for the loss of an arm or a leg, for example, but compensatory damages help the patient or the patient's family recover from the loss.

General damages include compensation for pain and suffering, for loss of a bodily member or faculty, for disfigurement, or for other similar direct losses or injuries. The fact of the losses must be proven, but the monetary value does not.

Special damages are those injuries or losses that are not a necessary consequence of the physician's negligent act or omission. These may include the loss of earnings or costs of travel. Both the fact of these losses and the monetary value must be proven.

Standard of Care

If a physician were to be held legally responsible for every unsuccessful result occurring in the treatment of a patient, no person would undertake the responsibility of practicing medicine. The courts hold that a physician must do the following:

- Use reasonable care, attention, and diligence in the performance of professional services
- Follow his or her best judgment in treating patients
- Possess and exercise reasonable skill and care that are commonly possessed and exercised by other reputable physicians in the same type practice in the same or a similar locality

Physicians who represent themselves as specialists must meet the standards of practice of their specialty. Whether or not they have met these requirements in treating a particular patient is generally a matter for the court to decide on the basis of testimony provided by an expert witness. Physicians are not required to possess extraordinary learning and skill, but they must keep abreast of medical developments and techniques, and they cannot experiment. They are also bound to advise their patients if they discover that the condition to be treated is one beyond their knowledge or technical skill.

In the worst of cases, a physician or medical facility may be faced with wrongful death litigation. A wrongful death **allegation** is one in which the physician or medical facility is being blamed for the death of a patient as a result of error or inappropriate treatment. A wrongful death suit is usually brought by the family of the **decedent** against the physician or others involved with the patient.

A medical assistant should treat every chart touched as if it will end up in a court of law. Handwriting must be implicitly clear and legible, information must be detailed, and absolutely no room must be left for errors. Never mark out, cross out, erase, or white-out a mistake. Always draw one line through the error, then initial and date it. Nothing should be committed to memory. Remember, if it is not in the chart, it did not happen!

Consent

A physician must have consent to treat a patient, even though this consent is usually implied by virtue of the patient's appearance at the office for treatment. This **implied consent** is sufficient for common or simple procedures that are generally understood to involve little risk. Phlebotomy and taking vital signs are examples of procedures that usually involve implied consent. When more-complex procedures are anticipated, the physician must obtain the patient's **informed consent.** A physician who fails to secure some formal expression of consent could be charged with the crime of **battery.**

The Health Insurance Portability and Accountability Act (HIPAA) was designed for two major purposes. First, a standardization of electronic data exchange was sought in hopes that the efficiency of the healthcare system would be improved. Second, HIPAA was developed to protect health information and secure the contents of patient medical records. In the past a section of the Health Insurance Claim Form (CMS-1500) was reserved for the patient to authorize the release of medical information to the insurance company so that the claim could be evaluated and paid. Today, because of the influence of HIPAA, many medical offices are moving toward the use of a general consent form that is signed before the physician sees the patient. This form allows the physician to not only treat the patient, but also to use and submit health information to third parties for reimbursement.

Informed consent involves a deeper understanding of the patient's condition and a full explanation of the plan for treatment. Informed consent is not satisfied merely by having the patient sign a form. A discussion must occur during which the physician provides the patient or the patient's legal representative with enough information to decide whether the patient will undergo the treatment or seek an alternative. After such discussion, the patient either consents to the proposed therapy and signs a consent form or refuses to consent. According to the AMA's standards for informed consent, the discussion should contain the following elements, at a minimum:

- The patient's diagnosis, if known
- The nature and purpose of a proposed treatment or procedure
- The risks and benefits of a proposed treatment or procedure

- Alternative treatments or procedures, regardless of the cost or the extent to which the treatment options are covered by health insurance
- The risks and benefits of the alternative treatment or procedure
- The risks and benefits of not receiving or undergoing a treatment or procedure

The discussion should be fully documented in the patient's medical record, and a copy of the signed form should be placed in the record. Treatment may not exceed the scope of the consent that the patient has given. Often the consent forms will be lengthy and mention excessive possibilities and complications. There may be language that attempts to be all-inclusive, such as "included, but not limited to" when risks are listed. It is wise to have an attorney review the forms that are used for informed consent, because those that are too broad or too specific can be detrimental to the physician in a medical professional liability case.

Patients cannot be forced to undergo any type of medical treatment or care. The ultimate decision regarding care must be left to the patient, and although medical professionals should disclose information to help the patient make a good, informed decision, the patient should never be persuaded to act in any manner or accept any treatment with which he or she does not agree. Should the patient decide not to undergo treatment that the physician feels is necessary, an informed refusal of treatment or care should be signed. This should be a statement similar to the informed consent but will indicate that the patient has elected not to undergo treatment. Some physicians will discontinue all treatment if a patient does not participate in the care that the physician recommends. This document, once signed, should be added to the patient's medical record.

CRITICAL THINKING APPLICATION

Barbara stresses to Samantha and Lynda that there may be times in their professional career when a patient asks for their advice as to whether he or she should undergo a certain procedure or treatment. Barbara explains that patients often consider advice from the medical assistants in the office to be an extension of the physician's opinions. How might they handle such questions from patients? Should a medical assistant offer any type of advice?

Giving Consent to Medical Procedures

Mentally competent adults are certainly able to consent to medical procedures. However, if an act is unlawful, then the consent is invalid. For instance, if an abortion is performed in a state where abortion is illegal, then the consent to that procedure is null. Consent is also invalid if it is given by a person who is unauthorized to do so or if it is obtained by misrepresentation or fraud.

In an emergency, one may render aid or care to prevent loss of life or serious illness or injury. However, implied consent in this circumstance lasts only as long as the emergency exists, and formal consent must be obtained for further treatment as soon as the emergency has passed.

Physicians are sometimes reluctant to render aid in an emergency to someone who is not their patient for fear that they will later be charged with negligence or abandonment. In 1959 California passed the first Good Samaritan Act, which provides immunity from liability to volunteers at the scene of an accident for any civil damages as a result of rendering emergency care. Today, the majority of states have either Good Samaritan or Volunteer Protection statutes. As long as the emergency care is given in good faith and without gross negligence, and the healthcare worker provides only emergency care that he or she has been trained to provide, the likelihood of a successful lawsuit against that individual is very slim.

Adults who have been found by a court to be insane or incompetent usually cannot consent to medical treatment. Consent must be obtained from the guardian except in emergency situations.

Generally, when the patient is a minor, consent for surgery or treatment must be obtained from a parent, guardian, or **guardian ad litem,** except in an emergency requiring immediate treatment. If the parents are legally divorced or separated, consent should be obtained from the custodial parent, but if the child is visiting the second parent, consent may be obtained from that parent, because in such a situation that parent has temporary custody.

Consent is not required for minors in the following circumstances:

- When consent may be assumed, such as in a life-threatening situation
- When a certain treatment is required by law, such as a vaccination or x-ray evaluation for school entry or safety
- When a court order has been issued, as in a situation in which parents withhold consent for a necessary treatment because of religious reasons

In many states, treatment of sexually transmitted diseases, drug abuse, alcohol dependency, or pregnancy or providing birth control measures does not require parental consent.

Emancipation is defined by statute and varies from state to state. An emancipated minor is a person younger than the age of majority (usually 18 to 21 years) who meets one or more of the following conditions:

- Is married
- Is in the armed forces
- Is living separate and apart from parents or a legal guardian
- Is self-supporting

Some states include a minimum age for emancipation. Unless a statute declares otherwise, a minor who has the right to consent to treatment is entitled to the protection of his or her confidences, even from parents.

Statute of Limitations

A statute of limitations is a period of time after which a lawsuit cannot be filed. The statute of limitations varies from state to state and differs for various types of litigation. Many states have a 2-year statute of limitations for medical malpractice issues. However, in some instances, the statute of limitations may be extended because of a delay in the discovery of an

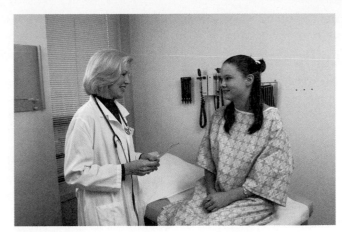

FIGURE 7-9 Patient confidentiality is the most important trust that exists between the physician and the patient.

injury. For example, a patient has surgery to replace a valve in the heart, and the surgery seems successful. Two years later, the patient undergoes a routine echocardiogram and the physician discovers that the surgeon mistakenly replaced the aortic valve when the surgery was intended for the pulmonary valve. Although 2 years have already passed, the statute of limitations begins at the point of discovery of the injury, so the patient could now bring suit against the surgeon for the error.

Confidentiality

Confidentiality is one of the most sacred trusts that the patient places in the hands of the physician and his or her staff (Figure 7-9). Breach of patient confidentiality is grounds for immediate dismissal of a healthcare professional. The strictest care must be taken when handling patient records and discussing information about patients.

In many special cases patient confidentiality plays a vital role. A patient who is human immunodeficiency virus (HIV) positive may face discrimination if the information about his or her medical condition surfaces. Physicians who treat such patients may wish to take extra care when leaving phone messages or sending mail. Instead of leaving a message for a patient from "Dr. Watson's office," the medical assistant could say that the message is from "Terry Watson's office." This could indicate an attorney, accountant, or real estate broker. Curious co-workers or relatives may not grow as suspicious as they might if they were to encounter a message from a physician's office.

Patients who are receiving treatment for substance abuse are protected by federal statutes. Confidentiality is also of utmost importance to patients receiving treatment for mental health issues, sexually transmitted diseases, sexual **assault,** and any type of abuse.

LAW AND MEDICAL PRACTICE

Law affects the day-to-day practice of the physician. Some of the ways in which the medical assistant will encounter legal issues in the physician's offices are discussed in this section. The medical assistant must comply with both state and federal laws and regulations while performing the duties associated with his or her job (Procedure 7-2).

Legal Disclosure

The physician is charged with safeguarding patient confidences within the constraints of the law, but according to state laws, which vary somewhat throughout the nation, certain disclosures must be made. Frequently the medical assistant is involved with the responsibility for reporting these events.

Births and deaths must be reported. In some states, detailed information about stillbirths is required. Physicians must also report cases that may have been a result of violence, such as gunshot wounds, knife injuries, or poisonings. Any death from accidental, suspicious, or unexplained causes must also be reported. In some states, occupational diseases and injuries must be reported within specific time limits.

Sexually transmitted diseases are reportable in every state. All 50 states require that patients who have confirmed cases of acquired immunodeficiency syndrome (AIDS) be reported by name to the local health department. However, just over 30 states require that patients who are HIV positive be reported. Individuals are reported either by name or by unique identifiers. A continuing controversy exists as to whether the reporting prompts patients to receive care or deters patients in high-risk groups from seeking care.

Child abuse is a leading cause of death among children younger than 5 years of age, and healthcare professionals are required by law to report any suspected cases of child abuse. The report should be made as soon as evidence is discovered that gives the physician "cause to believe" that abuse or neglect has occurred. Even if the evidence is uncertain, the physician should report the evidence and allow the government to investigate and determine what action to take to protect the child. However, it is essential to make every attempt to ensure that the report is legitimate, because it could lead to the child's being removed from the home and placed in foster care. Cases of spousal and elder abuse are difficult, because the person being abused is often reluctant to report the situation for fear of further mistreatment. The law requires that suspected cases of abuse of children, elderly persons, or any others at risk be reported to the authorities.

Local health departments publish lists of diseases that are reportable as well as the method that should be used in reporting. Often this can be done by telephone or mail. Appropriate forms must be used for mail reporting and are supplied by the health department or available on their websites. County and state health departments periodically issue bulletins that are sent to healthcare providers and provide information about disease outbreaks and various statistics. Local health departments should be consulted for specific procedures and reporting protocols.

PROCEDURE 7-2

Demonstrate Knowledge of Federal and State Health Care Legislation and Regulations

CAAHEP COMPETENCY: 3.c(2)(e)
ABHES COMPETENCY: 5.g

GOAL: *To be aware of federal and state legislation and regulations that apply to the employer's facility.*

EQUIPMENT and SUPPLIES

- Computer
- Access to organizational websites that have established legislation and regulations that pertain to medical facilities
- Information about changes to and new federal and state legislation and regulations

PROCEDURAL STEPS

1. Consistently review applicable legislation and regulations that apply to the facility.
   PURPOSE: To ensure compliance with the law.
2. Discover the federal and state ramifications of issues related to healthcare workers, such as:
   - Regulatory bodies
   - Education and credentials
   - Scope of practice
   - Job qualifications
   - CEU requirements
   - Loss of credentials
   PURPOSE: To ensure full compliance in the medical facility.

3. Review and understand federal and state legislation and regulations related to:
   - Americans with Disabilities Act
   - Controlled Substance Schedules
   - OSHA
   - Centers for Disease Control
   - Local Public Health Departments
   - Materials Safety Data Sheets (MSDS)
   PURPOSE: To ensure full compliance in the medical facility.
4. Review and understand accrediting agency requirements that affect the facility.
   PURPOSE: To ensure full compliance in the medical facility.
5. Stay aware of new state and federal legislation and regulations.
   PURPOSE: To ensure full compliance in the medical facility.
6. Always follow office policy when performing any action at the facility.
   PURPOSE: To ensure full compliance in the medical facility.

Patient Self-Determination Act

The Patient Self-Determination Act of 1990 brought the term *advance directives* to the forefront of medical care. This act requires healthcare facilities to develop and maintain written procedures that ensure that all adult patients receive information about living wills, durable powers of attorney for healthcare, and advance directives. These documents place the decision-making power into the hands of the patient and the patient's family, providing them with written notification of their right to consent to or refuse medical treatment.

Patients' Bill of Rights

In March of 1998, President Bill Clinton received the final report from the President's Advisory Commission on Consumer Protection and Quality in the Healthcare Industry. The Commission was created to advise the President on the current issues facing the healthcare industry and make recommendations that would assure that patients would receive high-quality healthcare services. The report, entitled *"Quality First: Better Healthcare for All Americans,"* led to the development of a Consumer Bill of Rights and Responsibilities for the healthcare industry. This is usually called the Patients' Bill of Rights. The document lists three specific goals:

- To strengthen consumer confidence by assuring the healthcare system is fair and responsive to consumer's needs, provides consumers with credible and effective mechanisms to address their concerns, and encourages consumers to take an active role in improving and assuring their health
- To reaffirm the importance of a strong relationship between patients and their healthcare professionals
- To reaffirm the critical role consumers play in safeguarding their health by establishing rights and responsibilities for all participants in improving their health

Most healthcare facilities have adopted a Patient Bill of Rights that provides a condensed version of the entire report, which contains eight sections. Often this information is presented to patients when they are admitted to healthcare facilities, or one might see it posted in a prominent place within the facility.

Because it is a patient's right to understand his or her diagnosis, prognosis, and all aspects of care, one must take special care when dealing with a patient with whom there may be a language barrier. If the patient's ability to understand is limited, an interpreter may be needed to ensure that communication from physician to patient is adequate.

Controlled Substances Act

On May 1, 1971, the Controlled Substances Act of 1970 became effective. In October 1973 a regulatory agency known as the Drug Enforcement Administration (DEA) became a part of the U.S. Department of Justice. The DEA works with local, state, federal, and international agencies and organizations to address and regulate the serious issues of drug use and abuse in the United States.

Before administering, prescribing, or dispensing any drugs, a physician is required to register with the regional office of the DEA. This registration is renewable every 3 years. If a physician

---

Patients' Bill of Rights

I. Information Disclosure

You have a right to receive accurate and easily understood information about your health plan, healthcare professionals, and healthcare facilities. If you speak another language, have a physical or mental disability, or just don't understand something, assistance will be provided so you can make informed healthcare decisions.

II. Choice of Providers and Plans

You have the right to a choice of healthcare providers that is sufficient to provide you with access to appropriate high-quality healthcare.

III. Access to Emergency Services

If you have severe pain, an injury, or sudden illness that convinces you that your health is in serious jeopardy, you have the right to receive screening and stabilization emergency services whenever and wherever needed, without prior authorization or financial penalty.

IV. Participation in Treatment Decisions

You have the right to know all your treatment options and to participate in decisions about your care. Parents, guardians, family members, or other individuals that you designate can represent you if you cannot make your own decisions.

V. Respect and Nondiscrimination

You have a right to considerate, respectful, and nondiscriminatory care from your doctors, health plan representatives, and other healthcare providers.

VI. Confidentiality of Health Information

You have the right to talk in confidence with healthcare providers and to have your healthcare information protected. You also have the right to review and copy your own medical record and request that your physician amend your record if it is not accurate, relevant, or complete.

VII. Complaints and Appeals

You have the right to a fair, fast, and objective review of any complaint you have against your health plan, doctors, hospitals, or other healthcare personnel. This includes complaints about waiting times, operating hours, the conduct of healthcare personnel, and the adequacy of healthcare facilities.

---

works from more than one office, he or she must register each individual office. Regulations regarding the writing, telephoning, and refilling of prescriptions vary according to which schedule is involved.

Under the Controlled Substances Act, drugs are categorized into Schedules I, II, III, IV, and V. Drugs in Schedule I have the highest potential for abuse and addiction, and those in Schedule V have the lowest abuse potential.

Schedule I substances are those that have no accepted medical use in the United States. Examples include heroin and lysergic acid diethylamide (LSD). Only the physician who is involved in conducting research with such drugs is concerned with Schedule I substances.

Schedule II drugs have a high abuse potential, with severe risk of mental and physical dependence. They include certain narcotic, stimulant, and depressant drugs, such as opium, morphine, codeine, and methylphenidate (Ritalin). Controlled substances in Schedule II can be obtained only with a federal triplicate order form obtained from the DEA. A special inventory must be maintained on controlled substances and retained for 2 to 3 years, depending on state requirements. When a controlled substance is removed from inventory, it must be recorded. The record must show the date, the name of the drug, the dosage, and the name of the patient, physician, and employee involved. Schedule III, IV, and V substances do not require triplicate forms.

Schedule III substances have an abuse potential that is lower than that of the first two schedules. They include compounds that contain limited quantities of certain narcotic drugs combined with nonnarcotic substances. Examples include acetaminophen (Tylenol) with codeine, hydrocodone, butalbital with aspirin and caffeine (Fiorinal), and several steroids.

Schedule IV substances have still lower potential for abuse. Phenobarbital, diazepam (Valium), propoxyphene (Darvon and Darvocet), alprazolam (Xanax), chlordiazepoxide (Librium), and pentazocine lactate (Talwin) are examples.

Schedule V substances have lower abuse potential than those in Schedule IV but still warrant control. They include preparations that contain moderate quantities of certain narcotics as may be found in cough medicines and antidiarrheal products.

The physician may call a prescription to the pharmacist, but the pharmacist must transcribe it in writing before filling it. With permission from the physician, the medical assistant may orally transmit a prescription for controlled substances only in Schedules III, IV, or V, and the dispensing pharmacist must put the prescription into writing before filling it. The medical assistant cannot under any circumstances orally transmit a prescription for a Schedule II drug. These prescriptions must be presented in writing to the pharmacist on the appropriate form.

Stored controlled substances must be kept in a locked cabinet or safe. Any loss of controlled drugs by theft must be reported to the regional office of the DEA at the time the theft is discovered. If a physician discovers that his or her DEA number is being used in the unauthorized prescribing of controlled substances, he or she should report the incident to the DEA, to the state regulatory agency, and to the local police authorities. This is especially important in the case of employees whose employment has been terminated and who are suspected of drug theft in the office. There have been numerous cases of retaliation by fired employees who report to the DEA exactly what they have actually taken, yet accuse the physician or other staff members of taking the controlled substances. This results in messy investigations and months of follow-up, so any suspected employee drug use or abuse should be documented and reported to the local authorities. Periodic drug testing of employees is one way to help prevent office drug abuse. Many states now have laws to prevent the filing of false reports, so if the physician is wrongly accused by a disgruntled employee, the physician often has some **recourse.**

A physician who discontinues medical practice must return the registration certificate and any unused order forms and triplicate prescription pads to the nearest office of the DEA. The regional DEA office will advise the physician on the disposition of any controlled drugs still on hand.

CRITICAL THINKING APPLICATION

Barbara explains the importance of reporting any employee who is suspected of using drugs or taking drugs from the office. This may be difficult, because co-workers are often friendly with one another and may hesitate to report such acts. Discuss ways to handle this situation.

Uniform Anatomical Gift Act

The Uniform Anatomical Gift Act was approved by the National Conference of Commissioners on Uniform State Laws in 1968. Although many states had passed laws before this time that permitted living persons to make a gift of their body or portions of it after death, the laws were so different from state to state that arrangements for a donation in one state might not be recognized in another. All states have adopted the Uniform Anatomical Gift Act or similar legislation.

Essentially, the model law for donation states the following:
- Any person of sound mind and 18 years of age or older may give all or any part of his or her body after death for research, transplantation, or placement in a tissue bank.
- A donor's valid statement of gift is paramount to the rights of others except when a state autopsy law may prevail.
- If a donor has not indicated an intent to donate during his or her lifetime, his or her survivors, in a specified order of priority, may do so.
- Physicians who accept organs or tissues, relying in good faith on the documents, are protected from lawsuits. The physician attending at the time of death, if acquainted with the donor's wishes, may dispose of the body under the Uniform Anatomical Gift Act.
- The time of death must be determined by a physician who is not involved in the transplantation, and the attending physician cannot be a member of the transplant team.
- The donor may revoke the gift, or the gift may be rejected by the proposed recipient.

The most important clause of the act permits the donation to be made by a will (without waiting for probate) or by other written or witnessed documents, such as a card designed to be carried by the person or a Uniform Donor Card (Figure 7-10). The Uniform Donor Card is considered a legal document in all 50 states. Many states now list donor preference on the driver's license as well.

The provisions of the Uniform Anatomical Gift Act are so designed that the offer is exercised only after death. Therefore

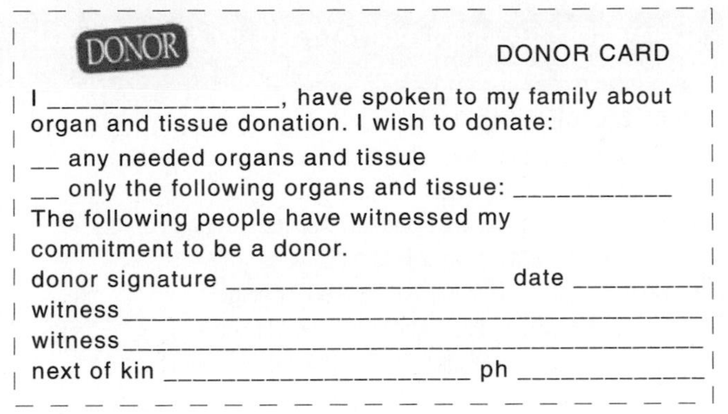
DONOR

DONOR CARD

I ________________, have spoken to my family about organ and tissue donation. I wish to donate:

__ any needed organs and tissue

__ only the following organs and tissue: ____________

The following people have witnessed my commitment to be a donor.

donor signature ____________________ date __________

witness ____

witness ____

next of kin ______________________ ph _____________

FIGURE 7-10 Organ donation card.

donors should reveal their intentions to as many of their relatives and friends as possible and to their physician. Because the human body and its parts are not commodities in commerce, no money can be exchanged in making an anatomic donation itself. Fees are charged for performing the transplant and various procedures, but organs cannot be bought and sold. It is also important to note that family members should be prepared to receive the body of the person who has donated his or her entire body to research once the research facility has completed its study. This can often be a traumatic experience, rekindling the grief process once again, so the procedures and final disposition of the body should be decided at the time of the donation to avoid this difficult situation.

Health Insurance Portability and Accountability Act

HIPAA was signed into law on August 21, 1996, and all healthcare providers were required to comply with HIPAA's privacy standards by April 2003. Its history began in the Clinton healthcare reform proposals. HIPAA was designed for several purposes, with many goals in mind. Limiting administrative costs of healthcare and privacy issues, as well as prevention of fraud and abuse, are of primary importance within the HIPAA regulations. The law has two provisions, which include Title I (Insurance Reform) and Title II (Administration Simplification). The use of electronic transmissions ideally lowers the administrative costs of providing healthcare, but this led to problems with privacy regarding health information. The law also had to provide security and confidentiality guarantees for the individual patient. Extensive privacy rules, including the use of unique identifiers, have shaped the law.

The final regulations regarding the privacy legislation sections of HIPAA were published in December 2000, after HCFA reviewed more than 50,000 comments on and concerns about this important subject. All healthcare organizations that transmit any health information electronically must comply with HIPAA; fines as well as prison terms can be imposed on those who do not comply with the regulations.

HIPAA has had a tremendous effect on the healthcare industry. All healthcare providers, clearinghouses, and health plans that use electronic information must comply with HIPAA regulations. The benefits of HIPAA compliance include the following:

- Lower administrative costs
- Increased accuracy of data
- Increased patient and consumer satisfaction
- Reduced revenue cycle time
- Improved financial management

HIPAA's Title I, which deals with insurance reform, includes several provisions that protect individuals and their insured dependents in the event that they change jobs or lose a job. Preexisting condition clauses are limited, and an individual cannot be discriminated against for a poor health history when changing insurance coverage. HIPAA also ensures that an individual can renew health insurance coverage even if he or she has a health condition that is covered under the policy. In many cases, individuals are guaranteed the right to purchase health insurance coverage after the loss or change of a job.

Title II details the process of administrative simplification. The standardization of the exchange of healthcare data is one way in which HIPAA promotes computer-to-computer transactions. This standardization process helps to reduce the number of forms and methods used in the claims processing cycle, including electronic transactions, standard code sets (such as diagnosis, procedure, and supply codes), and the provision for unique identifiers for providers, employers, health plans, and patients. These unique identifiers use alphanumeric systems to ensure privacy. Title II also details the implementation of privacy and security procedures designed to prevent the misuse of health information by ensuring confidentiality. Security standards were required to be in place by April 2005. Medical professionals who access medical information must use log-in and password systems that prevent unauthorized individuals from accessing protected health information.

Occupational Safety and Health Act and the Bloodborne Pathogens Standard

In 1970 President Nixon signed the Occupational Safety and Health Act, which created what we know today as the Occupational Safety and Health Administration (OSHA). OSHA is a division of the U.S. Department of Labor, and since its creation workplace injuries, illnesses, and fatalities have been significantly reduced. OSHA's mission is to ensure workplace safety and a healthy environment within the workplace.

Although OSHA is commonly thought of as the regulatory agency that requires steel-toed boots and hard hats, the medical industry moved into the OSHA spotlight in the late 1980s, when the threat of HIV infection extended to healthcare workers. Hepatitis and other pathogens were already of concern to healthcare workers, but when HIV, the virus that causes AIDS, was identified, action was needed to better protect the individuals who cared for patients with these infectious diseases. OSHA's Final Ruling on Bloodborne Pathogens became fully effective in July 1992, and since that time various additions have been made to update the regulations in light of new information learned about blood-borne pathogens.

The law requires medical facilities to comply with the Bloodborne Pathogens standard and to be able to prove that compliance to OSHA inspectors if necessary. The actual standard can be found in the 29 **Code of Federal Regulations**

(CFR) 1910.1030. The following information details the legal requirements of the OSHA Standard as it pertains to the physician's office.

General Duty Clause

No law can cover every single situation that may arise in the course of daily living. Because of this, OSHA's general duty clause is a catch-all regulation that fits almost any situation not specified in any other section of the law. The general duty clause simply states that a workplace must be free of any hazard that might cause serious harm or death. For example, one breach of the general duty clause is the "failure of a facility to provide reasonable security procedures at a retail store." Although not a specific breach of any regulation, this fits nicely into the general duty clause.

Occupational Safety and Health Administration Regulations as Performance-Based Standards

OSHA regulations are considered performance-based standards. This means that adequate compliance depends largely on what happens in the facility. For instance, the same regulations may not apply to two offices located right next to each other. Would it be possible that a family practitioner could be fined for not having sharps containers, whereas a surgeon in the office next door, inspected by the same OSHA inspector, does not receive a fine for not having sharps containers? It is possible if the surgeon does not perform any invasive, surgical, or any other procedures that involve blood in the office! Some surgeons perform all procedures at facilities other than the office.

This is one reason that employees must be trained in their individual facilities. Even if training was done 1 month before a job change, the employee must be trained again in the new facility. Offices and procedures are different from place to place, and the employee must have adequate training to function successfully in the medical office.

OSHA inspectors can recommend fines when a facility is found to be out of compliance with an OSHA standard. One of the most common infractions is that the facility has an Exposure Control Plan in the facility but is not using it or following the procedures and policies set forth within it. This could lead to an inspector's declaring the facility to be willfully negligent. Willful negligence exists when "an employer representative was aware of the requirements of the [OSHA] Act, or the existence of an applicable standard or regulation, and was also aware that the condition or practice was in violation of those requirements, and did not abate the hazard." Fines for noncompliance can quadruple for willful negligence.

Exposure Control Plan

The Exposure Control Plan can be a part of the regular safety plan written for the medical facility or may be a stand-alone document, but it must cover all of the elements required by OSHA. This plan must be in writing and be reviewed annually, and there must be written documentation that the plan was reviewed and updated or revised, if needed. A hard copy must be provided to employees on their request within 15 working

---

Common Occupational Safety and Health Administration Violations

- No eyewash facilities available
- No labeling or improper labeling of hazardous chemicals
- No MSDS for each hazardous chemical
- Storage of contaminated laboratory coats with clean ones
- Not communicating hazards to employees
- No documentation of initial employee training
- No documentation of annual employee training
- No annual hazard assessment performed
- Having an Exposure Control Plan but not following it
- No proof of destruction of hazardous waste
- No Emergency Action Plan in the facility
- No written Exposure Control Plan
- OSHA Form 300A not posted during required period
- No records of hepatitis B vaccinations or declination forms

MSDS, Material Safety Data Sheets; *OSHA*, Occupational Safety and Health Administration.

---

days, and the plan must be available at all times in the workplace.

The plan must delineate the tasks that employees perform where risk of blood exposure is present. It must also classify jobs within the facility according to the likelihood of exposures. For instance, some job duties would always expose the employee to blood or **other potentially infectious materials (OPIM)**, often on a daily basis. Some duties would only occasionally expose the employee, and other duties would never expose the employee to blood or OPIM. Employees must be told which category they are a part of and what duties they will perform that could lead to exposures. In addition, there must be a clear follow-up procedure in place that details how the medical facility will track employee exposures. The employee cannot be abandoned after an exposure incident. Periodic counseling must take place in which the facility determines and documents the progress of the employee who has had an exposure, including laboratory tests and medical treatment received.

The Exposure Control Plan must contain a Waste Management section that details how waste is removed from the facility and destroyed. Most medical offices contract with companies that specialize in removing and destroying medical waste. The office must keep the receipts given by the company that prove that the waste was taken away from the facility and then incinerated or otherwise destroyed.

The plan must also contain a section on Hazardous Materials Communication, which explains what substances in the facility are hazardous and how to handle a spill or exposure to those products. Only the manufacturer of a chemical can determine whether it is hazardous, and Material Safety Data Sheets (MSDS) must be kept on almost all chemicals and reagents in the facility. Recent rulings have exempted some chemicals, but without the MSDS information, a medical assistant could not determine what type of health, reactivity, flammability, or other risks the chemical could have.

If the facility has equipment for x-ray studies, a Radiation Safety Plan must also be written and followed. All facilities should have an Emergency Action Plan in place, which provides procedures in case of tornadoes, fires, floods, or any other type of emergency that might occur in the office. This plan should contain floor plans of the facility, diagrams depicting the most efficient exits from the building, and the chain of command in an emergency. Diagrams with exit routes should be posted in every room of the medical office. At least annually, a hazard assessment must be performed on the entire facility. The hazard assessment is an inspection for problem areas in which the facility might be out of compliance. The facility must have documentation that the hazard assessment was done.

Occupational Safety and Health Administration Record Keeping Regulations.

An injury or illness is considered to be work related when an event or exposure in the work environment contributed to or caused the condition or significantly aggravated a preexisting condition. OSHA made several changes in the regulations concerning work-related injury record keeping to simplify forms, protect employee privacy, encourage employee involvement, and enable computer usage for meeting OSHA requirements. The revised rules took effect on January 1, 2002. Three basic forms are now used to keep records regarding injuries, accidents, and illnesses related to the workplace. The forms are as follows:

- OSHA Form 300–Log of Work-Related Injuries and Illnesses (Figure 7-11): Information is posted on form 300 regarding work-related deaths and every work-related injury or illness that involves loss of consciousness, restricted work activity or job transfer, days away from work, or medical treatment beyond first aid. An OSHA Form 301 (Injury and Illness Incident Report) should be completed for each entry on the log.
- OSHA Form 300A–Summary of Work-Related Injuries and Illnesses (Figure 7-12): Form 300A must be completed even if no injuries or illnesses occurred during the year that were work related. It must be posted in a common area for viewing by all employees, and provides the total number of accidents, illnesses, and injuries in the facility for the previous year. The length of time that this information must be posted has increased from 1 month to 3 months, specifically from February 1 to April 30 each year. An additional change is the certification of the form. A company executive must examine the document and certify that it is accurate.
- OSHA Form 301–Injury and Illness Incident Report (Figure 7-13): Form 301 is used to report what actually happened when an employee suffers a work-related injury or illness. This form, or an acceptable substitute, such as a state worker's compensation form, must be completed within 7 calendar days after notification of the illness or injury. The form should be completed as quickly as possible so that an exact recollection of events can be documented. Now that the new record-keeping regulations have become effective, employees are

guaranteed access to their OSHA 301 forms for the first time.

The log and summary forms must be kept on file for a minimum of 5 years. Only the Summary should be posted during the specified time period from February 1 to April 30 each year, reflecting information from the previous calendar year. The forms are not sent to OSHA unless specifically requested.

CRITICAL THINKING APPLICATION

Barbara quickly realizes that the office is using older versions of OSHA Forms 300 and 301. Where might she look or go to find updated information and forms?

It is wise to keep a communication log of calls to OSHA in which questions were asked or information verified. Note the day and time called, the first and last name of the person spoken to, the person's title, and the question asked and response given. Take detailed notes while discussing the issue on the phone. This log could be invaluable if a question ever arises about a subject discussed with a local OSHA official. It may make the difference when an OSHA inspector suggests a hefty fine. If the medical facility can show documentation that a certain procedure was discussed with an OSHA official and decisions were made based on that discussion, the facility may have sufficient evidence that the law was considered and the facility did its best to comply.

Needlestick Safety and Prevention Act

An estimated 600,000 to 800,000 injuries occur annually among healthcare workers. One third of these injuries happen during the disposal process. In an effort to reduce these injuries, which can lead to exposure to HIV, hepatitis B virus (HBV), or other blood-borne pathogens, OSHA revised its Bloodborne Pathogens standard to comply with the Needlestick Safety and Prevention Act, which became law on November 6, 2000. The regulations became effective on April 18, 2001.

Employers are now required to involve employees in the selection of needle safety devices. The facility must be able to prove that consideration was given to various types of devices that promote needle safety, what led to the decision to choose the device currently in use, and which employees were involved in these decisions. A list should be kept of which employees contributed to the selection decisions. Minutes from meetings, copies of employee response forms, and the forms used to solicit input are good methods of proving that employees were involved in the selection process.

CRITICAL THINKING APPLICATION

Barbara needs input about the needle safety devices being used in the facility. Should she call a meeting of the entire office, or are there specific employees who should be present? If so, discuss who should have input in these decisions.

A needlestick and sharps injury log must also be kept in the medical facility. At a minimum, the log must include the following information:

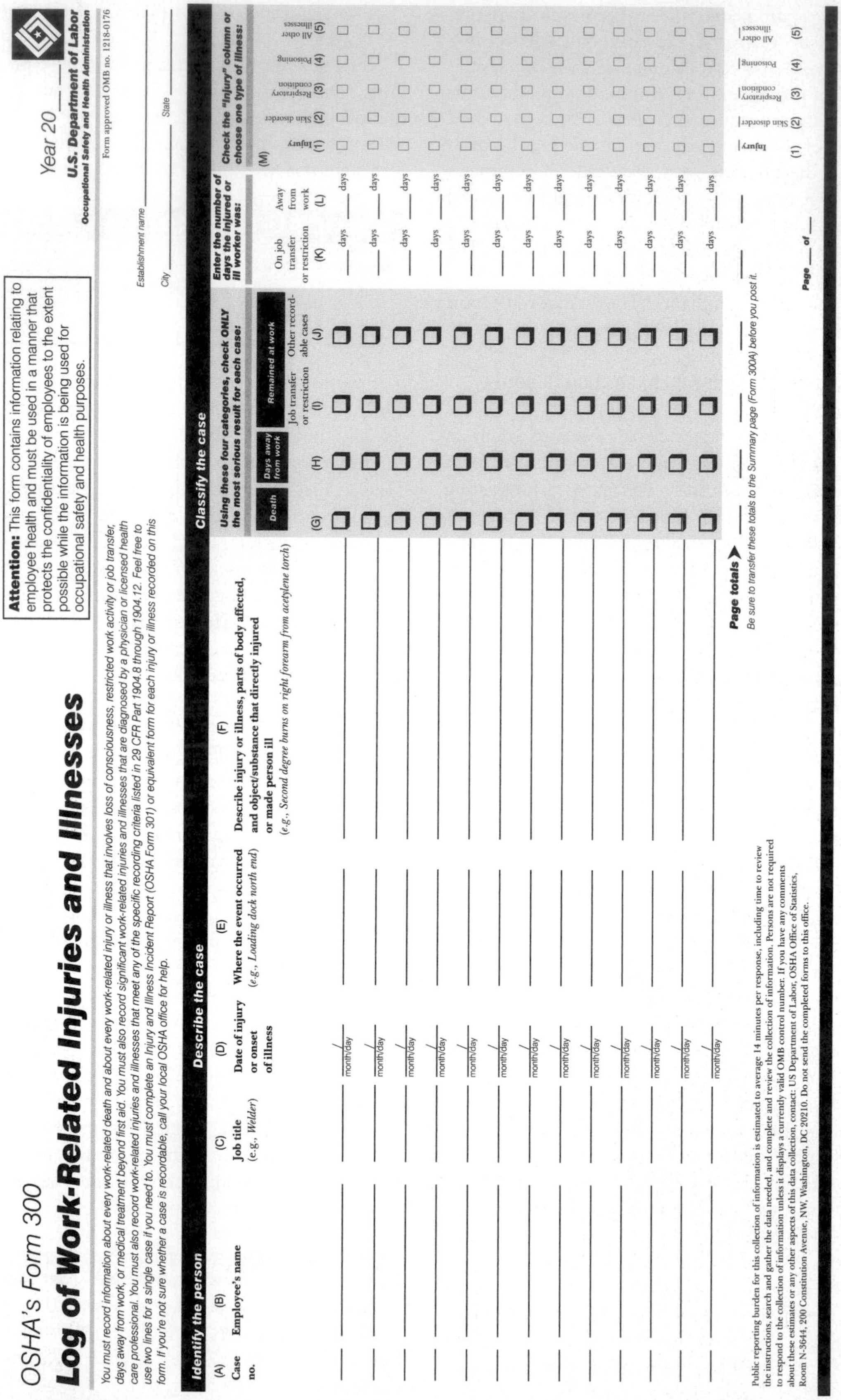

OSHA's Form 300

Log of Work-Related Injuries and Illnesses

You must record information about every work-related death and about every work-related injury or illness that involves loss of consciousness, restricted work activity or job transfer, days away from work, or medical treatment beyond first aid. You must also record significant work-related injuries and illnesses that are diagnosed by a physician or licensed health care professional. You must also record work-related injuries and illnesses that meet any of the specific recording criteria listed in 29 CFR Part 1904.8 through 1904.12. Feel free to use two lines for a single case if you need to. You must complete an Injury and Illness Incident Report (OSHA Form 301) or equivalent form for each injury or illness recorded on this form. If you're not sure whether a case is recordable, call your local OSHA office for help.

Attention: This form contains information relating to employee health and must be used in a manner that protects the confidentiality of employees to the extent possible while the information is being used for occupational safety and health purposes.

Year 20____

U.S. Department of Labor
Occupational Safety and Health Administration

Form approved OMB no. 1218-0176

Establishment name _____
City _____   State _____

Page ____ of ____

FIGURE 7-11 OSHA Form 300—Log of Work-Related Injuries and Illnesses. (From U.S. Department of Labor, Occupational Safety and Health Administration.)

OSHA's Form 300A

Summary of Work-Related Injuries and Illnesses

Year 20__ __

U.S. Department of Labor
Occupational Safety and Health Administration

Form approved OMB no. 1218-0176

All establishments covered by Part 1904 must complete this Summary page, even if no work-related injuries or illnesses occurred during the year. Remember to review the Log to verify that the entries are complete and accurate before completing this summary.

Using the Log, count the individual entries you made for each category. Then write the totals below, making sure you've added the entries from every page of the Log. If you had no cases, write "0."

Employees, former employees, and their representatives have the right to review the OSHA Form 300 in its entirety. They also have limited access to the OSHA Form 301 or its equivalent. See 29 CFR Part 1904.35, in OSHA's recordkeeping rule, for further details on the access provisions for these forms.

Number of Cases

Total number of deaths	Total number of cases with days away from work	Total number of cases with job transfer or restriction	Total number of other recordable cases
___(G)	___(H)	___(I)	___(J)

Number of Days

Total number of days of job transfer or restriction	Total number of days away from work
___(K)	___(L)

Injury and Illness Types

Total number of . . .
(M)

(1) Injuries ___

(2) Skin disorders ___

(3) Respiratory conditions ___

(4) Poisonings ___

(5) All other illnesses ___

Post this Summary page from February 1 to April 30 of the year following the year covered by the form.

Public reporting burden for this collection of information is estimated to average 50 minutes per response, including time to review the instructions, search and gather the data needed, and complete and review the collection of information. Persons are not required to respond to the collection of information unless it displays a currently valid OMB control number. If you have any comments about these estimates or any other aspects of this data collection, contact: US Department of Labor, OSHA Office of Statistics, Room N-3644, 200 Constitution Avenue, NW, Washington, DC 20210. Do not send the completed forms to this office.

Establishment information

Your establishment name _____

Street _____

City _____ State ____ ZIP ____

Industry description (e.g., Manufacture of motor truck trailers) _____

Standard Industrial Classification (SIC), if known (e.g., SIC 3715) ___ ___ ___ ___

Employment information (If you don't have these figures, see the Worksheet on the back of this page to estimate.)

Annual average number of employees _____

Total hours worked by all employees last year _____

Sign here

Knowingly falsifying this document may result in a fine.

I certify that I have examined this document and that to the best of my knowledge the entries are true, accurate, and complete.

Company executive _____ Title _____

Phone (___) ___ - ___ Date ___/___/___

FIGURE 7-12 OSHA Form 300A—Summary of Work-Related Injuries and Illnesses. (From U.S. Department of Labor, Occupational Safety and Health Administration.)

OSHA's Form 301
Injury and Illness Incident Report

U.S. Department of Labor
Occupational Safety and Health Administration

Form approved OMB no. 1218-0176

Attention: This form contains information relating to employee health and must be used in a manner that protects the confidentiality of employees to the extent possible while the information is being used for occupational safety and health purposes.

This *Injury and Illness Incident Report* is one of the first forms you must fill out when a recordable work-related injury or illness has occurred. Together with the *Log of Work-Related Injuries and Illnesses* and the accompanying *Summary*, these forms help the employer and OSHA develop a picture of the extent and severity of work-related incidents.

Within 7 calendar days after you receive information that a recordable work-related injury or illness has occurred, you must fill out this form or an equivalent form. Some state workers' compensation, insurance, or other reports may be acceptable substitutes. To be considered an equivalent form, any substitute must contain all the information asked for on this form.

According to Public Law 91-596 and 29 CFR 1904, OSHA's recordkeeping rule, you must keep this form on file for 5 years following the year to which it pertains.

If you need additional copies of this form, you may photocopy and use as many as you need.

Information about the employee

1) Full name _____

2) Street _____
   City _____ State ____ ZIP ____

3) Date of birth ___ / ___ / ___

4) Date hired ___ / ___ / ___

5) ☐ Male
   ☐ Female

Information about the physician or other health care professional

6) Name of physician or other health care professional _____

7) If treatment was given away from the worksite, where was it given?
   Facility _____
   Street _____
   City _____ State ____ ZIP ____

8) Was employee treated in an emergency room?
   ☐ Yes
   ☐ No

9) Was employee hospitalized overnight as an in-patient?
   ☐ Yes
   ☐ No

Completed by _____

Title _____

Phone (____) ____ - ____   Date ___ / ___ / ___

Information about the case

10) Case number from the Log _____ *(Transfer the case number from the Log after you record the case.)*

11) Date of injury or illness ___ / ___ / ___

12) Time employee began work _____ AM / PM

13) Time of event _____ AM / PM   ☐ Check if time cannot be determined

14) **What was the employee doing just before the incident occurred?** Describe the activity, as well as the tools, equipment, or material the employee was using. Be specific. *Examples:* "climbing a ladder while carrying roofing materials"; "spraying chlorine from hand sprayer"; "daily computer key-entry."

15) **What happened?** Tell us how the injury occurred. *Examples:* "When ladder slipped on wet floor, worker fell 20 feet"; "Worker was sprayed with chlorine when gasket broke during replacement"; "Worker developed soreness in wrist over time."

16) **What was the injury or illness?** Tell us the part of the body that was affected and how it was affected; be more specific than "hurt," "pain," or sore." *Examples:* "strained back"; "chemical burn, hand"; "carpal tunnel syndrome."

17) **What object or substance directly harmed the employee?** *Examples:* "concrete floor"; "chlorine"; "radial arm saw." *If this question does not apply to the incident, leave it blank.*

18) **If the employee died, when did death occur?** Date of death ___ / ___ / ___

Public reporting burden for this collection of information is estimated to average 22 minutes per response, including time for reviewing instructions, searching existing data sources, gathering and maintaining the data needed, and completing and reviewing the collection of information. Persons are not required to respond to the collection of information unless it displays a current valid OMB control number. If you have any comments about this estimate or any other aspects of this data collection, including suggestions for reducing this burden, contact: US Department of Labor, OSHA Office of Statistics, Room N-3644, 200 Constitution Avenue, NW, Washington, DC 20210. Do not send the completed forms to this office.

FIGURE 7-13 OSHA Form 301—Injury and Illness Incident Report. (From U.S. Department of Labor, Occupational Safety and Health Administration.)

- Description of the incident
- The type and brand of device used when the incident took place
- Location of the incident

The regulations that took effect in 2001 require all needlestick and sharps injuries to be reported and documented, not just the ones that result in injury or illness.

Occupational Safety and Health Administration Training Requirements

All employees, including full-time, part-time, and temporary employees with a risk of occupational exposure, must receive training within the facility in which they are employed at two very specific times. Initial training must be conducted before commencement of any work-related duties by a new employee. In addition, training must be conducted on an annual basis to update and inform employees about new regulations and procedures related to OSHA compliance. The initial training requirement is one of the most frequently breached regulations, yet it is critical for the safety of the employee.

Training must include the following:

- Making accessible a copy of the regulatory text of the standard and explanation of its contents
- General discussion of blood-borne diseases and their transmission
- Universal precautions and body substance isolation
- The Exposure Control Plan
- Engineering and work practice controls, including handling of needles and sharps
- Personal protective equipment
- Hepatitis B vaccine
- Response to emergencies involving blood
- Potential sources of infection and tasks that might preempt exposure
- Written schedules for cleaning
- Handling of contaminated laundry
- How to handle exposure incidents and spills
- The postexposure evaluation and follow-up program
- Reading of MSDS, signs, labels, and color-coding (Figure 7-14), and locations of these items

There must be an opportunity for questions and answers, and the trainer must be knowledgeable about the subject matter. Documentation of the training sessions should be kept in each employee's personnel file or a special file for OSHA-related information.

CRITICAL THINKING APPLICATION

Barbara reviews the employee files and finds that neither Samantha nor Lynda received OSHA training when they were initially hired. How might Barbara rectify this, and what documentation would be helpful?

Hepatitis B Vaccination

The hepatitis B vaccination series must be offered to employees at risk of occupational exposures at no cost to the employee. The employee cannot be asked to pay in advance for the vaccination and be reimbursed, nor can the employee be asked to put the vaccination series on his or her personal health insurance policy. It must be made available to the employee within 10 working days of initial hire or assignment. The vaccination series can be declined by the employee, who must sign a declination form. If at any time the employee decides to receive the vaccination series, this must still be offered at no cost. The employee does not have to offer a reason for the declination. Prescreening or postvaccination serologic tests cannot be required.

The vaccination series is completed within a 6-month period. The second vaccination is given 1 month after the first, and the third 5 months after the second. Documentation should be provided to the employee for each vaccination received. Currently a booster dose of the hepatitis B vaccination is not required. However, if a routine booster is recommended by the U.S. Public Health Service in the future, it must be made available at no cost to employees.

CRITICAL THINKING APPLICATION

Lynda has not disclosed to anyone at the facility that she has had a case of hepatitis. Should she discuss this matter with Barbara? Is Lynda required to discuss this matter with Barbara? Is Lynda placing her patients at risk? If Lynda declines the hepatitis vaccination, must she explain why on the declination form?

Clinical Laboratory Improvement Amendments

The Clinical Laboratory Improvement Amendments (CLIA) was a result of the Congressional investigation of **physician office laboratories (POLs)** and the deficiencies in the quality of the services and results provided by these laboratories. A set of minimum standards for laboratories was established and involved quality improvement in test procedures. Quality control and assurance, as well as personnel and proficiency testing, are of utmost importance to the facility complying with CLIA.

CLIA regulations set the minimum standard for laboratory practice and quality. Remember that CLIA is not a governmental agency, but a law. CLIA is enforced by the Department of Health and Human Services (HHS). OSHA is a law (Occupational Safety and Health Act), but also an agency (Occupational Safety and Health Administration). This is an important difference between the two.

Some tests conducted in the laboratory are exempt from CLIA standards. These tests include the following:

- Nonautomated dipstick or tablet urinalysis
- Fecal occult blood
- Ovulation using visual color comparison
- Urine pregnancy using visual color comparison
- Erythrocyte sedimentation rate
- Hemoglobin by copper sulfate method
- Spun microhematocrit
- Blood glucose using certain devices cleared by the FDA for home use
- Specialized self-contained hemoglobin tests

Offices that perform only these tests may obtain a certificate of waiver and will not be routinely inspected for CLIA compliance. Tests of moderate or high complexity must be performed by trained personnel with education and experience

Material Safety Data Sheets communicate hazards to employees about the products and chemicals used in the medical office. They also inform the employee as to what to do in case of an exposure. OSHA requires that MSDS sheets are kept on all hazardous chemicals, unless exempted. Only the manufacturer can determine if a product is hazardous. MSDS sheets can be obtained from either the manufacturer or the medical supply company from which the product was ordered. They must be provided after requested from the manufacturer within 30 days. Keep copies of requests to prove that an attempt has been made to obtain the MSDS information.

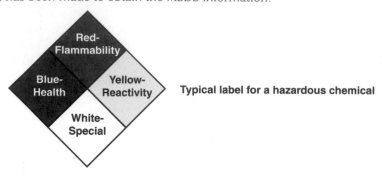

Typical label for a hazardous chemical

The appropriate number should be placed inside each box that applies in the figure above. Most offices use the National Fire Protection Association Rating System. Many MSDS sheets provide the labeling information on the sheet. Others must be read thoroughly to determine how the labels should be completed. If the MSDS says that a chemical has a "moderate to high" hazard, label it high. If it says "low to moderate," label it moderate. Never guess at the numbers used for the label—always consult the MSDS. If individual containers are labeled, the facility is said to always be out of compliance, because it is easy to miss a container that may have just arrived in a shipment. Many medical facilities place labels on a permanent fixture next to where the product is stored, but it must be permanently stored in that area.

Simple Rating Guide

0—no hazard
1—slight hazard
2—moderate hazard
3—high hazard
4—extreme hazard

NFPA Rating Summary

Health (Blue)			Reactivity (Yellow)		
4	Danger	May be fatal on short exposure. Specialized protective equipment required.	4	Danger	Explosive material at room temperature.
3	Warning	Corrosive or toxic. Avoid skin contact or inhalation.	3	Danger	May be explosive if shocked, heated under confinement, or mixed with water.
2	Warning	May be harmful if inhaled or absorbed.	2	Warning	Unstable or may react violently if mixed with water.
1	Caution	May be irritating.	1	Caution	May react if heated or mixed with water but not violently.
0		No unusual hazard.	0	Stable	Not reactive when mixed with water.
Flammability (Red)			**Special Notice Key (White)**		
4	Danger	Flammable gas or extremely flammable liquid.	W		Water reactive.
3	Warning	Flammable liquid flash point below 100° F.	Oxy		Oxidizing agent.
2	Caution	Combustible liquid flash point of 100° to 200° F.			
1		Combustible if heated.			
0		Not combustible.			

FIGURE 7-14 Labeling and the National Fire Protection Association (NFPA) Rating System. (Courtesy the National Fire Protection Association.)

in the test areas in which they are working. A list of the moderate- and high-complexity procedures can be found in the July 26, 1993, issue of the *Federal Register,* and updates are periodically published that detail any changes in the list or regulations regarding testing procedures. Laboratories apply for a CLIA certificate through their local health departments and will be periodically inspected for compliance.

Americans with Disabilities Act

In 1990, the Americans with Disabilities Act (ADA) was signed into law with the intent of eliminating discrimination against individuals with disabilities. The act is comprehensive legislation that addresses many areas in which a person might experience discrimination, including telecommunications, housing, public transportation, air carrier access, voting accessibility, education, and rehabilitation. Physician offices fall under the category of public accommodations, which is defined as a private entity that owns, lease, lease to, or operates public facilities.

Public accommodations must comply with basic nondiscrimination requirements that prohibit exclusion, segregation, and unequal treatment. They also must comply with specific requirements related to architectural standards for new and altered buildings; reasonable modifications to policies, practices, and procedures; effective communication with people with hearing, vision, or speech disabilities; and other access requirements. Additionally, public accommodations must remove barriers in existing buildings where it is easy to do so without much difficulty or expense, given the public accommodation's resources.

These regulations affect the physician office because those individuals with disabilities must be able to enter and exit the facility without difficulty. This means that a person in a wheelchair would need a ramp to enter and exit the building. They must also be able to navigate throughout the office without major barriers. Any facility with 15 or more employees must comply with the Americans with Disabilities Act. To be protected by the ADA, one must have a disability or have a relationship or association with an individual with a disability. An individual with a disability is defined by the ADA as a person who has a physical or mental impairment that substantially limits one or more major life activities, a person who has a history or record of an impairment, or a person who is perceived by others as having an impairment. The ADA does not specifically name all of the impairments that are covered. Every medical facility must comply with the Americans with Disabilities Act (1990). This law requires that public medical facilities must allow persons with disabilities to easily and safely do the following

- Reach door handles for opening and closing
- Enter and exit buildings
- Move through doors and hallways
- Use drinking fountains, phones, and restrooms
- Move from floor to floor (elevators are required for multilevel buildings)
- Do everything that the general public is able to do in a public place

PHYSICIAN LICENSURE AND REGISTRATION

A graduate of a medical school must be licensed before beginning the practice of medicine. Licensure is regulated by state statutes through the Medical Practice Acts. It is important for a medical assistant to understand licensing and other laws and regulations that are intended to protect patients, physicians, medical assistants, and other healthcare workers.

Medical Practice Acts

Medical practice acts existed as early as colonial days. However, these acts were later repealed, and in the mid-nineteenth century practically none of the states had laws governing the practice of medicine. As one might expect, a rapid decline in professional standards followed. The general welfare of the people was endangered by medical **quackery** and inadequate care. By the beginning of the twentieth century, medical practice acts were established by statute and were again in effect in every state. The purpose of the medical practice acts is as follows:

- To define what is included in the practice of medicine within that state
- To govern the methods and requirements of licensure
- To establish the grounds for suspension or revocation of license

Licensure

A Doctor of Medicine (MD), Doctor of Osteopathy (DO), or Doctor of Chiropractic (DC) degree is conferred on graduation from medical or chiropractic school. The license to practice medicine or chiropractic is granted by a state board, frequently known as the State Board of Medical Examiners or Board of Registration. Licensure may be accomplished by examination, reciprocity, or endorsement.

Examination

Every state requires medical doctors to pass a written examination. The Federation of State Medical Boards and the National Board of Medical Examiners agreed in 1990 to establish a single licensing examination—the Federation Licensing Examination (FLEX)—for graduates of accredited medical schools. Medical graduates in the United States must pass either the FLEX examination, the U.S. Medical Licensing Examination (USMLE), or the National Board of Medical Examiners' Examination (NBME). Osteopathic physicians pass the National Board of Osteopathic Medical Examiners' Comprehensive Osteopathic Medical Licensing Examination (COMLEX).

Reciprocity

Some states grant the license to practice medicine by reciprocity; that is, they automatically recognize that the requirements of the state in which the license was granted meet the standards required by the second state.

Endorsement

Most graduates of medical schools in the United States have been licensed by endorsement of the National Board certificate. To explain in simpler terms, a state will offer a license to a physician based on the examinations taken to grant the license, not by virtue of the license granted from another state. Licensure by endorsement is granted on a case-by-case basis. Graduates who have not been licensed by endorsement are required to pass a state board examination.

In all states, graduates of foreign medical schools who are seeking licensure by endorsement must meet the same requirements as graduates of medical schools in the United States, in addition to various other qualifying factors.

Exemptions

Some graduates may not wish to engage in the practice of medicine; their interests may lie in research or administration, or even in the practice of law with a special interest in medical liability. In such instances licensure is not required. Licensed physicians in the Armed Forces, Public Health Service, or

Veterans Administration facilities need not be licensed in the state in which they are employed. However, the Department of Defense is encouraging states to require full licensure of military personnel.

Registration and Reregistration

After a license is granted, periodic reregistration is necessary annually or biennially. A physician can be **concurrently** registered in more than one state. The issuing body notifies the physician when reregistration is due. A medical assistant can aid the physician by being aware of when the registration fees are due, thereby preventing a possible lapsing of the registration.

Many states require proof of continuing education in addition to payment of a registration fee. Continuing education units (CEUs) are granted to physicians for attending approved seminars, lectures, scientific meetings, and formal courses in accredited colleges and universities. A total of 50 hours per year is the average requirement for a license renewal. A medical assistant may be expected to help the physician arrange for completing the required units for license renewal.

Revocation or Suspension

Under certain conditions, the license to practice medicine may be revoked or suspended. Grounds for revocation or suspension of the license to practice medicine fall within one of three categories:

- Conviction of a crime: This may include felonies such as murder, rape, larceny, and narcotic violations.
- Unprofessional conduct: Failure to uphold the ethical standards of the medical profession may be indicated by betrayal of patient confidence, giving or receiving rebates, and excessive use of narcotics or alcohol.
- Personal or professional incapacity: Such incapacity is difficult to label or prove. For example, advanced age or an injury may reduce the apparent capacity of some physicians. Certain illnesses can affect the memory or judgment necessary to practice medicine.

A physician studies many years to learn the profession before becoming licensed by the state to practice medicine. A medical assistant is not licensed to practice medicine and must never prescribe or attempt to diagnose a patient's ailment. This is the illegal practice of medicine. For this reason a medical assistant must use great care in discussing the patient's complaints and treatment with them because patients identify the medical assistant's remarks as being the opinion of the physician.

CLOSING COMMENTS

The majority of patients never entertain the thought of taking legal action against their physicians, and a medical assistant should not develop an attitude of skepticism. However, a medical assistant can play an important role in preventing medical claims.

Give scrupulous attention to the needs of each patient and avoid leaving them alone for long periods. This especially applies to young children and elderly patients. Always avoid criticism of other physicians or healthcare facilities. Never give out any information about the patient without written consent, and verify the identity of anyone asking for information about a patient.

Use discretion in phone and office conversations. One never knows who is standing just around the corner. Be aware of tone of voice and attitude during spoken conversations. Communicate office policies and procedures to patients clearly in advance of treatment whenever possible.

Keep accurate records that show exactly what was done to the patient and when it was done. The medical assistant must never make any promises as to the outcome of treatment. Record cancelled and no-show appointments and record the facts if a patient discontinues treatment.

Check office equipment often to ensure that it is working properly. Keep drug samples and prescription pads out of sight. Never diagnose, prescribe, or offer a prognosis. Perform only the tasks for which you are trained and keep abreast of new findings and procedures in healthcare. Correctly follow all federal and state regulations.

Play a positive part in the prevention of medical liability claims. Take care of the patient in a compassionate and competent way, and malpractice will not be a frequent issue in the medical facility.

SUMMARY OF SCENARIO

Barbara is enthusiastic about her new job and duties. She is confident about appearing in court to represent Dr. Patrick and discuss the contents of the medical record of the patient suing his surgeon. Dr. Patrick is not a party to the lawsuit but has a physician-patient relationship with the patient just the same. An offer existed, as well as the acceptance of that offer. The relationship was based on legal subject matter, and the physician and the patient had the legal capacity to enter into a contract. Consideration existed as well, because the patient paid for services and the physician treated the patient. Both received something of value. Samantha and Lynda would like to accompany Barbara to the court proceedings to watch and learn.

Even if a patient does not pay for treatment, a contract still exists. The physician may elect to terminate the physician-patient relationship if the patient does not pay, but the trust that the patient places in the physician can be considered a thing of value. Patients should understand their role in their treatment, and their responsibilities to the physician. Often this information is communicated in the patient policy brochure or may be verbally discussed with the patient. Physicians are not required to accept all patients; for instance, not all

SUMMARY OF SCENARIO—cont'd

physicians deliver babies. Some physicians do not treat patients with worker's compensation claims. The physician does have the right to see the types of patients he or she wishes and is competent to treat but should never discriminate on the basis of race, sex, or any other protected status. A physician may not always be correct in his or her diagnoses, but this does not mean that the physician has committed malpractice. However, if expert witnesses feel that the physician should have made a different diagnosis based on the case, then the physician might be held liable for negligence. If an employee has information about a case that is damaging to the physician, he or she is ethically obligated to report the information, but rarely legally liable to speak up unless a law has been broken.

Samantha and Lynda have learned many new concepts about law from Barbara and are anxious to follow the court proceedings. They will learn more by seeing the actual process of law at work. Barbara looks forward to sharing more knowledge with the employees as they continue to work together.

Medical assistants can help the physician comply with legal regulations in the office by making certain that they understand the policies and procedures that are required by the facility. Rules are set in place in order to assure compliance so that both patients and employees are kept safe and risks in the office are at a minimum. Patient confidentiality is one of the most important

rules to remember. New graduates can learn about the laws that affect medical facilities in their area by discussing them with their supervisors and by attending seminars and training. Much information is available on the Internet regarding legal issues. Trust is a critical factor in avoiding medical professional liability lawsuits. When the patient trusts the physician, he or she is much more likely to work through issues that might otherwise lead to legal action against the physician. Keeping accurate patient records and documenting all information required in the patient chart will help to prove that the physician adequately cared for the patient. Clearly legible handwriting is vital in this process.

The medical assistant may find that the physician is not in compliance with certain rules and regulations. Never jump to conclusions and assume that the physician has no intention of complying. There are various reasons for noncompliance, and any issues should be brought to the attention of the office manager or the physician for clarification. It is the medical assistant's responsibility to question noncompliance and make every effort to bring the facility into compliance with the cooperation of supervisors, co-workers, and the physician. As a team, medical professionals can remain in compliance and deliver excellent care to all patients.

SUMMARY of LEARNING OBJECTIVES

1. Define, spell, and pronounce the terms listed in the vocabulary.
   - Spelling and pronouncing medical terms correctly adds credibility to the medical assistant. Knowing the definition of these terms promotes confidence in communication with patients and co-workers.
2. Distinguish among an act, a statute, and an ordinance.
   - Different types of laws and regulations affect us, depending on the origination of the law. Acts are introduced at the federal level and must be passed by Congress. State legislative bodies develop statutes, and local governments create ordinances.
3. Know the two types of law.
   - Criminal law governs violations that are punishable as offenses against the state or government. Civil law is concerned with acts that are not criminal in nature but involve relationships between individuals and other individuals, groups, or government agencies.
4. Explain the three basic categories of criminal law.
   - Misdemeanors are minor crimes punishable by a fine or imprisonment in a city or county jail. Felonies are major crimes, such as rape, murder, or burglary. Most felonies carry punishment of imprisonment for at least 1 year, and they are divided into subgroups, usually first-, second-, and

third-degree felonies. Treason is an attempt to overthrow the government. High treason constitutes a serious threat to the stability of the government—for example, an attempt on the life of the president.

5. Distinguish which type of civil law deals with medical professional liability.
   - Tort law is the division of civil law that deals with medical professional liability. Tort law provides relief for those who have suffered harm from the actions of others. The plaintiff must establish duty, breach of duty, damages as a result of the breach of duty, and the extent of the damages suffered.
6. Explain the four essential elements needed for a valid contract.
   - Four elements are essential to a valid, legal contract: (1) there must be a "meeting of the minds" or manifestation of assent; (2) the contract must involve legal subject matter; (3) the parties to the contract must have the legal capacity to enter into a contract; and (4) some type of consideration must be offered.
7. Distinguish between interrogatories and depositions.
   - Interrogatories are lists of questions directed from each party of a lawsuit to the other. Interrogatories are answered under oath and directed only to the parties actually named in the

Continued

SUMMARY of LEARNING OBJECTIVES

Continued

lawsuit. Depositions, however, can be taken from any witness or party to the lawsuit. They are also taken under oath, and often witnesses are subpoenaed to offer a deposition.

8. List three things to remember when testifying in court.
   - Testifying in court can sometimes be an intimidating experience, but good preparation beforehand will alleviate many anxieties. Discussing potential questions with the attorney will help prepare the witness for giving testimony. Always tell the truth to avoid charges of perjury. Speak clearly and distinctly, and do not hesitate to ask the attorney to repeat a question. A brief pause to think about an answer causes no harm. Dress conservatively, know the location and room of the court in advance, and always arrive on time. Credibility is critical in a medical professional liability trial.

9. Discuss the advantages of arbitration.
   - Arbitration is a popular alternative to court trials. It involves the use of a third party familiar with law or the issues at hand. It is recognized by statute in most states and provides a faster, confidential, fair, and less expensive resolution to a dispute.

10. Differentiate among malfeasance, misfeasance, and nonfeasance.
   - Malfeasance, misfeasance, and nonfeasance are types of negligence often involved in medical professional liability cases. Malfeasance is performing an act that is completely wrong or unlawful. Misfeasance, comparable to a mistake, is the improper performance of a lawful act. Nonfeasance is the failure to perform some act that should have been performed.

11. Explain the "four D's" of negligence.
   - The four D's of negligence include the duty to care for the patient; dereliction or failure to perform that duty; proof that this failure was the direct cause of a patient's injury; and proof that the patient suffered damages from the injury.

12. Define the types of damages.
   - Nominal damages are token compensations for invasion of a legal right. Punitive damages are designed to punish an offender and discourage repetition of an act. Compensatory damages are designed to compensate for the actual damages suffered, whereas general damages include compensation for pain and suffering, loss of a body member, disfigurement, and other similar losses. Special damages can include such losses as earnings or travel costs.

13. Explain the importance of informed consent.
   - Informed consent gives the patient a full understanding of the condition that has been diagnosed, including what could happen if the patient undergoes treatment, refuses treatment, or delays treatment. It provides the patient with information on the advantages and risks of a medical procedure and alternative treatments that the patient may wish to consider. Informed consent places the control in the hands of the patient, who is given the opportunity to make the decisions about his or her healthcare. Patients can never be forced to undergo any type of procedure or treatment.

14. List several legal disclosures the physician must make.
   - Several disclosures must be made by the physician with regard to a patient's health that do not require patient consent. Information about births and deaths, injuries or illnesses as a result of violence, accidental or suspicious deaths, sexually transmitted diseases, and any type of abuse are examples of legal disclosures that must be made by healthcare professionals.

15. Explain the importance of the Health Insurance Portability and Accountability Act.
   - Passage of HIPAA in 1996 offered the healthcare profession extensive privacy rules and regulations concerning the electronic transfer of information. The act also limited administrative costs by supporting the use of electronic transfer of information and presented fraud and abuse prevention guidelines. The privacy issues that surround HIPAA, however, have been the most discussed and debated topics related to this law.

16. Distinguish between OSHA and CLIA, explaining which of the two is an actual agency.
   - OSHA is an agency and a division of the U.S. Department of Labor. More than 2300 employees work for OSHA, and the agency runs on an annual budget of approximately $443 million as of 2002. Twenty-six states have their own OSHA programs, which adds an additional 3100 employees. The Occupational Safety and Health Act of 1970 created this agency to ensure safety in the workplace. CLIA is a law that regulates the quality of services provided by laboratories. CLIA is enforced by the HHS.

17. Discuss the three ways in which a physician can obtain a license to practice medicine.
   - Physicians may receive a license to practice medicine through examination, reciprocity, or endorsement. FLEX, USMLE, and NBME are all designed for graduates of accredited medical schools. Some states recognize the requirements of another state in which a license was granted, and through reciprocity will give a physician a license to practice medicine. Endorsement is the method of obtaining a license by recognition of the passed examinations, instead of by virtue of the license obtained in another state. Most physicians in the United States are licensed by endorsement, because they take the examination after graduating from medical school and this prompts the receipt of the license, after proper application and providing all required documentation. Practicing medicine without a license is illegal.

18. Discuss the ways that a physician might lose a license to practice medicine.
   - A physician may lose his or her license to practice medicine if convicted of a crime, if found guilty of unprofessional conduct, or as a result of personal or professional incapacity. An arrest will not cause the physician to lose the license, because this is an allegation not yet proven in court. Unprofessional conduct is usually determined by local medical societies or other organizations, such as a hospital, with which the physician is affiliated.

CONNECTIONS

 Study Guide Connection: Go to Chapter 7 Study Guide. Read the Case Study and Workplace Applications and complete the assignments. Do online research for answers to the questions in the Internet Activities associated with medicine and the law.

 CD Connection: Go to the Medical Assisting Competency Challenge CD and do the training activities under Legal Concepts.

 Evolve Connection: For more information related to medicine and the law, go to http://evolve.elsevier.com/kinn/admin and visit related weblinks for Chapter 7. Click on the Medical Assisting Exam Review and do the practice questions to sharpen your test-taking skills.

Computer Concepts

8

SCENARIO

Dr. Michael Bouchard is aware of the advantages of networking his office computers and having Internet access to meet the needs of his facility. Every day he sends and receives many important email messages to and from patients and colleagues. His staff members use the computer for communications and to access sources of online information. Patient tracking, accounting functions, and health information retrieval are immensely faster on a computer than with the use of a paper-based system. One other distinct advantage to Dr. Bouchard is the scheduling features of his software. Because the schedule is shared, everyone in the office knows the doctor's schedule and avoids double-booking and miscommunications. Dr. Bouchard sends his staff members for regular computer training so that all of them can use the computers in the best and most efficient ways possible.

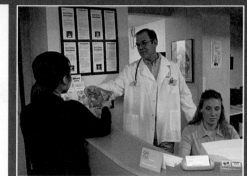

HIPAA requirements have altered the methods in which information may be used in medical facilities. No employee is allowed to access information in the clinic that is not necessary to that employee for patient care and assistance. Dr. Bouchard takes the HIPAA guidelines seriously and makes certain that all of his staff members understand the importance of keeping health information secure.

While studying this chapter, think about the following questions:

- How do computers help the physician's office to run more efficiently?
- Can an employee in the physician's office invade a patient's right to privacy by accessing medical records?
- How can information on the computer be kept secure from curious employees who do not need to access the information for the purpose of patient care?

- How does logging in and logging out of the office network help to ensure proper access to medical records?
- How could the computer be considered a co-worker in the medical office?

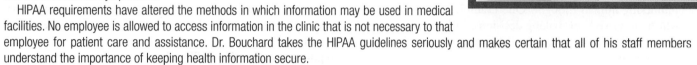

LEARNING OBJECTIVES

1. Define, spell, and pronounce the terms listed in the vocabulary.
2. List several ways that the computer can be effective in a medical office.
3. Explain the basic functions that a computer performs.
4. Explain the basic parts of a computer.
5. List the three elements that differentiate microprocessors.
6. Discuss the differences among various types of printers.

7. Explain the importance of a motherboard.
8. Explain and give examples of peripheral devices.
9. List and discuss several types of file formats.
10. Explain the concept of computer networking.
11. Define the function of browsers.
12. Discuss the importance of computer security.

National Accreditation Competencies and Content

CAAHEP COMPETENCIES

General
3.c.(4)(c). Utilize computer software to maintain office systems

ABHES COMPETENCIES

Communication
2.n. Application of electronic technology

Administrative Duties
3.d. Apply computer concepts for office procedures

Office Management
6.d. Evaluate and recommend equipment and supplies for practice

Financial Management
8.a. Use manual and computerized bookkeeping systems

VOCABULARY

application software Computer programs designed to perform specific tasks.

artificial intelligence The aspect of computer science that deals with computers taking on the attributes of humans, such as mimicking human thought. One example is expert systems, which are capable of making decisions, such as software that is designed to help a physician diagnose a patient, given a set of symptoms.

ASCII codes Acronym for American Standard Code for Information Interchange; a code representing English characters as numbers, where each is given a number from 0 to 255.

backup Any type of storage of files to prevent their loss in the event of hard disk failure.

banners Advertisements often found on a Web page that can be animated to attract the user's attention in hopes that he or she will click on the ad, be redirected to the advertiser's home page, and purchase from the site or gain information from the site.

bits The smallest units of information inside the computer, each represented by either the digit "0" or "1"; 8 bits equal 1 byte.

byte A unit of data that contains 8 binary digits, or bits.

cache (kash) A special high-speed storage that can either be a part of the computer's main memory or can be a separate storage device. One function of a cache is to store websites visited in the computer memory for faster recall the next time the website is requested.

CD burner A device that is capable of "writing" data onto a blank compact disk (CD) or copying data from one CD to a blank CD.

computer A machine that is designed to accept, store, process, and give out information.

cookies Messages sent to a Web browser from a Web server that identify users and can prepare custom Web pages for them, possibly displaying their name on return to the site.

cursor A symbol appearing on the monitor that shows where the next character to be typed will appear.

cyberspace The nonphysical space of the online world of computer networks in which communication takes place.

database A collection of related files that serves as a foundation for retrieving information.

device driver The program or commands given to a device connected to a computer that enable the device to function. For instance, a printer may come equipped with software that must be loaded onto the computer first, so that the printer will work.

digital subscriber line (DSL) High-speed, sophisticated modulation scheme that operates over existing copper telephone wiring systems; often referred to as "last-mile technologies," because DSL is used for connections from a telephone switching station to a home or office, and not between switching stations.

Digital video disk (DVD) An optical disk that holds approximately 28 times more information than a CD; a DVD is most commonly used to hold full-length movies. Compared with a CD, which holds approximately 600 megabytes, a DVD has the capacity to hold approximately 4.7 gigabytes. Also called a digital versatile disk.

disk A removable device shaped like a hard plastic square with a magnetic surface that is capable of storing computer programs; also called *diskettes*, and early versions were called *floppy disks*.

disk drives Devices that load a program or data stored on a disk into the computer.

ecommerce An abbreviation for electronic commerce; used to describe the sale and purchase of goods and services over the Internet; doing business over the Internet.

email Communications transmitted via computer or computer network.

environment The state of a computer, usually determined by the programs that are running as well as hardware and software characteristics.

fax Abbreviation for facsimile; also, a document sent using a facsimile (fax) machine.

flash Animation technology often used on the opening page of a website to draw attention, excite, and impress the user.

flash drive A small portable device that connects into the USB port that can carry 2 to 8 or more gigabytes of information.

List continues on next page

font A design for a set of type characters; a combination of typeface, spacing, pitch, and other qualities. Fonts are named; examples include Times Roman, Arial, and Garamond.

format To magnetically create tracks on a disk where information will be stored, usually done by the manufacturer of the disk.

gigabyte Approximately 1 billion bytes; abbreviated GB.

hard copy The readable paper copy or printout of information.

hardware The physical components of the computer system, such as the CPU, monitor, and printer.

HTML Acronym for HyperText Markup Language, which is the language used to create documents for use on the Internet.

HTTP Acronym for HyperText Transfer Protocol, which defines how messages are formatted and transmitted over the Internet. When a URL is entered into the computer, an HTTP command tells the Web server to retrieve the requested Web page.

hub A common connection point for devices in a network containing multiple ports, often used to connect segments of a LAN.

icons Pictures, often on the desktop of a computer, that represent programs or objects. By clicking on an icon, the user is directed to the program.

input Information entered into and used by the computer.

Java A commonly used object-oriented high-level programming language that is well suited for the Internet.

kilobyte Approximately 1024 bytes, abbreviated KB.

megabyte Approximately 1 million bytes; abbreviated MB.

megahertz The measuring device for microprocessors, abbreviated MHz. A megahertz is 1 million cycles of electromagnetic currency alternation per second and is used as a unit of measure for the clock speed of computer microprocessors. The hertz is a unit of measure named after Heinrich Hertz, a German physicist.

MIDI Acronym for Musical Instrument Digital Interface; a MIDI interface allows computers to record and manipulate sound.

modem A device that allows information to be transmitted over telephone lines, at speeds measured in bits per second (bps); short for modulator-demodulator. Modem speed is generally listed somewhere on the actual unit.

monochromatic Having or consisting of one color or hue.

multimedia The presentation of graphics, animation, video, sound, and text on a computer in an integrated way, or all at once. CD-ROMs are efficient multimedia devices.

output Information that is processed by the computer and transmitted to a monitor, printer, or other device.

queries Requests for information from a database.

router (rau'-ter) A device used to connect any number of LANs, which communicate with other routers and determine the best route between any two hosts.

scanner Device that reads text or illustrations on a printed page and can translate the information on that page into a form that the computer can understand.

search engines Programs that search documents for keywords and return a list of documents containing those words.

server A computer or device on a network that manages shared network resources.

sound card Device that allows a computer to output sound through speakers that are connected to the main circuitry board, or motherboard.

switch In networks, a device that filters information between LAN segments and decreases overall network traffic and increases speed and bandwidth usage efficiency.

system software The operating system and all utility programs that allow the computer to function and perform operations.

TCP/IP Acronym for Transmission Control Protocol/Internet Protocol; a suite of communications protocols used to connect users or hosts to the Internet.

telecommunications The science and technology of communication by transmission of information from one location to another via telephone, television, telegraph, or satellite.

terabyte Approximately 1 trillion bytes, abbreviated TB.

URL Acronym for Uniform Resource Locator; specifies the global address of documents or information on the Internet. The URL provides the IP address and the domain name for the Web page, such as microsoft.com.

virtual reality An artificial environment presented to a computer user that feels as if it were a real environment, often involving use of special gloves, earphones, and goggles to enhance the experience.

zip drive A small, portable disk drive that is primarily used for backing up information and archiving computer files. A 100-megabyte Zip disk will hold the equivalent of approximately 70 floppy disks.

COMPUTERS TODAY

Nearly 60 years ago, in 1946, the first electronic **computer** (ENIAC) was completed after 2½ years in the making. It weighed 30 tons, required a space of 15,000 square feet, and cost more than $1 million. Since that time, a computer explosion has taken place, and today our lives are affected by computers on a daily basis. Personal computers (PCs), laptop or notebook computers, and even cell phones that send and receive **email** are commonplace. Our world is now one of enhanced **telecommunications**, where faster processing of information is both needed and expected. Advances in technology happen daily; as soon as one "new and improved" device is on the market, its "better and faster" competitor is released. Most people venture into **cyberspace** on a daily basis, where a world of information is waiting with the simple click of a mouse!

For many years computers have been used in medical facilities, including physicians' offices. The development of software, the decrease in the cost of computer **hardware,** and the time savings that the computer brings to the office make it well worth the investment. Computers are now standard equipment in healthcare facilities (Figure 8-1). A medical assistant must have more than computer literacy; a good understanding of the way computers work and their capabilities is essential in a medical office.

Getting Started

Even with some basic knowledge of computer components and of what computers can do, without hands-on knowledge, the beginner may have some initial fear of the unknown. However, the computer is only a machine that takes its direction from the person operating it. It will perform the tasks that it is told to do. A computer can simulate the thought process and make decisions, but most computers found in medical facilities will wait for commands that prompt it to act. Dialog boxes appear that ask for **input** from the user. This is how the computer communicates with the person using it. Computers assist workers in medical offices in some of the following ways:

- Performing repetitive tasks
- Reducing errors
- Speeding up production
- Recalling information on command
- Saving time
- Reducing paperwork and storage space
- Allowing for more creative and productive use of workers' time

The more familiar a medical assistant becomes with the computer, the better skilled he or she will become in its use. Occasionally errors will be made, and the computer may respond with an error message. However, the monitor screen normally indicates what to do next. The computer will usually allow the operator the opportunity to figure out the correct information and input that information into the computer. A help menu can always be accessed, or the instruction manual can be consulted; help lines and technical support are available as well when problems occur. The problem may be with the software or with the computer itself. Usually it is fairly easy to determine which is causing the problem.

Rarely will the computer "break," although this is a common fear among new users. It is unlikely that records will be destroyed by accident; usually very specific commands are needed to delete stored information. However, a medical assistant must take care not to shut off the computer without saving the information that has been entered. By using a computer in the classroom and practicing at home or at a library, if possible, the medical assistant will gain familiarity with computer operation and confidence that it can be mastered. Mastery is accomplished only through practice.

With knowledge of computer terms, the ability to follow step-by-step instructions, and reasonable expertise with a keyboard, a medical assistant can rapidly learn and use almost any computer system. Although the computers and the software may vary from facility to facility, basic computer operation is similar, and if the instructions given by the computer are carried out, the user should be successful in the tasks attempted.

Although it seems elementary, the first step to computer use is to turn the system on. If nothing happens when the power button is pushed, the primary troubleshooting protocol is to make certain that the system is plugged into the power outlet. If it is, then check all of the cords that attach the hardware to determine if they are securely fastened. Once the power is on, the computer goes through a process called *booting*. The boot sequence is a set of operations that the computer performs that loads the operating system and prepares it for use.

Once the computer is on, the desktop will appear and the user will see several **icons.** To open a certain program, double-click on its icon. Once a program has been opened, many functions can be performed, such as creating a document, a spreadsheet, or a presentation or maintaining a **database.** Some of the basic computer functions include the following:

- *Formatting a* **disk**. Most of today's diskettes are purchased preformatted, but that formatting can be erased if the user desires. Formatting a disk prepares it for use on the system and divides it into sectors and tracks where information can be written by the computer.
- *Opening a document.* A document stored on the computer can be opened by clicking on its icon, if it is stored on the desktop. If the document is stored in a folder, open the folder and click on the document icon.
- *Saving a document.* Most toolbars have a button that allows a document to be saved to a folder or to the desktop. Click the button, then name the file so that it can be easily found when it is needed. Word processing programs usually have a "save as" option as well, so that a document can be saved and edited without changing the original file.
- *Creating a folder.* Folders in which documents can be stored are easily created. For instance, in a Windows **environment,** one can create a folder called "Study Guides" on the desktop. To do this, right-click on the desktop away from other files, folders, and icons, then select the command "new." When the second dialog box appears, select "folder." Click "folder" and a folder titled "new

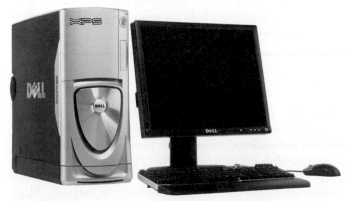

FIGURE 8-1 Computers are an invaluable tool for today's medical office. (Photo courtesy of Dell Corporation.)

folder" will appear on the desktop. To rename it, click twice on the words "new folder" and type in the words "Study Guides" or whatever title is to be used. The folder is now ready for use. To move documents into the folder, click on the document icon and hold the left mouse button down while dragging the document on top of the folder. This is called "drag and drop" or sometimes, "click and drag." To place documents that are not on the desktop into the folder, use the "save as" feature and save the document to the desired folder. Or the document can be saved to the desktop, after which the "drag-and-drop" feature can be used to place it in the desired folder.

- *Copying, moving, deleting, and renaming files.* Most word processing programs allow the user to copy, move, delete, and rename files. In Windows, a file may be copied easily by right-clicking on the document icon and then clicking "copy." Then, open the folder to which the file is to be copied, right-click inside the folder, and click "paste." A copy of the file will appear in the folder. Moving files from one place to another can be accomplished by using the drag-and-drop method. To delete a file, right-click on the document icon and click "delete." A dialog box will open that will confirm the user's choice to delete the file. The file will remain in the recycle bin on the desktop for a brief period of time once deleted, so if a mistake has been made and the file is needed, the user should look to see if it is still available. Renaming files is as simple as clicking twice on the filename and typing in the new one. The user can also right-click on the document icon and select "rename," which will allow the user to change the name of the document.

- *Cutting, copying, and pasting text.* Text can be moved from one place to another by cutting and pasting. First, highlight the text that is to be moved, then press the "cut" button. This function can also be accomplished by right-clicking the mouse and selecting "cut." Next, place the **cursor** at the point where the text should be inserted, then click the "paste" key or right-click the mouse and select "paste." Copying text is done in the same manner. Instead of clicking the "cut" button, press the "copy" button. These functions allow the user to be more efficient when creating documents.

- *Finding files.* Computers have a "search" mechanism that will allow the user to search for a file with certain keywords or extensions. In the Windows environment, click the "start" button, then click on "search." The dialog box that appears will ask the user what to search for, whether it be a picture, audio file, document, or other file type. An option to search all files and folders is also available. Enter keywords that pertain to the desired file, and click "search."

- *Copying an entire disk.* It is possible to copy an entire diskette or compact disk (CD). First, click on "start" and then click on "my computer." Find the drive that contains the diskette or CD and right-click on that icon. Then, click on "copy." Open the folder to which the contents should be copied, then click "paste." The actual diskette or CD could also be opened, then under the "edit" drop-down menu, the user can choose "select all." This also allows all of the files on the diskette or CD to be copied or permanently moved to another location.

- *Exiting a program.* Press the "x" key on the upper right corner of the document to exit a program. If the work has not yet been saved, the user will be prompted to either save the document or cancel the action. The user can also exit the program by clicking on "file" then "exit."

Once the user is finished with the computer for the day, it should always be shut down properly. To accomplish this, click the "start" icon, then click "turn off computer." The dialog box that appears will allow the user to turn the computer off, restart the computer, stand by, or cancel the action. The restart function is helpful when the computer "freezes" or fails to function as it should. This takes the computer back through the booting sequence and will often correct problems and allow the user to continue working. Never attempt to fix problems on the computer that are beyond the medical assistant's scope of knowledge. Often a technical assistance desk will be able to walk the user through various steps to correct basic issues. Always report computer malfunctions to the proper person or department.

Computer systems have user manuals that can be consulted when functions do not perform as they should or when a user is working with an unfamiliar system. Tutorials may be available that will help the new user to learn the system or to refresh the skills of the experienced user.

COMPUTER BASICS

A computer is a machine that is designed to accept, store, process, and provide information (Figure 8-2). Computers serve the following basic functions:

- *Input:* Input includes any information that enters the computer. It can take a variety of forms, from commands that are entered from the keyboard to data from another computer or device, such as a **scanner.** The device that feeds data into a computer, such as a mouse, scanner, keyboard, or voice recognition system, is called an *input device.*

- *Processing:* Processing is the act of manipulating the data that are currently inside the computer to carry out a certain task.

- *Output:* **Output** is anything that exits the computer. Output can appear in many forms, such as binary numbers, characters, pictures, printed pages, or a simple image on the computer screen. Output devices include monitors, speakers, printers, scanners, and modems.

- *Storage:* The act of retaining data or applications is called *storage.* Data can be stored on disks, on CDs, or on separate drives, such as a **zip drive** or a **flash drive.** The type of storage device used depends on the amount of information that needs to be saved and where it needs to be used. CDs and flash drives are common portable storage devices used in the business world.

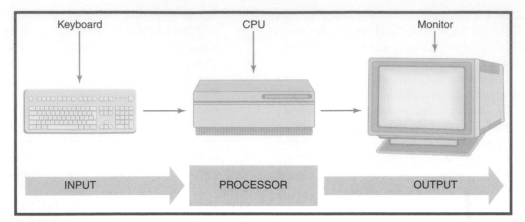

FIGURE 8-2 Input devices allow data to be entered into the computer, where they are processed; output is available in several different forms.

CRITICAL THINKING APPLICATION

- Dr. Bouchard plans to send two of his employees to a training class on using a new software program designed to perform all computer functions needed for his practice. Although he can send only two employees, how can the others learn the system?
- Would it be beneficial or detrimental to close the office for a day to educate the other employees about the system? What should the physician consider before losing a day of patient visits?

TYPES OF COMPUTERS

Various types of computers meet the needs of staff in today's physician office. The most common type is the desktop computer, which consists of a central processing unit (CPU), monitor, mouse, and keyboard, in most cases. The laptop, notebook, and personal digital assistant (PDA) have grown in popularity because they are compact and portable (Figures 8-3 and 8-4). Some physicians and office employees carry the computer from room to room while treating patients. Information can be entered directly into the computer, which saves time and is much more efficient than handwritten or transcribed notes. The PDA is small enough to carry in a pocket or purse. Physicians may use this device when treating patients or making hospital rounds, as it is lighter and even more convenient than a laptop. The PDA also organizes personal information, such as addresses and phone numbers, and most models allow the user to access the Internet and read email messages. The user can also use the PDA as a day planner, keeping track of appointments, meetings, and other important events.

Embedded computers are those that are inside another device, such as an ultrasound unit or electrocardiograph (ECG). These computers allow for data input and output and usually analyze information. A mainframe is a large, expensive computer that is capable of processing huge amounts of information. These computers are usually found in large companies and government institutions.

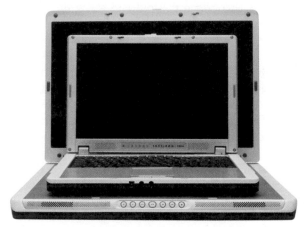

FIGURE 8-3 Laptop computers vary in size and weight and are easily portable. (Photo courtesy of Dell Corporation.)

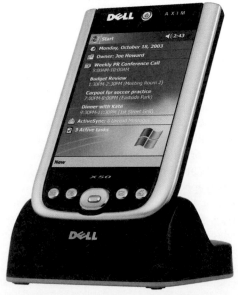

FIGURE 8-4 The PDA is a hand-held device that usually contains an address and phone book and a personal organizer and allows the user to access the Internet. (Photo courtesy of Dell Corporation.)

PARTS OF THE COMPUTER

A medical assistant must understand the function of the different parts of a computer. The physical pieces that can be touched and seen are called *hardware.* Computers using Windows software have an option in the control panel for adding hardware. This shortcut makes adding new equipment easy and provides instruction all along the way. Hardware provides the medium on which software can be used. Most PCs have a microprocessor, monitor, keyboard, and mouse and many are connected to a printer.

Microprocessor

Inside the casing of the main computer hardware, the microprocessor is housed. The microprocessor is the central unit of the computer that contains the logic circuitry, which carries out the instructions of a computer's programs. It is considered the most important piece of hardware in a computer system. Microprocessors act as the brain of the computer and interpret instructions from a program. Microprocessors, sometimes called CPUs, are differentiated by three basic elements:

- *Bandwidth:* Bandwidth describes how much information can be sent over a connection at one time, or how many **bits** can be processed in one single instruction. Bits, short for binary digits, are the smallest pieces of information on the computer. Eight bits make up 1 **byte.** A **kilobyte** is approximately 1024 bytes, and a **megabyte** is approximately 1 million bytes. A **gigabyte** consists of approximately 1 billion bytes. A **terabyte** provides a huge amount of storage, consisting of approximately 1 trillion bytes.
- *Clock speed:* Clock speed determines how many instructions per second that the processor can handle. Clock speed is measured in **megahertz** (MHz). One megahertz equals 1 million cycles per second, so a processor that operates at 300 MHz executes 300 million cycles per second.
- *Instruction set:* The instruction set is the set of instructions that the microprocessor can execute.

The higher the bandwidth and clock speed, the faster and more powerful the microprocessor. For instance, a 32-bit microprocessor that runs at 50 MHz is more powerful than a 16-bit microprocessor that runs at 25 MHz.

A microprocessor contains memory consisting of electronic and magnetic cells, each of which contains information. Two kinds of memory exist: read-only memory (ROM) and random-access memory (RAM). ROM is internal memory that contains a portion of the operating system and computer language. This is sometimes known as *main memory.* Data that have been "burned" onto a ROM chip cannot be removed and can only be read, similar to a CD-ROM, unless the CD is a "rewriteable" type. With this permanent memory, much less information has to be transferred from a disk to start the computing process. ROM cannot be overwritten and is not erased when the power is shut off. RAM can be thought of as an internal scratch pad for the computer. It contains the program instructions and the data that are currently processing. RAM is normally erased when the power is shut off.

Monitor

A monitor, which looks very much like a television (TV) screen, is a device used to display computer-generated information. A few are **monochromatic,** but most monitors today are color, capable of being adjusted for brightness, sharpness, and other settings of the user's choice. Many are high-definition monitors that rival the best plasma TV screens. Color monitors allow for a high-quality display, and the more advanced models have resolutions capable of reproducing high-quality pictures good enough for viewing a **digital video disk (DVD).** By viewing the monitor, the user receives instant feedback on entries into the computer. Monitors are sometimes referred to as *displays* and are considered output devices.

Keyboard

For most computers the keyboard is the primary text input device. Keyboards contain special function keys, such as the escape key, tab key, cursor movement keys, numeric keys, shift keys, and control keys. Additional function keys, numbered F1 to F12, are used to perform specific word processing or other computer-related operations. Used alone, a function key may create bold print, underline, indent, or call up a help screen. Used in conjunction with the Ctrl, Alt, or Shift key, the function keys can produce other desired results, such as activating the printer, inserting the current date into a document, retrieving a file, or moving a designated block of text. Wireless keyboards are a popular alternative that allow the user to move around more freely while operating the computer. Wave keyboards, and others designed with ergonomics in mind, are also popular.

Mouse

The mouse first became a widely used computer tool when Apple Computers made it a standard part of the Apple Macintosh computer. It resembles a mouse because of its shape and the cord, which attaches it to the microprocessor. A wireless mouse allows the user to manipulate the cursor without a cord attached. The mouse is a pointing device with a ball on the bottom that is moved by rolling it on a flat tabletop or mouse pad. The optical mouse has a photosensor instead of the rolling ball device. Some computers, especially laptops, have a built-in device called a *trackball* that is moved with the finger or thumb and serves the same function as a mouse. Other computers have a touchpad or a track-point that is manipulated to control the cursor. The cursor is a pointer or flat bar appearing on the monitor that shows where the next character will appear, which is the insertion point. The mouse allows the user to navigate around the screen quickly and click on links to access websites.

Printer

Printers are output devices. Documents appearing on the monitor may be directed to a printer to produce a printout or **hard copy** of a document. Many printers are bidirectional, which means they print both from left to right and from right to left. The type of printer used should depend on the job being performed.

Dot matrix printers are inexpensive and produce a moderate-quality hard copy. They form letters or shapes that they are directed to print by arranging patterns of dots on the paper. They operate faster than letter-quality machines, but the print lacks the clarity generally desired for a professional look.

Inkjet printers use an ink cartridge that feeds an array of nearly microscopic tubes, each of which has a heating element that is energized during the printing process. The ink cartridge may be black and white or color. Inkjet printers cost less than laser printers, but the ink cartridges they use are fairly expensive and increase the operating cost.

Laser printers use xerographic technology similar to that in photocopiers, so the laser printer is able to produce an almost limitless variety of forms and sizes as well as complex graphics. One disadvantage of inkjet and laser printers is that they are incapable of producing multiple copies with carbon sets or multicopy forms, which are often used by insurance companies for their filing forms.

Some printers today are multifunctional, serving as printers, **fax** machines, scanners, and copiers. Although these are excellent for home offices, they may not be the best investment for offices that will use these machines often during the day.

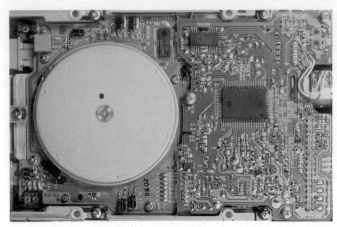

FIGURE 8-5 Hard drives store data and applications for fast and effective access and retrieval. Although a program installed on a hard drive can be removed, most programs are placed there for permanent use, such as Microsoft Office or Peachtree Accounting.

to the hard disk and stored there on the computer for use when needed. This is commonly called the *C drive.*

Floppy disks or diskettes are normally used in the computer's A drive, although the drives can have different names or labels, depending on the brand of computer. Floppy disks were so named because the original $5^1/_4$-inch variety was housed in a soft plastic cover that would "flop" if waved up and down. The $3^1/_2$-inch diskettes are less frequently used now because CDs have a higher capacity for holding information. Flash drives make transporting information from one computer to another quick and easy and are used more often today than diskettes.

CRITICAL THINKING APPLICATION

Dr. Bouchard has asked his office manager to perform a cost comparison on a printer for three of the office computers. He prefers that they have scanning and fax capability. What are some of the features that the office manager will be interested in knowing about these machines?

INSIDE THE COMPUTER

Basic knowledge of the parts of a computer and their function will help a medical assistant to deal with minor technical issues and easily communicate with technical support personnel.

Motherboard

A motherboard is the main circuit board for the computer, to which other devices can be attached. Usually it contains the processor, the memory, and other controllers and devices that allow the system to operate and function.

Disk Drives

Today's computers have various **disk drives** on which information can be stored or accessed. The hard disk or hard drive is a magnetic disk inside the computer that holds from approximately 10 megabytes to several hundred gigabytes of information (Figure 8-5). Application software is normally saved

---

CRITICAL THINKING APPLICATION

Dr. Bouchard mentions that he noticed CD-R disks on sale over the weekend. The price that he saw was $30 for 100 CD-Rs. One of the medical assistants noticed a 30-pack of CD-Rs for $9.99. Which is the better buy?

CD-ROM

Most of today's PCs are equipped with CD-ROM drives, which allow the storage of data on a CD. CDs hold much more information than floppy disks. A single CD can store as much information as approximately 700 floppy disks, which is the equivalent of about 300,000 text pages (Figure 8-6). A CD-RW is one on which data can be written, erased, and rewritten. Computers that have a **CD burner,** or CD-R drive, can take information from one CD or another source and write it to another CD. The computer must also have software that enables the burner to work. Software that is installed on a computer to allow a hardware device to function is called a **device driver.**

Expansion Boards

Expansion boards are devices that are inserted into a computer that give the computer added capabilities. For example, a **sound card** may be installed so that music or **MIDI** files can be heard from the unit. Other expansion boards are video adapters, internal modems, and graphics accelerators.

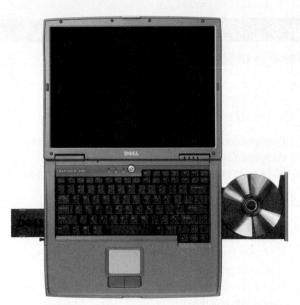

FIGURE 8-6 CD-ROMs allow the user to store and retrieve large amounts of information. Many computers are now equipped with CD-ROM burners, which allow copying of information from one CD to another, or from Internet files to CD-ROMs. (Photo courtesy of Dell Corporation.)

Software

Software is the programs and utilities that are loaded onto or inside the computer and used to carry out the work performed by the machine. There are two types of software: systems software and applications software. **System software** serves as the operating system of the computer and allows it to run and carry out the functions that the computer performs. For instance, Windows XP, Linux, and the now somewhat antiquated DOS are all types of operating system software. **Application software** refers to the programs loaded onto the computer that carry out the work for the actual users of the computer. Examples of application software are Microsoft Office, MediSoft, and Medical Manager. Applications (programs) are designed to perform specific tasks, such as word processing, billing, accounting, appointment setting, insurance form preparation, payroll, and **database** management. Many software applications are available for complete medical practice management (Procedure 8-1).

Modems

A **modem,** short for modulator-demodulator, is a device over which data can be transmitted via telephone lines and other media, such as a coaxial cable. Modems can be internal or external. An internal modem is built into or added to the inside of the computer casing. A cable modem operates over cable TV lines and uses the coaxial cable to provide faster Internet access. **Digital subscriber line (DSL)** modems operate over phone lines like normal modems, but they use a different frequency; therefore the telephone can be used while the computer is accessing the Internet. Often a filter is attached to the phone that removes other frequencies wherein the DSL is working, avoiding interference with the telephone line operation.

Speakers and Microphones

Some computers have external speakers to provide a higher quality sound from the computer. Many computers also have built-in speakers that provide a fair quality of sound. Microphones can be built in or attached so that the user can speak directly into the computer, even to someone on the other side of the world!

PERIPHERAL DEVICES

Peripheral devices are those that are not essential to the operation of the computer. For instance, the computer will operate without a modem, although a modem is necessary to access the Internet. A mouse is even considered a peripheral device, because everything that the mouse can access can also be reached by certain buttons on the keyboard, although often multiple keys have to be pressed at once. This section discusses some of the peripheral devices in use today.

Scanners

Scanners read text, illustrations, or photographs printed on paper and put them into a **format** that the computer can understand. Photographs can be placed into the scanner, saved on the computer, then used in a document. Some advanced scanners are used like highlighters and can collect notes from printed text.

Digital Cameras

Digital cameras use a charge-coupled device (CCD) to convert light into electrical charges. Digital cameras do not use film. Light strikes the surface of a photosite inside the camera, then filters add color and create the digital image. Many digital cameras can be attached directly to a computer or printer, and photos can be downloaded directly from the camera. Other cameras use a disk to load the pictures onto the computer.

CRITICAL THINKING APPLICATION

How might a digital camera be of use to a physician in his or her medical practice? What care should be taken when using the camera with a patient?

Zip Drives

A zip drive is a disk drive that has a very high storage capacity and is attached externally to a computer. It is usually used as a **backup** device for important data that should not be lost. Zip drives can hold between 100 and 250 megabytes of data and can even be stored somewhere other than the facility so that they are safe in case of fire or other destructive event.

ADDING A PROGRAM TO A COMPUTER

Adding or loading a program onto a computer is relatively easy. Most programs today come on a CD-ROM. The program will come with instructions as to how it should be loaded onto

PROCEDURE 8-1

Utilize Computer Software to Maintain Office Systems

CAAHEP COMPETENCY: 3.c(4)(c)
ABHES COMPETENCIES: 2.n, 3.d

GOAL: *To use the office computer system at maximum capacity to run the various aspects of the physician's office.*

EQUIPMENT and SUPPLIES

- Computer
- Computer software applications
- Software manuals
- Description of office systems
- Patient data
- Business data

PROCEDURAL STEPS

1. Determine the types of data that the physician's office needs to computerize.
   PURPOSE: To effectively plan the needs of the physician's office.
2. Discuss these needs with the physician and office manager.
3. Compile a budget for computer systems and/or upgrades.
   PURPOSE: Any large or capital purchases must be budgeted.

4. Research computer systems that can handle the tasks designated by the physician.
5. Invite sales representatives to present their options during a staff meeting.
   PURPOSE: The staff members may have significant questions that pertain to their particular area of concern.
6. Compare benefits and drawbacks of each system.
   PURPOSE: The comparison process will help in the decision as to which system should be used.
7. Ask sales representatives any questions that arise in the comparison process.
8. Discuss the final few choices with the physician and office manager.
9. Decide on a computer system or upgrade that best fits the needs of the office.
10. Purchase or lease the computer system.

---

the computer. Watch the monitor for steps to complete and information concerning the user's preferences, then follow all of the directions given.

In a Windows environment, the control panel provides an option to "add/remove programs." Once clicked, this will allow the program in the CD disk drive to be loaded onto the computer. At several points the computer may ask the user questions about his or her preferences for the program. Often the computer needs to be restarted after installation.

To remove a program from the computer, the "add/remove programs" **icon** should be accessed and the directions followed for removal of the program. This may be the only way to completely remove the program from the computer system.

FILE FORMATS

A file is a collection of data. Many types of files are related to computers. A text file, for example, contains some type of text, which is the main body of printed words or written matter on a page. Often an extension exists at the end of the filename that designates what type of file the document is. A file named manual.com might indicate that the file is some type of command file. A few of the common file extensions include the following:

- jpg: *JPEG* stands for Joint Photographic Experts Group and is a format often used for photographs.
- gif: *GIF* stands for Graphics Interchange Format, which supports color and is often used for scanned images and illustrations rather than photographs.

- doc: A file that includes the extension .doc is usually a file created by a word processor or word processing software; *doc* stands for document.
- txt: A text file usually has the extension .txt after its name. Characters in a text file are represented by their **ASCII codes.**
- rtf: *RTF* stands for Rich Text Format. This type of file combines ASCII codes with special commands that distinguish variations, such as a certain **font.**
- bmp: Bit-mapped graphics are indicated by the extension .bmp. These are compiled by a graphics image that is set in rows or columns of dots.

A medical assistant who is familiar with these types of files will be able to save and open them correctly and use the computer to the fullest advantage in the medical office.

COMPUTER NETWORKING

A network is a group of two or more computer systems that are linked together. Several types of networks exist:

- LAN: A LAN is a Local Area Network, or a computer network spanning a relatively small area. Most LANs are contained in a single building or group of buildings and are connected by a **router,** but LANs can be connected to other LANs even at a distance. A **hub** is a device that connects several computers or networks together, and a **switch** is designed to help the LAN run more efficiently by controlling local network traffic.
- MAN: A MAN is a Metropolitan Area Network. A MAN

spans an area that does not exceed a metropolitan area or city and connects several LANs.

- WAN: A WAN is a Wide Area Network, which spans a relatively large geographic area. Typically, a WAN consists of two or more LANs or MANs. These networks can be connected through public networks, such as a telephone system, or through leased lines or satellites. The largest WAN that exists is the Internet.
- HAN: A HAN is a Home Area Network, which connects computers inside a user's home.
- CAN: A CAN is a Campus Area Network, often used on college campuses and sometimes on military bases.

SERVERS

A **server** is important to the network, because it is the computer that manages the shared network resources. Several types of servers exist. When many computers are connected to one printer, often a print server manages these printers. File servers are used for file storage, and database servers are used to process database **queries.** Some servers are considered to be dedicated servers, meaning they perform tasks only as a server, although a server may also operate as a normal computer.

CLIENTS

A client is a computer that is configured to request access to resources from a server. Server applications, like access to the Internet, network printing, or email access, can run on a server and are accessed by the clients so that they can accomplish these tasks.

THE INTERNET

The Internet is a global network that connects millions of computers together. This fascinating structure has made the world a smaller place (Figure 8-7). Through chat programs one can talk with individuals literally on the other side of the world and be introduced to cultures that 20 years ago would never have been understood. Through Web pages we

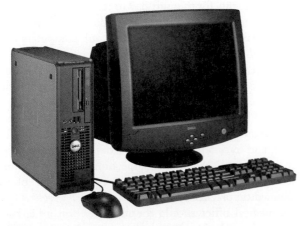

FIGURE 8-7 Computers in today's businesses can speak to one another from across the room or across the world. (Photo courtesy of Dell Corporation.)

can visit different parts of the world and learn and see many things that previously were impossible for the average person to experience. **Ecommerce** allows us to shop on the net, from the most exclusive shops in Beverly Hills to the corner grocery store. The Internet has changed the way we learn, do business, communicate, and entertain ourselves.

Each computer connected to the Internet is called a *host* and is independent of all the others. The users of each computer determine which services to make available to other users on the Internet. Often a company or organization also has an Intranet, which is a local network that uses Internet technology within a company or single location but does not have access to the Internet directly.

Internet service providers (ISPs) are companies that provide access to the Internet. Examples include America Online, Mindspring, Verizon, Earthlink, and Yahoo. ISPs issue each user an IP (Internet Protocol) address, which is a unique identifier for that user's particular computer on a Transmission Control Protocol/ Internet Protocol **(TCP/IP)** network. An IP address is a 32-bit number written as four numbers separated by a period. Each number can be zero to 255, so a valid IP address could be 10.145.32.254. Messages are defined and transmitted over the Internet when a Uniform Resource Locator **(URL)** is entered into the browser and a HyperText Transfer Protocol **(HTTP)** command tells the Web server to retrieve the requested Web page.

Domain names identify one or more IP addresses, such as microsoft.com or ama-assn.org. A limited number of top-level domains are available to which a domain name can be attached. Some of these top-level domains include .com (familiarly called *dot-com)* for commercial businesses; .org for organizations, usually nonprofit; .edu for educational institutions; .gov for government agencies; and .net for network organizations. Most Internet sites use a language called HyperText Markup Language **(HTML),** which was one of the first and is still one of the most popular languages used to create Web pages. **Java** is another popular language used in website creation.

Hotspots are locations that offer an access point providing public wireless broadband network services and are found in places such as airports, libraries, convention centers, and hotels. Users may be able to connect to the network for no charge or may be required to place a credit card number on file or make a deposit. This service is convenient for the medical professional who is traveling or attending events away from the office.

Many physicians and health organizations offer a website with information about their services. In today's data-driven society, this is an excellent way to educate the public about the services the organization offers and to provide all types of information to the audience that the organization wishes to reach. To obtain a domain name, one must pay a small fee to have the name registered and added to a central database, if the desired name is available. Companies such as register.com or verisign.com offer domain name registration services.

Websites often contain **banners,** which attract the eye of the user and tempt a click of the mouse, taking the user to a new website. They are similar to Internet commercials. These sites usually contain advertisements or surveys and can track the number of times a user views the site. These views are called "hits." Banners and website home pages sometimes use **Flash,** which is designed to grab the interest of the user with **multimedia** and encourage further exploration of a website.

A word of caution: Because most medical offices have some type of connection to the Internet, the medical assistant may be tempted to check personal email, "surf" the Web, or participate in instant messaging during working hours. Remember, personal business should not be conducted while at work. Supervisors appreciate the medical assistant who is honest with his or her time and spends it in productive, work-related activities.

BROWSERS

Web browsers are software applications that allow the user to locate and display Web pages. Two commonly used browsers are Netscape Navigator and Microsoft Internet Explorer. These browsers are able to display graphics as well as text and can also present multimedia information, the quality of which is dependent on the computer system in use and the Internet connection speed. Browsers also have a bookmark capability that allows the user to mark a certain Web page then easily return to it by clicking on its link in a drop-down box in the browser's menu. The **cache** allows quick retrieval of previously viewed sites because the computer remembers and saves the information on the hard drive. **Cookies** are stored information about individual users, like screen names and passwords.

Browsers and other websites also contain **search engines.** These are programs in which a topic, word, or group of words can be entered, and the engine will search the Internet for matches. A listing of those matches will appear, and the user can click on each match to reference information and complete research. Information on just about any subject can be found through using search engines.

CRITICAL THINKING APPLICATION

Dr. Bouchard wants all employees to have Internet access at his office but is still concerned that there will be occasional misuse of the computer. He does not want the staff to use the computer for personal business but does not mind if they check their personal email on a break or at lunch. What are some reasonable policies for office Internet use?

Popular Search Engines

www.alltheweb.com	www.lycos.com
www.altavista.com	www.metacrawler.com
www.ask.com	www.netscape.com
www.dogpile.com	www.search.aol.com
www.excite.com	www.search.msn.com
www.google.com	www.webcrawler.com
www.hotbot.com	www.yahoo.com

THE COMPUTER AS A CO-WORKER

The computer is a valuable tool in the medical office. It can assist in filing insurance claims by sending information from the computer in the office to the computers at the insurance company using a modem. Electronic processing of insurance claims not only saves time but also provides immediate information as to whether a claim will be accepted. Errors in coding or procedure are immediately evident, and many rejections can be avoided even before the claim is transmitted. Most insurance companies require that providers file claims electronically.

The demographics about a patient will appear on computerized patient ledgers, listing name, address, telephone number, and insurance information. As services are rendered, charges are entered into the computer, and payments will be displayed as well. This helps the medical facility to maintain an accurate balance of all patient accounts.

At the appropriate time each month, the computer can print a patient's billing statement, which shows a detail of charges, payments, adjustments, and the current balance. In addition, the computer can be programmed to age the accounts according to any criteria selected and to include this information on the billing statement. A series of collection letters can be developed and personalized for individual patients as they are needed.

Database software makes it possible to organize a large volume of information that can be used in a number of ways. One of the most practical uses is the organization of identifying information on each patient. The computer can also store clinical information about patients using much less space and with greater security than papers in a patient's chart. Access to records can be limited with passwords.

The computer has virtually replaced the appointment book in many medical offices today. Software for appointment-setting ranges from relatively simple programs to very sophisticated systems. An advantage to computer scheduling is that more than one person can access the system at one time, and the same information is available to all users.

Computers are even being used as marketing tools and virtual secretaries in some modern medical offices (Figures 8-8 and 8-9). Computers can be programmed to call all patients with appointments for the next day to remind them to visit the doctor, or perhaps to call all patients due for a 6-month eye or dental examination. As a marketing tool, computers can be programmed to call all phone numbers in a certain area code with a prerecorded message about a new procedure available at the office or a new physician in the area. Although many individuals are annoyed by the telemarketing concept and being called by a computer, the success rate is good. Computers can call thousands on thousands of phone numbers, relay a message, and track replies within a matter of hours. This could never be accomplished in the same time period by humans. These methods of using the computer open all kinds of doors for the medical practice of the future.

The medical office should routinely perform a file backup to be sure that valuable data can be retrieved in the event of a system failure. Many medical office computer programs have an

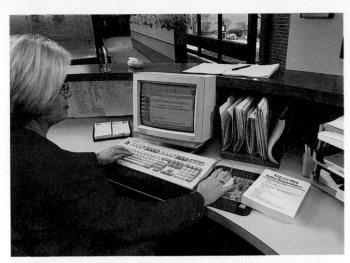

FIGURE 8-8 Computers assist the staff members and physicians of the medical office in numerous ways, making the office run in a more efficient manner.

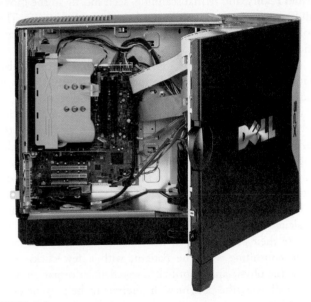

FIGURE 8-9 Inside a computer. Today's microprocessors are designed so that memory, additional drives, and other hardware can be easily added to the system. (Photo courtesy of Dell Corporation.)

automatic backup function, but some must be done manually. It is wise to keep backup copies of the database and other critical documents off the premises in case of fire or other tragedy.

COMPUTER SECURITY

Patients are entitled to the utmost confidentiality with respect to their medical records and the release of any information of a personal nature. Computer technology allows the accumulation and storage of a vast amount of data that may be accessible to a variety of individuals, making it imperative that guidelines be set up for the protection of such data.

Encryption is the translation of data into a code that is not readily understood by most users. It is one effective way to achieve data security. To access or read an encrypted file, the user must have a password that enables the code to be decrypted.

Once the code is decrypted, the file is then useable by the application. Encrypted data are called *cipher text.*

Some individuals attempt to access information in a computer without the owner's consent. These people may intend to use the information just for fun or may have a malicious intent, such as to steal or corrupt the data. Although these people are commonly called *hackers,* computer enthusiasts insist that the correct term for individuals who break into computers with dishonorable intent is *crackers.* The term *hacker* originally simply described a person who enjoyed learning about using computers and becoming proficient in that use.

Various ways may be used to protect computers and data from unauthorized access. Firewalls are systems designed for just such a purpose and can be implemented into both the hardware and the software of the computer. Firewalls are often used to prevent individuals from accessing private networks. Each message sent and received is examined, and the firewall blocks those that do not meet specific security criteria. Passwords, frequent password changes, and user logs also help protect data and the integrity of the database.

Viruses are programs or pieces of code that are loaded onto a computer, usually without the owner's knowledge, and can act like a physical virus in that they can make the computer "sick." Viruses can replicate themselves, copying themselves over and over again, and can be passed to other computers through emails, usually without the sender's knowing that a virus was passed along. Even simple viruses can quickly use all available memory and bring the system to a standstill; some can completely corrupt the computer's hard drive. More dangerous types of viruses can transmit over networks, bypassing security systems and destroying valuable data. This is why antivirus software is an important part of any computer system. Check for updates to the antivirus program at least weekly.

COMPUTERS AND THE HEALTH INSURANCE PORTABILITY AND ACCOUNTABILITY ACT

The Health Insurance Portability and Accountability Act (HIPAA) was developed in part to make certain that patient health information would be kept private and confidential. The wide use of computers in healthcare facilities sometimes makes this a difficult goal. The law limits who can look at and/or receive a patient's health information. Health information may be used and shared as follows:
- For patient care and treatment coordination
- To pay physicians and facilities for healthcare
- With family, friends, and relatives whom the patient has identified as being involved in the patient's healthcare
- To make certain that good care is provided in clean facilities
- To protect public health
- To make required reports to law enforcement officials

Health information cannot be shared or used without patient permission in most cases. Specifically, the provider cannot do the following:
- Give health information to a patient's employer
- Use or share health information for marketing purposes

- Share mental health information obtained in counseling sessions

The healthcare facility must take action to train those who use computer systems as to what information can and cannot be shared. Individual computer users should have their own log-in names and passwords that are not provided to anyone else. All users should be required to use the log-in name and password every time they use the computer system. Patient information must not be accessed unless the user needs to know the contents of the patient's file in order to provide patient care. Be careful when releasing any type of medical information to anyone. Questions should be directed to the office manager or to the physician. HIPAA will be discussed in more detail in Chapter 15, which covers Health Information Management.

ELECTRONIC SIGNATURES

A recently introduced convenience option is the electronic signature. Electronic signature programs are offered both as stand-alone products and as part of computerized medical record systems. After dictated reports are transcribed, a physician can use a password and personal identification number (PIN) to electronically "sign" the document by clicking on an icon after the document has been reviewed for accuracy. Once the document has been signed, it cannot be altered—only addenda are allowed.

COMPUTERS AND ERGONOMICS

The increased use of computers in the workplace has underscored the need to choose comfortable, safe furniture and equipment. Repetitive strain injury (RSI) accounts for the majority of work-related injury claims. This includes a number of conditions that are caused by repeatedly straining certain nerves, muscles, or tendons. Carpal tunnel syndrome is one example of RSI.

To avoid such injuries, office staff should use posture chairs that support the lumbar section of the back, with a correct angle of the knee and the feet resting on the floor. Of the many designs for keyboards available, one should be chosen that allows the correct angle at the elbow and the wrist to be held in a neutral position.

Eyestrain is another danger arising from continuous use of a computer. The monitor should be just below eye level and at an arm's length away. At least once each hour, the user should take a break from looking at the monitor.

CLOSING COMMENTS

Computers should be thought of as additional workers in the office. A medical assistant who learns how best to use the computer and discovers as many of its capabilities as possible will be a valuable employee.

Read the manuals that accompany equipment and programs and try new applications for old procedures. Computers are designed to save time, so look for ways to make the day's workload lighter by taking full advantage of the computer.

The future promises more rapid technologic advances; computer equipment can become archaic in as short a time as 6 months after purchase. **Artificial intelligence,** voice recognition, **virtual reality,** and retinal scanning, seen mostly in the movies, will become commonplace in our homes and businesses. These tools will make the work environment even faster and more efficient as the world becomes a smaller place.

The evolution of computers will continue to bring about changes in medical facilities of the future. Medical staffs will find themselves educating their patients about computer use, because numerous programs in development will allow patients to "check in" once they arrive at the office and verify their identity. A medical assistant will need patience to instruct these procedures and assure the patients that these new methods will increase their security as well as the protection of their medical records.

With the growing number of medical databases online, physicians can now use information on the Internet to help educate their patients about the illnesses that they are facing. While consulting with the patient, with a few clicks of the mouse the physician can print out excellent information, which often will assist the patient with referrals to help agencies and suggestions for better healthcare.

SUMMARY OF SCENARIO

Dr. Bouchard is a progressive physician who believes that the use of technology will assist him in the care of his patients and help his office to run more efficiently. The computer assists the staff to complete tasks in a timely manner and provides records of business transactions. Staff members are able to function much faster than when records were kept by hand. He understands the need to train his staff and keep them up to date on the latest versions of their computer software. His willingness to close his office for staff-wide training demonstrates his commitment. He is cost conscious and looks for the best available equipment for the investment he is willing to make.

Dr. Bouchard often uses digital camera equipment to take "before" and "after" pictures of his patients, but only with their special written consent. He also uses the computer to send his patients a monthly email newsletter with health information and special news about the practice.

He monitors his staff's Internet use but is reasonable about allowing them a small degree of personal access on breaks and at lunch. The doctor cautions his staff about accessing medical records that they are not actively involved with in patient care to avoid invading the patient's privacy. The computer system prints a daily log of all employees and what information they accessed throughout the day, so he stresses the importance of logging on and off the computer using their individual passwords and log-on IDs. Dr. Bouchard's employees realize the importance of keeping medical information private. Unless a staff member needs to know the information in the chart to care for the patient, he or she may be accused of invading the patient's privacy when accessing medical information.

He is very interested in new developments for healthcare facilities, such as those that will allow his patients to check themselves in and gain access to limited information about their own medical record. He has a vision that one day his patients will be able to download their statements or perhaps their child's immunization records from their home computers, reducing the staff's workload and providing instant access to some information for his patients. Insightful physicians like Dr. Bouchard see the computer as a co-worker in the medical facility.

SUMMARY of LEARNING OBJECTIVES

1. Define, spell, and pronounce the terms listed in the vocabulary.
   - Spelling and pronouncing medical terms correctly adds credibility to the medical assistant. Knowing the definition of these terms promotes confidence in communication with patients and co-workers.
2. List several ways that the computer can be effective in a medical office.
   - The computer can be an effective tool in the medical office. It performs repetitive tasks, reduces errors, speeds up production, recalls information on command, saves time, reduces paperwork, and allows for more creative and productive use of workers' time.
3. Explain the basic functions that a computer performs.
   - The computer performs four basic functions: input, processing, output, and storage. Input includes information that is put into the computer, and output is information that comes out of the computer. Processing is in-between, and is the actual manipulation of data. Storage is the retention of data inside the computer or on storage media.
4. Explain the basic parts of a computer.
   - Several basic parts make up a computer system. The microprocessor is the brains of the system that interprets the instructions given to it by an application program. The monitor allows the user to see immediate output on a screen, and printers allow the output to be printed to a hard copy. The keyboard and mouse serve as input devices.

5. List the three elements that differentiate microprocessors.
   - Three elements differentiate microprocessors. The bandwidth describes the amount of information that can be sent over a connection at one time, and the clock speed determines the number of instructions per second that the processor can handle. The instruction set is the instructions that the microprocessor can execute.
6. Discuss the differences among various types of printers.
   - Three main types of printers are in use in today's medical offices. Dot matrix printers produce output of moderate quality but are inexpensive. Inkjet printers use a cartridge and a heating element to produce an image on a page. A laser printer uses technology similar to a photocopier.
7. Explain the importance of a motherboard.
   - The motherboard is the main connection board to which all other devices are connected inside the computer. It contains all of the essential wiring and expansion devices needed to operate the computer, as well as the battery that keeps the clock and calendar running when the computer is turned off.
8. Explain and give examples of peripheral devices.
   - Peripheral devices, such as scanners, Zip drives, and other devices, are not necessary to the function of the computer but perform special functions.
9. List and discuss several types of file formats.
   - File format refers to the extension just after the filename and describes the method used to save the file. This also helps to

Continued

SUMMARY of LEARNING OBJECTIVES
Continued

identify the type of file on the computer. For example, a JPEG file is often used for photographs, a GIF file is used for scanned illustrations or images, and a TXT file is usually specifically for text for a printed page.

10. Explain the concept of computer networking.
    - Computer networks are groups of two or more computers linked together. These networks can be local or can cover a city or wide geographic area. Some are limited to a few buildings. Networks often share resources, such as printers.

11. Define the function of browsers.
    - Browsers are software applications that allow a user to find information on the Internet. They are able to show graphics, and often multimedia, such as videos. Commonly used browsers include Internet Explorer and Netscape Navigator.

12. Discuss the importance of computer security.
    - Computer security is critical, especially because confidential patient information is stored on computers in medical facilities. Several methods may be used to enhance computer security, such as the use of firewalls and antivirus programs. Restrictions on who may log in and the use of passwords also will assist the facility to ensure that only authorized individuals have access to confidential information.

CONNECTIONS

 Study Guide Connection: Go to Chapter 8 Study Guide. Read the Case Study and Workplace Applications and complete the assignments. Do online research for answers to the questions in the Internet Activities associated with computers in the medical office.

 CD Connection: Go to the Medical Assisting Competency Challenge CD and review the content of the training activities. These will be referred to throughout the textbook to enhance your learning experience.

 Evolve Connection: For more information related to computers in the medical office, go to http://evolve.elsevier.com/kinn/admin and visit related weblinks for Chapter 8. Click on the Medical Assisting Exam Review and do the practice questions to sharpen your test-taking skills.

Telephone Techniques

9

SCENARIO

Ashlynn McDowell is a recent graduate of a medical assisting program and has begun her first position as a receptionist in an obstetrician's office. It has been Ashlynn's lifelong goal to work in obstetrics, and she is determined to perform to the best of her abilities. However, Ashlynn has never held a job in a professional office. She knows that she will need to practice all of the skills she learned in school with regard to being an effective receptionist.

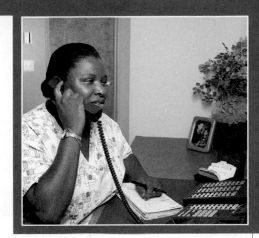

Ashlynn works for Dr. Stella Frank, who is customer service oriented and wants her patients to feel special and cared for. She insists that all of their concerns be taken seriously. Ashlynn is anxious to build trust with the patients and offer them help with the problems they encounter that fall into her realm of responsibility.

She knows that she will be required to speak clearly and distinctly and be adept at follow-up skills. She plans to dress professionally each day so that she projects the right image to the patients with whom she comes in contact. Ashlynn will strive to be the type of employee who presents a willingness to learn, an ability to adapt, and a heart full of compassion for the patient. She is a team player who sincerely wishes to cooperate with other staff members that might need her help.

Dr. Frank is pleased that she has found such an eager person to add to her staff and will provide assistance and guidance to Ashlynn as she learns how to make her patients feel a part of her clinic family. Ashlynn's self-esteem has increased because she feels she is making a great contribution to healthcare.

While studying this chapter, think about the following questions:

- How can Ashlynn's telephone demeanor convince patients that she wants to help them?
- Why does the tone of voice play an important role in patient perception?
- How does the medical assistant speaking to patients on the telephone strike a balance between too much and too little time?
- How can the medical assistant reduce patient frustration with telephone issues?

LEARNING OBJECTIVES

1. Define, spell, and pronounce the terms listed in the vocabulary.
2. Determine and discuss the source of incoming and outgoing calls to a physician's office.
3. Describe how one develops a pleasing telephone voice.
4. Demonstrate the correct way to hold a telephone handset.
5. Explain why courtesy is so important when speaking on the telephone.
6. Discuss different ways to handle callers who wish to speak to the physician.
7. List the seven items needed to take a telephone message correctly.
8. Explain how angry callers might be handled.
9. Discuss how the medical assistant should handle callers who have a complaint.
10. List several questions to ask when handling an emergency call.
11. Discuss several useful sections of the introductory pages of the phone directory.
12. Demonstrate the correct way to answer the telephone in the office.
13. Demonstrate the correct way to accurately record a message and take a request for action.
14. Demonstrate the most efficient way to call in a prescription or a prescription refill to a pharmacy.

National Accreditation Competencies and Content

CAAHEP COMPETENCIES

General

3.c.(1)(b). Recognize and respond to verbal communication
3.c.(1)(d). Demonstrate telephone techniques
3.c.(2)(a). Identify and respond to issues of confidentiality
3.c.(3)(a). Explain general office policies
3.c.(3)(d). Identify community resources

ABHES COMPETENCIES

Professionalism

1.h. Be courteous and diplomatic

Communication

2.a. Be attentive, listen, and learn
2.b. Be impartial and show empathy when dealing with patients
2.c. Adapt what is said to the recipient's level of comprehension
2.d. Serve as liaison between physician and others
2.e. Use proper telephone techniques
2.h. Receive, organize, prioritize, and transmit information expediently
2.k. Principles of verbal and nonverbal communication
2.l. Recognition and response to verbal and nonverbal communication
2.m. Adaptation for individualized needs
2.n. Application of electronic technology

Administrative Duties

3.a. Perform basic secretarial skills

VOCABULARY

clarity The quality or state of being clear.

competent Having adequate abilities or qualities; having the capacity to function or perform in a certain way.

cultivate To foster the growth of; to improve by labor, care, or study.

diction The choice of words especially with regard to clearness, correctness, or effectiveness.

enunciation (e-nun-se-a'-shun) Utterance of articulate, clear sounds.

inflection (in-flek'-shun) A change in pitch or loudness of the voice.

invariably (in-var'-e-uh-buh-le) Consistently; not changing or capable of change.

jargon The technical terminology or characteristic idiom of a particular group or special activity.

monotone A succession of syllables, words, or sentences in one unvaried key or pitch.

multitasking Performing multiple tasks at the same time.

pitch The property of a sound, especially a musical tone, which is determined by the frequency of the waves producing it; the highness or lowness of sound.

provider Individual or company that provides medical care and services to a patient or the public.

salutation (sal-yu-ta'-shun) An expression of greeting, goodwill, or courtesy by words or gestures.

screen Something that shields, protects, or hides; to select or eliminate through a screening process.

STAT Medical abbreviation for immediately; at this moment.

tactful Having a keen sense of what to do or say to maintain good relations with others or to avoid offense.

tedious (te'-de-yus) Tiresome because of length or dullness.

The telephone is the lifeline of a medical practice as well as a powerful public relations tool. The majority of patients who are seen in a medical facility make their initial appointments by telephone. When used appropriately, the telephone can help build a medical practice from its beginning and throughout its life (Figure 9-1). If used inappropriately, it can destroy a flourishing practice. Always remember that the voice on the other end of the line is that of the patient, and telephone calls can never be considered an interruption of the work day.

Most incoming calls are from the following sources:

- Established patients calling for appointments or to ask questions

- New patients making a first contact with the physician's office
- Patients and medical workers reporting treatment results or emergencies
- Other physicians who are making referrals or discussing a patient
- Laboratories reporting vital patient information

EFFECTIVE USE OF THE TELEPHONE

Active Listening

Although great emphasis is placed on rules for speaking, the importance of active listening is often overlooked. The same

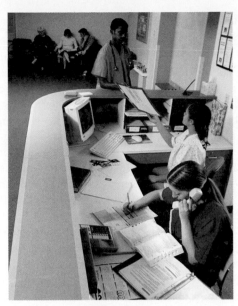

FIGURE 9-1 The telephone plays a vital role in the success of a medical practice.

attention should be given to a telephone conversation that would be given to a face-to-face conversation. Concentration is not always easy for a medical assistant who is juggling several duties at once in the medical office, so he or she must practice focusing on the call at hand. Effective active listening also provides vital information about the nature of the call—whether the caller is distressed, is agitated, or has a concern that needs to be addressed immediately.

Developing a Pleasing Telephone Voice

Individuals who call a physician's office should hear a pleasant, friendly voice when they are greeted. It is a common sales technique to be sure that the caller "hears a smile." Customer service is critical in today's medical offices, and this technique is quite useful for medical assistants because they are likely to be the caller's first point of contact with the practice. Be sure to enunciate words clearly, pronouncing them separately and distinctly. **Diction, pitch,** and **clarity** are important as well. Avoid speaking in a **monotone;** instead, use **inflection,** or a change in the pitch and loudness of the voice when speaking. This helps the speaker to emphasize certain points during the conversation.

When a telephone call is received from a stranger, one usually tries to visualize that person's appearance and perhaps will form an opinion of his or her personality. The caller may sound mature, somewhat worried, well educated, or frantic. As discussed in Chapter 5, communication is a two-way street, so the caller will be forming an impression of the person answering the phone at the same time. Sometimes these impressions are incorrect, but much can be inferred from what is heard on the telephone.

The tone of voice used by the medical assistant, as well as other medical staff members, plays a role in the attitude of the patient. A study conducted by Harvard University claims that the tone of voice used by surgeons has a direct link to medical professional liability claims. How something is said to a patient

is just as important as what is said. Always use a friendly and warm tone of voice and project confidence when speaking with patients. Be courteous and **tactful** and choose words carefully. Every caller should be made to feel that the medical assistant has time to attend to his or her wishes. A small mirror placed near the telephone will serve as a reminder to smile. If the medical assistant is rushed to pick up the telephone, he or she should wait a few seconds until able to answer graciously without seeming breathless or impatient.

Be alert and interested in the person who is calling. Always give full attention to the caller, and do not allow distractions to interfere with the conversation. Build a pleasant, friendly image for the office. Talk naturally and avoid repetition of mechanical words or phrases, such as "uh huh" and "you know." Avoid the use of professional **jargon,** such as referring to *otalgia* when the patient is reporting an earache. Using correct grammar adds to the caller's favorable impression. Speak distinctly; clear pronunciation and **enunciation** are vital. Move the lips, tongue, and jaw freely. Talk directly into the mouthpiece. Never answer the telephone when eating, drinking, or chewing gum. A well-modulated voice carries best. Use a normal tone of voice, neither too loud nor too soft. Talk at a moderate rate, neither too quickly nor too slowly. Be expressive, and vary the tone of voice. This will bring out the meaning of sentences and add color and vitality to what is said.

CRITICAL THINKING APPLICATION

Ashlynn has a tendency to speak a little fast in her normal conversations. How will she need to adjust as she is answering phones in the medical office? She is also a friendly person and enjoys talking on the phone. What precautions should she take so that this does not become an issue on the job?

Holding the Telephone Handset Correctly

A medical assistant must develop professional telephone habits and correct the more casual ones that are used at home. Consider how the handset is held. It should be placed so that the medical assistant's voice is relayed distinctly and accurately. Practice holding the handset around the middle, with the mouthpiece approximately 1 inch from the lips and directly in front of the teeth (Figure 9-2). Never hold it under the chin. Check the proper distance by taking the first two fingers and passing them through sideways in the space between the lips and the mouthpiece. If the fingers just squeeze through, then the lips are the correct distance from the telephone and the voice will go over the line in as close to its natural tone as possible. When using a headset, speak directly into its mouthpiece, positioning it the same distance from the mouth as a regular telephone.

Speak directly into the telephone immediately after removing it from its cradle. When turning to face another part of the room, make sure the handset moves, too; otherwise, the voice will be lost. A medical assistant who speaks too fast, enunciates poorly, or fails to speak directly into the transmitter may not be easily understood by the person on the other end of the receiver.

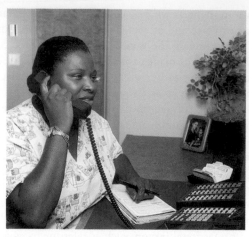

FIGURE 9-2 The handset should be held in the center, with the mouthpiece approximately 1 inch in front of the lips.

Maintaining Confidentiality

Keep in mind that all communications in a healthcare facility are confidential. If others are nearby, use discretion when mentioning the name of the caller. Be careful about being overheard when repeating any symptoms or other information received by telephone. Never use a speaker phone to listen to voicemail or to hold a phone conversation within the hearing range of others. Do not place patients on speakerphone at any time. Another individual may hear private medical information, which is a violation of HIPAA regulations.

CRITICAL THINKING APPLICATION

Ashlynn hears two employees speaking on the intercom in a derogatory manner about a patient who just left the office. How should she handle this situation? To whom should Ashlynn report this activity, if anyone, and why? What problems could be caused when staff members are overheard talking in this manner?

Thinking Ahead

It is always helpful to think ahead when an important call must be made. Have the patient's chart or the bill in question at hand before dialing the phone. Write down a list of questions to ask or goals for the conversation. Keep the call short and simple, then free the line for other calls.

Most offices keep a list of frequently called phone numbers both for staff use and to offer to patients. A list of local pharmacies, hospitals, and their departments is helpful. All of these are time-savers that will help the medical assistant to better serve patients.

TECHNIQUES FOR INCOMING TELEPHONE CALLS

Many incoming calls will be received in the medical office during the course of a single day. Each one deserves the medical assistant's complete and **competent** attention.

Answering Promptly

Whenever possible, answer the telephone on the first ring, and always by the third ring. If the facility has several incoming lines or more than one telephone, it will sometimes be necessary to interrupt a conversation to answer another call. It is courteous to say, "Excuse me just a moment; the other line is ringing." Answer the second call and determine who is calling. If it is not an emergency, ask that person to hold while the first call is completed. If possible, get the phone number of the second caller, but do not allow that request to turn into a lengthy conversation. Do not make the mistake of continuing with the second call while the first caller waits. Return to the first call as soon as possible and apologize briefly for the interruption. Think of what would happen during a face-to-face conversation. A second person who approaches people involved in a conversation should not expect to interrupt and be heard at length. However, if the second call is an emergency, take a moment to return to the first line and alert the caller that he or she will have to be kept waiting or be called back.

Never answer a call by saying, "Please hold" without first finding out who is calling. The call could be an emergency, and this type of greeting is extremely discourteous. It takes only a moment to be polite. If the call is an emergency, prompt attention to it could save a life.

Keep the focus on the call. Do not attempt to multitask while answering the telephone because this practice takes attention away from the patient. Callers can hear keyboard strokes and other office activity; therefore a caller might assume that the medical assistant is not giving full attention to the person on the phone. Treat the phone call just as if the patient were standing in the office face to face (Procedure 9-1).

Identifying the Facility

The medical assistant should identify the facility first, then state his or her name to the caller. Numerous telephone greetings can be used. Discuss which are best with the physician or office manager. Examples of telephone greetings include the following:
- "This is Dr. Frank's office, Miss McDowell speaking. How may I help you?"
- "Frank Maternal Health Clinic, this is Miss McDowell. How may I help you?"
- "Stella Frank's office, this is Miss McDowell. How may I help you?"

Some physicians avoid using the title "Doctor" so that they may protect their patient's confidentiality. For instance, if a physician needs to call a work number and leave a message for a patient, curious co-workers might attempt to investigate what type of physician is being seen. Dropping the "Doctor" when leaving messages and when answering the telephone can be an effective means of protecting patient privacy. However, merely saying "Hello" is unsatisfactory. The caller will **invariably** ask if he or she has reached the physician's office, so time is wasted, and the opportunity to create a favorable impression of your facility has been lost.

The use of a **salutation** in telephone identification is optional. Sometimes the addition of "Good morning" or

PROCEDURE 9-1

Demonstrate Telephone Techniques: Answer the Telephone

CAAHEP COMPETENCY: 3.c.(1)(d)
ABHES COMPETENCY: 2.e

GOAL: *To answer the telephone in a physician's office in a professional manner and respond to a request for action.*

EQUIPMENT and SUPPLIES

- Telephone
- Message pad
- Pen or pencil
- Appointment book
- Notepad

PROCEDURAL STEPS

1. Answer the telephone by the third ring, speaking directly into the mouthpiece, which should be positioned 1 inch from the mouth.
   PURPOSE: Answering promptly conveys interest in the caller. Proper positioning of the handset allows for audible tone and carries the voice well.
2. Speak distinctly with a pleasant tone and expression, at a moderate rate, and with sufficient volume for the calling party to understand every word.
3. Identify the office and/or physician and yourself.
   PURPOSE: The caller will know that the correct number has been reached and the identity of the staff member.
4. Verify the identity of the caller.
   PURPOSE: To confirm the origin of the call.
5. Triage the call, if necessary.
   PURPOSE: To determine if the caller has an emergency and needs immediate attention or a referral to the emergency department of a hospital.
6. Determine the needs of the caller, and provide the requested information or service, if possible. Provide the caller with excellent customer service. Be as helpful as possible.
   PURPOSE: The medical assistant can handle many calls and conserve the time and energy of the physician or other staff members.
7. If unable to assist the caller, transfer the call to the appropriate person. Before transferring the call, provide the person to whom the call is being transferred with as much information as possible about the caller and his or her needs.
   PURPOSE: To provide good customer service and be as helpful to the caller as possible.
8. Take a proper message for further action, if required.
   PURPOSE: Not all calls can be responded to immediately.
9. Terminate the call in a pleasant manner, and replace the receiver gently. Always allow the caller to hang up first.
   PURPOSE: To promote good public relations, provide excellent customer service, and ensure that the caller has no further questions.

"Good afternoon" to the identification is awkward. A rising inflection or a questioning tone of voice indicates interest and a willingness to assist and eliminates the need for an additional greeting. When the type of greeting to use has been decided, practice until it can be said easily and smoothly. It is critical that the greeting not be rushed so that all callers can clearly understand exactly what is being communicated.

CRITICAL THINKING APPLICATION

Most offices dictate how the phone is to be answered. What should Ashlynn do if she is very uncomfortable with the way she is being asked to answer the phone? Who should ultimately make the decision as to how the phone is answered?

Identifying the Caller

If the caller does not identify himself or herself, ask who is calling. It is helpful to write the name down immediately on a pad of paper or phone message form. Repeat the caller's name by using it in the conversation as soon as possible. Individuals like to hear their own names, and name repetition assures the

patient that he or she has been correctly identified. Try to use the person's name at least three times during the call, and remember other courteous expressions, such as "thank you," "please," and "you're welcome" as often as possible. However, if other patients are within the range of your voice, remember that the caller's privacy must be respected.

Occasionally a caller will refuse to identify himself or herself to the medical assistant and may be quite insistent on speaking with the physician. The individual could be a patient, so every attempt to identify the patient and assist him or her should be made. Such callers may also be salespersons who are fully aware that if their identity is revealed, they will never get the opportunity to speak to the physician. These people may be firmly told, "Dr. Frank is busy with a patient and has asked that we take messages for her. If you will not leave a message, you may wish to write a letter to her and mark it 'personal.'"

Screening Incoming Calls

Most physicians expect the medical assistant to **screen** all telephone calls. The physician and office manager will provide guidance as to the type of calls that should be routed to the physician and those that he or she will want to return at a later

STAYING IN CONTROL OF CALLS

The Dartnell Corporation publishes a newsletter entitled "Effective Telephone Techniques" that is an excellent tool for building good customer relations while using the phone. One issue suggests ways to control calls and keep them from becoming too lengthy. Try the tips below to keep callers on track and make all phone time productive.

- Ask the caller, "How may I help you today?"
- If the caller becomes sidetracked, say "You were describing the pain in your side?"
- When making a call, get right to the purpose of it after the initial greeting by saying "I was calling you about…"
- Keep explanations short and direct.
- Type information directly into the database, if used, while speaking on the phone.
- Keep personal and friendly comments to a minimum, or only one per call.
- Once the business is concluded, say "If there are no other questions…" and bring the conversation to a close.

FIGURE 9-3 Several tips to stay in control of the telephone calls in the medical office.

time. The medical assistant should become familiar with their preferences and also use good judgment, much of which comes with experience, in deciding whether to put a call through to the physician (Figure 9-3).

If it is the policy of the office, put calls from other physicians through at once. If the physician is busy and cannot possibly come to the telephone, explain this briefly and politely, then say that the physician will return the call as soon as possible.

Many callers will ask, "Is the doctor in?" or "May I speak to the doctor?" Avoid answering this question with a simple "Yes" or "No" or by responding with the question, "Who is calling, please?" If the physician is not in, say so before asking the identity of the caller. Otherwise, the impression may be created that the physician is just not willing to talk with this person.

If the physician is away from the office, the rule of offering assistance still holds. The medical assistant may say, "No, I am sorry, Dr. Frank is not in. May I take a message?" or "No, I am sorry, but Dr. Frank will be at the hospital most of the morning. May I ask her to return your call after 1 o'clock?"

If the physician is in and is available for telephone calls, a typical response would be, "Yes, Dr. Frank is in; may I say who is calling, please?"

When physicians prefer to keep telephone calls to a minimum, say, "Yes, Dr. Frank is in the office, but she is not free to come to the phone. May I take a message, please?" By responding in this way, the physician is not committed to taking the call.

During the time that a physician is examining a patient, he or she will not wish to be interrupted with a routine call. In such cases you might say, "Yes, Dr. Frank is in but is with a patient right now. May I help you?" or "Yes, Dr. Frank is in but is with a patient right now. Is there anything you would like me to ask her?"

Try to guard against being overprotective. A patient should be able to talk with the physician when necessary; but unless it is an emergency, the patient is probably willing to do so at the convenience of the physician. The medical assistant who answers the telephone acts as a screen, not a roadblock.

Find out exactly how calls are to be handled when the physician is out of the office and under what circumstances he or she can be interrupted when the physician is on the premises. **Cultivate** a reputation for being helpful and reliable. A medical assistant will save the physician many interruptions if patients develop confidence in the medical assistant's ability to help them and have faith in his or her promises to take messages and deliver them properly.

CRITICAL THINKING APPLICATION

Ashlynn answers the phone and a male pharmaceutical representative who has been visiting the clinic for several months is on the phone. She cheerfully greets him and asks if he is calling to make an appointment. He states that he wants to make an appointment with Ashlynn—for a date. How should she handle this call? What problems could arise if this were a patient and Ashlynn were to accept the date?

Minimizing Wait Time

When a call cannot be put through immediately, ask, "Would you prefer to wait, or should I call you back when Dr. Frank is free?"

If the caller elects to wait, remember that waiting with a silent telephone can be irritating and **tedious.** The waiting time always seems long, no matter how brief it really is. Many of today's phones are equipped with timers that tell the caller exactly how long they have been waiting on hold. The longer they wait, the more irritated they may become. Let no more than 1 minute pass without breaking in with some reassuring comment. For instance: "I'm sorry, Dr. Frank is still busy. Would you like to continue to hold?" or "I'm sorry to keep you waiting so long, Ms. Hughes. Would you prefer to have me return your call when Dr. Frank is free?" If the wait is longer than expected, the caller may wish to reconsider and call back at another time or have the call returned. By going back on the line at frequent intervals, the medical assistant allows the caller an opportunity to express such concerns.

Try to give the caller some estimate of when he or she may expect the return call. In any event, be considerate and remember that irritation can be lessened each time the medical assistant returns to the call by saying, "Thank you for waiting, Ms. Hughes."

When it is necessary to leave the telephone and obtain information, ask the caller, "Will you please wait while I get the information?" Listen for a reply. If it will take longer than a few seconds to get the information, give some estimate of the time required and offer to call back. When returning to the telephone, always thank the caller for waiting. Requests that might require pulling the patient's chart from the files are best handled with a call back to the patient.

Remember that leaving a person on hold ties up one of the physician's telephone lines, and an emergency call could be coming through, or new patients might be attempting to call. The majority of phone calls that come in to a physician's office during the day are important, so the lines should be kept clear as much as possible.

Transferring a Call

Always ask the patient's permission to place him or her on hold and to transfer the call. Identify the person on the phone when a call is transferred to the physician or another person in the facility. It is considered poor customer service to transfer the call to a co-worker's voicemail without warning the caller that the person is not available. Any person who refuses to give a name should not be put through unless the medical assistant has been specifically instructed to do so. If the person is not immediately available, ask the caller whether he or she would prefer to be put through to voicemail. Some callers simply believe their call will receive more attention if a human takes the message. If the caller insists, take a written message and deliver it to the proper person as soon as possible.

All medical assistants should learn "who does what" in the medical facility. Knowing about the functions of the office and which person is responsible for which areas will make a significant difference in the customer service provided to the patient. For example, suppose that the medical office employs one insurance receptionist, named Sarah, and three insurance billers. Opel handles names that begin with A through G, David handles names that begin with H through P, and Andrea handles names that begin with Q through Z. If a call comes to the office and the patient has an insurance question, the medical assistant could put the call through to Sarah. However, better customer service dictates that the medical assistant ask the name of the patient and put the call through to the person who handles that patient's particular claims. If the patient's name is Rebecca Whitehead, the medical assistant should call Andrea and ask if she may transfer Ms. Whitehead's call to her. The fewer times the caller is transferred, the happier the caller.

When the caller is a patient, the physician or clinical medical assistant will probably need his or her medical record at hand during the conversation. Remember that it is vital to protect the patient's right to privacy. If others are within hearing range, take the chart to the person responsible for the call and say, "This patient is waiting on the telephone." Because physician offices are often hectic, most require that a message be taken so that the medical record can be reviewed, the patient's request considered, and the patient called back with questions or instructions from the doctor.

Taking a Telephone Message

Always have a pen or pencil in hand and a message pad nearby when answering the telephone. Several calls may be answered before an opportunity arises to relay a message or carry out a promise of action. The written message is a vital part of competent patient care (Procedure 9-2).

Many types of message pads are available today (Figure 9-4). Ordinary spiral-bound notebooks are inexpensive, sturdy, and well proportioned. These usually lie flat on a desk and can be filed for future reference. Never use small scraps of paper for messages; they are too easily lost. Message books should be kept indefinitely in the medical office, because they could be used as evidence in a court of law. A copy of a phone message could be added to the patient's chart once acted on, or at a minimum the information could be noted in the chart if it concerns the patient's medical care.

A minimum of seven items are needed to take a telephone message correctly:

- The name of the person to whom the call is directed
- The name of the person calling
- The caller's daytime, evening, and/or cellular telephone number
- The reason for the call
- The action to be taken
- The date and time of the call
- The initials of the person taking the call

Impression-sensitive message pads that provide a copy of each page ensure that no message will be forgotten and are the best way to keep track of messages. This also provides a copy of the message in the event that one is somehow lost, and will help to assure that all messages are acted on. The nature of the message will determine whether it should be reported immediately. The person who completes the call must sign and date the message. If the call is from a patient and relates in any way to the medical history, or if any instructions were given or queries answered, this information should be placed in the patient's chart. Message forms are available that have a self-adhesive backing and can be placed permanently in the patient's case history.

Taking Action on Telephone Messages

The message procedure is not complete until the necessary action has been taken. Notations on the memo pad should be carried over to the following day if they have not been completed, but this should be a rare occurrence. Do not trust to memory messages that were not attended to from previous days; always carry them forward in writing.

Make brief notations of patients' reactions while talking to them on the telephone. The physician does not require a character study, but it is helpful to know when a patient appears fearful, apprehensive, or nervous. If a patient shows such symptoms, it may be wise to consult with or transfer the call to the physician or clinical medical assistant.

Ending a Call

When a caller's requests have been satisfied, do not encourage inappropriate chatting or permit the call to monopolize your time unnecessarily. The telephone lines should be cleared for other calls. Allow the person who placed the call to hang up first, and be sure to thank him or her for calling. Close the conversation with some form of "good-bye," and replace the telephone on its cradle gently.

PROCEDURE 9-2

Demonstrate Telephone Techniques: Take a Telephone Message

CAAHEP COMPETENCY: 3.c(1)(d)
ABHES COMPETENCY: 2.e

GOAL: *To take an accurate telephone message and follow up on the requests made by the caller.*

EQUIPMENT and SUPPLIES

- Telephone
- Message pad
- Pen or pencil
- Notepad

PROCEDURAL STEPS

1. Answer the telephone using the guidelines in Procedure 9-1.
   PURPOSE: Answering promptly and courteously conveys interest in the caller and promotes good customer service.
2. Using a message pad or notepad, take the phone message, obtaining the following information:
   - The name of the person to whom the call is directed
   - The name of the person calling
   - The caller's telephone number
   - The reason for the call
   - The action to be taken
   - The date and time of the call
   - The initials of the person taking the call
   PURPOSE: Accurate information allows the staff member to address the caller's issues quickly and efficiently.
3. Repeat the information back to the caller after the message is recorded on the message pad.
   PURPOSE: To verify that all information taken has been recorded accurately.
4. Provide the caller with an approximation of the time and date that he or she will be called back, if possible.
   PURPOSE: To be considerate of the patient's time and to keep him or her from sitting next to the phone awaiting a call.
5. End the call and wait for the caller to hang up first.
6. Deliver the phone message to the appropriate person. Separate trays or slots for each staff member are helpful.
7. Follow up on important messages.
   PURPOSE: To make certain that important issues are addressed in a timely manner.
8. Keep old message books for future reference. Carbonless copies will allow the facility to keep a permanent record of phone messages.
   PURPOSE: To have a permanent source of messages in case a number is needed after the paper message has been discarded.
9. File pertinent phone messages in the patient's chart.
   PURPOSE: To keep a permanent record of important information in the patient's chart.

Retaining Records of Telephone Messages

Each office must develop a policy regarding retention of telephone message records. Many offices elect to keep message pads for the same period that the statute of limitations exists for medical professional liability cases. Remember, phone records would include telephone bills, especially those that detail long-distance charges. Keeping message records can be of assistance in proving any number of claims, including the number of times that patients called the office and the fact that calls to the patient were returned. Be sure that accurate telephone records are kept to ensure good patient care and customer service.

TYPICAL INCOMING CALLS

One reason for having a medical assistant answer incoming calls is to spare the physician unnecessary interruptions during visits with patients. Many calls relate to the administrative aspects of the office and can actually be better handled by the medical assistant. The policy regarding how calls are to be handled should be clearly set forth in the office procedures manual.

New Patients and Return Appointments

Procedures for handling appointments for new patients and scheduling return appointments are discussed in the chapter on appointment scheduling. Always provide excellent customer service to the caller. Remember that the routine questions that may be asked should be answered in a polite and cheerful manner. Health matters are important to the individual patients whom the practice serves. Follow the designated office procedure as to what information should be gathered and recorded when appointments are made.

Directions

Each office should have a clear set of directions written out that can be read to the caller who requests directions. Prepare them from various points in the area; for instance, one set would guide a patient who is coming from the north, and another set would be for a patient coming from the south. Place these directions close to the telephone so that all employees can access them easily. Not all employees live close to the clinic or are familiar with the area, so the written set of directions will be helpful to all staff members and those who call the facility. Place a map on the office website and direct patients there for printable instructions.

Inquiries about Bills

A patient may ask to speak with the physician about a recent bill. Ask the caller to hold for a moment while the ledger is obtained. If nothing irregular is found on the ledger, return to the telephone and say, "I have your account in front of me now.

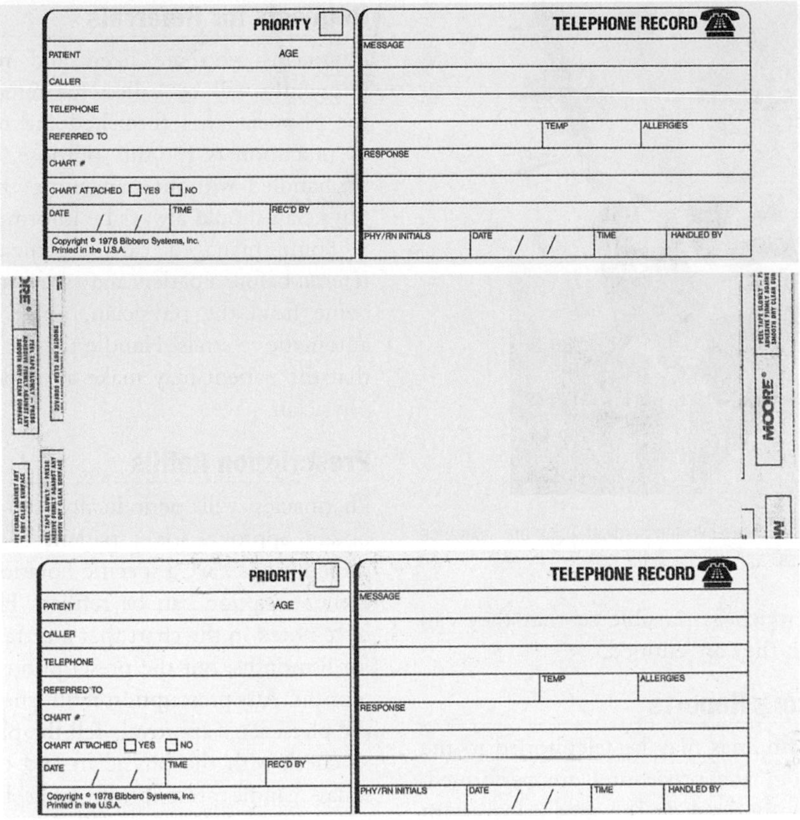

PRIORITY ☐

PATIENT AGE

CALLER

TELEPHONE

REFERRED TO

CHART #

CHART ATTACHED ☐ YES ☐ NO

DATE / / TIME REC'D BY

Copyright © 1978 Bibbero Systems, Inc. Printed in the U.S.A.

TELEPHONE RECORD

MESSAGE

TEMP ALLERGIES

RESPONSE

PHY/RN INITIALS DATE / / TIME HANDLED BY

PRIORITY ☐

PATIENT AGE

CALLER

TELEPHONE

REFERRED TO

CHART #

CHART ATTACHED ☐ YES ☐ NO

DATE / / TIME REC'D BY

Copyright © 1978 Bibbero Systems, Inc. Printed in the U.S.A.

TELEPHONE RECORD

MESSAGE

TEMP ALLERGIES

RESPONSE

PHY/RN INITIALS DATE / / TIME HANDLED BY

FIGURE 9-4 Phone message forms with self-adhesive backing make charting the call easier and more time efficient. (Courtesy Bibbero Systems, Inc., Petaluma, Calif.)

Perhaps I can answer your question." Most likely the caller will have some simple inquiry, such as whether the insurance has paid, or he or she may wish to delay making a payment until the next month. Not all patients realize that the medical assistant usually makes such decisions and is the best person with whom to discuss these matters.

A patient may have a question about a statement that was received in the mail. If billing matters are handled by another employee, tell the patient that the call will be transferred to the billing office. If you are responsible for billing, politely ask the patient to hold the line while you obtain the patient ledger. On returning to the line, thank the patient for waiting and explain the charges carefully. If an error has occurred, apologize and say that a corrected statement will be sent out at once. Always remember to thank the patient for calling. If patients are properly advised about charges at the time that services are rendered, the number of these calls will be considerably reduced.

Inquiries about Fees

Fees vary widely in each medical office, and it is very difficult to quote an exact fee before the patient is seen by the physician. However, a good estimate should be given to the patient as to what they should expect to pay, especially on the first visit. Asking a patient to just appear at the office without having any idea of the cost is unreasonable. Discuss with the physician or office manager what range should be quoted to the patient, then follow your quotes with the statement that the fees will vary, depending on the patient's condition and tests that the physician orders. If fees are regularly discussed on the telephone, write a suggested script in the policy manual. Do not be evasive. Have a schedule of fees available.

Participating Provider

Patients may call the office to inquire as to whether the physician is a participating **provider** with their particular insurance plan or managed care organization. The physician should keep a carefully updated list of which plans are valid. This is important, because insurance benefits vary for participating and nonparticipating providers.

Requests for Assistance with Insurance

In today's environment of managed care, copays, Medicaid, and Medicare, insurance claims will more than likely be completed and filed by the healthcare facility. Nevertheless, patients may call to inquire about their coverage or ask whether there has been any response to claims. A medical assistant or member of the staff who is responsible for insurance filing will have the knowledge to answer these inquiries (Figure 9-5). Be patient with these inquiries; insurance is a difficult subject to understand, even for those who are trained and familiar with the various forms and procedures to use. Some patients, especially elderly ones, are quite confused when dealing with insurance

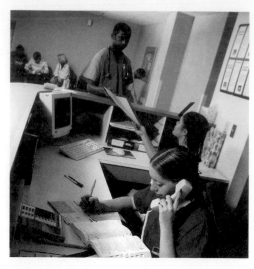

FIGURE 9-5 Many of the calls that come into the medical office are insurance questions, with which the medical assistant will assist the caller.

companies. Help them as much as possible so that they can collect the benefits to which they are entitled.

Radiology and Laboratory Reports

Laboratory and radiologic findings may be telephoned to the physician's office on the day the procedures are performed, when their results are urgently needed. The medical assistant should take these reports and relay them to the physician. Reports may also be faxed to the physician's office, especially if the test has been marked **"STAT,"** which means that the physician wants the results immediately. Original reports will usually be delivered by mail for the permanent record. Some facilities are equipped to receive laboratory results directly from the laboratory by computer.

Satisfactory Progress Reports from Patients

Physicians sometimes ask patients to phone the office to report on their condition a few days after the office visit. The medical assistant can take such calls and relay the information to the physician if the report is satisfactory. Assure the patient that you will inform the physician about the call. The physician should always be immediately informed about unsatisfactory progress reports. The doctor should provide instructions for the patient to follow in such situations.

Routine Reports from Hospitals and Other Sources

Routine calls may be received from hospitals and other sources reporting a patient's progress. Take the message carefully and make sure that the physician sees it. The message should then be placed in the patient's medical record.

Office Administration Matters

Not all calls concern patients. Calls may come from the accountant or the auditor or about banking procedures, office supplies, or office maintenance, most of which the medical assistant can handle or refer to the appropriate person. For some of these calls the medical assistant may need to gather additional information and return the call.

Requests for Referrals

Physicians who are liked and respected by their patients frequently will be called for referrals to other specialists. If the physician has furnished the medical assistant with a list of practitioners for this purpose, these inquiries can usually be handled without consulting the physician. However, the physician should always be informed of such requests.

Some managed care organizations require a physician referral before a patient may see a specialist. This referral should come from the physician, unless he or she has authorized automatic referrals. Handle these calls as quickly as possible so that the patient may make an appointment to see the referral physician.

Prescription Refills

Pharmacies will periodically call the physician's office to obtain approval for a patient to refill a prescription. Most prescriptions have a specific notation as to the number of times the prescription can be refilled. However, the physician may have noted in the chart that a certain medication is to be taken for 6 months, but the prescription was only written for 1 to 2 months. Any prescription refills should be authorized only with the physician's approval. Tell the pharmacist that you will have to check with the physician and call back. Many pharmacies today handle prescription refills by fax so that they have a written record that the refill was authorized. Be sure that state regulations and procedures are followed any time the medical assistant deals with prescription refills or calls (Procedure 9-3). Some medications cannot be called to the pharmacy and require a written prescription.

SPECIAL INCOMING CALLS

Patients Refusing to Discuss Symptoms

Occasionally patients will call and wish to talk with the physician about symptoms that they are reluctant to discuss with a medical assistant. Patients do have a right to privacy, but the physician cannot be expected to take numerous calls from patients who do not wish to speak to the medical assistant. If the patient refuses to discuss any symptoms, suggest that he or she make an appointment with the physician to discuss the problem in person.

Unsatisfactory Progress Reports

If a patient under treatment reports that he or she is still not feeling well or that the prescription the doctor provided is not helping, do not try to practice medicine by giving the patient medical advice. Make detailed notes about the patient's comments, then present them to the physician. He or she will make the decision as to whether the patient should return to the office or may make a medication change. Follow up with the patient, and convey the physician's instructions.

Requests for Test Results

When the physician orders special tests for the patient, the patient may be told to call the office in a couple of days for

PROCEDURE 9-3

Demonstrate Telephone Techniques: Call the Pharmacy with New or Refill Prescriptions

<u>CAAHEP COMPETENCY:</u> 3.c.(1)(d)
<u>ABHES COMPETENCY:</u> 2.h
GOAL: *To call in an accurate prescription to the pharmacy for a patient in the most efficient manner.*

EQUIPMENT and SUPPLIES

- Prescription
- Notepad
- Patient chart
- Telephone

PROCEDURAL STEPS

1. Receive the call from the patient requesting a prescription; use appropriate telephone technique.
   <u>PURPOSE:</u> To provide consistently good customer service when speaking with callers.

2. Obtain the following information from the patient:
   - Patient's name
   - Telephone number where he or she can be reached
   - Patient's symptoms and current condition
   - History of this condition
   - Treatments the patient has tried
   - Pharmacy name and telephone number
   <u>PURPOSE:</u> To have the information the physician will need to make a determination as to whether a prescription will be called in for the patient or whether he or she needs to come to the office to be seen by the doctor.

3. Write in the patient's chart the prescription that the physician wishes the patient to have. Be very careful to transcribe the information correctly. Read it back to the physician.
   <u>PURPOSE:</u> To have a permanent record of the prescription in the chart and to make certain that the prescription is exactly what the physician wants the patient to take, eliminating errors in medication name and dosage.

4. If the prescription is a refill, give the physician the patient's chart with the message requesting a refill attached, along with the information in procedure step 2.
   <u>PURPOSE:</u> To have the patient's chart as a reference and to provide the physician with the information needed to determine if the medication requested should be refilled.

5. Note the comments that the physician writes in the chart. If the prescription is written or a refill is approved, call the patient's pharmacy and ask to speak to a member of the pharmacy staff.

6. Ask the pharmacy staff member to repeat the prescription back to you.
   <u>PURPOSE:</u> To verify that the pharmacy staff member took the prescription down accurately.

7. Note in the chart the date and time that the prescription was called to the pharmacy.
   <u>PURPOSE:</u> To provide a permanent record of the medication being called to the pharmacy, along with the correct dose amounts and frequency of doses.

8. Call the patient to notify him or her that the prescription has been called in. Provide any information regarding the prescription doses, frequency, etc, that is requested by the physician. Tell the patient when to return to the office, if necessary. Ask the patient to write this information down.
   <u>PURPOSE:</u> To inform the patient as to the dosage and frequency, so that if an error is made by the pharmacy, the patient will notice a discrepancy and the error can be corrected before the patient takes any doses of the medication.

---

the results. Never assume that the patient will call for results. It is ultimately the responsibility of the physician to notify the patient of test results, especially if they are abnormal. Be certain that the physician has seen the results and has given permission before sharing the results with the patient. Patients do not always understand that the medical assistant does not have the privilege of giving out information without the permission of the physician. If the result is unfavorable, the physician should be the one to inform the patient and give further instructions. This call must be handled tactfully; otherwise, the patient may feel as if the staff is concealing information.

Most physicians prefer that medical assistants provide only normal test results to the patients. However, the medical assistant may provide abnormal test results to the patient if authorized by the physician. For example, when a patient has a questionable Pap smear, the medical assistant is usually the person who

calls the patient with the results and further instructions from the physician. If the patient then has any questions about the test results, he or she must be referred to the physician. The medical assistant will need good communication skills to relay information such as this without crossing the lines of practicing medicine without a license. Human immunodeficiency virus (HIV) test results should never be given on the telephone, and the physician should always inform the patient when an HIV test returns a positive result.

Patients who call the office for results of tests must be appropriately identified before the results are given. Some offices use a special code that is written in the chart, and knowledge of this code or password gives the person access to the information. Make sure the right individual is on the line before offering test results. Especially be careful in situations in which the family includes a "Senior" and "Junior." If the medical assistant calls and asks for Robert Smith, the elder Mr. Smith may answer, whereas the younger Mr. Smith is the one who came to the office for tests. Awkward situations can be created when the office staff does not accurately identify the patient.

Requests for Information from Third Parties

The patient must give written permission before any member of the physician's staff can give information to third-party callers. This includes insurance companies, attorneys, relatives, neighbors, employers, and any other third party. Releases of information will be discussed in more detail in Chapter 14.

Complaints about Care or Fees

A medical assistant may be able to offer a satisfactory explanation to a patient who complains about the care he or she received or the fee charged. If a patient seems angry, offer to pull the chart, research the problem, and if needed, discuss it with the physician. Four magic words often calm the angry patient: "Let me help you." This reassures the patient that someone is willing to talk about the problem. However, if you are unable to appease the patient easily, the physician or office manager may prefer to talk directly to the patient.

Calls from the Physician's Family and Friends

Personal calls to the physician from family members or friends are handled in accordance with instructions from the physician. If the physician does not wish to take the calls, the medical assistant must tactfully tell the caller that the physician cannot be disturbed at that time.

Calls from Staff Members' Family and Friends

The telephone lines should never be burdened with an excess of personal calls to the staff. A call is necessary in emergencies, but staff members should never monopolize the telephone for personal business and conversations. Emergency calls could be coming through, and the lines must be clear. Keep personal calls to an absolute minimum.

HANDLING DIFFICULT CALLS

Angry Callers

No matter how efficient you are on the telephone or how well liked your employer may be, sooner or later an angry caller will be on the line. There may be a legitimate reason for the anger, or the caller's irritation may have resulted from a misunderstanding. It is a real challenge to handle such calls. First, take the required action—even if it is to say that the matter will be discussed with the physician as soon as possible and the patient will be called back later. If answers are not readily available, a friendly assurance that the situation is important and that every attempt will be made to find the answer quickly will usually calm the angry feelings.

The medical assistant may find that lowering the tone of voice and volume of speech may force the angry caller to do the same in order to hear. This method does not always work, but it is usually true that when dealing with an angry person, calm promotes calm. There are always those who will misread

this method and become even angrier, thinking that their complaint is not being taken seriously. Interpersonal skills are critical when dealing with other individuals, because the more skilled the medical assistant becomes, the better able he or she is to deal with multiple types of personalities.

Always avoid getting angry in response, and try to get to the root of the real problem. Express interest and understanding, take careful notes, and follow through with the problem to the most appropriate resolution. Never "pass the buck" by saying, "That isn't my job," or "I am not the person who filed that insurance claim." No matter whose fault the problem is, it is best to deal with it and find a solution instead of placing blame.

CRITICAL THINKING APPLICATION

An angry caller raises his voice at Ashlynn over an issue that happened before she began to work at the facility. She suggests that he speak with the office manager, but he refuses and continues to berate Ashlynn. What choices does she have in this situation, and should she simply hang up on the patient?

Aggressive Callers

Aggressive callers insist that they receive whatever action they feel is necessary, and they usually insist on action immediately. Treat these callers with a calm, poised attitude, but do not allow the caller's aggression to initiate inappropriate action. Reassure the caller that the concern being shared is valid and will receive the full attention of the right person. Explain when the caller can expect a response from the office, and be sure to follow up that the appropriate action was taken on the call.

Unauthorized Inquiry Calls

Some individuals call the physician's office requesting information to which they are not entitled. These callers must be told politely but firmly that such information cannot be provided to them because of privacy laws. Insistent callers should be referred to the office manager or physician.

Sales Calls

Sales calls are often thought of as an interruption to the physician's busy day, but some salespersons may have important information on products, equipment, or services that the office uses regularly. Do not completely disregard salespersons, but do not allow them to monopolize time or telephone lines, either. Keep these calls quick and to the point. Most professional salespersons realize that the physician's and the staff's time is extremely valuable and will respect this. Developing a good rapport with representatives ("reps") from the companies whose products are frequently used in the practice may result in discounted prices and first news of sales and promotions. In turn, these people rarely waste the time of office personnel.

Physician Shopping

Some calls will be from prospective patients seeking information about the office and the types of illnesses or conditions that the physician treats. Consider these callers to be future patients, or as those who may refer patients to the office. Always be polite and answer questions respectfully. Remember, even if the caller does not become a patient, he or she may share his or her impressions of the practice with another prospective patient.

Complaints

When callers complain, use an approach similar to the one used with angry callers. Do not make an attempt to blame, and never argue with the patient. Find the source of the problem, then present the options to the caller as to how the situation can be resolved. Remember to treat callers in the same manner that you would wish to be treated. A complaint may seem small and insignificant to the office staff, but to the patient it could be paramount. Provide good customer service to patients, and complaints will be few and far between.

EMERGENCY CALLS

Many emergency calls require judgment on the part of the person answering the phone in the medical practice. Good judgment comes from experience and proper training by the physician with regard to what constitutes a real emergency in each type of practice and how such calls should be handled. If the physician is not immediately available, what should the staff do? The person answering the telephone should first determine whether the call is truly urgent. Emergency calls could include such conditions and/or symptoms as chest pain, profuse bleeding, severe allergic reactions, cessation of breathing, injuries resulting in loss of consciousness, and broken bones. Often, the physician will instruct the patient to go straight to the closest hospital emergency room or to call an ambulance. Office policy and procedure manuals should dictate the action to take in such emergency situations.

If the physician is in, the call should be transferred immediately. All offices should have a written plan of action for the times that the physician is not physically present in the office to handle the call. The physician and medical assistant may also jointly develop typical questions to ask the caller to determine the validity and disposition of an emergency. Some examples of questions to ask would include the following:
- At what telephone number can you be reached?
- Where are you located?
- What are the chief symptoms?
- When did they start?
- Has this happened before?
- Are you alone?
- Do you have transportation?

If the call is such that an ambulance is dispatched, the policy in most offices is to stay on the line until the paramedics or police arrive on the scene.

Triage Guidelines

In the facility with multiple employees, the physician may designate one individual as the triage nurse or assistant. Within the environment of managed care, every physician would be wise to have a written telephone protocol for handling urgent situations and emergencies. The protocol should state that the employees are bound by the written guidelines and that any giving of advice by unauthorized personnel may be grounds for dismissal.

A special sheet of instructions listing specific medical emergencies such as chest pain, heavy bleeding, fainting, seizure, and poisoning should be posted by each telephone. The phone numbers for the nearest poison control center, hospital, and ambulance should be listed. Such calls should be routed to a physician immediately. Additional instructions should include what action to take if no physician is available, such as sending the patient to an emergency department or calling an ambulance. Most offices have some means of constant contact with the physician, whether by pager, cell phone, or another method.

Getting the Information the Physician Needs

As the medical assistant gains experience and knows the physician better, he or she will begin to have a sense of the questions that the physician will have for patients that call the facility. For instance, the physician will be interested in how long the patient has had symptoms, what makes the symptoms better or worsens them, what remedies have been tried, what has worked and not worked, and other specifics about the condition the patient is experiencing. If the patient complains of painful urination, the medical assistant will learn to ask about pain in the back, blood in the urine and/or stool, and cramping. One way to learn about questions to ask is to listen to the physician carefully as he or she questions patients about their symptoms. This will help the medical assistant to learn more about signs and symptoms and will enable him or her to be a better assistant to the physician.

Remember to always be "patient with your patients." Those who call the medical office for help are almost never at their best. When feeling ill, people are often short-tempered and even display poor manners. Some can be verbally abusive. Care for patients as if they were family members, and they will feel care and compassion in the medical facility.

OUTGOING CALLS

The majority of the outgoing calls in a physician's office are responses to the incoming calls. The same rules regarding courtesy and diction apply to the calls being made from the office to patients, other individuals, or businesses.

It is helpful to plan outgoing calls in advance. For instance, if the medical assistant is placing an order for office supplies, a list should be made that includes the product, the price, the quantity needed, and a catalog page number, if applicable. Questions about the various products ordered should be noted so that they can be asked while the sales representative is on the phone.

Some medical assistants find it helpful to make all outgoing calls at once, when possible. This way the calls can be made one after another, and if a call back is necessary, it is likely that the medical assistant may still be by the phone. Organizing calls will help to increase office efficiency.

Never be rude to an individual on the phone. Remember to treat those on the other end of the phone as you would wish to be treated. Do not forget that the medical assistant is a representative of the physician and should behave in a professional manner at all times (Procedure 9-4).

TELEPHONES IN THE MILLENNIUM

Voicemail

Voicemail is widely used in today's business offices because it affords an around-the-clock method for receiving patient messages. Unfortunately, it can prove frustrating to those who find themselves speaking to an electronic device more often than with a human being. Voicemail allows the caller to hear a recorded message that may also provide information about what to do in case of an emergency. Similar to an answering machine, voicemail will record a caller's message that can later be retrieved. It often allows special temporary greetings when the user is away from the office. Keep patients happy by answering voicemail messages promptly.

Answering Machines

Answering machines do the same job as voicemail, but a machine is attached to the telephone rather than being an integral part of the office phone system. With the inexpensive cost of voicemail, most businesses have retired their answering machines and have chosen more modern methods of message-taking.

Answering Services

Because a physician's telephone is an all-important tool of the practice, there must be someone to answer it at all times—day and night, weekends and holidays. This presents no problem during weekdays, but nights and weekends require special attention. Most physicians subscribe to telephone answering services that provide round-the-clock coverage. Answering services normally provide an operator (rather than a recording device) to answer the phones, and this is often preferred over standard voicemail. Two types of operator-answered services exist. With the first type, physician-subscribers leave messages with, or obtain patients' messages from, a service whose number appears in the local telephone directory after the physician's

---

PROCEDURE 9-4

Demonstrate Telephone Techniques

CAAHEP COMPETENCY: 3.c.(1)(d)
ABHES COMPETENCY: 2.e

GOAL: *To project a professional image while handling telephone calls.*

EQUIPMENT and SUPPLIES

- Telephone
- Message Pad

PROCEDURAL STEPS

1. Answer incoming calls quickly and always by the third ring.
   PURPOSE: Individuals prefer prompt responses to their calls.
2. Greet the caller professionally, using words that identify the office.
   PURPOSE: To assure the caller that he or she has reached the right number.
3. Identify the caller and determine to whom the caller wishes to speak or what the caller needs from the office.
   PURPOSE: To be able to assist the caller and to direct the call to the right person.
4. Ask if you may put the caller on hold before transferring the call.
   PURPOSE: To show consideration for the caller's time.
5. Call the person to whom the call will be transferred, and explain that you will be transferring a call to him or her.
   PURPOSE: To make certain that the staff member is available to take the call to avoid wasting the patient's time and to prepare the staff member for the call, in case a file or other information is needed.
6. Go back to the caller, and tell him or her that you are prepared to transfer the call.
   PURPOSE: This process lets the caller know that you value his

or her time and have found the staff member who will be of assistance.
7. Transfer the call immediately.
   PURPOSE: To quickly and efficiently route the caller to the person to whom he or she wishes to speak.
8. If a second call comes in while you are speaking to the first caller, ask permission to place the first caller on hold.
   PURPOSE: Asking permission to place a caller on hold is polite and shows consideration for the caller's time.
9. Answer the second call and ask permission to place the call on hold. Listen for a response to make certain that the caller does not have an emergency.
   PURPOSE: Always listen for a response to make sure that the second caller does not need immediate attention.
10. Place the second caller on hold, and return to the first caller.
    PURPOSE: The first caller's needs should be addressed before moving to the second caller.
11. Address the first caller's needs, complete the call, and go back to the second caller.
    PURPOSE: Callers should be assisted in the order that the calls come to the office, barring any emergency.
12. Take a message if necessary, following the guidelines in Procedure 9-2.
13. Always allow the caller to hang up first.
    PURPOSE: To remain on the line in case the caller has a last comment or question.

number, with a notation to call the second number after hours. This form of service is somewhat inconvenient for the patient but is far better than no coverage at all. With the second type the answering service has a direct connection with the office telephone. When the telephone rings in the physician's office or at home, it also signals on the switchboard of the answering service. As long as the telephone is ringing, it will continue to signal at the answering service. If no one answers within a certain agreed-on number of rings (or immediately in some cases), the answering service operator takes the call. This method provides continuous live telephone coverage.

Even during the day, such an answering service can function effectively. There may be times when the staff members are assisting the physician and not available to answer the telephone. Not answering the telephone is extremely poor policy, so if the office has an agreement with the answering service, its operators will accept calls in such situations. With this direct-wire answering method, the operator answers the telephone in the same manner as the regular staff.

The answering service will greatly appreciate receiving a call every day from a member of the physician's staff before leaving the office with information as to where the physician will be during the evening or other special messages. The next morning, a staff member should call the service and ask for any messages that may have been taken. Usually there will be messages from patients who called after office hours but whose calls were not urgent enough to merit an emergency call to the physician. An answering service can act as a buffer for the physician and help eliminate too frequent, unnecessary calls during the late evening or night hours.

Automatic Call Routing

In automatic call routing, a call is answered by an automated operator's message that presents a list of options, such as "If you are calling about your account, press 1; to make an appointment, press 2; and so forth. The impersonal nature of automation does not lend itself well to answering the telephone in a private physician's office, but the medical assistant will encounter it frequently when placing outgoing calls. Some larger clinics and hospitals may use automatic call routing on a daily basis.

CRITICAL THINKING APPLICATION

Ashlynn has had many complaints from patients about the new call-routing system, because it takes so long to "get to a human being." How can she get her patients to be more accepting of modern call-routing systems? What methods might help elderly patients in dealing with automated call routing more easily?

Call Forwarding

Call forwarding allows the user to forward calls to another designated number, such as a cellular phone. Usually a code is entered, then the phone number to which the calls should be forwarded. This keeps the user from missing important calls when away from the main telephone.

Caller ID

Caller ID allows the user to see who is calling before picking up the handset to answer the phone. The caller's phone number and name appear on a screen, and the user can decide whether to take the call. If the user subscribes to call-waiting services, another benefit called *call-waiting caller ID* is often available. Call-waiting caller ID allows the user to see who is calling even when the user is already on the phone.

Cellular Phones

Considered a luxury item only 10 years ago, cellular (or cell) phones have become commonplace in today's world (Figure 9-6). Many people no longer have a home phone because of the expense of having two phones, and the cell phone is usually the better buy for the money. Several of the more popular cell phone companies offer free long-distance calls in the United States and may provide users free night and weekend minutes as a bonus. Some of today's advanced cell phones will even allow the user to access the Internet through the telephone, and the user can check email. Cell phone companies usually offer a text messaging service, which allows the user to type a message using the cell phone keys which is then sent directly to a cell phone number.

Pagers

The popularity of pagers has dwindled somewhat with the growth of cell phones. However, pagers are quite useful for reaching individuals to notify them that they are needed

---

CELL PHONE RULES OF ETIQUETTE

1. *Hang Up and Drive:* Take care when using the phone and driving. It is best to pull over and talk on the phone instead of trying to manipulate the car and carry on a conversation.
2. *Turn Off the Phone at the Right Time:* Never leave the phone on during meetings or at public events like movies and formal dinners.
3. *Respect Personal Space:* Most people do not want to hear personal or business conversations while they are in line for a movie or eating dinner. Step away when speaking on the cell phone in public.
4. *The Phone Is Not a Human:* Nothing is more rude than having dinner with a friend and taking a casual call on the cell phone. Pay attention to the human and turn the phone off until later.
5. *Keep it Charged:* It is very frustrating to speak to someone on a cell phone who cannot hear. Keeping the phone charged will cause less periods of static and more clarity when in use.

FIGURE 9-6 Etiquette rules for cellular phones.

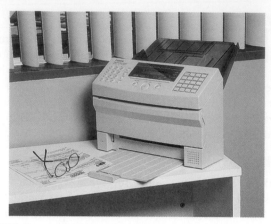

FIGURE 9-7 Fax machines allow the transfer of written data from one place to another with the simple dial of a telephone number.

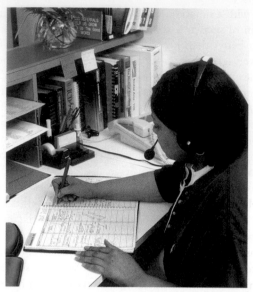

FIGURE 9-8 Using a headset helps the medical assistant keep hands free while using the telephone and is better ergonomically.

quickly. Physicians often carry pagers with them at all times. Many models allow the user to type into the pager a text message that is sent to the receiver electronically.

Fax Machines

A fax machine can be a great time and labor saver in conveying patient information from physician to physician or from physician to hospital. It allows its user to send and receive copies of printed documents over telephone lines to other facilities that have fax machines (Figure 9-7). Most offices find this machine indispensable. Unless precautions are taken to ensure security of information arriving by fax, the danger of loss of confidentiality is present. When sensitive material is sent, it is wise to telephone ahead to alert the receiver that this information will be arriving so that the appropriate person will be on hand to receive it. A fax cover sheet should be used that instructs individuals who receive faxes in error to destroy them and states that the information contained in the fax is strictly confidential.

Headsets

In today's world of **multitasking,** the headset helps a medical assistant to keep hands free while speaking on the phone. A popular headset is a very lightweight plastic earphone and microphone combination that allows the wearer to move about the room and to have the hands free (Figure 9-8). Some units weigh less than 1 ounce and are worn behind the ear or clipped to the wearer's glasses. Some headsets can be equipped with a cord that allows for easy mobility. Some also have a quick-disconnect feature that allows the user to separate the headset even during a call without breaking the connection.

USING LONG DISTANCE AND SPECIAL SERVICES

Long-distance calls are simple to place, usually inexpensive, and efficient. When information is needed in a hurry, it is much more expedient to telephone rather than wait for an exchange of letters. Before placing a long-distance call, have the correct number ready. This number often may be obtained from a letterhead or from other records. If you do not have the number,

you may obtain directory assistance by dialing the area code of the party you are calling, followed by 555-1212. In some areas you must dial 1 before the area code. Directory assistance is now an automated service in many regions, and you will be asked for the name of the city and the person you are calling. There is often a charge for using directory assistance.

One alternative to directory assistance is using the Internet to find phone numbers. A search for the business or physician the medical assistant is looking for may yield the information needed. There are also Internet services that allow the user to call long distance, and sometimes even internationally, through the computer with absolutely no long-distance charges.

Time Zones

The continental United States is divided into four standard time zones: Pacific, Mountain, Central, and Eastern (Figure 9-9). When it is noon Pacific time, it is 3 PM Eastern time. When calling from San Francisco to New York, plan to make the call no later than 2 PM if the call is to a business or professional office. When it is 2 PM on the West Coast, it is 5 PM on the East Coast.

International Service

International Direct Distance Dialing (IDDD) is available in many areas. International dialing codes are the same for all companies offering IDDD. Depending on the long-distance company, additional numbers or codes may preface the international access, country, and city codes. IDDD is still not available in all areas. If it is available, you may place international station-to-station calls by dialing the following in sequence:

1. International code 011
2. Country code
3. City code
4. Local telephone number
5. The pound sign (#) button if the telephone is touch-tone

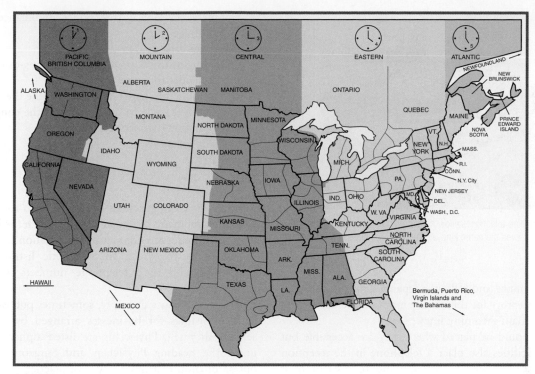

FIGURE 9-9 Time zones across the United States.

After dialing any international code, allow at least 45 seconds for the ringing to start. Consult the Internet for updates on international call procedures and country or city codes.

Wrong Numbers

One slip in direct distance dialing can mean a call to Los Angeles or New York instead of Dallas. If you reach a wrong long-distance number, be sure to obtain the name of the city and state that was called. Report this information promptly to the local operator, so the facility will not be charged for the call. If you are cut off before terminating a call, report this as well. The operator will either reconnect the call or make an adjustment of the charge.

Conference Calls

Conference telephone service is of great value to the medical profession in notifying and explaining to a family how a patient is progressing. It has exceptional value in family conferences, at which a quick decision by the entire family regarding a patient's condition is required.

This service can connect numerous points for a conference in which each person can hear or talk to all others participating. Conference calls may be local or long distance. Charges are added for the number of places connected, the distance between parties, and the length of the conversation.

Conference calls can be set up by a normal long-distance operator or through conference call services. To schedule a call, contact either an operator or the calling service and relay the pertinent information about time, date, and the individuals who are to be included in the call. Many businesses have conference call capabilities on their phone or computer systems. Notify everyone participating in the call of the time, date, number to call, and subjects to discuss. If prior arrangements are made with all parties, there is a better chance of reaching everyone and having a successful conference.

Operator-Assisted Calls and Services

Operator-assisted calls include the following:

- Person-to-person
- Billing to a third party
- Collect calls
- Requests for time and charges
- Certain calls placed from hotels
- Credit for wrong numbers
- Conference calls
- Some international calls

There is an initial charge and a service charge for operator-assisted calls provided through most phone service providers. Fewer and fewer calls are operator-assisted in today's business world, because the cost for these calls is often high. Try other alternatives before making an operator-assisted call.

OFFICE TELEPHONE EQUIPMENT NEEDS

Number and Placement of Telephones

Familiarity with a multiple-line telephone system is a must for medical assistants. Few healthcare facilities can get along with just one telephone line. Two incoming lines along with a private outgoing line with a separate number for the physician's exclusive use is the minimum recommended number of lines.

One medical assistant can handle no more than two incoming lines, so the addition of more lines may also involve additional staffing (Figure 9-10). If a staff member is assigned solely to

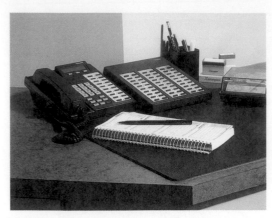

FIGURE 9-10 Multiline telephones allow numerous calls to come into the office at once. Each call deserves the same kind of attention and care from the medical assistant.

dealing with insurance and billing, a separate line and listing in the telephone directory for this service may considerably lessen the load on the main incoming lines.

Telephones should be placed where they are accessible but private. Some facilities also place a telephone in the reception room for the convenience of patients and to prevent their asking to use the facility's phones. However, recent trends suggest that a separate telephone line with a limited calling area for the convenience of patients who need to call out may be preferable. This telephone should not be in the reception room but in an area available to patients on request. It should be placed low enough for use by patients in wheelchairs. Wherever possible, other telephones should be placed on the wall to conserve desk space.

Equipment Selection

Selection of telephone equipment and services offers many options that differ from region to region. As with any major equipment purchase, research the availability and cost before making a purchase.

USING A TELEPHONE DIRECTORY

The primary purpose of the telephone directory is to provide lists of those who have telephones, their telephone numbers, and in most cases their addresses. In addition, the directory is an aid in checking the spelling of names and in locating certain types of businesses through the yellow pages. Some directories are color coded, with residence listings on white pages, business numbers on pink pages, and business by categories and advertisements on yellow pages. Often, federal, state, county, and city government listings are included as blue pages. Directories are usually organized into three sections:

- Introductory pages
- Alphabetic pages (white pages)
- Yellow pages

The introductory pages are sometimes entirely overlooked by subscribers. This section precedes the white alphabetic pages and provides basic information concerning the telephone services in the area, including the following:

- Emergency services (fire, police, ambulance, and highway patrol)
- Service calls
- Dialing instructions for local and long-distance calls
- Area codes for some cities

The introductory pages may also include the following:

- A survival guide for newcomers to the community
- Community service numbers
- Prefix locations
- Rates
- International calling information
- Time zones

Some directories include ZIP code maps for the local area. Take a few moments to become familiar with the local directory, then use it frequently for getting information fast.

The white pages are an alphabetic listing of telephone subscribers with their telephone numbers and often their addresses.

The yellow pages directory, sometimes published separately, contains listings for businesses arranged by the product or services they sell. Physicians are listed alphabetically, usually under the heading Physicians and Surgeons, and have the option of another listing by type of practice.

In some metropolitan areas, a street address and telephone directory is published that is arranged by street address, followed by the name and telephone number of the person or business at that address.

Organizing a Personal Phone Directory

Organize telephone numbers in a tabbed 3- × 5-inch desktop file or a rotary file. Binders with clear sheet protectors also work well as personal phone directories. Emergency numbers might be typed on a colored card or flagged with a color tab. A personal directory of telephone numbers should include all the numbers that are frequently called.

Identifying Community Resources

Patients will often call the physician's office looking for information on various community resources. Those who are fighting cancer may be interested in programs offered by the American Red Cross. Those who are diabetic may wish to know the options for ordering blood glucose testing supplies through online services. Some patients may benefit from Meals on Wheels. The medical assistant should be concerned with providing good customer service to patients and visitors with whom they come into contact. Therefore it is helpful to keep a list of the community resources that might be of assistance to patients. Often, information can be found in the first few sections of the telephone book. The physician may wish to keep a list of those services that are most often used by the patients of the clinic. Patients will appreciate staff members who try to offer assistance and resources outside the physician's office.

Using the Telephone to Educate Patients

Today's telephone systems allow physicians to educate patients while they are on hold; recordings may be played that offer health information on subjects from A to Z. These messages can be professionally recorded or custom designed by the physician and staff. Special events may be announced, with the option to press a certain number for more information about the event.

Some phone directories offer listings of health information in the introductory pages. A patient may call a main number, then press a second number to reach the subject of his or her choice. Such features help to address the needs of today's more information-oriented consumers of healthcare, who have an interest in healthy lifestyles and in gaining useful information immediately.

CLOSING COMMENTS

A telephone can be a tool to build a physician's practice, or one to break it apart. Medical assistants must become proficient in good telephone technique and must ensure that the caller hears compassion and patience in the voice of the medical assistant, even over the phone. A medical assistant must convey a genuine sense of caring for the patients who call the facility, just as if they were standing in the office face-to-face. By keeping this in mind, the medical assistant will play a major role in patient satisfaction, and the patients will find their medical care a pleasant process.

SUMMARY OF SCENARIO

Ashlynn is quickly becoming a part of the team at Dr. Frank's office and is developing into a well-liked asset to the staff. She has learned to slow down when speaking on the phone and to adjust her volume and pitch, depending on the patient with whom she is speaking. Although she tends to be quite talkative, she is balancing just the right amount of friendly chat with the business at hand. She does this by offering a friendly greeting to callers, getting to the business at hand, then being affable before ending the call. By expressing her concern and asking how she can be of help to the patients, Ashlynn shows them that she sincerely cares about their problems. She is careful about her tone of voice, realizing that patients may take her comments the wrong way if she does not treat them in a cordial manner. Dr. Frank is very pleased with her performance.

Ashlynn takes care when she speaks to patients and others on the phone so that she does not breach confidentiality in any way. She has become comfortable with the way she is to answer

the telephone. The pace of her speech and the wording are now a habit. Ashlynn is determined to maintain a professional relationship with all of the people related to her work environment. She is adept now at handling calls from angry patients and can maintain control with even the most aggressive callers. She leaves callers on hold for a minimum amount of time and reassures them frequently that she is attending to their situation. By treating callers as she would want to be treated, Ashlynn reduces frustration, and she feels that the office is more efficient in handling the large volume of calls that come into the office each day. She shows much promise for a long and rewarding career in the medical field and is satisfied with the track her career is on at the present time. As she continues to settle into her position, she looks forward to learning more about efficiency and time management. Her good attitude and desire to learn will only enhance her performance at work and make her an employee worth promoting and of great value in the facility.

SUMMARY of LEARNING OBJECTIVES

1. Define, spell, and pronounce the terms listed in the vocabulary.
   - Spelling and pronouncing medical terms correctly adds credibility to the medical assistant. Knowing the definition of these terms promotes confidence in communication with patients and co-workers.
2. Determine and discuss the source of incoming and outgoing calls to a physician's office.
   - Incoming calls to a physician's office come from a wide variety of sources. Established or new patients may be calling to set appointments. Insurance companies may be seeking information about a claim. Hospitals, nursing facilities, or other healthcare units may need to report the progress of a patient. Laboratory results may be coming in for a patient who is very ill. Routine sales calls and telemarketing calls also come to the

office, in addition to personal calls to the physician and staff members.
3. Describe how one develops a pleasing telephone voice.
   - A pleasing telephone voice is one that is friendly and conveys a favorable impression of the physician's practice. Enunciate words and pronounce them clearly and distinctly. Vary the pitch of your voice, avoiding a monotonous or droning manner. Always be courteous and use tact. Both incoming and outgoing calls should be businesslike and handled in a professional manner.
4. Demonstrate the correct way to hold a telephone handset.
   - The telephone handset should be held around the middle of the shaft, with the mouthpiece situated approximately 1 inch from the lips, in front of the teeth. Talk directly into the handset

SUMMARY of LEARNING OBJECTIVES

Continued

so the caller can clearly hear what is being said. Do not hold the mouthpiece beneath the chin, because the voice may not be heard clearly. Do not lean the head downward to hold the phone between the ear and the shoulder, to avoid sore muscles and neck problems.

5. Explain why courtesy is so important when speaking on the telephone.
   - It is vital to be courteous to patients and other callers. First impressions are important, and a medical assistant's phone manner sets the tone for the caller's perception of the physician's practice. Customer service is important to today's physician, because many patients have choices among their healthcare providers as to which physician provides their care, and the attitude of staff members may play a large part in such a decision. Good customer care to patients means that they will not only continue to see the provider, but they will also refer other patients to the physician. This is one of the best ways to help a practice grow.

6. Discuss different ways to handle callers who wish to speak to the physician.
   - The physician's time is valuable but is also centered around his or her patients. It would be physically impossible for the physician to take all of the calls from those who wish to talk each day. Therefore the medical assistant must screen the physician's calls and make decisions about which ones should be put through to the physician. The medical assistant should offer to take a message and attempt to find out exactly what the caller's needs are and how they can be resolved. The patient should not feel that the physician is totally inaccessible but must also understand that the patient in the office must have the physician's full attention.

7. List the seven items needed to take a telephone message correctly.
   - Seven distinct items are needed when taking a phone message, including the name of the person to whom the call should be directed and the name of the person calling. The caller's telephone number must be noted as well as the reason for the call. The medical assistant should describe the action to be taken. The date and time of the call should always be noted, as well as the initials of the person taking the call, so that if any question arises, that person can be identified and asked.

8. Explain how angry callers might be handled.
   - Never return anger when a caller is angry. Remain calm and speak in tones that are perhaps slightly quieter than those of the caller. This often prompts the caller to lower his or her tone of voice. Offer to help the angry person, and ask questions to gain control of the conversation, moving it toward resolution. Do not argue with angry callers.

9. Discuss how the medical assistant should handle callers who have a complaint.

   - Callers who have a complaint should be handled in a similar way as angry callers. Remain calm and offer to help. Take a serious interest in what the caller has to say. Let the caller know that his or her concerns are important to the staff and the physician. Find the source of the problem, and determine exactly what the caller wants or expects with regard to its resolution. Always follow up with complaints, and be sure that they were resolved as much to the caller's satisfaction as possible.

10. List several questions to ask when handling an emergency call.
    - Several questions should be asked when an emergency call comes to the medical office. First, obtain a phone number at which the caller can be reached in case of a sudden disconnection. Ask about the chief symptoms and when they started. Find out if the patient has had similar symptoms in the past and what happened in that situation. Determine whether the patient is alone, has transportation, or needs an ambulance dispatched to the location. In cases of severe emergencies, do not hang up the phone until the ambulance or police arrive.

11. Discuss several useful sections of the introductory pages of the phone directory.
    - The introductory pages of the telephone book contain several sections of useful information, such as area codes, emergency service information, long-distance calling information, time zones, government listings, and community service numbers. It may be helpful to tear these pages out, place them in clear sheet protectors, then add them to a binder for easy reference.

12. Demonstrate the correct way to answer the telephone in the office.
    - Medical assistants should answer the telephone promptly and professionally. The physician's image is affected by the way that telephone calls are handled. Be courteous and polite to all callers. The correct way to answer the telephone is addressed in Procedure 9-1.

13. Demonstrate the correct way to accurately record a message and take a request for action.
    - When taking a telephone message, strive for accuracy. Be sure to get all of the information that the physician will need to act. Repeat any words or numbers that are not heard clearly. The steps in taking an accurate telephone message are detailed in Procedure 9-2.

14. Demonstrate the most efficient way to call in a prescription or a prescription refill to a pharmacy.
    - The medical assistant should follow the office policy and procedure manual when calling new prescriptions or refills to a pharmacy. If a question ever arises as to what the physician meant, ask—do not guess. Mistakes with medication can cost a patient his or her life. Calling the pharmacy with new or refill prescriptions is explained in Procedure 9-3.

CONNECTIONS

 Study Guide Connection: Go to Chapter 9 Study Guide. Read the Case Study and Workplace Applications and complete the assignments. Do online research for answers to the questions in the Internet Activities associated with telephone techniques.

 CD Connection: Go to the Medical Assisting Competency Challenge CD and do the training activities under General Office Duties and Communication.

 Evolve Connection: For more information related to telephone techniques, go to http://evolve.elsevier.com/kinn/admin and visit related weblinks for Chapter 9. Click on the Medical Assisting Exam Review and do the practice questions to sharpen your test-taking skills.

Scheduling Appointments

10

SCENARIO

Ramona West is the medical assistant in charge of scheduling appointments for Dr. Charlotte Brown. Ramona is an extremely organized person who thinks quickly and creatively. One of her professional goals is to ensure that the office remains on schedule throughout each day and that patient wait time is kept to an absolute minimum. She is fortunate that Dr. Brown is cooperative and time oriented, so they work well together to reach this common goal.

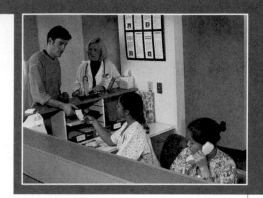

Ramona usually arrives at work at least 15 minutes early to begin her preparations for the day. She pulls patient charts each evening for the next day so that they will be easily accessible the next morning. She pays particular attention to the patients who arrive in the office as she completes her daily tasks. Ramona greets each patient by name and carries on a brief but cordial conversation. Patients appreciate that she goes the extra mile to remember something about them, and this promotes excellent patient relations.

Ramona leaves a little time in the morning and afternoon for emergency appointments. She calls or emails patients to confirm appointments in advance, and this increases her show rate. Her friendly, caring attitude makes her a favorite among the patients, and Dr. Brown is pleased with the relationship-building skills that Ramona has developed.

While studying this chapter, think about the following questions:

- How can the medical assistant contribute to an efficient daily routine?
- How does the medical assistant keep the daily schedule on track?
- How can the schedule be put back on track when emergencies disrupt the day?
- How does the flexibility of the medical assistant contribute to office efficiency?

LEARNING OBJECTIVES

1. Define, spell, and pronounce the terms listed in the vocabulary.
2. Discuss three items that must be considered when scheduling appointments.
3. Explain the features that should be considered when choosing an appointment book.
4. Discuss the advantages of computerized appointment scheduling.
5. Explain how self-scheduling would reduce calls to the medical office.
6. List and explain at least three methods of appointment scheduling.
7. Explain the basic procedure to follow when the office is behind schedule.
8. Discuss offering choices to patients when scheduling appointments.
9. Explain the importance of legible writing in the appointment book.
10. Discuss several methods of dealing with patients who consistently arrive late.
11. Name several reasons for failed appointments.

National Accreditation Competencies and Content

CAAHEP COMPETENCIES

Administrative

3.a.(1)(a). Schedule and manage appointments
3.a.(1)(b). Schedule inpatient and outpatient admissions and procedures

General

3.c.(1)(b). Recognize and respond to verbal communication
3.c.(1)(d). Demonstrate telephone techniques
3.c.(2)(a). Identify and respond to issues of confidentiality
3.c.(2)(d). Document appropriately
3.c.(3)(a). Explain general office policies
3.c.(3)(b). Instruct individuals according to their needs
3.c.(4)(a). Utilize computer software to maintain office systems

ABHES COMPETENCIES

Professionalism

1.h. Be courteous and diplomatic

Communication

2.e. Use proper telephone techniques
2.h. Receive, organize, prioritize, and transmit information expediently
2.k. Principles of verbal and nonverbal communication
2.l. Recognition and response to verbal and nonverbal communication
2.m. Adaptation for individualized needs
2.n. Application of electronic technology
2.p. Professional components

Administrative Duties

3.a. Perform basic secretarial skills
3.c. Schedule and monitor appointments
3.f. Manage physician's professional schedule and travel
3.g. Schedule inpatient and outpatient admissions

Legal Concepts

5.b. Document accurately

VOCABULARY

disruption An unexpected event that throws a plan into disorder; an interruption that prevents a system or process from continuing as usual or as expected.

established patients Patients who are returning to the office who have previously been seen by the physician.

expediency (ik-spe′-de-un-se) A means of achieving a particular end, as in a situation requiring haste or caution.

integral (in′-ti-grul) Essential; being an indispensable part of a whole.

interaction A two-way communication; mutual or reciprocal action or influence.

intermittent Coming and going at intervals; not continuous.

interval Space of time between events.

matrix Something in which a thing originates, develops, takes shape, or is contained; a base on which to build.

no-show A person who fails to keep an appointment without giving advance notice.

prerequisite (pre-re′-kwe-zut) Something that is necessary to an end or to carry out a function.

proficiency (pruh-fi′-shun-se) Competency as a result of training or practice.

socioeconomic Relating to a combination of social and economic factors.

triage (tre′-awzh) Process of evaluating the urgency of medical need and prioritizing treatment.

The physician's time is the most valuable asset of a medical practice. The person responsible for scheduling this time must understand the practice, be familiar with the working habits and preferences of the physicians, and have clear guidelines for time management within the practice.

Appointment scheduling is the process that determines which patients will be seen by the physician, the dates and times of appointments, and how much time will be allotted to each patient based on his or her complaint, as well as the physician's availability. Time management involves the realization that unforeseen interruptions and delays will always occur. Most providers of medical care find that efficient scheduling of appointments is one of the most important factors in the success of the practice. Many approaches to scheduling are available, and each facility must find what suits it best.

GUIDELINES FOR APPOINTMENT SCHEDULING

One of the most common complaints that patients make is the amount of money they pay for such short visits with the physician. A patient may say, "I only saw the doctor for 5 minutes and could not even remember all the questions I wanted to ask!" The patient must feel confident that the physician will take enough time to understand his or her concerns. Well-planned scheduling and adherence to that schedule will allow the physician to do more than run in and out of examination rooms, leaving little time for the patient to talk with the physician.

Some medical offices stick to a strict schedule, with little room for maneuvering, whereas many are more flexible in scheduling to meet the needs of the patients and the providers.

The key to good scheduling is organization and teamwork in the office. Without these, even the best-planned schedule will not succeed.

The person who is scheduling appointments must learn the physician's habits and desires. If the physician suggests scheduling patients every 15 minutes but always spends 20 to 25 minutes with a patient, the schedule must be adjusted. Talk with the physician and/or office manager and compromise so that the schedule is a workable one. Some physicians need prompting to end the patient visit and move to the next patient. The medical assistant who is assisting in the examination room can help the physician remain on schedule, because he or she teams with the scheduler and both work together for the efficient flow of patients through the office.

The scheduling system must be individualized to each specific practice. The following guidelines are general and can be applied to any practice, whether paper-based or computer-based. Three items must be considered when scheduling: patient need, physician preference and habits, and available facilities.

Patient Need

A major consideration in determining office hours and appointment times is the **socioeconomic** status of the area being served. The office staff should answer the following questions:

- Is the office located in a busy metropolitan area or a rural agricultural community?
- Are the patients young, middle-aged, or retirement age?
- Is the area more industrial or residential?
- What type of patients are seen? Are they of a specific age or gender? Do they have common diagnoses? Is the physician a general practitioner?
- Are evening and weekend appointments essential for most of the patients served?

After these items are considered, the scheduler must allot time based on the patient needs for each individual office visit. These needs can be assessed by determining the following:

- What is the purpose of this visit?
- What is the age of the patient?
- Will the patient require the physician's time for the entire visit, or will another staff member perform all or part of the service?
- Is the patient a parent who prefers to schedule appointments while the children are at school?
- Does the patient object to traveling after dark?
- Is the patient a day worker who cannot take time off from a job?
- Is the patient a child whose parents are both working during the day?

The office should make every attempt to meet the patient's needs while balancing the physician's preferences and available facilities.

Physician Preferences and Habits

The preferences and habits of the physicians in the practice must be considered before a scheduling plan can be established and followed. Consider the following:

- Does the physician become restless if the reception room is not packed with waiting patients?
- Does the physician worry if even one patient is kept waiting?
- Is the physician methodic and careful about being in the facility when patient appointments are scheduled to begin?
- Is the physician habitually late?
- Does the physician move easily from one patient to another?
- Does the physician require a "break time" after a few patients?
- Would the physician rather see fewer patients and spend more time with each one, or schedule more patients each day?

All of these preferences and habits become an **integral** part of the scheduling process (Figure 10-1). Keep in mind that the physician cannot spend every moment of the day with patients. The physician also has telephone calls to make and receive, reports to examine and dictate, meetings to attend, mail to answer, and many other business responsibilities that require his or her attention. An experienced staff can handle many—but not all—of these tasks.

CRITICAL THINKING APPLICATION

- Ramona has noticed that Dr. Brown is taking a little longer with patients than normal and that she is running consistently behind schedule by approximately 5 to 15 minutes. How can Ramona help to rectify this situation?
- Discuss ways of approaching the physician when he or she is the cause of the delays in the schedule. What opening remarks can the medical assistant use to start the discussion in a positive way?

Available Facilities

It is pointless to get a patient into the office at a time when no facilities are available for the services needed. For example, suppose that a two-physician office has only one room that can be used for minor surgery. You would not schedule two patients requiring minor surgery for the same time block even if both

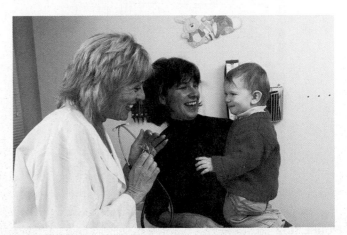

FIGURE 10-1 The habits and preferences of the physician must be considered when scheduling appointments for patients.

doctors could be available. If the office has only one electrocardiograph, you would not book two electrocardiographic procedures at the same time. As the medical assistant gains **proficiency** in scheduling, patient needs will be paired with the available facilities, according to the physician's preference. Major equipment that is frequently used or a certain room containing such equipment may need its own scheduling column in the appointment book or software system.

SELECTING THE METHOD OF APPOINTMENT SCHEDULING

The two most common methods of appointment scheduling are using an appointment book and computer-based scheduling. Each has advantages and disadvantages, and the physician's office should weigh the benefits and choose the method that best suits the physician and the staff.

Appointment Books

Office suppliers carry a variety of appointment book styles. Certain basic features should be considered when choosing an appointment book:

- The size should conform to the desk space available.
- It should be large enough to accommodate the practice.
- It should open flat for easy writing and reference.
- It should allow space for writing when, who, and why.

Some appointment books show an entire week at a glance, and many are color-coded, with a special color for each day of the week (Figure 10-2). This is very helpful when the physician asks the patient to return, for instance, in 2 weeks. If Wednesdays are colored yellow, the medical assistant can flip quickly to the correct day 2 weeks later and schedule the appointment. Multiple columns may be available to correspond

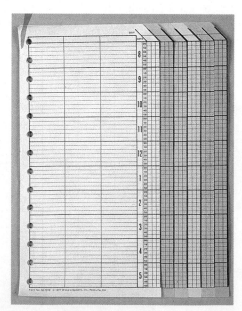

FIGURE 10-2 Color-coded appointment book pages help a medical assistant to flip to the right day of the right week quickly. Appointments for multiple physicians can be color-coded in the book.

with the number of doctors in a group practice, and the time can be divided according to their preferences.

Computer Scheduling

The computer has replaced the appointment book in many practices. Software for appointment scheduling ranges from relatively simple programs that merely display available and scheduled times to more sophisticated systems that perform several other functions. Many programs can display such information as the length and type of appointment required and day or time preferences. The computer can then select the best appointment time based on the information entered into the computer.

The computer can also be used to keep track of future appointments. For example, when a patient calls and inquires about an appointment, the system can search by his or her name to find the time and date. Printouts can also run to show the physician's daily schedule, including the patients' names and telephone numbers and the reason for the visit. Multiple copies of these schedules can be made, according to the needs of the practice.

One advantage of computer scheduling is that more than one person can access the system at one time, and the information is available to all operators. The medical assistant can generate a hard copy of the next day's appointments before leaving each evening. In some facilities, employees still maintain an appointment book as a backup to computer scheduling.

Self-Scheduling

The future of appointment scheduling includes self-scheduling, which is a method by which a patient can log on to the Internet and view a facility's schedule, then select his or her own appointment time and make the appointment right then. The system should allow for patient confidentiality by showing only available times. Other patients' names should never be visible on an online system.

Software is available that will allow the patient to self-schedule through secure links to the physician's appointment book. The software or Internet site for the physician's office should give the patient guidelines as to the amount of time needed for certain appointments or should allow only a certain length of time to be self-scheduled, such as 15 minutes. These systems will reduce calls to the office and are available to the patient 24 hours a day. Some of these systems will also send an automatic email reminder to the patient the day before the appointment, requesting a reply to confirm. These systems are less frustrating to patients, who do not have to wait on hold to speak to the person who does scheduling for the office. Appointments that are more lengthy or complicated should be scheduled through the office staff.

Although this type of appointment-setting system will appeal to most technologically savvy people, some patients will stringently reject online scheduling because it requires at least minimal computer skills that the patient may not be capable of or comfortable with performing. If this method is used, some allowance must be made for those who are computer illiterate. Other patients may object to online scheduling because they do not wish their name to be anywhere on the Internet. This is a valid issue and the office should allow these patients to schedule over the phone.

ADVANCE PREPARATION

Having chosen an appropriate method of appointment setting, some advance preparation should be done. This is sometimes called establishing the **matrix** (Procedure 10-1). Block off time slots when the physician is routinely not available to see patients, such as days off, holidays, lunch or dinner breaks, time for hospital rounds, and meetings. In the space in which a patient's name would normally be placed, note the reason the time is blocked off. Always try to account for every time period in each day. The medical assistant should also make a note of social or family engagements to help the physician remember these obligations. Because time is a valuable commodity for the physician and the office staff, the schedule is the tool that assists in making certain that the day runs smoothly.

TYPES OF APPOINTMENT SCHEDULING

Different types of appointment scheduling are used to meet the various needs of the medical facility, the providers, and the patients served. Some offices use a combination of methods to create the right mix of activity during the day and to ensure that the day runs smoothly and efficiently. The medical assistant should become proficient at managing appointments (Procedure 10-2).

Open Office Hours

When using the open office hours method, the facility is open at given hours of the day or evening, and the patients are "scheduled" by the physician by mentioning to the patient that he or she should return "in a couple of weeks" for follow-up. At **intermittent** times the patients come in, knowing in advance that they will be seen in the order of their arrival. Physicians who use this method say that it eliminates the annoyance of broken appointments and of the office running behind schedule. The open office hours method has also been referred

---

PROCEDURE 10-1

Schedule and Manage Appointments: Prepare Appointment Pages by Matrixing

CAAHEP COMPETENCY: 3.a.(1)(a)
ABHES COMPETENCY: 3.c

GOAL: *To establish the matrix of the appointment page and enter information according to office policy.*

EQUIPMENT and SUPPLIES

- Appointment book or computer
- Office procedure manual
- Information regarding physician office hours and availability
- Clerical supplies
- Calendar

PROCEDURAL STEPS

1. Determine the proper methods to use when scheduling an appointment by consulting the office procedure manual.
   PURPOSE: To follow prescribed office policy for appointment scheduling.
2. Become familiar with any software that is used for scheduling appointments.
   PURPOSE: To become proficient with the scheduling software used in the office.
3. Determine the hours that the physician(s) will not be available.
   PURPOSE: To make certain that patients are not scheduled when the physician is unavailable and to avoid rescheduling issues.
4. Make a column in the appointment book for each provider.
   PURPOSE: Some medical facilities have multiple providers who will maintain a schedule of patients—for example, many physicians employ physician assistants or nurse practitioners who also see patients.
5. Establish the matrix of the appointment book by blocking out the times that the physician(s) will be unavailable or the office will be closed.
   PURPOSE: To leave available only those time slots that can be used for patient appointments.
6. Allow buffer time in the morning and afternoon.
   PURPOSE: To allow for emergencies and short rest or catch-up times for the staff and providers.
7. Determine the number of available rooms for patient examinations, treatments, and procedures.
   PURPOSE: The number of available rooms affects the number of patients that can be seen during a day.
8. Establish a list of procedures that details the amount of time needed for an appointment.
   PURPOSE: To better gauge the amount of time that the physician will spend with patients.
9. Place the book in a convenient place for all employees who will schedule appointments.
   PURPOSE: To make certain that the appointment book is always readily available.

PROCEDURE 10-2

Schedule and Manage Appointments: Manage Appointments

<u>CAAHEP COMPETENCY:</u> 3.a.(1)(a)
<u>ABHES COMPETENCY:</u> 3.c

GOAL: *To manage appointments as they are cancelled, no showed, or rescheduled throughout the business day.*

EQUIPMENT and SUPPLIES

- Appointment book or computer
- Office procedure manual
- Appointment cards
- Clerical supplies
- Telephone

PROCEDURAL STEPS

1. Determine the names of patients who have appointments either the day before or the morning of the appointment.
   PURPOSE: To prepare the medical records for the patients who have appointments.

2. Confirm the appointments if required.
   PURPOSE: To make certain that the patient plans to keep the appointment and provide an opportunity to reschedule or call in a patient on the waiting list.

3. Make note of any patient arriving late in the appointment book. If this behavior has become a pattern, note it in the medical record as well.
   PURPOSE: Repeated behavior that disrupts the clinic schedule should be documented.

4. Document failure to arrive for an appointment in the appointment book or scheduling program and in the patient's medical record.

5. Call the patient to attempt to reschedule the appointment and obtain a reason for the no-show.
   PURPOSE: To document failure to comply with physician's recommendation to return.

6. Reschedule missed appointments if possible after talking with the patient.
   PURPOSE: To keep the patient on schedule for medical care.

7. Write the new appointment time, date, and day on an appointment card, or give the information to the patient over the telephone.
   PURPOSE: To ensure that the patient is aware of the new appointment time.

8. If the physician is running more than 15 minutes late, inform patients of the delay.
   PURPOSE: To offer the patients the opportunity to reschedule if necessary.

9. As patients arrive, place a check next to the name in the appointment book.

10. Offer the sign-in sheet to the patient for his or her signature.
    PURPOSE: To verify that the patient arrived in the clinic.

to as *tidal wave scheduling.* Some of these facilities allow online or telephone check-in, and patients are notified when it is close to their turn with the provider.

Few healthcare facilities in metropolitan areas have open office hours with no scheduled appointments, but this system is still found in some rural areas, where the way of life is governed not so much by the clock as by the needs of the people in the area. Many freestanding emergency clinics also offer open office hours, as do many laboratories and imaging facilities.

There can be many disadvantages to open office hours. The office may already be crowded when the physician arrives, resulting in an extremely long wait for some patients. Patients may arrive in waves throughout the day, which causes parts of the day to be very busy and parts to be slow. This makes it difficult to get other office duties accomplished. Without planning, the facilities and staff can be overburdened.

Other types of practices that have open office hours include emergency departments, many of which are open 24 hours a day. Although called *emergency departments,* many of these facilities deal with general practice cases.

Scheduled Appointments

Studies have shown that practitioners are able to see more patients with less pressure when their appointments are scheduled.

Unfortunately, the skill required for scheduling appointments is often not fully appreciated by the practitioner or office manager, resulting in the responsibility being delegated to the least-qualified medical assistant. An efficient, bright individual proficient at multitasking should be assigned to scheduling duties. Although the skill and attitude of the assistant who manages the appointment schedule is very important, the ultimate success of the system lies in the cooperation of the physicians.

Different procedures take varying amounts of time; the scheduler must understand how long it takes to draw blood, fill out new patient paperwork, weigh and check the patient in—all procedures, even the simplest ones, must have an associated amount of time that is necessary to complete the task. If the patient needs an average of 15 minutes to do new patient paperwork, then this time must be included in the schedule. (This is why many offices ask new patients to arrive 15 minutes early for their appointment.) If an allergy shot takes only 20 minutes from check-in to checkout and does not require the patient to see the physician, the scheduler knows that other patients can see the physician while the medical assistant gives the allergy shot. The scheduler cannot accurately set appointments without skill in knowing how long it takes to complete office procedures.

Remember, people other than patients will want to make appointments to see the physician or office staff members, such as pharmaceutical reps or office salespersons. They must make appointments and adjust to the physician's schedule. Patients should not be moved around to accommodate salespersons.

Flexible Office Hours

Most scheduling practices are carryovers from the days when expectant mothers of families with young children relied on one wage earner. Today families commonly have two working parents. As a result, many healthcare providers are turning to extended-day and flexible office hours. Staff hours are affected by these schedules, but this flexibility works to the advantage of the employee and the employer. For instance, if a medical assistant has decided to continue his or her education, morning class hours become available if he or she agrees to work evening hours. Scheduling evening and weekend hours may increase the size of the practice because of the convenience offered to patients.

CRITICAL THINKING APPLICATION

Dr. Brown would like to implement evening appointments 1 night each week and open the office every other Saturday morning. She feels this will better serve her patients with children who have difficulty making daytime appointments. If this is her primary goal, should other types of patients be seen during these time slots? Why or why not?

Wave Scheduling

Wave scheduling is an attempt to create short-term flexibility within each hour. Wave scheduling assumes that the actual time needed for all of the patients seen will average out over the course of the day. Instead of scheduling patients at each 20-minute **interval,** wave scheduling places three patients in the office at the same time, and they are seen in the order of their arrival. Therefore one person's late arrival will not disrupt the entire schedule.

Modified Wave Scheduling

The wave schedule can be modified in several ways. One method is to have two patients scheduled to come in at, for example, 10:00 AM, and a third at 10:30 AM. This hourly cycle is repeated throughout the day. Another application would have patients scheduled to arrive at given intervals during the first half of the hour, and none scheduled to arrive during the second half of the hour. Physicians can modify wave scheduling to best suit the clinic's needs. If a patient complains that more than one patient was scheduled for the same time, explain the method of scheduling used and its efficiency. Patients are usually more cooperative when they understand why tasks are completed a certain way in the office.

Double Booking

Booking two patients to come in at the same time, both of whom are to be seen by the physician, is poor practice. Of course, if each appointment is expected to take only 5 minutes, there is no harm in telling both to come at the same time and reserving a 15-minute period for the two. This is simply one method of wave scheduling. However, if each patient requires 15 minutes, two will require 30 minutes. This must be reflected in the scheduling. It is not considered double booking if a patient comes to the office to receive a treatment by someone other than the physician, such as a patient receiving a physical therapy modality or an allergy injection.

Grouping Procedures

Grouping or categorizing of procedures is another method of scheduling that appeals to many practitioners. For instance, an internist might reserve all morning appointments for complete physical examinations or a pediatrician for well-baby visits. A surgeon might devote one day each week to seeing only referral patients. Obstetricians often schedule pregnant patients on different days than gynecology patients. The physician and staff can experiment with different groupings until the plan that works best for the practice eventually becomes evident. In applying a grouping system of appointments, the medical assistant may find it helpful to color-code the sections of the appointment book being reserved for designated procedures.

Advance Booking

Often appointments are made months in advance. When any appointment is made, an appointment card should be completed and given to the patient. All appointment cards should mention that patients must give 24 hours' notice if they are unable to keep the time reserved for them. Most offices have some type of confirmation procedure by which patients are called the day before to verify that they will keep the appointment.

TIME PATTERNS

When booking appointments, a medical assistant should make it a policy to leave some open time during each day's schedule, so that if a patient calls with a special problem that is not an immediate emergency, there will be some time available to book the patient for at least a brief visit. It is also wise to keep one time slot available in the morning and afternoon specifically for emergencies. A busy physician will always be able to fill these open slots of time, and having them in the schedule will cause the least amount of **disruption** during the day. If possible, time should be set aside in the morning and afternoon for a break. Even 15 minutes will give the physician time to return calls from patients, verify prescription calls, or answer questions.

In the average medical practice, Mondays and Fridays are the most hectic days of the week. Patients may have been waiting the whole weekend to call for an appointment and expect to be seen immediately on Monday. Similarly, toward the end of the week, small problems that could magnify if left unattended over the weekend may prompt the patient to be anxious to see the physician on Friday. Incorporating more buffer time on these 2 days may be worthwhile.

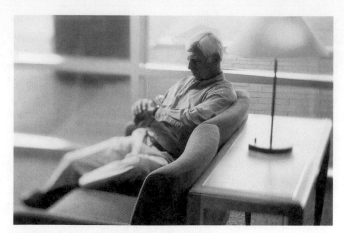

FIGURE 10-3 One of the most common patient complaints is the time spent in the reception area.

PATIENT WAIT TIME

Be conscious about the amount of time that the patient sits in the reception area. Ideally the patient's name will be called to go to the examination room precisely at the scheduled appointment time (Figure 10-3). However, the scheduling has failed if the patient then waits in the back office for 30 minutes to see the physician. Make it clear to the patient whether he or she is free to leave the office after the physician has finished the examination. Some patients mistakenly wait in the examination room until actually told that they are free to leave. Always make certain that the patient knows when to go where.

If a patient has waited more than 15 minutes in the reception area, the medical assistant should briefly explain the delay and offer to reschedule the appointment. The longer patients sit and wait, the more anxious and frustrated they become. Remember, some patients are there to see the physician for test results or may be expecting a negative diagnosis. Do not make their visit more stressful by forcing them to wait for a long time.

Of course, some delays are unavoidable. The physician may be delayed as a result of unforeseen circumstances, or there could be a patient with an emergency. Occasionally a physician becomes ill or must be unexpectedly absent from the office. Briefly explain the situation to the patient and allow him or her to decide whether to wait or reschedule. If a delay is forthcoming, attempt to call patients who may be en route to the office and inform them that there will be a delay. Again, offer to reschedule, or allow the patient to come in and wait to see the physician. Always ask for the patient's cell phone number for just such events.

CRITICAL THINKING APPLICATION

Ramona offers to reschedule patient appointments if the schedule ever falls more than 15 minutes behind. If a patient becomes belligerent about the delays, how can Ramona handle the situation in a professional manner?

TELEPHONE SCHEDULING

It is just as important for a medical assistant to be pleasant and express a desire to be helpful on the telephone as it is when meeting face to face. This is especially true when making appointments, because the telephone contact may be the patient's first impression of the facility. Often the manner in which the booking is made makes more of an impact than the convenience of the appointment time.

Be especially considerate if the time requested for an appointment must be refused. Briefly explain why the time is not available and offer a substitute date and time. Comply with the patient's desires as much as possible, and do not show any annoyance if the patient does not understand the scheduling process. Most people, however, understand the need for a well-managed office and are willing to cooperate.

Many offices offer the patient a choice when scheduling the appointment and let the patient decide which option is best for him or her. For example, the following dialog might take place during the scheduling call:

MA: Mrs. Thomas, Dr. Stern is available to see you in the office next Tuesday or Wednesday, January 6 or 7. Which day is better for you?

Patient: I will be working on Wednesday, so I would like to come on Tuesday.

MA: Do you prefer a morning or afternoon appointment?

Patient: The afternoon is best for me.

MA: Great. Would 1:30 or 3:30 be a better time?

Patient: I can be there at 1:30.

MA: Then Dr. Stern will see you at 1:30 next Tuesday, January 6. Thank you for calling, Mrs. Thomas. We'll see you then!

These small courtesies will give patients the feeling that they are in control of their time. Always repeat the time to reinforce the appointment, and do not hesitate to ask the patient if he or she has a pen with which to jot down the time and date. While repeating the information to the patient, check the appointment book or computer screen to ensure that it was posted correctly.

Write legibly when using an appointment book. These records could be called to court, and the medical assistant must be able to read his or her own writing if asked to testify. Form the habit of entering the patient's daytime telephone number after every entry. It may become necessary to cancel or rearrange the schedule in a hurry, and many precious minutes can be saved if the telephone number is handy. Cell phone numbers are also quite useful for tracking down a patient quickly.

SCHEDULING APPOINTMENTS FOR NEW PATIENTS

Arranging the first appointment for a new patient requires time and attention to detail (Procedure 10-3). This first encounter provides the first impression of the office and may set the tone for all subsequent visits. Tact, courtesy, and professionalism are extremely important. During the conversation with the new patient, request preliminary information to assist in deciding

PROCEDURE 10-3

Schedule and Manage Appointments: Schedule New Patients

CAAHEP COMPETENCY: 3.a.(1)(a)
ABHES COMPETENCY: 3.c

GOAL: *To schedule a new patient for a first office visit.*

EQUIPMENT and SUPPLIES

- Appointment book
- Scheduling guidelines
- Appointment card
- Telephone

PROCEDURAL STEPS

1. Obtain the patient's full name, birth date, address, and telephone number.
   NOTE: Verify the spelling of the name.
2. Determine whether the patient was referred by another physician.
   PURPOSE: You may need to request additional information from the referring physician, and your physician will want to send a consultation report.
3. Determine the patient's chief complaint and when the first symptoms occurred.
   PURPOSE: To assist in determining the length of time needed for the appointment and the degree of urgency.

4. Search the appointment book for the first suitable appointment time and an alternate time.
5. Offer the patient a choice of these dates and times.
   PURPOSE: Patients are better satisfied if they are given a choice.
6. Enter the mutually agreeable time in the appointment book, followed by the patient's telephone number.
   NOTE: Indicate that the patient is new by adding the letters NP.
7. If new patients are expected to pay at the time of the visit, explain this financial arrangement when the appointment is made.
   PURPOSE: The patient will be aware of the payment policy and can come prepared to pay at the time of the visit.
8. Offer travel directions for reaching the office as well as parking instructions.
   PURPOSE: To relieve any anxiety about being able to find the medical facility.
9. Repeat the day, date, and time of the appointment before saying goodbye to the patient.
   PURPOSE: To verify the patient understands the date and time of the appointment.

how much time to allot for the visit on the appointment schedule. The physician may also expect the medical assistant to give general instructions to patients seeking care for specific complaints. For example, the patient may be required to bring a urine specimen or to make certain that laboratory tests are completed before the appointment. Some offices obtain enough information to build a patient chart before the office visit; others wait until the patient actually arrives to construct the chart.

After the necessary information has been recorded, offer the first available appointment to the patient. Whenever possible, offer the patient choices between two dates and times. Ask the patient if he or she knows the directions to the office, or offer the physical address for those who wish to obtain exact directions from one of the many Internet sites, such as Mapquest. Tell the patient whether there are any special parking conveniences and whether the office will provide a token or parking validation. The options that the patient will have for the first payment should also be discussed. If payment is expected immediately, inform the patient. The office staff should expect patient concerns about the amount of the first bill and should address this issue in advance of the appointment so that there are no surprises or misunderstandings. Before ending the conversation, repeat the appointment date and time, then thank the patient for calling.

Some medical offices mail an information packet about their facility to new patients, especially if the appointment is several days away. With today's technology and the patient's email address, such information can also be sent via the Internet. This information should tell the patient about the nature of the practice, should introduce the medical staff, and should explain appointment policies and financial arrangements.

If another physician has referred the patient, the medical assistant may need to call the referring physician's office to obtain additional information before the patient's appointment. This information should be printed out and given to the attending physician in advance of the patient's arrival. Remember to send a thank-you note to anyone who refers a patient to the facility.

Many offices call each patient the day before the appointment as a reminder and a courtesy. This can be a time-consuming procedure, but most patients appreciate this service, and it may open appointments for others if the original patient cannot keep the scheduled time slot. Email and automatic dialers can also be programmed to call or send electronic reminders to patients about their appointments. This procedure can run automatically if the office has access to the proper equipment, which takes no time away from the medical assistant's other duties.

SCHEDULING APPOINTMENTS FOR ESTABLISHED PATIENTS

In Person

Most return appointments for **established patients** are arranged when the patient is leaving the office. It is a good policy for all patients to stop by the front desk before leaving, in case any information is needed from the patient or any outside scheduling must be done. The patient's chart can be reviewed to see whether the physician ordered any laboratory tests or procedures, and these can be scheduled and discussed with the patient. When making a return appointment, follow the same procedures as scheduling any appointment by phone, offering the patient choices in the day and time slots (Procedure 10-4). If a certain time is not available that the patient specifically requests, offer two alternatives. Always give the patient an appointment card and any necessary instructions at this time, along with a bright smile (Procedure 10-5). Never forget to provide excellent customer service to the patient.

By Telephone

Usually it is necessary only to determine when the patient is required to return and to find a suitable time on the schedule. Established patients do not usually need directions and parking information, unless the office has recently moved. If there has been a lengthy interval since the patient's last visit, the medical assistant should recheck certain information and enter any changes on the patient's chart. Be sure to ask whether insurance companies or benefits have changed, and it is always a good idea to verify the address and phone numbers of the patient. If an email address is not on file, obtain one for quick and easy notification of appointments and other events.

PROCEDURE 10-4

Schedule and Manage Appointments: Schedule Appointments with Established Patients or Visitors

CAAHEP COMPETENCY: 3.a.(1)(a)
ABHES COMPETENCY: 3.c

GOAL: *To schedule a general appointment either by telephone or in person.*

EQUIPMENT and SUPPLIES

- Appointment book or computer
- Office procedure manual
- Clerical supplies
- Appointment cards
- Telephone

PROCEDURAL STEPS

1. Know the proper methods to use when scheduling an appointment by consulting the office procedure manual.
   PURPOSE: To follow prescribed office policy for appointment scheduling.
2. Ask the name of the person wishing to make the appointment and obtain his or her phone number.
   PURPOSE: To be able to speak professionally with the individual and to identify the person in the patient database, if applicable. Ask for the phone number in case the line is disconnected or the appointment needs to be changed.
   Say: "To whom am I speaking, please?"
3. Ask the reason for making the appointment.
   PURPOSE: To determine the length of time needed for the appointment.
   Say: "What is the reason for making this appointment?"
4. Determine who the appointment is for, if necessary.
   PURPOSE: To schedule the individual with the right provider or person.
   Say: "Mr. Adams, would you like to see Dr. Blake, or would you like to see our office manager, Mrs. Jackson?"
5. Give the person a choice between 2 days of the week.
   PURPOSE: To allow the individual to choose a convenient time;

this decreases missed appointments. If the suggested days are not satisfactory, allow the person to suggest an alternate day.
   Say: "Would you prefer to come on Monday or Tuesday, Mr. Adams?"
6. Give the person a choice between a morning or an afternoon appointment.
   PURPOSE: To allow the individual to choose a convenient time of day.
   Say: "Would morning or afternoon be better for you?"
7. Give the person a choice between two specific times.
   PURPOSE: To allow the individual to choose the best time for his or her needs.
   Say: "Mr. Adams, would you prefer 9 am or 11 am?"
8. Write the name of the individual and the phone number on the appropriate line of the appointment book, or enter this information into the scheduling system.
   PURPOSE: To document the appointment and assure that the time is reserved.
9. Repeat the appointment day, date, and time back to the person being scheduled.
   PURPOSE: Repeating the appointment time reduces errors and misunderstandings.
   Say: "I have you scheduled for 9 am on Tuesday, March 14, Mr. Adams. If you are not able to keep your appointment, please let us know."
10. If the person scheduling the appointment is in the office instead of on the phone, give an appointment card to him or her.
    PURPOSE: Providing appointment cards reduces missed appointments.

PROCEDURE 10-5

Schedule and Manage Appointments: Prepare an Appointment Card

CAAHEP COMPETENCY: 3.a.(1)(a)
ABHES COMPETENCY: 3.c

GOAL: *To provide a written notation of the appointment for the convenience of the patient (or other individual making the appointment) and to reduce missed appointments.*

EQUIPMENT and SUPPLIES

- Appointment book or computer
- Office procedure manual
- Appointment cards
- Clerical supplies
- Telephone

PROCEDURAL STEPS

1. Make an appointment following the steps listed in Procedure 10-2.
   PURPOSE: The information about the appointment is necessary to complete the appointment card.

2. Copy the appointment information onto the appointment card directly from the appointment book or the computer, including the day, date, and time.
   PURPOSE: To provide a written record of the scheduled appointment.

3. Mention that a 24-hour notice is appreciated when canceling an appointment.
   PURPOSE: To allow others to fill the empty slot that a missed appointment creates.

4. Give the individual the appointment card.

SCHEDULING OTHER TYPES OF APPOINTMENTS

There are other appointments that a medical assistant will make and that will appear on the appointment schedule, such as surgeries the physician will be performing at a hospital or other facility, hospital rounds and consultations, appointments and meetings, and even house calls if the physician performs them. The physician must also have time to get from one location to another, so driving time must be considered when arranging all appointments.

Inpatient Surgeries

When scheduling a surgery, call the facility where the procedure will be performed as soon as the operation is planned. Most surgical departments and centers have a surgical secretary who makes these arrangements. Provide all necessary information as well as any special requests that the physician may have, such as the amount of blood to have available for the patient. The secretary may want all of the patient's insurance information and will certainly want a phone number so that the patient can be contacted before the surgery if necessary. Be sure that all of this information is handy before placing the call.

Some hospitals request that the patient complete a pre-admission form so that all records can be processed before the patient is admitted. In such cases it may be the medical assistant's responsibility to see that this is done. These are general guidelines only, because procedures vary in different areas and hospitals.

Outpatient and Inpatient Procedure Appointments

A medical assistant is often requested to arrange laboratory or radiography appointments for patients. Before calling the facility to schedule the appointment, be sure all necessary information is handy. When the patient is informed of the time and place for the appointment, relay any special instructions that may be necessary, then note these arrangements in the patient's chart. Some offices will make a reminder call to the patient, or a reminder email message can be sent.

Outpatient testing is common, because most physicians do not have extensive x-ray or laboratory equipment in their offices. Magnetic resonance imaging (MRI), computed tomography (CT) scans, numerous x-ray evaluations, ultrasonography, and simple blood tests all may need to be scheduled (Procedure 10-6). Provide the patient with the name, address, and phone number of the facility where the tests will be performed.

Some patients may require a series of appointments, such as at weekly intervals. Try to set up these appointments on the same day of each week at the same time of day. This considerably reduces the risk that the patient will forget an appointment.

In some cases the medical assistant may be responsible for scheduling inpatient admissions or inpatient surgical procedures (Procedures 10-7 and 10-8). This is similar to scheduling outpatient testing, but the medical assistant must coordinate with the hospital instead of with an outside facility.

Outside Visits

If the physician regularly makes house calls or visits patients in skilled nursing facilities, a special block of time will need to be reserved in the appointment schedule. The physician will need demographic information, such as addresses, room numbers, and the best route to each home or facility. Remember to allow for travel time. Although most physicians never make house calls because of the ease of seeing patients in the office, they may be necessary in certain situations. The physician's medical bag should always be prepared and well stocked before he or she has to make any outside visits.

PROCEDURE 10-6

Schedule Outpatient Admissions and Procedures

CAAHEP COMPETENCY: 3.a.(1)(b)
ABHES COMETENCY: 3.c

GOAL: *To schedule a patient for outpatient admission or procedure within the time frame needed by the physician, confirm with the patient, and issue all required instructions.*

EQUIPMENT and SUPPLIES

- Diagnostic test order from physician
- Name, address, and telephone number of diagnostic facility
- Patient demographic information
- Patient chart
- Test preparation instructions
- Telephone
- Consent form

PROCEDURAL STEPS

1. Obtain an oral or written order from the physician for the exact procedure to be performed.
   PURPOSE: To have a documented order for the procedure to be performed

2. Precertify the procedure with the patient's insurance company, if necessary.
   PURPOSE: To make certain that expected insurance benefits are valid and the procedure will be covered by the patient's insurance policy.

3. Determine the physician and patient availability.
   PURPOSE: To be certain that the patient will be able to comply with the arrangements for the test and that the physician is available, if he or she must be present for the procedure. The urgency of the needed test results affects the time and date of the appointment needed.

4. Telephone the diagnostic facility and schedule the procedure or test.
   - Order the specific test needed.
   - Provide the patient's diagnosis.
   - Establish the date and time.
   - Give the name, age, address, and telephone number of the patient.
   - Provide the demographic information for the patient, including insurance policy numbers and addresses for filing claims.
   - Determine any special instructions for the patient or special anesthesia requirements.
   - Notify the facility of any urgency for test results..
   PURPOSE: To schedule the procedure or admission and provide needed information.

5. Notify the patient of the arrangements, including:
   - Giving the name, address, and telephone number of the diagnostic facility
   - Conveying the date and time to report for the test
   - Giving instructions concerning preparation for the test (e.g., eating restrictions, fluids, medications, enemas).
   - Telling what preadmission testing will be necessary, if any
   - Asking the patient to repeat the instructions.
   PURPOSE: To be certain that the patient understands the preparation necessary and the importance of keeping the appointment. If time permits, issue written instructions to the patient.

6. Have the physician review the consent form with the patient. The patient should sign the consent form, and a copy should be placed in the chart. Note arrangements on the patient's chart.
   PURPOSE: To make certain that the patient understands the risks, benefits, and alternatives to the procedure. To ensure follow-up on diagnosis and/or treatment.

7. Place reminder on the physician's tickler or desk calendar, if needed. Be sure the information is listed on the office schedule. Check the postsurgical status of the patient. Follow up if results are not received in a timely manner.
   PURPOSE: To check whether the appointment was kept and a report was received from the testing facility.

SPECIAL CIRCUMSTANCES

Late Patients

Probably every medical practice has a few patients who are habitually late for appointments. This seems to be a problem for which no cure has been found. Emergencies and small delays can happen to anyone, but a patient who constantly arrives late can place a strain on the practice. Such patients can be booked as the last appointment of the day. Then, if closing time arrives before the patient does, the staff has no obligation to wait.

Some medical assistants tell the patient to come in 30 minutes before the appointment time that is actually scheduled. Make an attempt to work with patients who have occasional difficulties arriving on time, but do not allow the schedule to be constantly disrupted by late patients.

CRITICAL THINKING APPLICATION

Seth Jones is always late for his appointments. How might Ramona approach him about this? What can Ramona do to assist Mr. Jones in arriving for appointments on time?

PROCEDURE 10-7

Schedule Inpatient Admissions

<u>CAAHEP COMPETENCY:</u> 3.a.(1)(b)
<u>ABHES COMPETENCY:</u> 3.c

GOAL: *To schedule a patient for inpatient admission within the time frame needed by the physician, confirm with the patient, and issue all required instructions.*

EQUIPMENT and SUPPLIES

- Admission orders from physician
- Name, address, and telephone number of inpatient facility
- Patient demographic information
- Patient chart
- Any preparation instructions for the patient
- Telephone
- Admission packet for the patient

PROCEDURAL STEPS

1. Obtain an oral or written order from the physician for the admission.
   <u>PURPOSE:</u> To have a documented order for the admission.

2. Precertify the admission with the patient's insurance company, if necessary.
   <u>PURPOSE:</u> To make certain that expected insurance benefits are valid and the admission will be covered by the patient's insurance policy.

3. Determine the physician and patient availability if the admission is not an emergency.
   <u>PURPOSE:</u> To be certain that the patient will be able to comply with the arrangements for the admission and that the physician is available to care for the patient during the admission. The urgency of the admission affects the time and date of the appointment needed.

4. Telephone the diagnostic facility and schedule the admission.
   - Order any specific tests needed.
   - Provide the patient's admitting diagnosis.
   - Establish the date and time.
   - Convey the patient's room preferences.
   - Give the name, age, address, and telephone number of the patient.
   - Provide the demographic information for the patient, including insurance policy numbers and addresses for filing claims.
   - Determine any special instructions for the patient.
   - Notify the facility of any urgency for test results.
   <u>PURPOSE:</u> To schedule the admission and provide needed information.

5. Notify the patient of the arrangements, including:
   - Giving name, address, and telephone number of the facility
   - Conveying date and time to report for admission
   - Giving instructions concerning preparation for any procedures, if necessary (e.g., eating restrictions, fluids, medications, enemas)
   - Outlining preadmission testing that will be necessary, if any
   - Asking the patient to repeat the instructions
   <u>PURPOSE:</u> To be certain that the patient understands the preparation necessary and the importance of admittance. If it is your office policy to do so, give an admission packet to the patient that contains the orders and basic instructions for the admission.

6. Note arrangements and the admission on the patient's chart.
   <u>PURPOSE:</u> To ensure follow-up on diagnosis and/or treatment.

7. Place reminder on the physician's tickler or desk calendar, if needed. Be sure the information is listed on the office schedule. If the physician keeps a list of all inpatients, add the patient's name to that list.
   <u>PURPOSE:</u> To keep a record of the number of days the patient was seen in the hospital by the physician during rounds for insurance billing purposes.

Rescheduling Canceled Appointments

Changes sometimes must be made in the appointment schedule. Unexpected conflicts might arise that force a patient to change the appointment time. When rescheduling an appointment, be sure that the first appointment day and time is removed from the appointment book or database, then set the new appointment. Otherwise, the patient will be expected in the office on 2 days, and time will be wasted with calls and follow-up, only to find out that the appointment was rescheduled.

Emergency Calls

Periodically, emergency or urgent calls will come to the office and an appointment will need to be scheduled. To some extent, all calls that come to the office go through a **triage** process, and emergencies are prioritized to evaluate the urgency of the need to see the physician. Triage is an extremely important function that requires experience and knowledge of signs and symptoms, as well as tact.

Emergencies may include emotional crises as well as the more obvious physical problems. Patients with emergencies should be seen the same day. The urgency of the call can be initially determined by having a list of questions prepared for reference with the help of the physician. The physician should determine what is considered urgent. The patient may need to be referred directly to the emergency department of a hospital, or the physician may want to see the patient that day in the office. In many cases, the caller will consider the situation more urgent than his or her responses to the medical questions may indicate. Skillful handling of such situations requires

PROCEDURE 10-8

Schedule Inpatient Procedures

CAAHEP COMPETENCY: 3.a.(1)(b)
ABHES COMPETENCY: 3.c

GOAL: *To schedule a patient for inpatient surgery within the time frame needed by the physician, confirm with the patient, and issue all required instructions.*

EQUIPMENT and SUPPLIES

- Orders from physician
- Name, address, and telephone number of inpatient facility
- Patient demographic information
- Patient chart
- Any preparation instructions for the patient
- Telephone
- Consent form

PROCEDURAL STEPS

1. Obtain an oral or written order from the physician for the admission.
   PURPOSE: To have a documented order for the admission.
2. Precertify the admission with the patient's insurance company, if necessary.
   PURPOSE: To make certain that expected insurance benefits are valid and the admission will be covered by the patient's insurance policy.
3. Determine the physician availability if the surgery is not an emergency. Another physician may be the surgeon. If this is the case, the surgery will need to be coordinated with his or her office as well.
   PURPOSE: To be certain that the physician is available to care for the patient during the admission and the surgery. The urgency of the surgery affects the time and date of the appointment needed.
4. Telephone the hospital surgical department and schedule the procedure.
   - Order any specific tests needed.
   - Provide the patient's admitting diagnosis.
   - Establish the date and time.
   - Give the name, age, address, and telephone number of the patient.
   - Provide the demographic information for the patient, including insurance policy numbers and addresses for filing claims.
   - Determine any special instructions for the patient.
   - Notify the facility of any urgency for the surgery.
   PURPOSE: To schedule the surgery and provide needed information to the facility.
5. Notify the patient of the arrangements, if the patient is not already admitted to the hospital. Include:
   - Name, address, and telephone number of the facility.
   - Date and time to report for admission.
   - Instructions concerning preparation for any procedures, if necessary (e.g., eating restrictions, fluids, medications, enemas).
   - Tell what preadmission testing will be necessary, if any.
   - Ask the patient to repeat the instructions.
   PURPOSE: To be certain that the patient understands the preparation necessary and the importance of surgery. If it is your office policy to do so, give an admission packet to the patient that contains the orders and basic instructions for the surgery.
6. The physician should review the consent form with the patient. Have the patient sign a consent for the surgical procedure. Keep the original consent in the patient's chart and give a copy to the patient.
   PURPOSE: To ensure that the patient understands the risks, benefits, and alternatives to the surgical procedure.
7. Note arrangements on the patient's chart.
   PURPOSE: To ensure follow-up on diagnosis and/or treatment.
8. Place reminder on the physician's tickler or desk calendar, if needed. Be sure the information is listed on the office schedule. If the physician keeps a list of all inpatients, add the patient's name to that list. Follow up with the hospital after the procedure regarding the patient's condition as required by the physician.
   PURPOSE: To check on the patient's status and keep a record of the number of days the patient was seen in the hospital by the physician during rounds for insurance billing purposes.

---

considerable tact. Maintaining a caring and reassuring response will frequently alleviate the fear evidenced by the caller.

Acutely Ill Patients

There is sometimes a fine line between an emergency patient and an acutely ill patient, but the latter should be seen as soon as possible. At the very least, let the physician decide whether an appointment should be made for another day. For example, a patient may report having had flu symptoms for several days and now having an elevated temperature. The physician will probably want more information before deciding whether the patient should be seen immediately or whether some other course of action is appropriate. The 15- to 20-minute breather time saved in the middle of the morning may rescue the schedule and provide the needed time for the patient. Escort these patients to the examination room on their arrival if possible. Patients with symptoms of infection should be placed so as to prevent cross-contamination.

Physician Referrals

If another physician telephones and requests that a patient be seen today, most offices will honor that request if at all possible. It is important to keep a schedule that will not be intolerant of this type of request.

Patients Without Appointments

There must be a policy agreed to by the physician and carried out by medical assistants for patients without appointments. A patient who requires immediate attention will most likely be accommodated into the schedule somehow. If the patient does not need immediate care, a brief visit with the physician and a scheduled appointment at a later time may be the answer. The medical assistant may simply have to turn down the request. Follow established office policy.

The medical assistant should always make it clear, even when accommodating patients without appointments, that the office runs on an appointment basis. Try to convey the message that appointments save not only the physician's time but also the patient's time. Emphasize that the physician is able to give the patient full attention and more time if an advance appointment is made.

FAILED APPOINTMENTS

Why do patients fail to keep appointments? Some are simply forgetful. Once this tendency is detected in a patient, form the habit of telephoning or emailing a reminder the day before the appointment, or send a postcard timed to arrive 1 or 2 days in advance.

A patient who has been pressed for a payment may stay away because of his or her inability to pay for medical services. Do not make the mistake of classifying all such patients as "deadbeats." Many have every desire to pay, but they cannot afford to and feel embarrassed about their situation, so they avoid their appointments.

If the office consistently runs behind schedule, some patients may not be willing to waste any time waiting to see the physician. Time is a valuable commodity for patients as well, and every effort must be made to get patients in at their appointment time and out quickly.

One other reason for failed appointments that is often overlooked is a patient's state of denial regarding his or her condition. For instance, if a patient has been recently diagnosed as human immunodeficiency virus (HIV) positive, he or she may avoid doctor appointments, because going to see the physician forces the patient to face the reality of the disease. Take special care with such patients, and if denial is suspected, discuss this with the physician, who may wish to refer the patient for counseling.

It is important to determine the reason for failed appointments and do whatever is possible to remedy the situation. Telephone the patient to be sure no misunderstanding has occurred. If the patient's health is such that medical care must continue, write a letter and explain this to the patient. Send the letter by certified mail, with return receipt requested. Keep the letter in the patient's chart for legal protection.

No-Show Policy

Some patients may not realize the importance of keeping their appointments. The patient who does not arrive for a scheduled appointment or reschedule it is called a **no-show.** A busy practice must have a very specific policy on appointment no-shows and must enforce it effectively. The first time a patient fails to show, note the fact on the medical chart and/or ledger card. The second time, warn the patient, and if a third no-show occurs, consider dropping the patient by using the customary methods that provide legal protection for the physician.

The physician may wish to charge patients for not showing up or for rescheduling the appointment. Be understanding whenever possible, but do not let a patient take advantage of the physician's time. The office policy manual must state that patients may be charged for missed appointments, especially if the time slot could not be filled with another patient. Many physicians do not press this issue, but it is an available tool if needed.

Recording the Failed Appointment

When a patient fails to keep an appointment, a notation should be made in the patient's chart as well as in the appointment book or database. If the patient is seriously ill, the physician should also be told about the failure to show. In some cases it may be necessary to call or write the patient to remind that a missed appointment may have serious effects on the patient's health.

INCREASING APPOINTMENT SHOW RATES

Everyone benefits from a full schedule of appointments that are kept. Appointment show rates may be increased in several ways.

Appointment Cards

Most healthcare facilities use appointment cards to remind patients of scheduled appointments, as well as to eliminate misunderstandings about dates and times (Figure 10-4). Make a habit of reaching for an appointment card while writing an entry in the appointment book. After the date and time have been written on the card, double-check with the book to see that the entries agree.

Confirmation Calls

Patients who have made appointments in advance may appreciate a confirmation call to remind them that they have a time set aside to see the physician. Always note the phone number that the patient prefers the office to use for such calls. Many individuals now have home phone, cell phone, and work phone numbers; however, they may wish calls from the physician to go only to their home phone. The preferred phone number can be highlighted in the chart or on the computer. The office must use caution in making calls to patients because of the significance of privacy guidelines and standards. Some offices may wish to prepare a release form in which the patient grants the office staff permission to contact the patient. Many physicians insist

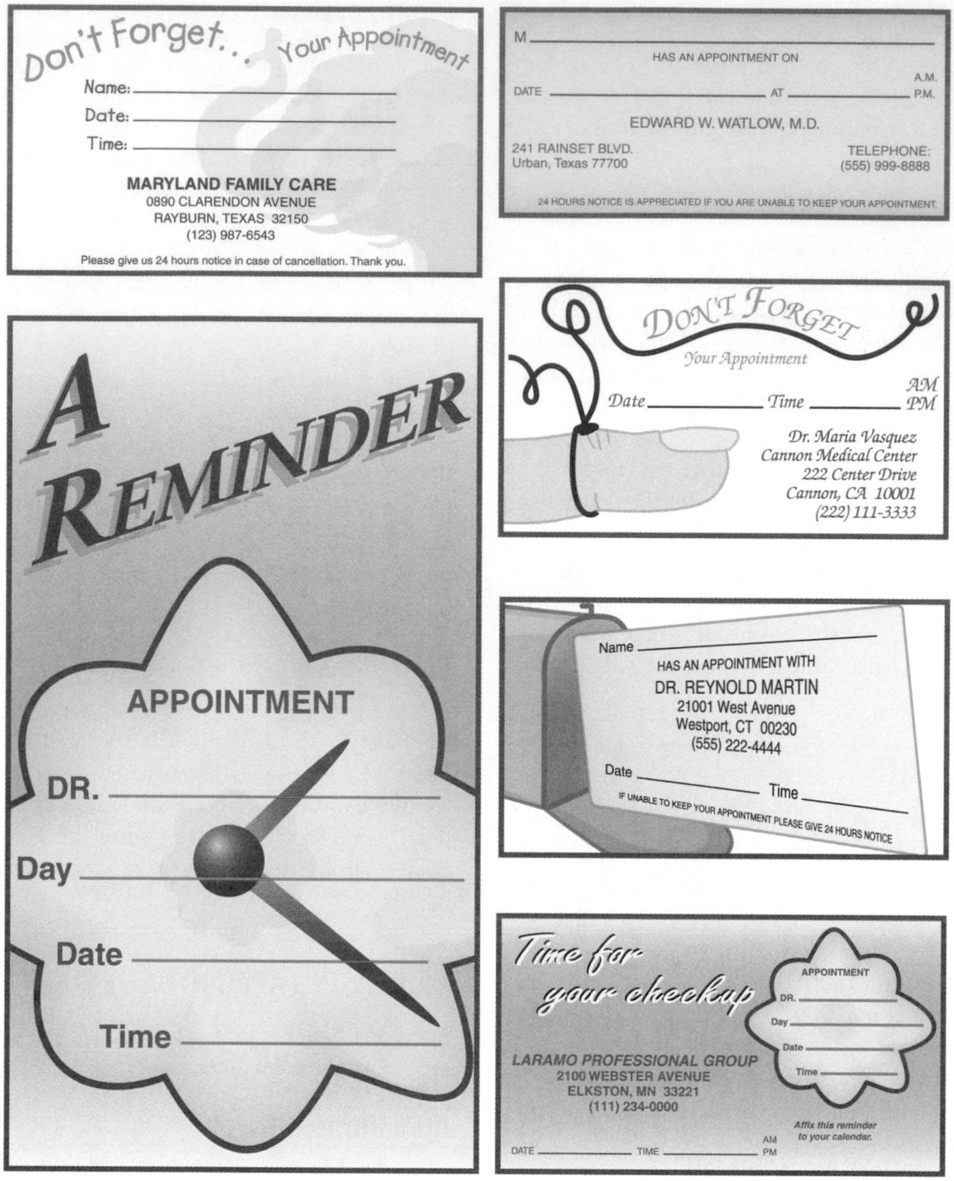

FIGURE 10-4 Examples of appointment cards.

that messages left on voicemail not mention the term "doctor" or "doctor's office" for confidentiality reasons. The medical assistant might say, "This is Pam at Robert Welch's office confirming your appointment tomorrow at 2:00 PM. Please call us if you cannot make the appointment. Our number is 555-212-0909. Thank you!"

If the patient has signed the privacy policy, and the policy states that messages may be left at certain numbers from the physician's office, then the office can certainly leave messages at that number and mention that the call is from the physician's office. Still, it is a good idea to have an established policy regarding leaving messages that does not breach any patient's confidentiality.

Email Reminders

Many computer scheduling programs have the capacity to send an email to patients to remind them of appointments the day before. This is a great timesaver for the office staff, because no time is taken to perform this duty, other than the original scheduling of the appointment.

Mailed Reminders

Mailed reminder cards may be sent to patients by the office staff. This method is a bit time consuming, but worth the effort if the patients show up for their appointments.

A patient who is due for an appointment but has not yet arranged a date and time may be sent a reminder. A simple way of handing this is to have a supply of postcards on hand, and while patients are still in the office, have them write their name and address on the postcard. Then place the card in a tickler file box under the date it is to be mailed.

Innovative Ideas

Knowing that time is valuable to patients as well as to the physician, many of today's offices try to make the time spent at the office as productive as possible for the patient. Some reception areas are equipped with computers, televisions, and even video games and movies for children. Often a small desk with a phone will allow the patient to do a limited amount of work, if needed, while waiting to see the physician. Keeping the patient's needs in mind makes the patient less likely to break an appointment.

HANDLING CANCELLATIONS AND DELAYS

When the Patient Cancels

Inevitably, some cancellations will occur. If a list is kept of patients with advance appointments who would like to come in sooner, the medical assistant can begin calling to try to get one of them in to fill the available opening. By keeping a list of patients willing to take the first cancelled appointment, the medical assistant can readily identify which patients to call to fill the vacancy. Each patient cancellation should be noted in the medical record, along with a note regarding why the appointment was cancelled, if that information is available. If the patient simply reschedules an appointment, it is not necessary to make a notation in the medical record, unless a pattern develops that might be significant to his or her medical treatment.

When the Physician Is Delayed

There will be days when the physician is delayed in reaching the office. If there is advance notice of the delay, start calling patients with early appointments and suggest that they come later. If some patients have already arrived before the office learns of the delay, explain that an emergency has detained the physician.

Show concern for the patient but avoid being overly apologetic, which might imply some degree of guilt. Most patients realize that a physician has certain priorities. The patient who is in the office may be inconvenienced, but it is not a life-or-death matter. If this kind of situation occurs frequently, however, consider devising a different scheduling system.

When the Physician Is Called for Emergencies

Physicians are conscious of their responsibilities for responding to medical emergencies, and most patients will be sympathetic to such occurrences if the medical assistant takes the time to explain what has happened. The medical assistant may say:

"Dr. Wright has been called away to answer an emergency. She asked me to tell you she is very sorry to keep you waiting. There will be at least a 1-hour delay."

Ask the patient:

"Do you wish to wait? If it is inconvenient, I'll be glad to give you the first available appointment on another day. Or perhaps you'd like to have some coffee or do some shopping and return in an hour."

As quickly as possible, call the patients who are scheduled for a later hour. In many offices, especially those of obstetricians, surgeons, and general practitioners, it sometimes is necessary to cancel a whole day's appointments. For this reason, it is particularly important to have the daytime telephone number of each patient available so that the appointment can be rescheduled.

If it is at all possible, cancel appointments before the patient arrives in the office to find that the physician is not available. The **expediency** of the office staff in contacting the patients who will be affected by an emergency will be most appreciated.

When the Physician is Ill or Out of Town

Physicians get ill, too, and the patients who are scheduled to be seen during the course of the physician's expected recovery period must be informed of this. They need not be told the nature of the illness. When the physician is called out of town for personal or professional reasons, the appointments will have to be canceled or rescheduled. It is customary to give the patient the name of another physician, or possibly a choice of several, who will be providing care during such absences. For security reasons, it is best to merely state that the doctor is unavailable. Stating over the telephone that the physician is out of town could lead to attempted burglary or other unauthorized intrusion of the premises.

OTHER TYPES OF APPOINTMENTS

There will be a wide range of other unscheduled callers with whom the physician will need to meet. Handle all of these individuals with care and courtesy.

Physicians

Another physician dropping into the facility should be ushered in to see the physician as soon as possible, regardless of the appointment schedule. If the physician is seeing a patient, explain the situation and, if possible, take the visiting physician into a private room to wait. Then notify the physician as soon as possible. Visits from other physicians are usually brief and do not appreciably affect the schedule.

Pharmaceutical Representatives

Also known as *detail persons* or *reps,* representatives from pharmaceutical companies are frequent visitors to physicians' offices and are generally welcomed when the schedule permits. They are well trained and bring valuable information on new drugs to the physician. The medical assistant is often expected to screen such visitors and turn away those whose products would not be used in that practice. If the representative or the pharmaceutical company is unknown to the office, ask for a business card, then check with the physician, who will decide whether to see the caller.

Specialists usually limit their conferences with pharmaceutical representatives to their line of practice. The medical assistant, together with the physician, can prepare a list of the representatives with whom the physician is willing to spend time, then let the list be the determining factor in future conferences. The medical assistant can say whether the physician will be available that day and give an estimate of the waiting time or suggest a later time at which the caller may return. The caller can then make a decision regarding whether to wait or return later. The pharmaceutical representative is usually quite understanding and cooperative and is willing to wait patiently a long while for just a brief visit with the physician. The medical assistant should in turn treat the representative with courtesy, showing as much cooperation as possible.

In some cases the representative will just leave literature or materials for the physician with the medical assistant. The detail person who is not on the calling list for a particular physician will also appreciate the time saved by knowing this in advance. Most representatives say they would rather be told outright if the physician does not wish to see them than to be given some evasive reply.

Salespersons

Salespersons from medical, surgical, and office supply houses call regularly at physicians' offices. Sometimes they will want to see the physician, but the office manager or the medical assistant who is in charge of ordering supplies usually is able to handle these calls.

Unsolicited salespersons can sometimes present a problem in the professional office. If the physician does not wish to see such callers, the medical assistant must firmly but tactfully send them away. Suggest that they leave their literature and cards for the physician to study and say that the physician will contact them if further information is desired.

Miscellaneous Callers

From time to time other callers appear in the medical office. Some are civic leaders seeking the physician's aid in community projects. Others may be church leaders, insurance representatives, solicitors for fund drives, and so forth. A general policy regarding seeing such callers should be established so that each incident does not require a separate discussion and decision.

Civic leaders should be treated with courtesy and consideration when they telephone or come into the office. Most physicians feel a responsibility to take an active part in community affairs, but no one can participate in all activities. The responsibility for accepting or refusing such community appointments is sometimes delegated to the office manager or medical assistant. In this event, one should use discretion and exercise great tact and courtesy. Turning away community leaders with a blunt refusal does not create good medical public relations.

When it is necessary to refuse requests for community projects, the medical assistant can explain that the physician is already participating in such community projects as, for example, the Boy Scouts, Girl Scouts, Kiwanis, and the Health Council and cannot accept additional responsibilities at this time. The practice of tact, courtesy, and consideration applies to every caller in the healthcare facility.

PLANNING FOR THE NEXT DAY

Before leaving at the end of the day, look over the appointments scheduled for the next day. Review the charts for scheduled patients. If laboratory tests or other procedures were scheduled on the patient's last visit, determine that the reports are available in the chart. If the patient is scheduled for specific procedures on this visit, make certain that everything that will be needed for the procedure is on hand and available. Planning can save many precious moments at the time of the patient visit.

CLOSING COMMENTS

The person charged with the responsibility for scheduling appointments will have a huge impact on the efficiency of the medical office. A friendly and helpful attitude is a **prerequisite** for cordial **interaction** with patients and the ability to make compromises that will benefit both the physician and the patient. The office that runs smoothly and stays on schedule indicates professionalism and competence and will be greatly appreciated by all who come into contact with the medical office.

Providing patients with an information booklet about the office will familiarize them with the policies and procedures of the office. Many physicians compile an extensive booklet that even provides tips as to when the physician should be called immediately, listing symptoms and signs of emergencies.

Educating the patient regarding office policies will help the facility to run smoothly from day to day. All patients should be familiar with the policies about appointments. This leads to fewer misunderstandings and conflicts over bills that might include a charge for a missed appointment.

If the facility offers Internet-based appointment scheduling, patients will have to be taught how to use the system. A printed pamphlet or information sheet will be helpful in providing instruction to the patient. It would be wise to have a special phone number that patients can call if they have problems with the scheduling system. For best results choose a program that is simple to use and easy to understand and one that does not breach patient confidentiality.

The appointment schedule may be used as a legal record and could be brought by subpoena into a court of law. Be sure that all handwriting in the book is completely legible and that information is routinely collected in a consistent manner for each entry. Do not fail to note a no-show in the patient's chart as well as the appointment schedule. This is often helpful when a physician must prove that the patient did not follow medical advice or that the patient contributed to his or her poor condition by missing appointments. Old appointment schedules should be kept for a time equal to the statute of limitations in the state in which the practice exists.

SUMMARY OF SCENARIO

Ramona is an asset to the medical office because her dedication and customer service skills help her to interact with patients in a positive way. She genuinely cares about the patients and makes every effort to meet their needs while following the preferences of her physician. She has found that her bright smile is a valuable tool to use when patients have been waiting and are growing restless.

Ramona cooperates with other staff members to get the patients seen as quickly as possible and to minimize wait time. She is flexible and can change the order of the patients seen, if needed, to maximize the use of time and facilities in the office. Because she is so cheerful and friendly, patients do not seem to mind when she asks for their cooperation. She keeps current phone numbers and cell phone information so that she can notify a patient quickly if Dr. Brown is running behind schedule. Ramona's proficiency on the computer also is an asset, and she makes frequent use of email to take care of patient problems or rescheduling desires.

Because of the cooperation she receives from staff and patients alike, Ramona successfully runs an efficient office. She contributes to that efficiency by constantly refining her knowledge about her job. She pays attention to the times during the day that don't run as smoothly as others, evaluates the problems at those times, and then corrects them. Ramona also keeps the schedule moving by communicating with the clinical medical assistants and keeping them informed about arriving patients, and those who have come early or are running late. She is able to quickly adjust and substitute a patient who has already arrived. Ramona has learned how to manipulate the schedule to accommodate an emergency. She knows that by making minor adjustments and keeping the waiting patients informed, the staff can handle any emergency. All medical assistants need to develop skills in flexibility. Through the establishment of a system that works and through correct use of it, patients and staff will be more content with their experience in the physician's office.

SUMMARY of LEARNING OBJECTIVES

1. Define, spell, and pronounce the terms listed in the vocabulary.
   - Spelling and pronouncing medical terms correctly adds credibility to the medical assistant. Knowing the definition of these terms promotes confidence in communication with patients and co-workers.
2. Discuss three items that must be considered when scheduling appointments.
   - When scheduling appointments, a medical assistant must consider the patients' needs, the physician's preferences, and the available facilities. Make every attempt to schedule a patient at his or her most convenient time. This will help to avoid no-shows. The physician will outline preferences, which should be of high priority to the medical assistant. However, most physicians are flexible and will make adjustments according to the needs of the office. The availability of facilities within the office is perhaps the most inflexible factor. If a certain room or piece of equipment is being used for one patient, it usually cannot be used for another.
3. Explain the features that should be considered when choosing an appointment book.
   - When choosing an appointment book, all of the needs of the office should be considered. If there are multiple physicians, the book should be arranged so that each physician is readily identified. Books that open flat on the surface of the desk are much easier to handle, but if not enough space is available to open the book entirely, another style might be better. The book should also provide enough space to write all of the patient information needed in the various time slots, such as the name, phone number, and reason for the visit.

4. Discuss the advantages of computerized appointment scheduling.
   - Computerized scheduling programs are in demand today because they are easy to operate, simplifying scheduling appointments and making changes to the schedule. The computer can find the first available time much more quickly than a person scanning through an appointment book. Most programs can prepare reports and even notify patients automatically by email of the impending appointment. Web-based self-scheduling programs are becoming popular: these allow a patient to see the physician's available appointments and book his or her own date and time.
5. Explain how self-scheduling would reduce calls to the medical office.
   - Self-scheduling would vastly reduce calls to the office, because a high number of everyday calls are requests to schedule appointments. Patients could make an appointment at midnight, if they desired.
6. List and explain at least three methods of appointment scheduling.
   - Open office hours allow patients to come to the physician's office when it is convenient and wait in turn to see the physician. Scheduling specific appointments is the most popular method for seeing patients. Flexible office hours allow patients to see the physician during the evening and often on weekends. Many of today's medical offices have some flexible scheduling, because most families now consist of two working parents. Wave scheduling brings two or three patients to the office at the same time, and they are seen in the order of their arrival. This type of scheduling can be modified in many ways to suit the needs of the facility. Other scheduling methods include double booking and grouping of like procedures.

Continued

SUMMARY of LEARNING OBJECTIVES
Continued

7. Explain the basic procedure to follow when the office is behind schedule.
   - When the office is running 15 minutes behind schedule, the medical assistant should briefly explain the delay to the waiting patients, then offer to reschedule their appointments. Keep the patients informed of wait times until the schedule resumes.

8. Discuss offering choices to patients when scheduling appointments.
   - Giving a patient a choice in appointment times to better meet his or her needs is a part of good customer service. Offering the patient a choice of 2 days, morning or afternoon, and two times helps to ensure that the patient will keep the appointment.

9. Explain the importance of legible writing in the appointment book.
   - Because the appointment schedule might be called into a court of law, it is vital that the handwriting in the book be completely legible. Even if the book is 5 years old, the person charged with testifying in court should be able to clearly read all entries. Scribbled, messy handwriting implies incompetence and reflects on the practice.

10. Discuss several methods of dealing with patients who consistently arrive late.
    - Patients who are habitually late for appointments might be told to arrive 15 minutes before the time written in the book. Some offices book these patients as the last appointment of the day, so that if they do not arrive promptly, they do not see the physician. Usually talking with the patient and gaining an understanding of why the patient arrives late will improve the situation. The office can work with the patient to choose the best times that will result in a show appointment.

11. Name several reasons for failed appointments.
    - Some patients forget the appointment with the physician, and some are habitually careless about remembering their scheduled time. Small emergencies often come up, and in today's busy business world, some patients just cannot get away from their own offices or other obligations to visit the physician. In some cases patients do not keep appointments because they do not want to deal with a health issue confronting them.

CONNECTIONS

 Study Guide Connection: Go to Chapter 10 Study Guide. Read the Case Study and Workplace Applications and complete the assignments. Do online research for answers to the questions in the Internet Activities associated with scheduling appointments.

 CD Connection: Go to the Medical Assisting Competency Challenge CD and do the training activities under General Office Duties.

 Evolve Connection: For more information related to scheduling appointments, go to http://evolve.elsevier.com/kinn/admin and visit related weblinks for Chapter 10. Click on the Medical Assisting Exam Review and do the practice questions to sharpen your test-taking skills. To learn more about office software, do the exercises for the Altapoint demo that is on the CD.

Patient Reception and Processing 11

SCENARIO

Most people enter the healthcare field for very specific reasons. Georgina Robertson recalls being in a serious car accident when she was 6 years old. As a result, her vision was temporarily impaired. She remembers seeing a woman in a white uniform who offered words of comfort. The woman seemed to have a haze around her that, when combined with the hospital lights, made her look as if she had wings. The vision of an angel never left Georgina's thoughts and led her into the medical field.

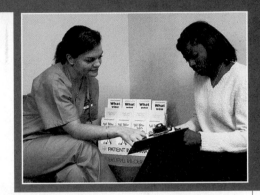

Today Georgina works for Dr. Stuart Wade, a cardiologist in a metropolitan city. Georgina is an experienced medical assistant, and she enjoys getting to know her patients. She makes notes on the chart that remind her of special events in the lives of the patients who visit Dr. Wade's office. The patients feel that she truly cares about them, aside from her duties at the clinic. Although she is efficient and time conscious, she always has a moment to share a warm smile or hear about a new grandchild. Georgina is a valued member of the medical team in her office. She is currently attending a state college in the evening hours, gaining credits toward her bachelor's degree. She plans to continue her education and apply to medical school in the future.

While studying this chapter, think about the following questions:

- What are some ways to develop good rapport with patients?
- Why is the sign-in register a potential breach of patient confidentiality?

- What is the value in knowing some information about patients' personal lives?

LEARNING OBJECTIVES

1. Define, spell, and pronounce the terms listed in the vocabulary.
2. Explain the purpose of the office mission statement.
3. List several patient amenities and why these are important additions to the medical office.
4. Describe how to prepare for patient arrivals.
5. Explain why it is important to use the patient's name as often as possible.
6. Discuss how the medical assistant may help the patient prepare for an examination.
7. List and explain two methods of chart placement.
8. Discuss how the medical assistant might deal with talkative patients.
9. Discuss ways to make the patient feel at ease and comfortable in the medical office.

National Accreditation Competencies and Content

CAAHEP COMPETENCIES

Administrative
3.a(1)(c). Organize a patient's medical record

General
3.c(1)(b). Recognize and respond to verbal communication
3.c(2)(a). Identify and respond to issues of confidentiality
3.c(2)(c). Establish and maintain the medical record
3.c(2)(d). Document appropriately
3.c(3)(a). Explain general office policies
3.c(3)(b). Instruct individuals according to their needs

ABHES COMPETENCIES

Communication
2.l. Recognition and response to verbal and nonverbal communication

Administrative
3.a. Perform basic secretarial skills
3.b. Prepare and maintain medical records

Legal Concepts
5.a. Determine needs for documentation and reporting
5.b. Document accurately
5.c. Use appropriate guidelines when releasing records or information

Instruction
7.a. Orient patients to office policies and procedures
7.b. Instruct patients with special needs

VOCABULARY

amenity (uh-me'-nuh-te) Something conducive to comfort, convenience, or enjoyment.

demographic (de-muh-gra'-fik) The statistical characteristics of human populations (as in age or income) used especially to identify markets.

depleted Lessened markedly in quantity, content, power, or value.

fervent Exhibiting or marked by great intensity of feeling.

flagged Marked in some way as to remind or remember that specific action needs to be taken.

harmonious Marked by accord in sentiment or action; having the parts agreeably related.

immigrant A person who comes to a country to take up permanent residence.

intercom A two-way communication system with a microphone and loudspeaker at each station for localized use.

perception A quick, acute, and intuitive cognition; a capacity for comprehension.

phonetic (fuh-ne'-tik) Constituting an alteration of ordinary spelling that better represents the spoken language, that employs only characters of the regular alphabet, and that is used in a context of conventional spelling.

progress notes Notes used in the patient chart to track the progress and condition of the patient.

sequentially (si-kwen'-shuh-le) Of, relating to, or arranged in a sequence.

The patient reception area should be an inviting place in which patients feel comfortable. Visits to the physician can be times of great stress, so the office staff must do everything possible to make the experience pleasant for patients. A patient usually has a choice of healthcare providers and should be given excellent customer service. Good patient relations will result in referrals to the physician, and this helps the practice grow. When patients have a good experience with a physician, they are likely to tell others. When the office staff is committed to making the patient feel welcome and the focus is on care of the patient, the success of the practice is inevitable.

THE OFFICE MISSION STATEMENT

Healthcare providers often have a **fervent** reason for entering the medical field. One physician remembers the heritage his **immigrant** grandfather left in his heart. The physician has fond memories of his grandfather's pride and thankfulness for the opportunities he found in America, after coming to the United States with nothing but the clothes on his back. The grandfather's dream was to see his grandson become a physician, and that is exactly what he did. Even on the most trying days, he can step into his office and see a picture of his grandfather. His memories helped him to find the strength and determination to care for his patients.

The office mission statement reflects this deep-seated desire by expressing the reasons for the existence of the practice (Figure 11-1). The physician develops the mission statement alone or may consult the office staff for input. Many offices display the mission statement prominently in the reception area and on printed material, such as patient information booklets. Whatever the contents, each employee of the facility should be

---

WADE CARDIAC CLINIC MISSION STATEMENT

The mission of the Wade Cardiac Clinic is fourfold:

- The staff of the clinic promotes the highest standards of ethical medical practice.
- The physician and staff members commit to serving their patients with respect and courtesy.
- All staff members shall promote a healthy lifestyle and preventative measures for the patients that present to the clinic.
- The clinic will support medical patient education, scientific research and development, community service, and community health promotion.

It is our desire to give the best customer service to our patients and care for them as if they were members of our own families.

FIGURE 11-1 The mission statement should be presented to all employees early in their tenure, and the staff should strive to meet the mission every day.

familiar with the statement and have a personal commitment to promoting the mission statement in everyday practice.

THE RECEPTION AREA

A first impression is lasting. Nowhere is this more important than in the healthcare facility, where the environment must appear orderly and faultlessly clean. The facility may be a physician's office, a hospital, a health maintenance organization, an insurance company, or one of the many other healthcare establishments. No matter what type of facility is involved, the appearance of the reception room and the front desk as well as a cordial greeting by the receptionist influence a patient's **perception** of the entire facility and the care that he or she will receive.

The reception room is just that—a place to receive patients and visitors. The area should be planned for the patients' comfort, made as attractive and cheerful as possible, and kept clean and uncluttered. Often a medical assistant has the opportunity to assist in the design and decoration of this very important area. Consider traffic flow; the movement of patients from place to place within the reception room—as well as in the rest of the office—should be unhindered and logical (Figure 11-2).

that is adequate to accommodate the peak load of patients seen each day, and arrange it in conversational groups. Individual chairs are best (Figure 11-4); people usually prefer to stand rather than sit next to a stranger on a sofa. Provide good lighting, ventilation, and regulated temperature, and the essentials are in place for an attractive, comfortable reception area. Reduce room clutter by providing a place to hang coats, rainwear, and umbrellas. Professional designers can be consulted regarding reception room décor and improvements or to solve a problem area that inhibits office traffic.

Most physicians' offices are well supplied with recent magazines, and some have various books. Publications with short items of popular interest are favorites, like *Reader's Digest*. Any reading material placed in the reception room should be of interest to the general public; *Good Housekeeping*, *U.S. News and World Report*, *Real Simple*, *Oprah*, and *People* are examples of interesting magazines that most people would enjoy reading. The reception room, incidentally, is not the place for the physician's professional journals.

A writing desk with writing paper in the reception area for the convenience of patients is a nice touch, as is restful music from a concealed speaker. A lighted aquarium or an educational display of some sort enhances the attractiveness and individuality of the reception area in the professional practice. Patients are often interested in health-related brochures. The physician may also have a videotape or healthcare book library that allows patients to check out items of interest to them. A telephone in the reception area is an asset and can be programmed by the phone company not to allow long-distance calls.

A television VCR or DVD player will help the time pass much faster, especially in pediatric offices. Children enjoy Disney movies and cartoon programs, and these hold their interest until it is time to see the physician. Young patients would be thrilled to find a video game system in the waiting area, although this may make them more uncooperative when called back to see the physician—they may want to continue playing the game! A children's corner equipped with small-scale furniture and some playthings works well (Figure 11-5). Youngsters who might otherwise get into mischief are kept pleasantly occupied. Toys should be easily cleanable; plastic washable items are especially good. Take extra care to ensure that no toy has sharp corners that could cause injury or small parts that could be swallowed. In selecting toys, make certain that they will not stimulate the child toward noisy activity. And no rubber balls, unless there is time to chase them around the room!

CRITICAL THINKING APPLICATION

Georgina feels that her patients enjoy a homelike atmosphere, which is less intimidating than the sterile, clinical feel of some medical offices. How might she accomplish giving her office a homelike feeling?

CRITICAL THINKING APPLICATION

Georgina has a few patients who bring young children to their appointments. Sometimes the children are a bit disruptive and make other patients feel uncomfortable. How might Georgina handle this problem in the medical office? Some children misbehave in public, and the parents do not respond or correct them. How might Georgina deal with this situation if it happens in her office?

Fresh, **harmonious** colors and cleanliness are the foundation of an attractive room (Figure 11-3). Select comfortable furniture

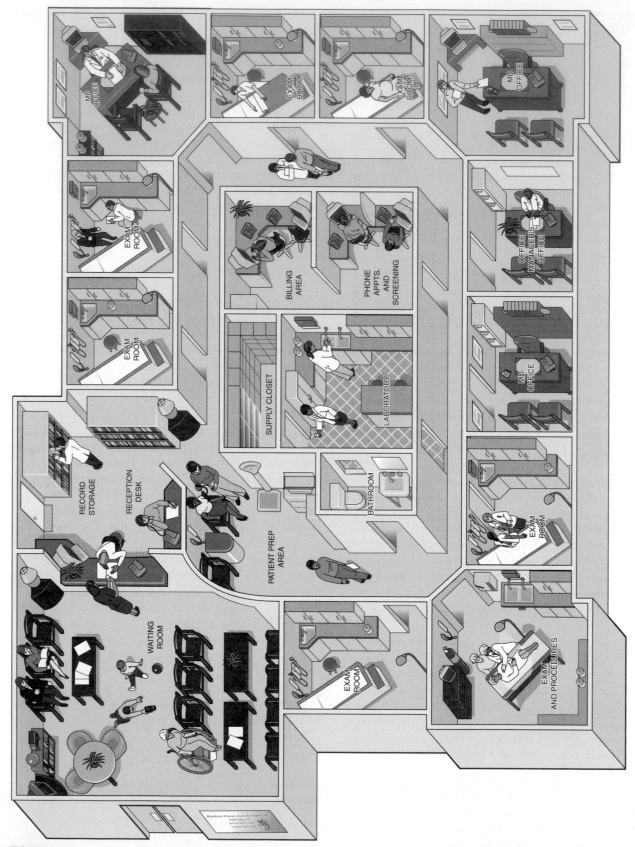

FIGURE 11-2 The medical office should be arranged so that the flow of traffic is conducive to the movement of patients throughout the office.

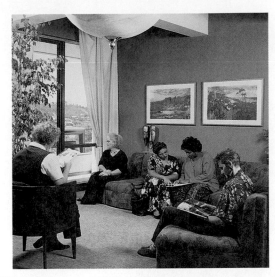

FIGURE 11-3 Patients appreciate cleanliness, restful colors, good ventilation, and light to read by when waiting in the reception area.

Many of today's modern offices offer a computer for patient use while waiting to see the physician. This is a wonderful **amenity** because the patient can make good use of his or her time while in the reception area. Some patients may bring their personal laptop computers and use their time in the waiting room to complete projects. An amazing amount of work can be done just by checking office email, so providing Internet access to patients is also helpful, whether it is wired or wireless. If patients are allowed to connect to the office wireless network, it is wise to provide one specific log-on name and password just for them, to maintain control over access to private health information.

Periodically, take an objective look around the reception room. Could it use a little brightening or freshening up? Try to look at the room as if seeing it for the first time. The receptionist is partly responsible for the appearance of the area by making

certain that the room remains neat and orderly throughout the day. Check the temperature and lighting for comfort. Scan the room at various intervals during the day to ensure that the room is in good order.

If the medical assistant's desk is in the reception area or in open view of the patients, it should be free of clutter. In particular, patients' medical and financial records should not be in sight. Keep computer monitors out of view to protect patient confidentiality. Some offices use privacy screens that allow only the user to see the monitor. Personal articles, coffee cups, and other personal items should not be on the receptionist's desk.

PREPARING FOR PATIENT ARRIVAL

Advance preparation helps to make the day go smoothly and contributes toward a more relaxed atmosphere for all concerned. Some offices prepare for the next day on the evening before, whereas others prepare each morning. The office should be consistent and should always perform the same routine so that important preparations are not left undone. More information about opening the office, closing the office, and its daily operation can be found in Chapter 12.

CRITICAL THINKING APPLICATION

There will always be housekeeping chores associated with preparing for each day in the physician's office. What are some ways that Georgina can divide these tasks fairly among the staff members? How should Georgina handle the employee who feels that general housekeeping duties are not a part of the job description?

Preparing Medical Records

Pull the medical records for the day (or the next day if this is done in the evenings), and check off the patient's name on a copy of the appointment schedule to be sure that all of the records have been located and are ready (Figure 11-6).

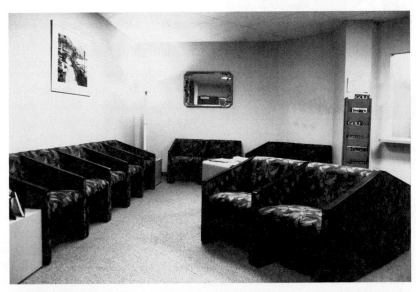

FIGURE 11-4 Patients tend to prefer individual seating. Comfortable seating helps patients relax and be at ease while waiting to see the physician. (Courtesy August Incorporated, Centerville, Ohio.)

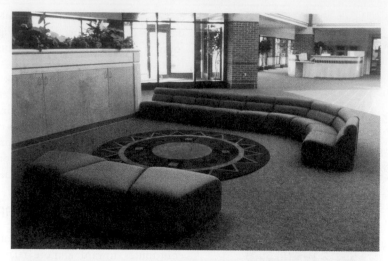

FIGURE 11-5 Furniture in a pediatrician's office should be durable and fun, child sized, and able to withstand the most active children. (Courtesy August Incorporated, Centerville, Ohio.)

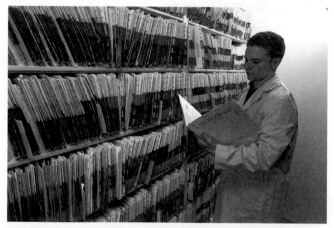

FIGURE 11-6 Charts should be pulled in advance for the patients arriving for appointments. Each chart should be checked to see whether it has adequate forms and is in good order for the physician's use.

Occasionally more than one patient may have the same or a similar name. Check the patient's social security number, date of birth, or other pertinent information to ascertain that the right medical record has been pulled. Review each record to verify that any recently received information, such as laboratory reports and radiograph readings, has been correctly entered into and permanently attached to the record (Procedure 11-1).

Arrange the medical records **sequentially** in the order in which the patients are scheduled to be seen. The medical assistant may be expected to place the records of all the patients to be seen that day on the physician's desk, but it is more likely that the physician will prefer to review each record just before entering the examination room. Be sure that there is enough space on the **progress notes** for the physician to write in the record. If not, place additional progress notes in the record.

Replenishing Supplies

Replenish supplies at the reception desk regularly. Stationery, appointment cards, charge slips, sharpened pencils, pens, telephone message pads, and any items likely to be needed should be on hand when the day begins. Discovering that supplies are **depleted** during a busy day can seriously interrupt the flow of patient care. One person should be in charge of checking the inventory of supplies on a regular basis and ordering as necessary. Inventories and supply ordering will be discussed in Chapter 12.

In a multiple-employee practice, a clinical assistant usually has the responsibility of checking clinical supplies and preparing the patient rooms; however, in a small practice there may be only one assistant available for all duties. Before patients begin to arrive, everything should be ready for the day so that the physician and medical assistant can give undivided attention to the patients' needs.

PROCEDURE 11-1

Establish and Maintain the Medical Record: Organize a Patient's Medical Record

CAAHEP COMPETENCY: 3.c(2)(c)
ABHES COMPETENCY: 3.b

GOAL: *To prepare patient charts for the daily appointment schedule and have them ready for the physician before the patients' arrival.*

EQUIPMENT and SUPPLIES

- Appointment schedule for current date
- Patient files
- Clerical supplies (e.g., pen, tape, stapler)

PROCEDURAL STEPS

1. Review the appointment schedule.
2. Identify full name of each scheduled patient.
3. Pull patients' charts for files, checking each patient's name on your list as each is pulled.
   PURPOSE: To determine that the correct charts have been pulled and that no charts have been omitted.
4. Review each chart.
   PURPOSE: To reaffirm that:

- The correct patient chart has been pulled
- Any previously ordered tests have been performed
- The results of the tests have been mounted or entered in the chart
- Forms have been replenished inside the chart, such as progress notes, and so forth

5. Annotate the appointment list with any special concerns.
   PURPOSE: To alert the physician regarding matters that should be checked or discussed with the patient.
6. Arrange the charts sequentially according to each patient's appointment.
7. Place the charts in the appropriate examination room or other specified location.

GREETING THE PATIENT

Every patient has the right to expect courteous treatment in a physician's office. No matter what the patient's economic or social status may be, each individual who enters the reception room should receive a cordial, friendly greeting (Figure 11-7). Using a personal touch, such as greeting the patient by name, is an easy way to develop patient rapport. Use the patient's last name and title unless the patient insists on using his or her first name.

"How are you today, Mr. Roberts?"

"Ms. Nelson, the doctor will be in to see you shortly."

If the office creates a policy of obtaining a copy of all patients' photo identification cards, such as the driver's license,

it can be used to identify patients and greet them by name, even if they do not visit the office often.

Patient Check-In

The reception desk should be in clear view of all visitors who come into the office. If only one medical assistant is present, it is sometimes impossible for each new visitor to be welcomed personally. Develop an announcement system that alerts staff when people enter the office. The patient who enters an empty reception room does not know whether to sit down, knock on the glass partition, or try to announce his or her presence in some other way. One solution would be a bell that the patient can ring on arrival. A sign placed in the reception room that reads, "Please sit comfortably. The receptionist will be with you shortly," will assure patients that their presence will be acknowledged.

The receptionist should check the reception room each time he or she has been away from the desk to see if additional patients have arrived. Greet these patients by name; if the staff member is unaware who has entered the reception area, ask the person his or her name. Use a sign-in register that promotes patient privacy. Patient confidentiality is violated when others can read the names on the register. The best registers allow the staff to remove the patient's name and information after he or she signs the document. Pressure-sensitive labels, printed with lines for the patient name, appointment time, and changes in insurance coverage, are a practical, inexpensive solution for confidential patient registers. The signed label can then be placed in a separate log book or even inside the patient's medical record. The office can order custom registers that work like a pegboard, making the identifying information invisible to

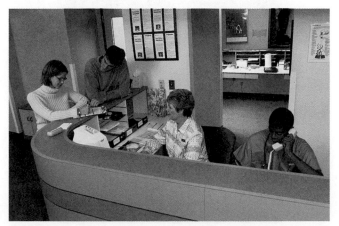

FIGURE 11-7 Greet all patients with a warm smile, and assist them with forms they need to complete for the chart.

subsequent patients. Patients should not be expected to provide details of the reason for their visit in a public area.

Knowing the Patients

Cultivate the habit of greeting each patient immediately in a friendly, self-assured manner. Establish eye contact and smile while introducing yourself to the patient. For example, "Good morning, I'm Elizabeth Parr, Dr. Wade's medical assistant." Remember to ask about the patient before asking about insurance coverage; no patient wants to feel that the physician's main interest in him or her is the collection of an insurance check.

Patients like to be acknowledged when they arrive. All staff members should review the day's schedule in the morning to be prepared to greet patients by name and to know whether the patient is new or established (Figure 11-8). Learn how to pronounce each patient's name correctly; incorrect pronunciations may offend or irritate some people. If the name is unusual, write the **phonetic** spelling on the record for reference. By using the patient's name often, the medical assistant ensures that he or she is treating the correct patient.

Make brief notes in the medical record about the current events in the patient's life. With this information, the medical assistant and the physician can read those notes before entering the examination room and share a short dialog with patients at the beginning of their visits. An example follows:

Georgina: Hello, Mrs. Williams, how are you today?

Mrs. Williams: I am doing very well, Georgina, how are you?

Georgina: I'm fine. How was the cruise you took with your husband last month?

Mrs. Williams: It was wonderful! The water was the bluest I have seen!

Georgina: You went to Cozumel, didn't you?

Mrs. Williams: Yes, we did! I'm surprised you remember, as many patients as you see each day!

This brief chat will confirm that the staff members care about the individual patients because they take an interest in their personal lives (Figure 11-9). Because the patient does not see the medical assistant or physician look at the notes before entering the patient room, the patient assumes that the information is being recalled from memory. This is an impressive customer service technique. Most patients appreciate the interest of the physician and the staff in their families, hobbies, and work.

Some state regulations prohibit information other than health details being placed in the medical record; however, most health professionals agree that the mental and emotional health of a patient is connected to his or her physical health. Details about what is happening in patients' lives provide clues to physical problems they are experiencing. As a simple example, a patient going through a divorce may experience depression that needs to be treated with medication. Without knowledge of the divorce, the physician would not have all of the information needed to make a sound medical decision. Physicians can treat patients more effectively when such information is available in the medical record.

REGISTRATION PROCEDURES

On a patient's first visit to the physician's office, the staff performs certain registration procedures (Procedure 11-2). Most physicians use a patient information form to gather **demographic** information about the patient. The form may

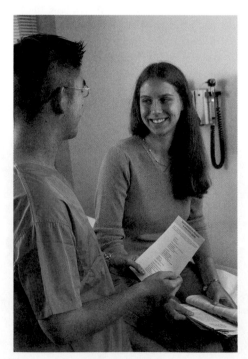

FIGURE 11-9 Patients appreciate being called by name and remembered from visit to visit.

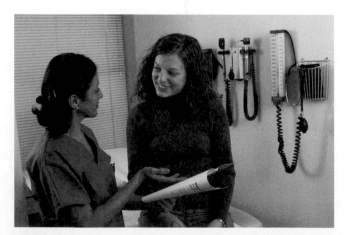

FIGURE 11-8 The medical assistant should develop a good relationship with the patient and be a caring advocate.

PROCEDURE 11-2

Establish and Maintain the Medical Record: Register a New Patient

<u>CAAHEP COMPETENCY:</u> 3.c.(2)(c)
<u>ABHES COMPETENCY:</u> 3.b

GOAL: *To complete a registration form for a new patient with information for credit and insurance claims, and to inform and orient the patient to the facility.*

EQUIPMENT and SUPPLIES

- Registration form
- Clerical supplies (pen, clipboard)
- Private conference area

PROCEDURAL STEPS

1. Determine whether the patient is new to the practice.
2. Obtain and record the necessary information:
   - Full name, birth date, name of spouse (if married)
   - Home address, telephone number (include ZIP and area codes)
   - Occupation, name of employer, business address, telephone number
   - Social Security number and driver's license number, if any
   - Name of referring physician, if any
   - Name and address of person responsible for payment
   - Method of payment
   - Health insurance information (photocopy both sides of insurance ID card)
   - Name of primary carrier

- Type of coverage
- Group policy number
- Subscriber number
- Assignment of benefits, if required
<u>PURPOSE:</u> This information is necessary for credit and insurance claims.

3. Review the entire form and confirm patient eligibility for insurance coverage.
   <u>PURPOSE:</u> To verify that the given information is complete and legible.
4. Determine that required referrals have been received, if applicable.
   <u>PURPOSE:</u> Insurance coverage may not be valid without referral.
5. Explain medical and financial procedures to patients.
   <u>PURPOSE:</u> The patient develops a comfort level and knows what to expect.
6. Collect co-payments or balance payment charges.
   <u>PURPOSE:</u> Keeps accounts current and prevents the necessity of mailing statements.

be attached to a clipboard and handed to the patient with instructions to complete sections. The medical assistant must be ready and willing to answer any questions (Figure 11-10). The patient's name should appear prominently at the top of the form, followed by other pertinent facts in logical order. Most information sheets contain the following:

- Patient's full name and date of birth
- Responsible person's name and relationship to the patient

FIGURE 11-10 The medical assistant should take the time to explain forms that the patient does not understand and always be willing to answer questions.

- Address and telephone number
- Name, address, and telephone number of spouse
- Occupation
- Place of employment
- Social Security number
- Driver's license number
- Nearest relative not living with patient, and his or her relationship
- Source of referral, if any

When the completed form is returned, check carefully to verify that all the necessary information has been provided.

CRITICAL THINKING APPLICATION

Often some time is needed to complete patient forms when a new patient arrives in the office. How might Georgina keep the office on schedule when new patients arrive, necessitating chart construction and form completion? What are some ways to trim time from these activities?

Obtaining a Patient History

The personal and medical history and the patient's family history may be obtained by asking the patient to complete a questionnaire; the physician can augment this information during the patient interview. Some experienced medical assistants conduct the interview to obtain the patient's personal and medical history, family history, and chief complaint. This is a specialized procedure, and the medical assistant should be specifically trained to perform it for the individual practice.

CONSIDERATION FOR PATIENTS' TIME

The patient expects to see the physician or practitioner at the appointed time. The medical assistant should get the patient into the examination room for treatment or consultation as near the appointment time as possible or explain delays. All patients want to be kept informed about how long they should expect to wait to see the physician. They will usually respond positively when the physician or the assistant comes to the reception area to apologize for any delay. Always consider the patient's time and make every effort to streamline the office visit.

In a solo or small practice there should seldom be more than three to five patients in the reception room. Patients complain that the wait time in medical facilities is one of the most frustrating aspects of the medical profession. The patient who complains about medical fees or the care received may have first become agitated during a long wait to see the physician. Many patients are fearful and tense; long wait times intensify these feelings. The medical assistant can often put patients in a better frame of mind with just a friendly smile and a show of concern.

A crowded reception room is not always an indication of a physician's popularity. It may simply mean that the physician or the assistant is inefficient in scheduling patients. Business people, for example, who are in the habit of making the most of their time, are particularly displeased at what may appear to them to be inefficient scheduling of appointments. Any delay of longer than 10 to 15 minutes should be explained to the person waiting. Some personal attention, such as offering a drink of water, a cup of coffee, or a new magazine, may help to calm a patient who appears irritated with the delay. However, be sure that the patient is allowed caffeine before offering coffee. Be careful that the refreshment offered does not go against the physician's orders or would interfere with scheduled blood testing or other procedures.

Patients with Special Needs

Some patients will be physically challenged, some very ill, and some severely uncomfortable. There may be language or cultural barriers. Observe the patient's appearance and behavior. Is the patient pale? Do the eyes or voice reflect pain or discomfort? Find out how the patient is feeling before suggesting that he or she be seated to wait for the physician. The patient may need to lie down in a cool room or perhaps be seen as an emergency case.

Patients with disabilities, such as those in a wheelchair or using a cane, walker, or crutches, may need extra attention. Some patients may need help in disrobing even when a disability is not obvious. Ask if the patient needs assistance.

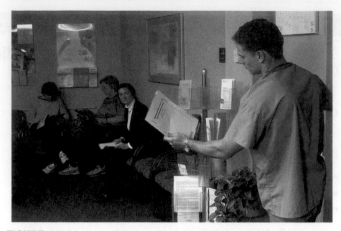

FIGURE 11-11 Pronounce the patient's name correctly, and use it often. This promotes good customer service and pleases the patient.

ESCORTING AND INSTRUCTING THE PATIENT

Patients prefer to be escorted while inside the physician's office rather than simply told where to go. This is usually the responsibility of the clinical medical assistant, but the task could be assigned to administrative staff, including the receptionist. Pronounce the patient's name correctly when he or she is called to the clinical area (Figure 11-11). If unsure of the pronunciation, ask the patient. Write the name phonetically on the medical record for quick retrieval at the next appointment.

Remember that to an employee of the practice the office surroundings may become as familiar as home. A stranger to the practice's environment may be confused or disoriented by all the hallways, doors, and rooms. Uncertainty creates anxiety. Take the time to personally escort the patient to the appropriate examination or treatment room; do not point to the room and expect the patient to find the way. If a urine specimen is needed, direct the patient to the restroom and always explain what to do with the specimen.

On arrival in the examination room, tell the patient if he or she needs to disrobe. Explain what garments, if any, can be left on, whether shoes are to be removed, whether jewelry needs to be removed, and any other necessary instructions. If a gown is to be worn, specify whether the opening should be in the front or back and tell the patient where he or she can hang up clothes if this is not obvious. An examination table should never be placed in such a position that the patient is exposed to passersby in the hallway if the door is opened. Imagine a patient ready for a Pap smear, facing the door as the physician enters! Allow patients a sense of modesty at all times, and make all instructions completely clear. Be equally clear when the examination has been completed. Do not assume that patients will know what is expected of them. Tell the patient whether he or she should go to the physician's office for consultation, or return to the reception area to wait, or whether he or she is free to check out with the front office and leave.

The medical assistant helps keep the schedule operating smoothly by immediately tidying each examination room and escorting the next patient in so that the physician has no idle moments waiting for a patient to be prepared. Try not to place a patient in an examination room just to clear out the reception area. It is especially inconsiderate to keep the patient waiting after being gowned, draped, and positioned on the examining table. Medical offices are often chilly or even cold, which will make a draped patient quite uncomfortable. A magazine rack on the wall of the treatment room is a welcome addition in some practices.

Remember that in today's litigious society, physicians prefer a second person in the room during examinations to avoid claims of sexual assault or harassment. The office may be equipped with a buzzer that alerts the medical assistant to enter the examination room after the physician has initially consulted with the patient. Be prompt in answering the buzzer, and provide assistance during the examination. Patients may be uncomfortable and uneasy, so it is appropriate to offer words of encouragement, a smile, and a pat on the shoulder.

MEDICAL RECORD PLACEMENT

Medical records should never be left in the examination room to be picked up and read by a patient. This can cause misunderstandings because patients rarely know medical terms and abbreviations. A number of different methods are used to signal that a patient is ready to be seen. Often there are file holders on the doors of the examination rooms, where the medical record can be placed horizontally when the patient is ready to be seen. Then the physician can signal the medical assistant that he or she is finished examining the patient by placing the chart in an upright position on leaving the examination room. Some offices have call systems, by which a physician can press a button to call the medical assistant for help with the examination. Others have a visual item outside the door that signals what that particular patient needs next.

Other offices place patients in examination rooms in a certain order, and the physician knows, for instance, that when he or she has finished with the patient in room one, the next patient will be waiting in room two. The office should develop a method that allows the most efficient use of time while providing high-quality care to the patients.

PROBLEM SITUATIONS

Talkative Patients

Problem patients exist in any professional office. Talkative patients, for example, take up far more of the physician's time than is justified. An alert medical assistant can usually spot this tendency during the initial interview. The patient's history can be **flagged** with a symbol to alert the physician. The medical assistant can buzz the physician's **intercom** and remind him that the next patient is ready. Once the medical assistant has learned which patients take extra time, they can be booked for the end of the day or more time can be allowed for them.

CRITICAL THINKING APPLICATION

Georgina has one patient who insists on sitting close to her desk and attempting to chat the entire time she is waiting to see the physician. What is worse, she comes to her appointments at least an hour early. How might Georgina subtly deal with this patient?

Children

Children frequently present special management problems, whether they are patients or they accompany a patient. Sometimes younger patients are escorted into the treatment room without the parent. Of course, this should be at the discretion of the physician and must be with the permission of the parent. The physician cannot force the parent to leave the examination room by any means. Although this practice of separating children from their parents to treat their needs is not always feasible, it sometimes can be applied with great success. In some offices a token of the physician's friendship, such as a trinket or toy, is given to the child at the completion of the visit.

Angry Patients in the Reception Area

Every medical assistant will eventually be confronted by an angry patient. The anger may simply be a reflection of the patient's pain or fear of what the physician may discover during the examination. If possible, invite the patient into another room out of the reception area. Usually it is best to let the patient talk out his or her anger. Pacify the patient using a calm attitude, and speak using a low tone of voice. Under no circumstances should the assistant return the anger or become argumentative.

Patient's Relatives and Friends

Patients are sometimes accompanied by a relative or well-meaning friend who may become restless while waiting for the patient and attempt to discuss the patient's illness. The medical assistant should sidestep any discussion of a patient's medical care, except by direction of the physician. Avoid a too-casual attitude, such as, "I'm sure there's nothing to worry about." A show of moderate concern and reassurance that "the patient is in good hands" usually takes care of the situation. Remember that health information cannot be released to anyone, including concerned friends and relatives, without patient consent.

PATIENT CHECKOUT

When the patient returns to the front office for checkout, greet him or her with a friendly smile and call the patient by name. Form the habit of asking patients if they have any questions. Check the medical record to determine when the physician wishes the patient to return to the office. Most physicians will note this information on the encounter form. Make the return appointment, remembering the technique of giving the patient choices as to which day they wish to come, morning or afternoon, and specific time. Then ask the patient for payment, using phrases such as, "Your co-pay today is $15, Mrs. Williams.

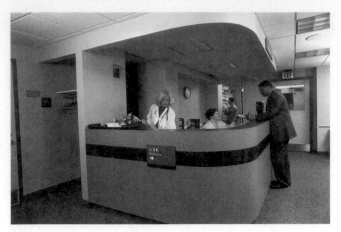

FIGURE 11-12 Always thank the patient for coming and wish him or her well.

Will you be writing a check or would you like to charge this visit to your Visa?"

Be sure to thank the patient for coming, and wish him or her well as they leave the office (Figure 11-12).

THE FRIENDLY FAREWELL

As soon as the visit with the physician has been completed, the medical assistant should be ready to assist the patient in dressing, if necessary, and make certain that any questions the patient may have are answered. Answer questions if they can be addressed ethically and legally; otherwise, direct the patient to the physician. Some questions can be answered only by the physician; in such cases the assistant can offer to get answers for the patient or bring the physician back to the examination room to answer the questions. Remember, patients view the medical assistant as an extension of the physician and the medical assistant must be very careful to avoid accusations of practicing medicine without a license.

The assistant can help convey a sense of caring by terminating the patient's visit cordially. If the patient is returning for another visit, the assistant can say something like, "We'll see you next week." If it is the patient's last visit, a pleasant "I certainly hope you'll be feeling fine from now on" is appropriate. The assistant may wish to tell a patient on a last visit that it has been a pleasure to make his or her acquaintance. Whatever words of goodbye are chosen, all patients should leave the facility with the feeling that they have received top-quality care and were treated with friendliness, respect, and courtesy.

CLOSING COMMENTS

A medical assistant must never offer medical advice to a patient unless specifically instructed to do so by the physician. The patient sees the medical assistant as an extension of the physician and tends to weigh advice and comments by the medical assistant with the same validity as if they came from the physician. Provide only information that the physician has approved or is included in the office policy and procedure manuals.

When a patient complains, listen carefully and attempt to resolve the problem or assure the patient that the issue will be discussed with the appropriate staff member to find a solution. If someone other than the patient asks for information about the patient, refrain from discussion unless the patient or physician has authorized the release of information.

A personal touch is vital to projecting a sense of care to the patients seen in the physician's office. Many medical offices are not concerned enough about the customer service aspect of the business. Patients talk about their experiences with their friends and relatives and may be an excellent source of referrals if they are treated with dignity and courtesy. If they have had a good experience, they will tell several people. If they have a poor experience, they tend to tell everyone they know! Be sure to have a part in each patient feeling a sense of satisfaction as they leave the office. All patients should feel that their time and money were well spent.

Georgina is a person who truly makes a difference in the healthcare profession. She takes her role as a patient advocate seriously and strives to make her patients feel comfortable in her physician's office. She keeps the mission statement posted close to her desk and rereads it often to keep her focus clear. She shares the vision with the other staff members, who are supportive and in agreement with the purpose for which the office exists.

Dr. Wade promotes continuing medical education and encourages his staff members to participate in courses and seminars that will assist them in being more effective patient advocates. The office sends birthday and Christmas cards to the

patients in the database, and at the annual holiday party the staff hand-signs each Christmas card. Georgina sends a monthly newsletter to the patients, some by mail and some by email, to keep the patients up to date on office policies and interesting health information. All of these activities indicate a strong caring attitude toward the patients. Georgina considers each one a customer of the clinic, and she is determined that they receive excellent customer service.

Wait times are at a minimum in Dr. Wade's office. Cell phone numbers and email addresses are gathered at registration and updated frequently so that the staff can quickly contact patients. Georgina offers new patients a form for evaluation of

SUMMARY OF SCENARIO—cont'd

the office so that they can provide input about the experience they had as a new patient. All of these efforts promote a trusting, caring relationship among physician, staff, and patients.

By treating patients as one would wish to be treated, the medical assistant will develop a strong rapport. Patients enjoy hearing their own names and being recognized by medical staff members. Georgina remembers to greet each patient on his or her arrival to the clinic and always asks the names of patients she does not know. She knows that having a bit of personal

knowledge about the patients will be of benefit to Dr. Wade, so the entire staff is cordial and friendly to all patients.

Georgina knows that she must keep the sign-in register confidential and uses a form that is HIPAA compliant. This prevents patients from obtaining private health information during check-in procedures. By protecting patient confidentiality, the office not only remains in compliance with federal regulations but also puts the patients' interests first, assuring that they can enter the office with confidence and trust.

SUMMARY of LEARNING OBJECTIVES

1. Define, spell, and pronounce the terms listed in the vocabulary.
   - Spelling and pronouncing medical terms correctly adds credibility to the medical assistant. Knowing the definition of these terms promotes confidence in communication with patients and co-workers.

2. Explain the purpose of the office mission statement.
   - The office mission statement is the philosophy of why the office exists. Often physicians themselves develop the mission statement, which outlines their vision and reasons for entering medical practice. Some physicians allow the office staff to assist in its development. All employees should become familiar with the mission statement and promote its ideas to all patients and visitors.

3. List several patient amenities and why these are important additions to the medical office.
   - Patient amenities include such things as a VCR, television, computer, telephone, and a desk where patients can sit and balance a checkbook or review work while away from the office. These features turn the time spent in the physician's office into productive minutes instead of wasteful ones.

4. Describe how to prepare for patient arrivals.
   - Some offices prepare for patient arrivals the evening before, and some in the morning. Patient charts must be pulled and should be reviewed, checking for completed laboratory tests and posting of results, and to ensure that progress notes for this visit are ample. Rooms should be checked and inventoried to make certain that sufficient supplies are on hand and that they present a clean, neat appearance.

5. Explain why it is important to use the patient's name as often as possible.
   - People like hearing their own names; a better relationship is built between the staff and patients when the names are used often. Patients feel that the office staff cares enough about them to acknowledge them, and this custom adds a personal touch.

6. Discuss how the medical assistant may help the patient prepare for an examination.
   - The medical assistant should escort the patient to the examination rooms and other areas of the office. Always tell the patient when to disrobe and exactly what should be removed. Offer to assist with disrobing if the patient needs extra help. Take care that the patient's purse or wallet is in a secure place. Be sure that doors do not open and expose the disrobed patient. Instruct the patient as to whether he or she may leave or should wait after seeing the physician. Ask whether the patient has any questions.

7. List and explain two methods of chart placement.
   - Some medical offices place patient charts in a door file, which alerts the physician that the patient is ready to be seen. The chart may be placed horizontally or vertically, one placement meaning that the patient is ready for the physician, and the other meaning that the doctor is finished with the patient. Other offices place the charts in door files in a certain order. For example, if examination rooms one, two, and three are available, patients are seen in that order by the physician.

8. Discuss how the medical assistant might deal with talkative patients.
   - Patients who are talkative may be lonely and enjoy the social interaction of their visits to the physician's office. Be as courteous as possible with talkative patients, expressing to them when necessary that another patient is waiting or that the physician needs assistance. When this is said with a smile, most patients understand.

9. Discuss ways to make the patient feel at ease and comfortable in the medical office.
   - The personal touch will help the patient to feel at home and comfortable in the office. An attractive reception area with various patient amenities will provide a warm atmosphere. Using the patient's name often and a gentle touch will impart a sense of caring as well.

CONNECTIONS

 Study Guide Connection: Go to Chapter 11 Study Guide. Read the Case Study and Workplace Applications and complete the assignments. Do online research for answers to the questions in the Internet Activities associated with patient reception and processing.

 CD Connection: Go to the Medical Assisting Competency Challenge CD and do the training activities under General Office Duties.

Evolve Connection: For more information related to patient reception and processing, go to http://evolve.elsevier.com/kinn/admin and visit related weblinks for Chapter 11. Click on the Medical Assisting Exam Review and do the practice questions to sharpen your test-taking skills. To learn more about office software, do the exercises for the Altapoint demo that is on the CD.

Office Environment and Daily Operations

12

SCENARIO

Kayla Kemper performed her externship at Dr. Richard Tarago's office, a general practice clinic located downtown that serves patients who do not have medical insurance. Some patients must pay a copayment of $5 to $25, and others pay no copayment, depending on their income level. Kayla's family is quite wealthy, and it was an eye-opening experience for her to see patients who live a very different life than she does. There were many days that she wanted to leave the clinic because she realized that many of the patients were unable to seek medical care when the illness first began, and when they finally came to the clinic they were in worse condition. Kayla is a caring person, and she saw the suffering that many of the patients experienced on a daily basis. She found it hard to see people who had difficulty obtaining healthcare, yet she realized that a large number of Americans have no insurance coverage at all. Kayla discussed her feelings with the clinic manager, Elaine Mays, and expressed her concern for the patients in the clinic. Elaine asked if Kayla would like to continue working with the patients, and Kayla admitted that she would, although it was not easy for her. Elaine then suggested that because Kayla's background was so different from the patients, she might

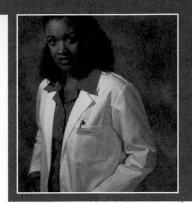

wish to stay at the clinic as a volunteer for a few months to add to her learning experience. She accepted the offer, and after Kayla worked for 3 months as a volunteer, Elaine hired Kayla to work in the clinical area full-time. The patients consistently commented on Kayla's compassion and considerate treatment while they were at the clinic. Kayla truly learned the meaning of giving as it relates to the medical profession, and her externship was the start of her full-time career.

While studying this chapter, think about the following questions:

- What are some of the issues that might prevent a medical assistant from showing compassion to all patients? How can these issues be resolved?
- Why is it a good practice to allow the person who uses a certain supply to order it?
- Why might outsourcing be less expensive than doing testing or procedures in the office?
- How might an extensive list of community resources be helpful to patients?

LEARNING OBJECTIVES

1. Define, spell, and pronounce the terms listed in the vocabulary.
2. List five actions that need to be taken before the office opens in the morning.
3. Explain why patient traffic flow is an important consideration in office design.
4. List some of the expenses involved in the operation of a medical practice.
5. Describe how prices can be compared for medical office supplies.
6. Describe the purpose of white noise.
7. List several ways to save money in the medical office.
8. Explain the difference between medical waste and regular waste.
9. Explain why keys and alarm codes should be shared with only a few people.

National Accreditation Competencies and Content

CAAHEP COMPETENCIES

General

3.c.(3)(a). Explain general office policies
3.c.(3)(b). Instruct individuals according to their needs
3.c.(3)(d). Identify community resources
3.c.(4)(a). Perform an inventory of supplies and equipment
3.c.(4)(b). Perform routine maintenance of administrative and clinical equipment

ABHES COMPETENCIES

Communication

2.m. Adaptation for individualized needs

Administrative Duties

3.a. Perform basic secretarial skills
3.e. Locate resources and information for patients and employers
3.f. Manage physician's professional schedule and travel

Office Management

6.a. Maintain physical plant
6.b. Operate and maintain facilities and perform routine maintenance of administrative and clinical equipment safely
6.c. Inventory equipment and supplies
6.d Evaluate and recommend equipment and supplies for practice

Instruction

7.a. Orient patients to office policies and procedures
7.b. Instruct patients with special needs

VOCABULARY

backorder An ordered item that has not been delivered when promised or demanded but will be supplied at a later date.

bookmarking Marking a document or a specific place within a document for later retrieval; a feature supported by most browsers that allows the user to save the address (or URL) so that the document can be located when it is needed again.

budget A plan for the coordination of resources and expenditures; the amount of money that is available or required for a particular purpose.

circumvent To manage to get around, especially by ingenuity or strategy.

discrepancies Differences among conflicting facts, claims, or opinions.

fiscal year An accounting period of 12 months during which a company determines earnings and profit; the fiscal year does not necessarily begin in January—instead, the beginning of the fiscal year is determined by the business.

incur To become liable or subject to; to bring down on oneself.

outsourcing The practice of subcontracting work to an outside company.

packing slip A list of items that are included in a shipment.

proactive Acting in anticipation of future problems, needs, or changes.

The physician's office is a busy environment where the medical assistant encounters new challenges each day. The more flexible the medical assistant is, the more valuable he or she becomes to the physician. By learning and refining adaptation skills, office efficiency increases and the schedule can handle interruptions and emergencies.

Chapter 11 covered patient reception and processing. Remember that the patient is the reason the office exists and is of primary importance to the office staff. However, various tasks demand attention in the daily operation of the medical office. This chapter explores many of the duties that the medical assistant performs throughout a typical day at work.

OPENING THE OFFICE

The employees arrive earlier than the patients so that the office can be prepared for the day ahead. Some office policies dictate that the office be readied for the next day on the evening before, but for the purposes of this chapter, assume that the policy requires that preparation be done in the mornings.

Although the physician may trust the employees, office policy should demand that supervisors be **proactive** in avoiding the risk of theft. Depending on the size of the clinic, a certain number of employees will have keys and will know the alarm codes to the facility. The best policy is to strictly monitor this access and information. When numerous keys are distributed, more employees will have after-hours access to the office. By limiting this access, the physician may **circumvent** losses by theft. Two items in particular make the physician's office a target—money and drugs. Usually only limited cash is found in the office, but some medications are narcotics, and many, even those that are not narcotics, can be addictive. These items must be protected, not only for safety but also to remain in compliance with the law.

PREPARING FOR THE DAY AHEAD

Once the employees have arrived for work, all of them will begin to prepare for patients and visitors. Each employee is responsible for his or her own work space, and employees may work as a team to prepare common areas of the office, such as the reception area. When each person understands the required duties and they are divided among the staff, work can be completed quickly and efficiently.

Several duties are completed before patient arrival. The answering service should be called to collect any messages that were left since the last time the staff was in the office (Figure 12-1). Make certain that the phone message book is handy when calling the answering service; write each message into the message book, and include all information necessary to properly respond to the message. This action ensures that copies of the messages are available if one happens to get lost. Patient records may need to be pulled so that the medical assistant can take action and follow up on the messages.

Make two copies of the day's appointments, and place one copy on the physician's desk. Use the other copy to pull medical records for the patients who will visit the office during the day. In multiphysician practices, a copy of the day's appointments should be made for each physician. Keep the medical records in a convenient, central area so that staff members can find them easily once the patients begin to arrive. Make certain that there is enough room in the progress notes section of the medical record for the physician to write the details of the office

visit. If not, add a new sheet of progress notes. Glance over the notes from the last visit to ascertain whether laboratory work or treatments were ordered, then verify that the results are available to the physician.

Patient examination rooms should be restocked with all of the regular supplies used in the individual rooms. Items such as cotton balls, adhesive bandages, gauze pads, patient gowns, and drapes need to be replenished daily. The medical assistant should never force the physician and patient to wait in the examination room while the medical assistant searches for supplies. Check the restrooms as well, to make sure that toilet paper, soap, and hand towels are available. If urine specimen cups are kept in patient restrooms, there should be enough available to last throughout the day.

Be sure that prescription pads are available for the physician, although they should not be left in open areas or on counters (Figure 12-2). Patients should never have access to the prescription pads, because an unscrupulous patient might try to forge a prescription. Take extra care that the pads are out of the patient's' sight.

Certain equipment may need to be turned on, such as computers, laboratory equipment, and copy machines. Lights should be turned on in all of the examination rooms. If quality-assurance tests need to be performed on any of the laboratory machines, run the tests and record the results.

Some specimens from previous days may need to be checked for results or additional testing; for example, a blood culture may be ready to view for growth after 1 or 2 days. Always record test results in the patient's medical record. Make certain that the physician sees all test results as dictated in the office policy manual, especially if they fall outside normal ranges. The physician may need to perform follow-up work or see the patient again if the results are not normal.

CRITICAL THINKING APPLICATION

Kayla realizes that there is no set method through which the medical assistants know that laboratory results are ready to be filed. How might she handle this, and what suggestions can Kayla make to Elaine?

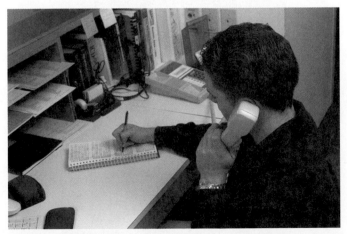

FIGURE 12-1 The telephone is the lifeline of a medical practice. The medical assistant will take several phone messages throughout the course of the day. (From Hunt SA: *Saunders fundamentals of medical assisting*, Philadelphia, 2002, Saunders.)

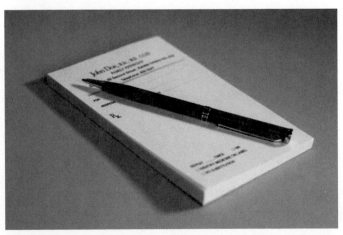

FIGURE 12-2 Keep a close watch on prescription pads so that patients do not have access to them.

The patient accounting software or day sheets should be prepared for the day. Secure enough encounter forms for each patient on the appointment book. Stock the patient checkout area with plenty of appointment cards. If the office gives small gifts to patients, like refrigerator magnets or coffee mugs, be sure that they are available for use. Many offices place the physician's business card just outside the receptionist's window or in the patient reception area. Because patients often take a card, this supply should also be checked.

Various specialty offices may need to prepare additional equipment, so make certain that everything necessary is available for the physician and staff members. Some offices use a checklist to ensure that all of the opening duties are completed. In others the staff knows each person's responsibilities by memorization and carries them out successfully each day. Whichever method is used, the day will go much more smoothly when the office is completely prepared for the patients. Once all of these duties are completed, the last task is to unlock the front door and begin welcoming patients to the practice.

PATIENT TRAFFIC FLOW

The design of the medical office is usually outside the realm of the medical assistant's control; however, the employees of the office can adapt to the physical design and determine the best room layout for efficient patient traffic flow. The reception area is the first room that most patients enter. Some physicians allow patients who are very ill to enter a back doorway or maintain a room separate from the reception area for these patients. This accommodation helps to prevent well patients from contracting a communicable disease.

CRITICAL THINKING APPLICATION

One of the older patients expresses concern that an ill child is coughing so much in the waiting area. How can Kayla help to alleviate the patient's concern? What can Kayla do to resolve the issue?

The fewer steps that patients have to walk as they work their way through the medical office, the better the traffic flow. Avoid making the patient backtrack over their previous steps, if possible. Many offices perform all procedures or treatments in the examination room. If the patient needs blood drawn, the medical assistant brings the equipment to the examination room where the patient is waiting. Some procedures, such as x-ray procedures, require that the patient go to another room. Move the patient from one room to another only when no other options exist.

When moving through hallways, the medical assistant should walk on the right side, leaving the left side for those traveling in the opposite direction—similar to the way people drive in the United States. The same principle applies to patients in wheelchairs or using some other form of walking assistance. Push or direct them along the right side of the hallway.

VISITORS TO THE OFFICE

Many people who are not patients visit the physician's office. Some of these people have appointments, and others stop by at random. The office policy manual should detail the procedure to follow when dealing with such individuals. Most physicians prefer that a specific time be set aside for pharmaceutical representatives (also called *detail persons*). Some will see one representative in the morning and one in the afternoon. Others will speak briefly to representatives in the hallway, then allow them to replenish the supply of drug samples in the storage area. Sometimes the representative will not need to speak to the physician; other times he or she will make an appointment to supply the entire office with lunch so that he or she can spend some time with the physician to explain new drugs. These professionals are usually quite competent in their knowledge of various drugs, and they should be treated with respect (Figure 12-3). Often, they leave giveaways for the staff and patients, such as pens, pencils, notepads, coffee mugs, videos relating to their products, pamphlets, and other novelty items. All of their efforts go toward convincing the physician to prescribe their drugs more often or to begin prescribing a new drug.

CRITICAL THINKING APPLICATION

One of the pharmaceutical representatives is extremely pushy. How can Kayla express that the physician cannot meet with the representative? What can Kayla do if the representative continues to be insistent about seeing the physician?

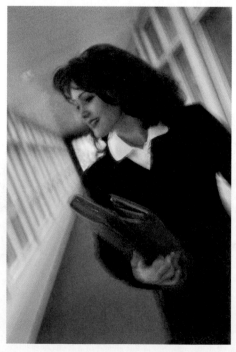

FIGURE 12-3 Pharmaceutical representatives are highly trained, knowledgeable professionals who can help the office staff understand the medications that patients are taking.

PROCEDURE 12-1

Explain General Office Policies

CAAHEP COMPETENCY: 3.c(3)(a)
ABHES COMPETENCY: 7.a

GOAL: *To effectively communicate office policies and procedures to employees, patients, and visitors in the office.*

EQUIPMENT and SUPPLIES

- Office policy manual
- Office procedure manual (if not included in policy manual)
- Patient information sheets (if needed)
- Patient information brochure

PROCEDURAL STEPS

1. Design an office policy manual and patient information brochure that contains general information for employees and patients. At a minimum the following information should be included:
   - Philosophy statement
   - Goals
   - Description of the medical practice
   - Location and/or map
   - Phone numbers
   - Pager numbers
   - Email and website addresses
   - Staff names and credentials
   - Services offered
   - Hours of operation
   - Appointment system
   For employees:
   - Vacation, sick leave
   - Confidentiality
   - Grievances
   - Benefits
   - Payroll information
   - Other employee information
   PURPOSE: To give the employees and patients a written document that details general information that can be used as a reference when needed.

2. Offer the brochure to new employees and patients or to any other employees and patients who do not have a current brochure.

3. Briefly discuss each section of the brochure with new employees and patients.
   PURPOSE: To acclimate the employees and patients to the contents of the policy manual and answer questions that might arise about each section.

4. Watch for verification of understanding from the employee or patient, both verbally and nonverbally.
   PURPOSE: By watching a patient's body language and listening to his or her questions, the medical assistant can determine whether the patient truly understands the information presented.

5. Ask the employee or patient if he or she has any questions.
   PURPOSE: To ensure understanding of the information presented.

6. Document that the employee or patient received the information in the medical record, if required.
   PURPOSE: This action is helpful in proving that an employee or patient was given certain information about policies and procedures.

Pharmaceutical representatives are not the only salespersons that may visit the physician's office. Sales people from office supply stores, medical equipment sellers, and others may stop by the office to make appointments or to take orders for various items. Usually the office manager can address the needs of salespeople and is authorized to place orders.

At times other physicians will stop by the office to see the doctor. They may not have an appointment, but the physician should be notified at once when another doctor is waiting in the reception area. If office policy allows, take the visiting physician to the doctor's office instead of forcing him or her to wait in the patient reception area. Usually the physician will agree to see the visiting doctor, if only for a few moments. Because doctors understand busy schedules, most will not stop by another doctor's office without having important information to share.

The physician's family members or friends may stop by the medical office, but they have usually been given restrictions by the physician as to when they can stop by and for what reasons. Never send family members or friends away without notifying the physician of their presence and asking whether he or she has time to speak to them.

USING THE OFFICE POLICY MANUAL

All employees should read the office policy manual when they begin to work in the physician's office. By reading the manual the medical assistant will become informed about the expectations of supervisors. However, the office policy manual is not used only for new employees (Procedures 12-1 and 12-2). The manual should be a daily source of information for all employees to reference whenever needed. The policy manual should be reviewed at least annually to make certain that all of the information contained within it is accurate and up to date. Whenever revisions are made, insert a page in the manual that tells the date that revisions became effective.

After review and acceptance of the revised manual, it is helpful to distribute a memo detailing what changes were made and where to look for the changes.

PROCEDURE 12-2

Instruct Individuals According to Their Needs

<u>CAAHEP COMPETENCY:</u> 3.c(3)(b)
<u>ABHES COMPETENCY:</u> 2.m

GOAL: *To effectively communicate office policies and procedures to employees, patients, and visitors in the office so that they understand instructions from the physician.*

EQUIPMENT and SUPPLIES

- Office policy manual
- Office procedure manual (if not included in policy manual)
- Patient information sheets (if needed)
- Physician orders, if applicable
- Patient information brochure

PROCEDURAL STEPS

1. Determine the communication needs of the employee, patient, or visitor.
   PURPOSE: To discover the best way to communicate information to an employee, patient, or visitor who may have special needs.
2. Arrange for an interpreter, if needed.
   PURPOSE: To make certain that information is communicated and received accurately.
3. Provide instructions to the employee, patient, or visitor.
4. Watch for verification of understanding from the patient, both verbally and nonverbally.
   PURPOSE: By watching body language and listening to questions, the medical assistant can determine whether the employee, patient, or visitor truly understands the information presented
5. Ask if there are any questions.
   PURPOSE: To ensure understanding of the information presented.
6. Document that the employee, patient, or visitor (if necessary) received the instructions in the medical record, if required.
   PURPOSE: This action is helpful in proving that an employee or patient was given certain instructions about policies, procedures, and expectations or directions regarding treatment.

The office policy manual should include sections that deal with several topics:

- Expected performance of the employee
- Tardiness and absenteeism
- Sexual harassment
- Confidentiality
- Vacations, sick time, paid time off
- Employee evaluation
- Continuing education
- Chain of command
- How to deal with certain patients and visitors

Some offices require that employees sign a document that states they have read and understand the policy in its entirety. The manual should be written in clear, concise language that is easily understood and should be used whenever a question about policy matters arises or the employee is unsure about why or how to proceed when completing a task. Often a procedure manual is combined with policy manuals. There should be no office tasks that are not detailed in either the policy manual or the procedure manual.

DAILY, WEEKLY, AND MONTHLY DUTIES

Develop a list of duties that are done daily, weekly, and monthly. Checklists are helpful when staff members want to make certain that all duties are completed. The lists help the supervisors divide chores evenly among staff members. Be specific on the checklist, and include every task that needs to be done, even the smallest ones. Staff members should cheerfully accept assignments they are given and should complete them quickly and efficiently. If one staff member is struggling with finishing her daily duties, other staff members should assist so that all required jobs are finished for the day. Usually, that employee will later help others complete their own duties when help is needed.

Constant Cleaning

Patients expect the physician's office to be immaculate. Nothing should be or appear dirty in any part of the facility. If the office is truly clean, it is less likely that germs and communicable diseases will spread, though not impossible. Effective cleaning products should be used on a daily basis, especially in high-traffic areas. There will never be a lack of equipment or furniture that could use a wipe down with a disinfectant or a light dusting. Countertops, sinks, door handles, and restrooms should be checked frequently and cleaned whenever needed. During slow periods between patients or during lengthy office visits, take a cloth and use a disinfectant on nearby counters and on the areas on doors near the handle. Look for things to clean in the office. By being conscientious about these things, the medical assistant will become more valuable to the physician. Supervisors and physicians will notice this productivity; good cleaning habits reflect positively on the medical assistant and will be important factors during employee evaluations.

Cleaning Services

Many offices employ a cleaning service that performs more intensive chores for the office. These professionals usually come

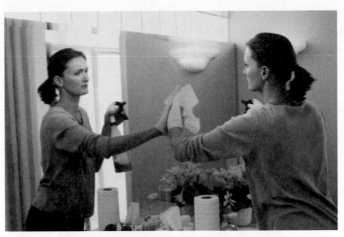

FIGURE 12-4 Cleaning services usually work in the evenings and keep the office looking professional and attractive.

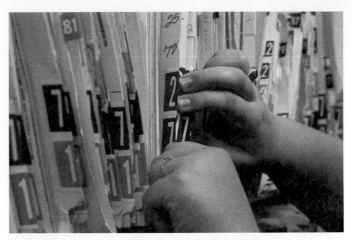

FIGURE 12-5 Filing is a critical job that must be done on a daily basis.

to the facility during the evening when patients and staff are not present. They clean and disinfect the bathrooms, vacuum, dust, empty trash, and may perform other specific tasks as required by the office staff (Figure 12-4). Some form of communication should exist between the office manager and the person who heads the cleaning team. Many offices leave a notebook for the cleaning crew that will detail what specific cleaning tasks should be performed in addition to the regular cleaning tasks. The office manager should delegate a staff member to be the contact person for the service. If any task is not completed in a satisfactory manner, the contact person should immediately contact the cleaning supervisor and resolve the problem. Make certain that a log is kept so that tasks are listed and a notation is made regarding whether they were completed or why they were not completed. Always inspect; the cleaning service must perform the jobs that they are being paid to do. Do not allow situations to go unresolved. Be open and frank with services that do not meet expectations.

CRITICAL THINKING APPLICATION

Kayla has noticed that on the days after the cleaning crew has come, sodas, plastic tableware, and other small items seem to be missing from the kitchen area. Today, she notices that an entire box of toilet paper is gone from the office. Kayla knows the box was there the day before, because she personally checked in the shipment. How can Kayla handle this situation? How is the situation complicated if one of the people who cleans the office at night is a co-worker's sister?

Filing

The medical assistant will rarely find a shortage of documents that are ready to file in the physician's office. Although this task is sometimes monotonous, filing is a critical job that must be completed accurately and in a timely manner (Figure 12-5). If a laboratory result is not placed in the right medical record, important information that may affect the patient's health could be lost. Chapter 14 explains rules that apply to the filing process and describes the equipment and supplies needed to perform this task.

SUPPLIES AND EQUIPMENT IN THE PHYSICIAN'S OFFICE

Physicians become frustrated when they reach for an item in an examination room and do not find it in its proper place. The medical assistant is responsible for stocking examination rooms and making certain that all supplies and equipment are available and in good working order. The following section describes the process of ordering and receiving medical supplies and equipment.

Identifying the Need for Specific Supplies

The medical assistant orders supplies periodically to ensure that the physician has everything he or she needs to treat patients. The office policy and procedure manual details the way that employees should identify the need for certain supplies, order them, check them in, and place them into the office inventory for use. Communication is the key to keeping supplies in stock. Once a method for ordering is established, all employees must adhere to the plan so that employees and patients are not affected by an item or product being out of stock.

Budgeting

Most offices operate using an annual **budget** to determine the amount of money that is to be spent on various categories of expenses (Figure 12-6). Some of the expenses that are involved in the operation of a medical practice include the following:

- Salaries
- Medical supplies
- Business equipment
- Medical equipment
- Utilities
- Rent or mortgage
- Insurance
- Maintenance
- Taxes
- Laboratory fees
- Office supplies

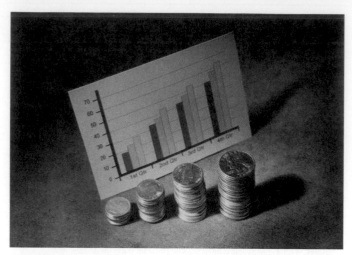

FIGURE 12-6 Smart budgeting is important to every physician.

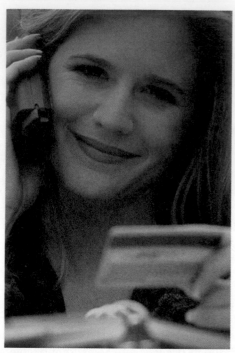

FIGURE 12-7 Compare prices before deciding on suppliers, then make a confident purchase.

Expense categories may be very specific and detailed or may constitute a more general list, such as the one above. A specific category listing would separate expenses for electricity, gas, and water, as opposed to grouping these expenses together as "utilities." These categories are important because most business expenses can be deducted on tax returns. Always keep receipts when shopping for items that will be used in the medical office and submit them in a timely manner to the office manager or other designated individual.

CRITICAL THINKING APPLICATION

Elaine has asked Kayla to prepare a budget for next year for her department. Kayla has never done this before. How can she get through her first challenging task?

The majority of people operate their households using some type of budget. The process of planning the coordination of resources and expenditures defines budgeting. Businesses usually plan expenses for the year in advance, allocating expected income into various categories of expenses. Then, on at least a monthly basis, expenses are logged onto a ledger or spreadsheet and separated into specific categories. This process allows tracking of expenses to make certain that a category is not over budget. If a specific category of expenses is over budget, adjustments may need to be logged to allow more funds in that category, or spending may need to be stopped in that category until the next year. It is not necessarily uncommon for budgets to exceed allowed amounts, but good business practice dictates that budgets be very close to estimations made at the beginning of the budget year. When a category goes over budget, money must often be taken from another budget category to cover the amount. This reduces the money available in the second category. Employees should not be allowed to spend money needlessly or wastefully. The physician should designate a minimum of persons authorized to make purchases on behalf of the facility.

Comparing Prices

A good shopper is an asset to the physician's office. Compare prices when shopping for supplies and equipment. Make it clear to salespersons that comparisons will be conducted and that price will be a strong consideration when the time comes to make a purchase (Figure 12-7). However, price may not be the only consideration. Warranties, bulk purchase opportunities, maintenance agreements, and other factors may influence the best deal available on a certain item. Quality is another important factor; the physician may be willing to pay more for an item based on its quality and durability. Personal preference also influences purchasing decisions. The clinical medical assistant may prefer one brand of needles over another even though they are the same price. In most circumstances, the person or persons who regularly use a certain item should be allowed to make decisions as to the brand, model, or other specifics before the item is purchased.

Most companies use a catalog, whether it is a paper catalog or one that is available online. Once a need is identified, compare the prices from at least three sources before placing an order. For instance, if 70% isopropyl alcohol is the product, and a stock is needed to last for 6 months, first determine how much is needed. Suppose that approximately one 16-ounce bottle of the alcohol is used per month in each of five treatment rooms. Further suppose that the following prices are listed:

Smith's Medical Supply	1 dozen bottles	$10.53
Argosy Medical and Dental Supply	2 dozen bottles	$17.44
Walgreen's	1 bottle	$0.53
Gibson's Pharmacy	1 gallon	$6.12

By comparing these prices, assuming that all other aspects of the products are equal, it is clear that buying bottles of alcohol at Walgreen's is a better deal than buying one or two dozen at either Smith's Medical Supply or Argosy Medical and Dental Supply. The alcohol at Smith's costs approximately $0.87 per bottle, and at Argosy a bottle costs approximately $0.72. Is the gallon a better buy? The alcohol can always be poured into containers from the gallon bottle. However, because there are 128 ounces in a gallon, only eight bottles with 16 ounces each could be divided from the gallon container. This means that the cost of the eight bottles is approximately $0.76 each. Walgreen's offers the best price. Still, if the only Walgreen's location is 35 miles away, the gas used in getting the product may make the overall cost to obtain the alcohol higher than driving 2 miles to Argosy. In addition, consider delivery, shipping, and handling charges that might be added to the total cost of the order. Some suppliers may cut the cost on certain items to get the order, either meeting or beating the deal offered by another supplier. Examine all costs before awarding the order to a supplier.

Ordering Supplies

The responsibility for ordering supplies in the medical office should be assigned to one person. The medical assistant who assumes this task can use various methods to track the supplies that are needed and place orders to replenish them. The simplest method is to develop a spreadsheet listing all of the products and supplies that need to be ordered periodically. Post the sheets in areas where supplies are stored. When staff members take supplies from storage, they should make a note on the spreadsheet. When it is time to place an order, the sheets are gathered and used to determine which supplies need to be replenished. Some offices use software to prepare orders, and others use a computer system to enter products that are taken from the supply area. Still others may use a sticker system, whereby a coded sticker is removed when a product is used and placed on a card or form, then that amount is charged to the patient. Others use a notecard system, wherein a notecard is prepared for each supply item and after inventory is performed; orders are completed based on the needs reflected on the note cards (Procedure 12-3). The physician should use the system that works best in that particular office. After determining the items that need to be ordered, browse medical or office supply catalogs to shop for the best prices. The order may need to be divided and offered to two different suppliers if certain items can be obtained at a better rate (Procedure 12-4).

Remember that the Internet is a source for shopping for supplies, too. Often businesses can find excellent prices by ordering online. Some physicians and office managers may be hesitant to use credit card accounts online; however, if an account is established with an online supply company, they will hold payment information or perhaps extend credit, and the company credit card need not be used. Investigate this helpful source, and use it to lower costs wherever possible.

Ordering Equipment

Ordering equipment is more involved than ordering simple supplies. Much of the equipment acquired for the physician's office is considered a capital purchase. Before purchasing this type of equipment, compare price, features, and benefits.

The physician is almost always involved in the purchase of capital equipment. Different businesses use different monetary amounts to classify capital purchases; some use $1000, whereas others may consider a capital purchase to be one that is over $5000. Physicians consult with accountants to determine limits on capital purchase amounts. At least three estimates should be obtained before making a major equipment purchase.

The physician and staff members who will use the equipment will have questions about the features and benefits, as well as the cost to purchase and the cost to use in the facility. Sometimes, the cost to use certain equipment may exceed the cost of **outsourcing.** For instance, the cost to perform a complete blood count (CBC) in the office may be $10. If the test can be outsourced and sent to an outpatient lab, resulting in a cost of $8, the physician could avoid equipment and maintenance costs. In addition, if the physician continues to charge $10, he will make a profit of $2 on every CBC performed. Physicians should not order unnecessary testing, but it is certainly ethical to make a profit on procedures and treatments performed. Remember, the physician's office is a business, and there is nothing unethical about making a profit.

CRITICAL THINKING APPLICATION

Kayla is talking with a patient who tells her husband that she doesn't know how they will afford the laboratory tests the doctor wants run. When Kayla walks by them, they stop talking. How can Kayla help the patient in this situation?

The medical assistant has numerous options when looking for equipment to purchase. Local suppliers offer catalogs detailing the products and equipment available, and the suppliers' sales representatives will be able to answer questions. Investigate whether used equipment might be for sale from the supplier. Physicians who are selling their practice or retiring might have equipment for sale. Research the Internet, even eBay, to find bargains on quality equipment (Figure 12-8). Obviously,

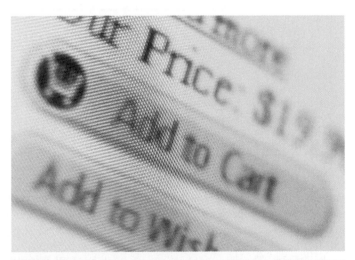

FIGURE 12-8 Check prices on the Internet and compare with those of local suppliers.

PROCEDURE 12-3

Perform an Inventory of Supplies and Equipment

CAAHEP COMPETENCY: 3.c.(4)(a)
ABHES COMPETENCY: 6.c

GOAL: *To establish an inventory of all expendable supplies in the physician's office and follow an efficient plan or order control using a card system.*

EQUIPMENT and SUPPLIES

- File box
- Inventory and order control cards
- List of supplies on hand
- Metal tabs
- Pen or pencil

PROCEDURAL STEPS

1. Write the name of each item on a separate card (Figure 1*).
   PURPOSE: To establish a record of all items in inventory.
2. Write the amount of each item on hand in the space provided.
   PURPOSE: To establish beginning inventory.
3. Place a reorder tag at the point where the supply should be replenished (Figure 2*).

PURPOSE: The tag will serve as an alert that supply is low.
4. Place a metal tab over the *order* section of the card.
   PURPOSE: The metal tab will be a reminder to include this item in the next order.
5. When the order has been placed, note the date and quantity ordered and move the tab to the *on order* section of the card.
6. When the order is received, note the date and quantity in the appropriate column, remove the tab, and refile the card.
   NOTE: If the order is only partially filled, let the tab remain until the order is complete.

*Courtesy of Colwell Systems, Champaign, Illinois.

FIGURE 1

ORDER	(ITEM NAME)	3-ply Disposable Drape Sheets (white) 7459									ON ORDER
ORDER QUANTITY	300					REORDER POINT	100				

ORDER	QTY	REC'D	COST	PREPAID	ON ACCT	ORDER	QTY	REC'D	COST	PREPAID	ON ACCT
1/25	300	2/10	64.95	X							

INVENTORY COUNT

	JAN	FEB	MAR	APR	MAY	JUNE	JULY	AUG	SEPT	OCT	NOV	DEC
20 00	200											
20 00												

ORDER SOURCE
The Colwell Company
201 Kenyon Road
Champaign, IL 61820

UNIT PRICE
100 - $23.95
300 - $64.95

FORM 2450 COLWELL CO., CHAMPAIGN, ILLINOIS

RED FLAG RE-ORDER TAG

when this inventory point is reached, it's time to reorder

Product Identification

The Colwell Company
Champaign, Illinois

FIGURE 2

some items should be purchased only from a medical supplier, but many great deals are available from various sources.

Receiving an Order

When an order arrives from a supplier, notify the person in charge of inventory. Boxes should be opened only if there is enough time to check them in properly. Carefully open the package, and look for the **packing slip.** A packing slip is a list of items ordered and items shipped. Occasionally, an ordered item will not be included in the package because it has been placed on **backorder.** The item may be out of stock but will be sent to the physician as soon as it becomes available. Compare the items listed on the packing slip with the items found inside the box. If any **discrepancies** are found, bring them to the attention of the supplier immediately. Discourage other employees from taking items from the package before they are checked against the packing slip. Once the order is checked in, make a note on the packing slip that the package was received as expected, then place new stock in the proper place.

Warranty Information

Many purchased items include a warranty. The medical assistant should always mail warranty information to the manufacturer. Warranty cards usually resemble a postcard and contain several

PROCEDURE 12-4

Prepare a Purchase Order

CAAHEP COMPETENCY: 3.c(4)(a)
ABHES COMPETENCY: 6.c

GOAL: *To prepare an accurate purchase order for supplies or equipment.*

EQUIPMENT and SUPPLIES

- List of current inventory
- Purchase order
- Pen
- Phone
- Fax machine

PROCEDURAL STEPS

1. Review the current inventory and determine what items need to be ordered.
   PURPOSE: To determine what is needed so that the office will not be overstocked or understocked.

2. Complete the purchase order accurately, filling in all applicable spaces and blanks with the information requested.
   PURPOSE: An accurately completed purchase order helps to eliminate mistakes in the order and in shipments.

3. List the items to be ordered, including quantity, item numbers, size, color, price, and extended price. Be sure that all applicable information is included.
   PURPOSE: To help ensure accurate orders.

4. Provide the physician's signature, DEA certificate, and medical license when needed.
   PURPOSE: Some items require these documents to verify that the physician is eligible to order them.

5. Call in, fax, mail, or electronically submit the order to the vendor. Keep a copy for your records. Keep any verification provided that the order was received.
   PURPOSE: To document exactly what was ordered on what date and provide proof that the order was received.

6. Note on the inventory which items are on order.
   PURPOSE: To keep other staff members from preparing duplicate orders.

7. Keep a copy of the order in the appropriate place in the office filing system.
   PURPOSE: To reference the order if needed and have a copy of the items ordered to compare with the packing list once the items arrive at the office.

---

questions about the purchaser. By completing the warranty card and mailing it, the manufacturer will be able to contact those who have purchased a certain product if defects are discovered. The warranty period begins on the date of purchase and usually lasts 1 year but can be lengthier, depending on the item purchased. Keep a copy of the completed warranty in a file that contains other information on the specific product or piece of equipment, such as the receipt of purchase, expense records, owner's manuals, and maintenance records.

Invoices and Statements

An invoice is an itemized list of goods shipped that specifies price and the terms of a sale. A statement is a summary of a financial account that shows the balance due, as well as transactions that affect the account. Invoices precede statements. A medical supplier may send an invoice when a sale has been completed, and statements are mailed whenever a balance exists on an account. Some invoices request payment on receipt, and some allow a certain period of time to make a payment (Figure 12-9). Read invoices and statements carefully and make certain that there are no errors before making payment.

Troubleshooting Equipment Failure

When equipment fails to function properly, consult the owner's manual to determine the steps for troubleshooting. The owner's manual is usually found in the package that the product was in when purchased. Many are published on the Internet, which allows

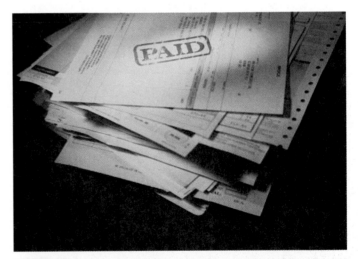

FIGURE 12-9 Invoices and statements must be compared carefully with orders actually received at the physician's office.

for quick access to details about the item. The owner's manual includes contact information so that the purchaser can reach the manufacturer if necessary. Today, purchasers have additional contact options, such as email and chat rooms; both offer fast access for problems that need to be quickly solved. Remember to consider the reasonable, simplest solutions first—is the equipment plugged in? Does the computer need to be rebooted? Often, the solution is a straightforward one that can be easily deduced.

PROCEDURE 12-5

Perform Routine Maintenance of Administrative and Clinical Equipment

<u>CAAHEP COMPETENCY</u>: 3.c.(4)(b)
<u>ABHES COMPETENCY</u>: 6.b

GOAL: *To ensure that all office equipment is in good working order at all times.*

EQUIPMENT and SUPPLIES

- Notecard or spreadsheet containing information on each piece of office equipment, including serial number and periods that the equipment needs servicing
- Pen or pencil
- Computer
- Access to all office equipment

PROCEDURAL STEPS

1. Gather information about each piece of equipment. The following information is needed at a minimum:
   - Name of equipment
   - Type of equipment
   - Manufacturer or maker's name
   - Address of manufacturer
   - Contact phone numbers for technical support
   - Contact phone numbers for main office
   - Date purchased
   - Cost of product
   - Original receipt showing where the item was purchased
   - Date warranty begins and ends
   - Addresses to send equipment if under warranty
   - Number of times the equipment needs service in a year
   - Last date of service
   - Explanation of what was done during last servicing
   - A number assigned by the office manager to identify the equipment

PURPOSE: To give the medical assistant all of the information needed for maintenance and service for the equipment.

2. Place all of the information about each piece of equipment into a document or spreadsheet.
   PURPOSE: This provides a written recording of all information about each piece of equipment.

3. Make a list containing each month of the year. Note which equipment needs servicing in which months.
   PURPOSE: To provide a calendar for servicing equipment.

4. On the first of each month, check the spreadsheet and list to determine which equipment needs servicing that month.

5. Schedule servicing and maintenance for equipment during the current month.
   PURPOSE: To provide a specific time that the equipment will be available for servicing.

6. Check with co-workers to make certain that servicing dates work with all schedules, especially if a piece of equipment will be out of service for any length of time.
   PURPOSE: To prevent scheduling conflicts during times when the equipment is needed by the staff.

7. Oversee scheduling appointments to make certain they are kept.

8. Record new information on the document or spreadsheet to reflect new times for servicing and any additional information.
   PURPOSE: To ensure that the most accurate information is on file about every piece of equipment in the physician's office.

Equipment Maintenance

Medical office equipment must be maintained regularly, especially machines that perform testing procedures. The Clinical Laboratory Improvement Act (CLIA) requires that controls and calibrations be performed, and all of these requirements are designed to ensure that patient testing is accurate and that the results are reliable. The maintenance process is similar to maintaining a car in good working condition. Periodically, oil, filters, and tires must be changed, brake pads must be removed and replaced, and engines must be kept clean. Similarly, medical office machines must be kept in good repair and working condition (Procedure 12-5).

Maintenance guidelines are found in most owners' manuals, and they should be the basis of any maintenance plan. The medical assistant can develop a maintenance schedule to ensure that all office equipment receives proper, timely attention. Keep all information about each equipment item in a separate file, and add maintenance records to it as they are produced.

PREVENTING WASTE

Waste prevention reduces or eliminates waste before it is generated. Companies can reduce the cost of waste management, reduce long-term liability for disposal of hazardous waste materials, and become more efficient to enhance profit margins. The key to successful waste management is the cooperation of employees—unless they are willing to participate in waste management efforts, the efforts will be unsuccessful.

Physician office employees can reduce waste while saving money in the following ways:

- Use solar powered calculators and battery rechargers
- Use refillable pens, pencils, and tape dispensers
- Use refillable calendars
- Use two-way envelopes
- Reuse file folders and binders
- Refurbish office equipment
- Use bulletin boards

- Change to cloth towel dispensers
- Reuse printer toner and ribbon cartridges
- Retrofit exit sign bulbs
- Convert to high efficiency fluorescent lighting
- Reuse dishware
- Use reusable forced air filters
- Eliminate single-use cups
- Reuse paper printed on only one side

Avoiding waste and being conservative with products at the office will save money and may result in an increase in employee wages and benefits. Always participate in efforts to preserve products and be open to trying new conservation methods.

LUNCH AND BREAK ETIQUETTE

Even though the physician's office is a busy place and often hectic, all staff members should take a morning and afternoon break, as well as a lunch period. Many offices close between noon and 2:00 PM so that the staff can have lunch and use the moments to rest, refocus, and catch up (Figure 12-10). Try to alternate lunch times so that some assistants go to lunch during the first hour and some during the second hour. Be respectful of lunch hours and break times by leaving and returning at the appropriate time. Remember to clean any dishes used and put them away, as well as food items that should be returned to the refrigerator. Medical supplies that need to be refrigerated cannot be stored with food. Leftovers should be removed at least once a week. All employees should have a hand in keeping the lunch or break area clean.

SENDING AND RECEIVING EMAIL

Electronic communications are sent and received frequently throughout the business day. Email messages are similar to memos, and when used in the professional office they should

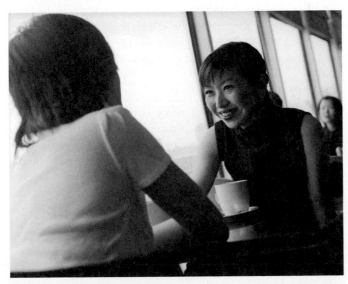

FIGURE 12-10 Use lunch periods and breaks to relax. Don't skip lunch or breaks, because this practice can lead to burnout.

project a professional tone. More information about the format of emails is available in Chapter 13. Use the office email system for work-related messages only. Never forward comic email or messages that are sexual in nature using the office email system. A good general rule to follow is to refrain from sending any email at the workplace that supervisors should not read. Remember that the information services staff of a facility can often find emails and other improper files on computers even if they have been deleted. A file is not completely gone from a computer until another file is written over it. In addition, computers can be monitored in real time, with every keystroke recorded and every website visited logged. Several free email sites allow the user to create an email account with substantial storage space. Use the separate, personal email address for non–business-related information. The medical assistant should treat email information as confidential if it relates to a patient.

INTERNET RESEARCH

The medical assistant may be asked to research various types of information using the Internet. If a word or phrase is entered into a search engine, it produces a results screen containing links to various websites that contain the word or phrase in the search. The medical assistant can then enter the websites and look for the required information. Not all of the articles found on the Internet are reliable; some are completely false and others are simply one person or group's opinion. Look for information from sites that can be trusted, such as the American Heart Association or the American Medical Association. Once a good, informative site is found, read through it carefully, because it may lead to more sites that will provide additional information. **Bookmarking** the site allows it to be easily referenced at a later time. In the Internet Explorer environment, a site is bookmarked by clicking on "Favorites" then clicking on "Add to favorites."

Various types of information can be found on the Internet, such as the following:

- Company reports
- Financial information
- Company profiles
- Conference proceedings
- Seminar announcements
- Law, government announcements, and parliamentary debates
- News and current affairs
- Databases of reference material
- Places to discuss topics and ask for help

Before beginning a search online for information, jot down several keywords that are relevant to the research topic. For instance, consider the subject "medical office management." A search for those three words on www.yahoo.com reveals over 37,000,000 sites with information on the topic. Once a listing has been obtained, the medical assistant can begin to research the sites and determine which ones contain pertinent information. When writing a paper using information contained on websites, be sure to cite the website in the proper place at the end of the paper.

TRAVELING FOR BUSINESS PURPOSES

Throughout the course of a **fiscal year,** employees may attend seminars or workshops to gain additional information, learn new techniques or procedures, and obtain continuing education units (CEUs), which may be needed to maintain certification (Figure 12-11). There is more to these workshops than registering and attending. Shifts must be covered for employees attending the seminar, and travel arrangements must be secured.

Seminars and Workshops

Both physicians and office staff members will periodically attend seminars or workshops to participate in continuing education events or learn new skills. Physicians are required to accumulate a certain number of continuing education credits each year, and medical assistants may need continuing education credits as well, depending on the type of certification that he or she has earned. When planning to attend a seminar, consider not only the cost of the sessions, but also the cost of travel to and from the seminar and hotel, gas, and food costs. Invitations to attend seminars often arrive in the mail, although some arrive by email. Watch for enrollment deadlines, and make certain that registration is done before the deadline date. Some seminars offer great discounts if registration is completed early.

Scheduling Travel, Hotel Rooms, and Car Rentals

The location of the event will often dictate the type of travel arrangements that should be made (Procedure 12-6). Distant locations usually require an airline flight. A travel agent is sometimes used to book flights and hotel rooms, but companies are booking their own flights using the Internet more than ever

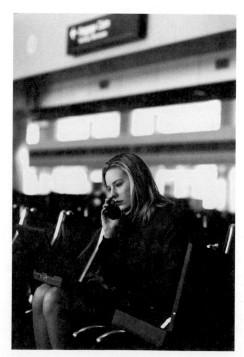

FIGURE 12-11 The medical assistant may need to travel to attend seminars or workshops.

before. Other trips involve car travel. Staff members who travel by car are entitled to reimbursement for mileage expenses. In fact, if staff members **incur** any reasonable business expense, they should be reimbursed by the company.

The brochures for many events that the physician and staff will attend list suggested hotels. If the physician has a preference for a certain hotel, reservations should be made at that location if possible. However, do not hesitate to suggest a different hotel if one is closer to the event or offers a better price for the same amenities.

A car rental may be necessary so that staff members can travel from place to place while attending the seminar. Take care when using a debit card to pay for rentals or deposits. Many establishments will place a hold on the estimated total balance due, even when the balance is paid in cash. This process could place a hold on available funds until the payment actually clears.

BASIC SAFETY AND SECURITY IN THE MEDICAL OFFICE

No one knows when our safety and the security we enjoy will be jeopardized. The saying "Better safe than sorry" has never been truer than today. Don't think that any place of business is immune to crime.

Suspicious Persons

If a suspicious person enters the office, make every effort to keep a distance. Staff members should stay behind the counter or desk so that the person cannot grab or gain control of one of the employees. When feeling serious concern about a suspicious individual, attempt to notify another employee early in the conversation. Pick up the telephone and dial the office manager's extension. Plan a code in advance for different emergency situations. For instance, use the phrase "Norman is here to see you," which relates to Norman Bates of the *Psycho* films, an individual who was at least frightening. This will alert the office manager that there is a potential problem at the front desk and the police should be called. Even if it isn't a life-threatening emergency, the police would rather respond to a false alarm than arrive to find a situation that is out of control.

Robbery

Although physician's offices rarely have an excess of cash on hand, thieves may assume that there is money to steal or, more likely, narcotics. Do not argue or fight with such people. Give them what they want—the object is to get them out of the office as quickly as possible. Once they are out, lock the doors and call the police. Do not touch any items that the criminals touched so that the crime scene is preserved. When such a situation occurs, the employees will clearly be under stress, but make every effort to remember basic identifying markers, such as the following:

- Height
- Weight
- Hair color and length

PROCEDURE 12-6

Locate Resources and Information for Patients and Employers:
Make Travel Arrangements

ABHES COMPETENCY: 3.f

GOAL: *To make travel arrangements for the physician or another staff member.*

EQUIPMENT and SUPPLIES

- Travel plan
- Telephone
- Telephone directory
- Typewriter or computer
- Typing paper

PROCEDURAL STEPS

1. Verify the dates of the planned trip. Consider the following:
   - Desired date and time of departure
   - Desired date and time of return
   - Preferred mode of transportation
   - Number in party
   - Preferred lodging and price range
   - Preferred ticketing method (electronic or paper).

2. Telephone a trusted travel agency to arrange for transportation and lodging reservations, or book the trip using Internet resources.
   PURPOSE: A travel agent might be better suited to answer questions involving regulations for international travel. The Internet is an easy way to book trips on your own.

3. Arrange for traveler's checks, if desired.
   PURPOSE: Traveler's checks are a better alternative than carrying large sums of cash and can be easily replaced if lost or stolen.

4. Pick up tickets or e-receipts or arrange for their delivery.

5. Check tickets to confirm conformance with the travel plan.
   PURPOSE: To avoid any error resulting from misunderstanding and to verify compliance with requests.

6. Check to see that hotel and air reservations are confirmed.

7. Prepare an itinerary, including all the necessary information:
   - Date and time of departure
   - Flight numbers or identifying information for other modes of travel
   - Mode of transportation to hotel(s)
   - Name, address, and telephone number of hotel(s), with confirmation numbers if available
   - Name, address, and telephone number of travel agency
   - Date and time of return.
   PURPOSE: The itinerary provides the details of the entire trip at a glance and is a more organized way to keep up with times, dates, confirmation numbers, and other details all on one document.

8. Place one copy of itinerary in the office file, and give one to the office manager.
   PURPOSE: It may be necessary to contact the traveler or to forward mail.

9. Give several copies of the itinerary to the traveler.
   PURPOSE: The traveler may wish to have extra copies for family or friends.

- Clothing, especially the color
- Race
- Distinctive marks (scars, tattoos, etc.)

Make the observations as subtly as possible; criminals who think they are being sized up for later identification may not react well!

If the criminals don't leave the office and the situation escalates, make every effort to find out what they want that will prompt them to leave. Remain as calm as possible throughout the ordeal. If the employee remains calm, a criminal will usually remain calm as well. Unfortunately, this is not always the case, but most criminals want to leave the crime scene as opposed to being present when the authorities arrive. Review the general safety tips for employees in Figure 12-12.

Office Security

Various items of value can be found in the medical office. Narcotic medications are stored in a locked cabinet, and cash and checks are kept in the office as well. For these reasons the office must always be secure.

Alarm systems are often used to protect the medical office; such systems either are monitored or simply sound an alarm when tripped. Monitored alarms go off when a door or window is opened and the security code is not entered into the unit. When the alarm is tripped, an employee of the alarm company will attempt to call the office to determine if there is a true emergency. If no one answers, the alarm company will send police to the facility. An alarm that sounds will also be active until a code is entered, but these systems allow a short period of time for the alarm code to be entered before the main alarm begins to ring. Occasionally a false alarm will sound and prompt the police to investigate; however, many alarm companies charge the business a fee when the alarm is not a valid emergency.

Only a few staff members need to know the alarm code. The office manager and those who open and close the facility need to know the code, as does the physician. The fewer people who know the code, the better. A combination of letters and numbers is best for alarm codes, instead of a strictly numeric or alphabetic code.

General Safety Tips for Employees

- Be sure to always lock the car when leaving it, no matter how short a visit to the destination.
- Park in a well-lighted area and have the car key in hand when approaching the vehicle.
- Attempt to walk out of the office with another person. If there is no choice but to walk alone, walk confidently and with determined stride.
- Be aware of the surroundings. Walk in the middle of parking lanes, not too close to cars on the left or right to avoid being pulled in between two vans or SUVs.
- Take a good look at the vehicle on approach, including underneath, if possible. Once the door is open, glance around the vehicle. If parked in a well-lit area, it is easier to see into the back seat.
- Once inside the vehicle, immediately lock the doors, start the car, and leave. Don't perform menial tasks, such as balancing a checkbook, applying makeup, or talking on the phone, while sitting in a parking lot.
- Never leave valuable items lying in the car in plain sight, such as iPods, cell phones, CD players, laptop computers, etc.
- Don't be afraid to ask security personnel to provide an escort when leaving for the day, if security is available.
- Report all suspicious activity immediately; don't wait until the next day.

FIGURE 12-12 General safety tips for employees.

Smoke Alarms and Fire Extinguishers

Smoke alarms should be installed in every physician's office. The two basic types of smoke alarms are photoelectric and ionization alarms. If nuisance alarms continually sound (for instance, from cooking popcorn in the lounge area), changing alarm types may solve the problem. Smoke alarm batteries must be changed twice a year; the best time to do this is when daylight savings time begins and ends. Although the old batteries may not be dead, new ones will be fresh and will certainly last for 6 months.

Fire extinguishers must be readily available in the office and must be prominently mounted in a visible, convenient place. The extinguishers must be serviced annually by a fire professional who holds a valid certificate to perform inspections. In addition, staff members should be trained in the use of fire extinguishers; most fire departments offer this training either free or for a nominal charge. A multipurpose ABC fire extinguisher is appropriate for a small business. Staff members can remember the basic use of the fire extinguisher by memorizing the mnemonic device PASS:

P—pull the pin
A—aim the hose
S—squeeze
S—sweep the nozzle

To determine whether a physician's office is safe, answer the following questions:

- Are all exit ways accessible and unobstructed?
- Are all of the fire extinguishers operational and properly locatable?
- Are all of the emergency lighting units and exit signs operational?
- Are any extension cords or multiplug adaptors in use?
- Is there an escape plan with two ways out, and do employees know how to use it?
- Are the fire alarms and sprinkler system functioning correctly and easily accessible?
- Is all storage neat and orderly and not obstructing sprinkler heads?
- Are all flammable liquids and materials stored away from heat sources?
- Are all plumbing, mechanical, and electrical systems functioning properly?

Fire Exits and Exit Routes

At least two exits must be designated as fire exits in the medical facility. These exits must be clearly marked and easily accessible. The exit doors must remain unlocked during business hours so that people can get out in case of a fire or other emergency. For security reasons, doors can be locked on the outside, yet have an exit bar on the inside that allows exit by pushing on the exit bar.

An escape plan must be posted in several areas of the facility, and employees should have regular drills that allow them to practice evacuating the building. If escape plans are posted in every room, then the escape from that particular room can be diagrammed. Two escape routes should be posted from each room—a primary route and a secondary route. Before exiting through a door, touch it and determine whether it feels warm. If it does, then use another route. If the facility is two stories tall, have ladders ready that attach to a window and unfold to allow escape. Buildings with two or more stories should have stairwells that can also be used in case of fire.

Locked Storage Areas

Several items in the medical office must be kept in locked cabinets or storage areas. Narcotic drugs and other prescription medications should be secured, and employees should have limited access to them. Because some over-the-counter medications are readily available, such as pseudoephedrine (an ingredient in common cold medication), most pharmacies and discount stores have begun limiting the number of packages of the medicine that one person can purchase.

Narcotics must be logged when a dose is used. More details about the requirements when administering a dose of medication can be found in Chapter 32. Prescription pads should also be kept under lock and key unless the physician is using the pad. Most doctors are protective of prescription pads because they realize that patients, or even employees, sometimes steal them.

WASTE STORAGE AND DESTRUCTION

Two basic types of waste are found in physicians' offices: medical waste and regular waste. Medical waste includes anything that was once a part of the human body. Most offices use a trash service to remove regular waste, whether it is contracted or a service provided by the city. Removing medical waste is

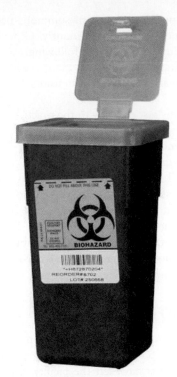

FIGURE 12-13 OSHA requires that medical waste be disposed of properly and that the office keep records of waste removal and incineration.

somewhat more complicated (Figure 12-13). The Occupational Safety and Health Administration (OSHA) requires records that prove that (1) medical waste was collected by the removal waste service, and (2) the same waste was destroyed by the waste service. The medical waste service usually comes every few days; the waste is picked up, then destroyed by incineration.

Regular trash is usually collected twice a week. Holiday weeks may result in additional trash, and that may mean additional fees. Trash pickup will occur two or three times per week; make certain that all trash is brought to the predetermined location for disposal outside. Do not place trash outside early, as it may attract animals and insects.

ERGONOMICS

Ergonomics is the applied science concerned with designing and arranging things people use so that the people and the things interact efficiently and safely. OSHA developed a four-pronged approach to quickly and efficiently address musculoskeletal disorders in the workplace. The approach includes a combination of industry-specific and task-specific guidelines, outreach, enforcement, and research. Since these measures have been implemented, OSHA has seen significant improvement in these areas. A plethora of information on ergonomics is available online, both through a general search and on the OSHA website.

ACOUSTICS AND WHITE NOISE

Acoustics is defined as the science that deals with the production, control, transmission, reception, and effects of sound. Acoustics

differ from room to room. When acoustics are good, sound reception is sharp and clear. In a room that has poor acoustics, the sound seems to be more muffled.

Acoustics are important in the medical office because they can affect confidentiality. Most people have visited a medical office in which a patient sitting in an examination room could hear every word spoken in the next room. If the diagnosis is revealed and overheard by another patient, then patient confidentiality has been broken. Medical professionals must be aware of the acoustics in the office and attempt to work with them, guarding patients' right to confidentiality.

Although the technical definition of *white noise* is long and complicated, for the purposes of this text, the shortened definition will help students understand the term. White noise is commonly used with architectural acoustics, where it "masks" undesirable noises, such as multiple conversations in interior spaces, by generating a low level of background noise that is used as background sound. It is also used on some sirens for emergency vehicle use because of its ability to cut through background noise; one benefit of this ability is that the siren is easier to distinguish as a separate sound and it does not create an echo, so it is easier to determine the direction from which the siren sound is coming.

White noise is often used in medical offices because the stark quiet of the facility can be unnerving for patients. Most people have no idea that white noise is being generated. Even if soft music is playing in the office, white noise can be in the background. Sometimes white noise sounds like a soft static. Some businesses use a CD of white noise, and they can contain the sounds of waterfalls, thunderstorms, rushing water, jungle sounds, and many others, all designed to make the office visit less frightening and more relaxing and to absorb distracting noise.

IDENTIFYING AND SHARING COMMUNITY RESOURCES

The medical assistant must be able to identify community resources so that he or she can assist patients with needs that are not office related, and possibly not medically related. At various times, patients need help with meals, rehabilitation, Medicare issues, exercise groups, and other services. Grocery stores that deliver are a great convenience resource for the older patient. Get to know the people in the community, trade information, and refer patients when they need help with a particular issue. Figure 12-14 includes some of the more common community resources in which patients may be interested. This can be used to create a phone directory for a local community resource list (Procedure 12-7). To expand the knowledge base as to what resources are available in the community, get involved in various organizations, especially health industry councils and organizations for medical assistants or other office staff members. Make introductions, and be prepared to talk about the services that the clinic offers. Ask questions about other facilities. Exchange business cards, if they are available. Stay in touch with community resource contacts to make certain that information being provided to patients is accurate. Patients

Community Resources

Check with these organizations for services available in the local area.

Alcoholics Anonymous
Alzheimer Support Organizations
American Cancer Society
American Heart Association
American Red Cross
Child Protective Services
Civic Organizations
Council on Aging
Family Services
Homeless Organizations
Hospice Services
Legal Aid Societies
Mental Health and Mental Retardation Services
Public Health Department
United Way

FIGURE 12-14 Examples of community resources.

appreciate that the office staff can refer them to local resources and can assist them in gathering information.

Emergency Phone Numbers

Every medical facility should keep a list of emergency and frequently called numbers close to each telephone in the office.

The list should include 911, which summons police and fire departments in most areas in the country. Other numbers on the list might include those for the following:

- Local hospitals
- Local pharmacies, including extensions to the emergency room
- All physicians associated with the practice
- All employees
- Nonemergency police services
- Physicians who are periodically on call

Each office will have different numbers on the emergency phone numbers list. The physician and office manager often provide input about the numbers that are included. Periodically the numbers will need to be updated. If the list is kept on a computer, a new one can be printed and distributed each time a phone number changes. Because the list is used in emergencies, it must be current and accurate at all times.

CLOSING THE OFFICE

When the day comes to an end, several duties must be completed before the doors are locked and the office is closed. First, check to see that all patients have left the facility. Walk through all examination rooms and treatment areas to make certain that they are empty. At the same time, straighten the examination rooms so that they are ready for the next day's patients. Because the rooms are tidied in between patients, they should be easy

PROCEDURE 12-7

Identify Community Resources

CAAHEP COMPETENCY: 3.c.(3)(d)
ABHES COMPETENCY: 3.e

GOAL: *To help patients find organizations that can assist with their needs beyond the physician's office and to establish a listing of community resources that can be used for referral purposes.*

EQUIPMENT and SUPPLIES

- Phone book
- Internet access
- Library access
- Newspapers
- Local volunteer guides
- Computer
- Pen or pencil
- Notepad

PROCEDURAL STEPS

1. Research the resources available in the local community using the Internet, phone book, newspapers, and other guides.
   PURPOSE: To become familiar with various agencies that provide services in the local area.
2. Open a document on the computer, either using a word-processing program or a spreadsheet. Create a list of the

resources within the document. Include the following information on the list:
   - Name of agency
   - Purpose or mission of agency
   - Physical address
   - Mailing address, if different
   - Phone numbers
   - Contact name
   - Hours of operation
   - Services offered or performed
   PURPOSE: To make information readily available.
3. Update the information whenever a change is needed.
   PURPOSE: To provide the most accurate information possible.
4. Provide referrals to agencies when patients, their friends, or their families ask for it or when the physician recommends referral.
   PURPOSE: To get patients the help that they need.

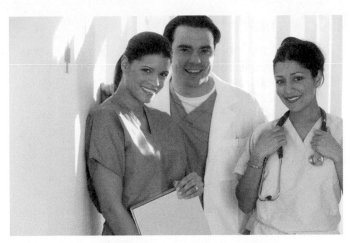

FIGURE 12-15 Teamwork is vital to ensure successful completion of the workday in the physician's office.

to clean at day's end. Work with fellow employees as a team to accomplish all of the tasks that are required each day (Figure 12-15).

Other duties include locking patient file cabinets, placing laboratory specimens in the outside lockbox for pickup, performing general housekeeping duties, running accounting reports, balancing the day sheet, and preparing the bank deposit. The phones will need to be turned over to the answering service or voicemail. Using a mnemonic device, as discussed in the last chapter, helps the medical assistant to remember closing duties. Remember the safety tips for leaving offices and returning to vehicles. The saying bears repeating: "Better safe than sorry."

CLOSING COMMENTS

Although the tasks discussed in this chapter include duties that are done on a daily basis, the medical assistant should not be lazy about completing them. When the physician sees that employees are competent about completing small duties, he or she will consider the medical assistant to be competent in completing more difficult tasks. By consistently proving to be a skilled, dependable worker, the medical assistant will be promoted to higher levels of responsibility.

Always keep in mind that the patient is of primary concern in the physician's office. The medical assistant's efforts should be directed at making the patients feel more at ease and encouraging them to follow the treatment plan devised by the physician. Therefore even the smallest of office duties plays a part in the health and well-being of the patient.

SUMMARY OF SCENARIO

Kayla learned much more on her externship than she thought she would. She saw patients who had few belongings and no health insurance coverage. Her experience helped her to realize just how difficult it is to obtain medical care without insurance. Kayla is happy that her clinic sees these patients and allows the patients to pay what they can to obtain medical care. She feels slightly guilty that she has had such an easy life as she listens to her patients' stories and their problems.

Kayla has developed a sense of caring for the people she helps in the clinic. She does not treat the patients disrespectfully; on the contrary, she treats them as individuals who deserve dignity. She understands that although she might not connect with all patients, she can make a difference to the ones who enter the clinic by expressing an emotion that she truly feels—compassion.

Elaine allowed Kayla to order many of the supplies that she needs, because Kayla is the primary user of those items. This allows Kayla to use the items she has found perform the best and with which she is most comfortable. Kayla suggested that the clinic outsource some of their laboratory tests because of the expense of buying the supplies to run the tests. This has allowed the clinic to keep their prices lower, a great help to the patients.

Kayla found that most of the patients who come to the clinic are in need of referrals, whether it be for food, clothing, other medical services, child care, or other issues. She designed a lengthy list of community resources, and she can tell patients where to go to receive help with various problems. The patients appreciate Kayla's willingness to help them. Even though Kayla comes from a completely different background, the patients have accepted her as a medical assistant who truly cares.

SUMMARY of LEARNING OBJECTIVES

1. Define, spell and pronounce the terms listed in the vocabulary.
   - Spelling and pronouncing medical terms correctly adds credibility to the medical assistant. Knowing the definition of these terms promotes confidence in communication with patients and co-workers.
2. List five actions that need to be taken before the office opens in the morning.
   - Before the medical office is opened in the morning, several tasks must be completed. The office should be clean, whether it is done the evening before or as one of the morning duties. Examination rooms should be checked for supplies and replenished, if necessary. The phone should be taken off of voicemail or the answering service called to inform them that the office staff has arrived for the day. Make two copies of the appointment book, placing one on the physician's desk and using the other to pull the medical records of the patients who have appointments. Individual offices may assign additional duties to the medical assistants who work in the office.
3. Explain why patient traffic flow is an important consideration in office design.
   - Patient traffic flow is important because patients should not have to repeatedly retrace their steps as they move throughout the clinic. Furnishings should be arranged so that it is easy to get from one place to another without having to dodge objects in the room.
4. List some of the expenses involved in the operation of a medical practice.
   - Many types of expenses affect the operation of a physician's office. Lease or mortgage payments are one of the largest expenses. Utilities, payroll, equipment and supplies, professional organization dues, insurance, maintenance, and taxes are all examples of items that must be worked into the annual budget.
5. Describe how prices can be compared for medical office supplies.
   - Compare unit prices by determining what each individual item costs. If a bulk package of eight containers of correction fluid

costs $9.99, then each individual bottle costs $1.25. If another company offers the same product at 10 for $12.00, then the individual cost is $1.20, which is the better buy of the two. However, the cost to buy the product, meaning the gas to get to the store, or the shipping and handling costs, if any, may increase the price. Be aware of these situations and figure all costs possible before placing an order.

6. Describe the purpose of white noise.
   - White noise is used to absorb sound and mask undesirable noises. It creates a low-level noise so that a conversation in one room won't be heard in the next room. White noise can also be in the form of CDs that play sounds of waterfalls, thunderstorms, rain, and other nature sounds.
7. List several ways to save money in the medical office.
   - Physicians can save money in several ways when purchasing items for the office. Make sure that trash bags are completely full before taking trash out. Use refillable print cartridges and solar-powered calculators and adding machines. Print on both sides of paper when possible. Monitor ordering to determine where budget cuts could be made. Watch carefully for areas where money could be saved or items could be bought in bulk.
8. Explain the difference between medical waste and regular waste.
   - Medical waste includes any disposed-of item that was once a part of the human body or used to clean up blood or body fluids. Regular waste is any other trash that does not have to go into a biohazard waste container.
9. Explain why keys and alarm codes should be shared with only a few people.
   - The fewer people who know alarm codes and have keys, the easier it is to keep track of them. In addition, if fewer people have the codes and keys, there is less chance that someone will use them to enter the office and steal equipment and supplies.

CONNECTIONS

Study Guide Connection: Go to Chapter 12 Study Guide. Read the Case Study and Workplace Applications and complete the assignments. Do online research for answers to the questions in the Internet Activities associated with the office environment and daily operations.

CD Connection: Go to the Medical Assisting Competency Challenge CD and do the training activities under General Office Duties.

Evolve Connection: For more information related to the office environment and daily operations, go to http://evolve. elsevier.com/kinn/admin and visit related weblinks for Chapter 12. Click on the Medical Assisting Exam Review and do the practice questions to sharpen your test-taking skills. To learn more about office software, do the exercises for the Altapoint demo that is on the CD.

Written Communications and Mail Processing

13

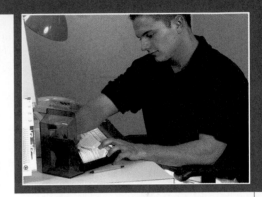

Brandon Tipps is a medical assistant working with his father, Dr. Rick Tipps. Brandon has considered continuing his education to become a doctor, but he is not sure whether he would like to be a medical doctor, an osteopathic physician, or a chiropractor. He decided to spend his summer off from college working in his father's family practice so that he could get a closer look at the inner workings of a physician's office.

Brandon has assisted with every procedure in the clinic, including the administrative skills required in the front office. The staff has been impressed with Brandon's ability to do any task, no matter how small, as if it were the most important task in the office. He continuously moves from employee to employee to ask what he can do to help. When the administrative medical assistant working in the front office, Darla Grover, was injured in a car accident and had to be off work for a while, Brandon stepped right in to do her job and quickly learned her duties. His help enabled the office to continue to run smoothly even with one employee absent for several weeks.

Brandon has an excellent command of the English language and types about 60 words per minute. He is organized and efficient, so he is able to handle the enormous amount of incoming and outgoing mail with very little assistance from the office manager. He is also able to answer phones and schedule appointments. He speaks clearly and is an expert at customer service. Many of Dr. Tipps' patients have known Brandon since he was a small child, and they enjoy seeing him helping in his father's office. The patients and staff alike will certainly miss him once he returns to college.

While studying this chapter, think about the following questions:

- What types of difficulties are faced when a physician's family member works at the office?
- How do proofreader's marks help the medical assistant to save time?

- What types of impressions could be formed by the receiver of mail from a physician's office?
- Explain why any written communication discussed in this chapter should be worded in a professional manner.

LEARNING OBJECTIVES

1. Define, spell, and pronounce the terms listed in the vocabulary.
2. Discuss the responsibility of the medical assistant with respect to equipment and supplies.
3. List the four common sizes of letterhead stationery.
4. Explain the various parts of speech.
5. Name some of the essential references for the medical assistant's library.
6. List several steps to complete before answering a business letter.
7. Discuss the process of developing and the value of keeping a communications portfolio.
8. Discuss the differences in the four letter styles.
9. Explain the four standard parts of a business letter.
10. List several ways to save money when mailing.
11. Open, sort, and annotate incoming mail.
12. Compose, proofread, and mail a business letter.
13. Properly send a fax.
14. Process incoming mail.
15. Address an envelope according to Postal Service optical character reader guidelines.

National Accreditation Competencies and Content

CAAHEP COMPETENCIES

General

3.c.(1)(a). Respond to and initiate written communications
3.c.(1)(b). Recognize and respond to verbal communications
3.c.(1)(c). Recognize and respond to nonverbal communications
3.c.(2)(d). Document appropriately

ABHES COMPETENCIES

Communication

2.g. Use appropriate medical terminology
2.h. Receive, organize, prioritize, and transmit information expediently
2.i. Recognize and respond to verbal and nonverbal communication
2.j. Use correct grammar, spelling, and formatting techniques in written works
2.k. Principles of verbal and nonverbal communication
2.l. Recognition and response to verbal and nonverbal communication
2.o. Fundamental writing skills

Administrative Duties

3.a. Perform basic secretarial skills
3.d. Apply computer concepts for office procedures

Legal Concepts

5b. Document accurately

VOCABULARY

academic degree A title conferred by a college, university, or professional school on completion of a program of study.

amiable (a′-me-uh-buhl) Having qualities that make one liked and easy to deal with.

annotating Furnishing with notes that are usually critical or explanatory.

archaic (ar-ka′-ik) Of, relating to, or characteristic of an earlier or more primitive time.

archived To have filed or collected records or documents.

bond A durable, formal paper used for documents.

categorically Placed in a specific division of a system of classification.

clauses Groups of words containing a subject and predicate and functioning as a member of a complex or compound sentence.

collect on delivery (COD) Method of payment used when an article or item is delivered and payment is expected before it is released.

concise (kun-sis′) Expressing much in brief form.

condescending Assuming an air of superiority.

continuation pages The second and following pages of a letter.

curt Marked by rude or peremptory shortness.

disseminate (di-se′-muh-nat) To disperse throughout.

domestic mail Mail that is sent within the boundaries of the United States and its territories.

flush Directly abutting or immediately adjacent, as set even with an edge of a type page or column; having no indention.

girth A measure around a body or item.

grammar The study of the classes of words, their inflections, and their functions and relations in the sentence; a study of what is to be preferred and what avoided in inflection and syntax.

international mail Mail that is sent outside the boundaries of the United States and its territories.

intrinsic (in-tri′-zik) Belonging to the essential nature or constitution of a thing; indwelling, inward.

mailpiece A piece of mail.

microfiche (mi′-kro-fish) A sheet of microfilm containing rows of microimages of pages of printed matter.

portfolio A set of pictures, drawings, documents, or photographs either bound in book form or loose in a folder.

ream A quantity of paper weighing 20 lb or consisting of, variously, 480, 500, or 516 sheets.

recipient The receiver of some thing or item.

stationers (sta′-shuh-nerz) Sellers of stationery.

substance number A number based on the weight of a ream of paper containing 500 sheets.

superfluous (suh-puhr′-flu-uhs) Exceeding what is sufficient or necessary.

watermark A marking in paper resulting from differences in thickness usually produced by the pressure of a projecting design in the mold or on a processing roll and visible when the paper is held up to the light.

Entrepreneur and co-founder of the Amway Corporation, Rich de Vos, believed in a simple principle regarding the many business papers that crossed his desk on a daily basis. He believed that each paper should be handled only once. Whatever the news, information, or action required, the paper should be dealt with immediately, and this resulted in the most efficient use of his time. This excellent idea is beneficial for any business, including the medical office.

Written correspondence and mail processing consumes a large part of the administrative medical assistant's day. Many physicians, when queried about the skills they most desire in an administrative assistant, say that a person who can spell accurately and write a good letter is a valuable addition to the medical office. When a physician delegates the responsibility of composing letters or reports that have the potential to reflect positively or negatively on the practice, he or she is expressing confidence in that medical assistant's abilities.

IMPORTANCE OF WRITTEN COMMUNICATIONS

Written communications offer the perfect opportunity for making a good impression on others, but they do not just happen. They require thought, preparation, skill, and a positive attitude. Written communications take many forms in the medical office. The medical assistant needs skills in creating various forms of communication.

Written communications include original letters, memorandums, replies to inquiries, responses to requests for information, telephone messages, email, transcriptions, orders for supplies, instructions for patients, and a variety of other forms. Communications that are courteous to the reader, correct in content, and **concise** without being **curt** are most appreciated. Communication is truly an art as well as a skill. The ability to communicate effectively is extremely important to the administrative medical assistant who wishes to succeed and advance his or her career.

CRITICAL THINKING APPLICATION

Brandon has just found a small backlog of correspondence that accumulated during the first 3 days that Darla was out of the office. A large amount of mail comes to the office each day. How can Brandon manage the daily mail and clear the pile of communications that accumulated over those 3 days?

WRITTEN COMMUNICATION AS A PUBLIC RELATIONS TOOL

Public relations involves "telling the organization's story." The public relations department or director of any organization exists to present a business in the best possible light and to communicate to the public and other interested parties all of the positive aspects of a business. With this understanding, it is easy to see why written communications are so important. These documents can present a professional image or a very poor image to the receiver. Individual medical offices rarely employ public relations professionals, so each member of the staff must be conscientious about the documents and materials that are present within and that leave the office. An envelope addressed carelessly or a patient information sheet that has been photocopied over and over insinuates that the office personnel are not concerned about the appearance of documents that leave the office. If the staff is careless in this respect, many patients will assume that the staff is careless with everything, including patient care.

REFLECTION ON THE PHYSICIAN

Everything that happens in the medical office is a reflection on the physician or physicians who practice there. Letters with misspelled words or errors will give the reader a negative impression of the physician and the practice itself. Great care must be taken to ensure that each document in the office and sent from the office is well written and grammatically correct. Table 13-1 lists proofreader's marks. Although these marks are usually used in copyediting, medical assistants who take the time to learn them will be able to process written communications twice as fast as those who make lengthy notes on documents that need revision or need an answer. Tables 13-2 and 13-3 list frequently misspelled and misused words.

WRITING SKILLS AND COMPOSING TIPS

Business letters are much different from the social letters that the medical assistant may have written. Social letters tend to be long and chatty and do not necessarily follow any organized plan. Most business letters should be less than one page in length and carefully organized (Procedure 13-1, p. 229). This takes practice and preparation. Every person who writes letters develops his or her own personal style.

The medical assistant should carefully read the letter to be answered. Make note of or underline any questions asked or materials requested. Then decide on the answers to the questions and verify the information. This is called **annotating.** Draft a reply, proofread it, then rewrite for clarity (Procedure 13-2, p. 230). Keep most of the sentences short. Put only one idea in each sentence, and eliminate **superfluous** words. Be careful about using medical terms in correspondence with patients. Instead, use language that the reader will easily understand.

Most physicians conform to a highly professional and formal style in their dictation. The medical assistant who is given the responsibility of composing correspondence for the medical office should strive for the same degree of formality used by the physician. It would be inappropriate for the assistant to write in a breezy, informal style when acting as the representative of an employer who has a more formal approach. The principal point to remember is that every letter produced in your office should project the image of the physician regardless of who composes or signs the letter.

Grammar Review

Good **grammar** is essential to writing effective, professional business letters. Medical assistants need an understanding of the elements of acceptable grammar and writing skills.

TABLE 13-1 Proofreader's Marks

Symbol or Margin Notation	Meaning	Example
ℒ or ℸ or ⅁	Delete	take it out
⌒	Close up	print as o ne word
ℒ	Delete and close up	cloₛse up
∧ or > or ⋏	Insert	insert here ⌐ (something
#	Insert a space	put one here
eg#	Space evenly	space evenly ∧ where indicated
stet	Let stand	let marked text stand as set
tr	Transpose	change order the
[	Set farther to left	⌐ too far to the right
]	Set farther to right	too⌐ far to the left
¶	Begin a new paragraph	the same is true. ¶In conclusion
(sp)	Spell out	set 5 lbs as five pounds
cap	Set in CAPITALS	set nato as NATO
lc	Set in lowercase	set South as south
ital	Set in *italic*	set oeuvre as *oeuvre*
bf	Set in **boldface**	set important as **important**
∨	Superscript or superior	∨ as in πr^2
∧	Subscript or inferior	∧ as in H_2O
⌄	Comma	red blue, and yellow
⌄	Apostrophe	Calvin's lizard was green.
⊙	Period	The end is near ⊙
; or ;/	Semicolon	1, this; 2, that
: or ⊡	Colon	is the following :
⸌⸍ or ⸜⸝	Quotation marks	He said, I did it.
( )	Parentheses	Run (fast) now.

Parts of Speech

Nouns. A noun is a person, place, or thing. Nouns can also be thoughts, ideas, or concepts, as in *freedom* or *courage*. Common nouns name general persons, places, or things, such as *teacher* and *city*. Proper nouns are specific, such as *Mrs. Adams* and *New York City*.

Pronouns. Pronouns replace nouns and provide the writer with shortcuts so that proper nouns do not have to be constantly repeated. Pronouns include words such as *it, you, he, she, her, his, them, mine, you, yours, its, ours,* and *theirs.*

Verbs. Verbs are action words that express movement, such as *runs, drove,* or *typed.* Linking verbs express a condition or state of being and include *is, am, are, was, be,* and *been.* Linking verbs also express the senses, as in *smell, hear, taste, touch, feel,* and *look.*

Adjectives. Adjectives are words that describe nouns and pronouns or may show which one, how many, and what kind

TABLE 13-2 One Hundred and Fifty Frequently Misspelled or Misused English Words

absence	corroborate	inimitable	persistent	ridiculous
accede	definitely	inoculate	personal	sacrilegious
accessible	description	insistent	personnel	seize
accommodate	desirable	irrelevant	possession	separate
achieve	despair	irresistible	precede	siege
affect	development	irritable	precedent	similar
agglutinate	dilemma	judgment	predictable	sizable
all right	disappear	labeled	predominant	stationary
altogether	disappoint	led	predominate	stationery
analyses (pl.)	disastrous	leisure	prerogative	subpoena
analysis (s.)	discreet	license	prevalent	succeed
analyze	discrete	liquefy	principal	suddenness
anoint	discriminate	maintenance	principle	superintendent
argument	dissatisfaction	maneuver	privilege	supersede
assistant	dissipate	miscellaneous	procedure	surprise
auxiliary	drunkenness	mischievous	proceed	tariff
balloon	ecstasy	misspell	professor	technique
believe	effect	necessary	pronunciation	thorough
benefited	eligible	newsstand	psychiatry	tranquility
brochure	embarrass	noticeable	psychology	transferred
bulletin	exceed	occasion	pursue	truly
category	exhilaration	occurrence	questionnaire	tyrannize
changeable	existence	oscillate	rearrange	unnecessary
clientele	February	paid	recede	until
committee	forty	pamphlet	receive	vacillate
comparative	grammar	panicky	recommend	vacuum
concede	grievous	parallel	referring	vicious
conscientious	height	paralyze	repetition	warrant
conscious	incidentally	pastime	rheumatism	Wednesday
coolly	indispensable	perseverance	rhythmical	weird

of. *A, an,* and *the* are special types of adjectives called articles. Examples of adjectives include a *golden* sunset, a *mangy* dog, and a *crooked* nose.

   Adverbs. Just as adjectives describe nouns, adverbs describe verbs, adjectives, or other adverbs. Adverbs specify when, where, to what extent, or how. Examples include *unusually* warm, *never* won, and *quite* cold.

   Prepositions. Connecting words that show a relationship between nouns, pronouns, or other words in a sentence are called prepositions. Examples of prepositions include *by, from, of, to, in, at, with, into,* and *on.*

   Conjunctions. Conjunctions join words or phrases. These helpful words include *and, or, nor,* and *but.*

   Interjections. Interjections show strong feeling. They are often followed by an exclamation point and sometimes by a comma. *"Ouch! That really hurt!"* is a sentence that uses an interjection.

Making Sense of Sentences

Sentence structure is important when writing a professional letter or document. The medical assistant should know the basics of good sentence structure so that written documents will make sense and represent the medical facility and staff in a positive way.

   Types of Sentences. The four basic sentence types are as follows: declarative, interrogatory, imperative, and exclamatory. Declarative sentences make a statement, whereas interrogatory sentences ask a question. Imperative sentences state a command or request. Exclamatory sentences express strong feeling. An example of each type follows:

TABLE 13-3 Frequently Misspelled Medical Words

abscess	defibrillator	intussusception	parietal	pruritus
additive	desiccate	ischemia	paroxysmal	psoriasis
aerosol	ecchymosis	ischium	pemphigus	pyrexia
agglutination	effusion	larynx	percussion	respiratory
albumin	epididymis	leukemia	perforation	rheumatic
anastomosis	epistaxis	malaise	pericardium	roentgenology
aneurysm	eustachian	malleus	perineum	sagittal
anteflexion	fissure	melena	peristalsis	sciatic
arrhythmia	flexure	mellitus	peritoneum	scirrhous
bilirubin	glaucoma	menstruation	petit mal	serous
bronchial	gonorrhea	metastasis	pharynx	sessile
cachexia	graafian	neurilemma	pituitary	sphincter
calcaneus	hemorrhage	neuron	plantar	sphygmomanometer
capillary	hemorrhoids	occlusion	pleura	squamous
cervical	homeostasis	optic chiasm	pleurisy	staphylococcus
chromosome	humerus	oscilloscope	pneumonia	suppuration
cirrhosis	idiosyncrasy	osseous	polyp	trochanter
clavicle	ileum	palliative	prophylaxis	venous
curettage	ilium	parasite	prostate	wheal
cyanosis	infarction	parenteral	prosthesis	xiphoid

Declarative — *She was the last person here.*
Interrogatory — *Are we going to the fair today?*
Imperative — *Clean your room before dinner.*
Exclamatory — *I am so excited for you!*

Sentence Structure. Sentences, when written correctly, follow certain patterns. Three very basic patterns are used in constructing sentences. These patterns are as follows:

- Subject-predicate
- Subject-object
- Subject-complement

The subject of a sentence is usually a noun and is the word or group of words in a sentence that acts, is acted on, or is described by the verb. The predicate is the part of the sentence that contains the verb and tells what the subject is doing or experiencing or what is being done to the subject. The object is a noun, pronoun, or group of words functioning as a noun or pronoun that receives the action of the verb. The complement is a word or group of words in the predicate of a sentence that renames or describes a subject or object in that sentence.

Sentence Errors. Three main sentence errors plague most writers. These include the sentence fragment, the run-on sentence, and the comma splice.

A sentence fragment is an incomplete thought or a portion of a sentence that is punctuated as though it were a complete sentence. An example follows:

Although the doctor had seen the patient.

A run-on sentence contains independent **clauses** without a semicolon, comma, or conjunction between them. These sentences are also called *run-together* or *fused* sentences. An example follows:

The office was clean when the staff left on Friday the doors were locked.

A comma splice is a sentence in which a comma alone joins independent clauses. An example follows:

The storm grew worse, it began to snow.

Personal Tools

Competent handling of written communications requires a basic knowledge of composition. A personal reference library that includes an up-to-date standard dictionary, a medical dictionary, a composition handbook, an English-language reference manual, and a thesaurus will be a tremendous help. The book *English Grammar for Dummies* by Geraldine Woods is actually used in many masters-level English courses and is extremely easy to understand. This helpful book would be a good addition to a personal tools list.

For those who have difficulty with spelling, keep a small loose-leaf indexed notebook or card index of words that are troublesome. When it is necessary to look up a word in the dictionary for spelling, record the word in the notebook or card index for quick reference. The physician or a medical assistant who is familiar with the practice might compile a basic list of frequently used medical terms and abbreviations as a reference.

PROCEDURE 13-1

Respond to and Initiate Written Communications: Compose Business Correspondence

CAAHEP COMPETENCY: 3.c.(1)(a)
ABHES COMPETENCY: 2.j

GOAL: *To compose a letter that will convey information in an accurate and concise manner and that is easy for the reader to comprehend.*

EQUIPMENT and SUPPLIES

- Computer or word processor
- Word processing software
- Draft paper
- Letterhead
- Printer
- Pen or pencil
- Highlighter
- Envelope
- Correspondence to be answered
- Other pertinent information needed to compose a letter
- Electronic or paper dictionary and thesaurus
- Writer's handbook
- Portfolio

PROCEDURAL STEPS

1. Determine the purpose of initiating correspondence or read through any correspondence to be answered, and highlight the specific questions that should be addressed.
   PURPOSE: To make certain that all of the issues raised in the correspondence are addressed or answered.
2. Make any necessary notes on the letter or a copy of the letter. A scrap sheet of paper may be used.
3. Prepare a draft of the letter using good grammar, and save it in the computer or word processor.
   PURPOSE: To put the thoughts on paper for later revision and make the letter easy to understand for the reader.
4. Proofread a printed copy of the letter, using proofreader's marks to make corrections.
   PURPOSE: To see the document as it will look once printed and to speed the process by using proofreader's marks.
5. Make any necessary corrections.
6. Allow the physician or other interested parties to proofread the letter, if the medical assistant is not the person whose signature will appear at the bottom.
   PURPOSE: To give the physician an opportunity to correct the letter and add additional thoughts, if desired.
7. Make any final changes, then print the letter on stationery. Allow the person whose name appears at the bottom to sign the letter.
8. Address the envelope using OCR guidelines, and place the letter and any supporting documents inside. (See Procedure 13-5 for using postal OCR guidelines.)
9. Mail the letter using correct postage.
   PURPOSE: Using incorrect postage or guessing can delay the arrival time of the document.

EQUIPMENT AND SUPPLIES

To create a favorable impression with letters, the medical assistant must use good equipment and high-quality supplies. Whatever kind of equipment is available, it is the medical assistant's responsibility to know how to use it to the best advantage and to keep it in good working condition. If the equipment manual is available, study it and keep it handy for reference when problems occur. Know how to maintain equipment so that the effort made in composing the correspondence results in a high-quality appearance.

Equipment

Computers

Computers have made composing correspondence simple. Various letters and documents may be saved and reused time after time by changing the name and basic information contained within the text. Computers can add graphics to text, compute figures, and use multimedia in communications—all of which enhance the appearance and effectiveness of the document.

Word Processors

Word processors are used mainly for letter writing and simple documents. The word processor has taken a backseat to today's desktop and notebook computers.

Typewriters

Typewriters, too, are becoming **archaic,** given the versatility of the computer. Most typewriters use correctable film ribbons that pass through the spool only one time. However, if the typewriter uses a cotton or silk ribbon that becomes lighter with use, be sure to change the ribbon before the resulting type impression becomes too light. The typewriter keys need to be cleaned frequently in typewriters that use a cotton ribbon.

Copiers

Maintain the copier so that copies are crisp and clear. The toner cartridge must be changed when necessary and can be expensive. Multiple copies of documents are usually made on a copier rather than printed from the computer.

PROCEDURE 13-2

Respond to and Initiate Written Communications: Proofread Documents for Accuracy

CAAHEP COMPETENCY: 3.c.(1)(a)
ABHES COMPETENCY: 2.j

GOAL: *To compose a clearly written, grammatically correct business letter that is easily understood by the reader, and to eliminate spelling and grammatic errors.*

EQUIPMENT and SUPPLIES

- Stationery
- Computer or typewriter
- Correspondence to be answered or notes
- Proofreader's marks guide

PROCEDURAL STEPS

1. Scan through the letter to be answered or the notes about the correspondence to be written and highlight any questions that should be answered or points to be made.
   PURPOSE: To ensure that the goals of the correspondence are fulfilled and no important points are omitted.
2. Write the letter using good grammar.
3. Print a draft copy of the letter. Read it carefully and highlight changes to be made or note any additions to be made. Use proofreader's marks.

PURPOSE: Seeing a hard copy of a letter is more conducive to finding errors and grammatic mistakes.

4. Revise the letter using the notes and proofreader's marks.
5. Read the letter once again on the screen. Complete spelling and grammar checks if those tools are available on the computer.
   PURPOSE: To locate any missed errors or misspelled words.
6. Print a final draft. Read the letter word for word, and check once again for errors.
7. Have another person proofread correspondence that is especially important.
   PURPOSE: Often another person can locate missed errors quickly.
8. Complete the final preparations for mailing the letter. Address the letter using guidelines for OCR and fast processing at the post office.

Scanners

Occasionally documents are scanned and sent by email. Scanners provide high resolution and can produce images of written text and photos. Scanners are often used to create images so that older documents can be stored, much like the **microfiche** systems of the past.

Supplies

Stationery

The quality of paper unquestionably affects the reader's total impression of the communication. **Stationers** or printing companies are qualified to advise on the selection of paper, which can range from all-sulfite (a wood pulp) to all-cotton fiber (sometimes called *rag)*. Letterhead paper is usually on **bond** with a 25% or higher cotton fiber content.

The weight of paper is described by a **substance number.** This number is based on the weight of a **ream** consisting of 500 sheets of 17- × 22-inch paper. The larger the substance number, the heavier the paper. If the ream weighs 24 lb, the paper is referred to as *Sub 24* or *24-lb weight.* Letterhead stationery and matching envelopes are usually 16-, 20-, or 24-lb weight. This is often abbreviated as 16#, 20#, or 24#.

Sizes and Types of Letterhead Paper. Letterhead paper is available in four basic sizes:

Standard or letter	$8^{1}/_{2} \times 11$ inches
Monarch or executive	$8^{1}/_{2} \times 10^{1}/_{2}$ inches
Baronial	$5^{1}/_{2} \times 8^{1}/_{2}$ inches
Legal	$8^{1}/_{2} \times 14$ inches

Standard letterhead is used for general business and professional correspondence. Monarch is often used by professional people for informal business and social correspondence. Baronial, which is a half-sheet of standard, is used for very short letters or memoranda. Legal, as its name indicates, is used for the lengthy documents presented in court or of a legal nature. Each size of letterhead should have its matching envelope.

Letterhead should be well designed and of a high-quality paper. The letter represents the sender, and the letterhead paper should be carefully chosen to promote the image that the sender wishes to convey. The paper itself makes a strong statement about the business or person it represents and can help the receiver form an impression of the professionalism of the business.

Bond paper has a felt side and a wire side. When a sheet of letterhead is picked up and held to the light, a design or letters can be read from the printed side. This design is called a **watermark** and is an indication of quality. The side from which the watermark can be read is the felt side of the paper and is the side on which printing or typing should be done. The watermark should always read across the page in the same direction as the typing.

Paper with a linen finish is so named because it is similar to fine cloth, with finely spaced lines crossing each other at right angles. Wove is a smooth paper that is normally inexpensive. Antique finish has a semismooth texture, and laid has a finish similar to that of corduroy. All of these paper finishes can make a very professional, impressive letterhead.

CRITICAL THINKING APPLICATION

Brandon realizes that his father's office does not have a method of logging letters sent by certified mail. This forces the receptionist to dig through a patient's file to determine if a certified mail was actually sent and the notice of delivery received. How can this issue be resolved?

Continuation Pages. The second and continuing pages of a letter are placed on plain bond that matches the letterhead in weight and fiber content and are called **continuation pages.** The stationery used for continuation pages should be an exact match to the letterhead, only without the letterhead printing. It is considered unprofessional to use different paper for the continuation pages.

Envelopes. Envelopes are usually made of the same paper as the letterhead stationery. Just as the continuation pages should be the same type of paper as the letterhead, so should the envelopes.

Envelopes also come in the following basic sizes or types:

- No. 10
- No. 6¾
- Window

No. 10 envelopes are the general business size used for letter and legal stationery. No. 6¾ envelopes and window envelopes are often used for statements.

LETTER STYLES

A business letter is usually arranged in one of three styles: block, modified block or standard, or modified block indented. A fourth style, called *simplified,* is occasionally used. The block and modified block styles are most commonly used in the physician's office.

Block Letter Style

When block letter style is used, all lines start **flush** with the left margin (Figure 13-1). This style is considered the most efficient but is less attractive on the page.

Modified Block Letter Style

The dateline, the complimentary closing, and the typewritten signature all begin at the center when typing in modified block letter style. All other lines begin at the left margin (Figure 13-2).

Modified Block Letter Style with Indented Paragraphs

The modified block letter style with indented paragraphs is identical to the block style except that the first line of each paragraph is indented five spaces (Figure 13-3).

Simplified Letter Style

With the simplified letter style, all lines begin flush with the left margin (Figure 13-4). The salutation is replaced with an

Elizabeth Blackwell, M.D.
223 Orange Avenue, N.W.
Cottonwood, UT 84121

January 26, 20—

Mr. Richard Fluege
3678 North Willow Avenue
Palm Beach, FL 33480

Dear Mr. Fluege:

Please send me full particulars on the professional suites you expect to offer for sale or rent in the Medical Arts Professional Annex.

In about six months, I will be ready to open my practice, and I am interested in locating in Florida. My preference is a street-level suite of approximately 2,000 square feet.

After I have had an opportunity to study the information you send me, I will write or telephone you if I have further questions.

Very truly yours,

Elizabeth Blackwell, M.D.

EB:mek

FIGURE 13-1 Block letter style.

MEDICAL ARTS PROFESSIONAL ANNEX
3678 North Willow Avenue
Palm Beach FL 33480

January 29, 20—

Elizabeth Blackwell, M.D.
223 Orange Avenue, N.W.
Cottonwood, UT 84121

Dear Doctor Blackwell:

We have two remaining street-level suites available for occupancy about July 1. These are marked on pages 3 and 4 of the enclosed descriptive brochure. If one of these suites appeals to you, we will be pleased to customize it for your practice.

Please feel free to call me collect at the number on the brochure for further discussion of your needs.

Sincerely yours,

Richard Fluege
Business Manager

RF:ab
Enclosure

FIGURE 13-2 Modified block letter style.

WILLIAM OSLER, M.D.
1000 South West Street
Park Ridge, NJ 07656

January 26, 20—

Robert Koch, M.D.
398 Main Street
Park Ridge, NJ 07656

Dear Doctor Koch:

Mrs. Elaine Norris

Thank you for referring your patient, Mrs. Elaine Norris, for consultation and care. She was examined in my office today.

FINDINGS: The patient complained of pain in the left lower quadrant and some abdominal tenderness. She had a temperature of 100.2 degrees.

RECOMMENDATIONS: The patient was placed on a soft, low-residue, bland diet, antibiotics, and bed rest for a few days. Upper and lower gastrointestinal x-rays will be performed next week.

TENTATIVE DIAGNOSIS: Diverticulitis of large bowel.

Mrs. Norris has been asked to return here for reevaluation in about ten days.

Sincerely yours,

William Osler, M.D.

WO:gm

FIGURE 13-3 Modified block letter style with indented paragraphs.

ROBERT KOCH, M.D.
398 Main Street
Park Ridge, NJ 07656

January 30, 20—

William Osler, M.D.
1000 South West Street
Park Ridge, NJ 07656

ANNABELLE ANDERSON

You will be pleased to know, Bill, that Mrs. Anderson is progressing nicely. Her wound is healing. Her temperature has returned to normal, and she is beginning to resume her usual activities.

Mrs. Anderson has an appointment to return here for one more visit next week. At that time, I will ask her to return to you for any further care.

ROBERT KOCH, M.D.

RK:hb

FIGURE 13-4 Simplified letter style.

all-capital subject line on the third line below the inside address. The body of the letter begins on the third line below the subject line. The complimentary closing is omitted. An all-capital typewritten signature is entered on the fifth line below the body of the letter.

Types of Punctuation for Letter Styles

Traditionally the punctuation pattern is selected on the basis of letter style. Normal punctuation is always used within the body of a business letter. The other parts use either standard or open punctuation.

When standard punctuation is used, a colon is placed after the salutation, and a comma is placed after the complimentary closing. This is the punctuation pattern most commonly used. It is appropriate with the block or modified block letter styles. When open punctuation is used, no punctuation is used at the end of any line outside the body of the letter unless that line ends with an abbreviation. This pattern is always used with the simplified letter style.

SPACING AND MARGINS

Generally a letter centered on a page is the most attractive. Accomplishing this is easy with today's computer programs, such as Microsoft Word or WordPerfect. Business letters are almost always single-spaced. If a letter consists of only a few lines, double-space both the inside address and the message and indent the first line of each paragraph five spaces.

The first typed entry, which is the date on the first page of the letter, is usually placed on the third line below the letterhead or on line 13 if there is no letterhead. The typing on continuation pages begins 1 inch from the top.

On standard letterhead, the side margins are usually $1\frac{1}{2}$ inches to 1 inch on each side. The appearance of a very short letter is improved by increasing the width of all margins.

A 1-inch bottom margin is the minimum. This can be increased if the letter is to be carried over to a second page. Never use a second page to type only the complimentary closing and signature. Carry over a minimum of two lines of the body of the letter onto a continuation page.

PARTS OF LETTERS

The structure of a letter and its placement on a page have been fairly well standardized into the following four main parts:
- Heading
- Opening
- Body
- Closing

Heading

The heading includes the letterhead and the dateline. The printed letterhead is usually centered at the top of the page and includes the name of the physician or group and the address. It may include the telephone number and the medical specialty or specialties. In a group or corporate practice, the names of the physicians may also be listed. Occasionally, the heading also includes the name of an office manager.

The dateline consists of the name of the month written in full, followed by the day and year. The date should not be abbreviated, nor should ordinal numbers (e.g., 1st, 2nd, and 3rd) be used after the name of the month.

Opening

The opening consists of the inside address, the salutation, and the attention line, if there is one. The inside address has two or more lines, starts flush with the left margin, and contains at least the name of the individual or firm to whom the letter is addressed and the mailing address. When the letter is addressed to an individual, the name is preceded by a courtesy title, such as Dr., Mr., Mrs., Miss, or Ms. When addressing a letter to a physician, omit the courtesy title and type the physician's name followed by his or her **academic degree,** such as *Rick P. Tipps, MD.* The name could also be written as *Dr. Rick P. Tipps.* Do not use both a courtesy title and a degree that means the same thing, as in *Dr. Rick P. Tipps, MD.* Although this construction is often seen, even on the sign in front of physician's' offices, it is wrong to write a doctor's name in this manner.

CRITICAL THINKING APPLICATION

Brandon has noticed that some of the correspondence leaving the office is signed incorrectly, with "Dr. Rick P. Tipps, MD" in the typed signature line. This is an uncomfortable situation because Brandon realizes that the person who is typing the signature this way is the office manager.

- How might he approach her so that the mistake can be corrected?
- Is it wise to approach the office manager, or should Brandon go to his father? Why or why not?

The salutation is the letter writer's introductory greeting to the person being addressed; it is typed flush with the left margin on the second line below the last line of the address and is followed by a colon unless open punctuation is used. The words in the salutation vary depending on the degree of formality of the letter.

The attention line, if used, is placed on the second line below the inside address. If the name of the person for whom the letter is intended is known, that person's name is used in the inside address and he or she is addressed personally. If the letter is being addressed to a company or organization and directed to a division or department within the company, the division or department name is placed on the attention line.

Body

The body of a letter includes the subject line, if one is used, and the message. In medical office correspondence, the subject of a letter is frequently a patient; in that instance, the patient's name is used as the subject line. Because the subject line is considered to be a part of the body of the letter, it is placed on the second line below the salutation. It may start flush with the left margin or at the point of indentation of indented paragraphs, or it may be centered. The word subject, followed by a colon, may be used or omitted entirely.

Begin typing the message on the second line below the subject line or on the second line below the salutation if there is no subject line. The first line of each paragraph may be indented five spaces or may start flush with the left margin, depending on the chosen letter style.

Closing

The closing includes the complimentary closing, the typed signature, the reference initials, and any special notations.

The complimentary closing is the writer's way of saying goodbye. This closing is placed on the second line below the last line of the body of the letter and is followed by a comma unless open punctuation is used. Only the first word is capitalized. The words used are determined by the degree of formality in the salutation. For example, if the salutation is *Dear Herb,* the closing might be *Cordially, Very truly yours,* or *Sincerely yours* with consistent punctuation. If the letter is addressed to a business, the complimentary closing most used is *Sincerely.*

A typewritten signature is a courtesy to the reader, especially if the name does not appear on the printed letterhead or if the personal signature is difficult or impossible to decipher. The typewritten signature is placed on the fourth line directly below the complimentary closing.

Reference initials that identify the typist are placed flush with the left margin on the second line below the typewritten signature. If the writer's name is included on the signature line, the writer's initials need not be included in the reference block unless desired. The writer's initials, if used, should precede the typist's initials and are separated by a colon or diagonal line. Examples include *mek, GB:mek,* and *GB/mek.*

Special notations are sometimes needed to indicate that enclosures are included with the letter or that copies of the letter are being distributed to others. If the letter indicates an enclosure, type the word *Enclosure* or *Enc.* on the first line below the reference initials. If there is more than one enclosure, specify the number (e.g., *Enclosures 3*). If copies are to be sent to others, type this notation in the same manner as the enclosure notation or after it if both notations are needed. The copy notation is usually written as *cc:* or *copy to:* followed by the name or names of those to whom a copy will be sent. If the person to whom the letter is addressed is not to know that copies are being distributed to others, use the notation *bc:* for "blind copy" on all copies except the original. Place this notation either in the upper left of the letter at the margin or below the last notation at the lower left margin.

Postscripts

Although a postscript may sometimes be used to express an afterthought, it is often used to place emphasis on an idea or statement. Begin the postscript on the second line below the last special notation. Follow the style of the letter, indenting the first line if paragraphs were indented in the body of the letter or starting at the margin if indentation was not used in the letter.

Continuation Pages

If the letter requires one or more continuation pages, the heading of the second and subsequent pages must contain the following three items of information:

- The name of the addressee
- The page number
- The date

The heading should begin on the seventh line from the top of the page. Continuation of the body of the letter begins on the tenth line or the third line below the heading. The three accepted forms for the continuation page heading are as follows:

RICK P. TIPPS, M.D.

Page 2

July 5, 2003

Rick P. Tipps, M.D.

Page 2

July 5, 2003

Subject: Susan Clemmons

Rick P. Tipps, M.D.   -2-   July 5, 2003

Signing the Letter

Some physicians prefer to compose and sign all letters that leave their offices. The majority are more than pleased to delegate to a competent assistant the responsibility of composing and signing letters of a business nature. Although not all authorities agree on the form to be followed, most recommend that a woman's typewritten signature includes a courtesy title (Miss, Mrs., or Ms.) and that the title not be enclosed in parentheses. It is not necessary to include the courtesy title in the handwritten signature.

In general, the physician signs all of the following:

- Letters that deal with medical advice to patients
- Letters to officers or committees of the medical society
- Referral and consultation reports to colleagues
- Medical reports to insurance companies
- Personal letters

The medical assistant usually composes and signs letters dealing with the following matters:

- Routine matters such as arranging or rescheduling appointments
- Orders for office supplies
- Notification to patients about surgery or hospital arrangements
- Collection of delinquent accounts
- Letters of solicitation

CRITICAL THINKING APPLICATION

One of the employees has brought an urgent letter to Brandon that Brandon's father neglected to sign before leaving the office for the

Continued

day. The letter is to another physician reporting his findings on a referred patient. The employee asks Brandon to sign the letter. What should he do? What are some ways to resolve this situation, if the letter must leave in the mail today?

MORE TYPES OF WRITTEN COMMUNICATIONS

There are many types of written communications other than a business letter. Remember, every piece of written communication that leaves the office is a reflection on the office. Make certain to follow the rules of grammar even when sending a simple business email.

Telephone Messages

One of the most common types of written communications in the medical office is the telephone message. Seven items must be recorded when taking a phone message, including the following:

- The name of the person to whom the call is directed
- The name of the person calling
- The caller's daytime and/or cell phone number
- The reason for the call
- The action to be taken
- The date and time of the call
- The initials of the person taking the call

Email Messages

Email is a very popular way to send written communications in today's computer-literate society. Email messages can be saved, printed for the patient's chart, and **archived** for storage. Emails that are pertinent to the patient's care or a conflict situation should be printed, and a copy placed in the patient's medical record. Emails that show a pattern of cancelled appointments should also be added to the patient's medical record. Any email sent in a professional capacity from the physician's office or by a physician's representative should adhere to proper rules of grammar and should use accurate spelling. People tend to classify email as casual communication, but because it is so frequently used in business, it should be considered just as professional as a mailed letter. Use of the proper letter format, including the inside addresses and date, is not necessary. However, the rest of the email should read similarly to a letter. Some emails are only one-line responses, but they can still be grammatically correct.

The medical assistant should also avoid the tendency to immediately answer an email that is derogatory, accusatory, or negative in some other way. Print the email and go through it calmly, marking what needs to be addressed. Because attitude is often easily detectable in an email, avoid any hint of negativity in the response. Once a professional response has been crafted, then type and send it. In this situation, it is often best to cc: the office manager, either openly or blindly, depending on the situation. By doing this the medical assistant is including the supervisor in the conflict and keeping him or her aware of the brewing situation. If necessary the office manager will get involved, or he or she may just monitor the situation and how it is handled by the medical assistant.

Faxed Messages

Faxes are another form of written communication. All faxes should have a cover sheet that states that the information contained within it is of a confidential nature and is intended only for the person to whom the fax was sent (Procedure 13-3). Use correct grammar in all faxed messages. Use a fax only when absolutely necessary or when the information sent would not breach patient confidentiality. This helps to avoid other individuals on the receiving end from reading faxed information.

Memorandums

Most offices **disseminate** various memorandums throughout the business week (Figure 13-5). These written documents must also be clear, concise, and grammatically correct. Remember that people reading memos, emails, faxes, and letters can often detect attitudes in written communications, so make the document sound professional, even if the subject matter is frustrating or difficult.

When sending emails to employees, make certain that the important points are all included and presented in a way that does not sound **condescending**. Sometimes, it is wise to include a supervisor's initials on memos that might not receive a positive response, so that employees realize that the writer's supervisor is aware of and supports the information in the memo. This action sometimes avoids a rush to the boss's office to complain about the contents of a memo.

CRITICAL THINKING APPLICATION

- Email is used more and more often to communicate with employees. Brandon has noticed that very few printed memos circulate throughout the office. What are the advantages and disadvantages of communicating through email with employees?
- The office manager has given Brandon information to disseminate to all of the employees of the clinic. She did not specify whether to give out the memo by hand or by email but did state that the information was very important. Which would be the best method?

DEVELOPING A PORTFOLIO

Letter composition can be sped up by developing a **portfolio** of sample letters to suit the various situations that frequently arise. As the physician approves letters, add them to the office portfolio. Suppose, for instance, a letter is needed for a patient who wishes to change an appointment. Compose a letter that is clear, concise, and courteous—and make an extra copy to place in the portfolio of letters. Alternatively, if using a computer, store the letter on a disk or on the computer's hard drive. If letters and other documents are stored on the hard drive, be sure to back the files up on disk or a zip drive. Do this each time a new kind of letter is written. Soon the medical assistant will be able to select a letter from the portfolio and change it slightly to suit the current situation. This will make letter writing in the medical office quick and easy.

PROCEDURE 13-3

Respond to and Initiate Written Communications: Prepare a Fax for Transmission

CAAHEP COMPETENCY: 3.c.(1)(a)

GOAL: *To send a fax from the medical office and ensure that it arrives at its destination in a confidential manner.*

EQUIPMENT and SUPPLIES

- Fax machine
- Fax cover sheet
- Correspondence to be sent

PROCEDURAL STEPS

1. Fill out a fax cover sheet. Include the name of the person sending the fax and that person's phone number. List the name of the person to receive the fax and the fax number to which the document is being sent. Use cover sheets that contain a confidentiality statement.
   PURPOSE: To identify a fax that has been misdirected and to ensure that it goes to the right person when it arrives.

2. Note the number of pages that are being sent, including the cover page.
   PURPOSE: To ensure that all pages are received.

3. Turn the last page upside down, and write the fax number on the top of the document. Many machines require the documents to be in place before the fax is started. This allows the user to see the number without having to memorize it and make an error.
   PURPOSE: To see the fax number clearly once the pages have been placed in the fax machine.

4. Follow the instructions for individual fax machines.

5. Be sure the machine is set to provide a verification that the fax went through. Print the verification and attach it to the fax. Verify the arrival of critical fax documents by phone.
   PURPOSE: To document that the fax arrived at its destination.

6. File the fax and verification sheet in the appropriate location.
   PURPOSE: To maintain a record of information sent via fax.

INTEROFFICE MEMORANDUM

TO   All Staff

FROM   Office Manager

DATE   December 1

SUBJECT   Holiday Schedule

Our entire facility will be closed on December 24, December 25, December 31, and January 1. The office will be on reduced staff during the days of December 26, 27, 28, 29, and 30. Assignments will be based on seniority of staff members. Please submit your preferences as soon as possible.

A

MEMO TO: George Walker

FROM: Stanley Barr

DATE: February 8

SUBJECT: Office rental

We are experiencing unexpectedly rapid growth in our business office and will soon need additional space for our increased number of employees. Do you have a larger facility available in this building? If so, I would like to hear from you regarding the location, square footage, and anticipated rental costs.

B

FIGURE 13-5 Examples of memorandums. Memos are intended to be short, specific, and to the point.

U.S. POSTAL SERVICE

The U.S. Postal Service (USPS) is an independent establishment of the executive branch of the U.S. government. The organization is not a part of the government but was established by the government and operates independently. Established on July 26, 1775, by the Second Continental Congress, the organization we know as the USPS is the second oldest federally established department or agency in the United States.

The Postal Service has transformed from messages sent to neighbors in colonial times to a service dedicated to providing mail service to every single home and business in the United States. Today, many operations can be done online at www. usps.com.

MAIL PROCESSING

Incoming Mail

Each day, a great variety of mail comes into the professional office and must be processed. Common items in the daily mail include the following:

- General correspondence
- Payments for services
- Bills for office purchases
- Insurance claim forms to be completed
- Laboratory reports
- Hospital reports
- Medical society mailings

- Professional journals
- Promotional literature and samples from pharmaceutical houses
- Advertisements

In large clinics and medical centers the mail is opened by specially designated people in a central department to speed up this daily task. In the average medical office, however, a medical assistant, often the receptionist, opens the mail using the ordinary letter-opener method.

Opening the Mail

Before opening any mail the medical assistant should have an agreement with the physician as to what procedure to follow regarding incoming mail—in other words, what letters should be opened and what pieces, if any, the physician prefers to open personally. For example, the physician may prefer to open any communications from an attorney or accountant, even when they are not marked personal. If there is any doubt with regard to opening an envelope, do not open the item and forward it to the person to whom it is addressed. Even a simple procedure such as opening the daily mail can be done with more efficiency if a good system is followed (Procedure 13-4).

Annotating

Annotating the mail is an additional service the medical assistant can perform. Reading each letter through, underlining the significant words and phrases, and noting in the margin any action required make taking action on the mail much easier. If the letter needs no reply, code it for filing at this

PROCEDURE 13-4

Respond to and Initiate Written Communications: Process Incoming Mail

CAAHEP COMPETENCY: 3.c.(1)(a)
ABHES COMPETENCY: 2.h

GOAL: *To efficiently sort through the mail that arrives in the medical office on a daily basis.*

EQUIPMENT and SUPPLIES

- Computer or word processor
- Draft paper
- Letterhead stationery
- Pen or pencil
- Highlighter
- Staple remover
- Paper clips
- Letter opener
- Stapler
- Transparent tape
- Date stamp

PROCEDURAL STEPS

1. Clear a working space on the desk or countertop.
2. Sort the mail according to importance and urgency:
   - Physician's personal mail
   - Ordinary first-class mail
   - Checks from insurance companies and patients
   - Periodicals and newspapers
   - All other pieces, including drug samples.

   PURPOSE: To prioritize the mail for the physician so that the most important issues can be addressed first.

3. Open the mail neatly and in an organized manner.
4. Stack the envelopes so that they are all facing in the same direction.
5. Pick up the top one and tap the envelope so that when you open it you will not cut the contents.
   PURPOSE: To avoid damaging any of the contents inside the envelope.
6. Open all envelopes along the top edge for easiest removal of contents.
7. Remove the contents of each envelope, and hold the envelope to the light to see that nothing remains inside.
8. Make a note of the postmark when this is important.
9. Discard the envelope after you have checked to see that there is a return address on the message contained inside. Some offices make it a policy to attach the envelope to each piece of correspondence until it has received attention.
10. Date-stamp the letter, and attach any enclosures.
    PURPOSE: The date stamp identifies when the envelope and its contents was received at the office.
11. If there is an enclosure notation at the bottom of the letter, ensure that the enclosure was included. If it is missing, indicate this on the notation by writing the word *no* and circling it. This may be as far as your employer will want you to proceed with handling the correspondence.

---

time. A highlighter that does not photocopy may be used for annotating. When mail refers to previous correspondence, obtain this from the file and attach it or a copy. If the patient's chart is needed when replying to an inquiry, pull the chart and place it with the letter.

There should be a specific place for the opened and annotated mail in the medical office. This will probably be some area on the physician's or office manager's desk. After sorting, opening, and annotating the mail, place those items that the physician will wish to see in the established place, with the most important mail on top. Personal mail, of course, is to remain unopened. If a piece of personal mail addressed to the employer is opened in error, fold and replace it inside the envelope, and write across the outside *opened in error,* followed by the initials of the person who opened the mail. Use the same procedure with a piece of mail addressed to another office that may have been opened in error. In such cases reseal the envelope with transparent tape and hand it to the mail carrier.

Responding to the Mail

In some offices, the physician and the medical assistant go over the mail together. Once the medical assistant gains

confidence, he or she will find it easy to draft a reply to most inquiries. Usually, the physician is very pleased to delegate this responsibility, especially for matters that do not relate to patient care.

Letters of referral from other physicians should be carefully noted so that an answer can be sent after the patient has been seen and the physician can give a report. If considerable time may pass before such information can be sent, it is a courteous gesture to write a letter to the referring physician advising that a detailed report will follow. Some physicians send printed cards expressing thanks for referrals; others prefer to write thank-you letters to professional colleagues.

Mail Requiring Special Handling

Payment Receipts

Payments from patients and insurance companies will come to the office on a daily basis. All payments should be separated and recorded immediately in the day's receipts. A payment received on Monday should be recorded on Monday. Most patients consider their cancelled check as a receipt; if the patient requests a receipt, one should be mailed. Otherwise, the receipt may be placed in the patient's chart for delivery on a future office visit.

Insurance Information

Insurance information should be put in a predetermined place for handling by the billers. Documents relating to insurance should be passed to the appropriate person immediately to avoid delays and time limitations that might cause the claim to go unpaid.

Drug Samples

Sample drugs and related literature are usually delivered by pharmaceutical representatives and may occasionally arrive in the mail. Determine from the physician what types of literature and samples should be saved. Most physicians keep pertinent new samples in a locked sample storage area, along with the accompanying literature for immediate reference. Other drug samples are **categorically** stored. Drugs should never be tossed into the trash.

Vacation Mail

When the physician is away from the office, it is generally the responsibility of a medical assistant to handle all mail. In this event, all pieces should be examined carefully. The medical assistant can then decide how to handle each piece based on the following questions:

- Is this important enough that I should phone or fax the physician?
- Shall I forward this for immediate attention?
- Shall I answer this myself or send a brief note to the correspondent, explaining that there will be a slight delay because the physician is out of the office?
- Can this wait for attention until the physician returns, or would that give the appearance of negligence?

If the medical assistant is unable to contact the physician or to forward important mail, he or she should always answer the sender immediately, explaining the delay and requesting cooperation. Instead of forwarding an original piece of mail and risking possible loss, make a copy for forwarding. Then, if the physician wishes the letter answered, notations can be made on the copy and then the copy may be returned to the office staff for answering and returned without defacing the original letter.

When the physician is traveling from place to place, the envelopes for all communications sent to him or her should be numbered consecutively. Doing this enables the physician to easily determine whether any mail has been lost or delayed. By keeping a record of each piece of mail sent out, with its corresponding number, anything that might be lost can be identified and remailed if necessary.

Correspondence not requiring immediate action that the medical assistant is unable to answer until the physician returns should be placed in a special folder marked *Requires Attention* and placed on top of other accumulated mail. Mail that the medical assistant can compose but that requires the physician's approval before mailing should be put into another special folder marked *For Approval*. When the physician returns, these letters can be rapidly checked and signed.

Any letters marked *Personal* may be acknowledged to the return address on the envelope. The brief acknowledgment should state that the physician is out of town for a certain length of time and will attend to the letter immediately on returning. This acknowledgment should also offer help in any way possible in the meantime.

Discard any mail that would ordinarily not be brought to the physician's attention. Some promotional literature falls into this category. Make certain that mailings from professional organizations are saved.

There may be rare periods during which the entire facility is closed. In such cases the post office can be contacted to hold mail until the facility reopens. The postal carrier cannot accept an oral request, so a formal written request must be made. Never leave mail unattended to gather outside a mailbox or clutter up a doorway in a hall. Even mail slots may become filled, or magazines may become stuck in them, causing important mail to pile up outside the slot. Far too much money and mail of a confidential nature are sent to physicians' offices to take chances on mail theft or destruction.

Outgoing Mail

Folding and Inserting Letters

Standard ways of folding and inserting letters are used so that the letter fits properly into the envelope and so that it can be easily removed without damage (Figure 13-6).

No. 10 Envelope. Bring the bottom third of the standard-sized letter up and make a crease. Fold the top of the letter down to within about $3/8$ inch of the creased edge, and make a second crease. The second crease goes into the envelope first.

No. $6^3/4$ Envelope. For a standard-sized letter, bring the bottom edge up to within about $3/8$ inch of the top edge and make a crease. Then, folding from the right edge, make a fold a little less than one third of the width of the sheet and crease it. Folding from the left edge, bring the edge to within about $3/8$ inch of the previous crease. Insert the left creased edge into the envelope first.

Window Envelope. To fold a letter for insertion into a window envelope, bring the bottom third of the letter up and make a crease, then fold the top of the letter back to the crease you made before. The inside address should now be facing forward. This method is often followed for mailing statements.

Addressing the Envelope

Delivery Addresses. The USPS attempts to have all mail in standard-sized envelopes read, coded, sorted, and canceled automatically at regional sorting stations where mail can be

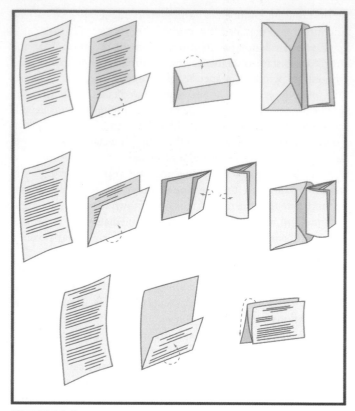

FIGURE 13-6 Correct methods of folding letters.

processed at a rate of over 30,000 letters per hour. The success of automatic sorting depends on the cooperation of mailers in preparing envelopes in a format that can be read by automatic equipment (Procedure 13-5).

Many regulations affect delivery addresses, because this is the most important information on the envelope. The goal of the **mailpiece** is to get delivered.

The Postal Service provides three special sets of abbreviations: (1) state names; (2) long names of cities, towns, and places; and (3) names of streets and roads and general terms, such as University or Institute. The information can be obtained from the Postal Service, or a program can be purchased for the computer. When these abbreviations are used, it is possible to limit the last line of any **domestic mail** address to 27 strokes. The next-to-last line in the address block should contain a street address or post office box number.

The address block should start no higher than 2³/₄ inches from the bottom. Leave a bottom margin of at least ³/₈ inch and left and right margins of at least 1 inch. Nothing should be written or printed below the address block or to the right of it.

The regulations for addressing envelopes were developed mainly for volume mailers with computerized mailing lists (Figure 13-7, p. 243). Some exceptions are acceptable to the Postal Service and its scanning equipment. For example, the traditional style of typing an address in lower case with initial capital letters is readable by the optical scanners. Also, if the ZIP code cannot fit on the line with the city and state, it can be placed on the line immediately below. When using a suite number, most people place it after the delivery address, which is fine. However, if it does not fit in that space, it should be placed *above* the delivery address, not below it.

Return Addresses. Always place a complete return address on the envelope. If there is no stamp on the envelope or if the stamp falls off and there is no return address, it will go to the dead letter office. There, the postal employees will open the mail in an attempt to identify the sender, but huge time delays may make the mail useless on delivery. If an address is found for the sender, the mail will be returned in an official envelope with a notice of postage due. If an address is not found for the sender, the mail is destroyed.

Notations. Any notations on the envelope directed toward the addressee, such as Personal or Confidential, should be typed and underlined on line 9 or on the third line below the return address, whichever is lower. Align it with the return address on the left edge of the envelope.

Any notations directed toward the Postal Service, such as special delivery or Certified Mail, should be typed in all capital letters on the upper right side of the envelope immediately below the stamp area. If an address contains an attention line, it should be typed above the organization line or on the line immediately above the street address or post office box number.

Sealing and Stamping Hints

Here is a suggestion for speeding up the sealing of a number of envelopes—at statement time, for example, when many envelopes go into the mail at one time:

- Fan out unsealed envelopes, address side down, in groups of six to 10.
- Draw a damp sponge over the flaps, and starting with the lower piece, turn down the flaps and seal each one.

Do not use too much moisture because this may cause the glue to spread and several envelopes to stick together. A similar process simplifies stamping several letters at one time if not using a postage meter. If possible, purchase stamps by the roll. Tear off about ten stamps from the roll. Fanfold the stamps on the perforations so that they separate easily. Fan the envelopes address side up. Wet a strip of stamps with the sponge and, starting at one end of the fanned envelopes, attach the stamp at the end of the strip, tear it off, and proceed to the next envelope. Automated sealers and stampers are also available to make this procedure easier and more efficient.

Cost-Saving Mailing Procedures

Using ZIP Codes. The ZIP code is a very important part of an address, just as the area code is a very important part of a telephone number. ZIP codes start with the number 0 on the East Coast and gradually increase to number 9 on the West Coast and in Hawaii.

The five-digit ZIP code was introduced in 1961. The first three digits identify a major city or distribution point, and all five digits identify an individual post office, zone of a city, or other delivery unit. The Postal Service later developed the nine-digit ZIP code, consisting of the original five digits followed by a hyphen and four additional digits that further identify the addressee's street location. The ZIP code is electronically transformed into a bar code. The office computer may have this

Basic U.S. Postal Service Delivery Address Guidelines

- Always put the address and the postage on the same side of your mailpiece.
- On a letter the address should be parallel to the longest side.
- Use the following:
  - All capital letters
  - No punctuation
  - At least 10-point type
  - One space between city and state
  - Two spaces between state and ZIP code
  - Simple type fonts
  - Left-justified format
  - Black ink on white or light paper
  - No reverse type (white printing on a black background)
- If your address appears inside a window, make sure there is at least ⅛ inch clearance around the address. Sometimes parts of the address slip out of view behind the window, and mail processing machines can't read the address.
- If you are using address labels, make sure you don't cut off any important information. Also make sure your labels are on straight. Mail processing machines have trouble reading crooked or slanted information.

More Tips

- Always put the attention line on top—never below the city and state or in the bottom corner of your mailpiece.
- If you can't fit the suite or apartment number on the same line as the delivery address, put it on the line *above* the delivery address, *not* on the line below.

From the U.S. Postal Service website.

- Words like "east" and "west" are called *directionals* and they are *very* important. A missing or a bad directional can prevent your mail from being delivered correctly.
- Use the free ZIP code Lookup and the ZIP+4 code lookup on the Postal Service website to find the correct ZIP codes and ZIP+4 codes for your addresses.
- Almost 25% of all mailpieces have something wrong with the address—for instance, a missing apartment number or a wrong ZIP code. Can some of those mailpieces be delivered in spite of the incorrect address? Yes. But it costs the Postal Service time and money to do that.
- When a first-class-mail letter weighs 1 oz or less and the address is parallel to the shortest side, the piece may be nonmailable or will be charged the nonmachineable surcharge.
- Sometimes it is not important that your mailpiece reach a specific customer, just that it reach an address. One way to do this is to use a generic title such as "Postal Customer" or "Occupant" or "Resident," rather than a name, plus the complete address.
- Fancy fonts such as those used on wedding invitations do not read well on mail processing equipment. Fancy fonts look great on your envelopes but also may slow down your mail.
- Use common sense. If you can't read the address, then automated mail processing equipment can't read the address.
- Some types of paper interfere with the machines that read addresses. The paper on the address side should be white or light in color. No patterns or prominent flecks, please! Also, the envelope shouldn't be too glossy—avoid shiny, coated paper stock.

---

capability. The Postal Code claims that the ZIP-plus-4, when used with the automated letter-sorting machinery, can eliminate 20 mail-handling steps and result in considerable savings. This saving is passed on to bulk mailers on mailings of 250 or more pieces that have typewritten addresses in machine-readable format along with the nine-digit ZIP code.

Presorting. Bulk mailers can get a discount on postage for presorting their mail. A discounted presort rate is charged on each piece that is part of a group of 10 or more pieces sorted to the same five-digit code or a group of 50 or more pieces sorted to ZIP codes with the same first three digits. The USPS uses the words "presorting" and "bulk" interchangeably.

Using Correct Postage. Although mailing fees are still one of our better bargains, the mailing costs for even a small office are a sizable item in the annual budget, and carelessness can cause them to soar. If the facility does not have a postage meter that dispenses postage exactly, then be sure that you are not putting too many stamps on your outgoing mail. Use an accurate postage scale and remember that only the first ounce requires the base rate; additional ounces are at a lower rate. Remember, the USPS will not deliver mail without postage.

Getting Faster Mail Service

Postage Meters. The postage meter is the most efficient way of stamping the mail in a large business office (Figure 13-8, p. 244). It can print postage onto adhesive strips that are then placed onto the envelopes or packages, or it can print the postage directly onto an envelope. Metered mail does not have to be canceled or postmarked when it reaches the post office. This means that it can move on to its destination faster. Meters vary in size and capabilities. Consult an office-equipment dealer for information on postage meters.

CRITICAL THINKING APPLICATION

- Brandon knows that the mail processing would go much faster if the office invested in a postage meter. The office manager states that she has mentioned this to Brandon's father several times, but he did not purchase a meter. How might Brandon approach his father about this issue?
- What should Brandon do before discussing the postage meter with his father?

PROCEDURE 13-5

Respond to and Initiate Written Communications: Address an Envelope According to Postal Service Optical Character Reader Guidelines

CAAHEP COMPETENCY: 3.c(1)(a)
ABHES COMPETENCY: 2.j

GOAL: *To correctly address business correspondence so that the mail arrives at and is processed by the U.S. Postal Service as efficiently as possible.*

EQUIPMENT and SUPPLIES

- Envelopes
- Computer or typewriter
- Correspondence

PROCEDURAL STEPS

1. Place the envelope into the printer or typewriter.
2. Enter the word processing program, such as Microsoft Word, and check the "Tools" section for envelopes. If this is not available in the word processing program or if a typewriter is being used, judge the area on the envelope that can be read by the optical character reader (OCR). The address block should start no higher than $2^3/_4$ inches from the bottom. Leave a bottom margin of at least $5/_8$ inch and left and right margins of at least 1 inch. Nothing should be written or printed below the address block or to the right of it.
   PURPOSE: To ensure the correct placement of the address for accurate reading by the OCR.
3. Use dark type on a light background and no script or italics, and capitalize everything in the address.
   PURPOSE: To ensure that the OCR can read the address.
4. Type the address in block format, using only approved abbreviations and eliminating all punctuation. If a suite number is to be included, type it above the delivery address on a separate line.
5. Type the city, state, and ZIP code on the last line of the address.
6. No line should have more than 27 total characters, including spaces.
7. Leave a $5/_8$-inch by $4^3/_4$-inch space blank in the bottom right corner of the envelope.
   PURPOSE: To allow for bar code scanning (BCS).
8. Mail addressed to other countries includes the city and postal code on the third line, and the name of the country on a fourth line.

Mailing Practices. For large mailings, local letters should be separated from out-of-town letters. Letters or packages that need to be rushed should be taken directly to the post office for mailing. Others can be placed in street boxes or the building's mail chute for pickup. Packages should always be taken to a post office and weighed for proper postage. Place a letter tray on the desk or some other convenient place so that all outgoing mail is kept together until it is ready to leave the office.

Classifications of Mail

Mail is classified according to type, weight, and destination. The ounce and pound are the units of measurement. Domestic mail is sent to a destination within the United States and its territories, and **international mail** is sent to a destination outside the United States. Letters to distant points of the globe are in almost all cases sent by air and can be expected to reach their destination within a few days. The rates for international mail are based on increments of $1/_2$ to 1 ounce. A table of rates can be obtained from the post office.

Express Mail. Express Mail is available 7 days per week, 365 days per year for items weighing up to 70 lb and measuring 108 inches in combined length and **girth.** This includes delivery on Sundays and holidays. It is the fastest mail service offered by the USPS. Service features include the following:

- Noon delivery between major business markets
- Merchandise and document reconstruction insurance
- Express mail shipping containers
- Shipment receipt
- Optional return receipt service
- Optional **collect-on-delivery (COD)** service
- Waiver of signature option
- Collection boxes
- Optional pickup service

First-Class Mail. First-class mail includes sealed or unsealed handwritten or typed material, such as letters, postal cards, postcards, and business reply mail. Postage for letters weighing 13 ounces or less is based on weight, in 1-ounce increments. Envelopes larger than the standard No. 10 business envelope should have the green diamond border to expedite first-class delivery. The minimum quantity to mail at discount prices is 500 mailpieces. First-class mail over 13 ounces automatically becomes Priority Mail. At the time of this publishing, first-class stamps cost $0.39 cents.

Priority Mail. First-class mail weighing over 13 ounces is classified as Priority Mail, and the postage is calculated on the basis of weight and destination, with the maximum weight being 70 lb. A few tips about Priority Mail include the following:

- If using an envelope or box not purchased from the USPS, make certain to mark it *Priority Mail.*
- Priority mail drop shipment is a special way to get mail delivered sooner. Sacks or trays of standard mail are sent to the post office nearest the zip code for delivery, then sent via standard mail.

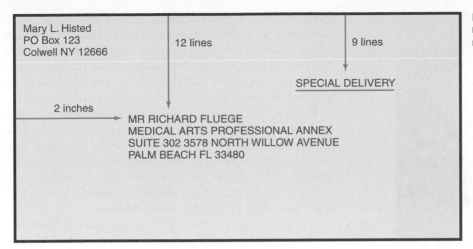

Mary L. Histed
PO Box 123
Colwell NY 12666

12 lines

9 lines

Placement of return address, mailing address, and mailing notation on 6³/₄ envelope

SPECIAL DELIVERY

2 inches

MR RICHARD FLUEGE
MEDICAL ARTS PROFESSIONAL ANNEX
SUITE 302 3578 NORTH WILLOW AVENUE
PALM BEACH FL 33480

Placement of mailing address and personal notation on No. 10 envelope

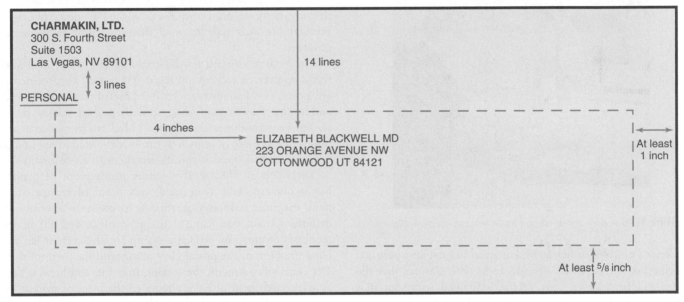

CHARMAKIN, LTD.
300 S. Fourth Street
Suite 1503
Las Vegas, NV 89101

14 lines

3 lines

PERSONAL

4 inches

ELIZABETH BLACKWELL MD
223 ORANGE AVENUE NW
COTTONWOOD UT 84121

At least 1 inch

At least ⁵/₈ inch

FIGURE 13-7 Addressing envelopes.

* Priority mail parcels that weigh more than 15 lb and are larger than 84 inches in combined length and girth are charged a balloon rate.

Bound Printed Matter. Bound printed matter consists of advertising, promotional, directory, or editorial material (or any combination of such material). It must be securely bound by permanent fastenings such as staples, spiral binding, glue, or stitching, and cannot have the nature of personal correspondence. Loose-leaf binders and similar fastenings are not considered permanent. Mail in this class cannot weigh over 15 lb.

Media Mail. Media mail is used for books, film, manuscripts, printed music, printed test materials, sound recordings, play scripts, printed educational charts, loose-leaf pages and binders consisting of medical information, videotapes, and computer recorded media such as CD-ROMs and diskettes. Media mail cannot contain advertising, and it cannot weigh over 70 lb.

Special Services

Insured Mail. Insurance for coverage against loss or damage is available for Priority Mail, first-class mail, and parcel post.

Registered Mail. Mail of all classes, particularly that of unusually high value, can be additionally protected by registering it. The sender may request evidence of its delivery. Registering a piece of mail also helps to trace delivery, if necessary. The Hope Diamond, worth an estimate of up to $250,000,000, was sent via Registered Mail from New York City to the Smithsonian Institute in Washington, D.C. when Harry Winston donated it to the museum.

When sending a registered letter, it is necessary to go to the post office and fill in the required forms. All articles to be registered must be thoroughly sealed with USPS tape. Cellophane tape is not permitted. On receipt of the item, the **recipient** is required to sign a form that acknowledges delivery. A registered letter may be released to the person to whom it is

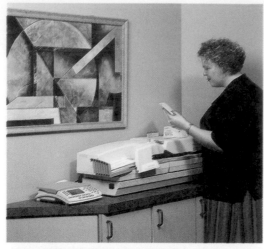

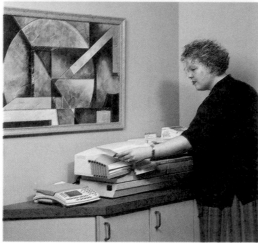

FIGURE 13-8 Postage meters help the mail processing run more efficiently.

addressed or to his or her agent. For an additional fee a personal receipt may be requested (Figure 13-9). This ensures that the letter will be released only to the individual to whom it is addressed. Such pieces bear the label *To Addressee Only.*

Registered Mail is accounted for by number from the time of mailing until the time of delivery and is transported separately from other mail under a special lock. In case of loss or damage, the customer may be reimbursed up to certain limits, provided that the value of the registered article has been declared at the time of mailing and that the appropriate fee has been paid.

Postal Money Orders. Postal money orders are a convenient way of mailing money, especially for the individual who does not have a personal checking account. They may be purchased in amounts as high as $700.

Special Delivery. Mail of any class that has been marked *special delivery* is charged at the special-delivery rate. Such pieces may be regular first- or second-class, registered, insured, or COD pieces. The special-delivery designation generally does not speed up the normal travel time between two cities but does ensure immediate delivery of the item when it arrives at the designated post office.

Special Handling. Third- and fourth-class mail sent by special handling receives the fastest service and ground transportation practicable—about the same as that for first-class mail. The special-handling fee is in addition to required postage and is determined according to weight. This fee does not include insurance or special delivery at the destination, but special delivery, if desired, is available at an added cost. If a parcel is sent by Priority Mail, special handling is of no additional advantage because it is already traveling at the greatest possible speed.

Certified Mail. Any piece of mail without **intrinsic** value and on which postage is paid at the first-class rate will be accepted as Certified Mail. Such items as contracts, deeds, mortgages, bank books, checks, passports, insurance policies, money orders, and birth certificates that are not themselves valuable but that would be difficult to duplicate if lost should be certified. Certified Mail is also often used as an aid in debt collection.

Regular postage in addition to a Certified Mail fee must be affixed. For an additional fee a receipt verifying delivery can be requested (Figure 13-10). Certified Mail can be sent special delivery if the prescribed fees are paid. A record of delivery of Certified Mail is kept for 2 years at the post office of delivery; however, no record is kept at the post office of origin. Furthermore, this type of mail does not provide insurance coverage.

The medical assistant should keep a supply of Certified Mail forms and return receipts on hand. These may be obtained at any post office. Full instructions are included on the forms. Fees and postage may be paid using ordinary postage stamps, meter stamps, or permit imprints. Certified Mail can be mailed at any post office, station, or branch or can be deposited in mail drops or in street letter boxes if specific instructions are followed.

Certificate of Mailing. If a sender needs proof of mailing but is not especially concerned with proof of receipt of an item, the most economic method is to obtain a certificate of mailing. Obtain this form at the post office and fill in the required information. Attach a stamp for the current fee and hand the form to the postal clerk along with the piece of mail. The clerk will postmark the receipt, initial it, and hand it back as acknowledgment of having received the piece of mail at the post office. This is sometimes used when mailing tax reports or other items that must be postmarked by a certain date.

Private Delivery Services

Not all mail is delivered by the USPS. Actually, the USPS delivers only about 44% of the mail in the United States. Many private services pick up and deliver mail overnight. Among these are Federal Express, United Parcel Service, Emery, Airborne Express, and DHL. These services are highly advertised and competitive. All large cities and many smaller communities have centralized points where packages can be dropped off for the service of the sender's choice. Pickup service is also available in many communities.

CRITICAL THINKING APPLICATION

■ The office has always used FedEx for sending packages. However, Brandon is curious as to whether FedEx offers the best rates. How might he gather this information?

■ What should be considered when choosing a private delivery service?

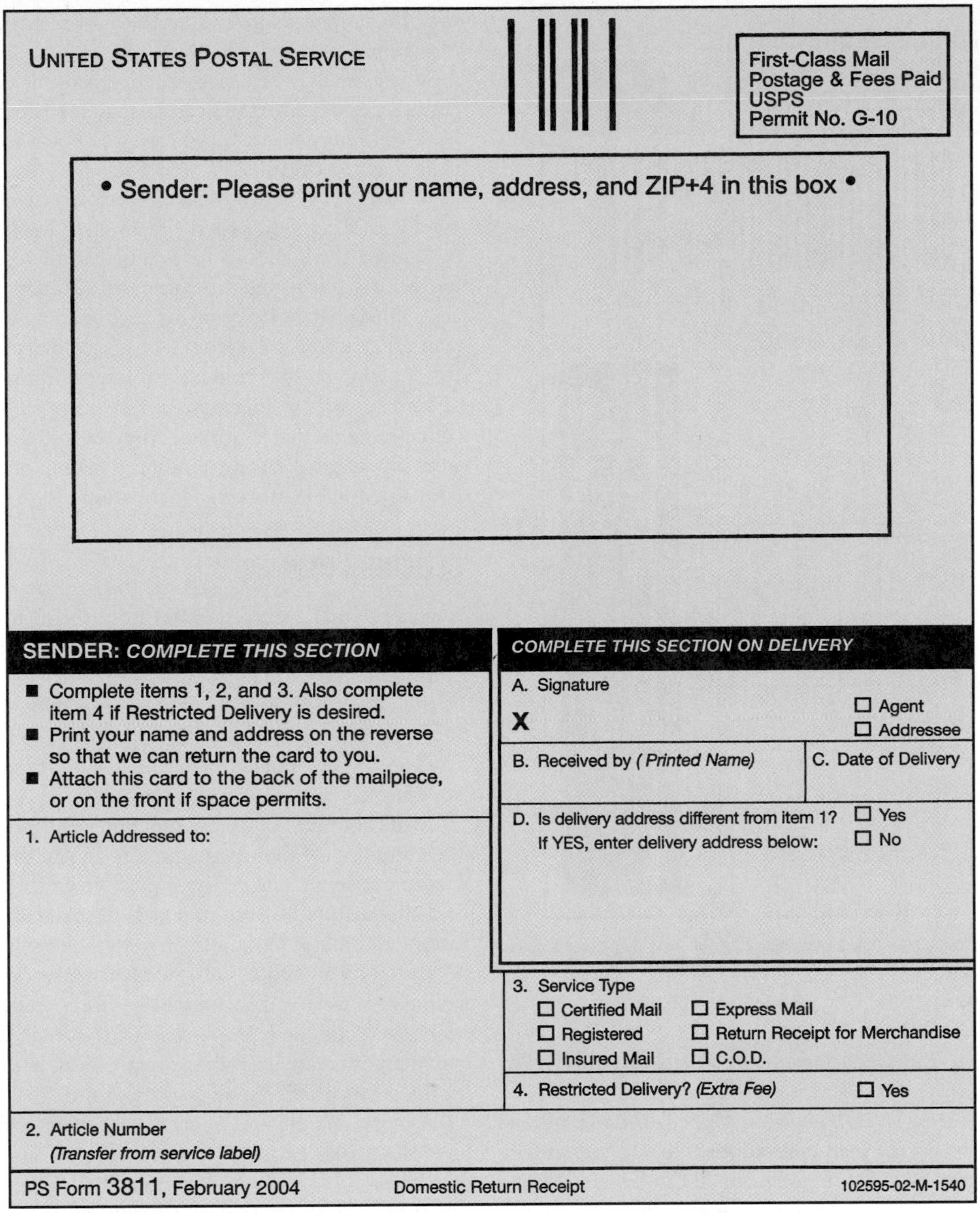

UNITED STATES POSTAL SERVICE

First-Class Mail
Postage & Fees Paid
USPS
Permit No. G-10

• Sender: Please print your name, address, and ZIP+4 in this box •

SENDER: ***COMPLETE THIS SECTION***

- Complete items 1, 2, and 3. Also complete item 4 if Restricted Delivery is desired.
- Print your name and address on the reverse so that we can return the card to you.
- Attach this card to the back of the mailpiece, or on the front if space permits.

1. Article Addressed to:

COMPLETE THIS SECTION ON DELIVERY

A. Signature
X ☐ Agent ☐ Addressee

B. Received by (*Printed Name*) C. Date of Delivery

D. Is delivery address different from item 1? ☐ Yes
If YES, enter delivery address below: ☐ No

3. Service Type
☐ Certified Mail ☐ Express Mail
☐ Registered ☐ Return Receipt for Merchandise
☐ Insured Mail ☐ C.O.D.

4. Restricted Delivery? (*Extra Fee*) ☐ Yes

2. Article Number
(*Transfer from service label*)

PS Form 3811, February 2004 Domestic Return Receipt 102595-02-M-1540

FIGURE 13-9 Delivery receipts for Certified Mail, Registered Mail, and insured mail. Attach to the back of the article, and endorse the front with the phrase *return receipt requested* adjacent to the article number.

Handling Special Situations

Forwarding and Obtaining a Changed Address. By marking a piece of mail with the notation *Forwarding Service Requested*, the U.S. Post Office will forward mail to the new address if it is sent within 12 months of the change or if the receiver has left a forwarding order with the post office. At that time the forwarding order is expired unless the receiver requests that it be continued. Between 12 and 18 months, the piece will be returned to the sender with the new address noted. After 18 months, mail is usually returned with the reason for nondelivery noted. There is no charge for forwarding when priority or first-class mail is used.

If the mailer wants to know an addressee's new address, this service can be obtained from the post office by placing the words *Address Correction Requested* beneath the return address on the envelope. This can be handwritten, stamped, typewritten, or printed. The new address will be noted on a sticker and returned to the sender, and there is no charge for this if the item is sent priority or first-class mail. The post office charges a weighted fee for this service for standard mail and packages. If the envelope is marked *Change Service Requested*, the post office will dispose of the piece of mail and return a card to the sender showing the forwarding address of the addressee. If the piece was sent priority or first class, no charge is incurred for the service unless

FIGURE 13-10 Receipt for Certified Mail. Attach the bottom portion of the receipt to the top of the envelope, just to the right of the return address.

the notification is sent electronically, in which case there is a small charge.

Recalling Mail. If a letter has been dropped in the mailbox by mistake, do not ask the mail collector to give it to you; he or she is not permitted to do so. However, mail can be recalled by making written application at the post office, together with an envelope addressed identically to the one being recalled. If the letter has already left the local post office, the postmaster, at the sender's expense, can notify the postmaster at the destination post office to return the letter. However, there is no guarantee that the letter will be retrieved.

Returned Mail. If a letter is returned to the sender after an attempt has been made to deliver it, it cannot be mailed again without new postage. It is best simply to prepare a new envelope

with the correct address, affix the proper postage, and place it in the mail.

When mail is returned to the medical office, be sure to correct the database, indicating that mail to a certain patient has been returned, so that postage is not wasted sending mail to that address again.

Tracing Lost Mail. Receipts issued by the post office, whether for money orders, Registered Mail, Certified Mail, or insured mail, should be retained until receipt of the item has been acknowledged. If after an adequate time elapses no acknowledgment of receipt for such mailing arrives, notify the post office to trace the letter or package. Regular first-class mail is not easily traced, but the post office will make every attempt to find it for you. In tracing a lost letter or package, the post office requires that a special form be filled out; information from any original receipt should be written on this form, along with any other identifying information.

CLOSING COMMENTS

Remember that every letter sent from the medical office should project a professional image. Use neat handwriting when correspondence is not typed or generated on a computer. All of the office staff must be able to read items written years ago. It is worth the time and effort to brush up on English skills so that writing documents becomes as comfortable as setting an appointment or assisting in a procedure.

Medical offices often use brochures and printed material for the education of their patients. It is critical that these materials look professional and reflect a positive image for the physician and the facility. Be sure that copied material is clean without streaks and that it looks attractive to the eye. If the information is written by an office staff member, make certain that correct grammar is used and that several office members proofread the work for errors and proper use of the English language. It is wonderful to make a good first impression, but every impression in the medical office is an important one.

A copy should be kept of all communications leaving the office that relate to patient care. If any information is handwritten, it must be completely legible to the patient. Certainly, everyone should be able to read his or her own handwriting, even years later.

Because the appointment book is also considered a communications tool, the information entered by hand in the book must also be clear and easy to read. Take enough time to write legibly so that there is no confusion when the document is referred to at a later date. In legal battles, all written documentation must be concise and must not promote questions about the content.

SUMMARY OF SCENARIO

 Brandon has been a tremendous help to the office staff over the summer months. He has learned about every area of the medical clinic and has mastered several of the office procedures, both clinical and administrative. He has a greater understanding now of the business aspect of the medical office.

His duties as a temporary administrative medical assistant have opened his eyes to the value and importance of the administrative personnel. He can easily see that everyone—from the receptionist to the scheduler to the insurance billers—plays a vital role in the smooth operation of the facility.

Toward the end of the summer, the office staff honored Brandon with a going-away party. He announced with a smile that he had decided that he wished to become a pediatrician, based on his experience in his father's family practice. He expressed to the staff that he planned to hire them all away from his father! Then on a serious note, he thanked all the employees for their patience and for their willingness to let him learn from them. Everyone expects Brandon to be a complete success.

Sometimes it is difficult to work with a member of the physician's family. Employees should understand that family members often have as much at stake on the success of the practice as the employee. Make every attempt to get along with family members, even when they are less than **amiable.**

By learning proofreader's marks the medical assistant will find that it is much easier and faster to work through a document that needs revision or simple grammatic corrections. The marks are simple to use, once learned, and will be helpful throughout the medical assistant's career.

All documents make an impression, and that impression may be negative or positive. Each document that is generated by the medical assistant needs to make a positive impression. Proofread everything, including emails and memos, and look for ways in which the wording can be made more accurate or more fitting for the message that is being communicated. Because of the reflection on the physician, all documents must be professional—each one, each day, every single time.

SUMMARY of LEARNING OBJECTIVES

1. Define, spell, and pronounce the terms listed in the vocabulary.
   - Spelling and pronouncing medical terms correctly adds credibility to the medical assistant. Knowing the definition of these terms promotes confidence in communication with patients and co-workers.
2. Discuss the responsibility of the medical assistant with respect to equipment and supplies.
   - The medical assistant is responsible for making certain that equipment is in good working order. Warranties should always be mailed when new equipment is purchased, and the correct maintenance procedures should be followed to keep machines working at an optimal level. Supplies should be ordered before they run out, and prices should be compared to find the best quality for the best price available.
3. List the four common sizes of letterhead stationery.
   - Letterhead stationery comes in four basic sizes. Standard or letter stationery, which is most commonly used for business purposes, is $8\frac{1}{2} \times 11$ inches. Monarch or executive stationery is $8\frac{1}{4} \times 10\frac{1}{2}$ inches and is used for informal business correspondence. Baronial stationery is $5\frac{1}{2} \times 8\frac{1}{2}$ inches, whereas legal stationery is $8\frac{1}{2} \times 14$ inches.
4. Explain the various parts of speech.
   - The medical assistant should be familiar with the various parts of speech and the way to use them correctly in a sentence. Nouns name something, such as a person, place, or thing; pronouns are substitutes for nouns. Verbs are action words and express movement, a condition, or a state of being. Adjectives usually describe nouns, whereas adverbs usually describe

   verbs. Prepositions are connecting words, as are conjunctions. Interjections show strong feelings and are often followed by an exclamation point.
5. Name some of the essential references for the medical assistant's library.
   - It is quite helpful to develop a personal tool collection that will assist the medical assistant with written communications in the medical office. An up-to-date dictionary, a medical dictionary, a composition handbook, an English-language reference manual, and a thesaurus will be valuable additions to the tool library.
6. List several steps to complete before answering a business letter.
   - Before any type of correspondence is answered, the piece should be read carefully. Often a highlighter is used for marking questions that must be answered, or notes may be written on the correspondence in pencil. A draft of the reply should be written first, then the correspondence should be rewritten in its final draft.
7. Discuss the process of developing and the value of keeping a communications portfolio.
   - Subsequent letters will be much easier to draft if the medical assistant develops a portfolio that contains sample letters and other types of communications. Once a letter is written, it can be saved on the computer hard drive or on a disk, or it can be printed and placed in a binder for easy viewing. If the letter is printed in a binder, it is wise to note on each example the file name as it is saved on the computer so that the document can be easily found again when needed. This is an excellent way to save time in the busy medical office.

Continued

SUMMARY of LEARNING OBJECTIVES
Continued

8. Discuss the differences in the four letter styles.
   - Block is an efficient but less attractive letter style wherein all lines begin flush with the left margin of the paper. Modified block is similar, but some lines begin at the center of the page instead of the left margin. Modified block with indented paragraphs is identical to block style, with the exception of the indention of the paragraphs. Simplified letter style contains lines that begin flush at the left margin, but other items, such as the salutation and complimentary closing, are omitted.

9. Explain the four standard parts of a business letter.
   - The four standard parts of a business letter include the heading, the opening, the body, and the closing. The heading includes the letterhead and dateline, whereas the opening includes the inside address and any attention or salutation line. The body is the message of the document, and the closing includes the signature, complimentary closing, reference initials, and special notations.

10. List several ways to save money when mailing.
    - Money can be saved by consulting the post office when mailing, checking for better rates, and using ZIP codes. Consult a local post office when mailing in bulk to obtain the best rates.

11. Open, sort, and annotate incoming mail.
    - Mail is one of the most common types of communication used in the physician's office. The process for responding to and initiating written correspondence is outlined in Procedure 13-1.

12. Compose, proofread, and mail a business letter.
    - Business letters must look professional and contain sentences that are grammatically correct. The process for proofreading a business letter or publication for accuracy is outlined in Procedure 13-2.

13. Properly send a fax.
    - Transmissions sent by fax must arrive at their destination in a confidential manner. The process for preparing a fax for transmission is outlined in Procedure 13-3.

14. Process incoming mail.
    - Most physician offices have a process for dealing with mail that arrives at the facility. The method for processing incoming mail is outlined in Procedure 13-4.

15. Address an envelope according to postal service optical character reader guidelines.
    - Addresses should be written in such a way that they are quickly and efficiently read by postal service machines. The process for addressing an envelope according to Postal Service optical character reader guidelines is outlined in Procedure 13-5.

CONNECTIONS

 Study Guide Connection: Go to Chapter 13 Study Guide. Read the Case Study and Workplace Applications and complete the assignments. Do online research for answers to the questions in the Internet Activities associated with written communications and mail processing.

 CD Connection: Go to the Medical Assisting Competency Challenge CD and do the training activities under Communication.

 Evolve Connection: For more information related to written communications and mail processing, go to http://evolve.elsevier.com/kinn/admin and visit related weblinks for Chapter 13. Click on the Medical Assisting Exam Review and do the practice questions to sharpen your test-taking skills.

Medical Records Management

14

SCENARIO

Susan Beezler has just begun her career in the medical assisting profession. She is attending medical assisting school in the morning hours and works part-time for a family practitioner in the afternoons as a clerical record assistant. Susan is eager to learn about medicine and looks forward to taking on more responsibility at the office.

The practice is growing swiftly and recently added a new physician, Dr. Alex Thomas. Dr. Thomas has enjoyed working with Susan and feels that her energy will be just what his patients need. He has taken a special interest in Susan and often lets her assist him with patients when her other duties allow.

Susan knows that although she is a beginner in the office, she will gain trust from her supervisors and patients as long as she projects a teachable attitude. She cheerfully performs filing and often does transcription for Dr. Thomas. The other staff members are pleased with her willingness to perform the most mundane tasks. Her warm personality and caring way with patients ensure that she has a great chance at a long career in this medical office.

Susan enjoys sharing her experiences with the other students in her class. She is the only person who is currently working in the medical field, so the other students ask many questions about what Susan has experienced in the real world of medicine. She is very careful not to breach patient confidentiality as she discusses situations in general, never mentioning any patient names.

Susan feels a great sense of pride that she is already a member of the healthcare team and able to make a positive contribution to the lives of her patients.

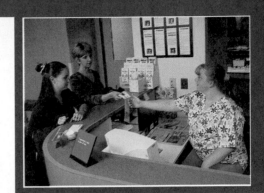

While studying this chapter, think about the following questions:

- How can the medical assistant help to alleviate patient concerns about electronic medical records?
- How can the medical assistant earn the patient's trust so that he or she is comfortable revealing the very private information contained in health histories?
- Why is the simple task of filing such a critical action in the physician's office?

LEARNING OBJECTIVES

1. Define, spell, and pronounce the terms listed in the vocabulary.
2. State several important reasons for keeping accurate medical records.
3. Discuss the ownership of records.
4. Explain the difference between a traditional medical record and a problem-oriented medical record.
5. Illustrate the difference between subjective and objective information.
6. Discuss changing an entry in the patient record and the importance of following correct procedures.
7. List and discuss the basic equipment used in a filing system.
8. Describe the steps in filing a document.
9. List and discuss application of the basic filing systems.
10. Explain how color-coding of files can be useful in a medical facility.
11. Establish a patient's medical record.
12. Prepare an informed consent for treatment form.
13. Add supplementary items to an established patient record.
14. Prepare a record release form.
15. Transcribe a machine-dictated letter using a computer or word processor.
16. File medical records and documents using an alphabetic system.
17. File medical records and documents using a numeric system.
18. Color-code medical records.
19. Document appropriately and accurately.

National Accreditation Competencies and Content

CAAHEP COMPETENCIES

Administrative
3.a.(1)(c). Organize a patient's medical record
3.a.(1)(d). File medical records

General
3.c.(2)(c). Establish and maintain the medical record
3.c.(2)(d). Document appropriately

ABHES COMPETENCIES

Communication
2.j. Use correct grammar, spelling, and formatting techniques in written works
2.n. Application of electronic technology
2.o. Fundamental writing skills

Administrative Duties
3.b. Prepare and maintain medical records
3.h. File medical records

Legal Concepts
5.a. Determine needs for documentation and reporting
5.b. Document accurately
5.c. Use appropriate guidelines when releasing records or information
5.d. Follow established policy in initiating or terminating medical treatment

VOCABULARY

alphabetic filing Any system that arranges names or topics according to the sequence of the letters in the alphabet.

alphanumeric Of or relating to systems made up of combinations of letters and numbers.

audit A formal examination of an organization's or individual's accounts or financial situation; a methodic examination and review.

augment To make greater, more numerous, larger, or more intense.

caption A heading, title, or subtitle under which records are filed.

chronologic order Of, relating to, or arranged in or according to the order of time.

continuity of care Continuation of care smoothly from one provider to another, so that the patient receives the most benefit and no interruption in care.

dictation (dik-tay′-shun) The act or manner of uttering words to be transcribed.

direct filing system A filing system in which materials can be located without consulting an intermediary source of reference.

gleaned Gathered bit by bit (e.g., information or material); picked over in search of relevant material.

indirect filing system A filing system in which an intermediary source of reference, such as a card file, must be consulted to locate specific files.

microfilm A film bearing a photographic record on a reduced scale of printed or other graphic matter.

numeric filing The filing of records, correspondence, or cards by number.

objective information Information that is gathered by watching or observation of a patient.

obliteration (uh-bli-tuh-ra′-shun) Act of making undecipherable or imperceptible by obscuring or wearing away.

OUTfolder A folder used to provide space for the temporary filing of materials.

OUTguide A heavy guide that is used to replace a folder that has been temporarily moved from the filing space.

power of attorney A legal instrument authorizing one to act as the attorney or agent of the grantor.

pressboard A strong, highly glazed composition board resembling vulcanized fiber; heavy card stock.

procrastination (pruh-kras-tuh-na′-shun) The intentional postponement of doing something that should be done.

provisional diagnosis A temporary diagnosis made before all test results have been received.

quality control An aggregate of activities designed to ensure adequate quality, especially in manufactured products or in the service industries.

requisites (re′-kwuh-zuhts) Entities considered essential or necessary.

retention schedule A method or plan for retaining or keeping medical records, and their movement from active, to inactive, to closed filing.

shelf filing A system that uses open shelves rather than cabinets for storing records.

shingling A method of filing whereby one report is laid on top of the older report, resembling the shingles of a roof.

subjective information Information that is gained by questioning the patient or taken from a form.

tickler file A chronologic file used as a reminder that something must be taken care of on a certain date.

transcription To make a written copy of, either in longhand or by machine.

vested Granted or endowed with a particular authority, right, or property; to have a special interest in.

A medical records management system is only as good as the ease of retrieval of the data in the files. Because the pace of the medical office is usually quite rapid, patient medical records must be found quickly and also be functional, so that the information inside is easily obtainable.

Few phrases are more frustrating to the patient than "we cannot locate your records." Patients have every right to question the competence of the medical care they are receiving if the office has problems simply finding a chart. Organization and adherence to set routines will help to ensure that medical records are accessible when they are needed.

WHY MEDICAL RECORDS ARE IMPORTANT

Medical records exist for four basic reasons. First, the medical record assists the physician in providing the best possible medical care for the patient. The physician examines the patient and enters the findings on the patient's medical record. These findings are the clues to diagnosis. The physician may order many types of tests to confirm or **augment** the clinical findings. As the reports of these tests come in, the findings fall into place like the pieces of a jigsaw puzzle. Then, with the confirmation data to support the diagnosis, the physician can prescribe treatment and form an opinion about the patient's chances for recovery, assured that every resource has been used to arrive at a correct judgment. The medical record provides a complete history of all of the care given to the patient.

The medical record also provides critical information for others. By reading through the record and discovering the methods used to treat the patient, healthcare professionals can provide a **continuity of care.** Each person knows what the patient has experienced and can provide continued care, even from one facility to another. For example, when a patient is transferred from a hospital to a skilled nursing facility, the information from the patient's hospital record will help the nursing facility staff to better care for the patient. When patients move from place to place or caregivers change, copies of the pertinent information should move with the patient to provide this continuity of care.

The second reason for keeping medical records is to offer legal protection for those who provided care to the patient. A documented medical record is excellent proof that certain procedures were performed or medical advice was given. An accurate record is the foundation for legal defense in cases of medical professional liability. This is one reason that it is critical to write legibly in the record and document exactly what happens to the patient. Remember: *If it isn't charted, it didn't happen.*

Third, medical records provide statistical information that is helpful to researchers. The patient's record provides information about medications taken and the reactions to them. Medical records may be used to evaluate the effectiveness of certain kinds of treatment or to determine the incidence of a given disease. Often, physicians take part in drug studies that track adverse reactions and side effects. The effects of various treatments and procedures can also be tracked and statistics **gleaned** from the information gathered from patient records.

Correlation of such statistical information may result in a new outlook on some phases of medicine and can lead to revised techniques and treatments. The statistical data from medical records are also valuable in the preparation of scientific papers, books, and lectures.

Fourth, medical records are vital for financial reimbursement. The information in the medical record supports claims for reimbursement and is required by most third-party payors.

OWNERSHIP OF THE MEDICAL RECORD

Who actually owns the medical record? Patients often assume that because the information contained in the medical record is about them, the ownership of the record rightfully belongs to the patient. However, the owner of the physical medical record is the physician or medical facility, often called the "maker," that initiated and developed the record. The patient has the right of access to the information within but does not own the physical chart or other documents pertaining to the record. The patient has a **vested** interest and therefore has the right to demand confidentiality of all of the information placed in the chart.

The actual medical record should never leave the medical facility from which it originated. Even the physician should refrain from taking the record from the office to the hospital or nursing facility. If information from the record is needed, copies can be placed in a file, and progress notes written on-site and returned to the original record later. Patient records should be kept in a locked room or locked filing cabinets when the office is closed.

CRITICAL THINKING APPLICATION

On Susan's third day at work, a man comes into the office and demands to see his mother's medical chart. Susan pulls the chart and sees an entry stating that the mother does not wish the son to have any information about her. What should Susan do in this situation? Are there any viable reasons why the son should have access to the mother's medical information?

CREATING AN EFFICIENT MEDICAL RECORD MANAGEMENT SYSTEM

The medical record management system used in the medical office should provide an easy method for retrieving information. The files should be organized in an orderly fashion, and all of the information within the record must be completely legible to the average reader. The information must also be accurate, and corrections should be made and documented properly. The wording in the record should be easily understood and grammatically correct. An efficient method of adding documents to the chart must be in place so that the physician or other provider always has the most up-to-date information.

Above all, the medical record management system must be one that works for the individual facility. Attempting to adopt a method used by another facility may not always be best. The system should be adapted to the needs of the facility and the provider.

Types of Records

The two major types of patient records include the paper-based medical record and the computer-based medical record. As computer technology advances, the paper-based medical record seems more and more inefficient. It is difficult to use a paper-based record for multiple purposes. In most cases, only one person can use the paper-based record at any given time, and the record is not available to others who need it when it is in use by a single person. Misfiled information is common, and the entire record can be misfiled as well. Data cannot be accessed easily for research and **quality control,** and in facilities with multiple departments the information is difficult to share. The paper-based record is a good evidence of patient care, but it not nearly as useful in other capacities.

The computer-based medical record (also called the *electronic health record)* is much more efficient than the paper-based record. The book *Electronic Health Records: Changing the Vision* offers the following definition:

> An electronic health record is any information relating to the past, present, or future physical/mental health, or condition of an individual which resides in electronic systems used to capture, transmit, receive, store, retrieve, link, and manipulate multimedia data for the primary purpose of providing healthcare and health related services.

Some healthcare professionals distinguish between a computer-based medical record and an electronic health record. To simplify a difficult definition, consider the computer-based medical record as one in which the bulk of information is entered via computer but there are still paper aspects to the record. For instance, an x-ray film may not be included in a patient's computer-based record. The x-ray film may still be filed in a room among all other patient x-ray films. However, using an electronic health record, all healthcare information is stored in one format. This means that x-ray studies, bone scans, magnetic resonance imaging (MRI) studies, and so on would be scanned into the electronic health record and become a permanent part of the record.

Granted, not all physicians today have the means or desire to convert to a total electronic health record. The cost of such a conversion would be tremendous. However, physicians who are just opening and establishing their practices may look more toward the future and plan for an electronic medical practice. Even today, many physicians use laptop computers, or smaller electronic units, to record patient information during office visits.

Be aware that for a medical assistant, learning never stops. As facilities grow, medical assistants will be asked to make changes and learn new ways of completing tasks. Be willing to move into the future and embrace new ideas. Those who balk and complain about change will find themselves left behind as technology advances.

The computer-based medical record is a great improvement over the paper-based record, but it is not without its disadvantages. Patient confidentiality is critical and sometimes difficult to maintain with computer-based records. Many providers worry about computer malfunctions that would inhibit access to the record in an emergency.

Still, the advantages of the computer-based record seem to far outweigh the disadvantages. Information can be accessed in a variety of physical locations, and more than one person can see the record at any given time. The patient database usually allows various types of statistical information to be recalled, which is a valuable tool. Patient information is available quickly in an emergency, even when the patient is not in his or her hometown. All of these advantages mean that the computer-based record will continue to be a key tool in the future.

CRITICAL THINKING APPLICATION

Some of the patients who visit Dr. Thomas have expressed concern that computer-based medical records may not be private enough. They are worried that unauthorized individuals could somehow access their information on the computer and somehow cause the patients harm. How might Susan alleviate the patients' fears? What disadvantages regarding confidentiality are associated with the computer-based patient record? Should a patient be allowed to decide whether his or her records will be kept on computer or on paper?

ORGANIZATION OF THE MEDICAL RECORD

Source-Oriented Records

The traditional patient record is source oriented; that is, observations and data are cataloged according to their source—physician, laboratory, radiology department, nurse, technician—with no recording of a logical relationship among them. Forms and progress notes are filed in reverse **chronologic order** (most recent on top) and filed in separate sections of the record by the type of form or service rendered—all laboratory reports together, all x-ray reports together, and so on.

Problem-Oriented Medical Records

The problem-oriented medical record (POMR) is a radical departure from the traditional system of keeping patient records. It is sometimes referred to as the *Weed system,* because it was originated by Dr. Lawrence L. Weed, a professor of medicine at the University of Vermont's College of Medicine. The POMR is a record of clinical practice that divides medical action into four bases:

- The database includes chief complaint, present illness, patient profile, review of systems, physical examination, and laboratory reports.
- The problem list is a numbered and titled list of every problem the patient has that requires management or workup. This may include social and demographic troubles as well as strictly medical or surgical ones.
- The treatment plan includes management, additional workups needed, and therapy. Each plan is titled and numbered with respect to the problem.
- The progress notes include structured notes that are numbered to correspond with each problem number.

Several companies have developed file folders for the organization of patient data consistent with the POMR (Figure 14-1). The problem list is entered on the divider cover for

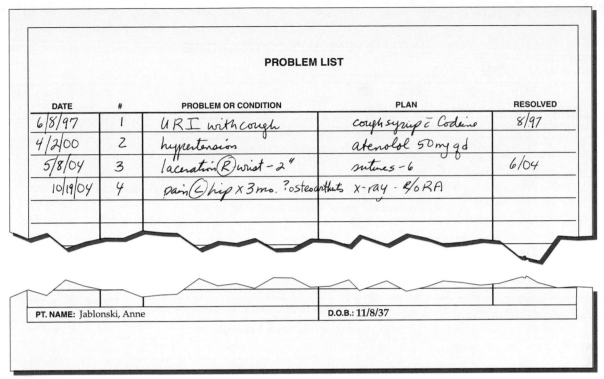

FIGURE 14-1 A chart designed for a problem-oriented medical record (POMR). Some charts are specifically adapted to the POMR. (Courtesy Bibbero Systems, Inc., Petaluma, Calif. 94954, (800) 242-2376, www.bibbero.com.)

laboratory reports. Special sections are provided for current major and chronic problems and for inactive major or chronic problems. The divider cover for progress notes is a chart for listing medications and other therapeutic modalities. Progress notes follow the SOAP approach. SOAP is an acronym for the following:

- *S*ubjective impressions
- *O*bjective clinical evidence
- *A*ssessment or diagnosis
- *P*lans for further studies, treatment, or management

Some medical offices also used an "E" in the record, to represent "Evaluation." This section is used to record an assessment of the patient's understanding of and possible compliance with the treatment plan. As this is not used in every practice, the medical assistant may never see or use it to complete a patient record.

The POMR has the advantage of imposing order and organization on the information added to a patient's medical record. The records are more easily reviewed, and the likelihood of overlooking a problem is greatly reduced. The SOAP method essentially forces a rational approach to patient problems and assists in formulating a logical and orderly plan of patient care (Figure 14-2).

CRITICAL THINKING APPLICATION

Dr. Thomas wants Susan to thoroughly understand the SOAP method of charting. How would Susan explain each aspect of this method to a classmate? Distinct differences exist between the SOAP method and the POMR. Help Susan distinguish between the two. Which method seems easier and more efficient to you?

Popularity of the POMR has continued to grow since its introduction in the 1960s, and it is especially advantageous in clinics, group practices, and hospitals, where more than one person must be able to find essential information in the chart.

CONTENTS OF THE COMPLETE CASE HISTORY

The medical case history is the most important record in a physician's practice. For completeness, each patient's record should contain **subjective information** provided by the patient and **objective information** provided by the physician. If all entries are completed, the case history will stand the test of time. No branch of medicine is exempt from the necessity of keeping patient history records.

Subjective Information

Personal Demographics

The patient's case history begins with routine personal data, which the patient usually supplies on the first visit (Procedure 14-1). Most patients are required to complete a patient information form (Figure 14-3). The basic facts needed are the following:

- Patient's full name, spelled correctly
- Names of parents if patient is a child
- Patient's sex
- Date of birth
- Marital status
- Name of spouse, if married
- Number of children, if any
- Home address, telephone number, and email

OUTLINE FORMAT PROGRESS NOTES

Patient Name __Fletcher, LeRoy_____

Page __1__

Prob. No. or Letter	DATE	**S** Subjective	**O** Objective	**A** Assess	**P** Plans
2	01/26/06	Patient complains of two days of severe high epigastric pain and burning, radiating through to the back. Pain accentuated after eating.			
			On examination there is extreme guarding and tenderness, high epigastric region. No rebound. Bowel sounds normal. BP 110/70		
				R/O gastric ulcer, pylorospasm.	
					To have upper gastrointestinal series. Start on Cimetidine, 300 mg. q.i.d. Eliminate coffee, alcohol, and aspirin. Return in two days.

Start each Progress Note (Subjective, Objective, through the intervening columns to the right   Assessment and Plans) at the appropriate margin of the page.   shaded column to create an outline form. Write

ANDRUS/CLINI-REC® PRIMARY CARE CHARTING SYSTEM FORM NO. 26-7115, ©1976 BIBBERO SYSTEMS, INC., PETALUMA, CA.

FIGURE 14-2 SOAP progress notes. The SOAP method keeps information organized and in a logical sequence. An actual progress note would include the physician's signature or initials after this entry. (Courtesy Bibbero Systems, Inc., Petaluma, Calif. 94954, (800) 242-2376, www.bibbero.com.)

PROCEDURE 14-1

Establish the Medical Record

<u>CAAHEP COMPETENCY:</u> 3.a(1)(c), 3.c.(2)(c)
<u>ABHES COMPETENCY:</u> 3.b

GOAL: *To initiate a medical file for a new patient that will contain all the personal data necessary for a complete record and any other information required by the facility.*

EQUIPMENT and SUPPLIES

- Computer or typewriter
- Clerical supplies (pen, clipboard)
- Information on the agency's filing system
- Registration form
- File folder
- Label for folder
- Identification (ID) card if using numeric system
- Cross-reference card
- Financial card
- Routing slip
- Private conference area

PROCEDURAL STEPS

1. Determine that the patient is new to the office.
2. Obtain and record the required personal data.
   <u>PURPOSE:</u> Complete information is necessary for credit and insurance claim processing.
3. Type the information onto the patient history form.

4. Review the entire form.
   <u>PURPOSE:</u> To confirm that the information is complete and correct.
5. Select a label and folder for the record.
   <u>EXPLANATION:</u> If color-coding is used, a decision must be made regarding the appropriate color for the patient name.
6. Type the caption on the label and apply it to the folder.
   <u>EXPLANATION:</u> Use the patient's name for alphabetic filing or appropriate number for numeric filing.
7. For a numeric filing system, prepare a cross-reference card and a patient ID number.
   <u>PURPOSE:</u> Numeric filing is an indirect system and requires a cross-reference to a patient's name for locating the chart. The patient will use the number of the ID card when arranging appointments or making inquiries.
8. Prepare the financial card, or place that patient's name in the computerized ledger.
9. Place the patient's history form and all other forms required by the agency into the prepared folder.
10. Clip an encounter form on the outside of the patient's folder.

- Occupation
- Name of employer
- Business address and telephone number
- Employment information for spouse
- Healthcare insurance information
- Source of referral
- Social Security number

Personal and Medical History

The personal and medical history, which is often obtained by having the patient complete a questionnaire, provides information about any past illnesses or surgical operations that the patient may have had and includes data about injuries or physical defects, whether congenital or acquired (Figure 14-4). It also includes information about the patient's daily health habits. The presence of allergies, advance directives, and other information can be easily indicated on the front of the medical record by the use of stickers (Figure 14-5). These are useful when important facts about the patient need to be on the forefront of the health professional's mind while treating the patient.

Patient's Family History

The family history is composed of the physical condition of the various members of the patient's family, any illnesses or diseases that individual members may have experienced in the past, and a record of the causes of death. This information is

important, because a hereditary pattern may be present in the case of certain diseases.

Patient's Social History

The patient's social history includes information about the lifestyle the patient lives. If the patient drinks, how many drinks per day or per week are consumed? If the patient uses cigarettes, how many packs a day are smoked? Drug use and even marital information can be considered part of the social history.

CRITICAL THINKING APPLICATION

While taking a medical history from a patient, Susan asks about the social history. She questions the patient as to whether he drinks alcohol. The patient immediately becomes defensive and accuses Susan of getting too personal about his affairs. How might Susan explain her reasons for asking these questions? What options are available if the patient refuses to discuss the social history with Susan? Could this opposition to questions about the social history raise suspicion in Susan's mind? What might she suspect?

Patient's Chief Complaint

The patient's chief complaint is a concise account of the patient's symptoms, explained in the patient's own words. It should include the following:

Thank you for selecting our health care team!
To help us meet all your health care needs, please
fill out this form completely in ink. If you have any questions
or need assistance, please ask us - we will be happy to help.

Welcome

Patient # _____

Soc. Sec. # _____

Date _____

Patient Information (CONFIDENTIAL)

Name_____ Birth date _____ Home phone _____

Address_____ City _____ State_____ Zip _____

Check appropriate box: ☐ Minor ☐ Single ☐ Married ☐ Divorced ☐ Widowed ☐ Separated

If student, name of school/college _____ City _____ State __ ☐ Full time ☐ Part time

Patient's or parent's employer _____ Work phone _____

Business address _____ City _____ State_____ Zip _____

Spouse or parent's name _____ Employer _____ Work phone _____

Whom may we thank for referring you? _____

Person to contact in case of emergency _____ Phone _____

Responsible Party

Name of person responsible for this account _____ Relationship to patient _____

Address _____ Home phone _____

Driver's license # _____ Birth date _____ Financial institution _____

Employer_____ Work phone _____ SSN# _____

Is this person currently a patient in our office? ☐ Yes ☐ No

Insurance Information

Name of insured _____ Relationship to patient _____

Birth date _____ Social Security # _____ Date employed _____

Name of employer_____ Union or local # _____ Work phone _____

Address of employer _____ City _____ State_____ Zip _____

Insurance company_____ Group # _____ Policy/ID # _____

Ins. co. address _____ City _____ State_____ Zip _____

How much is your deductible? _____ How much have you used? _____ Max. annual benefit _____

DO YOU HAVE ANY ADDITIONAL INSURANCE? ☐ Yes ☐ No   IF YES, COMPLETE THE FOLLOWING:

Name of insured _____ Relationship to patient _____

Birth date _____ Social Security # _____ Date employed _____

Name of employer_____ Union or local # _____ Work phone _____

Address of employer _____ City _____ State_____ Zip _____

Insurance company_____ Group # _____ Policy/ID # _____

Ins. co. address _____ City _____ State_____ Zip _____

How much is your deductible? _____ How much have you used? _____ Max. annual benefit _____

I authorize release of any information concerning my (or my child's) health care, advice and treatment provided for the purpose of evaluating and administering claims for insurance benefits. I also hereby authorize payment of insurance benefits otherwise payable to me directly to the doctor.

X _____   _____

Signature of patient or parent if minor   Date

FIGURE 14-3 The patient information form provides all of the information that the medical assistant needs to construct a patient chart.

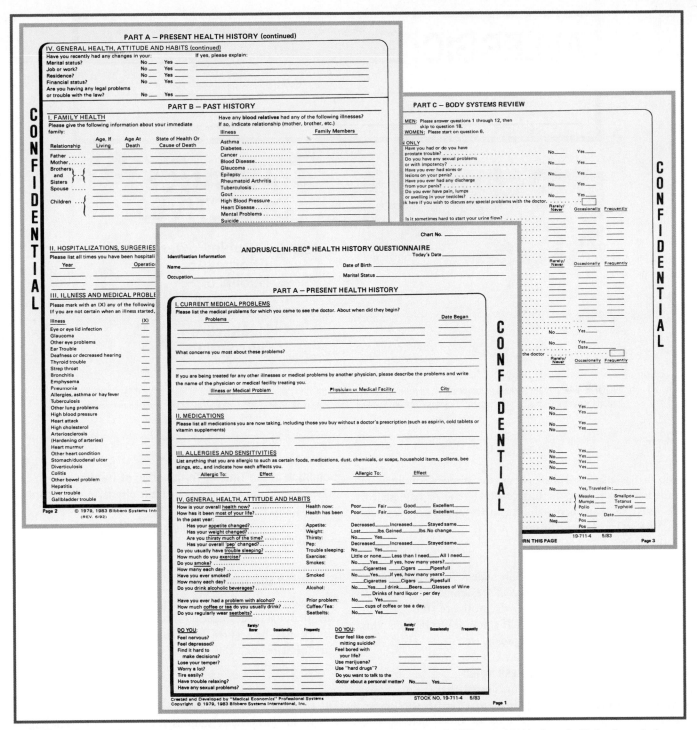

FIGURE 14-4 Database self-administered general health history questionnaire. Lengthy questionnaires should be completed by the patient before he or she is seen by the physician. Either mail the information to the patient in advance or ask the patient to come in early to complete the paperwork. (Courtesy Bibbero Systems, Inc., Petaluma, Calif. 94954, (800) 242-2376, www.bibbero.com.)

- Nature and duration of pain, if any
- Time when the patient first noticed symptoms
- Patient's opinion as to the possible causes for the difficulties
- Remedies that the patient may have applied before seeing the physician
- Other medical treatment received for the same condition in the past

Objective Information

Objective findings, sometimes referred to as *signs*, become evident from the physician's examination of the patient.

Physical Examination and Findings and Laboratory and Radiology Reports

This section of the case history varies greatly with the specialty of the physician and the complaint of the patient. After the

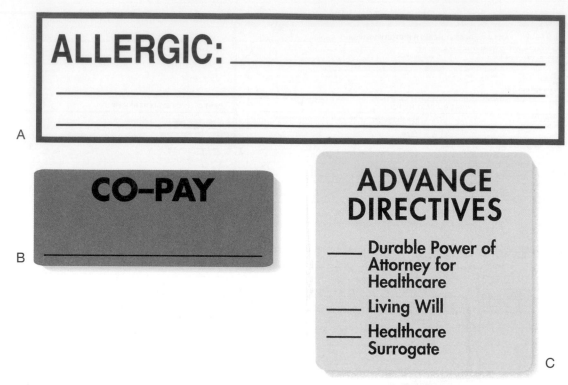

FIGURE 14-5 Chart stickers. Information on stickers on the outside of the chart allows the physician and medical staff to quickly see important information about the patient. (Courtesy Bibbero Systems, Inc., Petaluma, Calif. 94954, (800) 242-2376, www.bibbero.com.)

physician has examined the patient, the physical findings are recorded in the history. Results of other tests or requests for these tests are then recorded or, if they appear on separate sheets, are attached to the history.

Diagnosis

The physician, on the basis of all evidence provided in the patient's past history, the physician's examination, and any supplementary tests, places the diagnosis of the patient's condition on the medical record. If some doubt remains, this may be termed a **provisional diagnosis.**

Treatment Prescribed and Progress Notes

The physician's suggested treatment is listed after the diagnosis. Generally, instructions to the patient to return for follow-up treatment in a specific period of time are noted here as well. If surgery or other treatment is needed, the patient must sign a consent form (Procedure 14-2).

On each subsequent visit the date must be entered on the chart and information about the patient's condition and the results of treatment added to the history, on the basis of the physician's observations. Notations of all medications prescribed or instructions given, as well as the patient's own progress report, should be placed in the record. Any home visits are noted. If the patient is hospitalized, the name of the hospital, the reason for the admission, and the dates of admission and discharge are recorded. Much of this information may be obtained from the hospital discharge summary.

Condition at the Time of Termination of Treatment

When the treatment is terminated, the physician will record that information. For example:

August 18, 2006. Wound completely healed. Patient discharged.

Obtaining the History

The medical assistant usually secures the routine personal data. The personal and medical history and the patient's family history may be secured by asking the patient to complete a questionnaire, with the physician augmenting the information provided during the patient interview (see Procedure 27-1).

The Medical Assistant's Role

When the medical assistant is responsible for recording the patient's history, care must be exercised to ensure that the patient's answers are not heard by others in the reception room. If privacy is not possible, it is better to give the patient a form to fill out, then to transfer this information to permanent records later. When privacy is available, the medical assistant may ask the patient questions and at the same time write or type the answers directly on the record. This method offers an opportunity to become better acquainted with the patient while completing the necessary records. In facilities where lengthy questionnaires are to be completed by the new patient, the questionnaire may be mailed to the patient with a request that it be completed and returned to the physician before the appointment. If the record

PROCEDURE 14-2

Establish and Maintain the Medical Record: Prepare an Informed Consent for Treatment Form

CAAHEP COMPETENCY: 3.c.(2)(d)
ABHES COMPETENCY: 3.b., 5.a

GOAL: *To adequately and completely inform the patient regarding the treatment or procedure that he or she is to receive, and to provide legal protection for the facility and the provider.*

EQUIPMENT and SUPPLIES

- Pen
- Consent form

PROCEDURAL STEPS

1. After the physician provides the details of the procedure to be done, prepare the consent form. Be sure that the form addresses the following:
   - The nature of the procedure or treatment
   - The risks and/or benefits of the procedure or treatment
   - Any reasonable alternatives to the procedure or treatment
   - The risks and/or benefits of each alternative
   - The risks and/or benefits of not performing the procedure or treatment

   PURPOSE: To make certain that the patient is fully informed about the procedure or treatment and the risks and/or benefits of having or not having it performed.

2. Personalize the form with the patient's name and any other demographic information that the form lists.
   PURPOSE: To correctly identify the patient and the procedure.

3. Deliver the form to the physician for use as the patient is counseled about the procedure.

PURPOSE: To avoid charges of practicing medicine without a license. The physician should explain procedures, risks, benefits, and alternatives and answer all of the patient's questions.

4. Witness the signature of the patient on the form, if necessary. The physician will usually sign the form as well.

5. Provide a copy of the consent form to the patient.
   PURPOSE: To make certain that the patient is fully informed regarding the procedure and has a copy of the information for his or her personal records.

6. Place the consent form in the patient's chart. The facility where the procedure is to be performed may require a copy.
   PURPOSE: To maintain a permanent copy of the signed consent form.

7. Ask the patient if he or she has any questions about the procedure. Refer questions that the medical assistant cannot or should not answer to the physician. Be sure that all of the questions expressed by the patient are answered.
   PURPOSE: To make certain that the patient is fully informed.

8. Provide information regarding the date and time for the procedure to the patient.

---

is to be computerized, requesting the information ahead of time gives the office staff the opportunity to transfer information to the computer before the new patient's visit.

The patient's chief complaint may have been indicated to the medical assistant, but the physician will question the patient in more detail. Many practitioners write their own entries on the chart in longhand. Some may key the findings directly into the computer. Others may dictate the material, either directly to the medical assistant or by using a recording device. If the material is dictated and typed, the physician should check each entry then initial the entry to verify accuracy. For a chart to be admissible as evidence in court, the person dictating or writing the entries must be able to attest that they were true and correct at the time they were written. The best indication of that is the physician's signature or initials on the typed entry.

MAKING ADDITIONS TO THE PATIENT RECORD

As long as the patient is under the physician's care, the medical history is building. Each laboratory report, radiology report, and progress note is added to the record, with the latest information always on top (Procedure 14-3). Although each item is important, the most recent is usually of greatest significance to the patient's care. Again, the physician should read and initial each of these reports before it is placed in the record.

Laboratory Reports

Different colors of paper are often used for reporting different procedures. For example, urinalysis report forms may be yellow, blood count forms pink, and so on. When laboratory slips are smaller than the history form, they should be placed on a standard $8^{1}/_{2}$- × 11-inch sheet of colored paper. Type or print the patient's name in the upper right corner; then, with transparent tape, fasten the first report even with the bottom of the page. The second laboratory report will be taped or glued in place on top of and approximately $^{1}/_{2}$ inch above the first slip, allowing the date to show on the first report. By this method, called **shingling,** the latest report always appears on top (Figure 14-6). When checking previous reports, it is necessary only to run a finger down the slips until the desired date is found; then flip up the slips above. Laboratory report carrier forms with adhesive strips may be purchased.

PROCEDURE 14-3

Establish and Maintain the Medical Record: Add Supplementary Items to Established Patient Records

CAAHEP COMPETENCY: 3.c.(2)(c)
ABHES COMPETENCY: 3.b

GOAL: *To add supplementary documents and progress notes to patient histories, observing standard steps in filing, while creating an orderly file that will facilitate ready reference to any item of information.*

EQUIPMENT and SUPPLIES

- Assorted correspondence, diagnostic reports, and progress notes
- Patient files
- Computer or typewriter
- Mending tape
- FILE stamp or pen
- Sorter
- Stapler

PROCEDURAL STEPS

1. Group all papers according to patients' names.
   PURPOSE: To expedite the filing process.
2. Remove any staples or paper clips.
   PURPOSE: Staples in the file folders are hazardous; paper clips are bulky and may become inadvertently attached to other materials.
3. Mend any damaged or torn records.
4. Attach any small items to standard-size paper.
   PURPOSE: Small items are easily lost or misplaced in files.
5. Group any related papers together.
6. Place your initials or FILE stamp in the upper left corner.
   PURPOSE: To indicate that the document is released for filing.
7. Code the document by underlining or writing the patient's name in the upper right corner.
   PURPOSE: To indicate where the document is to be filed.
8. Continue steps 2 through 7 until all documents have been conditioned, released, indexed, and coded.
9. Place all documents in the sorter in filing sequence.
   EXPLANATION: Sorter can be taken to file cabinet or shelf for placing documents in patient folders.

Radiology Reports

Radiology reports are usually typed on standard letter-size stationery. They are placed in the patient's history folder, with the most recent report on top. All radiology reports may be stapled together or kept behind a special divider in the chart.

Progress Notes

Reports on the patient's progress are continually being added to the medical record. Each visit of the patient should be entered on the chart, with the date preceding any notations about the visit. The medical assistant can type or stamp the date on the chart when readying the charts for the patient's visits. Every instruction, prescription, or telephone call for advice should be entered with the correct date. It is always advisable to initial each entry, especially when several persons are handling and making entries on a patient's record. This aids in tracing entries about which there may be some question.

MAKING CORRECTIONS AND ALTERATIONS TO MEDICAL RECORDS

Sometimes it is necessary to make corrections to medical records. Erasing, using correction fluid, or any other type of **obliteration** is never acceptable. To correct a handwritten entry, follow these three steps:

1. Draw a line through the error.
2. Insert the correction above or immediately after the error.
3. In the margin, write *correction* or *Corr.*, the initial of the person correcting the entry, and the date.

Errors made while typing are corrected in the usual way. However, an error discovered in a typed entry at a later date is corrected in the same manner as described for a handwritten entry. Never attempt to alter medical records without using this specific correction procedure, because this alteration of records may indicate a fraudulent attempt to cover up a mistake made by a staff member or the physician. Do not hide errors. If the error could in any way affect the health and well-being of the patient, it must immediately be brought to the attention of the physician.

Additions to electronic health records must be made by making an additional entry. Never delete a previous entry or change it, unless it was entered seconds ago. A good rule of thumb is to avoid changing any electronic entry after the initials of the maker have been added. This, of course, should happen immediately after the note is placed into the record. Once this has happened, a new entry must be made to correct information in a previous entry.

CRITICAL THINKING APPLICATION

Susan has been using an incorrect abbreviation for several weeks and is having a difficult time remembering the right abbreviation. After taking a call from Mrs. Johnston, she remembers that she used the incorrect abbreviation in her chart last week. When Susan pulls the

Continued

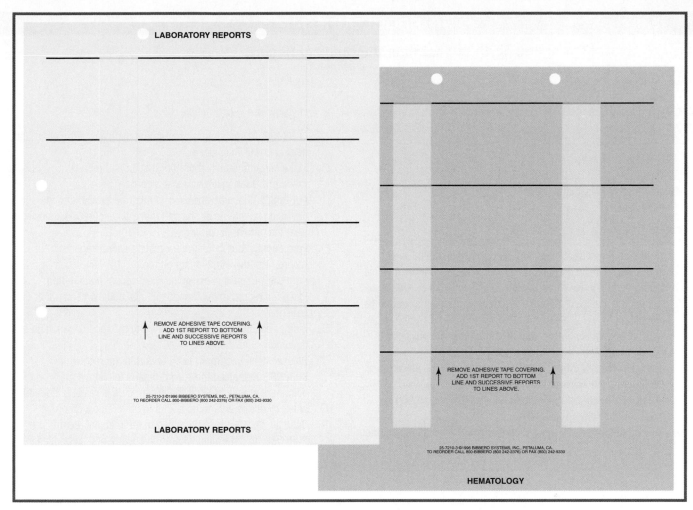

FIGURE 14-6 Shingled laboratory report forms. These forms make filing laboratory reports easy and provide a good adhesive so that the reports will not fall out of the chart if they are not standard size. (Courtesy Bibbero Systems, Inc., Petaluma, Calif. 94954, (800) 242-2376, www.bibbero.com.)

chart, she notices that entries have been made after the ones that Susan made on Mrs. Johnston's last visit. How does Susan correct her error?

KEEPING RECORDS CURRENT

One of the greatest dangers to good record keeping is **procrastination.** The record must be methodically kept current (Procedure 14-4). The medical assistant is responsible for seeing that this is done.

Case histories and reports may accumulate on the physician's or the medical assistant's desk during the day. After the last patient has gone, check each history to make certain that all necessary information has been recorded and that each entry is sufficiently clear for future understanding. Give the physician all abnormal reports to read and initial so that action can be taken and they may be filed in the patient's case history folder. Some physicians will want to see every laboratory report, whether it is normal or abnormal. Follow the requirements as set forth in the office policy and procedure manual.

While the physician is reviewing these reports, pull the histories of any patients seen outside the office that day, as well as those of patients who have been given special instructions by telephone or for whom prescriptions were ordered. These entries are made in the same manner as for an office visit, but the type of call is explained in parentheses after the date.

A prescription pad, printed on no-smear, carbonless paper, is available for a timesaving, write-it-once system. By placing the prescription blank over the patient's record, the prescription is automatically copied on the record as it is written. Prescription carriers with adhesive strips are also available for the physician who uses duplicate prescription blanks (Figure 14-7).

The patient record should not leave the office. A physician's pocket call record can be used for outside calls, and the information can be transferred to the chart in the office (Figure 14-8). Notations should be made of any missed appointments or of refusals to cooperate with instructions as they occur.

After all records have been reviewed for the day, they should be placed in a file tray and locked away for the night if there is insufficient time to file them. Do not leave histories out in view at night, especially if the facility has a cleaning service. On

Maintain the Medical Record

CAAHEP COMPETENCY: 3.c(2)(c)
ABHES COMPETENCY: 3.b

GOAL: *To make certain that the medical record is maintained and usable by all parties involved in patient care.*

EQUIPMENT and SUPPLIES

- Patient medical record
- Various forms used inside the medical record
- Results and reports, if applicable
- Clerical supplies

PROCEDURAL STEPS

1. Verify that the correct medical record has been pulled.
   PURPOSE: To make certain that all items placed into the medical record pertain to the right patient.
2. Inspect the medical record to determine which forms need to be added.
   PURPOSE: To make certain that the forms that the physician needs are available at all times.
3. Add all necessary forms to the record to enable the physician to document the office visit properly.
   PURPOSE: To make certain that the forms that the physician needs are available at all times.
4. Attach the forms to the record permanently or according to office policy.

PURPOSE: To keep information from falling out of the chart and getting lost or misplaced.

5. Make certain that all laboratory results and reports are available to the physician in the medical record.
   PURPOSE: All results and reports must be available to the physician so that he or she can make an accurate diagnosis and treat the patient accordingly.
6. Permanently attach laboratory results and/or reports in the record, with the most recent on top.
   PURPOSE: To easily access the most recent patient data.
7. Place the record in the designated place to await arrival of the patient.
8. If other documents are to be added to the record, condition each document.
9. Release each document to be added to the record.
   PURPOSE: Releasing the record means to place a mark on the document to indicate that the information is ready to be filed.
10. Index all documents to be added to the medical record.
11. Code all documents to be added to the medical record.
    PURPOSE: To determine where the document is to be filed.

---

arrival the next morning the medical assistant can index the histories for filing. Attach extra reports and information sheets. Always attach material to the chart permanently—do not simply drop forms into the folders. When this has been done, the records are ready for filing.

The physician may prefer to dictate progress notes rather than write them in longhand. At appropriate times during the day, everything is dictated: patient histories, physical examination findings, medications prescribed, follow-up findings, and summaries of telephone conversations. At the end of the day, the recorded information is given to the medical assistant for transcribing onto the records.

A great deal of time may be saved in transcribing these notes by using a continuous roll or pages of self-adhesive strips. When the **transcription** has been completed, the physician may wish to check the notes, underline important points, and initial each entry before returning the notes to the medical assistant for insertion into the charts to verify that they are correct in the event of **audit** or litigation. The use of self-adhesive strips saves removing the sheet from a chart that may be bound with metal fasteners, inserting the sheet into the typewriter, and putting the sheet back into the folder (Figure 14-9). It also simplifies the physician's part in checking and initialing the notes, because only the transcribed material is handled, not the bulky charts.

TRANSFER, DESTRUCTION, AND RETENTION OF MEDICAL RECORDS

Regular Transfer of Files

In most medical offices, records are filed according to three classifications:

- Active files are those of patients currently receiving treatment.
- Inactive files generally are those of patients whom the doctor has not seen for 6 months or longer. When such individuals return for care, their folders are replaced in the active file.
- Closed files are records of patients who have died, moved away, or otherwise terminated their relationship with the physician.

Some system must be established for regular transfer of files from active to inactive status or possibly destruction. The yearly expansion of charts and the file space available can influence the transfer period. Charts for patients who are currently hospitalized may be kept in a special section for quick reference, then placed in the regular active file when the patient is discharged from the hospital. In a surgical practice there frequently is a specific date on which the patient is discharged from the physician's care, and

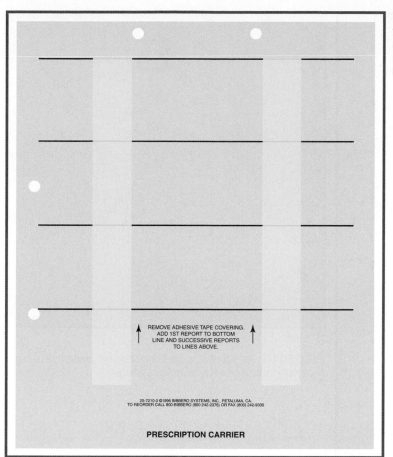

REMOVE ADHESIVE TAPE COVERING.
ADD 1ST REPORT TO BOTTOM
LINE AND SUCCESSIVE REPORTS
TO LINES ABOVE.

25-7210-3 ©1996 BIBBERO SYSTEMS, INC., PETALUMA, CA.
TO REORDER CALL 800-BIBBERO (800 242-2376) OR FAX (800) 242-9330

PRESCRIPTION CARRIER

FIGURE 14-7 Filing copies of prescriptions. The self-adhesive on this form allows a copy of the prescription to be filed inside the patient's chart, and saves time over handwriting the information a second time. (Courtesy Bibbero Systems, Inc., Petaluma, Calif. 94954, (800) 242-2376, www. bibbero.com.)

PHYSICIANS POCKET CALL RECORD		DATE				
NAME	ADDRESS OR REMARKS	SYMBOL	MONEY RECEIVED	HOME CHARGES	HOSPITAL CHARGES	
	Post these TOTALS to office book daily. ☞					

FIGURE 14-8 Physician pocket call record. The pocket call record may be used to record information about patients seen away from the clinic, such as skilled nursing facility patients or hospital patients.

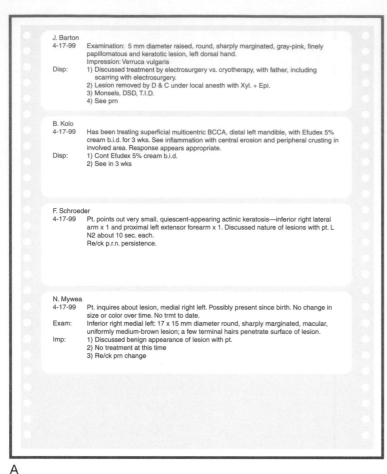

J. Barton
4-17-99   Examination: 5 mm diameter raised, round, sharply marginated, gray-pink, finely
           papillomatous and keratotic lesion, left dorsal hand.
           Impression: Verruca vulgaris
Disp: 1) Discussed treatment by electrosurgery vs. cryotherapy, with father, including
              scarring with electrosurgery.
           2) Lesion removed by D & C under local anesth with Xyl. + Epi.
           3) Monsels, DSD, T.I.D.
           4) See prn

B. Kolo
4-17-99   Has been treating superficial multicentric BCCA, distal left mandible, with Efudex 5%
           cream b.i.d. for 3 wks. See inflammation with central erosion and peripheral crusting in
           involved area. Response appears appropriate.
Disp: 1) Cont Efudex 5% cream b.i.d.
           2) See in 3 wks

F. Schroeder
4-17-99   Pt. points out very small, quiescent-appearing actinic keratosis—inferior right lateral
           arm x 1 and proximal left extensor forearm x 1. Discussed nature of lesions with pt. L
           N2 about 10 sec. each.
           Re/ck p.r.n. persistence.

N. Mywea
4-17-99   Pt. inquires about lesion, medial right left. Possibly present since birth. No change in
           size or color over time. No trmt to date.
Exam: Inferior right medial left: 17 x 15 mm diameter round, sharply marginated, macular,
           uniformly medium-brown lesion; a few terminal hairs penetrate surface of lesion.
Imp: 1) Discussed benign appearance of lesion with pt.
           2) No treatment at this time
           3) Re/ck prn change

A

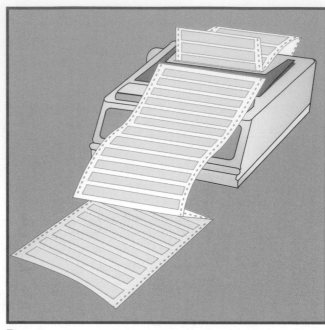

B

FIGURE 14-9 Self-adhesive progress notes. Progress notes can be quickly filed into the chart when self-adhesive forms are used.

the notation made on the chart "Return prn" (for the Latin pro re nata, "as the occasion arises" or "when needed"). This record may safely be placed in the inactive file. In a general practice office, the outside of the folder may be stamped with the date of the visit each time the patient is seen. It will then be a simple matter to determine when the chart should be transferred to the inactive status. This is called the *perpetual transfer method.*

Retention and Destruction

Physicians have an obligation to retain patient records that may reasonably be of value to a patient, according to the American Medical Association (AMA) Council on Ethical and Judicial Affairs. There is no standard, nationwide rule to follow in establishing a records **retention schedule** at this time.

Medical considerations are the primary basis for deciding how long to retain medical records. For example, operative notes and chemotherapy records should always be part of the patient's chart. The laws regarding the retention of medical records vary from state to state, and many governmental programs, such as Medicare and Medicaid, have their own guidelines for records retention. These guidelines range anywhere from 3 years to permanent retention. When no restriction exists for the retention of medical records, it is best to keep the records for a 10-year period. However, when retaining the records of a minor, the facility should keep the records until the minor reaches the age of majority, plus an additional 3 years.

If a particular record no longer needs to be kept for medical reasons, the physician should check state law to see whether there is a requirement that records be kept for a minimum length of time (most states do not have such a provision). The time is measured from the last professional contact with the patient.

In all cases, medical records should be kept for at least as long as the length of time of the statute of limitations for medical malpractice claims, which may be 3 or more years, depending on state law. In the case of a minor the statute of limitations may not apply until the patient reaches the age of majority.

The records of any patient covered by Medicare or Medicaid must be kept at least 6 years. The Health Insurance Portability and Accountability Act (HIPAA) recommends that records for patients who have died should be kept for at least 2 years.

Before old records are discarded, patients should be given an opportunity to claim a copy of the records or have them sent to another physician, if it is feasible to give the patient that opportunity. To preserve confidentiality when discarding old records, the documents should be destroyed by shredding or through a professional document destruction service.

Protection of Records

Releasing original case histories to anyone outside the healthcare facility should be avoided. Instead, prepare a summary or photocopy the materials needed for reference and retain the original in the physician's office. With the facsimile machine becoming standard equipment in business facilities, as well as in many of our homes, the transfer of information is simplified and the records remain in safekeeping. Often only certain aspects of the record are requested by colleagues or others, and these can easily be supplied by faxing the required pages, observing precautions for confidentiality.

Occasions may arise when records are temporarily out of the office, although this should be an extremely rare occurrence. Some physicians release case histories to their colleagues, or an original record may be subpoenaed by the court. In such instances, a colored **OUTfolder** should be inserted in the file in place of the regular folder and a notation made of the name, date, and to whom the record was released. Interim papers may be placed in the OUTfolder until the original is returned.

Long-Term Storage

Large healthcare facilities may find it advisable to **microfilm** records for storage. Another option is the transfer of paper records by laser beam onto optical disks. Microfilm and optical disk technology are both expensive and probably are not practical for any but a very large group practice or health maintenance organization.

Facilities that have computerized the patient records will be able to keep those records indefinitely on disk. Scanners can convert a paper record into an image on the computer screen, resulting in an electronic medical record. Records can be scanned and stored in electronic format on writeable CD-ROM or DVD-ROM. The bulky paper files can then be put in storage or eliminated. There is no longer a need to fill hundreds of square feet of storage space or search through stacks of storage file boxes for an inactive or closed file.

RELEASING MEDICAL RECORD INFORMATION

The medical facility must be extremely careful when releasing any type of medical information. The patient must sign a release for information to be given to any third party (Procedure 14-5).

Often a family member will call to inquire about a patient, but without the patient's specific request or release, no information may be given. Some offices have a "code" system whereby the patient gives the facility a code word that must be used by a family member to receive medical information about the patient.

Requests for medical information should be made in writing (Figure 14-10). It is unwise to accept a faxed request for medical information or a faxed release of information from a patient. Even requests from the patient's attorney or third-party payors must be cleared by the patient to receive information. Some attorneys may present a legal document called a **power of attorney,** which authorizes them to see the records. Still, this document is signed by the patient, so it is a release in itself.

PROCEDURE 14-5

Establish and Maintain the Medical Record: Prepare a Record Release Form

<u>CAAHEP COMPETENCY:</u> 3.c.(2)(c)
<u>ABHES COMPETENCY:</u> 5.c

GOAL: *To provide a legal document that indicates the patient's consent to the release of his or her medical records to another provider or healthcare facility.*

EQUIPMENT and SUPPLIES

- Medical record release form
- Pen
- Envelope

PROCEDURAL STEPS

1. Explain to the patient that a medical record release form will be necessary to obtain records from another provider. If the patient is having records sent to another provider, a release for that will also be required.
   <u>PURPOSE:</u> To ensure the patient's understanding of the record release procedure and purposes.

2. Review the record release form with the patient and ask if the form is understood or if the patient has any questions about the form.
   <u>PURPOSE:</u> To provide the opportunity for questions and to ensure the patient's understanding of the form.

3. Have the patient sign the form in the space indicated. If other demographic information is required, such as a social security number or other names used, complete that information as well.
   <u>PURPOSE:</u> The patient must sign the form for records to be released by any medical facility.

4. Make a copy of the form for the file, then mail it to the appropriate facility. Note the date that the form was sent. Provide a copy to the patient if requested.
   <u>PURPOSE:</u> To provide a record that the information or documents were actually requested on a certain date

5. Follow up to ensure that the requested records actually arrived.
   <u>PURPOSE:</u> To make certain that the records needed by the physician to accurately and competently treat the patient are available in a timely manner.

6. Check the patient's medical record to determine if a signed, current privacy policy document is on file. If not, have the patient sign one, and place it in the record.
   <u>PURPOSE:</u> To ensure that all patients are notified of the office privacy policy.

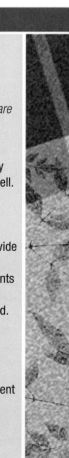

RECORDS RELEASE AUTHORIZATION

TO _____
Doctor or Hospital

_____
Address

I HEREBY AUTHORIZE AND REQUEST YOU TO RELEASE TO:

ALL RECORDS IN YOUR POSSESION CONCERNING _____

_____ILLNESS AND/OR

TREATMENT DURING THE PERIOD FROM _____TO _____.

NAME _____TEL. _____

ADDRESS_____

SIGNATURE _____DATE _____
(If relative, state relationship)
WITNESS_____DATE _____

25-8104 © 1973 BIBBERO SYSTEMS, INC., PETALUMA,, CA.

FIGURE 14-10 Authorization to release medical records. All requests for medical records should be in writing, and the request should be kept in the patient chart. (Courtesy Bibbero Systems, Inc., Petaluma, Calif. 94954, (800) 242-2376, www.bibbero.com.)

CRITICAL THINKING APPLICATION

Susan has never seen a power of attorney and is curious about this type of document. How might she investigate and learn more about them? Whom should Susan approach first for this information? The physician has an attorney that Susan has met once. Should she call him and ask about the document without notifying the physician? Why or why not?

The time may come when a patient decides that he or she no longer agrees to the release of medical information. In this case the patient should sign a revocation form, and it must be made a part of the medical record (Figure 14-11).

Sometimes the patient will want to view his or her own record. They certainly have a right to see this information, but some patients may not understand the terminology used in the record. A staff member should always remain with the patient who is viewing his or her medical record. Remember, the original medical record should never leave the medical facility.

When a release is presented to the office, copy only the records requested in the release. Do not provide additional information that is not requested. It is acceptable to charge reasonable copying fees to the person requesting the information.

DICTATION AND TRANSCRIPTION

Administrative medical assistants may find that transcribing **dictation** is one of the job requirements they perform periodically. Transcription can be performed from handwritten notes, such as those in shorthand, or from machine dictation. In a healthcare facility, the medical transcriptionist is a part of the team. Smooth operation of the facility may depend on the timely and accurate performance of assigned responsibilities, such as record documentation and the preparation of special reports.

The transcriptionist will find that accuracy and speed are primary **requisites,** as well as a strong grasp of medical knowledge, especially anatomy and physiology (Figure 14-12). Income depends on the transcriptionist's productivity, which may be measured by the number of pages, characters, or lines typed. The person who intends to do transcribing exclusively should take a special course in transcription techniques. Certification is available through the American Association for Medical Transcriptionists.

Machine Transcription

Three stages of activity are involved in the process of dictation and transcription:

FIGURE 14-11 Revocation of release of medical records. (Courtesy Bibbero Systems, Inc., Petaluma, Calif 94954, (800) 242-2376, www.bibbero.com.)

REVOCATION OF AUTHORIZATION TO RELEASE MEDICAL RECORDS

_____ , who resides at _____
          Name   Street Address

_____ , hereby revokes authorization to the physician, hospital, clinic,
          City/State/Zip

lab, radiology center or other healthcare provider listed below:

_____
                              Name

_____
                          Street Address

_____
                          City/State/Zip

to disclose information from the medical records of:

_____
                              Name

_____
                          Street Address

_____
                          City/State/Zip

My revocation extends to the data or documents I have initialed below:
_____ Records of visits (all visits)
_____ Record of visit for a specific date or dates, including or limited to _____
_____ Copies of records or reports provided to the above named (i.e. hospital, lab, etc.)
_____ Statements of charges or payments
_____ Mental health, alcohol and/or drug abuse treatment _____
_____ HIV information
_____ Hepatitis information
_____ Other (specific) _____

This revocation is given freely with the understanding that:

1. Disclosures made in good faith may have already occured based upon my previously issued authorization and that this renovation cannot apply retroactively to such disclosures. I also understand that the disclosure of health information may be required by law in some instances, such as for the reporting of communicable diseases.
2. The facility, it's employees, officers, and physicians are hereby released from any legal responsibility or liability for disclosure of the information I authorized previously.

_____   _____   _____
   Patient's Printed Name   Social Security # (for identification purposes only)   Date

_____   _____
 Patient's Signature (or Guardian, if for a minor)   Revocation Date (if other than 60 days from date above)

_____   _____
          Witness   Date

#25-8402 • 12/02 • BIBBERO SYSTEMS, INC • PETALUMA, CA   TO REORDER FORMS: (800) BIBBERO (800 242-2376) OR FAX: (800) 242-9330 MFG IN U.S.A.

FIGURE 14-11 Revocation of release of medical records. (Courtesy Bibbero Systems, Inc., Petaluma, Calif 94954, (800) 242-2376, www.bibbero.com.)

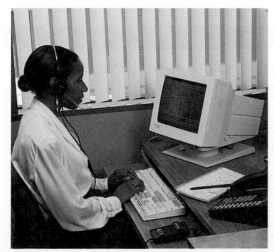

FIGURE 14-12 Medical transcriptionists must have excellent typing skills and good hearing. They must be accurate and use good grammar while completing transcription duties.

- Dictating into a dictation unit
- Listening to what has been dictated
- Keyboarding the dictated text to a printed document using correct format and required punctuation

Dictation Unit

A dictation unit is used by the physician to record material to be typed. Dictation units vary in design and capabilities. A desktop dictation unit is common in an office setting. This may be a combination unit used for both dictation and transcription. Alternatively, a machine used only for dictation may remain at the physician's desk; a separate transcription unit, including headphones and a foot pedal, remains at the transcriptionist's station. A lightweight, portable, handheld dictation unit may be used for times when the physician wishes to dictate while traveling or attending meetings away from the office. Digital dictation machines are now available; these are lightweight and portable and hold more information than standard dictation recorders. Physicians in a larger setting may install transcribing equipment that they can access by telephone wherever they may be. Many hospitals have this arrangement. All produce a recording that the transcriptionist listens to while keyboarding the text.

CRITICAL THINKING APPLICATION

Susan would like to practice transcription skills at home, but she does not have a transcription unit. How could she do this without the proper equipment? Medical terminology is important to the medical assistant who does transcription. What are some ways Susan can improve her medical terminology skills?

Transcriber Unit

The unit operated by the transcriptionist may use magnetic tape, a cassette, or a disk. A desktop unit using minicassettes, microcassettes, or standard cassettes is typical in the physician's office.

There are many types and manufacturers of transcribing equipment, but most units contain certain standard features. Before using any equipment, the medical assistant should study the manufacturer's instruction manual. Most transcription units have at least the following features:

- Stop and start control, with backup and fast-forward ability
- Speed control
- Volume control
- Tone control
- Indicator for locating special instructions and determining the document length

A beginning transcriptionist tends to listen to a few words, stop the machine, type those words, then restart the transcriber unit. Through practice, the transcriptionist learns to coordinate keyboarding activity with listening skills and listen ahead, thereby retaining in memory more and more of the dictated material so that it becomes unnecessary to stop and start the machine for this purpose.

Keyboarding Unit

The most important piece of equipment for the transcriptionist is the typewriter or computer on which the printed text will be produced (Procedure 14-6). Many improvements have occurred within the past few years. Computers have attachable foot pedals and headphones that allow the medical assistant to perform transcription directly onto the unit. A variety of computer programs are available to assist with transcription duties.

FILING EQUIPMENT

The vertical four-drawer steel filing cabinet, used with manila folders with the patient's name on the tab, was the traditional system of choice for years. The most popular system today is color-coding on open shelves. Rotary, lateral, compactable, and automated files are also available. Some records are kept in card or tray files. Regardless of the type or style of equipment, the best quality is always an economy. Some of the considerations in selecting filing equipment are as follows:

- Office space availability
- Structural considerations
- Cost of space and equipment
- Size, type, and volume of records
- Confidentiality requirements
- Retrieval speed
- Fire protection

Drawer Files

Drawer files should be full suspension; they should roll easily, close securely, and be equipped with a locking device. The best cabinets have a center trough at the bottom of each drawer with a rod for holding divider guides. Floor space of twice the depth of the drawer must be allowed so that the drawer can be pulled out to its full extent. A drawback of the vertical four-drawer files is that only one person can use a file cabinet at any given time. Filing is also slower because the drawer must be opened and closed each time a file is pulled or filed. Drawer files are

---

PROCEDURE 14-6

Transcribe a Machine-Dictated Letter Using a Computer or Word Processor

CAAHEP COMPETENCY: 3.c.(1)(a)
ABHES COMPETENCIES: 2.j, 2.n, 2.o

GOAL: *To transcribe a machine-dictated letter into a mailable document without error or corrections, using a computer or word processor.*

EQUIPMENT and SUPPLIES

- Transcribing machine
- Word processor or computer with appropriate software
- Stationery
- Reference manual

PROCEDURAL STEPS

1. Assemble supplies.
2. Set up format for selected letter style.
3. Keyboard the text while listening to the dictated letter.
4. Edit the letter on the monitor.
   PURPOSE: The letter should be in mailable form before printing.
5. Execute a spell check.
6. Direct the letter to the printer.

relatively easy to move, but for safety reasons they should be bolted to the wall or to one another.

File cabinets are heavy and can tip over, causing serious damage or injury unless reasonable care is observed. Open only one file drawer at a time, and close it when the filing has been completed. A drawer left even slightly open can cause injury to a passerby.

Shelf Files

Shelf files should have doors to protect the contents. A popular type of shelf file has doors that slide back into the cabinet; the door from a lower shelf may be pulled out and used for work space. Approximately 50% more material per square foot of floor space may be filed in shelf files when compared with the four-drawer file. Open shelf units hold files sideways and can go higher on the wall because there is no drawer to pull out (Figure 14-13). File retrieval is faster because several individuals can work simultaneously.

Open shelf units without doors are the most economic but offer little protection or confidentiality to the records. They are susceptible to water and fire damage. Shelf files are available in many attractive colors and can add a decorative note to the business office. Special storage or shelf space should be provided for x-ray films, if many films are stored.

Rotary Circular Files

Rotary circular files can hold a large volume of records. They save space and clerical motion. The files revolve easily; some come with push-button controls. Several persons can work at one rotary file and use records at the same time. One disadvantage is that they afford less privacy and protection than files that can be closed and locked.

Lateral Files

Lateral files are good for personal files and are especially attractive for the physician's private office. They use more wall space than the vertical file but do not extend out into the room

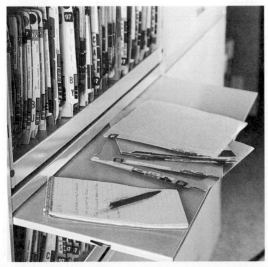

FIGURE 14-13 Open shelf filing is an efficient method, especially for color-coded filing systems. The shelf doors can often be used as workspace.

so far. The folders are filed sideways in the lateral file, left to right, instead of front to back as in a vertical file. Some have a pull-out drawer, as the vertical file does; others have doors that slide into the cabinet, exposing the filing space.

Compactable Files

The office with little space and a great volume of records might use compactable files, which are a variation of open shelf files. The files are mounted on tracks in the floor, and the units slide along the tracks so that access is gained to the needed records. The rolling may be either automated or manual. One drawback is that not all records are available at the same time.

Automated Files

Automated files are very expensive initially and require more maintenance than do the other types of filing equipment. They will probably be found only in very large installations such as clinics or hospitals. These files bring the record to the operator instead of the operator going to the record. When the operator presses a button indicating the appropriate shelf, the shelf automatically moves into position in front of the operator for record retrieval. The automated or power file is fast and can store large numbers of records in a small amount of space. Only one person can use the unit at one time.

Card Files

Almost every office has some occasion to use a card file. This may be for patient ledgers, a patient index, a library index, an index of surgical tray setups, telephone numbers, or numerous other records. A good-quality steel box or tray is a sound investment.

Special Items

Metal framework is available that can convert a regular drawer file into suspension-folder equipment. The assistant with a great deal of filing may wish to purchase a portable filing shelf that fits on the side of an opened drawer and can be moved from place to place as needed. Another special filing item is a sorting file, which can be a great time saver. A portable file cart for the temporary filing of unbilled insurance claims may be quite useful. It may also be used for the preliminary sorting of charts to be refiled. This is sometimes called a *suspense file*.

SUPPLIES

Divider Guides

Each file drawer or shelf should be equipped with plenty of dividers or guides. Some authorities recommend one guide for approximately each $1\frac{1}{2}$ inches of material, or every eight to ten folders. Guides should be of good-quality **pressboard** or strong plastic. Economy guides will soon become bent and frayed and have to be replaced. Divider guides have a protruding tab, which either may be an integral part of the card or may be made of metal or plastic. The guides reduce the area of search and serve as supports for the folders. They are available in single, third, or fifth cut (one, three, or five different positions). The guide may have a projection at the bottom edge with a ring or hole through which a rod may go. This type of guide card is used in drawers that have a trough for the projection and a rod to hold the guides in place.

OUTguides

An **OUTguide** is a heavy guide that is used to replace a folder that has been temporarily removed (Figure 14-14). It should be of a distinctive color for quick detection. This makes refiling simpler and alerts the file clerk that a file is missing. Several colors may be used, each color designating the temporary location of the file. The OUTguide may have lines for recording information, or it may have a plastic pocket for inserting an information card.

Chart Covers of Folders

Most records to be filed are placed in covers or tabbed folders. The most commonly used is a general-purpose third-cut manila folder that may be expanded to $3/4$ inch. These are available with a double-thickness reinforced tab that will greatly lengthen the life of the folder. Folders kept in drawers have tabs at the top; those kept on shelves have tabs at the side. Many variations of folder styles are available for special purposes.

The vertical pocket, which is of heavier weight than the general-purpose folder, has a front that folds down for easy access to contents and is available with up to a $3^{1}/_{2}$-inch expansion. These are used for bulky histories or correspondence.

Hanging or suspension folders are made of heavy stock and hang on metal rods from side to side in a drawer. They can be used only with files equipped with suspension equipment.

Binder folders have fasteners with which to bind papers within the folder. These offer some security for the papers, but filing the materials is time consuming.

The number of papers that will fit in one folder depends on the thickness of the papers. Near the bottom edge of most folders are one or more score marks, which should be used as the contents of the folders expand. If folders are refolded at these score marks, the danger of their bending and sliding under other folders is reduced, and a neater file results. Papers should never protrude from the folder edges, and they should always be inserted with their tops to the left. When papers start to ride up in any folder, the folder is overloaded.

Labels

The label is a necessary filing and finding device. Use labels to identify each shelf, drawer, divider guide, and folder. A label on

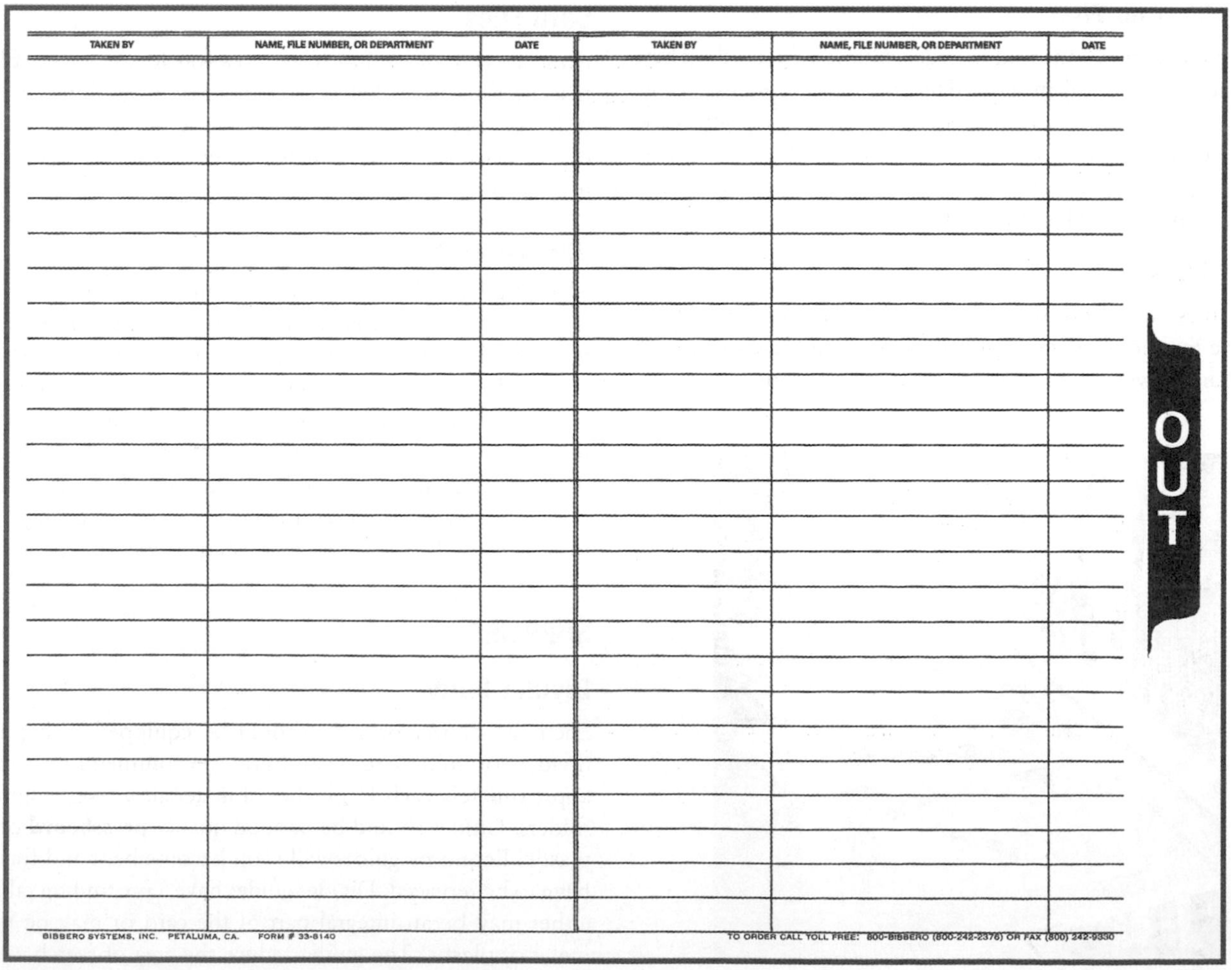

FIGURE 14-14 OUTguides provide tracking for files that are not in their proper location. The guide gives information as to where the file can be located. (Courtesy Bibbero Systems, Inc., Petaluma, Calif. 94954, (800) 242-2376, www.bibbero.com.)

the drawer or shelf identifies the nature of its contents. It should also indicate the range (alphabetic, numeric, or chronologic) of the material filed in that space.

The label on the divider guide identifies the range of folder headings following that divider guide up to the next divider; for example, BaBo. The label on the folder identifies the contents of that folder only. This may be the name of the patient, subject matter of correspondence, a business topic, or anything at all that needs to be filed. Label a folder when a new patient is seen or existing folders are full or when materials need to be transferred within the filing system.

Paper labels may be purchased on rolls of gummed tape; another type has adhesive backs that are peeled from a protective sheet. Labels are available in almost any size, shape, or color to meet the individual needs of any facility. Visit a stationer and study the catalogs to find the best product to meet the needs of the facility.

A narrow label applied to the front of the folder tab is the easiest to use and is satisfactory for folders kept in a drawer file. Labels for **shelf filing** should be identifiable from both front and back. Always type the label before separating it from the roll or protective sheet. Type the **caption** on the label in indexing order.

FILING PROCEDURES

Filing of all materials involves five basic steps: conditioning, releasing, indexing and coding, sorting, and storing and filing.

Conditioning

Conditioning of papers involves removing all pins, brads, and paper clips; stapling related papers together; attaching clippings or items smaller than page-size to a regular sheet of paper with rubber cement or tape; and mending damaged records.

Releasing

The term *releasing* simply means that some mark is placed on the paper indicating that it is now ready for filing. This will usually be either the medical assistant's initials or a FILE stamp placed in the upper left corner.

Indexing and Coding

Indexing means deciding where to file the letter or paper, and coding means placing some indication of this decision on the paper (Table 14-1). This may be done by underlining the name or subject, if it appears on the paper, or writing the indexing subject or name in some conspicuous place. If there is more than one logical place to file the paper, the original is coded for the main location and a cross-reference sheet prepared, indicating this location and coded for the second location. Every paper placed in a patient's chart should have the date and name of the patient on it, usually in the upper right corner.

Sorting

Sorting is arranging the papers in filing sequence. Sort papers before going to the file cabinet or shelf. Do any necessary

INDEXING RULE	NAME	UNIT 1	UNIT 2	UNIT 3
1	Robert F. Grinch	Grinch	Robert	F.
	R. Frank Grumman	Grumman	R.	Frank
2	J. Orville Smith	Smith	J.	Orville
	Jason O. Smith	Smith	Jason	O.
3	M. L. Saint-Vickery	Saint-Vickery	M.	L.
	Marie-Louise Taylor	Taylor	Marielouise	
4	Charles S. Anderson	Anderson	Charles	S.
	Anderson's Surgical Supply	Andersons	Surgical	Supply
5	Ah Hop Akee	Akee	Ah	Hop
6	Alice Delaney	Delaney	Alice	
	Chester K. DeLong	Delong	Chester	K.
7	Michael St. John	Stjohn	Michael	
8	Helen M. Maag	Maag	Helen	M.
	Frederick Mabry	Mabry	Frederick	
	James E. MacDonald	Macdonald	James	E.
9	Mrs. John L. Doe (Mary Jones)	Doe	Mary	Jones (Mrs John L.)
10	Prof. John J. Breck	Breck	John	J. (Prof.)
	Madame Sylvia	Madame	Sylvia	
	Sister Mary Catherine	Sister	Mary	Catherine
	Theodore Wilson, M.D.	Wilson	Theodore (M.D.)	
11	Lawrence W. Sloan, Jr.	Sloan	Lawrence	W. (Jr.)
	Lawrence W. Sloan, Sr.	Sloan	Lawrence	W. (Sr.)
12	The Moore Clinic	Moore	Clinic (The)	

TABLE 14-1 Application of Indexing Rules

stapling of papers at the desk or filing table. Invest in a desktop sorter with a series of dividers, between which papers are placed in filing sequence. One general-purpose sorter has six means of classification: alphabetic sections, numbers 1 to 31, days of the week, months of the year, numbers in groups of five, and space on the tabs for special captions to be taped when desired. In the preliminary sorting, place the papers in the appropriate division in the sorter. Then it is comparatively simple to arrange these groups into the proper sequence for filing.

Storing and Filing

In storing or filing papers in the folder, items should be placed face up, top edge to the left, with the most recent date at the front of the folder. Lift the folder 1 or 2 inches out of the drawer before inserting new material, so that the sheets can drop down completely into the folder. It is best to permanently attach items to the file folder. When refiling completed folders, arrange them in indexing order before going to the file cabinets.

Locating Misplaced Files

Unless files are promptly replaced after use, they may become lost. Papers may be misfiled, requiring a thorough search to find them, which wastes valuable time. After a methodic and complete search through the proper folder, there are several places one may look for a misplaced paper: (1) in the folder in front of and behind the correct folder; (2) between the folders; (3) at the bottom of the file under all the folders; (4) in a folder of a patient with a similar name; or (5) in the sorter.

Indexing Rules

Indexing rules are fairly well standardized, based on current business practices. The Association of Records Managers and Administrators takes an active part in updating the rules. Some establishments adopt variations of these basic rules to accommodate their needs. In any case the practices need to be consistent within the system.

1. Last names of persons are considered first in filing; given name (first name), second; and middle name or initial, third. Compare the names beginning with the first letter of the name. When a letter is different in the two names, that letter determines the order of filing. For example:

   ab*e*
   ab*i*
   ab*m*
   ab*x*
   ac*l*
   ac*m*
   ad*a*
   ad*e*
   ad*i*

2. Initials precede a name beginning with the same letter. This illustrates the librarian's rule, "Nothing comes before something." For example:

   Smith, J.
   Smith, Jason

3. Hyphenated personal names. The hyphenated elements of a name, whether first name, middle name, or surname, are considered to be one unit. For example:

   Carlotta Freeman-Duque is filed as
   Freemanduque, Carlotta
   Cindy-Jean Green is filed as Green, Cindyjean

4. The apostrophe is disregarded in filing. For example:

   Andersons' Surgical Supply
   Andersons Surgical Supply

5. When indexing a foreign name when you cannot distinguish the first and last name, index each part of the name in the order in which it is written:

   Cau Liu
   Talluri Devi

   If you can make the distinction, you should use the last name as the first indexing unit:

   Liu, Jason

6. Names with prefixes are filed in the usual alphabetic order, with the prefix being considered as part of the name. For example:

   von Schmidt is filed as Vonschmidt
   DeLong is filed as Delong
   LaFrance is filed as Lafrance

7. Abbreviated parts of a name are indexed as written if that is the form generally used by that person. For example:

   Ste. Marie is filed as Stemarie
   St. John is filed as Stjohn
   Wm. is filed as Wm
   Edw. is filed as Edw
   Jas. is filed as Jas

8. Mac and Mc are filed in their regular place in the alphabet:

   Maag
   Mabry
   MacDonald
   Machado
   MacHale
   Maville
   McAulay
   McWilliams
   Meacham

If the files contain a great many names beginning with Mac or Mc, some offices file them as a separate letter of the alphabet for convenience.

9. The name of a married woman is indexed by her legal name (her husband's surname, her given name, and her middle name or maiden surname). For example:

> Doe, Mary Jones (Mrs. John L.)
> not Doe, Mrs. John L. (unless first name is unknown)

10. Titles, when followed by a complete name, may be used as the last filing unit if needed to distinguish from another identical name. For example:

> Mr. James D. Conley
> Conley James D Mr.
> Dr. James D. Conley
> Conley James D Dr.

Titles without complete names are considered the first indexing unit:

> Madame Sylvia
> Sister Theresa

11. Terms of seniority, or professional or academic degree, are used only to distinguish from an identical name. For example:

> Theodore Wilson, PhD
> Theodore Wilson, Sr.
> Theodore Wilson, Jr.
> Theodore Wilson, MD
> These examples would be filed in the following order:
> Theodore Wilson, Jr.
> Theodore Wilson, MD
> Theodore Wilson, PhD
> Theodore Wilson, Sr.

12. Articles such as The and A are disregarded in indexing:

> Moore Clinic (The)

FILING METHODS

The three basic methods of filing used in healthcare facilities are these:

- Alphabetic by name
- Numeric
- Subject

Patient charts are filed either alphabetically by name or by one of several numeric methods. Subject filing is used for business records, correspondence, and topical materials.

Alphabetic Filing

Alphabetic filing by name is the oldest, simplest, and most commonly used system. It is the system of choice for filing patient records in the majority of physicians' offices. If the medical assistant can find a word in the dictionary or a name in the telephone directory, then he or she already knows some of the rules.

The alphabetic system of filing is traditional and simple to set up, requiring only a file cabinet or shelf, folders, and some divider guides (Procedure 14-7). It is a **direct filing system,** in that the person filing need know only the name in order to find the desired file. Alphabetic filing does have some drawbacks:

- The correct spelling of the name must be known.
- As the number of files increases, more space is needed for each section of the alphabet. This results in periodic shifting of folders from drawer to drawer or shelf to shelf to allow for expansion.
- As the files expand, more time is required for filing or retrieving each folder because of the greater number of folders involved in the search. The time can be greatly reduced by color-coding.

Numeric Filing

Some form of **numeric filing** combined with color and shelf filing is used by practically every large clinic or hospital. Management consultants differ in their recommendations; some recommend numeric filing only if there are more than 5000 charts, more than 10,000 charts, or in some cases more than 15,000 charts. Others recommend nothing but numeric filing. Numeric filing is an **indirect filing system,** requiring the use of an alphabetic cross-reference to find a given file. Some people object to this added step and overlook the advantages, which are as follows:

- It allows unlimited expansion without periodic shifting of folders, and shelves are usually filled evenly.
- It provides additional confidentiality to the chart.
- It saves time in retrieving and refiling records quickly. One knows immediately that the number 978 falls between 977 and 979. By contrast, an alphabetic system, even with color-coding, requires a longer search for the exact spot.

There are several types of numeric filing systems. In the straight or consecutive numeric system, patients are given consecutive numbers as they visit the practice. This is the simplest of the numeric systems and works well for files of up to 10,000 records. It is time consuming, and the chance for error is greater when filing documents with five or more digits. Filing activity is greatest at the end of the numeric series.

In the terminal digit system, patients are also assigned consecutive numbers, but the digits in the number are usually separated into groups of twos or threes and are read in groups from right to left instead of from left to right. The records are filed backward in groups. For example, all files ending in 00 are grouped together first, then those ending in 01, etc. Next the files are grouped by their middle digits so that the 00 22s come before the 01 22s. Finally the files are arranged by their first digits, so that 01 00 22 precedes 02 00 22.

Middle-digit filing begins with the middle digits, followed by the first digit and finally by the terminal digits.

Some practices use the last four digits of each patient's Social Security number to file patient records. However, there is no

PROCEDURE 14-7

File Medical Records and Documents Using the Alphabetic System

CAAHEP COMPETENCY: 3.a.(1)(d)
ABHES COMPETENCY: 3.h

GOAL: *To file records efficiently using an alphabetic system and ensure that the records can be easily and quickly retrieved.*

EQUIPMENT and SUPPLIES

- Medical records
- Physical filing equipment
- Cart to carry records, if needed
- Alphabetic file guide
- Staple remover
- Stapler

PROCEDURAL STEPS

1. Using alphabetic guidelines, place the records to be filed in alphabetic order. If a stack of documents is to be filed, place them in alphabetic order inside an alphabetic file guide or sorter. Use rules for filing documents alphabetically.
   PURPOSE: To organize the filing process and file the record or document quickly without retracing steps and skipping from letter to letter.

2. Go to the filing storage equipment (shelves, cabinets, or drawers), and locate the correct spot in the alphabet for the first file.

3. Place the file in the cabinet or drawer in correct alphabetic order.

4. If adding a document to a file, place it on top so that the most recent information is seen first. This puts the information in the file in reverse chronologic order.
   PURPOSE: To provide access to the most pertinent and recent information.

5. Securely fasten documents to the chart. Do not just drop the documents inside the chart.
   PURPOSE: To keep vital information from falling out of the chart and being lost.

6. Refile the chart in its proper place.

---

legal requirement that every U.S. resident have a Social Security number; if a patient does not, a "pseudo number" would have to be issued.

Numeric filing requires more training, but once the system is mastered, fewer errors occur than with alphabetic filing (Procedure 14-8).

CRITICAL THINKING APPLICATION

Susan is unsure whether alphabetic or numeric filing is best in the medical office. What are some advantages and disadvantages of each method?

Subject Filing

Subject filing can be either alphabetic or **alphanumeric** (A 1-3, B 1-1, B 1-2, and so on) and is used for general correspondence. The main difficulty with subject filing is indexing, or classifying—deciding where to file a document. Many papers require cross-referencing. All correspondence dealing with a particular subject is filed together. The papers within the folders are filed chronologically, the most recent on top. The subject headings are placed on the tabs of the folders and filed alphabetically.

Color-Coding

When a color-coding system is used, both filing and finding are easier, and misfiled folders are kept to a minimum (Procedure 14-9). The use of color visually restricts the area of search for a specific record. A misfiled chart is easily spotted even from a distance of several feet. In color-coding, a specific color is selected to identify each letter of the alphabet. The application of the principle may be through using colored folders, adhesive colored identification labels, or various combinations of these. Any selection of colors may be used, and the division of the alphabet is determined by one's own needs. However, studies have shown that there is wide variation in the frequency with which different letters occur.

Alphabetic Color-Coding

There are several ways of color-coding files. One alphabetic system uses five different colored folders, with each color representing a segment of the alphabet. The second letter of the patient's last name determines the color.

As medicine continues to consolidate into larger facilities, with more patients under one management, the filing of patient charts becomes more complicated and color-coding becomes more useful. Several color-coding systems use two sets of 13 colors—one set for letters A-M, and a second set of the same colors on a different background for the letters N-Z.

Many ready-made systems are available (e.g., Bibbero, Colwell, Kardex, Remington Rand, Smead, TAB, VisiRecord). Self-adhesive colored letter blocks with either two or three letters in the specific colors are supplied in rolls. The color blocks with the appropriate letter are placed on the index tab of the folder, along with the patient's full name. The letters are in pairs so that they can be seen from either side of the chart.

PROCEDURE 14-8

File Medical Records and Documents Using the Numeric System

CAAHEP COMPETENCY: 3.a.(1)(d)
ABHES COMPETENCY: 3.h

GOAL: *To file records efficiently using a numeric system and ensure that the records can be easily and quickly retrieved.*

EQUIPMENT and SUPPLIES

- Medical records
- Physical filing equipment
- Cart to carry records, if needed
- Numeric file guide
- Staple remover
- Stapler
- Paper clips

PROCEDURAL STEPS

1. Using numeric guidelines, place the records to be filed in numeric order. If a stack of documents is to be filed, write the chart number on the document. Use rules for filing documents alphabetically.
   PURPOSE: To organize the filing process and file the records or documents quickly without retracing steps and skipping from letter to letter.

2. Go to the filing storage equipment (shelves, cabinets, or drawers) and locate the numeric spot for the first file.

3. Place the file in the cabinet or drawer in correct numeric order.

4. If adding a document to a file, place it on top so that the most recent information is seen first. This puts the information in the file in reverse chronologic order.
   PURPOSE: To provide access to the most pertinent and recent information.

5. Securely fasten documents to the chart. Do not just drop the documents inside the chart.
   PURPOSE: To keep vital information from falling out of the chart and being lost.

6. Refile the chart in its proper place.

PROCEDURE 14-9

Establish and Maintain the Medical Record: Color-Code Medical Records

CAAHEP COMPETENCY: 3.a.(1)(d)
ABHES COMPETENCY: 3.h

GOAL: *To color-code patient records using the agency's established coding system to effectively facilitate filing and finding.*

EQUIPMENT and SUPPLIES

- List of patient medical records to code
- File folders
- Information on agency's coding system
- Full range of color tabs

PROCEDURAL STEPS

1. Assemble patient records.

2. Arrange records in indexing order.
   PURPOSE: When records have been color-coded, they will be in filing order.

3. Pick up the first record, and note the second letter of the patient's surname.

EXPLANATION: For the purpose of this activity, the color-coding system described in the text will be used.

4. Choose a tab of the appropriate color.

5. Type the patient's name on the label in indexing order, and apply tab to the folder tab.
   PURPOSE: To identify the sequence of folders in the filing system.

6. Repeat steps 4 and 5 until all records have been coded.

7. Check the entire group for any isolated color.
   PURPOSE: If the order and color of the folders are correct, all charts of the same color within each letter of the alphabet will be grouped together.

Strong, easily differentiated colors are used, creating a band of color in the files that makes it easy to spot out-of-place folders (Figure 14-15).

Numeric Color-Coding

Color-coding is also used in numeric filing. Numbers 0 through 9 are each assigned a different color. In a terminal digit filing system, the colors for the last two numbers would be affixed to the tab. If the number 1 is red and 5 is yellow, all files with numbers ending in 15 form a red and yellow band. Usually a predetermined section of the number is color-coded.

Other Color-Coding Applications

There are many other ways to make color work for the efficient medical office. Small pressure-sensitive tabs in a variety of colors may be used to identify certain types of insured patients and

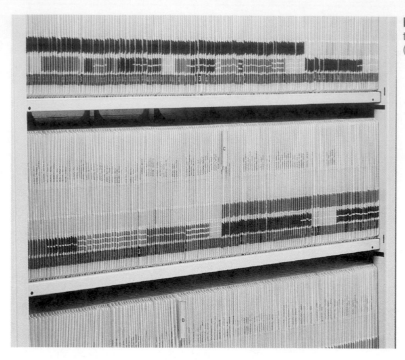

FIGURE 14-15 Color-coding patient charts makes it easy to see a file that is misplaced. (Courtesy Bibbero Systems, Inc., Petaluma, Calif. 94954, (800) 242-2376, www.bibbero.com.)

other specific information. For example, a red tab over the edge of the folder may identify a patient on Medicaid; a blue tab may identify a CHAMPUS patient; a green tab may identify a workers' compensation patient; matching tabs may be attached to the insured's ledger card; research cases may be identified by a special color tab; and brightly colored labels on the outside of a patient chart can indicate certain health conditions, such as drug allergies. In a partnership practice, a different color folder or label may identify each physician's patients. Color can also be used to differentiate dates—one color for each month or year.

Business records may also use color-coding. Main divider guide headings may be in one color, subheadings in a second color, and subdivisions in a third color. A fourth color might be used for personal items.

The use of color in filing is limited only by the imagination. One word of caution: Every person in the facility who uses the files must know the key to the coding, and the key should also be written in the facility's procedures manual.

ORGANIZATION OF FILES

It is very difficult for a physician to study a disorganized history. Some systematic method must be followed in placing items in the patient folder. The content of the patient record has already been discussed. From the filing standpoint, it should be emphasized that when a patient record is not in actual use, it should be in only one place—in the filing cabinet or on the shelf. Many precious hours can be lost in searching for misplaced or lost records that were carelessly left unfiled.

The patient's full name, in indexing order, should be typed on a label, and the label attached to the folder tab. A strip of transparent tape can be placed on the label to prevent smudging if this is a problem. The patient's full name should also be typed on each sheet within the folder.

Health-Related Correspondence

Correspondence pertaining to patients' medical records should be filed with the case history. Other medical correspondence should probably be filed in a subject file.

General Correspondence

The physician's office operates as a business as well as a professional service. There will be correspondence of a general nature pertaining to the operation of the office. In all likelihood, a special drawer or shelf will be set aside for the general correspondence. The correspondence is indexed according to subject matter or names of correspondents. The guides in a subject file may appear in one, two, or three positions, depending on the number of headings, subheadings, and subdivisions.

Practice Management Files

The most active financial record is, of course, the patient ledger. In facilities that still use a manual system, this will be a card or vertical tray file, and the accounts will be arranged alphabetically by name. There will be at least two divisions:

- Active accounts
- Paid accounts

Miscellaneous Folder

Papers that do not warrant an individual folder are placed in a miscellaneous folder. Within the folder, all papers relating to one subject, or with one correspondent, are kept together in chronologic order, with the most recent on top, then filed alphabetically with other miscellaneous material. Related materials may be stapled together. Never use paper clips for this purpose. When as many as five papers accumulate with one correspondent or subject, a separate folder should be prepared.

Other business files include records of income and expenses, financial statements, income and payroll tax records, canceled checks, and insurance policies. These papers may be filed chronologically.

Tickler or Follow-Up Files

The most frequently used follow-up method is that of a **tickler file,** so called because it tickles the memory that something needs to be done or followed up on a particular date. The tickler file is always a chronologic arrangement. In its simplest form, it consists of notations on the daily calendar. If information, such as an x-ray report or laboratory report, is expected concerning a patient who has an appointment to come in, the medical assistant might make a note on the calendar or tickler file a day ahead to check on whether the report has arrived.

The tickler file is often a card file with 12 guides for the names of the months and 31 guides printed with numbers 1 through 31 for the days of the month. The guide for the current month, followed by the 31-day guides, is placed at the front of the file. Notations of actions to be taken are placed behind the guides for specific days of the current month. Notations for future months are placed behind the guide for that month. To be effective, the tickler file must be checked the first thing each day.

CRITICAL THINKING APPLICATION

Susan is responsible for checking the tickler file on a daily basis. What types of documents and duties might she find inside these files?

The tickler file can be used in many ways. It is a useful reminder for recurring events such as payments, meetings, and so forth. On the last day of each month, all the notations from behind the next month's guide are distributed among the daily numbered guides, and the guide for the month just completed is placed at the back of the file.

Transitory or Temporary File

Many papers are kept longer than necessary because no provision is made for segregating those that have a limited usefulness. This situation is avoided by having a transitory or temporary file. For example, if a medical assistant writes a letter requesting a reprint, the file copy is placed in the transitory folder. When the reprint is received, the file copy is destroyed. The transitory file is used for materials that have no permanent value. The paper may be marked with a T and destroyed when the action is completed.

CLOSING COMMENTS

Just as in every aspect of the medical profession, advances in medical records management are occurring rapidly, allowing physicians and other caregivers to perform their duties in a more efficient and accurate way. A medical assistant must constantly be willing to learn and to adapt to changes that result from legislation and technologic strides. Because patients are fast becoming more computer literate, computers will become more generally accepted as a viable means of recording medical information. This is a positive change, because many patients and providers were not in favor of computer-based medical records when the concept was first presented to the general public.

The medical assistant should always explain to the patient any paperwork that he or she may be required to complete. Patients do not like to be told to simply "sign here." Take the time to explain any form that needs completion or a signature, so that the patient will understand the reason for collecting the information and the necessity for the information to be available to the medical facility.

Many forms are similar, and patients may complain about answering the same questions on multiple forms. It can be frustrating for patients when they must list their address and phone numbers on each of several forms. Review and revise the forms used in the office often so that they are user-friendly for the office and patient alike.

Patients may need reassurance that each staff member in the physician's office is committed to complete patient confidentiality. Always be open to answering questions regarding the patient medical record.

The authority to release information from the medical record lies solely with the patient unless required by law by subpoena. Ownership of the record is often a subject of controversy. The record belongs to the physician; the information belongs to the patient.

When a medical record is used as evidence in a court case, the person who entered information in the chart must be able to read it, no matter how much time has elapsed since the entry was created. When a chart is corrected, the proper method must be followed, and the record should never be obliterated.

Be sure to understand the laws concerning records retention. Records should be kept through the period of the statute of limitations, and possibly longer in certain situations. Take care with the medical chart, as it is the lifeline of patient care in the medical facility. When a chart is corrected, the proper method must be followed, and the record should never be obliterated (Procedure 14-10).

PROCEDURE 14-10

Document Appropriately and Accurately

CAAHEP COMPETENCY: 3.c(2)(d)
ABHES COMPETENCY: 5.b.

GOAL: *To document appropriately and accurately on all patient medical records and other office paperwork that concerns the patient.*

EQUIPMENT and SUPPLIES

- Any medical document
- Clerical supplies
- Computer or word processor
- Office policy and procedure manual

PROCEDURAL STEPS

1. Determine the information that needs to be added to the patient's medical record, appointment book, telephone message, or other office paperwork that concerns the patient.
   PURPOSE: To place pertinent, accurate information into the document.

2. Make certain that the information is factual, timely, and accurate.
   PURPOSE: To ensure that the information is usable.

3. Write or type the information into the document.

4. Re-read the information to make certain that it is legible.
   PURPOSE: To be sure that the information can be read even after several years by anyone who needs to access the information.

5. Date and sign the entry, if necessary.
   PURPOSE: To authenticate the entry.

6. Make certain that the entry meets any local, state, or federal guidelines that may apply to the information contained in the document.
   PURPOSE: To remain in compliance with local, state, and federal rules and regulations.

7. Make certain that the entry is written in compliance with office policies and procedures.
   PURPOSE: To comply with office policy.

8. If the entry needs to be corrected, draw one line through the entry, and make the new entry below or in the required place within the document.
   PURPOSE: To correct the document according to office policy and procedure guidelines.

9. Place the date and initial the corrected entry.
   PURPOSE: To authenticate the correction.

10. Make certain that the correction has not obliterated any part of the medical record or documentation that affects the patient.
    PURPOSE: TNo obliteration is acceptable in any part of the medical record.

SUMMARY OF SCENARIO

 Susan looks forward to attending her medical assisting classes each day and works diligently to perform to the best of her ability in the classroom. She strives to do well on each procedure check-off and each examination that she completes. Her instructors provide excellent feedback and appreciate her contributions to the classroom experience.

Susan has the attitude that everything she is allowed to do in the medical office is a learning tool. She regularly asks for additional responsibilities and is always ready to assist a co-worker. Dr. Thomas has recognized that she has the desire to learn, and he gives her many opportunities to glean more knowledge through the everyday activities in the office.

Although she is new to the medical profession, Susan learns quickly and thinks logically. She knows the rules and regulations regarding patient confidentiality and is always careful about the information she provides to those who request it. She is never hesitant about asking her office manager for guidance if she is unsure about any aspect of her duties. Susan is understanding and respectful when patients are concerned about their privacy. Her confidence and warm personality play a role in the trust that she earns from the patients at the clinic.

Susan is willing to admit when she has made an error and has sought advice from Dr. Thomas and her office manager when an error needed correction. Although filing is not one of her favorite duties, she can be counted on to do her best while completing this important task. She realizes that filing is a critical task, because the documents contained in the patient's medical record direct the care provided to the patient. An abnormal laboratory report that is missing may make a crucial difference in the patient's care. She takes pride in her work and is efficient and accurate where medical records are concerned. When she is faced with a task that is new to her, she considers it a learning experience and seeks help when she is not completely certain about the way to handle a given situation.

Susan's co-workers are supportive and always willing to assist her as she learns to be the best medical assistant that she can possibly be. Her future as a professional medical assistant will certainly be laden with opportunity and advancement. Just as important, the patients extend their trust to Susan. She has alleviated patient concerns about electronic medical records by taking the time to explain privacy policies and exactly what information will be accessible to third parties. This trust also gives patients the confidence to reveal personal information and know that it will be held in the strictest confidence, not just by Susan, but by each employee at the physician's office.

SUMMARY of LEARNING OBJECTIVES

1. Define, spell, and pronounce the terms listed in the vocabulary.
   * Spelling and pronouncing medical terms correctly adds credibility to the medical assistant. Knowing the definition of these terms promotes confidence in communication with patients and co-workers.

2. State several important reasons for keeping accurate medical records.
   * Medical records must be accurate primarily so that the right care can be given to the patient. The record also helps to provide continuity of care between providers so that there is no lapse in treatment of the patient. The record serves as indication and proof in court that certain treatments and procedures were performed on the patient, so it can be excellent legal support if it is well maintained and accurate. Medical records also aid researchers with statistical information.

3. Discuss the ownership of records.
   * The physician owns the physical medical record, whereas the patient owns the information contained within it.

4. Explain the difference between a traditional medical record and a problem-oriented medical record.
   * The POMR categorizes each problem that a patient has and elaborates on the findings and treatment plan for all concerns. Detailed progress notes are kept for every individual problem. This method separates each of the patient's concerns and addresses them separately, whereas a traditional record may address all problems and concerns at one time. The POMR helps to assure that all individual problems are addressed.

5. Illustrate the difference between subjective and objective information.
   * Very simply, subjective information is provided by the patient, whereas objective information is provided by the physician or provider. Subjective information includes items such as the patient address, social security number, insurance information, and the patient's explanation of the condition he or she is experiencing. Objective information is obtained through the questions the physician asks and the observations made during the examination.

6. Discuss changing an entry in the patient record and the importance of following correct procedures.
   * Correct procedures must be followed when making corrections to a patient chart. A single line should be drawn through the incorrect information, then initialed and dated. Some offices require a notation of "Corr." or "correction" on the chart as well. A medical assistant should never try to alter the medical record or cover up an error in charting.

7. List and discuss the basic equipment used in a filing system.
   * Several types of equipment and supplies are necessary when managing patient records. A variety of shelving units and filing containers is available. Open shelving allows the maximized use of color-coded charts, which make finding misfiles quick and easy. Many file folder styles are available, and several types of forms can be used within the patient charts. The preference of the physician and staff members who use these tools is important, as well as concerns such as cost and availability. A medical assistant should be conservative when ordering supplies and purchasing equipment, ordering only the number needed to save on office supply costs.

8. Describe the steps in filing a document.
   * Five basic steps are involved in filing documents. The papers are conditioned, which is the preparatory stage for filing. Releasing the documents means that they are ready to be filed because they have been reviewed or read, and some type of mark is placed on the document to indicate this. Indexing involves the decision as to where the document should be filed, and coding is placing some type of mark on the paper relative to that decision. Sorting is placing the files in filing sequence. The last step is the actual filing and storing of the document.

9. List and discuss application of the basic filing systems.
   * Alphabetic filing is a simple and traditional filing system whereby documents are filed in alphabetic order. Numeric filing systems use a number code to give order to the files. An alphanumeric system is a combination of the two.

10. Explain how color-coding of files can be useful in a medical facility.
    * Color-coding is an excellent way to keep patient charts in order and swiftly locate those charts that have been misfiled. The medical assistant can tell at a glance when a chart is out of place. Color-coding also makes retrieval and refiling of files quick and easy.

11. Establish a patient's medical record.
    * The patient's chart must be organized so that the components are easy to find. The process for establishing the medical record is outlined in Procedure 14-1.

12. Prepare an informed consent for treatment form.
    * Patients must sign an informed consent for treatment form so that the physician can perform specific treatments and/or procedures. The process for preparing an informed consent for treatment form is outlined in Procedure 14-2.

13. Add supplementary items to an established patient record.
    * Items must be periodically added to patient records when test results arrive or new information becomes available. The process for adding supplementary items to an established medical record is outlined in Procedure 14-3.

14. Prepare a record release form.
    * Records cannot be released without the express permission of the patient. The process for preparing a record release form is outlined in Procedure 14-5.

15. Transcribe a machine-dictated letter using a computer or word processor.
    * At times, the medical assistant will be required to transcribe information from a recorder or other device into a medical record. The process for transcribing a machine-dictated letter using a computer or word processor is outlined in Procedure 14-6.

Continued

SUMMARY of LEARNING OBJECTIVES
Continued

16. File medical records and documents using an alphabetic system.
    - Some offices use an alphabetic filing system. The process for filing records and documents using an alphabetic filing system is outlined in Procedure 14-7.
17. File medical records and documents using a numeric system.
    - Some offices use a numeric filing system. The process for filing records and documents using a numeric filing system is outlined in Procedure 14-8.

18. Color-code medical records.
    - Color coding records is a great help in filing accurately. The process for color coding records is outlined in Procedure 14-9.
19. Document appropriately and accurately.
    - All medical documentation must be correct and complete. The process for documenting appropriately and accurately is outlined in Procedure 14-10.

CONNECTIONS

 Study Guide Connection: Go to Chapter 14 Study Guide. Read the Case Study and Workplace Applications and complete the assignments. Do online research for answers to the questions in the Internet Activities associated with documentation and medical records management.

 CD Connection: Go to the Medical Assisting Competency Challenge CD and do the training activities under General Office Duties: The Medical Record.

 Evolve Connection: For more information related to documentation and medical records management, go to http://evolve.elsevier.com/kinn/admin and visit related weblinks for Chapter 14. Click on the Medical Assisting Exam Review and do the practice questions to sharpen your test-taking skills. To learn more about office software, do the exercises for the Altapoint demo that is on the CD.

Health Information Management

15

SCENARIO

Laura Kelly graduated from her medical assistant training 1 year ago and is now employed at a regional hospital in the quality-assurance department as an administrative assistant. She enjoys working with statistics, is very detail oriented, has excellent computer skills, and is able to comprehend the lengthy regulatory text, such as that set forth in the Health Insurance Portability and Accountability Act (HIPAA) rules and guidelines. She has proven to be a valuable employee and her efforts help the hospital to comply with privacy laws.

Laura thought that quality assurance involved only patient satisfaction when she began working for the hospital. She has learned that this is just a small part of the total quality picture of the facility. The hospital has developed a patient questionnaire to solicit input from patients, and she enjoys talking with them about their experiences. Laura rarely encounters complaints, and she is proud to work for a medical facility that employs individuals who are concerned about giving exceptional care to patients. She understands that there are many aspects to providing quality in a healthcare facility.

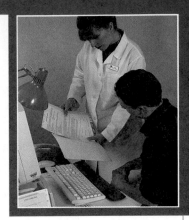

Laura also realizes that health information encompasses much more than the patient's medical record. She knows that health statistics are vital to research and that physicians rely on statistical information when prescribing drugs, giving treatments, and performing other services. Providers frequently contact Laura to determine how many cases of a certain disease or disorder occurred at the hospital during a given period. The hospital database is very sophisticated and allows her to access many types of statistics quickly. Her office also monitors who enters the database and what information is accessed. This is one method of ensuring that privacy is maintained.

Laura has attended continuing education workshops that allow her to gain information and help the staff stay in compliance with the numerous regulations that govern the facility. She is eager to learn and assist her employers in keeping the hospital safe for all patients and visitors.

While studying this chapter, think about the following questions:

- How is health information used in today's medical facilities?
- What can the individual medical assistant do to improve the quality of care given in his or her employer's facility?
- Why is quality management an important aspect of today's healthcare industry?
- How do statistics impact healthcare?

LEARNING OBJECTIVES

1. Define, spell, and pronounce the terms listed in the vocabulary.
2. Describe several ways that health information is used.
3. Contrast the nine characteristics of quality health data.
4. Explain the four concerns of quality assurance.
5. Discuss the importance of the Health Insurance Portability and Accountability Act (HIPAA).
6. Explain the functions of the National Center for Health Statistics (NCHS).
7. Discuss the types of statistics kept by the NCHS.
8. Define total quality management.
9. Explain the function of the Joint Commission on Accreditation of Healthcare Organizations (JCAHO).
10. Discuss the importance of healthcare standards in medical facilities.

National Accreditation Competencies and Content

CAAHEP COMPETENCIES

General

3.c.(2)(a). Identify and respond to issues of confidentiality

3.c.(2)(b). Perform within legal and ethical boundaries

3.c.(2)(d). Document appropriately

3.c.(2)(e). Demonstrate knowledge of federal and state health care legislation and regulations

ABHES COMPETENCIES

Professionalism

1.b. Maintain confidentiality at all times

1.d. Be cognizant of ethical boundaries

Legal Concepts

5.a. Determine needs for documentation and reporting

5.b. Document accurately

5.c. Use appropriate guidelines when releasing records or information

5.g. Monitor legislation related to current healthcare issues and practices

5.h. Perform risk management procedures

VOCABULARY

authenticated Proved; with regard to medical records, it applies to a signature, initials, or computer keystroke by the maker of the record to verify that the record is correct.

circumvent (suhr-kuhm-vent′) To manage to get around, especially by ingenuity or stratagem.

contraindications (kahn-truh-in-duh-ka′-shuns) Factors, such as symptoms or conditions, that make a particular treatment or procedure inadvisable.

disparities (di-spar′-uh-tez) Fundamentally different and often incongruous elements; elements that are markedly distinct in quality or character.

encrypted (in-kript′-ed) Encoded; converted from one system of communication to another.

erroneous (eh-ro′-ne-uhs) Containing or characterized by error or assumption.

gradients Changes in response with distance from a stimulus.

nosocomial (no-suh-ko′-me-uhl) Originating or taking place in a hospital.

quality assurance Activities designed to increase the quality of a product or service through process or system changes that increase efficiency or effectiveness.

sentinel events Unexpected occurrences involving death or serious physical or psychologic injury, or the risk thereof.

standards Models or examples established by authority, custom, or general consent; something set up and established by authority as a rule for the measure of quantity, weight, extent, value, or quality.

transposed Altered in sequence; interchanged.

Before the 1990s, practitioners in the healthcare field were barely familiar with the term *health information management.* Today, this well-respected profession employs thousands of individuals across the United States. As more medical facilities move toward computer-based medical records, more trained health information management professionals are needed. The medical assistant may wish to pursue employment in this growing field.

The health information management profession is supported by a national organization called the *American Health Information Management Association.* This association's House of Delegates developed a statement in 1994 that defines the profession. The statement reads:

> *"Health information management is the profession that focuses on healthcare data and the management of healthcare information resources. The profession addresses the nature, structure, and translation of data into usable forms of information for the advancement of health and healthcare of individuals and populations. Health information professionals collect, integrate, and analyze primary and secondary healthcare data; disseminate information; and manage information resources related to research, planning, provision, and evaluation of healthcare services."*

EVOLUTION OF THE PROFESSION

In 1928 the American College of Surgeons realized that accurate medical records promoted good medical care. This desire for quality led to the establishment of the Association of Record Librarians of North America. Years later in 1970 the organization changed its name to the American Medical Record Association. Medical records professionals found employment in hospitals, health clinics, insurance companies, and other organizations that used medical records.

In 1991 the organization became known as the *American Health Information Management Association.* Advances in technology have brought the health information management profession from a paper-based environment into a highly sophisticated computer age, where physicians can access patient and statistical data in seconds.

In 2005, nearly a quarter of U.S. physicians used some form of electronic patient record, according to the CDC. Most experts agree that electronic records can reduce medical errors by keeping prescriptions, allergies, and other information organized, as well as reduce costs by avoiding duplicate tests. Electronic records may also reduce staffing needs, since fewer personnel are needed to manage them. The CDC agrees that progress has been made toward a presidential goal of having digital health data for every American by 2014, but states that there is still a long way to go toward meeting that goal.

THE USE OF HEALTHCARE DATA

Many people and various organizations use healthcare data in a multitude of ways (Figure 15-1). Primarily, healthcare data are used to plan care for patients and ensure that they receive continuity of care from one healthcare provider to another. However, the information provided through healthcare records is useful in other capacities.

For example, when a drug is being evaluated, statistics must be kept to help the manufacturers of the product determine its effectiveness. Information on side effects and other **contraindications** is reviewed and used to make the product safer and more marketable. Sometimes the drug must be changed then returned to clinical trials.

Healthcare organizations gather information on the number of patients who enter the facility with the same diagnosis. This and other information helps them to plan what types of equipment will be needed to meet the needs of the patient population. For instance, if the geographic area where the facility is located contains a large number of patients with cardiac disease, a hospital may need to add a cardiac intensive care unit. If the facility is located in a neighborhood where there are many young families, the obstetrics and pediatrics departments may be expanded. Healthcare data and statistics guide planning for the needs of next week and for the next decade.

Third-party payors use healthcare information to determine whether claims should be paid. The data provide proof that a certain procedure or treatment was medically necessary and therefore its cost should be reimbursed (Figure 15-2). Government and regulatory agencies use data to make certain that healthcare facilities are in compliance with the various statutes and **standards** that govern them. Data also are used by facilities in determining whether high-quality healthcare is being provided to patients.

WHAT ARE HIGH-QUALITY DATA?

The information that is contained in a database is only as reliable as the person who entered it into the computer. Most database systems require information to be saved after it is entered by clicking an additional button. Unless the data information is saved, the time and effort spent in entering the data have been wasted.

Health Information: Management of a Strategic Resource* identifies nine characteristics of quality health data. These characteristics are validity, reliability, completeness, recognizability, timeliness, relevance, accessibility, security, and legality.

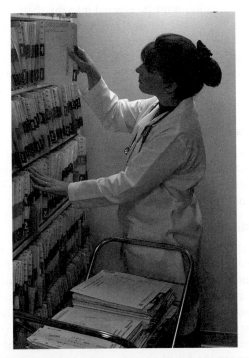

FIGURE 15-2 Healthcare providers often rely on statistics when treating their patients. Most statistical information is gleaned from patient charts.

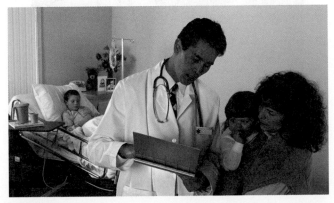

FIGURE 15-1 Physicians rely on health information to provide high-quality care to their patients.

Validity

The validity of health data is synonymous with accuracy. Accuracy is one of the most important characteristics of data, whether in paper-based or computer-based records. Great care must be taken when characters are typed on the keyboard, so that letters or numbers are not **transposed.**

Reliability

The healthcare professional must be able to rely on the data presented. If a patient's medical chart is marked to indicate that he or she has no allergies, the medical assistant must be able to trust that information and give an injection with the confidence that the patient is not allergic to the medication. Reliability also pertains to the degree to which the information in the database can be trusted.

Completeness

The information not only must be accurate; it also must be complete. If the medical assistant gives an injection yet fails to document it in the patient's chart, then the record is incomplete. If a computer system is designed to upload new information into the database every night and the system malfunctions, there is a strong possibility that the records contained within the system are incomplete, possibly lacking vital information needed to care for the patient.

Recognizability

All users of health information must be able to interpret the data that are presented in the health record. The facility should have a consistent use of abbreviations so that no misunderstandings occur when reviewing a patient's chart.

Timeliness

Health information must be entered into the chart or database as soon as it is available. The medical assistant should never commit information to memory intending to enter it later. Reports from laboratories or medical tests also should be placed in the chart as soon as the information is reviewed by the physician, so that decisions made are supported by the latest information about the patient's condition.

Relevance

The information contained in the database must be relevant to be useful. Needless and meaningless statistics about patient treatments or drug interactions do not benefit providers and users of health information.

Accessibility

One of the advantages of a computer-based patient record is that it is accessible to multiple users at the same time. The facility must take care to provide access only to individuals who are authorized to view the records. The computer should have a login system that prompts for a password. In addition, the computer system should keep records of who accesses information by time and date. Paper-based patient records should be returned to their proper place when they are not in use so that they will be accessible to all staff members.

Security

Although only certain employees are allowed to access health information, precautions must be taken to prohibit access to intruders. Firewalls are similar to filters that allow only certain types of data to enter or exit. Information can be **encrypted,** which means that it is changed into a code that can be read only after it has been unencrypted. These precautions are necessary because of the sensitivity of patient information. Also, care must be taken to ensure that no one can change the information already contained in the record.

Legality

Many statutes govern medical records. The laws concerning record retention vary from state to state. Medical records cannot be altered but should be corrected according to accepted guidelines. The record must be completely legible and **authenticated** properly (Figure 15-3).

CRITICAL THINKING APPLICATION

■ One of Laura's duties involves making sure that medical records have been authenticated. Why is the authentication of records important?

■ One physician, Dr. Anthony, is consistently careless about record authentication. How can the hospital encourage him to complete this critical duty?

THE CHALLENGES OF QUALITY-ASSURANCE PROBLEMS

Many of the larger medical facilities today have entire departments that are devoted to **quality assurance.** *Quality*

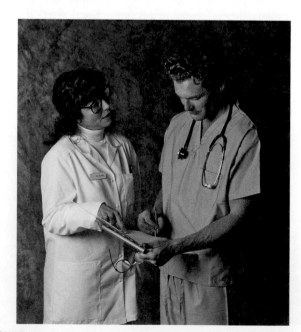

FIGURE 15-3 Physicians must authenticate medical records by initialing or signing their entries. Some computer systems automatically authenticate records.

assurance is defined as the activities designed to increase the quality of a product or service through process or system changes that increase efficiency or effectiveness. Although many people assume that quality is determined solely by the patient, much more is involved in quality assurance than just the patient's satisfaction with services rendered. Quality assurance also is concerned with the overuse, underuse, misuse, and variations in use of different healthcare services.

Healthcare services that are excessive and unnecessary cause costs to rise. Treatments and services that are overused include hysterectomies, tympanostomy tubes, and antibiotics. Medical studies have shown that up to 16% of all hysterectomies performed in 1993 were unnecessary and up to 23% of tympanostomy tube operations performed between 1991 and 1992 were unnecessary. Antibiotics are prescribed widely for common colds and acute bronchitis, but the drugs do not benefit patients with these illnesses.

The underuse of services and treatments can be equally costly. Mammograms and cervical cancer screening tests can detect medical problems yet are not taken advantage of by enough at-risk patients (Figure 15-4). The use of beta-blockers has been proven to reduce mortality in patients who have had heart attacks by as much as 43%, but often they are not prescribed for these patients. Diabetic patients should have their eyes checked regularly, but many do not. All of these are examples of the underuse of services that can affect the quality of healthcare.

CRITICAL THINKING APPLICATION

- How might a hospital employee encourage patients to have screening tests done, such as mammograms and for cervical cancer?
- What marketing strategies could Laura assist in developing that will result in more patients taking advantage of health screening opportunities?
- How do these services benefit the health facility?

Some healthcare services are misused. These errors can cause death, delay of correct diagnosis, unnecessary injuries,

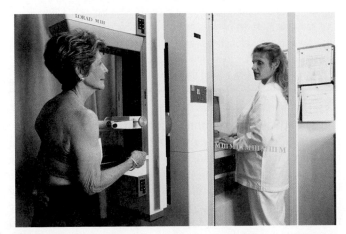

FIGURE 15-4 Healthcare professionals must encourage at-risk patients to have screening tests done, such as those for breast and cervical cancer.

and increased healthcare costs. Examples of misuse can include laboratory tests that provide **erroneous** results. Medication errors can be fatal to patients or can cause complications to illnesses that are already present. Hospital injuries and **nosocomial** infections promote further complications. A study at the Harvard School of Public Health published in 1994 estimated that up to 180,000 needless deaths occurred each year as a result of preventable errors.

Wide variations exist in services in different parts of the country. Discharge rates (which indicate that the patient left the hospital without expiring) are higher in some areas of the United States than others. Individuals who seek medical care are more conscientious and likely to seek health services in different geographic areas. All of these issues contribute to the concept of high-quality healthcare.

Health Insurance Portability and Accountability Act

As technology advanced and more health records became computerized, legislation dealing with privacy became imperative. The Health Insurance Portability and Accountability Act (HIPAA) 1996 was developed, in part, to help ensure the confidentiality of medical records. The statute, which became law in August 1996, applies to those records that are created or maintained by healthcare providers, health plans, and healthcare clearinghouses that engage in certain electronic transactions. The Office for Civil Rights, a division of the Health and Human Services Department, regulates HIPAA.

In August 2002, the Department of Health and Human Services Secretary Tommy Thompson announced the final ruling relating to HIPAA's privacy act, which became effective April 14, 2003. Under the privacy rule the following apply:

- Patients must give specific authorization before entities covered by the regulation could use or disclose protected information in most nonroutine circumstances—such as releasing information to an employer or for use in marketing activities. Doctors, health plans, and other covered entities would be required to follow the rule's standards for the use and disclosure of personal health information.

- Covered entities generally will need to provide patients with written notice of their privacy practices and patients' privacy rights. The notice will contain information that could be useful to patients choosing a health plan, doctor, or other provider. Patients would generally be asked to sign or otherwise acknowledge receipt of the privacy notice from direct treatment providers.

- Pharmacies, health plans, and other covered entities must first obtain an individual's specific authorization before sending marketing materials. At the same time, the rule permits doctors and other covered entities to communicate freely with patients about treatment options and other health-related information, including disease management programs.

- Specifically, improvements to the final rule strengthen the marketing language to make clear that covered entities cannot use business associate agreements to **circumvent** the rule's marketing prohibition. The improvement explicitly prohibits pharmacies and other covered entities from selling personal medical information to a business that would market its products or services under a business associate agreement.

• Patients generally will be able to access their personal medical records and request changes to correct any errors. In addition, patients generally could request an accounting of nonroutine uses and disclosures of their health information.

Many healthcare organizations have concern about the costs of implementing and maintaining measures that will comply with the privacy regulations. However, the benefits of the act far outweigh the inconveniences of remaining in compliance. Patients have the right to expect complete confidentiality with regard to their health records (Figure 15-5).

CRITICAL THINKING APPLICATION

■ Laura is concerned about the number of employees in her facility who are allowed to access patient information. For instance, all nurses have access to health information on all patients. Is this a good policy? Why or why not?

■ Should all physicians have access to all patient records? Why or why not?

National Center for Health Statistics

The National Center for Health Statistics (NCHS) is a division of the Centers for Disease Control and Prevention. The agency is the primary provider of health information statistics used to guide the actions and policies that relate to the health of the American public. The functions of the NCHS include the following:

• Documentation of the health status of the population and of important subgroups
• Identification of **disparities** in health status and use of healthcare by race, ethnicity, socioeconomic status (SES), region, and other population **gradients**
• Description of experiences with the healthcare system

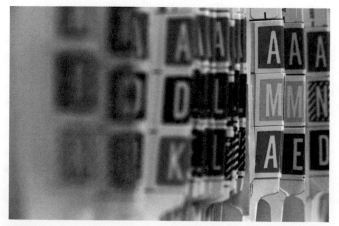

FIGURE 15-5 Patients must have the assurance that their medical records are accessed only by authorized individuals.

• Monitoring of trends in health status and healthcare delivery
• Identification of health problems
• Support for biomedical and health services research
• Provision of information for making changes in public policies and programs
• Evaluation of the impact of health policies and programs

Statistics are of vital importance to many entities that are interested in the healthcare industry. Some of the statistics available through the NCHS are related to the following:

• Teenage pregnancy
• Incidence of human immunodeficiency virus (HIV) infection
• Alcohol and drug use
• Births
• Deaths
• Communicable diseases
• Infant health and mortality
• Leading causes of death
• Life expectancy
• Sexually transmitted diseases
• Suicide

Total Quality Management

Total quality management is management and control activities based on the leadership of top-level management, supported by the involvement of all employees and departments from planning and development to sales and service. These management and control activities focus on quality assurance. Ideally, qualities that satisfy the customer are built into products and services as they receive care or services from providers.

For total quality management practices to be effective, all employees must make a commitment to provide patients with the best care possible. This includes top-level management as well as the staff members who work directly with the patients.

CRITICAL THINKING APPLICATION

■ Laura has noticed that many employees are frustrated when confronted with quality-assurance regulations. Often employees complain that the policies are a waste of time. How can Laura convince these employees that the regulations are important, and how can she foster cooperation from these people?

■ Should adherence to quality-assurance policies be a mandatory part of the employee's job description?

The Total Quality Management Concept

Much of the thrust of today's interest in total quality management originated from the teachings of W. Edwards Deming. Deming obtained a doctorate in mathematical physics from Yale University in 1928. He is perhaps best known for the work he did with Japanese managers and engineers regarding quality management. Deming compiled 14 points for managers to institute that were designed to place the emphasis on quality rather than quantity.

The following is an excerpt from Deming's book *Out of the Crisis* and briefly describes the Fourteen Points for Management.

- Create constancy of purpose toward improvement of product and service, with the aim to become competitive, to stay in business, and to provide jobs.
- Adopt the new philosophy. Western management must awaken to the challenge, must learn their responsibilities, and take on leadership for change.
- Cease dependence on inspection to achieve quality. Eliminate the need for inspection on a mass basis by building quality into the product or service in the first place.
- End the practice of awarding business on the basis of price tag. Instead, minimize total cost. Move toward a single supplier for any one item, on a long-term relationship of loyalty and trust.
- Constantly improve the system of production and service, to improve quality and productivity, and thus constantly decrease costs.
- Institute training on the job.
- Institute leadership. The aim of supervision should be to help people and machines and gadgets to do a better job. Supervision of management is in need of overhaul as well as supervision of production workers.
- Drive out fear, so that everyone may work effectively for the company.
- Break down barriers between departments. People must work as a team, to foresee problems of production and in use that may be encountered with the product or service.
- Eliminate slogans, exhortations, and targets for the work force asking for zero defects and new levels of productivity. Such exhortations only create adversarial relationships. Eliminate quotas and substitute leadership. Eliminate management by objective. Eliminate management by numbers and numerical goals. Substitute leadership.
- Remove barriers that rob the hourly worker of his right to pride of workmanship. The responsibility of supervisors must be changed from sheer numbers to quality.
- Remove barriers that rob people in management and in engineering of their right to pride of workmanship. This means the abolishment of the annual merit rating and of management by objective.
- Institute a vigorous program of education and self-improvement.
- Put everybody in the company to work to accomplish the transformation. The transformation is everybody's job.

Deming believed that these points would assist managers in bringing quality to the facility or business in which they were used (Figure 15-6). They are widely used in countless business and service organizations today.

Joint Commission on Accreditation of Healthcare Organizations

The Joint Commission on Accreditation of Healthcare Organizations (JCAHO) is a nonprofit organization that assists healthcare facilities by providing accreditation services. The

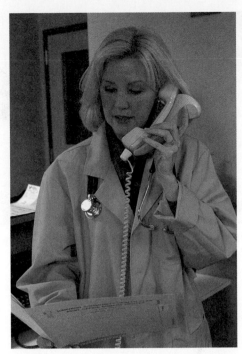

FIGURE 15-6 Quality management is a vital part of accreditation of healthcare organizations, and all physicians should be dedicated to providing optimal, high-quality care to patients.

facilities participate in obtaining accreditation voluntarily, but over 17,000 healthcare facilities in the United States are accredited by JCAHO and comply with its standards.

For many years, healthcare facilities were interested in meeting the minimum standards that would reflect quality healthcare. Recently, there has been a shift from simply meeting minimum standards to exceeding standards and providing optimal healthcare to patients (Figure 15-7). Standards are a set of criteria that the facility must adhere to, and the facility must be able to prove such compliance.

Risk Management

A risk is any occurrence that could result in patient injury or any type of financial loss to the healthcare facility. The policies and procedures that facilities develop are designed to manage risk and prevent situations that can cause harm to persons or property for which the healthcare facility could be held liable.

Risk management programs in healthcare facilities should focus on financial loss prevention and reduce the possibility of negative publicity resulting from **sentinel events.** JCAHO defines a sentinel event as an "unexpected occurrence involving death or serious physical or psychological injury, or the risk thereof." Sentinel events must be investigated thoroughly and their contributing factors rectified so that they are avoided in the future. Records are kept of the sentinel events that happen in a facility, especially those that involve injury to patients.

CLOSING COMMENTS

Health information management is a critical aspect of today's healthcare facility. Although regulations may seem stringent,

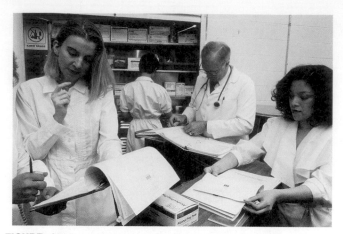

FIGURE 15-7 Accreditation of a healthcare facility takes teamwork and a commitment to quality assurance.

the value of protecting the patient's privacy is immeasurable. Patients have the right to expect their health information to be kept confidential. The medical assistant should focus on meeting privacy guidelines and should take great care when working with medical records and information.

Many patients may have questions about HIPAA and the extent of their rights to limit access to their records. Be prepared to answer these questions or guide such patients to the right source for information.

The medical assistant must be familiar with the laws surrounding privacy issues and be able to guide patients as concerns arise. Seminars that will target the compliance issues that affect the physician's office often are available to the medical assistant. Most employers are willing to pay for such seminars so that the office can remain in strict compliance with legal issues. Remember that the medical profession is one of constant change. The medical assistant must have a positive attitude about the learning process, especially when new rules and regulations take effect.

SUMMARY OF SCENARIO

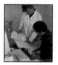

Laura is learning more about health information management each day that she goes to work. She has earned the respect of her supervisors, who often give her a lengthy, complicated document concerning regulations and ask her to read and summarize it for the staff. She has a knack for weeding out the actual requirements amid the excess of legalese.

Laura has developed good relationships with many of the staff physicians at the hospital. She has approached several of them about record authentication, and her bright personality helps to foster a sense of cooperation between the medical staff and the hospital staff. She has even begun to give coupons good for one lunch in the cafeteria when physicians form the habit of authenticating their records in a timely manner. The physicians appreciate the recognition for completing their duties on schedule.

Laura has given thought to continuing her education in the health management field and possibly gaining certification in this area. She knows that this will lend credibility to the knowledge that she has gained on the job. Her supervisors are pleased with her performance, and know they can count on Laura to complete any task she is assigned on time with accurate results. Laura looks forward to a long career at the hospital and being of service to the patients and staff alike in the years to come.

Health information is used on a daily basis in medical facilities. The patient record is probably the most common source of health information that healthcare professionals use, but they also access databases that provide statistical and other information that impacts patient care. Laura knows that she can contribute to quality healthcare by making certain that records are accurate, complete, and reliable for the medical professionals who use them. Providing quality healthcare is mandatory in today's society, because physicians are susceptible to lawsuits and complaints when patients feel that they did not receive optimal care. Additionally, patients have the right to choose their healthcare providers and they deserve and insist upon quality healthcare.

Laura has noticed that today's patients are more sophisticated and knowledgeable about health-related issues, primarily because of the ease of looking up their health issues on the Internet. Patients often tell the doctor what they think their diagnosis is, based upon their own Internet research. This is proof that even patients are using healthcare information. Statistical information helps Laura's employer determine the diseases and disorders that are most likely to affect patients in their hospital. Computers are an invaluable tool that allows healthcare providers and facilities to share information that will result in quality patient care.

SUMMARY of LEARNING OBJECTIVES

1. Define, spell, and pronounce the terms listed in the vocabulary.
   - Spelling and pronouncing medical terms correctly adds credibility to the medical assistant. Knowing the definition of these terms promotes confidence in communication with patients and co-workers.

2. Describe several ways that health information is used.
   - Both physicians and employees of medical facilities use health information in many ways. The information helps to ensure continuity of care from provider to provider. It assists manufacturers in determining side effects of drugs. It provides statistical information regarding primary and secondary diagnoses. Health information also helps the medical facility plan for future needs and capital equipment.

3. Contrast the nine characteristics of quality health data.
   - High-quality health data have nine characteristics. Validity refers to the accuracy of the information, and reliability means that the information can be counted on to be accurate and that medical decisions can be made based on the information. Completeness simply means that the information is available in its entirety, and recognizability refers to the data being understood by the users. Timely information allows the provider to make decisions based on the latest data about a patient or a treatment. Relevance refers to the usefulness of the health information, and accessibility means that the information is easily available to the provider when it is needed. Security encompasses the effort to keep unauthorized people from accessing health information. Legality refers to the correctness of the information and its authentication by the healthcare provider.

4. Explain the four concerns of quality assurance.
   - Four concerns that surround quality assurance include the overuse, underuse, misuse, and variations in use of healthcare services. Overused services are excessive and cause cost increases. An example includes using the emergency room for nonemergencies. Underuse means that patients do not take advantage of many services they should be using, especially if they are at-risk patients. Misuse of services often reflects errors, such as laboratory errors or misdiagnoses. Variations in services simply means that in various parts of the country, individuals use services in different ways, which can influence the quality of care overall in the United States.

5. Discuss the importance of the Health Insurance Portability and Accountability Act (HIPAA).
   - HIPAA is a milestone in support of patient privacy issues. The act has several facets, but the most widely publicized sections deal with the right to patient privacy. The act will give a degree of control to patients and allow them information about who accesses their records. Patients must also give specific authorization for the use and dissemination of the information contained in the medical record.

6. Explain the functions of the National Center for Health Statistics (NCHS).
   - The NCHS is a part of the Centers for Disease Control and Prevention. Health statistics are important, because they enable providers to better treat their patients. For instance, if a certain area has a high number of outbreaks of a particular disease, the physician may be better prepared to cope with patients with the symptoms of that disease, treating them faster and promoting a full recovery. Health statistics provide information about these types of issues. The NCHS helps to compile information such as the number of HIV infections, the number of teen pregnancies, and other vital health data that are useful to medical professionals.

7. Discuss the types of statistics kept by the NCHS.
   - Some of the statistics kept by the NCHS include alcohol and drug use information, births, deaths, communicable diseases, infant health and mortality, and life expectancy.

8. Define total quality management.
   - Total quality management is management and control activities based on the leadership of top-level management, supported by the involvement of all employees and departments in an effort to provide quality assurance.

9. Explain the function of the Joint Commission on Accreditation of Healthcare Organizations (JCAHO).
   - JCAHO is a nonprofit organization that offers accreditation services to healthcare facilities that wish to excel in healthcare services. Accreditation is voluntary; however, more than 17,000 healthcare facilities in the United States are accredited by this agency.

10. Discuss the importance of healthcare standards in medical facilities.
    - Without strong healthcare standards, quality cannot exist. The focus of quality assurance has shifted in recent years from just meeting the minimum standards to providing optimal quality. People expect high-quality healthcare when they get treatment. Today's organizations that seek accreditation or focus their efforts on quality will exceed standards, not just meet them.

CONNECTIONS

Study Guide Connection: Go to Chapter 15 Study Guide. Read the Case Study and Workplace Applications and complete the assignments. Do online research for answers to the questions in the Internet Activities associated with health information management.

CD Connection: Go to the Medical Assisting Competency Challenge CD and do the training activities under Patient Care and General Office Duties.

Evolve Connection: For more information related to health information management, go to http://evolve.elsevier.com/kinn/admin and visit related weblinks for Chapter 15. Click on the Medical Assisting Exam Review and do the practice questions to sharpen your test-taking skills.

Privacy in the Physician's Office 16

SCENARIO

Sabrina Ragland, a medical assistant with 12 years' experience, works for a gastroenterologist, Dr. Tim Taylor. She comes from a family heavily involved in the medical field. Her father was a surgeon and her mother was his office assistant. Two of Sabrina's sisters are nurses, and her brother is a respiratory therapist. Her husband, Joe, is a biomedical technician, and his mother, Elsa Ragland, has been an RN for 40 years. For more than half of her career, Elsa has worked for a local internist, Dr. Royce Berry. A casual comment at the Ragland family picnic resulted in a medical professional liability lawsuit based on violation of patient privacy. Sabrina and Elsa's careers were jeopardized by a simple exchange of what seemed to be innocent information.

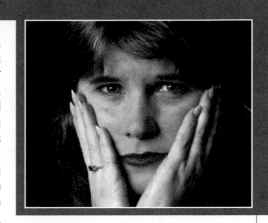

Vivian Adams, a 42-year-old hospital insurance biller, saw Dr. Berry in his office for pain located in her lower left quadrant. Ms. Adams was not a new patient but had not visited the office in approximately 2 years. When she arrived for her visit, she was presented with the office privacy policy and was asked to sign the document. Vivian glanced through it, signed it, and saw the doctor. He performed an examination and found that Vivian was likely suffering from irritable bowel syndrome and prescribed medication. Ms. Adams called the physician 1 week later complaining that she was no better. Dr. Berry changed her medication without seeing her and did not hear from her again, other than her requests for refills of the medication. After 6 months with no improvement, Ms. Adams went to Dr. Taylor; after several diagnostic tests, she was told that she had colon cancer and was given a bleak prognosis. She told Dr. Taylor that she blamed Dr. Berry for not being more thorough in his testing. Sabrina was in the room and heard the comment.

That weekend at the picnic, Sabrina mentioned Ms. Adams to her mother-in-law and stated that the patient might sue Dr. Berry, although the patient never said those words. Elsa defended Dr. Berry and proclaimed that he was a good doctor, then expressed her hope that Ms. Adams would not sue her employer. One week later, Elsa was in a grocery store and saw Ms. Adams. Elsa immediately expressed her sympathy about her diagnosis, and then asked if there was anything she could do. Her intent was to be kind and try to avert litigation against Dr. Berry. Her gesture might have been well received had Ms. Adams' daughter, Terri, not been standing with her. Terri was not yet aware that her mother had been diagnosed with cancer. Ms. Adams had told no one about her illness at that point. After the incident at the grocery store the first person Ms. Adams told was her attorney.

While studying this chapter, think about the following questions:

- When can the medical assistant discuss a patient, and with whom, and under what circumstances?
- What has HIPAA done for the medical industry and the patients it serves?
- When new policies and procedures are implemented, how can the staff embrace the changes and make the transitions easier?
- What happens if the patient refuses to sign the privacy policy?

LEARNING OBJECTIVES

1. Define, spell, and pronounce the terms listed in the vocabulary.
2. Explain how the HIPAA Privacy Rule benefits the healthcare industry and patients.
3. List what must be included on a Notice of Privacy Practices.
4. Explain the difference between Title I and Title II of the HIPAA Privacy Rule.
5. List the rights that patients have under the Privacy Rule.
6. Briefly explain what is expected of healthcare providers in relation to the Privacy Rule.
7. Describe an incidental disclosure.
8. List the three instances when a parent is not considered the child's representative.
9. Explain why a provider can discuss protected health information with a patient's friends and family.
10. Discuss the role of the Notice of Privacy Practices in emergencies.

National Accreditation Competencies and Content

CAAHEP COMPETENCIES

General

3.c.(2)(a). Identify and respond to issues of confidentiality
3.c.(2)(b). Perform within legal and ethical boundaries
3.c.(2)(d). Document accurately

ABHES COMPETENCIES

Professionalism

1.b. Maintain confidentiality at all times
1.d. Be cognizant of ethical boundaries

Legal Concepts

5.a. Determine needs for documentation and reporting
5.b. Document accurately
5.c. Use appropriate guidelines when releasing records or information
5.g. Monitor legislation related to current healthcare issues and practices
5.h. Perform risk management procedures

VOCABULARY

business associates Individuals or organizations that perform or assist a covered entity in the performance of a function or activity that involves the use or disclosure of individually identifiable health information.

complainant (kuhm-pla′-nuhnt) Person making a complaint against a person or organization.

covered entity An organization that transmits information in an electronic form during a transaction, as defined by HIPAA.

divulge (duh-vuhlj′) To make known, as a confidence or secret.

due diligence Also known as *due care;* the effort made by an ordinarily prudent or reasonable party to avoid harm to another party or himself; doing everything possible to prevent something from happening.

electronic media Means of electronic transmission, including the Internet, private networks, dial-up phone lines, and fax modems; includes information moved from one place to another while stored on an electronic device.

healthcare providers Providers of medical or health services, individually or as organizations, that furnish, bill for, or are paid for services or products.

individually identifiable health information Any part of a patient's health record that is created or received by a covered entity.

infer To derive as a conclusion from facts and premises.

Office for Civil Rights (OCR) The division of the federal government that enforces privacy standards.

Office of Inspector General (OIG) Established to protect the integrity of the Department of Health and Human Services (HHS), the office conducts audits, investigations, and inspections involving the laws that pertain to HHS.

personal health information The patient's own information that pertains to his or her health.

preclude To rule out in advance.

prevalent Generally or widely accepted, practiced, or favored.

privacy officer A person designated to ensure compliance with privacy standards for a covered entity.

protected health information (PHI) Any individually identifiable health information that is transmitted and/or maintained in electronic form.

transactions As defined by HIPAA, transmissions of information between two parties to carry out financial or administrative activities related to healthcare.

verbiage A manner of expressing oneself in words.

One of the most valuable character traits that the medical assistant develops is the ability to adjust to change and be flexible. The medical profession evolves rapidly, and advances in technology allow medicine to progress. Think of how few computers were found in physician's offices 40 years ago. Today, computers adorn almost every desk. Change is a concept that many individuals resist.

The creation of privacy and security laws was a huge step toward more efficient healthcare and faster reimbursements. Technology often forces organizations to move forward somewhat quickly. Healthcare facilities with already strapped budgets sometimes view such innovations as a hindrance. Compliance officers at larger facilities may wonder if additional federal regulations are necessary.

Many healthcare workers feel that they can say nothing to anyone, about any patient, at any time. By understanding the compliance that HIPAA requires, the employees of the physician's office can feel secure about their dealings with the patients and other individuals who frequent the facility.

THE HEALTH INSURANCE PORTABILITY AND ACCOUNTABILITY ACT

The Health Insurance Portability and Accountability Act (HIPAA) was introduced in Chapter 7. HIPAA, enacted in 1996, is a group of laws that affect both employees of a healthcare facility, insurance company, or other **covered entity** and the patients the organizations serve. The federal government required all covered entities to be in compliance with HIPAA by April 14, 2003 (small healthcare plans received an extra year to comply, extending their deadline to April 14, 2004).

Effect of the HIPAA Privacy Rule

The HIPAA Privacy Rule creates national standards to protect individuals' medical records and other personal health information. This is the first time that such a group of laws has been enacted to protect patient privacy. The creation of the HIPAA Privacy Rule provides benefits to both patients and their **healthcare providers:**

- Patients have more control over their medical records.
- Patients are able to make informed choices regarding how their personal health information is used.
- Boundaries are set on the use and release of health records.
- Safeguards are established that healthcare providers must achieve to protect the privacy of health information.
- Violators are held accountable and face both civil and criminal penalties if patient privacy rights are compromised.
- The Privacy Rule protects public health by striking a balance when public responsibility supports disclosure of personal health information.

Under the few laws that existed before the HIPAA Privacy Rule, personal health information could be distributed to others without either notice or authorization from the patient, even if the reason for the exchange of information had nothing to do with the patient's medical treatment or healthcare reimbursement. A health plan could pass patient information to a financial lender, who might then deny the patient a home mortgage or credit card based on his or her health history. Employers could obtain health information and use it in personnel decisions. Because computers make information exchange so much easier, laws had to be enacted to protect patient privacy (Figure 16-1).

Title I and Title II Provisions

HIPAA contains two provisions, Title I and Title II. Title I regulates insurance reform, and Title II deals with administrative simplification. Title I limits the use of preexisting health

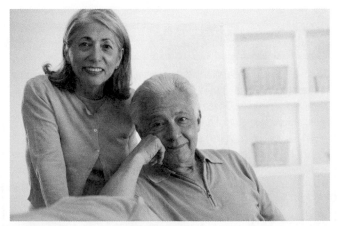

FIGURE 16-1 The HIPAA Privacy Rule was created in part to give patients more control over their personal health information.

conditions that in the past prevented or limited an employee from obtaining health insurance coverage. If an individual left a job with insurance coverage and attempted to secure new coverage, a preexisting health condition would often **preclude** that person from obtaining coverage for that illness. Many individuals were refused any coverage at all, especially if the condition was a serious one, such as a heart condition or high blood pressure. Today, because of HIPAA laws, discrimination against individuals who are in poor health now or were in the past is prohibited. The regulations limit the use of preexisting condition exclusions and guarantee that certain individuals can purchase healthcare insurance after leaving or losing a job.

The goal of Title II is to reduce administrative costs in the healthcare industry. Often goals sound simple, but to reach a goal, many actions are necessary. The medical assistant who enters school sets graduation as his or her goal. However, in order to graduate, he or she must study, pass tests, arrange for childcare, sacrifice sleep, adjust working hours, readjust to the school environment, and make any number of other adjustments to reach the goal. Likewise, to simplify the administrative costs involved in patient care, many different objectives must be met.

Provisions of Administrative Simplification

If given a choice to use a computer or an electric typewriter to write a report, most individuals would likely choose the computer. Because computers can perform so many duties much more rapidly than those that were performed manually, they have become indispensable to the healthcare profession. **Electronic media** is used daily in modern physician offices and healthcare facilities. However, as computers have become **prevalent,** patients have begun to express concerns about who sees **protected health information (PHI)** and what is done with that information. Title II contains two parts:

- Development and implementation of standardized electronic **transactions** using Standard Code Sets
- Implementation of privacy and security procedures to prevent the misuse of health information by ensuring confidentiality

The second part of the administrative simplification provision deals with privacy, confidentiality, and security of PHI and is the focus of this chapter.

Patient Rights

Separate from the Patients' Bill of Rights, HIPAA provides for several patient rights. These include the following:

- The right to notice of a facility's privacy practices
- The right to have access to, view, and obtain a copy of their PHI
- The right to restrict certain parts or uses of their PHI
- The right to request that communications from the facility be kept confidential
- The right to request the facility to amend the PHI
- The right to receive notice of all disclosures of their PHI

These patient rights are the heart of the HIPAA Privacy Rule. These rights must be protected by those involved in the healthcare profession and are explained in more detail in the following section.

Right to Notice of Privacy Practices

Patients have the right to a copy of the Notice of Privacy Practices used in the physician's office (Figure 16-2). A copy of the Notice of Privacy Practices must also be prominently displayed in the office. This policy is developed by the individual facility and must be written in terminology that the patient will understand. Patients should be given a copy of the Notice of Privacy Practices and sign an acknowledgement that they received the copy. If a patient refuses to sign the acknowledgement, the medical assistant can note that the document was offered to the patient and he or she refused to sign. This proves **due diligence** on the part of the office and that a good faith effort was made to provide the patient with privacy information. Most patients will sign the document. Be prepared to explain the Notice of Privacy Practices to the patients.

The Notice of Privacy Practices must include the following:
- How PHI is used and disclosed by the facility
- The duties of the provider to protect health information
- Patient rights regarding PHI
- How complaints can be filed if patients believe their privacy has been violated
- Whom to contact at the facility for more information
- The effective date of the Notice of Privacy Practices

Right to Access Protected Health Information

Patients must be allowed access to their personal health information. The maker, not the patient, owns the record; however, the HIPAA Privacy Rule grants patients the right to access, inspect, and obtain a copy of their health information. Most physicians' offices require patients to request access in writing and act on that request within 30 days (Figure 16-3). HIPAA does restrict access to psychotherapy notes, information compiled for use in legal proceedings, and information exempted from disclosure by the Clinical Laboratory Improvement Amendment (CLIA).

Right to Request Restrictions on Certain Uses and Disclosures of Protected Health Information

Patients can request restrictions on the use of their PHI. For instance, if a patient had an abortion many years ago and does not want that information released, she has the right to ask a provider not to **divulge** that information. The provider does not have to agree to the request but must review it and give a good reason for the restriction not to be honored. An appeal process should be in place for instances when the provider does not agree with the restriction.

Right to Request Confidential Communications

Patients have the right to express where they wish to receive communications from the provider. The patient may prefer to be contacted on a cell phone instead of a home phone, or through email. Providers must accommodate reasonable requests. Suppose a married female patient comes to the clinic for a pregnancy test. Further suppose that her husband has had a vasectomy. Clearly, a call to her home phone number with test results could initiate personal and private difficulties for the patient. Make certain that the preferred method of communication is used when contacting any patient (Procedure 16-1).

Right to Request Amendment of Protected Health Information

Patients can request that changes be made to their medical record, if they inspect it and find an error. This request should be made in writing. Providers must review the request and act on it in a timely manner, generally within 60 days. The request may be denied if the provider was not the creator of the record, as in the case of records provided by a consulting physician. Or, the provider may believe that the information is correct and complete. A review process must be in place by which such requests can be considered.

Right to Receive an Accounting of Disclosures of Protected Health Information

Patients may request that the physician provide an accounting of all disclosures of the patient's PHI that are nonroutine (as defined in the facility's Notice of Privacy Practices). Patients are entitled to receive this accounting annually without charge, but the provider can charge patients for additional accountings.

Responsibilities of Providers or Health Plans

The responsibilities placed on providers and health plans seems extensive when one reads the actual **verbiage** of the law. Do not be intimidated when reading a publication written by the federal government. These documents are rarely written for ease of understanding and may need to be reread several times before the reader grasps the meaning of a regulation.

In general, the HIPAA Privacy Rule requires activities such as the following.
- Notifying patients of their privacy rights
- Explaining how their health information might be used
- Development of privacy procedures in the facility
- Implementation of those privacy procedures
- Training employees so that they understand the procedures in place

---

Seven Components of HIPAA Compliance Offered by the Office of Inspector General

To simplify compliance with HIPAA regulations, the **Office of Inspector General (OIG)** has developed seven components of an effective compliance program. These components are as follows:
- Conducting internal monitoring and auditing
- Implementing compliance and practice standards
- Designating a compliance officer or contact
- Conducting appropriate training and education
- Responding appropriately to detected offenses, and developing corrective action
- Developing open lines of communication
- Enforcing disciplinary standards through well-publicized guidelines

WALNUT HILL FAMILY AND PREVENTIVE MEDICINE CLINIC, PA
1701 W. Walnut Hill Lane, Suite 200
Dallas, Texas 75229
214-549-1111   214-549-1222 (FAX)
info@walnuthillclinic.com

NOTICE OF PRIVACY PRACTICES

THIS NOTICE DESCRIBES HOW MEDICAL INFORMATION ABOUT YOU MAY BE USED AND DISCLOSED
AND HOW YOU CAN GET ACCESS TO THIS INFORMATION.
PLEASE REVIEW IT CAREFULLY.

YOUR MEDICAL RECORD (CHART) contains your symptoms, examination, and test results, diagnoses, treatment, and plan for follow-up. This is protected health information (PHI), and is used for many reasons. Your medical record serves as a

- basis for planning your care and treatment (this includes scheduling and appointment reminders)
- means of communication among the many health professionals who contribute to your care
- legal document describing the care you received
- means by which you or a third-party payer can verify services billed
- tool in educating health professionals
- source of data for quality control programs and medical research
- source of information for public health officials (by law, certain illnesses must be reported)

YOUR HEALTH INFORMATION RIGHTS
Although your medical record (chart) is the physical property of the clinic, the information contained within the record belongs to you. You have the right to:

- request a restriction on certain uses and disclosures of your information
- obtain a paper copy of this notice
- inspect and obtain a copy of your medical record as provided in our office policy manual
- amend your health record (requests must be made in writing)
- request communications of your health information by alternative means or at alternative locations
- revoke your authorization to use or disclose health information except to the extent that action has already been taken
- obtain an accounting of any non-routine disclosures of your health information

OUR RESPONSIBILITIES
The Walnut Hill Family and Preventative Medicine Clinic is required to:

- maintain the privacy of your medical record (chart)
- abide by the terms of this notice
- notify you if we are unable to agree to a requested restriction
- accommodate reasonable requests you may have to communicate health information by alternative means or at alternative locations or phone numbers

We reserve the right to change our practices and to make new provisions effective for all protected health information we maintain. We will post a copy of our current notice in a visible location at all times. We will not use or disclose your protected health information without your authorization, except as described in this notice.

FOR MORE INFORMATION OR TO REPORT A PROBLEM
Please contact Sue Singer or Ron Rachels during regular office hours at 214-549-1111 or you can email or mail questions or complaints to Dr. Robbie Speasak at the above address. If you believe that your privacy rights have been violated, you can file a complaint with the Secretary of the Department of Health and Human Services. You will not be penalized in any way for filing a complaint.

FIGURE 16-2 Notice of Privacy Practices.

REQUEST TO ACCESS MEDICAL RECORD

Patients have the right to access their personal health information. We will be happy to accommodate any patient who wishes to exercise this access to inspect or obtain a copy of the record. Please provide the information requested on this form. This request will be acted upon within thirty (30) days. Standard copy charges will apply.

Patient Name _____

Date of Birth _____ Phone _____

Address _____

City _____ State _____ Zip_____

Email Address _____

Date of Last Office Visit _____

Please note below what information should be copied or provided:

_____

_____

_____

Please note below the following change(s) that need to be addressed:

_____

_____

I wish to receive a regular accounting of non-routine disclosures of my protected health information.

❐ Yes   ❐ No

_____   _____
Patient Signature   Date

FOR OFFICE USE ONLY

Date Copied _____ Date Mailed _____

Certified Mail # _____

FIGURE 16-3 Request to access a medical record.

PROCEDURE 16-1

Identify and Respond to Issues of Confidentiality

CAAHEP COMPETENCY: 3.c(2)(a)
ABHES COMPETENCY: 1.b

GOAL: *To become proficient at identifying issues involving confidentiality and respond to them in the manner prescribed by office policy.*

EQUIPMENT and SUPPLIES

- Office policy manual
- Office procedure manual, if separate
- Release of information forms
- Notice of Privacy Practices
- Clerical supplies
- Patient medical records

PROCEDURAL STEPS

1. Review office policy regarding release of patient information and confidentiality in the facility.
   PURPOSE: To make certain that office policy is stringently followed and that the office remains in HIPAA compliance.
2. Review the Notice of Privacy Practices for the facility.
   PURPOSE: To be sure that the office's privacy policies are followed.
3. Review the facility's Authorization to Release Medical Records form.

4. Thoroughly read the request for information that is presented to the facility.
   PURPOSE: To determine what information is being requested.
5. Determine if the document is valid.
   PURPOSE: No information should be released if the requesting documents are not valid.
6. Determine the exact information that is being requested.
   PURPOSE: Only the exact information being requested should be released.
7. Make certain that the release of information form either is one designed by the facility or contains all of the same information.
8. Make the requestor complete one of the facility's request forms, if necessary.
9. Forward only the information requested to the person or organization that presented the authorization for release of information.
   PURPOSE: No information that has not been requested can be released without additional consent by the patient.
10. Release the information by mail or to the agent of the requestor.

- Designating an individual to be responsible for implementation
- Securing medical records so that they are not available to those who do not need them

PERMISSION TO DISCLOSE PROTECTED HEALTH INFORMATION

Once the patient has signed the Notice of Privacy Practices, the physician may disclose PHI in the manner that is described on the policy. Virtually all of the daily operations that involve PHI are covered under the Notice of Privacy Practices.

Some offices ask patients to sign a receipt of privacy practices annually. Others simply post the current policy prominently in the office, and state where it can be found on the original notice that the patient signs. Using either method, every current medical record should contain a signed Notice of Privacy Practices, an acknowledgement that the patient received the Notice of Privacy Practices, or a statement that the patient refused to sign the notice. Physicians also use separate release of information forms that detail exactly where to call a patient, whether the patient prefers email communications, and/or specific releases for human immunodeficiency virus (HIV)–related and psychotherapy information (Figures 16-4 and 16-5).

At times, conflicting permissions may be an issue when disclosing PHI. Suppose that a patient requests that a copy of his or her medical record be sent to a third party, such as an

attorney. The patient signs the release at an office visit. Before the medical record is copied and sent, the attorney forwards a signed release for just the progress notes. Call the patient first and attempt to verify what he or she wishes sent. Another option is to adhere to the most restrictive request; in this case, send only the progress notes. Always document any form of communication about the patient's preference in writing. The medical assistant may find it necessary to ask the patient to sign a new permission form. Do not hesitate to contact the patient if any question arises about what he or she wishes to be released.

Identifying the Patient

Providers see numerous patients each day and the medical assistant may not know each one by sight. Always insist on identification when releasing any type of health information to anyone. A state-issued drivers license or identification card is the best method of identification, but alternates may be necessary for those who do not have that particular document. The office policy manual should list acceptable forms of identification. When making any type of disclosure, make certain to note why the person has the authority to request and receive the PHI.

Patient Names and Sign-In Sheets

A staff member in a physician's office may call out a patient's name when it is time to see the physician. Sign-in sheets that list patient names may also be used. Covered entities are permitted to make such incidental disclosures if they comply with the

Patient Consent to the Use and Disclosure of Health Information
for Treatment, Payment, or Health Care Operations

I understand that as part of my health care, the practice originates and maintains paper and/or electronic records describing my health history, symptoms, examination and test results, diagnoses, treatment, and any plans for future care or treatment. I understand that this information serves as:

- A basis for planning my care and treatment,
- A means of communication among professionals who contribute to my care,
- A source of information for applying my diagnosis and treatment information to my bill,
- A means by which a third-party payer can verify that services billed were actually provided,
- A tool for routine health care operations, such as assessing quality and reviewing the competence of staff.

I have been provided the opportunity to review the *"Notice of Patient Privacy Information Practices"* **that provides a more complete description of information uses and disclosures. I understand that I have the following rights:**

- The right to review the *"Notice"* prior to acknowledging this consent,
- The right to restrict or revoke the use or disclosure of my health information for other uses or purposes, and
- The right to request restrictions as to how my health information may be used or disclosed to carry out treatment, payment, or health care operations.

Restrictions:

I request the following restrictions to the use or disclosure of my health information:

_____

_____

May discuss treatment, payment, or health care operation with the following persons:

(Please check all that apply)   Spouse [   ]   **Your Children** [   ]   **Relatives** [   ]   **Others** [   ]   **Parents** [   ]

Please list the names and relationship, if you checked "Relatives" or "Others" above

_____

_____

Messages or Appointment Reminders: (Please check all that apply)

May we leave a message on your answering machine at home [   ] or at work [   ]. **Do not leave a message** [   ]

May we leave a message with someone at your **home** using the doctor's name or the practice name: Yes [   ]   No [   ]

May we leave a message with someone at your **work** using the doctor's name or the practice name: Yes [   ]   No [   ]

Messages will be of a nonsensitive nature, such as appointment reminders.

I understand that as part of treatment, payment, or health care operations, it may become necessary to disclose health information to another entity, i.e., referrals to other health care providers, labs, and/or other individuals or agencies as permitted or required by state or federal law.

I fully understand and accept the information provided by this consent.

_____   _____   _____
Signature   Print name of person signing   Date

*If other than patient is signing, are you the parent, legal guardian, custodian, or have Power of Attorney for this patient for treatment, payment, or health care operations? Yes [   ]   No [   ]

_____

FOR OFFICE USE ONLY
[   ] Patient refused to sign the consent form.
[   ] Restrictions were added by the patient (see restrictions listed above)
[   ] "Consent form" received and reviewed by _____ on (date) _____
[   ] "Consent form" placed in the patient's medical record on (date) _____

FIGURE 16-4 Example of HIPAA-compliant patient disclosure form. (From Klieger DM: *Saunders textbook of medical assisting,* St Louis, 2005, Saunders.)

GENERAL MEDICAL HEALTH CARE

AUTHORIZATION FOR RELEASE OF MEDICAL INFORMATION

I, _____ ____/____/____ _____ hereby authorize
  Print Patient's Name   Date of Birth   Social Security Number

General Medical Health Care 1234 Riverview Road, Anytown, FL 33333

to release medical, including HIV Antibody Testing, Psychiatric/Psychological, Alcohol and/or Drug Abuse, information records to:

To: _____

Address _____
        (Street)   (City)   (State)   (Zip)

For the purpose of: 1. Drs. appointment on: _____

                       2. Other: _____

                       _____
                           Please Specify Reason for Disclosure

I understand that if I consent to the release of any of my medical records, the results of any HIV Antibody Testing, Psychiatric/Psychological, Alcohol and/or Drug Abuse information will be released.

I understand this consent may be cancelled upon written notice to the hospital, except that action by the hospital has been taken in reliance on this authorization, and that this authorization shall remain in force for a 90-day period in order to effect the purpose for which it is given. Alcohol and drug abuse information, if present, has been disclosed from records whose confidentiality is protected by Federal Law. FEDERAL REGULATIONS (42CFR, part II) prohibit making any further disclosure of records without the specific written authorization of the undersigned, or as otherwise permitted by such regulations. The confidentiality of HIV antibody test results is protected by Florida Law [Fla. Stat.ANN. 381.609 (2) (F)], which prohibits any further disclosure by a person to whom this information has been disclosed, without specific written consent of the undersigned or as otherwise permitted by state law.

_____ From: _____ To: _____
(Date of Authorization)   (Dates to be Released)

_____
Patient's Signature

_____
Parent, Legal Guardian, or Authorized
Representative Signature

_____
Relationship to Patient

_____
Witness

FIGURE 16-5 Example of HIPAA-compliant patient disclosure form containing HIV and psychologic information release. (From Klieger DM: *Saunders textbook of medical assisting,* St Louis, 2005, Saunders.)

HIPAA MINIMUM NECESSARY STANDARD
[45 CFR 164.502(b), 164.514(d)]

Background

The minimum necessary standard, a key protection of the HIPAA Privacy Rule, is derived from confidentiality codes and practices in common use today. It is based on sound current practice that protected health information should not be used or disclosed when it is not necessary to satisfy a particular purpose or carry out a function. The minimum necessary standard requires covered entities to evaluate their practices and enhance safeguards as needed to limit unnecessary or inappropriate access to and disclosure of protected health information. The Privacy Rule's requirements for minimum necessary standards are designed to be sufficiently flexible to accommodate the various circumstances of any covered entity.

How the Rule Works

The Privacy Rule generally requires covered entities to take reasonable steps to limit the use or disclosure of, and requests for, protected health information to the minimum necessary to accomplish the intended purpose. The minimum necessary standard does not apply to the following:

- Disclosures to or requests by a health care provider for treatment purposes.
- Disclosures to the individual who is the subject of the information.
- Uses or disclosures made pursuant to an individual's authorization.
- Uses or disclosures required for compliance with the Health Insurance Portability and Accountability Act (HIPAA) Administrative Simplification Rules.
- Disclosures to the Department of Health and Human Services (HHS) when disclosure of information is required under the Privacy Rule for enforcement purposes.
- Uses or disclosures that are required by other law.

The implementation specifications for this provision require a covered entity to develop and implement policies and procedures appropriate for its own organization, reflecting the entity's business practices and workforce. While guidance cannot anticipate every question or factual application of the minimum necessary standard to each specific industry context, where it would be generally helpful we will seek to provide additional clarification on this issue in the future. In addition, the Department will continue to monitor the workability of the minimum necessary standard and consider proposing revisions, where appropriate, to ensure that the Rule does not hinder timely access to quality health care.

http://www.hhs.gov/ocr/hipaa/

FIGURE 16-6 HIPAA's Minimum Necessary Standard Overview.

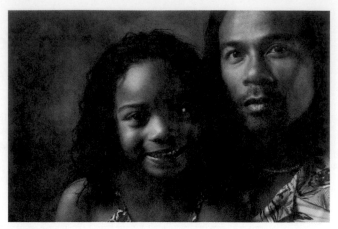

FIGURE 16-7 In most cases the parent is considered the child's representative and is allowed to view 'the child's medical records.

Privacy Rule is not intended to impede customary and necessary healthcare communications or practices or to require that all risk of incidental use or disclosure be eliminated to satisfy the Privacy standards. Disclosures that could occur as a byproduct of engaging in healthcare communications or practices may be considered acceptable under the Privacy Rule.

Incidental disclosures could include the following:
- Confidential conversations between providers or with patients, if a possibility exists that they may be heard (e.g., by hearing the patient and physician talking through the wall when in an adjacent examination room)
- Seeing other patient names when signing in
- A person not authorized to see PHI walks by medical equipment and sees material containing **individually identifiable health information** (e.g., seeing a patient's name on an ultrasound screen)
- Physicians speaking with patients in semiprivate hospital rooms
- Healthcare staff orally coordinating patient care services at a nurse's station or central location within an office
- A pharmacist discussing a patient with a physician on the phone when another person is standing nearby

Most physician offices have implemented sign-in sheets that ideally allow only one patient to sign in at a time and prevent them from seeing other patient names. Sign-in sheets that use pressure-sensitive stickers are a good example. The patient signs in on the form, then the sticker is removed and placed either in the patient's medical record or on a log sheet. Some offices are more technologically advanced and have a computer sign-in system. The patient arrives and goes to the computer screen, sees his or her name, and then presses "enter" to signify that he or she has arrived for the appointment. The patient name appears only for 15 minutes or so before the appointment and for 15 minutes after. If the name is not on the screen, the patient is directed to see the office staff. This subtly teaches the patient to be on time for appointments. These devices save time, although the patient must receive brief training on how to use the system. The short time that the patient's name is viewable on the screen is an incidental exposure but is acceptable through HIPAA guidelines as explained previously.

minimum necessary requirements of HIPAA (Figure 16-6). An incidental use or disclosure is a secondary use or disclosure that cannot reasonably be prevented, is limited in nature, and occurs as a result of another use or disclosure that is permitted. The

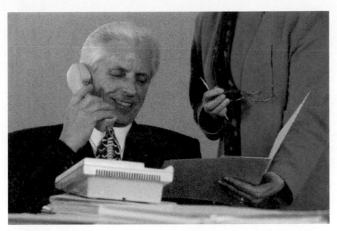

FIGURE 16-8 The telephone remains one of the most vital tools for communication with patients.

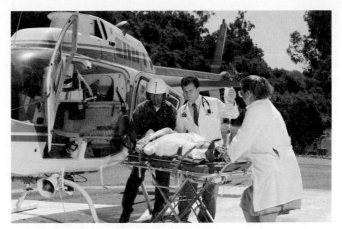

FIGURE 16-9 In emergencies the Notice of Privacy Practices does not have to be offered until it is practical to do so.

Placement of Patient Medical Records

Many physician offices place medical records inside a wall folder just outside of the examination room. By turning the record so that the name cannot be seen by someone passing through the hallway, the facility meets the minimum necessary requirement in protecting patient privacy. The hallway area should be supervised, and nonemployees should be escorted when in the clinical area of the office.

Children's Health Records

The Privacy Rule does allow parents to see the medical records of their children as long as this is not inconsistent with state law. In most cases the parent is the child's personal representative under the Privacy Rule (Figure 16-7). However, several instances exist in which the parent is not considered the child's personal representative. These instances include the following:

- When the minor is the one who consents to care and the consent of the parent is not required under state or other applicable law (for example, in the case of an emancipated minor)
- When the minor obtains care at the direction of a court or a person appointed by the court
- When the parent agrees that the minor and healthcare provider can have a confidential relationship

Discussing Information with Friends and Family

The Privacy Rule specifically permits covered entities to share information that is directly relevant to the patient's care with a spouse, family members, friends, or other persons identified by a patient. The covered entity may also share relevant information with the family and these other persons if it can reasonably **infer,** based on professional judgment, that the patient does not object or that the action is in the best interest of the patient. Remember that if the patient has requested that such information not be shared with others, the provider must honor that request unless it is deemed unreasonable.

Both covered entities and **business associates** can discuss a patient's bill with a person other than the patient to obtain reimbursement. No limit is placed on to whom such a disclosure may be made. However, the Privacy Rule does require a covered entity or business associate to reasonably limit the amount of information disclosed for such purposes to the minimum necessary and to abide by reasonable requests for confidential communications and restrictions that the patient has requested.

Telephone Messages and Faxes

Medical assistants must communicate with patients, and that communication is often initiated with a telephone call (Figure 16-8). At times the patient is not at home or available and the medical assistant must use professional judgment about leaving a message, as well as about how much information to disclose to the person who answers the telephone. Even leaving a message on an answering machine can be questionable, because no one is sure who will hear a message containing PHI.

If the patient has requested that the provider or provider's employees communicate only in a confidential manner, such as by alternative means or at an alternative location, the provider must honor that request if it is reasonable. For instance, requests to receive calls at work instead of at home are reasonable requests, unless there are extenuating circumstances.

A fax can be sent containing PHI to another healthcare provider for treatment purposes or to another individual as requested by the patient. Use reasonable care in sending a fax, such as verifying the correct numbers, directing the fax to a certain person, and using cover sheets that stress confidentiality. All fax machines should be located in secure areas to prevent unauthorized access to PHI. Information used for treatment purposes can be shared by fax, email, or telephone with other healthcare providers.

Emergencies

Healthcare providers and facilities, such as hospitals, with a direct treatment relationship with individuals are not required to provide their Notices of Privacy Practices to patients at the time they are providing emergency treatment (Figure 16-9). In such situations the HIPAA Privacy Rule requires only that providers give patients a notice when it is practical to do so after the emergency situation has ended. In addition, the Privacy Rule does not require that providers make a good faith effort to obtain the patient's written acknowledgement of receipt of the notice.

Complaints about Privacy Violations

When a patient has a complaint regarding his or her privacy information, the first person he or she should seek out is the **privacy officer** at the facility where the incident took place. If the complaint is not resolved, patients should be directed to the office manager or physician. In the event that the patient's issue has still not been resolved, he or she has the option to file a written complaint either on paper or electronically with the **Office for Civil Rights (OCR).** The complaint must be filed within 180 days of when the **complainant** knew or should have known that the act had occurred (Figure 16-10). The OCR may waive the 180-day time limit if good cause is shown.

Complaints must meet the following criteria:
- They must be filed in writing, either on paper or electronically.
- They must name the entity that is the subject of the complaint.
- They must describe the acts or omissions believed to be in violation of the Privacy Rule.
- They must be filed within 180 days of the incident.
- They must apply to an incident that occurred after April 14, 2003 (2004 for small health plans).

OCR has 10 regional offices, and each one covers certain states. Complaints must be filed with the correct regional office that has jurisdiction over the state in which the incident occurred. A complaint form is available on the OCR website. The **Office of the Inspector General (OIG)** conducts investigations and audits when there is a question regarding privacy laws.

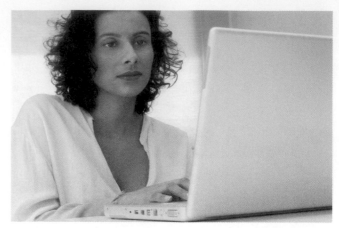

FIGURE 16-10 The time may come when a patient files a complaint against a provider for a violation of privacy practices.

CLOSING COMMENTS

Every employee of the physician's office must read the policy and procedure manual to make certain that he or she has a firm understanding of the HIPAA Privacy Rule and how it relates to the individual office (Figure 16-11). The medical assistant is responsible for learning and following the guidelines set forth by HIPAA. If uncertain about any situation, contact the privacy officer in the organization for direction or research the question on the HIPAA website. Never assume that a patient will not mind if certain information is disclosed. Always check the medical record to determine patient preferences. Keep current on changes to HIPAA regulations and continue to function in a state of constant learning. Embrace changes designed to improve patient care and treatment.

Guidelines for HIPAA Privacy Compliance

1. Consider that conversations occurring throughout the office could be overheard. The reception area and waiting room are often linked, and it is easy to hear the scheduling of appointments and exchange of confidential information. It is necessary to observe areas and maximize efforts to avoid unauthorized disclosures. Simple and affordable precautions include using privacy glass at the front desk and having conversations away from settings where other patients or visitors are present. Health care providers can move their dictation stations away from patient areas or wait until no patients are present before dictating. Phone conversations by providers in front of patients, even in emergency situations, should be avoided. Providers and staff must use their best professional judgment.

2. Be sure to check in the patient medical record and in the computer system to see if there are any special instructions for contacting the patient regarding scheduling or reporting test results. Follow these requests as agreed by the office.

3. Patient sign-in sheets are permissible, but limit the information requested when a patient signs in, and change it periodically during the day. A sign-in sheet must not contain information such as reason for visit because some providers specialize in treating patients with sensitive issues. Showing that a particular individual has an appointment with the physician may pose a breach of confidentiality.

4. Make sure patients sign a form acknowledging receipt of the NPP. The NPP allows the physician to release the patient's confidential information for billing and other purposes. If the practice has other confidentiality statements and policies besides HIPAA mandates, these must be reviewed to ensure they meet HIPAA requirements.

5. Format policies for transferring and accepting outside PHI must address how the office keeps this information confidential. When using courier services, billing services, transcription services, or email, ensure that transferring PHI is done in a secure and compliant manner.

6. Computers are used for a variety of administrative functions, including scheduling, billing, and managing medical records. Computers typically are present at the reception area. Keep the computer screen turned so that viewing is restricted to authorized staff. Screensavers should be used to prevent unauthorized viewing or access. The computer should automatically log off the user after a period of being idle, requiring the staff member to reenter their password.

7. Keep usernames and passwords confidential, and change them often. Do not share this information. An authorized staff member such as the PO will have administrative access to reset passwords if they are lost or if someone discovers the password. Also, practice management software can track users and follow their activity. Do not ever give out a password. Safeguards include password protection for electronic data and storing paper records securely.

8. Safeguard the work area; do not place notes with confidential information in areas that are easy to view by nonstaff. Cleaningservices will access the building, usually after business hours; ensure that PHI is protected.

9. Place medical record charts face down at reception areas so the patient's name is not exposed to other patients or visitors to the office. Also, when placing medical records on the door of an examination room, turn the chart so that the identifying information faces the door. If medical record are kept on countertops or in receptacles, ensure that non-staff persons will not access the records. Handling and storing medical records will certainly change because of HIPAA guidelines.

10. Do not post the health care provider's schedule in areas viewable by non-staff individuals. The schedules are often posted for professional staff convenience, but this may be a breach in patient confidentiality.

11. Fax machines should not be placed in patient examination rooms or in any reception area where non-staff persons may view incoming or sent documents. Only staff members should have access to the faxes.

12. Direct mail and phone calls only to the appropriate staff members.

13. Recognize, learn, and use HIPAA TCS if involved in coding and billing.

14. Send all privacy-related questions or concerns to the appropriate staff member.

15. Immediately report any suspected or known improper behavior to supervisors or the PO so that the issue may be documented and investigated.

16. Direct all questions to the supervisors or PO.

FIGURE 16-11 Guidelines for HIPAA Privacy Compliance. (From *Quick Guide to HIPAA for the physician's office*, St Louis, 2004, Saunders.)

SUMMARY OF SCENARIO

Sabrina and Elsa will experience many challenges as a result of the information exchange they shared at the family picnic. Their conversation probably began like any other, but once Sabrina told Elsa the details of Ms. Adams' visit, they violated patient privacy laws. Their future in the medical field is now uncertain.

Ms. Adams suffered emotionally after the breach of privacy. Her daughter, Terri, does not understand why her mother did not tell her about the illness. The relationship between the mother and daughter is now stressful, an interference with their normal bond during this critical time. The family questions whether to pursue the matter legally or spend the time they have left together in more productive ways. They have many decisions to make.

Dr. Taylor placed Sabrina on probation for 3 months. Before this incident, she had never received any type of disciplinary action. Elsa was not formally disciplined, largely because of her long-standing relationship with Dr. Berry. Still, there is sharp tension between them in the office now, as he faces a possible medical professional liability lawsuit, as well as complaints

about the privacy of Ms. Adams' PHI. Neither Sabrina nor Elsa will look at their jobs the same way as before the incident—for them, everything is different. They both feel that they have disappointed their employers, their patients, and themselves.

The medical assistant must remember that patients should be discussed only with others who are directly involved in the patient's medical care. The HIPAA Privacy Rule has made great strides in protecting patient privacy and in simplifying administrative processes. However, the rule is effective only if office policies are established and practiced. New policies may be difficult to implement, but gaining an understanding of the reason for the policy and its major goals will help the medical assistant embrace changes more readily.

Patients may not agree with the privacy practices or may not understand them. Make an effort to help the patient see the benefit in the policies that the office has established, reminding the patient that such policies are designed for their protection. The patient does not have to agree with the policy or sign it as long as the staff members make a good faith effort toward this end.

SUMMARY of LEARNING OBJECTIVES

1. Define, spell, and pronounce the terms listed in the vocabulary.
   - Spelling and pronouncing medical terms correctly adds credibility to the medical assistant. Knowing the definition of these terms promotes confidence in communication with patients and co-workers.
2. Explain how the HIPAA Privacy Rule benefits the healthcare industry and patients.
   - As a result of the HIPAA Privacy Rule, patients have more control over their medical records. They are able to make informed choices as to how their personal health information is used, and boundaries are set on the use and release of health records. Safeguards are established that healthcare providers must achieve to protect the privacy of health information. Violators are held accountable and face both civil and criminal penalties if patient privacy rights are compromised. The HIPAA Privacy Rule also protects public health by striking a balance when public responsibility supports disclosure of personal health information.
3. List what must be included on a Notice of Privacy Practices.
   - A Notice of Privacy Practices must include details as to how PHI is used and disclosed by the facility; the duties of the provider to protect health information; patient rights regarding PHI; how complaints can be filed if patients believe their privacy has been violated; whom to contact at the facility for more information; and the effective date of the Notice of Privacy Practices.

4. Explain the difference between Title I and Title II of the HIPAA Privacy Rule.
   - Title I of the HIPAA Privacy Rule regulates insurance reform. It limits the use of preexisting health conditions that in the past would have prevented or limited an employee from obtaining health insurance coverage. If an individual left a job with insurance coverage and attempted to secure new coverage, a preexisting health condition would often preclude that person from obtaining coverage for that illness. Title II deals with administrative simplification. This section is the source of privacy and security laws that affect the patient. The goal of Title II is to reduce administrative costs in the healthcare industry.
5. List the rights that patients have under the Privacy Rule.
   - Patients have several rights under the Privacy Rule, including the right to notice of a facility's privacy practices; the right to have access to, view, and obtain a copy of their PHI; the right to restrict certain parts or uses of their PHI; the right to request that communications from the facility be kept confidential; the right to request the facility to amend the PHI; and the right to receive notice of all disclosures of their PHI.
6. Briefly explain what is expected of healthcare providers in relation to the Privacy Rule.
   - Healthcare providers are expected to notify patients of their privacy rights; explain how their health information might be used; develop privacy procedures in the facility; implement

Continued

SUMMARY of LEARNING OBJECTIVES
Continued

those privacy procedures; train employees so that they understand the procedures in place; designate an individual to be responsible for implementation; and secure medical records so that they are not available to those who do not need them.

7. Describe an incidental disclosure.
   - An incidental disclosure is a secondary use or disclosure that cannot reasonably be prevented, is limited in nature, and occurs as a result of another use or disclosure that is permitted.

8. List the three instances when a parent is not considered the child's representative.
   - A parent is not considered the child's representative in any of three instances: when the minor is the one who consents to care and the consent of the parent is not required under state or other applicable law (e.g., in the case of an emancipated minor); when the minor obtains care at the direction of a court or a person appointed by the court; or when the parent agrees that the minor and healthcare provider can have a confidential relationship.

9. Explain why a provider can discuss protected health information with a patient's friends and family.
   - A provider can discuss PHI with a patient's friends and family unless the patient has limited disclosure and requested that he or she receive only confidential communication with the provider. Unless the patient makes this request, which should be in writing, the provider is able to discuss the patient with others as long as good judgment is used and the communication is related to the patient's treatment.

10. Discuss the role of the Notice of Privacy Practices in emergencies.
    - Healthcare providers and facilities, such as hospitals, with a direct treatment relationship with individuals are not required to provide their Notices of Privacy Practices to patients at the time they are providing emergency treatment (Figure 16-9). In such situations the HIPAA Privacy Rule requires only that providers give patients a notice when it is practical to do so after the emergency situation has ended.

CONNECTIONS

 Study Guide Connection: Go to Chapter 16 Study Guide. Read the Case Study and Workplace Applications and complete the assignments. Do online research for answers to the questions in the Internet Activities associated with privacy in the physician's office.

 CD Connection: Go to the Medical Assisting Competency Challenge CD and do the training activities under Legal Concepts.

 Evolve Connection: For more information related to privacy in the physician's office, go to http://evolve.elsevier.com/kinn/admin and visit related weblinks for Chapter 16. Click on the Medical Assisting Exam Review and do the practice questions to sharpen your test-taking skills.

Basics of Diagnostic Coding

17

Carline A. Dalgleish
Alexandra Patricia Young

SCENARIO

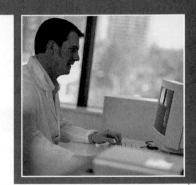

Mike Simeone has been employed with Drs. Shuman and Taylor in their gastroenterology practice for the last 2 years. He works as an administrative assistant in medical records and simultaneously has been enrolled in the medical assistant program at his local college. Since he has become more knowledgeable, Mike has been given more responsibility in both diagnostic and procedural coding tasks. Diagnostic coding is a system of numeric codes used in insurance claims processing and for statistical purposes. To perform diagnostic coding, Mike uses a manual called the International Classification of Diseases, Ninth Revision, Clinical Modification, or ICD-9-CM.

Mike's experience from working in medical records gives him an understanding of the importance of correct and thorough documentation. His strong skills in reading and understanding physician's orders, treatment plans, chart notes, and diagnostic statements will prove invaluable as Mike learns more about diagnostic coding and refines his coding skills.

Mike is aware of the legalities and importance of proper billing as it affects reimbursement. Now he will use his experience and hopes to advance his position within the office. He knows that the practice is committed to compliance with all of the regulations affecting the operation of the facility and he knows that the patient charts are well documented, making his new tasks easier to accomplish. Mike is a conscientious worker and looks forward to success in his new role and the exposure to more aspects of the medical assisting profession.

While studying this chapter, think about the following questions:

- How do the format, layout, and conventions of the ICD-9-CM manual help the medical assistant search for the most accurate and specific diagnostic code?
- Why is medical record documentation so critical in relationship to diagnostic coding?

- Why does the medical assistant need to know the steps for performing diagnostic coding?
- What are the benefits of using diagnostic codes found in the ICD-9-CM?

LEARNING OBJECTIVES

1. Define, spell, and pronounce the terms listed in the vocabulary.
2. Identify three purposes of the ICD-9-CM.
3. Explain the proper use of the ICD-9-CM.
4. Understand and apply the basic coding rules in the use of the ICD-9-CM.
5. Understand the importance of the Tabular Index, which contains the most specific coding information.

6. Comprehend and use instructional terms and symbols as defined in the ICD-9-CM.
7. Explain the use of V and E codes.
8. Properly perform basic diagnostic coding.

National Accreditation Competencies and Content

CAAHEP COMPETENCIES	ABHES COMPETENCIES
Administrative 3.a.(3)(d). Perform diagnostic coding	**Administrative Duties** 3.v. Perform diagnostic coding
General 3.c.(2)(d). Document appropriately	**Legal Concepts** 5.a. Determine needs for documentation and reporting 5.b. Document accurately
	Financial Management 8.b. Implement current procedural terminology and ICD-9 coding

VOCABULARY

ancillary diagnostic services Services that support patient diagnoses (e.g., laboratory or radiology services).

ancillary therapeutic services Services that support patient treatment (specialists or surgery).

"and" In the context of ICD-9-CM, the word *and* should be interpreted as *and/or.*

chapters Broad sections of the ICD-9-CM coding manual grouped by disease or illness, (e.g., Chapter 10 contains diagnostic codes for diseases of the genitourinary system).

"code also" Used when more than one code is necessary to fully identify a given condition, "code also" or "use additional code" is used.

coding Converting verbal or written descriptions into numeric and alphanumeric designations.

diagnosis The determination of the nature of a disease, injury, or congenital defect.

etiology The cause of the disorder; a claim may be classified according to etiology.

"excludes" Exclusion terms are always written in italics, and the word "excludes" is often enclosed in a box to draw particular attention to these instructions. Exclusion terms may apply to a chapter, a section, a category, or a subcategory. The applicable code number usually follows the exclusion term.

"includes" This term appearing under a subdivision, such as a category (three-digit code) or two-digit procedure code, indicates that the code and title include these terms. Other terms also classified to that particular code and title are listed in the Alphabetic Indexes.

International Classification of Diseases, Ninth Revision, Clinical Modification (ICD-9-CM) System for classifying disease to facilitate collection of uniform and comparable health information, for statistical purposes and indexing medical records for data storage and retrieval.

International Statistical Classifications of Diseases and Related Health Problems, Tenth Revision, Clinical Modifi- cation **(ICD-10-CM)** System containing the greatest number of changes in ICD history. To allow more specific reporting of disease and newly recognized conditions, the ICD-10-CM contains approximately 5500 more codes than ICD-9.

manifestation The signs and symptoms of a disease.

notations Notations, also known as instructional notations, are found in both the Alphabetic Index and the Tabular Index as instructions or guides in classification assignments, defining category content or the use of subdivision codes.

primary diagnosis Initial identification of the condition or complaint that the patient expresses in the outpatient medical setting.

"see" A direction given to the coder to look in another place. This term must always be followed and is found in the Alphabetic Index, Volumes 2 and 3.

"see also" A direction given to the coder to look elsewhere if the main term or subterm (or subterms) for that entry are not sufficient for coding the information. If a code number follows, "see also" is enclosed in parentheses. If there is no code number, "see also" is preceded by a dash.

"see category" A direction given to the coder to see a specific category (three-digit code). This must always be followed.

"use additional code" This term appears only in Volume 1 in those subdivisions in which the user should add further information by means of an additional code to give a more complete picture of the diagnosis. In some cases you will find "if desired" following the term. For the purpose of coding, the "if desired" phrase will not be used. When the term "use additional code...if desired" appears, disregard "if desired" and assign the appropriate additional code.

"with" In the context of ICD-9-CM, the terms "with," "with mention of," and "associated with" in a title dictate that both parts of the title be present in the statement of the diagnosis order to assign the particular code.

To facilitate accurate medical record keeping and the processing of claims, it is essential to identify appropriate services and descriptions of diseases, injuries, and procedures. The **International Classification of Diseases, Ninth Revision, Clinical Modification** (ICD-9-CM) statistically classifies elements of a subject according to diseases, injuries, and operations. The ICD-9-CM is used by healthcare providers for **coding** and reporting clinical information, as required for participation in Medicare and Medicaid programs. In addition, the ICD-9-CM is used for tracking healthcare statistics. Practice management software and third-party payors recognize these codes, which simplify the reimbursement process and speed payment to healthcare providers.

GETTING TO KNOW ICD-9-CM

What Is Diagnostic Coding?

Diagnostic coding is described as the translation or transformation of written descriptions of diseases, illnesses, and injuries into numeric codes. Accurate use of the ICD-9-CM manual is essential for accuracy in translating the medical record's diagnostic statement(s) into numeric codes. The medical assistant facilitates accurate medical record keeping and the efficient processing of claims by using the ICD-9-CM, which identifies the disease or injury for which a patient was treated by code. ICD-9-CM codes are used in the claims submission process to request reimbursement from payors, to track the diagnoses treated by the physician, and to provide statistical data for research and other purposes.

Why Use ICD Codes?

There are several pertinent reasons for the use of ICD-9-CM codes, including:

- Standardizing a system of diagnostic coding accepted and understood by all parties in the reimbursement cycle
- Creating a more convenient method of data storage and retrieval
- Assisting in the maximization of reimbursement
- Shortening the claims-processing time
- Facilitating and measuring guideline and usage compliance
- Assisting in measuring the appropriateness and timeliness of medical care

The Evolution of ICD Coding

Classification systems are used by healthcare organizations to organize health care data and make retrieval meaningful. The early Greeks were the first to group data by disease processes. Captain John Graunt of London was the first to publish mortality and morbidity statistics in his publication, *London Bills of Mortality (1662),* which was the first real attempt at studying disease processes from a statistical viewpoint. Later, in the 1830s, William Farr introduced uniformity in the use of statistics. His work helped classify diseases by anatomic site. He published the *International List of Causes of Death* and provided the foundation for current vital statistics.

In 1893 Dr. Jacques Bertillon developed the Bertillon Classification of Causes of Death. The American Public Health Association (APHA) recommended adoption of this classification system for Canada, Mexico, and the United States, and further recommended that the system be revised every 10 years. Subsequent revisions were called the *International Classification System of Causes of Death.* Revisions were completed in 1900, 1910, 1920, 1929, and 1938.

In the 1950s the U.S. Public Health Service published the *International Classification of Diseases,* which was adapted for indexing hospital records by diseases and operations (*International Classification of Diseases, Adapted* [ICDA]). Subsequent modifications made in 1962 provided greater detail and introduced a classification for surgical operations. In 1968, because of a need for even greater detail and specificity, the Eighth Revision of ICDA was adapted for use in the United States (ICDA-8). ICDA-8 provided a basis for coding morbidity and mortality statistics in the United States and served as a method of indexing all diagnoses and operative procedures in hospital records.

The ninth revision of ICD was published in 1975 and was renamed the *International Classification of Diseases, Ninth Revision* (ICD-9). In 1979 the National Center for Health Statistics (NCHS) developed a modification of ICD-9 for use in the United States. The modification is ICD-9-CM, which has been in use in the United States since that time.

At present, legislation is being written to formally adopt the Tenth Revision of the diagnostic coding manual for use within the United States. ICD-10 is a significant upgrade and improvement to the current Revision currently in use. See Appendix B for more information about the **International Statistical Classifications of Diseases and Related Health Problems, Tenth Revision, Clinical Modification,** also known as ICD-10-CM.

The ICD-9-CM Code

The ICD-9-CM code consists of a three-digit category code that represents a specific disease within a general disease category—for example, 250 is the disease classification for diabetes mellitus. Up to two additional digits can be used, which add further definition and specificity. These two additional digits are called the *fourth digit* or *subcategory* and the *fifth digit* or *subclassification,* respectively. The ICD-9-CM manual is used to assign a standardized numeric or alpha-numeric code to the diagnostic statement written by the provider of service, including those diagnostic statements found in operative reports, discharge summaries, history and physical (H&P) reports, **ancillary diagnostic services** and **therapeutic services**, or services that support the patient's diagnoses—for example, radiology, laboratory and pathology reports, as well as physical therapy or chemotherapy reports.

Using the diabetes classification code 250 example in Figure 17-1, a fourth digit can be added that describes any disease manifestation caused by the diabetes (e.g., renal, ophthalmic), and a fifth digit can be added that describes the type of diabetes (juvenile or adult, insulin-dependent diabetes mellitus [IDDM] or non–insulin-dependent diabetes mellitus [NIDDM]).

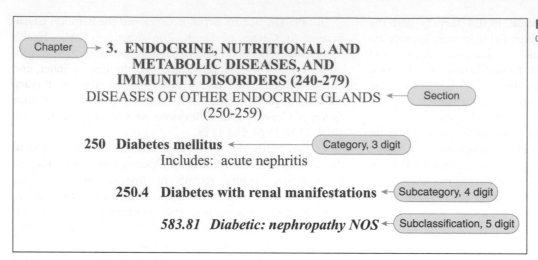

Figure 17-1 Example of Category, Subcategory, and Subclassification.

STRUCTURE OF THE ICD-9-CM

The ICD-9-CM is published in various media, including book, CD, and downloadable file. Depending on the publisher, the layout, symbols, color-coding, and some other features vary somewhat; however, the format, conventions, tables, appendixes, content, and basic structure remain the same. The basic ICD-9-CM manual contains three volumes. Volumes 1 and 2 are used for diagnostic coding by hospitals, physicians, and all other providers of service. Volume 1, also known as the *Tabular Index*, contains all of the diagnostic codes grouped into 17 classifications of disease and injury. Volume 2 is called the *Alphabetic Index* and is used in the same way an alphabetic index in any textbook is used except that it refers the user back to the category codes in the Tabular Index, rather than specific page numbers. Volume 3 is used by hospitals to code procedures and services performed within the hospital environment. Volume 3 is not used by most physician-providers.

Volume 1—Tabular Index

Volume 1, the Tabular Index, is a numeric listing of **diagnosis** codes and descriptions. A diagnosis is the determination of the nature of a disease, injury, or congenital defect. Volume 1 consists of 17 **chapters** that classify diseases and injuries; two sections containing supplementary classification codes (V and E), and five appendixes.

Each of the 17 chapters of the Tabular Index is further subdivided into four levels: section, category, subcategory, and subclassification. Refer back to Figure 17-1 for an example from the ICD-9-CM manual.

- Section: A group of three-digit code numbers describing a general disease category–e.g., 250-259 is the section for Endocrine, Nutritional and Metabolic Diseases. The section is also known as a chapter. This section, which includes codes 250 through 259, is also called Chapter 3.
- Category: A three-digit code representing a specific disease within the section–e.g., category 250 represents diabetes mellitus.
- Subcategory: A further breakdown of the category, assigning a fourth digit–e.g., in category 250, the fourth digit

describes whether any disease process or manifestation exists as a result of the diabetes mellitus.
- Subclassification: Five-digit code giving the highest level of specificity to the disease state. In this category the fifth digit specifies the type of diabetes mellitus–e.g., IDDM or NIDDM, controlled or uncontrolled.

Supplemental Classifications

The two supplementary classifications included in the Tabular Index are V codes, which describe factors influencing health status and which describe contact with health services that cannot be classified elsewhere, and E codes, which describe external causes of injury and poisoning.

V Codes. The V code is used on occasions when the patient is not currently ill or to explain problems that influence his or her current illness or injury. The *Supplementary Classification of Factors Influencing Health Status and Contact with Health Service* (V Code, V01-V85.4) is used in cases such as preventive vaccination or chronic disease states such as dialysis for renal disease.

E Codes. The E code classification, named the *Supplemental Classification of External Causes of Injuries and Poisoning,* is used to classify environmental causes of injury, poisoning, or other adverse effects on the body.

Appendixes

The five appendixes contained in Volume 1, Tabular Index, of the ICD-9-CM are as follows:

- Appendix A–Morphology (the form or structure) of Neoplasms. Morphology code numbers consist of five digits. The first four digits identify the histological type of neoplasm, and the fifth digit indicates its behavior. M codes are used for statistical data only and are not used in physician billing. This section of the appendix is used primarily by inpatient coders.
- Appendix B–Glossary of Mental Disorders. This glossary is an alphabetic listing of the psychiatric terminology that appears in Chapter 5 of Volume 1 (Tabular Index), entitled "Mental Disorders."
- Appendix C–Classification of Drugs. The adverse effects of drugs are coded according to the American Hospital

Formulary Service (AHFS) list. This section is used almost exclusively by pharmacies.

- Appendix D—Classification of Industrial Accidents. This appendix concerns the Statistics of Employment Injuries categorized by the type of industry where the accident occurred. This section is usually used by government organizations, such as the Occupational Safety and Health Administration (OSHA). It is seldom used by physician-providers.
- Appendix E—List of Three-Digit Categories. All of the three-digit category codes from the Tabular Index are listed in order, by chapter.

Conventions Used in Volume 1—the Tabular Index

Conventions refer to abbreviations, punctuation, symbols, instructional notations, and related entities that provide guidance to the medical coder in selection of an accurate and specific code. These conventions are found in Volume 1, the Tabular Index, of the ICD-9-CM. Understanding their meaning and using their guidance is crucial to accurate coding. Many different publishers offer the ICD-9-CM, and there may be some differences in the symbols, notations, colors, or other reference marks used for convenience or to convey specific meaning, depending on the publisher; however, the most common conventions are described here.

Abbreviations. There are two primary abbreviations used in the Tabular Index of the ICD-9-CM, NEC and NOS (Figure 17-2).

NOS—Not otherwise specified. This abbreviation is the equivalent of "unspecified" and means that the diagnostic statement does not provide more specificity or definition.

NEC—Not elsewhere classifiable. The category number for the term including NEC is to be used only when the coder lacks the information necessary to code the term to a more specific category. NEC means that the diagnostic statement contains specific wording but no specific classification exists to match the wording.

Punctuation. Four basic forms of punctuation are used in the Tabular Index: brackets, parentheses, colon, and braces (Figure 17-3). Each form serves a different purpose in the reading and understanding of code descriptions.

Symbols. Symbols are used to designate the requirement of a fourth and/or fifth digit, new entries, and revised text or codes. Other symbols may be found, depending on the publisher. Added symbols or other changes will be described completely in the Introduction to the ICD-9-CM, regardless of the publisher. The most common symbols are shown in Figure 17-4.

Other Conventions. Two other conventions used in both the Alphabetic Index and the Tabular Index are the use of bold and italic fonts.

Bold: Bold type is used for all codes and titles in the Tabular Index.

Italics: Italic type is used for exclusion notes and to identify any diagnosis that cannot be used as the **primary diagnosis.**

Instructional Notations. **Instructional notations** are notes included in the Tabular Index to provide additional guidance

---

NEC

Diagnosis: Pneumonia due to gram-negative bacteria

Index: **Pneumonia**
   gram-negative bacteria NEC 482.83

Tabular: **482.8 Pneumonia due to other specified bacteria**
   482.83 Other gram-negative bacteria

Code: 482.83 Pneumonia due to gram-negative bacteria

Code 482.83 identifies gram-negative bacterial pneumonia that cannot be classified more specifically into the other subclassifications. The other subclassifications within 482.8 are for anaerobes, *Escherichia coli [E. coli],* "other than gram-negative" bacteria, Legionnaire's disease, and other specified bacteria. None of these other subclassifications can be assigned to the diagnostic statement; therefore, 482.83 is the most appropriate choice.

NOS

Diagnosis: Bronchitis

Index: **Bronchitis** 490

Tabular: **490 Bronchitis, not specified as acute or chronic Bronchitis NOS**

Code: 490 Bronchitis

The diagnosis was not specified by the physician as acute or chronic; therefore, the "not otherwise specified" code 490 must be assigned. In this situation, it would be appropriate for the coder to request specificity from the practitioner.

Figure 17-2 Example of NEC and NOS Abbreviations. (Modified from Buck CJ: *Step by step medical coding,* St Louis, 2006, Saunders.)

[ ]	Brackets enclose synonyms, alternative wording, or explanatory phrases.
( )	Parentheses are used to enclose supplementary words, which may be present or absent in the statement of a disease or procedure. These supplementary words do not usually affect the code number selected, but instead provide further definition or specificity to the code description.
:	Colons are used in the Tabular Index after an incomplete term that needs one or more of the modifiers or adjectives that follow to make it assignable to a given category.
{ }	Braces enclose a series of terms, each of which is modified by the statement appearing to the right of the brace.

Figure 17-3 Example of punctuation usage in ICD-9-CM

when selecting a specific diagnosis code (Figure 17-5). The most common instructional notations include:

INCLUDES: A notation indicating that under a category or other subdivision separate terms can be found that will serve to further define, give examples of, or provide modifying adjectives, and sites or conditions.

☐ or ◯	The lozenge or circle symbol is found to the left of a disease code. The symbol will contain the number 4 or 5 and indicates that use of a fourth or fifth digit is required.
§	The section mark symbol is only used in the Tabular Index of Diseases and precedes a code denoting a footnote on the page.
•	The bullet symbol indicates a new entry.
△	The triangle symbol indicates a revision in the Tabular Index and a code change in the Alphabetic Index.

Figure 17-4 Symbols in the ICD-9-CM.

TUBERCULOSIS (010-018)

INCLUDES Infection by *Mycobacterium turberculosis* (human) (bovine)

EXCLUDES *Congenital tuberculosis (771.2)*
Late effects of tuberculosis (137.0-137.4)

006 Amebiasis

INCLUDES infection due to *Entamoeba histolytica*

EXCLUDES *amebiasis due to organisms other than Entamoeba histolytica (007.8)*

006.0 Acute amebic dysentery without mention of abscess
Acute amebiasis

Figure 17-5 Example of instructional notations. (Modified from Buck CJ: *Step by step medical coding,* St Louis, 2006, Saunders.)

EXCLUDES: Exclusion terms are enclosed within a box and are printed in italics. The excludes notation indicates that there are some code classifications that cannot be used with the code being selected.

NOTES: Notes are used to define terms and give coding instructions. They are often used to list the fifth-digit subclassification(s) for certain categories.

SEE: The SEE instruction follows a main term and indicates that a different term should be referenced.

SEE CATEGORY: This notation is a variation of the SEE instruction.

SEE ALSO: The SEE ALSO instruction is generally found following a main term in the Alphabetic Index and directs the coder to another area with additional index entries that may be useful.

CODE FIRST: This note directs the use of codes that are not normally intended to be used as a principal diagnosis or are not to be sequenced before the underlying disease.

USE ADDITIONAL CODE: This note indicates that a supplemental code should be used in addition to the one being selected. Using an additional code will help to give a more complete picture of the diagnosis.
Related Terms.

AND: The word *and* should be interpreted to mean either *and* or *or.*

WITH: The word *with* in the Alphabetic Index is sequenced immediately following a main term. It provides additional definition or specificity to the code description.

Volume 2—Alphabetic Index

The Alphabetic Index, Volume 2, consists of an alphabetic list of diagnostic terms and related codes; three supplementary sections (the Hypertension Table, Neoplasm Table, and Table of Drugs and Chemicals); and a separate Alphabetic Index for E Codes (Index to External Causes). In most published versions of Volumes 1 and 2, a Summary of the Additions, Deletions, and Revisions to the Tabular Index for the current year is included and is typically found at the end of the main Alphabetic Index. The Alphabetic Index structure includes main terms, subterms and carry-over lines.

- Main terms—appear in bold type
- Subterms—indented two spaces to the right under the main term
- Carryover lines—always indented two additional spaces from the level of the preceding line

A diagnostic statement from the physician may contain many medical terms, but there is typically only one main term that describes the patient's illness or injury. All accompanying words that further describe the main term are called modifiers. Modifiers are found in the Alphabetic Index indented below main terms. There are two types of modifiers: essential and non-essential. An essential modifier is indented under the main term. Essential modifiers affect code selection, and are used in the coding process only if they are specified in the diagnostic statement. A non-essential modifier is shown in parentheses after the term it modifies. These do not affect code selection.

Supplementary Sections of the Alphabetic Index

Three tables and one supplementary index are in the Alphabetic Index, the Hypertension Table, the Neoplasm Table, the Table of Drugs and Chemicals, and the Index to External Causes of Injuries and Poisoning (E codes). These tables and the index are discussed at length later in this chapter.

- Hypertension Table—The Hypertension Table lists types of hypertension and the manifestations and causes. The types of hypertension are further subdivided into three categories: malignant (a clinical course that progresses rapidly to death), benign (does not threaten health status significantly), and unspecified. Unspecified hypertension is used only when there is no documentation in the clinical record that the hypertension is malignant or benign.
- Neoplasm Table—The Neoplasm Table lists neoplasms by anatomic location. The neoplasms are further categorized into categories:

- Malignant Neoplasm—The malignant neoplasm category is broken down into three subclassifications: primary, secondary, and Ca (carcinoma) in situ.
  - Benign Neoplasm—Non-cancerous growth.
  - Unspecified Behavior
  - Uncertain Behavior
- Table of Drugs and Chemicals—This table contains a classification of drugs and other chemical substances to identify poisoning states and external causes of adverse effects.
- Index to External Causes of Injuries and Poisoning (E Codes)—E codes classify environmental events, circumstances, and other conditions as the cause of injury and other adverse effects.

Volume 3—Procedures: Tabular Index and Alphabetic Index

Volume 3 contains a Tabular Index and Alphabetic Index of procedures. Unlike Volumes 1 and 2, it is not used in a physician's office but is primarily used in hospitals and other facilities to code the procedures performed in those settings. The procedure codes are two digits, followed by a decimal and one or two additional digits. The Tabular Index of Volume 3 includes 16 chapters containing codes and descriptions for surgical, diagnostic, and therapeutic procedures performed in a hospital setting. The Alphabetic Index of Volume 3 is an alphabetic listing of the surgical, diagnostic, and therapeutic procedure codes used as a guide to finding a specific code or codes in Volume 3 of the ICD-9-CM.

BEGINNING THE CODING PROCESS

Medical Documentation

The steps for using the ICD-9-CM manual actually begin with interpretation and abstracting of the medical documentation. Information pertinent to code selection is culled from a variety of medical documents. Sources of diagnostic statements can include the following:

- Encounter form, also known as a *superbill, fee slip,* or *charge ticket*
- History and physical report (H&P)
- Discharge summary
- Treatment or progress notes
- Operative report
- Radiology, laboratory, or pathology report

The basic steps in diagnostic coding are to analyze and abstract the diagnosis or assessment documented in the medical record. To *abstract* means to create an outline or summary of information from a text or record. In diagnostic coding, an abstract is created to find all of the diagnostic statements performed during a patient encounter, and ensure nothing has been omitted or added to the encounter form or charge ticket that is not documented in the patient's medical record. When comparing the diagnosis, diagnostic statement, or even signs and symptoms, against any code description, all of the elements of that code must match, with nothing added or missing. These abstracted data are then broken down into main term(s) and any modifying or subterms, as described earlier in this chapter.

Main and Modifying Terms

The Alphabetic Index is organized by main terms—usually the condition, illness, or injury. Subterms, also known as modifying terms as described earlier, are terms that modify or act as adjectives. Subterms are below the main term and indented two spaces. These modifying terms further describe or add additional information or definition needed to narrow the search for an appropriate diagnostic code. Modifying terms affect the selection of appropriate codes; therefore it is important to review the list of modifying terms when selecting a code or code range.

A main term is typically the primary condition, disease, or injury, with any modifying terms providing further specificity, such as the anatomic site or additional manifestations of the condition. For example, in the diagnostic statement "atherosclerotic heart disease," the condition, and thus the main term, is "disease." The modifying term "heart" adds the anatomic location, and "atherosclerotic" adds the type of heart disease. Main terms can also be found by eponym, synonym, or acronym. An eponym describes a disease, condition or injury named after a person, such as Hodgkin's disease. Acronyms are abbreviations of words—for example, the acronym for an upper respiratory infection is URI. Synonyms are words that are similar in meaning and can be used interchangeably. It is important for the medical coder to have reference books on hand, including a medical dictionary that includes abbreviations, to assist in thoroughly understanding the diagnostic statement.

CRITICAL THINKING APPLICATION

Mike is sometimes confused as to which term is the main term and which are modifying terms. What documents can help him determine the main term? Who can he consult within the office to make certain he understands the main term?

Using the Alphabetic Index

Once the diagnostic statement has been abstracted from the medical record, and the main terms identified, the medical coder will begin the search for the best code in Volume 2, the Alphabetic Index, of the ICD-9-CM manual. The Alphabetic Index is a comprehensive, alphabetic listing of all procedures and services contained within the ICD-9-CM manual. The most important thing to remember about the Alphabetic Index is that it should be used only as an aid to finding the section, category, subcategory, or subclassification within the Tabular Index of the ICD-9-CM to evaluate and select the proper code. The Alphabetic Index is not a substitute for the main text, so the medical assistant must never code directly from the Alphabetic Index. Even if only one code is found in the Alphabetic Index, the code can be used only if a thorough review of the conventions and instructional notations in the Tabular Index, Volume 1, do not contraindicate the use of the code.

STEPS IN ICD CODING

Nine basic steps are required for accurate ICD-9-CM coding.

1. Abstract the diagnostic statement or statements from the encounter form and/or the patient's medical record.
2. Determine the main terms in the diagnostic statement describing the patient's condition.
3. Determine what modifying words describe the main term in the diagnostic statement.
4. Locate the main terms taken from the diagnostic statement in the Alphabetic Index of the ICD-9-CM manual.
5. Locate the modifying words listed under the main term in the ICD-9-CM manual.
6. Review any notes or cross-references (e.g., See and See Also) found with the main or modifying terms in the Alphabetic Index.
7. Choose a tentative code or codes found in the Alphabetic Index; and write them on a sheet of paper.
8. Verify the tentative code's accuracy in the Tabular Index. Carry the codes to their highest level of specificity (fourth and fifth digits if they are available).
   a. Review instructional notations
      i. Includes or Excludes statements
      ii. Code First, Code Also, Code Additional statements
      iii. "and", "or," and/or "with" statements
   b. Review conventions and punctuation
   c. Determine if a fourth or fifth digit is required
9. Assign the code selected from the Tabular Index as the appropriate code for the patient's condition. Document the code on the encounter form and/or the medical record.

Diagnostic Coding Decision Tree

A series of questions called a *decision tree* assists in navigating the Alphabetic and Tabular Index while the steps for diagnostic coding are performed. The decision tree for the main text is designed to guide the selection of the appropriate ICD-9-CM diagnostic code (Figure 17-6). Consider the following example for using the decision tree:

The medical documentation narrative describes the following disease: "ruptured abdominal cyst." Begin the search in the Alphabetic Index using the main term "Aneurysm" and the modifying terms "abdominal" and "ruptured." Through use of the decision tree and code selection steps, the code found in the Alphabetic Index should be 441.3.

In the Tabular List, code 441.3 is found in Chapter 7 of the ICD-9-CM, Diseases of the Circulatory System, in Category 441, aortic aneurysm and dissection, and subcategory 441.3. The code description for 441.3 is "aortic aneurysm, ruptured."

Decision Tree Question 1: Does the medical documentation entirely match the code description?

Answer: Yes. If the answer to Question 1 had been no, a new search in the Alphabetic Index using a different or synonymous main term would have been required.

Decision Tree Question 2: Does the code description add anything that is not documented in the medical record?

Examples of Steps in Diagnostic Coding

1. The diagnostic statement is "cholecystitis." There is only one main term: "Cholecystitis." In the Alphabetic Index, the main term "Cholecystitis" has a single code, 575.10. Turning to the Tabular Index, 575.10 states "Cholecystitis, unspecified." The surrounding codes all add information that is not contained in the diagnostic statement—for example: 575.1 does state "Cholecystitis," but a symbol convention to the left of the code contains the number 5, which means a fifth digit must be used for this diagnosis. Code 575.0 states "Acute cholecystitis." The diagnostic statement does not specify acute, therefore 575.0 adds inaccurate information. In the same way, codes 575.11, 575.12 and 575.2 add information that is not contained in the diagnostic statement. The final and most accurate code for the diagnostic statement "Cholecystitis," therefore, is 575.10.

2. Changing the diagnostic statement "cholecystitis" only slightly, by adding "with calculus (cholelithiasis)," changes the Alphabetic Index search, and the code as well. The main term remains "Cholecystitis," although "Cholelithiasis" could also be used as the main term. Choice of either as a main term guides the coder to the same place in the Tabular Index. Using "Cholecystitis" again as a main term guides the coder to 575.10; however, indented below the main term is the subterm "with calculus," followed by "See Cholelithiasis." The code for cholelithiasis is 574.2, but again indented below cholelithiasis is the subterm with cholecystitis and the code 574.1. In the Tabular Index, code 574.2 refers only to the cholelithiasis, code 574.1; however, it is a combination code that includes cholelithiasis with cholecystitis. There is one more step according to the symbol convention to the left of the code, which indicates a fifth digit must be added. At the beginning of the subcategory for cholelithiasis (574) an instructional note provides the fifth digit definitions: 0 means "without mention of obstruction," 1 means "with obstruction." Because the diagnostic statement did not mention an obstruction, the most specific and accurate code to choose from the Tabular Index is 574.11.

Answer: No. Had the answer to this question been yes, more evaluation would have been required—either returning to the Alphabetic Index to search further, or proceeding through the next questions to evaluate the instructional notations, punctuation, and other conventions in the Tabular Index.

Decision Tree Question 3: Read all the instructional notations for the section (chapter), category, subcategory, and, if necessary, subclassification. Are there any "includes," "excludes," "code first," or "code also" instructions?

Answer: In this case there are no instructional notations that affect the selection of code 441.3 for the diagnostic statement. If the answer had been yes, the medical assistant would have followed the instructions in the notes. Since the answer was no, the assistant would proceed to the next question.

Decision Tree Question 4: Evaluate the conventions and symbols. Is a fourth and/or fifth digit required?

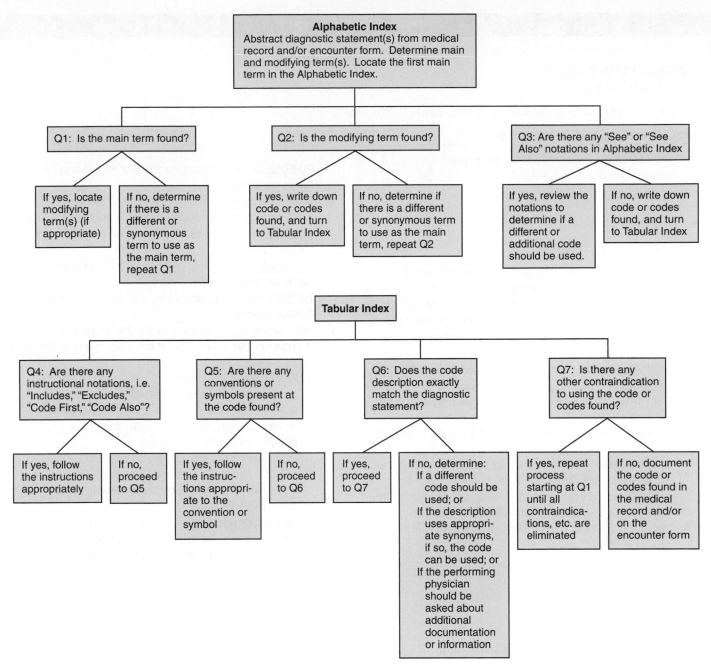

Figure 17-6 Decision Tree for ICD-9-CM Diagnostic Coding

Answer: No. In this case, 441.3 already has a fourth digit and there is no symbol showing a fifth digit is required. If the answer had been yes, the medical assistant should determine which additional digit is appropriate. Since the answer was no, proceed to next question.

Based on the answers to these questions, code 441.3 is the most accurate and specific code to use with the diagnostic statement *"ruptured abdominal aneurysm."* At this point, the diagnosis code should be documented on the encounter form and on the medical record next to the diagnostic statement.

Abstracting the diagnosis from the patient medical record or encounter form is only the first step in the coding decision

process. Procedure 17-1 describes the steps for using the Alphabetic and Tabular Index of the ICD-9-CM to guide the medical assistant in the selection of the most specific and accurate diagnosis code or codes.

CRITICAL THINKING APPLICATION

Mike is working with a medical record that contains the terms "cholelithiasis" and "acute cholecystitis with calculus." How will the coding steps and decision tree questions affect or change the selection of a diagnosis code?

PROCEDURE 17-1

Perform ICD-9 Coding

CAAHEP COMPETENCY: 3.a.(3)(d)
ABHES COMPETENCY: 3.v.

GOAL: *To perform accurate diagnosis coding using the ICD-9-CM manual*

EQUIPMENT and SUPPLIES

- ICD-9-CM manual, Volumes 1 and 2, current year
- Encounter form or charge ticket
- Medical record
- Paper
- Pen or pencil

PROCEDURAL STEPS

1. Abstract the diagnostic statement or statements from the encounter form and/or the patient's medical record.
   PURPOSE: To ensure all parts of the diagnostic statement are included on the encounter form, with nothing missing or added.

2. Determine the main terms in the diagnostic statement describing the patient's condition.
   PURPOSE: To provide a starting point for performing a search in the Alphabetic Index.

3. Determine what modifying words exist of the main term in the diagnostic statement.
   PURPOSE: To ensure further specificity of the codes found in the Alphabetic Index.

4. Locate the main terms taken from the diagnostic statement in the Alphabetic Index of the ICD-9-CM manual.
   PURPOSE: To find the code or codes which will be reviewed for accuracy and specificity in the Tabular Index.

5. Locate the modifying words listed under the main term in the ICD-9-CM manual.

PURPOSE: To ensure further specificity of the codes found in the Alphabetic Index.

6. Review any notes or cross-references (e.g., See and See Also) found with the main or modifying terms in the Alphabetic Index.
   PURPOSE: To ensure there are no additional searches needed in the Alphabetic Index.

7. Choose a tentative code or codes found in the Alphabetic Index; and write them on a sheet of paper.
   PURPOSE: To prevent backtracking and repeated searches in the Alphabetic Index.

8. Verify the tentative code's accuracy in the Tabular Index. Carry the codes to their highest level of specificity (fourth or fifth digits if they are available).
   a. Review Instructional Notes:
      i. Includes or Excludes statements
      ii. Code First, Code Also, Code Additional statements
      iii. Review "and," "or," and/or "with" statements
   b. Review conventions and punctuation.
   c. Determine if a fourth or fifth digit is required.
   PURPOSE: To ensure the most accurate and specific code is selected, and that there is no contraindication to use of the code or codes selected.

9. Assign the code selected from the Tabular Index as the appropriate code for the patient's condition. Document the code on the encounter form and/or the medical record.

SPECIAL CODING INSTRUCTIONS

Remember that all ICD-9-CM coding manuals, regardless of the publisher, will contain comprehensive instructional notes and conventions to aid the coder in selection of the most accurate diagnostic code or codes. When any discrepancy occurs between reference sources, including this text, the current year's ICD-9-CM coding manual is the final authority. This fact cannot be overemphasized. The medical assistant must always thoroughly review and refer to the conventions, instructional notations, code definitions, and other guidelines in the Tabular Index when coding. The following instructions are designed to provide some additional guidance in selecting diagnosis codes from various chapters within the ICD-9-CM; however, they are not to be considered a replacement for the ICD-9-CM manual, nor do they provide all the coding information, definitions, or explanations found in the manual. The steps for diagnosis coding found in Procedure 17-1 are the same for all chapters of the ICD-9-CM, but there are special rules and considerations for some chapters that must be considered during the coding selection process.

Signs and Symptoms

Signs and symptoms are coded only when the physician has not yet reached a determination of the final diagnosis. If the physician's notes contain terminology such as *"rule out"* or *"suspected,"* for example, the medical coder should use the patient's documented signs and symptoms, including subjective and objective findings. Subjective findings include the patient's chief complaint (CC) or statements regarding why the patient is seeing the physician. Objective findings are any measurable indicators found during the physical examination. Ill-defined conditions, signs, and symptoms are found in the ICD-9-CM manual in Chapter 16, of Volume 1, the Tabular Index. See Figure 17-7 for an illustration of Chapter 16's Signs and Symptoms Section.

- Use only if there is no final or determining diagnosis
- Use if "rule out" or "suspected" are included in the assessment or diagnostic statement.
- Signs and symptoms can be subjective and/or objective findings
  - Subjective: Chief complaint (CC) or patient's verbal statements
  - Objective: Any measurable indicators found during the physical examination
- Signs and Symptoms are found in Chapter 16, Ill-Defined Conditions, Signs and Symptoms, Volume 1 of the ICD-9-CM.

Figure 17-7 Rules for Coding Signs and Symptoms.

Suspected Conditions

When a diagnosis is stated as "questionable, probable, likely, or rule out," code the documented symptoms, signs, or chief complaint(s) of the patient. Do not code the suspected condition if there is no final assessment or diagnosis. If a patient is asymptomatic or has a family or personal history of a condition, a screening code from the Supplementary Classification of V Codes should be used.

Multiple Coding

Some single conditions require the use of more than one code. "Use additional code" means to use another code in conjunction with one selected; and "Code first" means that if more than one code is used, the code with the notation "Code first" should be the first or **primary diagnosis.** Multiple codes may be needed for late effects, complication codes, and obstetric codes, to more fully describe a condition. Always review the ICD-9-CM manual guidelines, instructional notes, and conventions to determine when it is appropriate to use multiple codes. A patient who is diagnosed with diabetic retinopathy with type I diabetes would require multiple codes. The first code, 362.01, represents the diabetic retinopathy, while 250.51 represents diabetes with ophthalmic manifestations. The subclassification of 1 designates Type I diabetes. Figure 17-8 shows an example of multiple coding.

Combination Codes

A combination code is used to fully identify when two diagnoses or a diagnosis with a secondary process (manifestation) or complication is included in the description of a single code number. Combination codes are identified by referring to the subterms in the Alphabetic Index (Volume 2) or the "inclusion" and "exclusion" terms in the Tabular Index (Volume 1). An example of a combination code from the ICD-9-CM is shown in Figure 17-9.

Late Effects

A late effect is a residual problem remaining after the acute phase of an illness or injury has terminated. There is no time limit on when a late effect code can be used. Coding of late effects generally requires two codes; the condition or nature of the late effect, such as hemiplegia, is coded first, and the code designating that the condition or nature is a late effect is coded second. A late effect will sometimes be described in the medical

---

Multiple Coding

Diagnosis: Diabetic retinopathy with type I diabetes

(Note: Retinopathy is the manifestation and diabetes is the etiology, or cause, of the retinopathy or retinal hemorrhage.)

Diagnosis: Index: **Retinopathy,** diabetic 250.5 [362.01]

The Index subterm "diabetic" identifies the code for the etiology as 250.5 and directs you to the code for the manifestation of [362.01] retinopathy. The italicized code is never sequenced first as the principal diagnosis but is used to identify a manifestation.

Tabular: **250 Diabetes mellitus**
              250.5 Diabetes with ophthalmic manifestations
                       Use additional code to identify manifestation
              250.51 Type I, not stated as uncontrolled

Note that the diagnosis of diabetes mellitus will always be reported with a five-digit code because the fifth digit indicates the type of diabetes. See the fifth-digit codes listed after code 250 in the Tabular Index of your ICD-9-CM.

  Code 250.51 is the correct code to describe the diabetes (etiology). The statement "Use additional code to identify manifestation…" directs you to assign a code that identifies the manifestation (retinopathy).

Tabular: **362. Other retinal disorders**

              362.0 Diabetic retinopathy
                       Code first diabetes (250.5)
              362.01 Background diabetic retinopathy

Note that the *"Code first diabetes"* directs you to the etiology code.

  Code: 250.51, 362.01 Diabetic retinopathy with type I diabetes.

The multiple codes fully describe the diagnostic statement. The guideline directs you to place the etiology code first, followed by the manifestation code.

Figure 17-8 Example of Multiple Coding. (Modified from Buck CJ: *Step by step medical coding,* St Louis, 2006, Saunders.)

---

documentation as old, residual, a sequela, or some other phrase that indicates the passage of time since the onset of the original condition. Be sure to distinguish between a late effect and a historical statement in a diagnosis. Whenever the statement uses the term "effects of old…," "sequela of…," or "residuals of…," then code as a late effect. If the diagnosis is expressed in terms of "history of…," then code using V codes to indicate a personal history of an illness or injury.

Impending or Threatened Conditions

When a condition is stated as "impending" or "threatened," it is coded only if there is a code specifically describing the condition in this way.

Combination Codes

Diagnosis: Acute cholecystitis with cholelithiasis

Index: **Cholecystitis** with calculus (stone in the gallbladder) directs you to *See* Cholelithiasis

Index: **Cholelithiasis** with, cholecystitis, acute 574.0

Tabular: **574 Cholelithiasis**

574.0 Calculus of gallbladder with acute cholecystis

A fifth-digit subclassification is indicated as 0 for a case without mention of obstruction and as 1 when there is obstruction; since there was no mention of obstruction, use the fifth digit 0.

Code: 574.00 Acute cholecystitis with cholelithiasis

The single code 574.00 fully describes the diagnosis of acute cholecystitis with cholelithiasis

Figure 17-9 Example of Combination Codes. (Modified from Buck CJ: *Step by step medical coding*, St Louis, 2006, Saunders.)

Infectious and Parasitic Diseases

Most often, multiple codes will be needed for coding infectious or parasitic diseases. The first code will identify the disease or condition, such as bacterial infection, and the second code will identify the organism causing the disease—for example, streptococcal bacteria. The basic coding principles regarding the use of either combination or multiple codes will apply throughout this section of the ICD-9-CM.

Coding Organism-Caused Diseases

Two categories for identifying the organism that is causing disease are found in other sections or categories. These codes, 041 and 079, may be used as either additional codes or as solo codes depending on the diagnostic statement. For example, for a urinary tract infection (UTI) caused by *Escherichia coli*, the UTI is coded first (599.0) and the *E. coli* is coded second (041.4).

Human Immunodeficiency Disease and Acquired Immune Deficiency Syndrome

It is essential first to understand the descriptions of the codes available. For coding, the key is whether or not the patient has symptoms.

- Human immunodeficiency virus (HIV)—This indicates only that the virus is present.
- Acquired immunodeficiency syndrome (AIDS)—A syndrome is defined as a "group of symptoms occurring together." AIDS is the manifestation(s) and/or symptoms that can occur as a result of having HIV.

Never code a patient as having HIV unless it is clearly documented as confirmed. Probable and suspected cases are never coded; instead, the signs and symptoms present should be coded. The code for a confirmed diagnosis of HIV is 042. The codes for illnesses and symptoms associated with Acquired Immune Deficiency Syndrome are primarily found in Chapter 3

Rules for Coding Impending or Threatened Conditions

1. If it did occur, code as a confirmed diagnosis.
2. If it did not occur, reference the Alphabetic Index to determine if the condition has a subentry term for "impending" or "threatened," and also reference main term entries for "impending" and for "threatened."
3. If the subterm "threatened" or "impending" is found, assign the given code.
4. If the subterm "threatened" or "impending" is not found, code the existing underlying condition(s), signs, or symptoms, and not the condition described as "threatened" or "impending."

of the ICD-9-CM manual. Remember that stringent restrictions are placed on the disclosure of medical information regarding patients with HIV infection and/or AIDS. Make certain that the patient has signed the appropriate release of medical information form before any disclosures are made to third parties.

Complications of Care

A complication of medical or surgical care generally results in additional procedures or services being ordered for a patient, but often the complication is not mentioned as part of the diagnostic statement, which results in reduced reimbursement. It is important to review the medical documentation to determine if a complication exists, and to code the complication in addition to the diagnostic statement.

- Postoperative complications that affect a specific anatomic site or body system are classified according to the appropriate ICD-9-CM chapter (1 through 16) of the Tabular Index.
- Postoperative complications that affect more than one anatomic site or body system are classified according to ICD-9-CM, Volume 1, Tabular Index, Chapter 17, Injury and Poisoning.
- If the Alphabetic Index does not provide a specific main term and/or subterm to identify a postoperative complication, classify the complication to categories 996 through 999, Complications of Surgical and Medical Care, Not Elsewhere Classified.

Etiology and Manifestation

Etiology refers to the underlying cause or origin of a disease. **Manifestation** describes the signs and symptoms of the disease. In the Alphabetic Index, the etiology and manifestation codes are listed together. The etiology code is listed first, with the manifestation listed beside it in italicized brackets. These italicized codes are always listed secondary to the etiology code.

Neoplasms

Neoplasm, or new growth, is coded by the site or location of the neoplasm and its behavior. The Table of Neoplasms (Figure 17-10) is located in the ICD-9-CM, Volume 2, or Alphabetic Index under the main term "Neoplasms." This table gives the

	Malignant					
	Primary	Secondary	Ca in situ	Benign	Uncertain Behavior	Unspecified
Neoplasm (continued)						
bone (periosteum)	170.9	198.5	—	213.9	238.0	239.2

Note—Carcinomas and adenocarcinomas, of any type other than intraosseous or odontogenic, of the sites listed under

"Neoplasm, bone," should be considered as constituting metastatic spread from an unspecified primary site and coded

to 198.5 for morbidity coding and to 199.1 for underlying cause of death coding.

acetabulum	170.6	198.5	—	213.6	238.0	239.2
acromion (process)	170.4	198.5	—	213.4	238.0	239.2
ankle	170.8	198.5	—	213.8	238.0	239.2
arm NEC	170.4	198.5	—	213.4	238.0	239.2
astragalus	170.8	198.5	—	213.8	238.0	239.2
atlas	170.2	198.5	—	213.2	238.0	239.2
axis	170.2	198.5	—	213.2	238.0	239.2
back NEC	170.2	198.5	—	213.2	238.0	239.2
calcaneus	170.8	198.5	—	213.8	238.0	239.2

Figure 17-10 Neoplasm Table. (Modified from Diamond MS: *Mastering medical coding*, St Louis, 2006, Saunders.)

code numbers for neoplasms by anatomic site in alphabetic order. Six possible code numbers exist for each anatomic site, depending upon whether the neoplasm is malignant or benign, exhibits uncertain behavior, or is of an unspecified nature. Malignant neoplasms are separated into three separate subclassifications: primary, secondary, and in situ.

Malignant Neoplasm Site and Behavior Definitions
- Primary: Identifies the originating anatomic site of the neoplasm. A primary malignancy is defined as the original site(s) of the cancer.
- Secondary: Identifies sites to which the primary neoplasm has metastasized (spread). A secondary malignancy defines a second location to which the cancer has spread from the primary location.
- In situ: Carcinoma in situ is defined as the absence of invasion of surrounding tissues. Tumor cells are undergoing malignant changes but are still confined to the point of origin without invasion of surrounding normal tissue. The In Situ column is used only if the physician uses that precise terminology.

Benign, Uncertain Behavior, and Unspecified Nature
- Benign: The growth is non-cancerous, nonmalignant, and does not invade adjacent structures or spread to distant sites.
- Of Uncertain Behavior: The pathologist is unable to determine whether the neoplasm is benign or malignant.

- Unspecified Nature: Neither the behavior nor the histologic type of neoplasm is specified in the diagnostic statement.

The ICD-9-CM instructional notes state that the behavior of the neoplasm should be determined first when coding. Most coding decisions for malignant neoplasms are between primary and secondary; in situ is used only when the diagnostic statement contains that exact phrase. Unspecified is used only when no pathology study has been done and the neoplasm is still described with a term such as *tumor* or *growth*. Uncertain is used only when the neoplasm's behavior is not malignant, the tumor is not in situ, or the behavior is unpredictable. Note that there is also a code beginning with M that is called the *morphology code*. The morphology code is not typically used by physicians or providers when coding diagnoses.

Five Steps for Coding Neoplasms
When coding for neoplasms, the additional steps shown below will assist in determining the most specific and accurate neoplasm diagnostic code. These should be considered in addition to the basic diagnostic steps.
1. Using the Neoplasm Table in the Alphabetic Index, determine the site (anatomic location) of the neoplasm, and select the row in the Neoplasm Table in which it appears.
2. Determine the neoplasm behavior, and select the Neoplasm Table column that best defines the behavior: Malignant, Benign, Of Uncertain Behavior, or Of Unspecified Nature.

3. If the neoplasm is malignant, determine whether the malignancy is primary, secondary, or in situ.
4. Link the appropriate Neoplasm Table column to the appropriate row to find the code.
5. Check the code in the Tabular Index to ensure the code complies with the guidelines, conventions, and instructional notations in the Tabular Index.

The ICD-9-CM manual also always provides additional information, definitions, and guidelines for coding neoplasms, just as it does for all other diseases, illnesses, and injuries.

Circulatory System

Physicians use a large variety of terms and phrases to identify components of the circulatory system. To accurately code disorders of the circulatory system, the coder must carefully review all inclusions, exclusions, conventions, guidelines, and instructional notations associated with each potential code selected. The major sections concerning the circulatory system are as follows:

Acute Rheumatic Fever	Category 390 to 392
Chronic Rheumatic Heart Disease	Category 393 to 398
Hypertensive Disease	Category 415 to 417
Ischemic Heart Disease	Category 410 to 414
Diseases of Pulmonary Circulation	Category 415 to 417
Other Forms of Heart Disease	Category 420 to 429
Cerebrovascular Disease	Category 430 to 438
Diseases of Arteries and Lesser Vessels	Category 440 to 448
Diseases of Veins and Lymphatics	Category 451 to 459

Ischemic Heart Disease

Ischemic heart disease is usually caused by a lesion on one of the coronary arteries that causes a lack of blood flow to the heart. The most common cause of heart disease is atherosclerosis, which is one type of arteriosclerosis. Both atherosclerosis and arteriosclerosis are coded to category 440, with the exception of certain specified arteries including, but not limited to, coronary, carotid, cerebral, pulmonary, and vertebral; coronary atherosclerosis, for example, is found at category 414.0.

Myocardial Infarction

A myocardial infarction (MI) is coded as acute if it is documented as such in the diagnostic statement or has a stated duration of 8 weeks or less. The MI is considered chronic if it is so stated in the diagnostic statement or if symptoms still are present after 8 weeks. If an MI is specified as "old" or "healed" without any current or presenting symptoms, it should be coded using category 412.

History of an MI uses code 412, which describes an "Old Myocardial Infarct." This code is used only if the patient has no symptoms and only if the old MI was diagnosed via an electrocardiogram. When the patient is symptomatic, code the underlying condition or symptoms only if the underlying condition is not known. Acute MIs are coded to category 410 for the first 8 weeks. If symptoms persist beyond 8 weeks, the chronic MI category code is used.

Arteriosclerotic Cardiovascular Disease

Arteriosclerotic cardiovascular disease (ASCVD) is classified to subcategory 429.2, with an additional code added to identify whether or not arteriosclerosis is present. For example, the diagnostic statement "generalized arteriosclerotic cardiovascular disease" should be coded using 429.2 followed by 440.9, "generalized and unspecified atherosclerosis."

Cerebrovascular Accident

The terms *stroke* and *cerebrovascular accident* (CVA) are often used interchangeably to refer to a cerebral infarction. When the patient is initially treated for CVA or stroke, use the code for the underlying condition that caused the stroke, and an additional code for any condition or deficit it caused if that condition or deficit is still present at discharge. These conditions or deficits may eventually resolve; sometimes they do not. When they persist they are considered residuals of the CVA. For coding purposes, this means there is now a late effect to take into consideration.

Hypertensive Disease

A distinction is made in the ICD-9-CM coding system between "elevated" and "high" blood pressure. High blood pressure is defined as hypertension. If a diagnostic statement does not contain the word *hypertension* or the phrase *high blood pressure*, it is coded as elevated blood pressure, not hypertension.

The Alphabetic Index contains a Hypertension Table (Figure 17-11) under the main term "Hypertension." Within the table are subterms that identify different types of hypertension and any complications caused by the hypertension. Hypertension is classified three ways: malignant, benign, and unspecified. Malignant hypertension is usually considered acute and life-threatening; benign hypertension, although considered dangerous, is not. Unless the diagnostic statement specifically states malignant or benign hypertension, hypertension should be classified as unspecified.

Hypertension is frequently the cause of various forms of heart and vascular disease; however, the mention of hypertension in the diagnostic statement does not mean that a combination code for hypertensive heart disease should be used. If there is a cause-and-effect relationship between the hypertension and the heart disease it should be clearly documented in the clinical record or diagnostic statement.

Coding for Complications of Pregnancy, Childbirth, and the Puerperium

Coding for the obstetric patient is like using a specialty codebook within the main codebook. This is challenging for those who do not code obstetrics often. Some important terminology regarding pregnancy includes the following: *antepartum* = pregnancy (as soon as there is a positive pregnancy test); *childbirth* = delivery; and *postpartum* = puerperium (6 weeks after delivery).

Obstetric Coding Guidelines

To begin searching for obstetric codes, start at either of the main terms "Pregnancy" or "Delivery." Look for a subterm regarding the condition, or start at the main term for the condition and

	Malignant	Benign	Unspecified
Hypertension, hypertensive (arterial) (arteriolar) (disease) (essential) (fluctuating) (idiopathic) (intermittent) (labile) (low rennin) (orthostatic) (paroxysmal) (primary) (systemic) (uncontrolled) (vascular)	401.0	401.1	401.9
with			
heart involvement (conditions classifiable to 428, 429.0-429.3, 429.8, 429.9 due to hypertension) (*see also* Hypertension, heart)	402.00	402.10	401.90
with kidney involvement – *see* Hypertension, cardiorenal			
renal involvement (only conditions classifiable to 585, 586, 587) (excludes conditions classifiable as 584) (*see also* Hypertension, kidney)	403.00	403.10	403.90
with heart involvement – *see* Hypertension, cardiorenal			
failure (and sclerosis) (*see also* Hypertension, kidney)	403.01	403.11	403.91
sclerosis without failure (*see also* Hypertension, kidney)	403.00	403.10	403.90
accelerated (*see also* Hypertension, by type, malignant)	401.0	—	—
antepartum – *see* Hypertension, complicating pregnancy, childbirth, or the puerperium			

Figure 17-11 Hypertension Table. (Modified from Diamond MS: *Mastering medical coding,* St Louis, 2006, Saunders.)

Benign, Malignant, and Unspecified Hypertension

- **Malignant** hypertension - acute and life-threatening;
- **Benign** hypertension - dangerous, but not life threatening
- **Unspecified** hypertension—use only if the diagnostic statement does not specify malignant or benign.

Use of Category 650 and V-Codes in Pregnancy Coding

- Use codes from Volume 1, Tabular Index, Chapter 11, of the ICD-9-CM in the range of 630 to 677. If the pregnancy is documented as a normal pregnancy or is unrelated to the reason for the physician encounter, use a V code, V22.2, in place of any Chapter 11 code.
- Chapter 11 codes are to be used only on the maternal record, not on the newborn record.
- Categories 640 to 648 and 651 to 676 require a fifth digit. These fifth digits indicate whether the encounter is antepartum or postpartum, or whether the delivery occurred.

look for a subterm that states "affecting pregnancy" or "during pregnancy." Normal, uncomplicated prenatal and postpartum care for the mother as well as routine visits for the baby are coded with V codes as long as there is no current problem. Some mothers have conditions that put them at high risk; these situations are also coded with V codes unless a problem manifests itself during the pregnancy.

Normal, uncomplicated delivery for the mother is coded using category 650. A normal, uncomplicated delivery is described as one in which no problem or complication occurred during the entire encounter and no procedures were performed other than those deemed "normal." The normal, uncomplicated procedures are episiotomy, amniotomy, administration of analgesia, fetal monitoring, and sterilization. The use of forceps or suction-assisted delivery is not considered normal for the purposes of ICD-9-CM coding.

Normal routine obstetric care does not use fifth digits; fifth digits are used only for obstetric patients with complications. The fifth digits divide the pregnancy into three different "time zones": before delivery (antepartum), delivery (the episode of care when the delivery occurs), and after delivery (postpartum). In addition, the delivery "time zone" is divided into two subclassifications. The fifth digit 1 describes delivery (birth) without postpartum complication; and the fifth digit 2 describes a delivery (birth) with postpartum complication(s).

If the baby has a problem while the mother is still pregnant, code it only if there is an impact on the mother's condition or management. Code the baby's problem on the mother's chart only if it creates a medical concern or a medical need for the mother to undergo testing or treatment. When it is appropriate to code a fetal condition that affects the mother's management, use codes for pregnant patients, not codes for babies.

Cesarean Delivery

Cesarean codes only define the reasons why a cesarean delivery was performed; they do not describe cesarean deliveries as separate from vaginal births. A cesarean delivery is considered the treatment for a problem or condition that exists at the time of delivery.

Outcome of Delivery and Liveborn Infant Codes

Other sets of V codes that must be discussed are the Outcome of Delivery codes and Liveborn Infant codes. The Outcome of Delivery codes (V27) are reported on the mother's health record after the delivery; the Liveborn infant code(s) (V30-V39) describe the condition of the baby at delivery (e.g., live or stillborn), and are reported on the newborn record.

Late Effects of Complication of Pregnancy

The Late Effect of Complication of Pregnancy code can be used any time after the 6-week postpartum period. Use this code following the code to represent the current problem to indicate that it is a residual effect of pregnancy complications.

Abortions

All of the codes for abortion require a fifth digit to indicate whether or not the abortion was complete before the admission. Remember that the term *abortion* applies to the termination of a pregnancy before 22 weeks, regardless of whether it was spontaneous or induced.

Newborn Coding

Babies are considered newborn or perinatal for the first 28 days. The codes used for these patients range from 760 to 779 in Volume 1, Tabular Index, Chapter 15 of the ICD-9-CM manual. After the twenty-eighth day of life, do not use codes that are specific to perinatal patients. Newborn codes are found in Chapter 15 of the ICD-9-CM. Codes from Chapter 15 should never be used on the maternal record. If a newborn is healthy, a code from the V code category 30 should be used in addition to any Chapter 15 code.

Liveborn Infant Category

The only time to use a fifth digit from the Liveborn Infant category is when the fourth digit of 0 is assigned. The fourth digit of 0 means that the baby was born in the hospital; the fifth digit then specifies whether the birth was cesarean. The other fourth digits, 1 and 2, represent births that occurred outside of the hospital. It is assumed no cesarean is performed outside of the hospital, and so no fifth digit is provided.

Injury

Injuries constitute a major section of ICD-9-CM. Injuries are classified first according to the type of injury, then by anatomic site. When coding injuries, separate codes should be assigned for each individual injury unless a combination code is provided. In cases in which a patient has multiple injuries, the most severe injury should be coded first. Superficial injuries such as abrasions or contusions are not coded when associated with more severe injuries of the same site. If an injury results in minor or major damage to peripheral nerves or blood vessels, the injury is coded first, with additional codes from categories 950 to 957, Injury to Nerves and Spinal Cord, and/or 900 to 904, Injury to Blood Vessels.

Coding Fractures

Fractures are coded first by anatomic site, then by type of fracture. The code category range for fractures is 800 to 829, in Volume 1, Tabular Index, Chapter 17, Injury and Poisoning. Fractures can be classified as either "open" or "closed." A fracture is said to be "open" when the skin has been broken and the bone protrudes outside the skin surface or when a wound, such as a puncture, enables the bone to be seen. In a "closed" fracture the bone does not have contact with the outside of the body. At any time if there is no indication as to whether the fracture is open or closed, it should be coded as if it were closed.

Burns

The same principles for combination and multiple coding apply here; code each burn separately unless specific combination codes are given in Volume 1, the Tabular Index. There are many combination codes. Because burns are coded by site and degree and by extent of body surface involvement, all burn cases should have at least two codes, and a third if they are infected. Other types of wounds, lacerations, punctures, and so on, use a different fifth digit to show that they are infected and therefore complicated. Burn codes use their fifth digits for other information, so an additional code is necessary to indicate infection.

Steps for Coding Burns

- Code the burn to the site by degree. Under the main term "Burn" find the subterm for the site, then the subterm for the degree. If the burn is stated to be at the same site but of a different degree, code to the highest degree. Omit the code for the lower level burn at the same site.
- Determine the percentage of body burned, using category 948 in the Tabular Index, Chapter 17, Injury and Poisoning. The fourth digit describes the total burned surface; the fifth digit describes the percent of only third-degree burns—for example, 50% of total body surface burned with 15% third-degree burns.
- If the burn is said to be infected, use code 958.3 as a third code to identify the infection.

E Codes

To describe the circumstances of an accident or injury, the ICD-9-CM manual provides E codes, which are listed in a separate Tabular Index and Alphabetic Index (Figure 17-12). E codes describe the following:

- Nature of an event (fire, fall, collision, abuse, etc.)
- Place of occurrence
- Late effect of an injury

Lund-Browder Chart for Determining Burn Percentages in Children

	0 yr	1 yr	5 yr	10 yr	15 yr
a—1/2 of head	$9^1/_2$	$8^1/_2$	$6^1/_2$	$5^1/_2$	$4^1/_2$
b—1/2 of 1 thigh	$2^3/_4$	$3^1/_4$	4	$4^1/_4$	$4^1/_4$
c—1/2 of lower leg	$2^1/_2$	$2^1/_2$	$2^3/_4$	3	$3^1/_4$

E CODE INDEX

Railway Accidents	E800-E807
Motor Vehicle Traffic Accidents	E810-E819
Motor Vehicle Nontraffic Accidents	E820-E825
Other Road Vehicle Accidents	E826-E829
Water Transport Accidents	E830-E838
Air and Space Accidents	E840-E845
Vehicle Accidents Not Classified Elsewhere	E846-E848
Place of Occurrence	E849
Accidental Poisoning by Drugs, Medicinal Substances, Biologicals	E850-E858
Accidental Poisoning by Other Solid and Liquid Substances, Gases, Vapors	E860-E869
Misadventure to Patients During Surgical/Medical Care	E870-E876
Surgical/Medical Procedures Cause of Abnormal Reaction of Patient or Later Complication, Without Mention of Misadventure at Time of Procedure	E878-E879
Accidental Falls	E880-E888
Accidents by Fire and Flames	E890-E898
Accidents Due to Natural/Environmental Factors	E900-E909
Accidents Caused by Submersion, Suffocation and Foreign Bodies	E910-E915
Other Accidents	E916-E928
Late Effects of Accidental Injury	E929
Drugs, Medicinal and Biological Substances Causing Adverse Effects in Therapeutic Use	E930-E949
Suicide and Self-Inflicted Injury	E950-E959
Homicide and Injury Purposely Inflicted by Other Persons	E960-E969
Legal Intervention	E970-E978
Injury Undetermined Whether Accidentally or Purposely Inflicted	E980-E989
Injury Resulting from Operations of War	E990-E999

Figure 17-12 Example of E Codes. (Modified from Diamond MS: *Mastering medical coding,* St Louis, 2006, Saunders.)

- Intent (self-inflicted, assault, accident, etc.)
- Drugs and chemicals that caused the injury or disease

E codes are never principal or listed first, because they are only supplementary information. They are most often used with injury codes but may be used with any condition that is the result of an external cause, such as a respiratory problem caused by smoke inhalation. The E code describing the initial incident is only used once, the first time the patient is treated for the condition. Some major categories of E codes include the following:

- Transport accidents
- Poisoning and adverse effects of drugs, medicinal substances, and biologicals
- Accidents and falls
- Accidents caused by fire and flames
- Accidents caused by natural and environmental factors
- Late effects of accidents, assaults, or self-injury
- Assaults or purposely inflicted injury
- Suicide or self-inflicted injury

It is correct to use as many E codes as necessary to describe all of the information provided by the record. It is acceptable to use non-physician documentation to support these codes, if they do not conflict with the physician documentation.

Table of Drugs and Chemicals

The Table of Drugs and Chemicals contains a classification of drugs and other chemicals. It is used to identify poisoning states and external causes of adverse effects. Each of the substances is assigned a code which is used based on the type of poisoning—for example, overdose, wrong substance given or taken, or intoxication. The table also contains a listing of external causes of adverse effects caused by the ingestion or exposure to a drug or chemical. The poisoning codes in the first column of the Table of Drugs and Chemicals should be determined and coded first, followed by the external cause (E-Code). There are five E-code headings in the Table of Drugs and Chemicals: accidental poisoning, therapeutic use, suicide attempt, assault, and undetermined cause.

E Codes Used with the Table of Drugs and Chemicals

An E code to identify a drug or chemical may be added to clarify the patient's circumstance whenever a drug or chemical is identified in the medical record as a causative substance. In addition to the E codes that identify the causative substances, the table includes a column for poisoning associated with each substance. These codes can be used with an E code from the other columns with one exception: a Poisoning code cannot be used with a Therapeutic Use code. Problems caused by correct substances properly used are considered "adverse effects," not poisoning.

V Codes: Classification of Factors Influencing Health Status and Contact with Health Service

V codes are used to describe circumstances or encounters with a physician or healthcare provider when no current illness or injury exists. V codes may stand alone or may be principal or secondary. Some codes have notation that they cannot be principal or stand-alone.

V Code Index for History Codes

Under the main term "History" in the Alphabetic Index, the subterm "personal" follows the main term. This means that

---

External Cause Codes (E-Codes) Used with Table of Drugs and Chemicals

- Accidental Poisoning (E850-E869). Accidental overdose of drug, wrong substance given or taken, taken inadvertently, accidents in the usage of drugs in medical and surgical procedures, and to show external causes of poisonings coded using Volume 1, Tabular Index, Chapter 17, Injury and Poisoning, category codes 980-989.
- Therapeutic Use (E930-E949). A correct substance properly administered in the proper dosage caused an adverse effect.
- Suicide attempt (E962). Self-inflicted injury or poisoning.
- Assault (E961-E962). Injury or poisoning inflicted by another person with the intent to injure or kill.
- Undetermined (E980-E982). To be used only when either accidental or intentional circumstances can not be determined.

Use of Fourth and Fifth Digit with Diabetes Mellitus

Fourth Digit Subcategories for Diabetes Mellitus
- 250.0 Diabetes mellitus without mention of complication
- 250.1 Diabetes mellitus with ketoacidosis (defined as a life-threatening condition in which ketones, which result from the breakdown of fat for energy, accumulate in the blood stream and the pH of the blood decreases)
- 250.2 Diabetes with hyperosmolarity (defined as a concentration of the body fluids that is abnormally increased)
- 250.3 Diabetes with other coma
- 250.4 Diabetes with renal manifestations
- 250.5 Diabetes with ophthalmic manifestations
- 250.6 Diabetes with neurological manifestations.
- 250.7 Diabetes with peripheral circulatory disorders
- 250.8 Diabetes with other specified manifestations
- 250.9 Diabetes with unspecified complication

Fifth Digit Subclassifications for Diabetes Mellitus
- 250.x0 = type II Adult onset (even if using insulin). Unspecified. Not stated as uncontrolled.
- 250.x1 = type I Juvenile type not stated as uncontrolled.
- 250.x2 = type II Adult onset (even if using insulin). Unspecified as to whether it is uncontrolled.
- 250.x3 = type I Juvenile type, uncontrolled.

---

the subterms are considered the patient's personal history. The subterm "family" indented two spaces under the "History" main term describes family history rather than personal history. Watch the subterm indentations closely to ensure that the code selected is for the proper history code.

Diabetes Mellitus

Diabetes mellitus codes always require use of a fourth and a fifth digit. The fourth digit describes any manifestations of the diabetes that may be present; and the fifth digit describes the type of diabetes. The fourth digit subcategories in Volume 1, Tabular Index, Chapter 3, Blood and Blood-Forming Organs, category 250, diabetes mellitus are divided by the presence or absence of complications and the nature of the complication. In the case of DM (diabetes mellitus) the word "with" is used rather than the words "due to." Words such as "with," "with mention of," "associated with," and "in" indicate that both elements in the title (of the code) must be present in the diagnostic statement. There are ten fourth digit subclassifications for manifestations of diabetes mellitus.

A fifth digit is also required for coding the type of diabetes mellitus. Determining the type of diabetes is critical to proper code assignment. There are two types of DM. Type I includes both juvenile-onset DM and IDDM (insulin-dependent diabetes mellitus). Type II DM is sometimes called *adult-onset diabetes mellitus.* Type II DM is not always treated with insulin, and is therefore also called *non–insulin-dependent DM.* When selecting the fifth digit it is important to remember that a patient has insulin-dependent diabetes only if he or she has type I diabetes.

There are four fifth digits to use, specifying the type of diabetes and whether it is under control.

MAXIMIZING THIRD-PARTY REIMBURSEMENT

The most important aspect to remember with ICD-9-CM is to code the diagnosis to the highest level of specificity, linking the ICD-9-CM code to the *Current Procedural Terminology, 4th Edition*

(CPT-4) code. CPT-4, or procedure and service coding, is further explained in the next chapter of this text, Chapter 18, Basics of Procedural Coding, and Chapter 20, The Health Insurance Claim Form.

Obtaining the correct reimbursement is important to the practice cash flow and depends on proper coding and billing techniques. Some other crucial points to remember when submitting diagnostic codes for claims are as follows:
- Use the current year ICD-9-CM manual, staying informed of all changes, revisions, and additions published for that year.
- Code accurately from documented information.
- Be sure the diagnosis corresponds to symptoms and treatment.
- Review data entry to ensure that no transposition of digits has occurred.
- Know the insurance carrier's rules and requirements for completion and submission of claims.
- Incomplete or inaccurate codes may result in delay or denial of reimbursement.

CLOSING COMMENTS

Medical assistants are entrusted by the physician and practice that employs them. To this extent, a medical assistant must be responsible and knowledgeable to ensure that no fraud takes place in the coding and claims submission process. Medical assistants are expected to adhere to ethical standards, assigning and reporting only codes that are clearly supported by concise documentation in the patient chart. When in doubt, a medical assistant should consult the attending healthcare provider for clarification. Maintaining and continually enhancing coding skills and keeping informed of changes in codes, guidelines, and regulations are necessary responsibilities for a coding professional.

SUMMARY OF SCENARIO

 Mike is enthusiastic about his position and enjoys learning more about the coding process. He knows that as he gains experience and earns his certificate, he will be even more valuable as an employee. As Mike progresses with diagnostic coding, he will also be able to help the physicians and nursing staff to be attentive to details in documentation of the patient chart.

Although using the superbill to enter the codes for billing is an easy tool, Mike has learned that knowing how to use the ICD-9-CM volumes is a necessary asset to ensure accurate coding. He also knows it is important when coding a diagnosis to ensure the medical documentation matches the encounter form, and that all elements of the diagnostic statement are included, and to ensure that the diagnosis listed on the encounter form is fully documented in the patient's medical record. In addition, Mike has learned that the layout and structure of Volumes 1 and 2 of the ICD-9-CM manual are designed to aid in the selection of the most specific and accurate diagnosis code. Every feature of the manual provides guidance in choosing and confirming a diagnostic code that matches the diagnostic statement on the encounter form, and in the medical record. The steps and decision tree for diagnostic coding ensure that Mike will be coding to the highest level of specificity and accuracy.

SUMMARY of LEARNING OBJECTIVES

1. Define, spell, and pronounce the terms listed in the vocabulary.
   - Spelling and pronouncing medical terms correctly adds credibility to the medical assistant. Knowing the definition of these terms promotes confidence in communication with patients and co-workers.
2. Identify three purposes of the ICD-9-CM.
   - The ICD-9-CM is used to track healthcare statistics, as well as to facilitate accurate medical record keeping and ease in processing claims. Use of the ICD-9-CM is mandatory for participation in many federal, state, and private insurance programs.
3. Explain the proper use of the ICD-9-CM.
   - Each of the three volumes of the ICD-9-CM has a specific use. Using Volume 2, the Alphabetic Index, look for the disease(s) documented in the clinical record. Proceed to the Tabular Index, Volume 1, to find and assign a code. Follow guidelines that are provided in the specific manual used for coding in the medical facility.
4. Understand and apply the basic coding rules in the use of the ICD-9-CM.
   - Several basic coding rules exist that will assist the medical assistant in coding. Be sure that the most recent ICD-9-CM manual is being used, and keep a medical dictionary handy. Proofread the claim, and be sure that it makes good sense. Avoid nonspecific codes, and use care when coding preexisting conditions.
5. Understand the importance of the Tabular Index, which contains the most specific coding information.

   - Never code directly from the index. The Tabular Index contains the most specific information. Check and recheck the codes, making certain that the documentation supports the codes that are used on the claim.
6. Comprehend and use instructional terms and symbols as defined in the ICD-9-CM.
   - The medical assistant should become familiar with all of the symbols used in the ICD-9-CM. Instructional notations should be read thoroughly and all directions followed while coding a claim.
7. Explain the use of V and E codes.
   - V or E codes may help to clarify a code or further explain the code. V codes are used when the patient is not currently ill but is being seen by health service professionals. E codes are used to explain that some external cause contributed to an adverse effect within the body.
8. Properly perform basic diagnostic coding.
   - The medical assistant's knowledge of accurate diagnostic coding contributes to the legal and financial health of the practice. In most cases ICD-9-CM codes are found on the provider's encounter form (or superbill) and/or in the practice management software. However, with literally thousands of current diagnostic codes, it may be necessary to code from the ICD-9-CM manual. Because these codes are updated yearly, they are an asset in coding compliance. The process for diagnosis coding is outlined in Procedure 17-1.

CONNECTIONS

 Study Guide Connection: Go to Chapter 17 Study Guide. Read the Case Study and Workplace Applications and complete the assignments. Do online research for answers to the questions in the Internet Activities associated with basics of diagnostic coding.

 CD Connection: Go to the Medical Assisting Competency Challenge CD and do the training activities under Health Insurance Activities.

Evolve Connection: For more information related to basics of diagnostic coding, go to http://evolve.elsevier.com/kinn/ admin and visit related weblinks for Chapter 17. Click on the Medical Assisting Exam Review and do the practice questions to sharpen your test-taking skills. To learn more about office software, do the exercises for the Altapoint demo that are on the CD.

Basics of Procedural Coding

Carline A. Dalgleish
Alexandra Patricia Young

18

SCENARIO

Kay James has excelled on her diagnostic coding examinations, and she now looks forward to learning procedural coding. The process for coding procedures and services will prove to be similar to that of ICD-9-CM and diagnostic coding, except she will use a different coding manual called *Current Procedural Terminology* (CPT-4) for most procedural coding. She will also use a manual called the *Healthcare Common Procedural Coding System*, or HCPCS (pronounced "*hixpix*"). As with the ICD-9-CM, accurate coding begins with the proper analysis of clinical information to abstract the correct data and accurately assign a procedure or service code. In the ICD-9-CM, she learned about coding conventions and guidelines. In the CPT-4, there are new conventions, symbols, guidelines, and formal steps specific to procedural coding that Kay will use to correctly assign procedure codes. Kay is beginning to fully understand the impact diagnostic and procedural coding has on reimbursement, and her responsibility to uphold ethical standards when coding to keep her employer in compliance with federal and state guidelines. She is excited to begin this new phase of her education and to have the opportunity to learn more skills in her goal of becoming an even morc valuable asset to the practice.

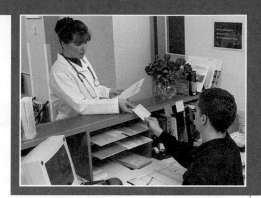

While studying this chapter, think about the following questions:

- What will Kay find similar to what she learned with the ICD-9-CM as she performs procedural coding?
- What will help Kay in selecting the most specific and accurate CPT-4 code?
- What are the differences between coding for the CPT-4 and coding for HCPCS?
- What will Kay learn about the legal and compliance implications of improper coding?

LEARNING OBJECTIVES

1. Define, spell, and pronounce the terms listed in the vocabulary.
2. Describe the steps for abstracting procedural data from clinical documentation.
3. Identify four purposes of the CPT-4.
4. List the main sections of the CPT-4, and describe their content.
5. Describe the coding conventions, guidelines, and layout of the CPT-4 manual and their importance.
6. Describe the process and steps for selecting the most accurate code based on clinical documentation.
7. Explain the importance of correctly assigning evaluation and management codes.
8. Discuss the importance of modifiers.
9. Define *upcoding*, and explain why it must be avoided.
10. Demonstrate an understanding of the process and procedures for code selection.
11. Demonstrate an understanding of main and modifying term selection.
12. Find codes in the Alphabetic Index of the CPT-4 manual.
13. Analyze and select codes using the CPT-4 main text.

VOCABULARY

abstract An outline or summary of the diagnostic statement and/or procedures and services performed. In procedural coding, the outline or summary assists in ensuring that all procedures and services are included in an insurance claim submission, and that nothing was omitted or added to the encounter form or charge ticket; to abstract also means to compile this outline or summary for use in procedural coding.

acronyms Abbreviations, such as ECG for electrocardiography.

add-on code A code that indicates additional or supplemental procedures carried out in addition to the primary procedure.

Alphabetic Index The reference section of the CPT-4 manual that is used to help find a code or code range.

bundled codes Codes designating procedures or services that are grouped together and paid for as one procedure or service.

categories Indented one level below a subsection in the CPT-4 coding manual, usually refers to a specific anatomic site or procedures and/or services.

category I code The primary procedure or service code selected when performing insurance billing or statistical research.

category II codes Special codes that can help providers track revenue and reimbursement.

category III codes Codes for a new or experimental procedure or service.

downcoding A change in code submitted for reimbursement, usually performed by the insurance company. This change generally occurs because the code submitted does not match in some way to the specifications of the insurance company.

eponyms Procedures, services, or diagnoses named after people, such as Mohs' micrographic surgery or Crohn's disease.

established patient (EP) A patient who has been seen by the same physician or same group of physicians over time. An established patient becomes a new patient if not seen by the physician or group in 3 years.

guidelines Found at the beginning of each of the six sections of the CPT-4. The guidelines define items that are necessary to appropriately interpret and report the procedures and services found in the section.

HCPCS Health Care Common Procedural Coding System; level II codes created to supplement procedures and services not covered in the CPT-4.

modifiers Code additions that explain circumstances that alter a provided service, or provide additional clarification or detail about a procedure or service.

new patient (NP) A patient who has his or her first encounter (visit) with a physician or physician group or who was an established patient with a physician or provider but has not been seen in 3 years.

patient status (PS) The state of a patient as either new or established; appears in the Evaluation and Management section of the CPT-4.

physical status The physical condition of the patient.

place-of-service (POS) codes Codes that indicate where a procedure or service was performed.

providers People who perform a medical procedure or service.

section The main divisions of the CPT-4 manual.

subsection Indented one level below a section, a subsection usually describes an anatomic site or organ system—e.g., integumentary system or cardiology.

subcategory Indented one level below a category, usually a procedure or service unique to a specific category.

unbundled codes Codes in which the components of a procedure are separated and reported separately.

upcoding A deliberate increase in a CPT-4 code, despite the lack of documentation, to the next highest reimbursable code in order to receive higher reimbursements.

Procedural coding is defined as the transformation of verbal descriptions of medical services and procedures into numeric or alphanumeric designations. As with diagnostic coding and use of the ICD-9-CM coding manual, accurate use of the American Medical Association's (AMA's) *Current Procedural Terminology* (CPT-4) and the *Healthcare Common Procedural Coding System* **(HCPCS)** is essential. The medical assistant facilitates accurate medical record keeping and the efficient processing of insurance claims by using the CPT-4 and HCPCS, which identify appropriate procedures and services common to the physician's office. CPT-4 and HCPCS are used in the claims submission process to receive reimbursement from payors as well as to track physician productivity, and provide statistical data for research and other purposes.

GETTING TO KNOW THE CPT-4

The Evolution of CPT-4 Coding

The CPT-4 manual is a listing of descriptive terms and identifying codes for reporting medical services and procedures performed by physicians in order to provide a uniform or standard language that will accurately describe medical, surgical, and diagnostic services and enhance reliable communication among physicians, patients, and third parties. The manual was developed after the AMA recognized a need for a standardized description of services that would be universally understood by physicians, hospitals, insurance companies, and everyone involved in the reimbursement or statistical data collection process.

The second edition of the CPT-4, published in 1970, presented an expanded system of terms and codes to designate diagnostic and therapeutic procedures in surgery, medicine, radiology, laboratory, pathology, and medical specialties. At that time the four-digit classification was replaced with the current five-digit coding system. The fourth edition was published in 1977 and represented significant updates in medical technology. At the same time a system of periodic annual updating was introduced to keep pace with the rapidly changing environment. The fourth edition is still in use today; however, at this writing, the AMA is in the process of developing the fifth edition of the CPT-4—the first major revision since 1977.

Purpose of CPT-4 Procedural Coding

According to the AMA, the CPT-4 contains a five-digit classification system that is designed to do the following:

- Encourage the use of standard terms and descriptors to document procedures in the medical record
- Help communicate accurate information on procedures and services to agencies concerned with insurance claims
- Provide the basis for a computer-oriented system to evaluate operative procedures
- Contribute basic information for actuarial and statistical purposes

Before continuing, keep this important fact in mind. There are roughly 150,000 procedure and service codes in the CPT-4 manual, and thousands more in the HCPCS manual. Memorizing the codes for each specific procedure and service would be impractical, if not impossible. Instead, learning how to use the coding manuals to find the most specific and accurate code based on interpretation of the medical record is the key to success. This requires a solid understanding of medical terminology, anatomy, and physiology and knowledge of how to use the CPT-4 manual and its symbols, conventions, **guidelines,** and notes. The goal of this chapter is to teach the skills, processes, and decisions required to use the CPT-4 and HCPCS manuals. The final authorities are always the CPT-4 and HCPCS manuals for the current year. The symbols, guidelines, conventions, and other instructions found in the CPT-4 manual contain all the information needed to select the correct code for the procedure or service documented in the medical record.

FORMAT OF THE CPT-4 CODING MANUAL

Each procedure or service is represented by a five-digit numeric code (Figure 18-1)—a type of medical shorthand that saves enormous amounts of time and effort and helps to ensure accuracy of information. Just imagine, for example, if a billing department had to describe, in writing, every single one of the medical procedures and services represented by the codes in the CPT-4 manual. Preparing one bill for one patient could take an hour or more and still affect reimbursement negatively when the health insurance or third-party payor has additional questions or, worse, reduces or even denies payment based on their interpretation of the written narrative. Using the five-digit CPT-4 codes eliminates the need, in most instances, for written descriptions, thus assuring clear communication, and the standardization of codes ensures that everyone in the reimbursement cycle understands exactly what procedure or service was provided to the patient. These codes also enable

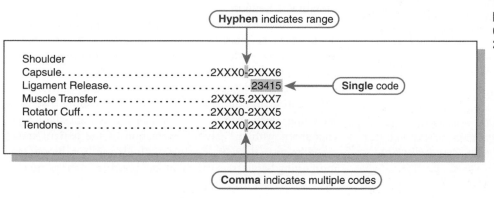

Figure 18-1 CPT code example. (From Buck CJ: *Step-by-Step medical coding,* 2006, St Louis, 2006, Saunders.)

automated computer processing of claims, which saves time and effort.

Modifiers

Modifiers provide a way for **providers** of service to indicate that a service or procedure performed has been altered by some specific circumstance but not changed in its definition. Two-digit alphanumeric modifiers, used in conjunction with a five-digit CPT-4 code, can also be used to add additional information or describe extenuating circumstances that affect the rendered procedure or service. Modifiers can be used, for example, to show that a procedure was performed bilaterally (on both sides of the body); in such a case, the modifier is -50. To describe a situation in which an assistant surgeon is needed for a surgical procedure, modifier -80 can be used to allow the assistant surgeon to submit charges for his or her time and services. Table 18-1 illustrates some commonly used modifiers.

CPT-4 Content

The CPT-4 manual includes the following content:
- Comprehensive instructions for use of the manual, including steps for coding
- A complete Alphabetic Index
- Main text (Tabular Index)
- Six **sections**
- Guidelines and notes
- Conventions
- Twelve appendixes
- Two addenda

CPT-4 Manual Structure

The CPT-4 contains two main divisions, the **Alphabetic Index** and the main text, also called the *Tabular Index*. The Alphabetic Index is like any other index within a textbook; it is simply a guide to finding data in the body of the textbook, however, instead of providing the page numbers where the information is located, as a typical index does, the CPT-4 Alphabetic Index lists the code or code ranges, which are then found in numeric order within each section of the main text.

The structure of the main text of the CPT-4 is as follows:
- Six sections divided into Evaluation and Management, Anesthesia, Surgery, Radiology, Pathology and Laboratory, and Medicine.

- Conventions, also called symbols
- Guidelines and notes
- Appendixes and other addenda

Sections of the CPT-4 Main Text

A **section** is a broad category in the main text of the CPT-4 manual, and each of the six sections is divided by the general type of service. The six sections of the CPT-4 main text are Evaluation and Management, Anesthesia, Surgery, Radiology, Pathology and Laboratory, and Medicine. Sections are subdivided into **subsections**, subsections are further divided into **categories**, and categories can be further subdivided into **subcategories**. Each level of a section provides more specificity regarding the procedure or service being performed, and the anatomical site or organ system involved. In most instances all four levels are found within a section, although this is not a hard and fast rule. See Table 18-2 for an illustration of a section, subsection, category, and subcategory.

The subsection of the CPT-4 manual is indented two spaces below a section, and typically describes an anatomical site or an organ system—for example, the heart, femur, or skull (anatomic site), or gastrointestinal, integumentary, or cardiology (organ system). Categories are indented two additional spaces below the subsection, and generally refer to a specific procedure or service, but can also be a more specific anatomical site—for example, esophagoscopy, incision and drainage, or cardiac catheterization (procedures); or mitral valve, distal femur, or occipital bone (specific anatomic site). Subcategories are the lowest level of code description and specificity. The subcategory is indented two spaces below a category, and provides even more specificity about an anatomical site, or procedure.

Evaluation and Management Section

The Evaluation and Management (E&M) section contains codes for the different types of encounters or visits patients have with providers, including office, hospital, and emergency room visits; consultations; and physician contact with patients in intensive care units, skilled nursing facilities, nursing homes, and other facilities. The code range within the E&M section is 99201 to 99499. The E&M section is further divided into subsections that include different types of services (e.g., office visits, hospital visits). The subsections, categories, and subcategories are written to further modify or describe the service or procedure performed.

Anesthesia Section

The Anesthesia section includes codes for anesthesia services rendered by anesthesiologists and anesthetists before, during, and after surgery. The code ranges within the Anesthesia section are 00100 to 01999 and 99100 to 99140. Codes are included for the types of anesthesia administered—for example, general, local, and sedation anesthesia administration; other support services, including preoperative and postoperative anesthesiologist encounters with the patient, evaluation of the **patient status,** the administration of anesthesia, fluids, and/or blood; and monitoring services, such as blood pressure, temperature, or electrocardiography (ECG).

TABLE 18-1 Example of CPT Code Modifiers	
MODIFIER	**DESCRIPTION**
-50	Bilateral procedure. If procedure was performed on both sides of the body (e.g., both knees, both eyes) and the code description does not indicate procedure or service was performed bilaterally, modifier -50 is used.
-62	Two surgeons. When two surgeons work together as primary surgeons performing distinct parts of a procedure, each surgeon should report the procedure he or she performed to the insurance carrier and use modifier -62. (This prevents the insurance carrier from possibly rejecting a surgical charge as a duplicate)

TABLE 18-2 Section, Subsection, Category, and Subcategory Illustration

SECTION	SUBSECTION	CATEGORY	SUBCATEGORY
Surgery	Musculoskeletal System	Application of Casts and Strapping	Body and Upper Extremity
Surgery	Cardiovascular System	Arteries and Veins	Embolectomy/Thrombectomy
Medicine	Physical Medicine and Rehabilitation	Modalities	
Medicine	Neurology and Neuromuscular Procedures	Sleep Testing	
Radiology	Diagnostic Radiology	Head and Neck	
Radiology	Vascular Procedures	Aorta and Arteries	

Surgery Section

The Surgery section, which is the largest section in the CPT-4, includes standardized codes for all invasive surgical procedures performed by physicians. Invasive procedures are defined as any medical procedure in which a bodily orifice or the skin must be penetrated by cutting, puncture, or other method. This section is divided into subsections typically identifying specific body systems, beginning with the integumentary (skin) system and ending with ophthalmologic (eyes) and otologic (ears) systems; in most instances each subsection is further divided into categories and subcategories, which describe procedures and services unique to that anatomic subsection.

Radiology Section

The Radiology section includes codes for diagnostic imaging, including x-ray studies and scans, as well as radiation therapy used in the treatment of cancer. The codes used in the Radiology section are in the range of 70000 to 79999.

Pathology and Laboratory Section

Codes are included for all diagnostic tests performed on bodily fluids and tissue, including urine, blood, sputum, and feces, as well as excised or biopsied cells, tissue, or body organs; and evaluation of those fluids and tissues to identify any pathology or disease present in those fluids or tissue. The code ranges for the Pathology and Laboratory section are 80010 to 89999.

Medicine Section

The codes for the Medicine section range from 90281 to 99199 and 99500 to 99602 (excluding anesthesia code ranges). The Medicine section includes many and varied subsections, categories, and subcategories. This section can be called a "catch-all" section, in that it includes codes for services and procedures that do not fit in any of the other sections of the CPT-4 manual. Medical specialties, such as ophthalmology, otolaryngology, and allergy, whose procedures and services vary greatly from the traditional office encounter, are grouped in the Medicine rather than the E&M section. In addition, noninvasive diagnostic tests are included here rather than in the Surgery section, which typically includes only invasive procedures.

Conventions of the CPT-4 Main Text

Conventions are special symbols used to provide additional information about certain codes. Seven conventions are used in the current CPT-4 manual. The most common conventions are shown in Figure 18-2.

Unlisted Procedure or Service Code

Occasionally, even with the best documentation and the coder's best efforts, an accurate, specific code will not be found in the CPT-4 manual that matches the procedure or service performed. In each section, and sometimes subsection, **category,** and/or **subcategory** of the CPT-4, nonspecific codes have been provided. These codes are called *unlisted procedures and services.*

Special Reports

When bills are submitted for services rendered or procedures performed, in most instances most insurance carriers or third-party payors require no additional information except for the procedure or service CPT-4 code. When a bill is submitted for a service that is unlisted, unusual, or newly adopted, the third-party carrier, in order to determine whether providing that service or procedure was medically appropriate, will require a special report.

Bundled and Unbundled Codes

Bundled codes are procedure codes designating procedures or services that are grouped together and paid for as one procedure or service. A good example of bundled codes are the Organ Panels found in the Laboratory and Pathology section. Each panel contains several different diagnostic tests that are "bundled" together under one code. **Unbundled codes** are codes which are separated into several components of a procedure. One procedure is separated into several different codes and reported separately.

Guidelines

Guidelines, found at the beginning of each section as well as some subsections of the CPT-4 manual, define items necessary to appropriately interpret and report the procedures and services contained in that section or subsection. For example, in the Medicine section specific instructions are provided for handling unlisted services or procedures, special reports, and supplies and materials provided to the insurance company or the patient (Figure 18-3). Guidelines are written specifically to assist in understanding when and under what circumstances codes may be used. It is important to thoroughly read and understand the guidelines provided throughout the main text. This is especially

⊘   **Modifier -51 exempt.** This symbol is used to specify when a code is exempt from use of the modifier -51. Modifier -51 allows coders to specify that one procedure was performed multiple times. Normally, in the instance when the same procedure has been performed more than once, reporting of modifier -51 would be required to indicate that the same procedure (with the same definition and code) was performed two or more times; however, when this symbol appears in front of the code, the code description already indicates the procedure was performed more than once, and therefore modifier -51 is not required.

+   **Add-on code.** An add-on code is used when more than one code must be used to completely describe a specific procedure or service. Some medical procedures are commonly carried out at the same time a primary procedure is being performed and are described as procedures performed by the same physician to include an additional treatment or procedure done at the same time or in conjunction with the main procedure being performed. Add-on codes can be readily identified by specific words used in the code description, such as additional digit(s), lesions(s), neurorrhaphy, etc. Add-on codes are always used in addition to the primary service or procedure and must never be reported as a standalone code.

•   **New code.** In healthcare, scientific research results in new emerging technology procedures and services. Once a new procedure or service is approved for use or judged to be effective, a temporary **category III** code is assigned. If the procedure or service is then adopted, and statistics bear out the integration of the new procedure with the more mainstream or traditional codes, then a permanent CPT-4 code is assigned, and the code is added to the main text of the CPT-4 manual.

▲   **Revised code.** In addition to the new codes added to the CPT-4 each year, many code descriptions are revised as well. The change may be only to clarify or improve the wording of the description, or, as is the case in most instances, it may be revised to add or remove terminology or information.

►◄   **New or revised text.** Text within the guidelines is often revised to add or remove information, correct grammar, or further clarify the content.

⊙   **Conscious sedation.** This is a new convention, added in 2005, to describe CPT-4 codes that include conscious sedation use. Codes with this convention do not require the use of separate Conscious Sedation codes from the Medicine Section of the CPT-4.

⚡   **FDA approval pending.** A symbol indicating that a CPT-4 category I code has been assigned to a vaccine product in anticipation of approval for use from the Food and Drug Administration (FDA)

Figure 18-2 CPT-4 main text conventions.

important when first learning to code, or working in a section of the CPT-4 that is rarely used. It is also important to reread the guidelines after the CPT-4 annual revisions, additions, and deletions are released in October of each year. Selecting a code without reading the guidelines will usually lead to selection of the wrong code; not only will this result in the potential for delayed or denied reimbursement, but continued inappropriate code selection can be considered fraud or abuse and can result in serious civil or criminal penalties.

Notes

Notes are typically found only in the category, subcategory, or code description area of the CPT-4. Notes apply only to the designated group of codes following the note, and not the whole section as guidelines do. Like guidelines, notes provide additional information to assist in the selection of specific codes.

Appendixes

Appendixes found in the CPT-4 are as follows:
- Appendix A: Modifiers. Lists all of the two-digit numeric or alphanumeric codes used to increase specificity and provide additional information about certain procedures and services.
- Appendix B: Summary of Additions, Deletions, and Revisions. At each annual update of the CPT-4, this appendix lists, for easy reference, all changes made to the CPT-4 from the previous year.

- Appendix C: Clinical Examples. Clinical examples are helpful narrative examples that aid in selection of the correct and most specific level of E&M codes.
- Appendix D: Summary of CPT-4 Add-on Codes. Services and procedures that require more than one code to fully describe the service or procedure rendered, or to identify a procedure that is performed concurrently with another procedure, are called *add-on codes*.
- Appendix E: Summary of CPT-4 Codes Exempt from Modifier -51. Lists all procedures and services exempt from the use of modifier -51.
- Appendix F: Summary of CPT-4 Codes Exempt from Modifier -63. Lists all procedures exempt from use of modifier 63. Modifier -63 is used to report procedures performed on infants less than 4 kg to identify the significantly increased complexity common to these patients. **Category I codes** that state specifically "Exempt from modifier -63" do not require use of this modifier.
- Appendix G: Summary of CPT-4 Codes that Include Moderate (Conscious) Sedation. Lists all procedure codes that include conscious sedation as part of the code description, thus eliminating the need to code the sedation separately.
- Appendix H: Alphabetic Index of Performance Measures by Clinical Condition or Topic. Used by providers in determining appropriate uses of optional **category II codes** (performance measurement codes).

99000—99116 Medicine

Miscellaneous Services

99000 Handling and/or conveyance of specimen for transfer from the physician's office to a laboratory

99001 Handling and/or conveyance of specimen for transfer from the patient in other than a physician's office to a laboratory (distance may be indicated)

99002 Handling, conveyance, and/or any other service in connection with the implementation of an order involving devices (e.g. designing, fitting, packaging, handling, delivery or mailing) when devices such as orthotics, protectives, prosthetics are fabricated by an outside laboratory or shop but which items have been designed, and are to be fitted and adjusted by the attending physician

(For routine collection of venous blood, use 36415)

99024 Postoperative follow-up visit, normally included in the surgical package, to indicate that an evaluation and management service was performed during a postoperative period for a reason(s) related to the original procedure

(As a component of a surgical "package," see **Surgery Guidelines**)

(99025 has been deleted)

Figure 18-3 Example of Miscellaneous Services in Medicine section.

- Appendix I: Genetic Testing Code Modifiers. Lists all modifiers, and their descriptions, unique to genetic testing.
- Appendix J: Electrodiagnostic Medicine Listing of Sensory, Motor, and Mixed Nerves. A listing of each sensory, motor, and mixed nerve conduction study code which can be used to assist in accurate use of codes 95900, 95903, and 95904.
- Appendix K: Product Pending FDA Approval. A list of vaccine products for which FDA approval is pending and that have already been assigned category I codes before approval.
- Appendix L: Vascular Families. A listing of the vascular system, grouped by families, starting from the aorta and branching from there. This appendix is designed to assist in coding for the Cardiology subsection of the Surgery and Medicine sections.

Other Addenda

Category II Codes

Category II codes are a relatively new addition to the CPT-4 manual. The AMA, in preparation for the release of the fifth edition of the CPT-4, added category II codes to the CPT-4 manual in 2004 in an effort to assist healthcare providers in development of automated statistical and reimbursement procedural tracking tools. Category II codes are optional "tracking" codes designed to help facilitate quality-of-care data collection, which can be used by the provider for practice performance measurement. They are not used for billing or reimbursement.

Category III Codes

Category III codes are temporary codes used to identify emerging technology, services, and procedures that have not been globally accepted or adopted as medically appropriate treatment or diagnostic procedures. They are to be used only when a category I code description does not match all the elements listed in the medical documentation but does match the category III code description.

BEGINNING THE CODING PROCESS

Medical Documentation

The steps for using the CPT-4 manual actually begin not in the CPT-4 coding manual but in the medical documentation. Information pertinent to code selection is taken from a variety of medical documents. Sources of information include the following:

- Encounter form, also known as a *superbill, fee slip,* or *charge ticket*
- History and physical report (H&P)
- Discharge summary
- Operative report
- Pathology report

Many physician offices have CPT-4 and even ICD-9-CM codes preprinted on the encounter forms or charge ticket; however it is important to review the medical record, and compile an **abstract**, which is a complete list of all the procedures and services performed. For instance, if, on the encounter form, the physician checked off the procedure for an EGD (esophagogastroduodenoscopy), but in the medical record the operative report states an EGD with biopsy was performed, the code selected, had the medical record not been reviewed, would have resulted in a loss of revenue because a code with a lower reimbursement amount was submitted to the insurance carrier. Update encounter forms annually to ensure that new code additions, changes, and revisions are documented on the preprinted forms.

When comparing the medical documentation against any code description, all of the elements of that code must match, with nothing added or missing. If a code is selected that doesn't fully describe the documented procedure or service, the procedure is "downcoded," and it can, and will, affect reimbursement. Consistent **downcoding** results in a loss of revenue, and it can also trigger an audit by the health insurance carrier, especially if the downcoding occurs in the Evaluation and Management section. If a code is selected that not only matches the procedure or service performed but also adds modifying information that is not in the medical documentation, the information is considered **"upcoded."** Consistent upcoding can result in legal charges of fraud or abuse as discussed earlier.

The steps and process outlined later in this chapter, including use of the Alphabetic Index and the main text of the CPT-4 are applicable to all of the text's sections. Some special considerations and differences apply to the E&M and Anesthesia sections and are also discussed later in this chapter.

Hint: Health Insurance Portability and Accountability Act

When abstracting medical records in preparation for coding, remember that patient-identifiable information must be safeguarded. Any handwritten notes that are not to be placed in the confidential patient record and that could identify the patient must be shredded.

The basic steps in medical coding are to read, analyze, and abstract the procedure or service documented in the medical record, and compare it with the encounter form or charge ticket to ensure all services and procedures have been recorded. The term abstract, used as a verb in this context, means to create an outline or summary of information from a text or record. In procedural coding, an abstract is created to find all of the procedures and services performed during a patient encounter, and ensure that nothing has been omitted or added to the encounter form or charge ticket that is not documented in the patient's medical record. The abstracted data are then broken down into main terms and modifying terms. A main term is defined usually as the primary procedure or service performed, with a modifying term further defining, or adding information to, a main term. Next, the main and modifying terms are used to find the code or code ranges in the Alphabetic Index, and last, the code selected is confirmed by reviewing the guidelines and conventions in the CPT-4 main text to verify that the most specific and accurate code was chosen.

USING THE ALPHABETIC INDEX

The Alphabetic Index is a comprehensive, alphabetic listing of all procedures and services contained within the CPT-4 manual. The most important thing to remember about the Alphabetic Index is that it should be used only as an aid to finding the area in the main text of the CPT-4 to evaluate for selection of the proper code. The Alphabetic Index is not a substitute for the main text. Even if only one code is assigned, the main text must be used to ensure that the code selection is accurate.

The Alphabetic Index of the CPT-4 is used as a guide to search for code(s) or code ranges. The index is similar to the index found in any textbook. It is an alphabetic list of major terms or concepts found within the main text of the book. Each term or concept found in the index then references a page or pages where detailed information can be found in the main text. The Alphabetic Index in the CPT-4 is used in the same way, except that the CPT-4 Alphabetic Index references code or code ranges, rather than pages. As discussed earlier, the main text of the CPT-4 is divided into sections, and the procedures and services are then listed in numeric order by the category I code.

The Alphabetic Index is organized by *main terms* that can stand alone or be further modified by up to four *modifying terms* indented under the main term. Do not confuse the two-digit modifiers discussed earlier in the chapter with modifying terms.

Modifiers are numeric supplements to a category I CPT-4 code, whereas modifying terms are words that add to or modify the meaning of the main term.

Modifying terms are indented below the main term. These modifying terms further describe or add additional information or definition needed to narrow down the search for an appropriate procedure or service code. A main term might be a procedure such as an *excision,* and each modifying term could provide further information about the anatomic location or organ being excised, the type of instrument used, or a special technique or whether other procedures were performed at the same time as the excision, such as the taking of biopsy tissue for examination. Modifying terms affect the selection of appropriate codes; therefore it is important to review the list of modifying terms when selecting a code or code range.

For example, look at Table 18-3. If the medical documentation contains the narrative description of a procedure as a diagnostic cystoscopy, the main term is "Cystoscopy" and the modifying term is "diagnostic," because it describes the type of cystoscopy performed. Another example is "esophagogastroscopy with biopsy and fulguration of lesions." In this example, the main term would be "Gastroscopy" (the procedure being performed), with the modifying terms being "esophago-" (it adds another anatomic site scoped at the same time as the gastroscopy was performed); "with biopsy" and "fulguration" (biopsy and fulguration are two additional procedures performed during the gastroscopy); and "lesions" (describes the object of the biopsy and fulguration).

Two rules should be followed when coding any procedure or service:

- Be as specific as possible in code selection, and use all pertinent words within the description given in your documentation.
- Never add any words, modifying terms, or descriptors to the procedure or service code description that are not documented.

Once the medical documentation has been abstracted to determine the procedures and services performed, and the main and modifying term or terms have been identified, the next step is to look for the terms in the Alphabetic Index. Use the Alphabetic Index to search for a code, code(s), or code range that best describes the procedure or service documented in the medical record. Using the code or codes found in the Alphabetic Index search, locate each in the appropriate section, subsection, category, or subcategory of the CPT-4's main text, and select the most specific code that best matches the medical record documentation. The steps for using the Alphabetic Index are as follows. Further steps for use of the main text are added later in the chapter.

Using the Alphabetic Index to Search

Begin the search by using one or all of the four primary classifications (or types) of main and modifying term entries:

- Procedure or service
- Organ or anatomic site
- Condition, illness, or injury
- Eponym, synonym, or acronym

TABLE 18-3 Main and Modifying Terms Identification in the Alphabetic Index

CODE	MAIN TERM(S)	FIRST MODIFYING TERM	SECOND MODIFYING TERM	THIRD MODIFYING TERM	FOURTH MODIFYING TERM
	Cystoscopy	Diagnostic			
	Gastroscopy	Esophago-	With biopsy	With fulguration	Of lesions
492000	**Cyst**	Abdomen Ankle Bartholin's gland Bile duct			
21030	**Excision**	Cheekbone			
23140		**Clavicle**			
23146				**With allograft**	
23147				With autograft	
27355-27758			Femur		
Cyst excision: 49200					
Cyst excision of clavicle: 23140					
Cyst excision of clavicle with allograft: 23146					

Acronyms are abbreviations of words—for example, the acronym for an electrocardiogram is either ECG or EKG; the acronym for a transurethral resection of the prostate is TURP; and the acronym for gastroesophageal reflux disease is GERD. **Eponyms** are procedures or services named after their inventor or developer. Examples of eponyms are *Mohs' micrographic surgery* and *Dupuy-Dutemps' operation.* Synonyms are words that are similar in meaning and can be used interchangeably.

Earlier in the chapter it was explained that the CPT-4 is divided into sections (E&M, Surgery, Radiology, and so on). The sections could first list the procedure (e.g., excision, incision, repair), the organ or anatomic site (e.g., clavicle, liver), or a condition (e.g., a fracture or laceration). Select a main term that is the procedure, anatomic site, or condition, or, if an acronym or eponym is used, search by the synonym, acronym, or eponym first.

Start the search by using the name of the performed procedure or service (anastomosis, splint, repair, stress test, therapy, vaccination); by the organ or other anatomic site of the procedure (tibia, colon, salivary gland, aorta); by the condition, illness, or injury (abscess, fracture, cholelithiasis, strabismus); or, if applicable, by the synonyms, eponyms, or abbreviations (ECG, Stookey-Scarff procedure, Mohs' micrographic surgery). Usually, but not always, it is helpful to begin by searching for the procedure.

Using "See" and "See Also" in the Alphabetic Index

The "See" statement in the Alphabetic Index points to another location in the Alphabetic Index to find the code or code range. The "See Also" statement points to additional code or code ranges in the Alphabetic Index that may be useful in addition to the code found in the original search.

Stand Alone Code and Code Ranges

When searching the Alphabetic Index, a procedure or service may list a single code—called a *stand alone code*—or may list a range

of possible codes that will match the medical documentation. Remember that the Alphabetic Index is an index—it is designed as a guide to the most suitable codes that match the documentation. It does not provide specificity; that is the purpose of the main text. At this point the search is only looking for the closest match or matches to the medical documentation.

Because some medical procedures and diagnostic tests can be quite complex, there may be a single code (standalone) or a code range that may include one main term but several variations—or modifying terms—of the main procedure or service. For example, the code for "Craterization, phalanges, toe" is 28124—a standalone code; however, using the same main term, "Craterization," this time of any of the phalanges (toes or fingers), yields a range of codes: 26235 to 29236. The range of codes is separated by a hyphen to indicate that all codes within that range could be appropriate. There will sometimes also be a standalone code and range of codes listed for the same service or procedure—for example, "Craterization, femur" lists both the range of codes 27070 to 27071 and the standalone code 27360. Once a standalone code or code range is found in the Alphabetic Index, the next step is to look up each code or code range found in the main text of the CPT-4 and select which code or codes most closely match the medical documentation (Table 18-4).

Steps for Using the Alphabetic Index

1. Using the Alphabetic Index, analyze the medical documentation to determine what procedures or services were provided.
2. Select main term classification to begin search in the Alphabetic Index.
3. Select modifying term(s), if needed, once main term is located, to narrow down search.
4. If no modifying term produces an appropriate code or code range, repeat steps 2 and 3 using a different main term classification.

TABLE 18-4 Comparing Codes in the Range of 52234 to 52250

CODE	MAIN TERM(S)	FIRST MODIFYING TERM	SECOND MODIFYING TERM	THIRD MODIFYING TERM	FOURTH MODIFYING TERM
52234	Cystourethroscopy	Treatment or fulgurations	Of a lesion or lesions	Using either cryosurgery or laser surgery	With or without a biopsy
52235/52240	Same	Same	Same except for size of lesions	Same	Same
52204	Cystourethroscopy	with biopsy			
52214	Cystourethroscopy	with fulguration	Of bladder, urethra or glands		
52224	Cystourethroscopy	with fulguration	No mention of specific urinary system structure or organ		

5. Find code or code ranges that include all or most of the medical record procedure or service description.

6. Disregard any code or code range containing additional descriptions or modifying terms not found in the medical record.

7. Write down the code or code ranges that best match the medical documentation.

CRITICAL THINKING APPLICATION

Kay is having trouble finding a procedure in the Alphabetic Index. What are some options and alternative ways Kay can perform an Alphabetic Index search?

Use of the Semicolon

If a main description is followed by a semicolon, this indicates that there are modifying terms and descriptions following it. Every indented description following a standalone code is related to that standalone code. Once there are no additional modifying terms for a main term, a new standalone description of a different procedure begins and is positioned flush left, without indentation.

Coding Decision Tree

A series of questions, sometimes called a decision tree, assists in navigating the Alphabetic Index and main text of the CPT-4. The decision tree for the main text is designed to guide the selection of the appropriate CPT-4 category I code or code range (Figure 18-4).

Following is an example of how to use the decision tree. The medical documentation narrative describes the following procedure: "excision of clavicular cyst." Begin the search in the Alphabetic Index using the main term "Excision" (procedure) and the modifying terms "clavicle" (anatomic site) and "cyst" (condition). Through use of the decision tree and code selection steps for the Alphabetic Index, the code found should be 23140.

In the main text, code 23410 is found in the Surgery section, the "musculoskeletal" subsection, the "excision" category, and finally the "shoulder" subcategory. The description of code 23410 is: "Excision or curettage of bone cyst or benign tumor of the clavicle or scapula."

Question 1: Does the medical documentation match the code description? Answer: Yes.

- The use of the word *or* between excision and curettage allows us to select "excision."
- The cyst is also included in the description.
- It states a bone cyst is acceptable; the clavicle is a bone.
- The use of the word *or* between clavicle and scapula allows us to select "clavicle."

Question 2: Does the code description add anything that is not documented in the medical record? Answer: No.

- Look above or below 23410, and read the descriptions. Notice that information is either missing or added to the documentation of "excision of clavicular cyst."
- Code 23145 is related to excision of a clavicular cyst but adds the description "with allograft," which is not in the documentation.
- The description for code 23130 directly above 23140 is "acromioplasty or acromionectomy, partial, with or without coracoacromial ligament release"—which certainly does not match the documentation in any way.

Question 3: Read the guidelines at the beginning of the Surgery section and before and after the subsection "musculo-skeletal system," the category "shoulder," and subcategory "excision." Is there anything in the guidelines that would prevent using code 23140 as the final code? Answer: No.

Question 4: Evaluate the conventions.

- Is there any indication that this is a revised or new code that might require a special report be sent with the insurance claim form? Answer: No.
- Is there an add-on code symbol, indicating that another procedure code should be used in addition to code 23140? Answer: No.
- Are any of the following conventions associated with code

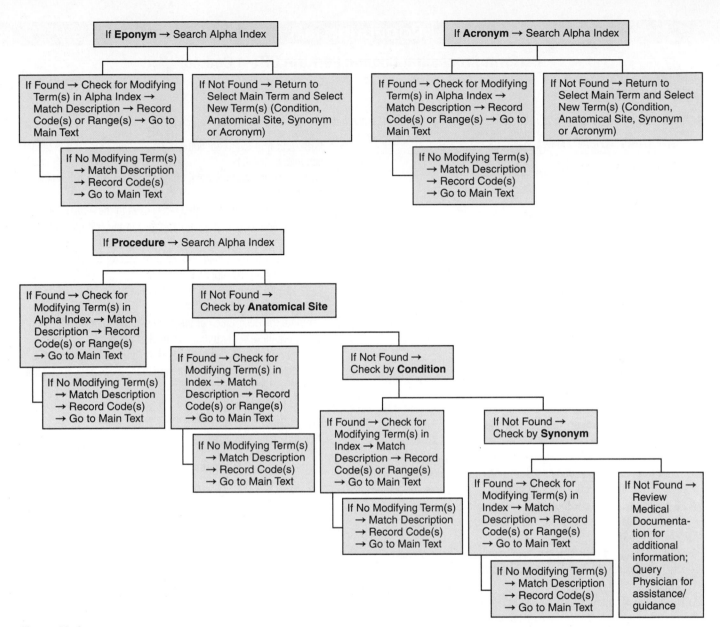

Figure 18-4 Decision tree for the CPT-4 main text.

23140: conscious sedation, exemption from modifier -63, or FDA approval pending? Answer: No.
- Code 23140 is not associated with any of the conventions or symbols that might require further action.

Question 5: Is there any indication in the medical documentation that a modifier might be required? Answer: No.

Based on these answers, 23140 is the most accurate and specific code to use with the medical narrative "excision of clavicular cyst."

Abstracting the procedure and service information from the patient medical record or encounter form is only the first step in the coding decision process. Procedure 18-1 illustrates the steps for using the Alphabetic Index and main text to guide the medical assistant to the selection of the most specific and accurate procedure or service code from the CPT-4 coding manual.

CRITICAL THINKING APPLICATION

If a patient was referred for epigastric pain and Dr. Shuman performed an ultrasound examination of the gallbladder, what would Kay need to consider to properly code this encounter for the ultrasound examination?

UNDERSTANDING EVALUATION AND MANAGEMENT

In order to properly code E&M services, it is important to understand how E&M services are classified. The E&M section is divided into broad subsections (Figure 18-5), such as "office visit," "emergency room visit," "hospital visit," and "consultation." These subsections are further divided into subcategories that include the place where the services were rendered—for example,

PROCEDURE 18-1

Perform Procedural Coding: Perform CPT-4 Coding

CAAHEP COMPETENCY: 3.a.(3)(c)
ABHES COMPETENCY: 3.v

GOAL: Use the steps for procedure and service coding to find the most accurate and specific CPT-4 category I code.

EQUIPMENT and SUPPLIES

- CPT-4 Coding Manual (current year)
- Encounter form (charge ticket)
- Medical record
- Paper
- Pen or pencil
- Medical dictionary or medical terminology reference book

PROCEDURAL STEPS

1. Read medical documentation to determine what procedures or services were provided.
   PURPOSE: To ensure all procedures and/or services are listed in the encounter form; that all procedures and services on the encounter form match the medical record; and that nothing documented in the medical record is missing from the encounter form.

2. Select main term classification to begin search.
   PURPOSE: To identify the term or terms to begin the search in the Alphabetic Index.

3. Select modifying term(s) if needed once main term is located.
   PURPOSE: To provide additional specificity and help narrow down the search for the code or code range in the Alphabetic Index.

4. If no modifying term produces an appropriate code or code range, repeat steps 2 and 3 using a different main term classification.
   PURPOSE: To aid in finding the most appropriate code or code range by using alternative methods of searching the Alphabetic Index.

5. Find code or code ranges that include all or most of the medical record procedure or service description.
   PURPOSE: To assist in directing the medical assistant to the proper section, subsection, category or subcategory of the main text of the CPT-4.

6. Disregard any code or code range containing additional descriptions or modifying terms not found in the medical record.

PURPOSE: To prevent upcoding or downcoding errors and other compliance issues.

7. Write down the code or code ranges that best match medical documentation.
   PURPOSE: To prevent repeated references to the Alphabetic Index by recording all possible matches to the code or code range being sought. It saves both time and redundant effort.

8. Turn to the main text, and find the first code or code range found while searching the Alphabetic Index.
   PURPOSE: To begin the process of finding the most specific and accurate code.

9. Compare the description of the code with the medical documentation. Verify that all or most of the medical record documentation matches the code description and that there is no additional element or information in the code description that is not found in the documentation.
   PURPOSE: To avoid upcoding and downcoding errors, and to ensure there are no contraindications to use of the code selected.

10. Read the guidelines for the section, subsection, and code to ensure there are no contraindications to the use of the code.
    PURPOSE: To ensure there are no instructions that would prevent use of the code selected.

11. Evaluate the conventions, especially add-on codes (+) and exemption from modifier -51.
    PURPOSE: To ensure there are no instructions that would prevent use of the code selected.

12. Determine if there are special circumstances that require the use of a modifier.
    PURPOSE: To select, if appropriate, modifiers that provide additional information for the code selected to explain certain circumstances or provide additional detail.

13. Record the CPT-4 code selected in the medical record documentation next to the procedure or service performed and in the appropriate block of the insurance claim form.

the provider's office, the emergency room, a skilled nursing facility, or the patient's home—and the patient status—that is, whether the patient is new or established.

The first two steps in choosing an E&M code are identifying the **place of service** (POS) and the patient status. The two most common place of service are "office" and "hospital." Table 18-5 provides a more complete list of POS locations and their two-digit identifying numbers. The patient status choices are new or established patient. A **new patient** (NP) is new to the practice or has not been seen by the physician or any of the physicians in

a group practice for more than 3 years. An **established patient** (EP) is one who has a continuing relationship with the practice and has been seen within the last 3 years.

Once the place of service and patient status are established, the next step in selection of an E&M code is determining the level of service provided. Three key components affect code selection: history, examination, and medical decision making. The findings of the history and physical examination, the complexity of the history and examination, and the complexity of medical decision making all factor into the level of E&M

►Initial Nursing Facility Care◄

New or Established Patient

When the patient is admitted to the nursing facility in the course of an encounter in another site of service (eg, hospital emergency department, physician's office), all evaluation and management services provided by that physician in conjunction with that admission are considered part of the initial nursing facility care when performed on the same date as the admission or readmission. The nursing facility care level of service reported by the admitting physician should include the services related to the admission he/she provided in the other sites of service as well as in the nursing facility setting.

Hospital discharge or observation discharge services performed on the same date of nursing facility admission or readmission may be reported separately. For a patient discharged from inpatient status on the same date of nursing facility admission or readmission, the hospital discharge services should be reported with codes 99238, 99239 as appropriate. For a patient discharged from observation status on the same date of nursing facility admission or readmission, the observation care discharge services should be reported with code 99217. For a patient admitted and discharged from observation or inpatient status on the same date, see codes 99234-99236.

(For nursing facility care discharge, see 99315, 99316)

►Typical unit times have not been established for 99304-99306.◄

►(99301-99303 have been deleted)◄

● **99304** Initial nursing facility care, per day, for the evaluation and management of a patient which requires these three key components:

■ **a detailed or comprehensive history;**

■ **a detailed or comprehensive examination; and**

■ **medical decision making that is straightforward or of low complexity.**

Counseling and/or coordination of care with other providers or agencies are provided consistent with the nature of the problem(s) and the patient's and/or family's needs.

Usually, the problem(s) requiring admission are of low severity.

Subsequent Nursing Facility Care

►All levels of subsequent nursing facility care include reviewing the medical record and reviewing the results of diagnostic studies and changes in the patient's status (ie, changes in history, physical condition, and response to management) since the last assessment by the physician.◄

● **99307** Subsequent nursing facility care, per day, for the evaluation and management of a patient, which requires at least two of these three key components:

■ **a problem focused interval history;**

■ **a problem focused examination;**

■ **straightforward medical decision making.**

Counseling and/or coordination of care with other providers or agencies are provided consistent with the nature of the problem(s) and the patient's and/or family's needs.

Usually, the patient is stable, recovering, or improving.

● **99308** Subsequent nursing facility care, per day, for the evaluation and management of a patient, which requires at least two of these three key components:

■ **an expanded problem focused interval history;**

■ **an expanded problem focused examination;**

■ **medical decision making of low complexity.**

Counseling and/or coordination of care with other providers or agencies are provided consistent with the nature of the problem(s) and the patient's and/or family's needs.

Usually, the patient is responding inadequately to therapy or has developed a minor complication.

● **99309** Subsequent nursing facility care, per day, for the evaluation and management of a patient, which requires at least two of these three key components:

■ **a detailed interval history;**

■ **a detailed examination;**

■ **medical decision making of moderate complexity.**

Counseling and/or coordination of care with other providers or agencies are provided consistent with the nature of the problem(s) and the patient's and/or family's needs.

Usually, the patient has developed a significant complication or a significant new problem.

Figure 18-5 Example of Evaluation and Management: new or established patient and place of service.

TABLE 18-5 Place-of-Service List

CODE	PLACE OF SERVICE	CODE	PLACE OF SERVICE
01	Pharmacy	41	Ambulance—land
03	School	42	Ambulance—air
04	Homeless shelter	49	Independence clinic
11	Office	50	Federally qualified health center
12	Patient's home	51	Inpatient psychiatric facility
13	Assisted-living facility	52	Partial hospitalization, psychiatric facility
14	Group home	53	Community mental health center
15	Mobile unit	54	Intermediate care facility/mentally retarded
20	Urgent care facility	55	Residential substance abuse treatment facility
21	Inpatient hospital	56	Psychiatric residential treatment center
22	Outpatient hospital	57	Nonresidential substance abuse treatment facility
23	Emergency department (ED) hospital	60	Mass immunization facility
24	Ambulatory surgery center (ASC)	61	Comprehensive inpatient rehabilitation facility
25	Birthing center	62	Comprehensive outpatient rehabilitation facility
26	Military treatment facility	65	End-stage renal disease treatment facility
31	Skilled nursing facility (SNF)	71	State or local public health clinic
32	Nursing facility	72	Rural health clinic
33	Custodial care facility	81	Independent laboratory
34	Hospice	99	Other unlisted facility

code selected. There are also contributing factors that aid in level of service determination: counseling, coordination of care, nature of presenting problem, and time.

The steps for finding a category I code for E&M services are quite different from those discussed earlier in this chapter (Procedure 18-2). The instructions include identifying the section, subsection, category, and subcategory of the procedure or service; reviewing the reporting instructions and guidelines for the code chosen; reviewing the level of E&M service; determining the extent of history obtained and examination performed; and determining the complexity of medical decision making.

Considerations for Evaluation and Management (E&M) Coding

Evaluation and Management Level of Service Components

There are seven components for determining the level of service for E&M: history, examination, medical decision making, counseling, nature of presenting problem, coordination of care, and time. The history, examination, and medical decision-making components are considered key. In other words, they are typically the three most important components for deciding the level of service. Counseling, coordination of care, nature of presenting problem, and time are secondary considerations and are called *contributing factors*.

Key Components

History. To understand the levels of history it is important to know the definition and components of the patient's history. The history relates to the patient's clinical picture and depends on the patient for answers to specific questions. The history is a subjective narrative account in the patient's own words. The history is composed of the following:

- Chief complaint (CC), or reason the patient is being seen: This is usually in the patient's own words.
- History of present illness (HPI): Identifies the location, severity, timing, modifying factors, quality, duration, context, and associated signs and symptoms relating to the chief complaint.
- Review of systems (ROS): The patient answers questions about the following systems and organs: constitutional; eyes; ear, nose, and throat (ENT), and mouth; cardiac; gastrointestinal; musculoskeletal; endocrine; neurologic; integumentary; psychiatric; genitourinary; allergic or immunologic; respiratory; and hematologic or lymphatic.
- Past medical, family, and social history (PMFSH): Patient's experiences with illness and surgery; whether they smoke or use illicit drugs and/or alcohol; whether the patient is married or has children; where the patient lives; and what diseases the patient's blood relatives have had play an extremely important part in determining risk factors for illness.

Levels of history.

- Problem-focused history: A problem-focused history concentrates on the chief complaint; it looks at the symptoms,

PROCEDURE 18-2

Perform Procedural Coding: Perform Evaluation and Management Coding

CAAHEP COMPETENCY: 3.a.(3)(c)
ABHES COMPETENCY: 3.v

GOAL: *Use the steps for Evaluation and Management (E&M) coding to find the most accurate and specific CPT-4 category I E&M section code.*

EQUIPMENT and SUPPLIES

- CPT-4 Coding Manual (current year)
- Encounter form (charge ticket)
- Medical Record
- Paper
- Pen or pencil
- Medical dictionary or medical terminology reference book

PROCEDURAL STEPS

1. Identify the place of service.
   PURPOSE: To determine where the procedure or service was performed.
2. Identify the patient status.
   PURPOSE: To determine if the patient is new or established.
3. Identify the subsection, category, or subcategory of service in the Evaluation and Management section.
   PURPOSE: To ensure that the correct place of service and patient status are used, as well as the appropriate level of service is selected.
4. Review the guidelines and notes for the selected subsection, category, or subcategory.

PURPOSE: To determine if there are any contraindications for use of the code selected.

5. Review the level of E&M service descriptions for each code in the subsection, category, or subcategory chosen.
   PURPOSE: To assist in selection of the appropriate level of service.
6. If needed, compare medical documentation against examples in Appendix C, Clinical Examples, of the CPT-4 manual.
   PURPOSE: To compare the medical documentation to the examples in Appendix C for assistance in selection of the appropriate level of service.
7. Determine the extent of history obtained.
   PURPOSE: To ensure the correct level of history is chosen.
8. Determine the extent of examination performed.
   PURPOSE: To ensure the correct level of examination is chosen.
9. Determine the complexity of medical decision making.
   PURPOSE: To ensure the correct level of medical decision making is chosen.
10. Select the appropriate level of E&M service code, and document it on the medical record or encounter form.

---

severity, and duration of the problem. It usually does not include an ROS or family and social history.

- Expanded problem-focused history: The physician proceeds as in the problem-focused history but includes a review of the systems that relate to the chief complaint. Usually past, family, and social histories are not included.
- Detailed history: The physician will document a more extensive history, ROS, and pertinent past, family, and social histories.
- Comprehensive history: The physician will document responses to all of the components listed previously. A comprehensive history is usually taken during an initial visit with patients who have a significant history of illness.

Examination. The examination is the objective part of the patient's visit. The physician examines the patient, obtains measurable findings, and makes notes referring to body areas and/or organ systems, as follows:

- Body areas: Head including face and neck; chest including breasts and axillas; abdomen; genitourinary (GU) system; back, including spine and extremities
- Organs and organ systems: Constitutional; eyes; ENT and mouth; cardiovascular; respiratory; gastrointestinal (GI); GU; musculoskeletal; skin; neurologic; psychiatric; and hematologic, lymphatic, and immunologic

The examination is divided into the following levels:

- Problem-focused examination: The examination is limited to the single body area or single system mentioned in the chief complaint.
- Expanded problem-focused examination: In addition to the limited body area or system, related body areas or organ systems are examined.
- Detailed examination: An extended examination is performed on the related body areas or organ systems.
- Comprehensive examination: A complete multisystem examination is performed.

Medical Decision Making. When a physician makes medical decisions, the decisions are based on many years of education and experience. Three elements comprise the medical decision-making process: number of diagnoses and management options; amount and complexity of data reviewed; and risk of complications and/or morbidity or mortality.

- Number of diagnoses and management options: The physician's notes during the history and examination should help identify whether the patient's problem is minor, acute, stable, or worsening. The medical documentation should also identify whether a new problem exists or whether the physician plans to order any diagnostic tests to further investigate the patient's illness or injury.

TABLE 18-6 Complexity of Medical Decision Making

NUMBER OF DIAGNOSES OR MANAGEMENT OPTIONS	AMOUNT AND/OR COMPLEXITY OF DATA TO BE REVIEWED	RISK OF COMPLICATIONS AND/OR MORBIDITY OR MORTALITY	TYPE OF MEDICAL DECISION MAKING
Minimal	Minimal or none	Minimal	Straightforward
Limited	Limited	Low	Low complexity
Multiple	Moderate	Moderate	Moderate complexity
Extensive	Extensive	High	High complexity

- Amount and complexity of data reviewed: The medical documentation should also identify what laboratory tests, x-ray diagnostic procedures, and other tests have been ordered or reviewed.
- Risk of complications and morbidity or mortality: Risk is often involved in medical care, either from the treatment given to the patient or from the lack of treatment and professional care. Morbidity, the relative incidence of disease, and mortality, which relates to the number of deaths from a given disease, is an integral part of the assessment of risks made by the physician.

Medical decision-making complexity levels. There are four levels of complexity in medical decision making: straightforward and low, moderate, and high complexity. See Table 18-6 for a description of each of the four levels.

- Straightforward: Minimal diagnosis and management options, minimal to no complex data to be reviewed, and minimal risk to the patient of complications or death if untreated
- Low complexity: Limited number of diagnoses or management options, limited data to be reviewed, and low risk to the patient of complications or death if untreated
- Moderate complexity: Multiple diagnoses or management options, moderate amount and complexity of data to be reviewed, and moderate risk to the patient of complications or death if untreated
- High complexity: Extensive diagnoses or management options, extensive amount and complexity of data to be reviewed, and high risk to the patient for complications and/or death if the problem is untreated

Contributing Factors

Counseling. Counseling is a discussion with a patient and/or family regarding diagnostic results, impressions, recommended diagnostic studies, prognosis, risks and benefits of management or treatment options, and instructions for management, treatment, and/or follow-up. Almost all E&M services contain a degree of counseling with the patient and/or the family. This is factored into the E&M code, and as long as this factor does not exceed 50% of the time spent with the patient, it is included in the E&M code. It can be considered a contributing factor when the counseling exceeds 50% of the encounter.

Coordination of care. Some patients need assistance in arranging for care beyond the visit or hospitalization. Some will need care in a skilled nursing facility or home health care. Others will need hospice care. The primary physician usually coordinates this care. Coordination of care is also factored into the E&M code and is a consideration for determining level of service only when it exceeds 50% of the patient encounter.

Nature of presenting problem. The presenting problem is usually explained in the chief complaint. It can range from something as simple as a cold in an otherwise healthy patient to a life-threatening problem. Unless the nature of the presenting problem exceeds half of the patient encounter, it is included in the E&M code description and is not a factor in selecting the level of service.

Time. Time is included in the E&M code descriptions only to assist physicians in selecting the most appropriate level of E&M service. The times expressed in the code descriptions are averages, and time is not a determining factor in code selection unless counseling exceeds more than 50% of the encounter. Only then can time be used as a determining component to code level selection.

Selecting a Level of E&M Service

1. Identify the category and subcategory of service.
2. Review the guidelines and reporting instructions for the selected category or subcategory.
3. Review the level of E&M service descriptions and examples.
4. If needed, compare medical documentation against examples in Appendix C: Clinical Examples to assist in selection of service level.
5. Determine the extent of history obtained.
6. Determine the extent of examination performed.
7. Determine the complexity of medical decision making.
8. Select the appropriate level of E&M service based on the following:
   a. All of the key components—history, examination, and medical decision making—must meet or exceed the stated requirements to qualify for the level selected if service is in the following category or subcategory:
      i. Office, new patient
      ii. Hospital observation service
      iii. Initial hospital care
      iv. Office consultations
      v. Emergency department services
      vi. Initial nursing facility care
      vii. Domiciliary care
      viii. New patient
      ix. Home, new patient
   b. Two of the three key components must meet or exceed

the stated requirements to qualify for the level selected if service is in the following category or subcategory:

    i. Office, established patient
    ii. Subsequent hospital care
    iii. Subsequent nursing facility care
    iv. Domiciliary care
    v. Established patient
    vi. Home, established patient

  c. Time may be considered one of the key components if counseling and/or coordination of care dominates more than 50% of the encounter.

Evaluation and Management (E&M) coding is difficult at first to understand and put into practice. The steps for E&M coding will act as a guide in determining the place of service, patient status, and the level of care provided in order to select the most accurate E&M code. Using Appendix C's clinical examples and comparing them to the medical documentation will also help provide a better understanding of E&M coding.

CRITICAL THINKING APPLICATION

Dr. Shuman performed a colonoscopy at the hospital on a patient, Cecil Matthews, who has been Dr. Shuman's patient for several years. Mr. Matthews came to the office with left lower quadrant pain and a history of colon cancer. What other factors or information would Kay need to know to properly code Mr. Matthews' office visit (encounter)?

ANESTHESIA CODING

The codes for anesthesia are listed in the Anesthesia section of the CPT-4 primarily, although codes for conscious sedation are found in the Medicine section. The codes are selected based primarily on the anatomic location of the surgery being performed—for example, code 00402 is for anesthesia during a reconstructive procedure on the breast in the integumentary system. In addition, there are categories and subcategories for radiologic procedures, burns, excisions, debridement, obstetric procedures, physiologic support during the harvesting of organs, and anesthesia delivered during nerve block procedures. The anesthesia codes include preoperative and postoperative visits, anesthesia care during the procedure, the administration of fluids and/or blood, and the usual monitoring services performed during anesthesia. The provider of anesthesia cannot bill separately for any of these services unless unusual circumstances exist. What makes anesthesia coding different from any other coding is the way in which anesthesia services are billed. There is a standard formula for payment of anesthesia services: basic units + time units + modifying units (B + T + M). This formula is also affected by two factors: the patient's **physical status** (PS), and any qualifying circumstances (QC). The steps for anesthesia coding are shown in Procedure 18-3.

Anesthesia Formula

Basic Unit Value (B)

The Anesthesia Society of America (ASA) publishes a *Relative Value Guide* (RVG), which lists the codes for anesthesia services.

The RVG compares anesthesia services with one another and assigns a numeric value to each service based on the level of complexity. This numeric value is called the *basic unit value*.

Time Unit (T)

Anesthesia services are provided based on the time during which the anesthesia was administered, in hours and minutes. Typically 15 minutes equals one time unit, although this can vary because insurance carriers make that determination independently. The time starts when the anesthesiologist begins preparing the patient to receive anesthesia, continues though the procedure, and ends when the patient is no longer under the personal care of the anesthesiologist. The hours and minutes during which anesthesia was administered are recorded in the patient record.

Modifying Unit (M)

Modifying units reflect circumstances or conditions that change or modify the environment in which the anesthesia service is provided. There are two modifying characteristics for anesthesia services: qualifying circumstances and physical status modifiers. A list and the descriptions of these modifiers are located in the Anesthesia section of the CPT-4. They are also shown in Table 18-7.

Qualifying Circumstances (QC)

Sometimes anesthesia is provided in situations that make the administration of the anesthesia more difficult. These types of cases include those performed in emergency situations, to patients of extreme age, during the use of controlled hypotension, and with hypothermia. There are four qualifying circumstances (QC) codes. Each of the five-digit codes is preceded by a + symbol, indicating that it is an add-on code, and is used in addition to the category I anesthesia code.

Physical Status Modifiers (PS)

The second type of modifying unit used in anesthesia coding is the physical status modifier. These modifiers are used to indicate the patient's physical condition at the time anesthesia was administered. There are five physical status modifiers, composed of two characters: first the letter P, followed by a ranking of 1 to 5 (e.g., P1, P2, P3). P1 represents a normal healthy patient, and P5 represents a brain-dead patient whose organs are being harvested.

Conversion Factors

A conversion factor is the dollar value of each basic unit value. Each third-party payor issues a list of conversion factors. The conversion factor for any given geographic location is multiplied by the number of basic unit values assigned to each procedure. See Figure 18-6 for a sample list of geographic conversion factors.

Calculating Anesthesia Services

Calculation of the fee for anesthesia services is performed using the anesthesia billing formula, B + M + T multiplied times the conversion factor (Figure 18-7).

PROCEDURE 18-3

Perform Procedural Coding: Perform Anesthesia Coding

CAAHEP COMPETENCY: 3.a.(3)(c)
ABHES COMPETENCY: 3.v

GOAL: *Use the steps to select the most accurate and specific anesthesia code, and perform the anesthesia formula calculation to determine the charge for the service.*

EQUIPMENT and SUPPLIES

- CPT-4 Coding Manual (current year)
- Encounter form (charge ticket)
- Medical record
- Conversion factor list (issued by an insurance carrier: for the purposes of this exercise, use the example in Figure 18-5).
- Paper
- Pen or pencil
- Calculator

PROCEDURAL STEPS

1. Read the medical documentation to determine what procedure or service was provided.
   PURPOSE: To ensure all procedures and/or services are listed on the encounter form; that all procedures and services on the encounter form are documented in the medical record; and that nothing documented in the medical record was omitted from the charge ticket.

2. Determine the anatomic site or organ system involved.
   PURPOSE: Anesthesia service codes use the anatomical site and organ system as a category.

3. In the Alphabetic Index, go to the heading "Anesthesia" and find the code or code range that includes all or most of the medical record procedure or service.
   PURPOSE: To avoid selecting a surgery or other type of procedure or service code other than anesthesia-related codes.

4. Write down the code or code range found in the Alphabetic Index, under the Anesthesia heading, that best matches the medical documentation.
   PURPOSE: To prevent repeated references to the Alphabetic Index by recording all possible matches to the code or code range being sought. It saves both time and redundant effort.

5. Turn to the main text, Anesthesia section, and find the code or code range found while searching the Alphabetic Index.

PURPOSE: To verify and select the most specific anesthesia code.

6. Read the guidelines and notes for the section, subsection, category, or subcategory.
   PURPOSE: To ensure the correct code is chosen and there are no instructions that prevent use of the code selected.

7. Evaluate the conventions, especially add-on codes (+) and exemptions from modifier -51.
   PURPOSE: To ensure the correct code is chosen and there are no contraindications to use of the code.

8. Document the code selected.
   PURPOSE: To determine the basic unit value and perform the anesthesia calculation to determine the charge.

9. Determine the Basic Unit Value from the Relative Value Guide.
   PURPOSE: Use to perform the anesthesia calculation to determine the charge for the anesthesia service.

10. Determine the patient's physical status, and document the appropriate modifier.
    PURPOSE: Used to perform the anesthesia calculation to determine the charge for the anesthesia service.

11. Determine if any qualifying circumstance modifier should be used. If yes, document the modifier.
    PURPOSE: Used to perform the anesthesia calculation to determine the charge for the anesthesia service.

12. Determine the total anesthesia time, divide by 15 (minutes) and document the time.
    PURPOSE: Used to perform the anesthesia calculation to determine the charge for the anesthesia service.

13. Select the appropriate geographic conversion factor.
    PURPOSE: Used to perform the anesthesia calculation to determine the charge for the anesthesia service.

14. Calculate the charge for the anesthesia service using the anesthesia formula.
    PURPOSE: To determine the charge for the anesthesia service or procedure.

15. Document the anesthesia charge and the code in the medical record and on the encounter form or charge ticket.

RADIOLOGY CODING

The Radiology section contains all diagnostic imaging codes, including not just x-ray studies, but also ultrasound, magnetic resonance imaging (MRI), and nuclear medicine procedures, as well as radiation oncology and several other types of diagnostic imaging procedures, services, and therapies. See Figure 18-8 for an illustration of the Radiology section from the CPT-4. The Radiology section is further subdivided into subsections,

such as head and neck, then chest, spine, and pelvis, upper and lower extremities, abdomen, gastrointestinal and urinary tracts, gynecologic, obstetric and vascular procedures. The next subdivision, categories, define the types or function of various procedures—e.g., diagnostic ultrasound, radiation oncology, hypothermia, and so on—that are unique to the anatomic site subsection. In addition to the radiology procedure codes, codes are included for physician supervision and interpretation of diagnostic imaging data; clinical and radiation treatment

TABLE 18-7 Anesthesia Physical Status and Qualifying Circumstances Modifiers

MODIFIER	DESCRIPTION
Physical Status Modifiers*	
P1	A normal healthy patient
P2	A patient with mild systemic disease
P3	A patient with severe systemic disease
P4	A person with severe systemic disease that is a constant threat to life
P5	A moribund patient who is not expected to survive without the procedure
P6	A declared brain-dead patient whose organs are being removed for donor purposes
Qualifying Circumstances Modifiers†	
99100	Anesthesia for patient of extreme age, under 1 year or over 70
99116	Anesthesia complicated by utilization of total body hypothermia
99135	Anesthesia complicated by utilization of total body hypothermia

*A physical status modifier is required for use in performing anesthesia calculations.
†Use a qualifying circumstances modifier code, if appropriate, in addition to the primary CPT category I Anesthesia code.

Locality Name	Anesthesia Conversion Factor
Manhattan, NY	19.49
NYC suburbs/Long I., NY	19.25
Queens, NY	18.97
Rest of state	16.16
North Carolina	15.56
North Dakota	15.25

Figure 18-6 Anesthesia conversion factors. (From Buck CJ: *Step-by-step medical coding,* 2006, St Louis, 2006, Saunders.)

Medical Narrative

A 25-year-old female patient in good physical condition has anesthesia services while undergoing laparoscopy (CPT-4 Code 00840). The time for the anesthesia administration was 2 hours. For the purposes of this example the RBV basic unit value will be 4.

Basic Unit Value = 4
+ Modifying Units: PS = 0
+ QC = 0
+ Time Units = 8
= 12 Total Units

The total units value of 12 is then multiplied by the conversion factor for the geographic location of the anesthesiologist's office. For the purposes of this exercise, the conversion factor for Manhattan, NY, will be $20.48, and for North Carolina, $15.77. For the office located in Manhattan, NY, multiply $20.48 by 12. The fee for the anesthesia services would be $245.76. For the office located in North Carolina, multiply 12 times $15.77, for a fee of $189.24.

Figure 18-7 Anesthesia formula and calculation example.

planning, and administration of contrast materials during radiologic procedures.

The coding steps for radiologic procedures are the same as those for other category I codes. When searching by main term in the Alphabetic Index, using "Radiology" as the main term, a "See" note directs the codes to the more specific subcategories of nuclear medicine, ultrasound, radiation therapy, and x-ray studies. As always, a thorough review of the conventions, guidelines, and notes in the CPT-4 main text is essential to accurate coding.

PATHOLOGY AND LABORATORY SECTION

The subcategories for the Pathology and Laboratory section include organ and disease panels, drug testing, therapeutic drug assays, evocative or suppression testing, consultations, urinalysis, chemistry, molecular diagnostics, infectious agents, microbiology, anatomic pathology, cytopathology, cytogenetic studies, and surgical pathology. Figure 18-9 is an illustration of the organ panels subsection of the Pathology and Laboratory section.

Organ or disease panels are groupings of numerous tests performed to diagnose the health or disease status of specific

Radiology

Diagnostic Radiology (Diagnostic Imaging)

Head and Neck

70010 Myelography, posterior fossa, radiological supervision and interpretation

70015 Cisternography, positive contrast, radiological supervision and interpretation

70030 Radiologic examination, eye, for detection of foreign body

70100 Radiologic examination, mandible; partial, less than four views

70110 complete, minimum of four views

70120 Radiologic examination, mastoids; less than three views per side

70130 complete, minimum of three views per side

70134 Radiologic examination, internal auditory meati, complete

70140 Radiologic examination, facial bones; less than three views

Figure 18-8 Radiology section of CPT-4.

Pathology and Laboratory

Organ or Disease Oriented Panels

These panels were developed for coding purposes only and should not be interpreted as clinical parameters. The tests listed with each panel identify the defined components of that panel.

These panel components are not intended to limit the performance of other tests. If one performs tests in addition to those specifically indicated for a particular panel, those tests should be reported separately in addition to the panel code.

80048 Basic metabolic panel

This panel must include the following:

Calcium (82310)

Carbon dioxide (82374)

Chloride (82435)

Creatinine (82565)

Glucose (82947)

Potassium (84132)

Sodium (84295)

Urea nitrogen (BUN) (84520)

(Do not use 80048 in addition to 80053)

80050 General health panel

This panel must include the following:

Comprehensive metabolic panel (80053)

Blood count, complete (CBC), automated and automated differential WBC count (85025 or 85027 and 85004)

Figure 18-9 Pathology and laboratory section of CPT-4.

organ systems. In order to use a panel code, all of the tests listed under the code selected must have been performed. Otherwise, the individual tests should be billed using a separate code for each. The codes for drug testing are qualitative—they are based on which *type* of drug is found. Quantitative assays on the other hand, are performed to determine the *amount* of drug found.

MEDICINE SUBSECTIONS

Immune Globulins

When coding immune globulins administration, identify the immune globulin product being administered and the method of administration using the codes in the "hydration, therapeutic, prophylactic, and diagnostic injections and infusions" subsection (Figure 18-10).

Immunization Administration for Vaccines or Toxoids

These codes are for the administration of vaccines and toxoids only and should be reported in conjunction with the appropriate codes in the "immunization administration for vaccine/toxoids" subsection (Figure 18-11).

Vaccines, Toxoids

These codes identify the vaccine product only. Codes in the Immunization Administration for Vaccines/Toxoids subsection must be used in addition to the vaccine or toxoid product codes. To meet the reporting requirements of immunization registries, vaccine distribution programs, and reporting systems the exact vaccine product administered needs to be reported on the insurance claim form.

Medicine

Immune Globulins

►Codes 90281-90399 identify the immune globulin product only and must be reported in addition to the administration codes 90765-90768, 90772, 90774, 90775 as appropriate. Immune globulin products listed here include broad-spectrum and anti-infective immune globulins, antitoxins, and various isoantibodies.◄

⊘ **90281**   Immune globulin (Ig), human, for intramuscular use

⊘ **90283**   Immune globulin (IgIV), human, for intravenous use

⊘ **90287**   Botulinum antitoxin, equine, any route

⊘ **90288**   Botulism immune globulin, human, for intravenous use

⊘ **90291**   Cytomegalovirus immune globulin (CMV-IgIV), human, for intravenous use

⊘ **90296**   Diphtheria antitoxin, equine, any route

⊘ **90371**   Hepatitis B immune globulin (HBIg), human, for intramuscular use

⊘ **90375**   Rabies immune globulin (RIg), human, for intramuscular and/or subcutaneous use

⊘ **90376**   Rabies immune globulin, heat-treated (RIg-HT), human, for intramuscular and/or subcutaneous use

Figure 18-10 Relationship of immune globulins and infusions in CPT-4.

Hydration, Therapeutic, Prophylactic, and Diagnostic Injections and Infusion

Hydration codes are intended to report a hydration intravenous (IV) infusion to consist of a prepackaged fluid and electrolytes but are not used to report infusion of drugs or other substances. When multiple drugs are administered, report the service(s) and the specific materials or drugs for each.

Psychiatric Diagnostic or Evaluative Interview Procedures

Psychiatric diagnostic interview examination includes a history, mental status, and a disposition and may include communication with family or other sources and ordering of and medical interpretation of laboratory or other medical diagnostic studies.

Psychiatric Therapeutic Procedures

Psychotherapy is the treatment for mental illness and behavioral disturbances in which the clinician attempts to alleviate the emotional disturbances, reverse or change maladaptive patterns of behavior, and encourage personality growth and development.

Dialysis

These codes are reported once per month to distinguish age-specific service related to the patient's end-stage renal disease

Immunization Administration for Vaccines/Toxoids

Codes 90465-90474 must be reported in addition to the vaccine and toxoid code(s) 90476-90749.

Report codes 90465-90468 only when the physician provides face-to-face counseling of the patient and family during the administration of a vaccine. For immunization administration of any vaccine that is not accompanied by face-to-face physician counseling to the patient/family, report codes 90471-90474.

If a significant separately identifiable Evaluation and Management service (e.g., office or other outpatient services, preventive medicine services) is performed, the appropriate E/M service code should be reported in addition to the vaccine and toxoid administration codes.

(For allergy testing, see 95004 et seq)

(For skin testing of bacterial, viral, fungal extracts, see 86485-86586)

►(For therapeutic or diagnostic injections, see 90772-90779)◄

90465   Immunization administration under 8 years of age (includes percutaneous, intradermal, subcutaneous, or intramuscular injections) when the physician counsels the patient/family; first injection (single or combination vaccine/toxoid), per day

(Do not report 90465 in conjunction with 90467)

+ 90466   each additional injection (single or combination vaccine/toxoid), per day (List separately in addition to code for primary procedure)

(Use 90466 in conjunction with 90465 or 90467)

Figure 18-11 Relationship of immune vaccines/toxoids and administration codes in CPT-4.

(ESRD) performed in an outpatient setting. Dialysis codes describe a full month of ESRD-related service provided in an outpatient setting.

Cardiology

Echocardiography

Echocardiography is an ultrasound examination of the cardiac chambers and valves, the adjacent great vessels, and the pericardium.

Cardiac Catheterization

Cardiac catheterization is a diagnostic medical procedure that includes introduction, positioning and repositioning of catheter(s), recording of intracardiac and intravascular pressure, obtaining blood samples for measurement purposes, cardiac output measurements with or without electrode catheter placement, and final evaluation and reporting of the procedure.

Intracardiac Electrophysiologic Procedures and Studies

Intracardiac electrophysiologic studies (EPS) are invasive diagnostic medical procedures that include the procedure itself, insertion and repositioning of electrode catheters, recording of electrograms before and during pacing or programmed stimulation of multiple locations in the heart, analysis of recorded information, and reporting of the procedure.

Peripheral Arterial Disease Rehabilitation

Peripheral arterial disease (PAD) rehabilitative physical exercise consists of a series of sessions, lasting 45 to 60 minutes per session, involving use of either a motorized treadmill or a track.

Noninvasive Vascular Diagnostic Studies

Vascular studies include patient care required to perform the studies, supervision of the studies, and interpretation of study results, with copies for patient records of hard copy output with analysis of all data.

Sleep Testing

Sleep studies and *polysomnography* refer to the continuous and simultaneous monitoring and recording of various physiologic parameters of sleep for 6 or more hours with physician review, interpretation, and report. The studies are performed to diagnose a variety of sleep disorders and to evaluate a patient's response to therapies such as nasal continuous positive airway pressure (NCPAP).

Nervous System

Central Nervous System Assessments and Tests

Codes for central nervous system assessments and tests are used to report the services provided during testing of the cognitive function of the central nervous system.

Health and Behavior Assessment and Intervention

Health and behavior assessment procedures are used to identify the psychologic, behavioral, emotional, cognitive, and social factors important to the prevention, treatment, or management of physical health problems.

Chemotherapy Administration

Chemotherapy administration codes apply to parenteral administration of specific drugs and agents that are provided for treatment of cancer and noncancer diagnoses.

Injection and Intravenous Infusion Chemotherapy

IV or intraarterial push is defined as an injection in which the healthcare professional who administers the substance or drug is continuously present to administer the injection and observe the patient, or as an infusion of 15 minutes or less.

Modalities

Modality codes apply to any physical agent applied to produce therapeutic changes to biologic tissue; this includes but is not limited to thermal, acoustic, light, mechanical, or electric energy.

Active Wound Care Management

Active wound care procedures are performed to remove devitalized and/or necrotic tissue and promote healing. The provider is required to have direct (one-on-one) patient contact to use these codes.

Acupuncture

Acupuncture is reported based on 15-minute increments of personal (face-to-face) contact with the patient, not the duration of acupuncture needle(s) placement. Only one code may be reported for each 15-minute increment.

Osteopathic Manipulative Treatment

Osteopathic manipulative treatment (OMT) is a form of manual treatment applied by a physician to eliminate or alleviate somatic dysfunction and related disorders.

Chiropractic Manipulative Treatment

Chiropractic manipulative treatment (CMT) is a form of manual treatment to influence joint and neurophysiologic function. The CMT codes include a premanipulation patient assessment. For purposes of CMT, the five spinal regions referred to are the cervical region, thoracic region, lumbar region, sacral region, and pelvic region.

Education and Training for Patient Self-Management

These codes are used to report education and training services prescribed by a physician and provided by a qualified, non-physician healthcare professional using a standardized curriculum to an individual or a group of patients for the treatment of established illness(s) or disease(s).

Home Health Procedures and Services

These codes are used by nonphysician health care professionals only. They are used to report services provided in a patient's residence (including assisted living apartments, group homes, nontraditional private homes, custodial care facilities, and schools).

HEALTHCARE COMMON PROCEDURE CODING SYSTEM (HCPCS)

HCPCS (pronounced *"hixpix"*), developed by CMS, is a collection of codes and descriptions that represent procedures, supplies, products, and services that are not covered by or included in the CPT-4. HCPCS codes, like CPT-4 codes, are updated annually. They are designed to promote standardized reporting and statistical data collection of medical supplies, products, services, and procedures. Figure 18-12 is an excerpt from the HCPCS that illustrates HCPCS codes and the HCPCS manual format.

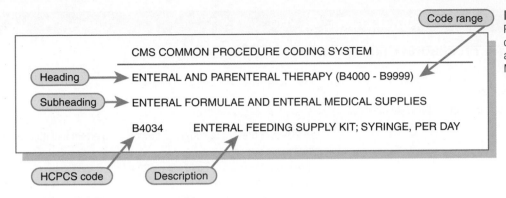

Figure 18-12 CMS's Healthcare Common Procedure Coding System (HCPCS), national codes. (Courtesy U.S. Department of Health and Human Services, Centers for Medicare and Medicaid Services.)

CODING LEVELS: CPT-4 VERSUS HCPCS

There are currently two levels of procedure codes:
- Level I: Developed by the AMA and contained in the current CPT-4 manual
- Level II: HCPCS codes developed by the Center for Medicare and Medicaid Services (CMS) to describe medical services and supplies not covered in the CPT-4

HCPCS Codes

The HCPCS Level II codes are five alphanumeric digits, beginning with one letter followed by four numerals. HCPCS also uses two alphabetic or alphanumeric character modifiers to add information or supplement the Level II Codes.

Conventions

HCPCS uses five conventions as shown in Figure 18-13.

HCPCS Manual

The HCPCS manual is divided into two parts; the Alphabetic Index and the Tabular Index. Procedures and services can be looked up in the Alphabetic Index as with CPT-4, then confirmed as the most accurate and appropriate code by using the Tabular Index. There are no subsections, categories, or subcategories in the HCPCS, only sections as outlined earlier. There is also an appendix of all the HCPCS modifiers and their descriptions for use.

The coding steps are almost identical to the steps for category I CPT-4 codes. A main term is determined, which is used to help find the procedure or service in the Alphabetic Index. The Alphabetic Index will list a code, codes, or code range. These codes or code ranges are then reviewed in the Tabular Index for specificity and accuracy. As with the CPT-4 codes, the clinical documentation is the starting point, and the final code selected should add nothing to nor omit any part of the medical documentation description. The final step is determining whether the code selected can stand alone or requires a modifier to further define or add needed information. Procedure 18-4 shows the coding steps in their entirety.

Coding using the HCPCS manual is essentially the same as coding for a CPT-4 procedure or service. The conventions,

⊙ **Special coverage instructions.** Indicates that there are instructions provided regarding circumstances in which the code might be included for reimbursement.

◆ **Not covered by or valid for Medicare.** These codes might result in reimbursement by private health insurance payors but not by Medicare. Their value may be only for statistical data collection but not for reimbursement.

✳ **Carrier discretion.** These codes may or may not be paid by health insurance carrier including Medicare.

▶ **New.**

⇒ **Revised.** The revised symbol is placed in front of codes with any data, payment, or miscellaneous change from the prior year.

Figure 18-13 Healthcare Common Procedure Coding System (HCPCS) conventions.

Upcoding and Downcoding "Penalties"

There are no legal consequences for undercoding procedures for reimbursement; however, not selecting the most accurate and complete code(s) will result in, at a minimum, a reduction in reimbursement to the performing provider. Always attempt to choose the most appropriate code using the available medical documentation, and to check the medical record to ensure that no primary or secondary procedures were accidentally omitted.

Upcoding is much more serious from a legal standpoint. Using higher-reimbursed codes without having the medical documentation can result in civil or criminal charges of fraud or abuse. The penalties for fraud or abuse can be monetary (fines), jail time, a loss of privilege to use Medicare, Medicaid, and other governmental insurance programs, and in some cases revocation of a provider's license to practice medicine.

layout, and format of the HCPCS manual are different, and there are only sections and subsections found in the HCPCS manual. The HCPCS codes can be used when a specific procedure or service is not found in the CPT-4 coding manual.

PROCEDURE 18-4

Perform Procedural Coding: Perform HCPCS Coding

<u>CAAHEP COMPETENCY:</u> 3.a.(3)(c)
<u>ABHES COMPETENCY:</u> 3.v

GOAL: *Use the steps for procedure and service coding to find the most accurate and specific HCPCS code.*

EQUIPMENT and SUPPLIES

- HCPCS Coding Manual (current year)
- Medical Record
- Encounter form (charge ticket)
- Paper
- Pen or Pencil

PROCEDURAL STEPS

1. Read medical documentation to determine what procedures or services were provided.
   <u>PURPOSE:</u> To ensure all procedures and/or services are listed in the encounter form; that all procedures and services on the encounter form match the medical record; and that nothing documented in the medical record is missing from the encounter form.

2. Select main term classification to begin search.
   <u>PURPOSE:</u> To identify the term or terms to begin the search in the Alphabetic Index.

3. Select modifying term(s) if needed once main term is located.
   <u>PURPOSE:</u> To provide additional specificity and help narrow the search for the code or code range in the Alphabetic Index.

4. If no modifying term produces an appropriate code or code range, repeat steps 2 and 3 using a different main term classification.
   <u>PURPOSE:</u> To aid in finding the most appropriate code or code range by using alternative methods of searching the Alphabetic Index.

5. Find code or code ranges that include all or most of the medical record procedure or service description.
   <u>PURPOSE:</u> To assist in directing the medical assistant to the proper section, subsection, category, or subcategory of the main text of the HCPCS manual.

6. Disregard any code or code range containing additional descriptions or modifying terms not found in the medical record.

<u>PURPOSE:</u> To prevent upcoding or downcoding errors and other compliance issues.

7. Write down the code or code ranges that best match medical documentation.
   <u>PURPOSE:</u> To prevent repeated references to the Alphabetic Index by recording all possible matches to the code or code range being sought. It saves both time and redundant effort.

8. Turn to the main text, and find the first code or code range found while searching the Alphabetic Index.
   <u>PURPOSE:</u> To begin the process of finding the most specific and accurate code.

9. Compare the description of the code with the medical documentation. Verify that all or most of the medical record documentation matches the code description and that there is no additional element or information in the code description that is not found in the documentation.
   <u>PURPOSE:</u> To avoid upcoding and downcoding errors, and to ensure there are no contraindications to use of the code selected.

10. Read the guidelines for the section, subsection, and code to ensure there are no contraindications to the use of the code.
    <u>PURPOSE:</u> To ensure there are no instructions that would prevent use of the code selected.

11. Evaluate the HCPCS manual conventions.
    <u>PURPOSE:</u> To ensure there are no instructions that would prevent use of the code selected.

12. Determine if there are special circumstances that require the use of a modifier.
    <u>PURPOSE:</u> To select, if appropriate, modifiers that provide additional information for the code selected to explain certain circumstances or provide additional detail.

13. Record the HCPCS code selected in the medical record documentation next to the procedure or service performed and in the appropriate block of the insurance claim form.

CLOSING COMMENTS

Medical assistants must be responsible and remain knowledgeable about CPT-4 to ensure that no fraud takes place in the coding and claims submission process. Medical assistants should also ensure that proper precautions are taken to avoid incorrect coding, data entry errors, and false claims submissions.

Codes or narratives should not be altered in patient chart documentation to increase insurance reimbursement or to accommodate policy coverage requirements. Deliberate misrepresentation may carry criminal and/or civil penalties.

Downcoding, in which lower level codes are used even when the diagnostic statement indicates a higher level procedure or service, usually affects reimbursement only by lowering the amount received, but may have civil and criminal penalty implications if it is done to skirt insurance policy restrictions or preexisting condition clauses. **Upcoding,** on the other hand, in which a higher level procedure or service code is used than is supported by the medical documentation, can result in civil and criminal penalties, including fines, loss of privileges as a participating provider, and even prison time.

SUMMARY OF SCENARIO

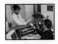

Kay has learned that procedural coding using the CPT-4 is similar in many ways to ICD-9-CM diagnostic coding. Both coding manuals have unique but similar steps, conventions, and guidelines. She has also learned that proper abstracting of procedural data from the medical record is just as important in both the ICD-9-CM and the CPT-4. Kay also discovered that HCPCS codes describe procedures and services not found in the CPT-4, such as medicines, ambulance services, and durable medical equipment. Kay now knows the legal implications of coding compliance errors, such as upcoding and downcoding.

Kay enjoys working toward becoming a medical assistant. As Kay progresses with learning procedural coding, she envisions herself as becoming more well rounded in her knowledge of the practice's administrative operations. The encounter form is a common document used to enter the procedure when a patient checks out, but knowing how to use the CPT-4 manual is essential when notes must be coded from procedures or services performed by Dr. Shuman or Dr. Taylor. As with diagnostic coding, Kay can pull the patient chart for research and documentation if any questions arise about a claim. Kay knows that coding to the highest level of specificity will help in accuracy and in obtaining maximum reimbursement. Kay continues to use the Internet to network and research. She stays informed of the changes in procedural coding by ordering the updated CPT-4 manual each year.

SUMMARY of LEARNING OBJECTIVES

1. Define, spell, and pronounce the terms listed in the vocabulary.
   * Spelling and pronouncing medical terms correctly adds credibility to the medical assistant. Knowing the definition of these terms promotes confidence in communication with patients and co-workers.

2. Describe the steps for abstracting procedural data from clinical documentation.
   * The medical assistant must thoroughly read clinical documentation and look for all of the procedures that were performed and should be charged to the patient. Most physician offices use the encounter form to document procedures and services, but there are instances when the medical assistant will need to read through the medical record to determine what was done to the patient and what charges should be made.

3. Identify four purposes of the CPT-4.
   * The CPT-4 is designed to encourage the use of standard terms and descriptors to document procedures in the medical record; to communicate accurate information on procedures and services to agencies concerned with insurance claims; to provide the basis for a computer-oriented system to evaluate operative procedures, and to contribute basic information for statistical purposes.

4. List the main sections of the CPT-4 and describe their content.
   * There are six sections in the main text: E&M, Anesthesia, Surgery, Radiology, Pathology and Laboratory, and Medicine. Each section contains subsections, categories, and subcategories that further define, modify, and describe the procedure or service codes.

5. Describe the coding conventions, guidelines, and layout of the CPT-4 manual and their importance.
   * The CPT-4 guidelines, symbols, conventions, notes, and steps are designed to guide a medical coder through the process of analyzing and translating clinical documentation and selecting the most accurate code for the procedure performed or the services rendered.
   * The CPT-4 contains a comprehensive Alphabetic Index, a main text listing of the category I CPT-4 codes, and several appendixes and addenda. The Alphabetic Index is composed of main and modifying terms that help provide specificity in selecting code or code ranges to evaluate in the main text.
   * The main text numerically lists all of the CPT-4 procedure and service codes and provides guidelines and conventions in selecting the most specific and most accurate code for insurance billing, reimbursement, and statistical data collection. Several appendixes and addenda provide lists of deletions, additions, and changes to the previous year's CPT-4, modifiers, category II and III codes, clinical examples for use of the E&M codes, add-on codes, exempt codes, codes that include conscious sedation, and drugs pending FDA approval.

6. Describe the process and steps for selecting the most accurate code based on clinical documentation.
   * To use the CPT-4 properly, the coder begins by reading and abstracting the medical documentation, then follows several specific steps using the CPT-4 Alphabetic Index to find a numeric, category I, CPT-4 procedure or service code, codes, or range of codes. The steps for using the Alphabetic Index include the following: (1) Read medical documentation; (2) Select main term classification to begin search; (3) Select modifying term(s) once main term is located; (4) If no modifying term produces an appropriate code or code range, repeat steps 2 and 3 using a different main term classification; (5) Find code or code ranges that include all or most of the medical record procedure or service description; (6) Disregard any code or code range containing additional descriptions or modifying terms not found in the medical record; (7) Write down the code or code ranges that best match medical documentation. Once the code, codes, or code range is found in the Alphabetic Index,

Continued

SUMMARY of LEARNING OBJECTIVES

Continued

the coder moves to the CPT-4 main text to further refine the search and find the appropriate code.

7. Explain the importance of correctly assigning evaluation and management codes.
   - The physician can only bill for services that are actually rendered to patients and must use the evaluation and management guidelines to determine the correct codes for each patient. The amount of time spent with the patient and the level of medical decision making, as well as the length and complexity of the history and examination process all affect the code choice that applies to that particular encounter with the patient.

8. Discuss the importance of modifiers.
   - Modifiers provide a way for the physician to indicate that a service or procedure was altered in some way but not changed in definition. Modifiers also allow the provider to add additional information or describe extenuating circumstances that affect the rendered procedure or service.

9. Define upcoding and explain why it must be avoided.
   - If a code is selected that not only matches the procedure or service performed but also adds modifying information that is not in the medical documentation, then the information is considered "upcoded." Consistent upcoding can result in legal charges of fraud or abuse.

10. Demonstrate an understanding of the process and procedures for code selection.
   - The medical assistant must understand the process for selecting the correct procedure codes that are used for billing

purposes. The selection directly influences the physician's total reimbursements. The process for code selection is outlined in Procedure 18-1.

11. Demonstrate an understanding of main and modifying term selection.
   - The Alphabetic Index is organized by main terms that can stand alone or be further modified by using modifying terms that are indented under the main terms. The medical assistant should be as specific as possible in code selections, using all pertinent words within the description as found in the medical documentation.

12. Find codes in the Alphabetic Index of the CPT-4 manual.
   - First, analyze the medical documentation to determine what services or procedures were performed. Select the main term from the documentation and search for it in the Alphabetic Index. Modifying terms will assist in finding the accurate code, which should then be located in the main text. Determine which code is the most accurate description for the procedure or service provided.

13. Analyze and select codes using the CPT-4 main text.
   - After the Alphabetic Index has been searched, turn to the appropriate codes in the main text to perform final coding steps. Read the section thoroughly to determine the most accurate code to assign to the procedure or service rendered to the patient. Code the procedure or service. The process for using the Alphabetic and main texts of the CPT-4 manual are detailed in Procedures 18-2, 18-3, and 18-4.

CONNECTIONS

 Study Guide Connection: Go to Chapter 18 Study Guide. Read the Case Study and Workplace Applications and complete the assignments. Do online research for answers to the questions in the Internet Activities associated with basics of procedural coding.

 CD Connection: Go to the Medical Assisting Competency Challenge CD and do the training activities under Health Insurance Activities.

 Evolve Connection: For more information related to basics of procedural coding, go to http://evolve.elsevier.com/kinn/admin and visit related weblinks for Chapter 18. Click on the Medical Assisting Exam Review and do the practice questions to sharpen your test-taking skills. To learn more about office software, do the exercises for the Altapoint demo that is on the CD.

Basics of Health Insurance

Carline A. Dalgleish
Alexandra Patricia Young

19

SCENARIO

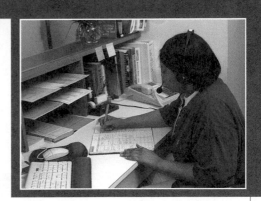

The instructor in Ann Grant's administrative medical assistant class, June Anderson, knows that working with medical insurance can be quite rewarding, and experienced billers find the field financially rewarding as well. Ms. Anderson works with Ann and her classmates, answering their questions and helping them to see that medical insurance is not as complicated as it seems.

The medical assistant who is able to pay attention to detail and likes paperwork will usually enjoy billing and coding activities. The person who performs these duties in the physician's office is a critical staff member, because the tasks that are done related to billing influence the physician's income. That income is used to pay clinic expenses and payroll, so all of the employees of the facility indirectly count on accurate and timely billing. The individual who contributes billing and coding skills, as well as an understanding of health insurance and reimbursement guidelines, will be an asset to the practice and can look forward to a long and rewarding career.

Ann will learn that when insurance billing is broken down into manageable segments of information and applied to real-life situations, it becomes an interesting task. She will learn about the importance of verifying insurance eligibility and the steps for obtaining authorization for referrals and procedures; and that those benefits differ among insurance carriers, whether a private, commercial, federal or state insurance payor.

While studying this chapter, think about the following questions:

- How will the medical assistant be able to remember all the benefits, exclusions, authorizations, and other required information for the multiple insurance carriers and third party administrators?
- Why is it important to verify insurance eligibility and benefits before the patient is seen in a provider's office?

- Why is it important to understand the procedures for obtaining referrals and authorizations?
- How does the medical assistant perform insurance deductible and co-insurance calculations?

LEARNING OBJECTIVES

1. Define, spell, and pronounce the terms listed in the vocabulary.
2. Discuss the purpose of health insurance.
3. Differentiate among the various types of insurance policies.
4. Explain the numerous classifications of insurance benefits available.
5. Explain how insurance benefits are determined.
6. Differentiate among the different types of managed care options.
7. List and discuss other major third-party payors.

8. Interpret the procedure for verifying insurance benefits.
9. Discuss the different types of fee schedules.
10. Obtain managed care referrals and precertifications.
11. Perform eligibility and verification of benefits procedures.
12. Perform a preauthorization procedure.
13. Demonstrate how insurance benefits are determined by calculating deductible and co-insurance payments.

National Accreditation Competencies and Content

CAAHEP COMPETENCIES

Administrative

3.a.(3)(a). Apply managed care policies and procedures
3.a.(3)(b). Apply third-party guidelines

General

3.c.(2)(b). Perform within legal and ethical boundaries
3.c.(2)(d). Document appropriately
3.c.(3)(a). Explain general office policies

ABHES COMPETENCIES

Administrative Duties

3.t. Apply managed care policies and procedures
3.u. Obtain managed care referrals and precertification
3.x. Use physician fee schedule

Legal Concepts

5.a. Determine needs for documentation and reporting
5.b. Document accurately

Instruction

7.a. Orient patients to office policies and procedures

Financial Management

8.c. Analyze and use current third-party guidelines for reimbursement

VOCABULARY

allowed charge (allowable amount) The maximum amount of money that many third-party payors allow for a specific procedure or service.

authorization A term used in managed care for an approved referral.

beneficiary Individual entitled to receive benefits from an insurance policy or program or a governmental entitlement program offering healthcare benefits. Also called a *participant, subscriber, dependent, enrollee,* or *member.*

benefits The amount payable by an insurance company for a monetary loss to an individual insured by that company, under each coverage.

birthday rule Under law, the rule stating that when an individual is covered under two insurance policies, the insurance plan of the policyholder whose birthday comes first in the calendar year (month and day, not year) becomes the primary insurance. This rule applies when there is a question as to whose insurance should be determined as primary, such as for a dependent child, and not used when the individual is the owner of one of the two policies, which would make that the primary policy.

capitation Payment method used by many managed care organizations wherein a fixed amount of money is reimbursed to the provider for patients enrolled during a specific period of time, no matter what services were received or how many visits were made.

carriers As related to insurance, companies that assume the risk of an insurance policy.

Civilian Health and Medical Program of the Uniformed Services (CHAMPUS) See TRICARE.

Civilian Health and Medical Program of the Veterans Administration (CHAMPVA) A health benefits program run by the Department of Veterans Affairs (VA) that helps eligible beneficiaries pay the cost of specific healthcare services and supplies.

co-insurance A policy provision frequently found in medical insurance whereby the policyholder and the insurance company share the cost of covered losses in a specified ratio (e.g., 80/20 means 80% is covered by the insurer and 20% by the insured).

commercial insurance Plans that reimburse the insured for expenses resulting from illness or injury according to a specific fee schedule as outlined in the insurance policy and on a fee-for-service basis. Sometimes called *private insurance.*

copayment A sum of money that is paid at the time of medical service; a form of co-insurance.

deductibles Specific amounts of money a patient must pay out of pocket before the insurance carrier begins paying. Usually this amount ranges from $100 to $500. This deductible amount is met on a yearly or per-incident basis.

dependents The spouse, children, and sometimes domestic partner or other individuals designated by the insured who are covered under a healthcare plan.

disability income insurance Insurance that provides periodic payments to replace income when an insured person is unable to work as a result of illness, injury, or disease.

effective date The date on which an insurance policy or plan takes effect so that benefits are payable.

eligibility A term which describes whether a patient's insurance coverage is in effect, and eligible for payment of insurance benefits.

exclusions Limitations on an insurance contract for which benefits are not payable.

explanation of benefits (EOB) A letter or statement from the insurance carrier describing what was paid, denied, or reduced in payment. It also contains information about amounts applied to the deductible, the patient's co-insurance, and the allowed amounts.

explanation of Medicare benefits (EOMB) The EOMB is the name for an explanation of benefits from Medicare. See explanation of benefits above for the definition.

fee for service An established schedule of fees set for services performed by providers and paid by the patient.

fiscal intermediary An organization that contracts with the government to handle and mediate insurance claims from medical facilities, home health agencies, or providers of medical services or supplies.

government plans Entitlement programs or healthcare plans that are sponsored and/or subsidized by the state or federal government, such as **Medicaid** and **Medicare**.

group policy Insurance written under a policy that covers a number of people under a single master contract issued to their employer or to an association with which they are affiliated.

guarantor The person who is responsible for paying a medical bill.

health insurance Protection in return for periodic premium payments that provides reimbursement of expenses resulting from illness or injury. Includes the following forms of insurance: accident, disability income, medical expense, and accidental death and dismemberment. Also known as *accident and health insurance* or *disability income insurance.*

Health Insurance Portability and Accountability Act (HIPAA) The Kassebaum-Kennedy Act, designed to improve portability and continuity of health insurance coverage; to combat waste, fraud, and abuse in health insurance and healthcare delivery; to promote the use of medical savings accounts; to improve access to long-term care services and coverage; to simplify the administration of health insurance; and to serve other purposes.

health maintenance organization (HMO) An organization that provides a wide range of comprehensive healthcare services for a specified group at a fixed periodic payment. HMOs can be sponsored by the government, medical schools, hospitals, employers, labor unions, consumer groups, insurance companies, and hospital-medical plans.

indemnity plans Traditional health insurance plans that pay for all or a share of the cost of covered services, regardless of which physician, hospital, or other licensed healthcare provider is used. Policyholders of indemnity plans and their **dependents** choose when and where to get healthcare services.

individual policy An insurance policy designed specifically for the use of one person (and his or her dependents), not associated with the amenities of a group policy, namely higher premiums. Often called *personal insurance.*

insured An individual or organization covered by an insurance policy according to the policy terms, usually the individual or group that pays the premiums. Blue Cross/Blue Shield refers to this person or group as the *subscriber.*

managed care plans An umbrella term for all healthcare plans that provide healthcare in return for preset monthly payments and coordinated care through a defined network of primary care physicians and hospitals.

medical savings accounts Tax-deferred bank or savings accounts that are combined with a low-premium, high-deductible insurance policy, designed for individuals or families who choose to fund their own healthcare expenses and medical insurance.

Medicaid A federal and state sponsored health insurance program for the medically indigent.

Medicare A federally sponsored health insurance program for those over 65 or individuals under 65 but disabled.

Medigap A term sometimes applied to private insurance products that supplement Medicare insurance benefits.

participating provider (PAR) A physician or other healthcare provider who enters into a contract with a specific insurance company or program, and by doing so agrees to abide by certain rules and regulations set forth by that particular third-party payor.

policyholder A person who pays a premium to an insurance company and in whose name the policy is written in exchange for the insurance protection provided by a policy of insurance.

preauthorization A process required by some insurance carriers where the provider obtains permission to perform certain procedures or services, or refer a patient to a specialist.

premium The periodic (monthly, quarterly, or annual) payment of a specific sum of money to an insurance company for which the insurer, in return, agrees to provide certain benefits.

primary care provider (PCP) A general practice, or non-specialist provider or physician responsible for the care of a patient for some health maintenance organizations. Also called a gatekeeper.

referral An insurance term used when a primary care provider wants to send a patient to a specialist. Typically, the provider must obtain authorization from the insurance carrier in advance to refer a patient.

remittance advice (RA) An explanation of benefits which comes from Medicaid. See explanation of benefits above for the definition.

resource-based relative value scale (RBRVS) A fee schedule designed to provide national uniform payment of Medicare benefits after being adjusted to reflect the differences in practice costs across geographic areas.

rider A special provision or group of provisions that may be added to a policy to expand or limit the benefits otherwise payable. It may increase or decrease benefits, waive a condition or coverage, or in any other way amend the original contract.

self-insured plan An insurance plan funded by an organization having a large enough employee base that it can afford to fund its own insurance program.

self-referral The act of a patient or insured individual who refers himself or herself to a specialist without requesting the referral from the primary provider, such as a woman seeking an annual gynecologic examination. Managed care guidelines may require the patient to report the self-referral.

service benefit plans Plans that provide benefits in the form of certain surgical and medical services rendered, rather than cash. A service benefit plan is not restricted to a fee schedule.

third-party administrator An organization that processes claims and performs other business-related functions for a health plan.

third-party payors Entities that make payment on an obligation or debt but are not parties of the contract that created the debt.

TRICARE A government-sponsored program wherein authorized dependents of military personnel receive medical care. This program was originally called *CHAMPUS*.

utilization review A review of individual cases by a committee to make sure that services are medically necessary and to study how providers use medical care resources.

workers' compensation Insurance against liability imposed on certain employers to pay **benefits** and furnish care to employees who are injured and to pay benefits to dependents of employees killed in the course of or arising out of their employment.

THE PURPOSE OF HEALTH INSURANCE

The purpose of **health insurance** is to help individuals and families offset the costs of medical care. Health insurance is defined as protection against financial losses resulting from illness or injury. This protection provides payment of monetary benefits for covered sickness or injury depending on the insurance policy purchased. There are various types of health insurance, such as accident insurance, **disability income insurance,** hospitalization, medical expense insurance, and accidental death and dismemberment insurance.

More and more of today's health insurance policies cover "preventative" care, which includes services provided to help prevent certain illnesses or lead to an early diagnosis. Health insurance typically covers services and procedures considered medically necessary. Most insurance policies do not cover "elective" procedures, such as certain cosmetic surgeries that are not considered medically necessary.

CRITICAL THINKING APPLICATION

There is so much to learn in the medical insurance field, and it seems that rules and regulations change on a daily basis. How can Ann keep current on healthcare issues that affect insurance? How can Ann advise patients to keep abreast of the changes in their own personal coverage, such as Medicare?

CYCLE OF HEALTH INSURANCE

The information that follows describes common types of insurance coverage and insurance carriers, the steps for obtaining insurance coverage information, and some of the terminology associated with obtaining insurance coverage and insurance billing. The **insured** or **policyholder,** defined as an individual, group, or employer, pays a set amount called a **premium.** A premium is the periodic (monthly, quarterly, or annual) payment of a specific sum of money to an insurance company for which the insurer agrees to provide certain benefits. This premium, in return, pays for an insurance policy that covers the insured for

a specific type(s) of coverage, such as basic and major medical coverage, accidental death or disability, and so on. When an insured or a covered **beneficiary** or **dependent** of the insurance policy becomes ill or suffers an injury, treatment is provided by a physician or other provider of service in a doctor's office, emergency room, or hospital.

Tasks Related to the Cycle of Health Insurance

The medical assistant's tasks related to health insurance processing are described in this section. These tasks are initiated when the patient encounters the provider, either by appointment, as a walk-in or in the emergency room or hospital. Each task will be discussed in more detail later in this chapter. Tasks completed by the medical assistant include:

- Obtain information from the patient and insured, including demographic, employment, and insurance data.
- Verify the patient's **eligibility** for insurance payment with the insurance carrier(s), as well as benefits available, exclusions, and whether special **authorization**s are needed to refer patients to specialists or perform certain services or procedures—for example, surgery or diagnostic tests.
- Perform diagnostic and procedural coding and review the encounter form or charge ticket for completeness once the patient is seen by the provider.
- Calculate insurance deductibles and co-insurance amounts and provide the patient with a statement showing the out-of-pocket expense amount owed by the patient.
- Obtain preauthorization for referral of the patient to a specialist or for special services or procedures that require advance permission. This information may be obtained verbally, but should also be documented in writing and should be obtained in advance of commencing any procedures or treatments.
- Complete an insurance claim form and submit it to the insurance company for reimbursement for services and procedures performed. In Chapter 20, detailed instructions are provided for completing a health insurance claim form.
- Post payments and adjustments on the patient ledger or account, and examine the **explanation of benefits (EOB), explanation of Medicare benefits (EOMB) or the remittance**

advice (RA) from the insurance company to identify what was paid, reduced, or denied, and includes deductible, co-insurance, and allowable amounts. Adjustments are made to the account, and the **allowable amount** is either written-off (adjusted) or passed on to the patient for payment.

- Bill the patient for any outstanding balance, or, if there is a secondary insurance, complete the secondary insurance claim form and submit it to the insurance company.
- Follow-up on any rejected or unpaid claims, and any requests from the insurance carrier for more information about specific claims are answered as soon as possible. Chapter 20 includes more information regarding insurance follow-up, as well as tips to help minimize claims rejections, reduce the number of requests for additional data, and maximize reimbursement.

Cost of Coverage

In this age of rising health care costs, most insurance **carriers** do not reimburse the full amount for services and procedures rendered. A carrier is an insurance company or third-party that pays for medical care. The insured, or beneficiary, in most instances will be required to pay certain "out-of-pocket" expenses such as **deductibles, copayment** or **co-insurance** charges, and costs for noncovered services.

A deductible is an amount a **policyholder** agrees to pay per claim or per accident toward the total amount of an insured loss before the insurance company will begin payment of benefits. A deductible amount is stated in the insurance contract and normally ranges from $100 to $500. Under most circumstances the deductible must be paid only one time per calendar year; however, some policies have a deductible per occurrence. The medical assistant should always verify the **effective date,** or date the insurance coverage began, on the patient's insurance card. An excellent policy for any provider's office is to call the insurance company to verify insurance eligibility, benefits, and **exclusions** before the patient's appointment or encounter with the provider. This verification is done by phone or fax and ensures that the insurance is in effect, and the patient is eligible for benefits. More about verification of benefits will be covered later in the chapter. Co-insurance is a policy provision frequently found in medical insurance whereby the policyholder and the insurance company share the cost of covered losses in a specified ratio, such as 80/20 (i.e., 80% of services are paid by the insurance carrier and 20% by the insured). Many plans now require a copayment, which is a type of co-insurance that is collected at the time of service. Copayments usually range from $10 to $25 for office visits but can vary according to the services rendered. Most **managed care plans** require a copayment. In addition, any services or procedures that are not covered under the terms of an insurance policy are the responsibility of the policyholder or insured.

TYPES OF HEALTH INSURANCE

Health insurance is available to the majority of persons in this country through group or individual plans. In addition, many people are covered by **government plans** or entitlement programs. However, although health insurance might be available, it is not always affordable. A recent survey revealed that more than 56 million Americans–roughly 21% of the population–have no regular source for obtaining medical care, and lack of health insurance was a major obstacle.

The types of health insurance available include group insurance, individual insurance, government-sponsored insurance, **self-insured plans,** and medical savings accounts. Government plans can be federal and/or state sponsored and include **Medicare, Medicaid, TRICARE, the Civilian Health and Medical Program of the Veterans Administration (CHAMPVA),** and **worker's compensation**.

Group Policies

Insurance written under a **group policy** covers a number of people under a single master contract issued to their employer or to an association with which they are affiliated. Group coverage usually provides greater benefits at lower premiums because of the large pool of people from whom premiums are collected. Physical examinations are normally not required, and preexisting conditions are often waived. Often the employee shares the cost of coverage through payroll deductions.

Individual Policies

Individuals who do not qualify for inclusion in a group or government-sponsored plan may apply to companies that offer individual policies, often called *personal insurance* or **individual policies.** The applicant is normally required to fill out an extended health questionnaire and undergo a physical examination before acceptance. Unlike with group policies, with personal insurance there is a risk that coverage may be denied, or the individual may have to accept a **rider,** or limitation, on benefits the policy will cover. Premiums are almost always higher with individual policies, and often the benefits are less.

Government Plans

Many large groups of people are covered by government plans or entitlement programs. A patient who is older than age 65 is covered by Part B of Medicare. A medically indigent patient may be eligible for Medicaid with or without Medicare. **Dependents** of military personnel are covered by **TRICARE** (formerly known as the **Civilian Health and Medical Program of the Uniformed Services** *(CHAMPUS);* surviving spouses and dependent children of veterans who died as a result of service-related disabilities are covered by CHAMPVA.

Some wage earners are protected against the loss of wages and the cost of medical care resulting from an occupational accident, disease, or disability through **workers' compensation** insurance. An individual may collect benefits for health expenses from an automobile policy if the injury is related to a car accident or other such loss.

TRICARE

The federal government first became responsible for insuring a large group of people in 1956 with passage of Public Law 569. This law authorized dependents of military personnel to receive treatment from civilian physicians at the expense of the government. The program administering these benefits became CHAMPUS, which today is known as *TRICARE* (discussed in detail later in this chapter).

Medicaid

In 1965 the federal government provided for another group—the medically indigent—through a program that is known as *Medicaid.* Title XIX of Public Law 89-97, under the Social Security Amendments of 1965, provided for agreements with states for assistance from the federal government to provide medical care for people meeting specific eligibility criteria.

Medicare

Established in 1965, Medicare is a federal health insurance program that provides health care coverage for individuals age 65 and older. The program also covers certain persons under age 65 with disabilities. The Medicare program was developed by the Healthcare Financing Administration (HCFA), now called the Centers for Medicare and Medical Services (CMS), as part of Title XVIII of the Social Security Act.

Workers' Compensation

All state legislatures have passed workers' compensation laws to protect wage earners against the loss of wages and the cost of medical care resulting from occupational accident or disease. State laws differ as to the classes of employees included and the benefits provided.

Self-Insured Plans

Many large companies or organizations have a big enough employee base that they choose to fund their own insurance program. This is called a **self-insured plan.** Technically, a self-funded plan is not insurance by true definition. The employer pays employee healthcare costs from the firm's own funds. Recent surveys indicate that about 40% of workers with employment-based health insurance are enrolled in plans that their employers self-insure. Usually benefits and premium costs under self-insured plans are similar to those under group plans. Self-funded plans tend to work best for companies that are large enough to offer good coverage and reasonable premium rates and are able to pay large claims for expensive medical services. Often a **third-party administrator** (TPA) or **fiscal intermediary** handles paperwork and claim payments for a self-insured group.

Medical Savings Account

In 1996 Congress made tax-free **medical savings accounts** (MSAs) available to 750,000 American workers and their families. This is a type of self-insurance. Under a provision of the Kassebaum-Kennedy health insurance reform bill, small companies (with 50 or fewer employees), self-employed persons, and the uninsured can purchase health insurance policies and make tax-free deposits to an MSA. They can use their MSA money to pay small and routine healthcare expenses, reserving a high-deductible medical insurance policy to pay large, catastrophic expenses. Money that remains in the account at year's end earns tax-free interest. People can also elect to use MSA money to pay their health insurance premiums during a job change,

which should reduce job lock, a situation in which people do not change jobs for fear of losing their health insurance.

There are both advantages and disadvantages to having an MSA, and it is wise to investigate them thoroughly to learn the values and limitations of these accounts.

CRITICAL THINKING APPLICATION

Ann understands how medical assistants can easily become intimidated by all of the regulations that affect insurance coverage. Discuss differences and similarities between the different types of insurance companies and insurance coverage. How can the medical assistant effectively keep up with all of the rules pertaining to policies that frequently are presented in the office?

TYPES OF INSURANCE BENEFITS

An insurance package is tailored to the needs of each individual or group policy, and the combinations of benefits are limitless. A policy may contain one or any combination of the following benefits as described here and in Table 19-1.

Hospitalization

Hospital coverage pays the cost of all or part of the insured person's hospital room and board and specific hospital services, such as the costs involved in having surgery in a hospital. Hospital insurance policies frequently set a maximum amount payable per day and a maximum number of days of hospital care. Some insurance companies require that the hospital be an accredited or a licensed hospital.

Surgical

Surgical coverage pays all or part of a surgeon's fee; some plans also pay for an assistant surgeon. Surgery includes any incision or excision, removal of foreign bodies, aspiration, suturing, and reduction of fractures. Surgery may be accomplished in a hospital, physician's office, or elsewhere. The insurer frequently provides the subscriber with a surgical fee schedule that establishes the amount the insurer will pay for commonly performed procedures.

Basic Medical

Basic medical coverage pays all or part of a physician's fee for nonsurgical services, including hospital, home, and office visits. Usually there is a deductible amount payable by the patient as well as a copayment or co-insurance payment each time service is received. The insurance plan may include a provision for diagnostic laboratory, radiology, and pathology fees. Some medical plans do not cover routine physical examinations or preventative health checkups such as mammograms or prostate examinations if the patient does not have a specific complaint or illness.

Major Medical

Major medical insurance (formerly called *catastrophic coverage*) provides protection against especially large medical bills

TABLE 19-1 Types of Health Insurance, Plan Benefits

BENEFIT	COVERED	PAYS
Hospitalization	Cost of all or part of the hospital room and board; and, specific hospital services, i.e., costs involved in having surgery in a hospital	Maximum amount per day and maximum number of days
Surgical	Any surgical procedure, including but not limited to: incision or excision; removal of foreign bodies; aspiration; suturing; reduction of fractures	Surgeon's fee Assistant surgeon's fee
Basic medical	Outpatient and/or physician office procedures and services	Physician's fees diagnostic, radiologic, laboratory, and pathology fees
Major medical (catastrophic)	Catastrophic or prolonged illness or injury	Takes over when basic medical, hospitalization and surgical benefits end
Disability	Accident or illness resulting in an inability for patient to work; can be paid whether work-related or non-work related.	Cash benefits paid in lieu of salary while patient is unable earn an income
Dental care	Preventative care and/or teeth and gum treatment and repair	Typically pays 100% for preventative care, 50% for repair and treatment
Vision care	Eye exam and glasses	Set benefit amount depending on vision care policy for examination and/or glasses
Medicare supplement	Deductible and co-insurance amounts unpaid by Medicare	Deductible and co-insurance amounts unpaid by Medicare
Special risk	Certain specific illnesses (cancer, heart failure) or accidents (automobile, airplane)	Typically pays a maximum benefit
Life insurance	Loss of life	Usually lump sum payment of life insurance benefit
Long-term care	Long-term skilled nursing or rehabilitation care	Set amount determined by policy benefits

resulting from catastrophic or prolonged illnesses. It may be a supplement to basic medical coverage or a comprehensive integrated program providing both basic and major medical protection.

Disability (Loss of Income) Protection

Weekly or monthly cash benefits are provided to employed policyholders who become unable to work as a result of an accident or illness. Many disability policies do not start payment until after a specified number of days or until a certain number of sick leave days have been used. Payment is made directly to the individual and is intended to replace lost income resulting from an illness or other disability. It is not intended for payment of specific medical bills, and it should not be confused with a regular insurance plan, entitlement program, or workers' compensation, in which compensation is provided for an employee who is injured on the job or cannot work as a result of a job-related illness or other disability.

Dental Care

Dental coverage is included in many fringe benefit packages. Some policies are based on a copayment and incentive program, in which preventive dental care (such as cleaning and x-ray films) is covered 100%, with most other coverage paid at 50%.

Vision Care

Vision care insurance may include reimbursement for all or a percentage of the cost for refraction, lenses, and frames.

Medicare Supplement

Many Medicare beneficiaries purchase a supplemental health insurance policy to help defray medical costs not covered, or only partially covered, by Medicare. Federal regulations now require that Medicare supplement contracts must be uniform in benefits to avoid confusion for the purchaser. Medicare supplements that cover Medicare recipients' out-of-pocket expenses, including the deductible and co-insurance payments, are called **Medigap** policies.

Special Risk Insurance

Special risk insurance protects a person in the event of a certain type of accident, such as an automobile or airplane crash, or for certain diseases, such as tuberculosis or cancer. There is usually a maximum benefit.

Liability Insurance

There are many types of liability insurance, including automobile, business, and homeowners' policies. Liability policies often include benefits for medical expenses payable to individuals who are injured in the insured person's home or car, without regard to the insured person's actual legal liability for the accident.

Life Insurance

Life insurance provides payment of a specified amount on an insured's death, either to his or her estate or to a designated beneficiary, or in the case of an endowment policy, to the policyholder at a specified date. Life insurance policies sometimes provide monthly cash benefits if the policyholder becomes permanently and totally disabled. Sometimes the proceeds from life insurance are used to meet the expenses of the insured person's last illness.

Long-Term Care Insurance

Long-term care insurance is a relatively new type that covers a continuum of broad-ranged maintenance and health services to chronically ill, disabled, or mentally retarded persons. Services may be provided on an inpatient basis (at a rehabilitation facility, nursing home, or mental hospital), on an outpatient basis, or at home. The **Health Insurance Portability and Accountability Act (HIPAA)** of 1996 gives some federal income tax advantages to people who buy certain long-term care insurance policies.

HOW BENEFITS ARE DETERMINED

Insurance benefits may be determined and paid in one of several ways:

- By indemnity schedules
- By **service benefit plans**
- By determination of the usual, customary, and reasonable (UCR) fee
- By relative value studies

Indemnity Schedules

Indemnity plans are traditional health insurance plans that pay for all or a share of the cost of covered services, regardless of which physician, hospital, or other licensed healthcare provider is used. Because physicians and other providers are paid for each office visit, test, procedure, or other service they deliver, indemnity plans are often called *fee-for-service plans*.

Policyholders of indemnity plans and their dependents choose when and where to get healthcare services. In exchange for premiums that members pay, the indemnity plan reimburses members or the provider when claims are filed. The subscriber is often given a schedule of indemnities (fee schedule), which explains the benefit payment amounts of the policy, when the policy is purchased. Indemnity benefits are usually paid to the person insured unless that person has authorized payment directly to the provider, which is a common practice.

Service Benefit Plans

In a **service benefit** plan the insuring company agrees to pay for certain surgical or medical services without additional cost to the person insured. There is no set fee schedule. In a service benefit plan, surgery with complications would warrant a higher fee than an uncomplicated procedure would. Premiums are sometimes higher for this type of coverage, but often payments are larger. Frequently payment of benefits is sent directly to the physician and is considered full payment for services rendered.

For example, the service benefit plan states it will pay $900 for a cholecystectomy. If Dr. Jones charges $1500 for this procedure, he has the right to either accept the $900 as payment in full and write off the balance due or to request payment for the remaining $600 balance from the patient or **guarantor**–the individual or group responsible for payment.

Usual, Customary, and Reasonable Fee

Some insurance companies agree to pay on the basis of all or a percentage of the physician's UCR fee. Charges for a specific service are compared with a database of charges for the same service to other patients by the same type of physician, and to patients by other physicians performing the same or similar services in the same geographic area. The insurance company determines whether the charge is UCR, and any amount over this **allowed charge** will not be paid.

Resource-Based Relative Value Scale

The **resource-based relative value scale (RBRVS)** is one of the outcomes of the Medicare Physician Payment Reform that was enacted in the Omnibus Budget Reconciliation Act of 1989 (usually called *OBRA '89*). Since the beginning of Medicare, Part B of the program has paid physicians using a fee-for-service system based on customary, prevailing, and reasonable charges that was similar in structure to the UCR fees described in the previous paragraph; however, implementation of the RBRVS, which came into effect in 1992, changed this system to a fee scale consisting of three parts: physician work, charge-based professional liability expenses, and charge-based overhead.

The physician work component includes the degree of effort invested by a physician in a particular service or procedure and the time it consumed. The professional liability and overhead components are computed by the Centers for Medicare and Medicaid Services (CMS). The fee schedule is designed to provide national uniform payments after being adjusted to reflect the differences in practice costs across geographic areas. The fee schedule includes a conversion factor, which is a single national number applied to all services paid under the fee schedule. Conversion factors are changed, usually annually, by Congress at the request of the CMS.

HEALTH INSURANCE PROVIDERS

Health insurance providers include managed care plans, Blue Cross/Blue Shield (BC/BS), **commercial insurance** companies, and federal and state government programs including Medicare, Medicaid, TRICARE, workers' compensation, and disability insurance.

Managed Care

Managed care is an umbrella term for all healthcare plans that provide healthcare in return for preset scheduled payments and coordinated care through a defined network of physicians and hospitals. Managed care refers to healthcare plans that provide healthcare in return for scheduled payments and coordinate healthcare through a defined network of **primary care providers** (PCPs), hospitals, and other providers.

The passage of the Health Maintenance Organization Act in 1973 provided for federal aid to health insurance prepayment plans that met certain criteria. This brought about a rapid growth of the **health maintenance organization** (HMO), which is an organization that provides comprehensive healthcare to an enrolled group for a fixed periodic payment. Some of these plans pay by **capitation,** which means that the provider is paid a fixed amount for each individual enrolled in the plan during a specified time period, regardless of the number of services provided to the patient. The provider still collects only the contracted rate, even if expenses cost much more than that rate for the time period (Procedure 19-1).

Managed care has been met with considerable controversy and has pros and cons that must be considered. It is important that medical assistants be well versed in the various types of managed care plans to fully understand their impact on healthcare costs.

Advantages of managed care include the following:
- Healthcare costs are usually contained.
- There are established fee schedules.
- Authorized services are usually paid for.
- Most preventive medical treatment is covered.
- Patients' out-of-pocket expenses tend to be less than with traditional insurance.

Disadvantages of managed care include the following:
- Access to specialized care and referrals can be limited.
- Physician choices in treatment of patients can be limited.
- The amount of paperwork may be increased.
- Treatment may be delayed because of preauthorization requirements.
- Reimbursement is historically less than that through traditional insurance.

Models of Managed Care

There are two basic models of managed care: the health maintenance organization (HMO) and the preferred provider organization (PPO). The HMO can be structured as an independent practice association (IPA), staff, or group model, or as an exclusive provider organization (EPO). Table 19-2 illustrates these HMO models.

Health Maintenance Organization. An HMO is a plan that contracts with a medical center or group of physicians to provide preventative as well as acute care for the insured. HMOs are state-licensed health plans that are regulated by HMO laws, which require them to include preventative care such as routine physical examinations and other services as part of their benefits package. HMOs always require referrals to specialists, precertification, and preauthorization for hospital admissions, outpatient procedures and treatments.

An HMO member is typically enrolled for a specified period of time (month, quarter, or year). The HMO receives a "per member per month" (pmpm) fee for each enrollee if they are on a capitation plan.

Providers receive payment in various structures. The two most common structures are **capitation** and **fee for service**. Capitation is payment in advance to the provider by the HMO for a contracted group of patients, regardless how often the patients are seen, and even if the patients are never seen by the provider. Fees charged for services to group members may be billed directly to the IPA rather than to the patient. Fees for services to nonmember patients are handled in the same manner as any other fee for service. The payment structure is based on the type of HMO model and the contract negotiated between the HMO and the provider(s). The most common models include the examples that follow.

Independent Practice Association. An independent practice association (IPA) consists of physicians with separately owned practices who formally organize a physician association and continue to practice in their own offices. The physician may be contracted with several IPAs. Payments to providers by an IPA can be structured either as a capitation or fee for service.

Staff model. A staff model HMO hires physicians and pays a salary to its physicians. Rather than contracting with physicians to create a network, the HMO owns the network. Medical care is given by, or authorized by, the patient's PCP. No capitation or fee for service payment structure is used with the staff model; however, the physicians may receive bonuses biannually or annually based on the number of patients treated and/or the cost savings.

Group model. A group model HMO contracts with a multispecialty medical group to deliver care to its members. It is similar to an IPA in that the multispecialty group may organize a physician association, but they typically practice together in one facility. The payment structure to the providers can be either capitation or fee for service.

Exclusive Provider Organization. An Exclusive Provider Organization (EPO) combines features of HMOs (e.g., an enrolled group or population, primary care providers, and an **authorization** system) and Preferred Provider Organizations (PPOs; e.g., flexible benefit design, and fee-for-service payments). It is referred to as "exclusive" because employers agree not to contract with any other plan. Members must choose medical care from network providers, with certain exceptions for emergency or out-of-area services. If a patient decides to seek care outside the network, he or she generally will not be reimbursed for the cost of treatment. Technically, many HMOs can be considered EPOs; however, EPOs are regulated under insurance statutes rather than federal and state HMO regulations.

Preferred Provider Organizations. The PPO model of managed healthcare preserves the fee-for-service concept that many physicians prefer. An insurer representing its clients contracts

TABLE 19-2 Comparison of HMO Models		
MODEL	**STRUCTURE**	**BILLING MODEL**
IPA	General or family practice physician or physician group that practices independently and may contract with several IPAs	Capitation or fee for service
Staff	Physician(s) hired by HMO	Salaried
Group	Multispecialty group with or without PCP (gatekeeper); may contract with several IPAs	Capitation or fee for service

PROCEDURE 19-1

Apply Managed Care Policies and Procedures

CAAHEP COMPETENCY: 3.a(3)(a)
ABHES COMPETENCY: 3.t

GOAL: *To act within the guidelines of the managed care contracts that the physician and/or medical facility has partnered.*

EQUIPMENT and SUPPLIES

- Managed care contracts
- Managed care handbooks
- Clerical supplies
- Forms from managed care organizations

PROCEDURAL STEPS

1. Determine which managed care organization the patient belongs to.
   PURPOSE: To make certain that the right information is applied to the right patient.
2. Read and study the policies and procedures that are set forth by the managed care organization.
   PURPOSE: To understand regulations and abide by them when working with patients that the regulations affect.
3. Obtain any forms that are needed to process patient claims.

PURPOSE: To submit the correct forms to the managed care organization.

4. Become familiar with the information in managed care policy manuals and handbooks.
   PURPOSE: By becoming familiar with handbooks and guidelines, the medical assistant will be able to assist patients in finding needed information.
5. Determine whom to contact in case of questions about the various managed care organizations.
   PURPOSE: To be able to refer patients to the best source of information when they have questions or concerns.
6. Attend seminars and workshops when offered by the managed care organizations.
   PURPOSE: To stay up-to-date on information and policies.
7. Use information gained on a daily basis when working with managed care organizations.

---

with a group of providers who agree on a predetermined list of charges for all services including those for both normal and complex procedures. Unlike HMOs, PPOs have no capitation or prepaid care. Typically there are deductibles or co-insurance payments of 20% to 25% of the predetermined charge that the patient pays, and the insurer pays the balance. A provider who joins a PPO does not need to alter the manner of providing care and continues to treat and bill the patients on a fee-for-service basis. When a patient covered under a PPO plan comes for treatment, the physician treats the patient and bills the PPO.

Technically PPOs are not HMOs, but they do have more patient care management than regular indemnity insurance plans. PPOs furnish their subscribers with a list of member-providers from which subscribers can receive healthcare at PPO rates. Rates are quite often lower than those charged to non-PPO patients. If a patient goes to a physician who is not in the PPO network, the out-of-pocket cost is higher.

CRITICAL THINKING APPLICATION

The physicians in the practice where Ann works are not members of a PPO that is often used in their geographic area. Many patients are confused when they have to pay a larger out-of-pocket fee for their medical services. How can Ann explain the reason for these higher fees to patients?

Blue Cross/Blue Shield

BC/BS is America's oldest and largest system of independent health insurers. It began in 1929 when an executive at Baylor University in Dallas came up with a plan for teachers to budget for their future hospital bills. The teachers paid $6 a year into a fund and were, in turn, guaranteed 21 days of free hospital care. Within 10 years the American Hospital Association officially embraced the concept of prepaid hospital care and symbolized their new program with a blue cross.

At the same time, workers in lumber camps in the Northwest developed a similar approach to deal with frequent logging accidents. Camp owners provided medical care for workers by paying physicians monthly fees, for which a physician would provide all the care the workers needed. Physicians formed groups, or medical service bureaus, which were linked to specific employers. The bureaus were identified with a blue shield, and they too quickly expanded in popularity.

BC/BS offers incentive contracts to healthcare providers. If the provider chooses to sign a member contract, he or she becomes a **participating provider (PAR).** The healthcare provider then agrees to accept BC/BS reimbursement as payment in full for covered services. In turn, BC/BS agrees to reimburse providers directly and in a shorter time.

BC/BS identification (ID) cards (Figure 19-1) carry the subscriber's name and ID number with a three-character alphabetic prefix. The letters are an important part of the number and must be included on the claim form.

Medicaid

Title XIX of Public Law 89-97 under the Social Security Amendments of 1965 provides for agreements with states for assistance from the federal government in providing healthcare for the medically indigent. All states and the District of Columbia

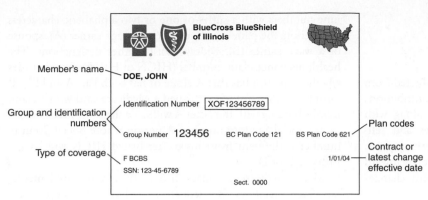

Figure 19-1 Blue Cross/Blue Shield identification card.

have Medicaid programs, but wide variations exist among these programs.

The federal government provides basic funding to the state, after which the states individually elect whether to provide funds for extension of benefits. The state determines the type and extent of medical care that will be covered within the minimum requirements established by the federal government. Some local areas and states are developing HMOs that serve only patients who qualify for Medicaid.

A physician may accept or decline to treat Medicaid patients. The physician who does accept Medicaid patients automatically agrees to accept Medicaid payment as payment in full for covered services. The patient cannot be billed for the difference between the Medicaid fee and the physician's normal fee. The patient can be billed for any services that are not covered by Medicaid. Eligibility for benefits is determined by the respective states.

Examples of individuals who qualify for benefits include the following:

- Persons who are medically needy
- Recipients of Aid to Families with Dependent Children (AFDC)
- Persons who receive Supplemental Security Income (SSI)
- Persons receiving certain types of federal and state aid
- For Qualified Medicare Beneficiaries (QMBs), Medicaid pays for Medicare Part B premiums, deductibles, and co-insurance for qualified low-income elderly
- Persons in institutions or receiving long-term care in nursing facilities and intermediate care facilities

Depending on the state in which the Medicaid is being administered, Medicaid recipients are identified with a benefits ID card (BIC), a monthly sticker, a label, or a letter, showing proof of eligibility. A BIC looks like a white credit card (Figure 19-2) and is verified by a point-of-service (POS) device similar to a credit card verification machine. The medical assistant must verify coverage each time the patient comes into the office regardless of the type of ID the recipient is issued.

Medicare

Medicare is a federal health insurance program for the following people:

- People 65 years of age and older
- People who are permanently disabled or blind

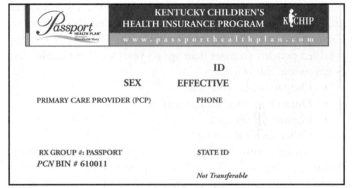

Figure 19-2 Medicaid benefits identification card.

- People receiving dialysis for permanent kidney failure or who have had a kidney transplant

On July 1, 1966, Medicare was established under the Social Security Administration as a national health insurance program for persons age 65 and older. Before Medicare only 50% of the nation's elderly had any health insurance. Today Medicare is the world's largest insurance program. It serves more than 38 million older and disabled Americans. The scope of coverage increased in 1973 to include disabled persons younger than age 65 receiving Social Security benefits, railroad retirees, and civil service retirees. This also included disabled workers of any age, disabled widows, disabled dependent widowers, adults disabled before age 18 whose parents are eligible or are retired on Social Security benefits, children and adults with end-stage renal disease, and living kidney donors (including all expenses related to the kidney transplant).

Medicare is administered by the Centers for Medicare and Medicaid Services (CMS), which was formerly known as the *Health Care Financing Administration (HCFA).* CMS is a division of the Department of Health and Human Services (DHHS), and the Medicare program is regulated by laws enacted by Congress. Medicare has two parts that cover healthcare services: Part A and Part B.

Part A is hospital insurance. Retired people 65 years of age and older and people who receive monthly Social Security or railroad retirement checks are automatically enrolled for hospital insurance benefits and pay no premiums for this insurance. Part A covers the following:

- Inpatient hospital care
- Skilled nursing facilities
- Home healthcare
- Hospice services

Part A is financed with special contributions deducted from employed individuals' salaries, with matching contributions from their employers. These sums are collected, along with regular Social Security contributions, from wages and self-employment income earned during a person's working years. There is a deductible that a hospitalized patient must pay toward hospital expenses. Typically the deductible amount changes annually by congressional enactment.

Part B is medical insurance. Persons who are eligible for Part A are also eligible for Part B, but they must apply for this coverage and pay a monthly premium. Some federal employees and former federal employees who are not eligible for Social Security benefits and Part A may still enroll in Part B. Certain disabled persons younger than age 65 years are also eligible. Part B covers the following:

- Outpatient hospital care
- Durable medical equipment
- Physicians' services
- Other medical services

A patient with Medicare Part B must meet an annual deductible before benefits become available, after which Medicare pays 80% of the covered, or allowed, benefits. Usually the physician accepts assignment of benefits for Medicare patients and is paid directly. In these cases the physician must accept the payment that Medicare allows and bills the patient for 20% of the charge allowed by Medicare. If the physician does not accept assignment, the patient must pay the entire bill (which cannot be greater than the limit set by Medicare for nonparticipating physicians), and the patient will receive a reimbursement check directly from Medicare.

Medicare health insurance cards (Figure 19-3) typically show nine numbers with a suffix of one or two alphabetic characters that denote the patient's status, such as wage earner (A), spouse of a wage earner (B), widow (D), or other designations. The health insurance claim number (HICN or HIC#) also identifies whether a person has Part A alone or has both Part A and Part B insurance. A patient who is issued a Medicare card with a claim number ending with the letter A will have the same HICN as his or her Social Security number. A person whose Social Security number is different from his or her issued HICN will have a suffix of B or D.

Many Medicare enrollees also carry private supplemental insurance that pays the deductible and the 20% copayment not covered by Medicare. If the supplemental policy pays the deductible and the 20% copayment, it is called a *Medigap policy.*

In 1997 a new option was added, called Medicare+Choice. This program is commonly referred to as *Part C,* although the Medicare administration does not label it as such. Medicare+Choice offers expanded benefits for a fee through private health insurance programs such as HMOs and PPOs that have contracts with Medicare. In 2004, as a result of congressional action to reform Medicare, Medicare+Choice was renamed Medicare Advantage.

In 2006, drug and prescription benefits were added, which are Part D of Medicare. In Medicare Part D, the Medicare recipient has the option to choose, at a reduced cost, a prescription drug plan that pays for prescription drugs with just a small copayment by the patient. Everyone with Medicare can get this coverage that may help lower prescription drug costs and help protect against higher costs in the future. Medicare Prescription Drug Coverage is insurance that is provided by private companies. Beneficiaries choose the drug plan and pay a monthly premium. Like other insurance, if a beneficiary decides not to enroll in a drug plan when they are first eligible, they may pay a penalty if they choose to join later.

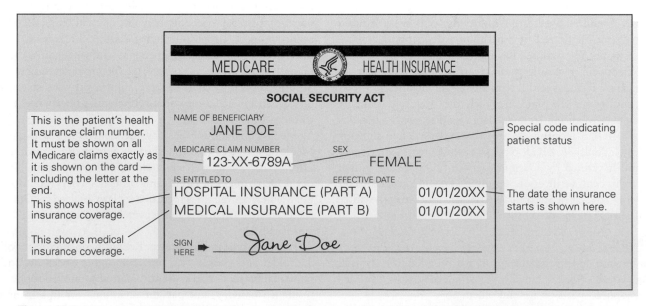

Figure 19-3 Medicare health identification card. (From Fordney MT: Insurance handbook for the medical office, ed 8, St Louis, 2004, Saunders.)

TRICARE (Formerly CHAMPUS)

TRICARE is the Department of Defense and the military's comprehensive healthcare program for family members of active duty personnel, military retirees and their eligible family members under the age of 65, and survivors of all uniformed services. Before January 1994, this program was known as *CHAMPUS,* created in 1966 under Public Law 89-614.

The TRICARE program is managed by the military in partnership with civilian hospitals and clinics. It is designed to expand access to healthcare, ensure high-quality care, and promote medical readiness. All military hospitals and clinics are part of the TRICARE program and offer high-quality healthcare at low costs to plan users.

To be eligible for TRICARE, an individual must be a TRICARE or CHAMPVA (covered later in this chapter) recipient, be entitled to retired, retainer, or equivalent pay, and be listed in the Defense Department's Defense Enrollment Eligible Reporting System (DEERS), which is a computerized database that lists all active and retired service members. Coverage is also available for a TRICARE-eligible spouse under age 65, and dependent, unmarried children under age 21, or age 23 if in college full-time. Eligible spouses and children of active-duty service members may enroll, as may TRICARE-eligible widows, widowers, and certain ex-spouses (who have not remarried).

There are three choices under TRICARE:
- TRICARE Prime: The Department of Defense's managed care option, similar to a civilian HMO
- TRICARE Extra: A preferred provider network option
- TRICARE Standard: A traditional fee-for-service option formerly known as *CHAMPUS*

Figure 19-4 illustrates the eligibility requirements and benefits of the three plans.

CHAMPVA

In 1973 a program similar to TRICARE was established for the spouses and dependent children of veterans suffering total, permanent, service-connected disabilities and for surviving spouses and dependent children of veterans who had died as a result of service-related disabilities. This program, CHAMPVA, is a health benefits program in which the Department of Veterans Affairs (VA) shares with eligible beneficiaries the cost of certain healthcare services and supplies. After eligibility for CHAMPVA has been determined and ID cards issued, the insured persons may obtain covered services and supplies from any provider who is appropriately licensed or certified to perform the services offered. Exceptions include certain mental health categories and freestanding ambulatory surgical centers.

Workers' Compensation

All state legislatures have passed workers' compensation laws to protect wage earners against the loss of wages and the cost of medical care resulting from occupational accident or disease. State laws differ as to the classes of employees included and the benefits provided.

No state's workers' compensation laws cover all employees. However, if a patient says that he or she was injured in the workplace or is suffering from a work-associated illness, the medical assistant should check with the patient's employer to verify the insurance coverage.

Compensation benefits include medical care benefits, weekly income replacement benefits for temporary disability, permanent disability settlements, and survivor benefits when applicable. The provider of service (e.g., doctor, hospital, therapist) accepts the workers' compensation payment as payment in full and does not bill the patient. Time limitations are set for the prompt reporting of workers' compensation cases. The employee is obligated to promptly notify the employer; the employer, in turn, must notify the insurance company and must refer the employee to a source of medical care.

In some states the employer and insurance company have the right to select the physician treating the patient. In essence, the purpose of workers' compensation laws is to provide prompt medical care to an injured or ill worker so that the person may be restored to health and return to full earning capacity in as short a time as possible.

Disability Programs

Disability income insurance is a form of health insurance that provides periodic payments to an individual to replace income (actual or presumed) when a sickness, injury, or disability that is not a work-related condition results in the insured being unable to work. A disability insurance policy can be obtained through employer-sponsored and/or government-funded programs, or private policies can be purchased through a commercial insurance company.

COMMERCIAL INSURANCE

Many people are covered by health insurance issued by private (commercial) insurance companies, such as Aetna, Connecticut General, Metropolitan, and Prudential. Physicians and medical societies control neither the premiums paid nor the benefits received from such policies. For traditional types of policies, payment is normally made to the subscriber unless the subscriber or insured has authorized that payment be made directly to the physician.

VERIFICATION OF INSURANCE BENEFITS

It is important to verify insurance benefits before providing services to patients. To verify benefits, the following steps should be taken (Procedure 19-2):
- When a patient calls for an appointment, identify what type of insurance the patient has or what managed care organization the patient belongs to.
- When the patient arrives for the appointment, photocopy both sides of the patient's ID card (because copayments or amounts to be paid may appear on the back for hospital, office, and the emergency department).
- Contact the insurance carrier to verify that the patient is eligible for benefits, and determine the basic benefits,

| ADFM = active duty family members
RFMS = retirees, family members and survivors | **Benefit and Coverage Chart** | | | | | |

Outpatient Services	**Programs and Beneficiary Costs**					
Program and Classification	**Tricare Prime**		**Tricare Extra**		**Tricare Standard**	
	ADFM	**RFMS**	**ADFM**	**RFMS**	**ADFM**	**RFMS**
Annual Enrollment Fee* (per fiscal year)	None	$230/person $460/family	None ⟶		None ⟶	
Annual Deductible (per fiscal year 10/1 to 9/30) (applied to outpatient services before cost-share is determined)	None (except when using Point-of-Service option)		E-4 and below $50/person $100/family E-5 and above $150/person $300/family	$150/person $300/family	E-4 and below $50/person $100/family E-5 and above $150/person $300/family	$150/person $300/family
Physician Services	None	$12	15% of contracted fee	20% of contracted fee	20% of maximum allowable charge	25% of maximum allowable charge
Ancillary Services (certain radiology, laboratory, & cardiac services)	None ⟶ (RFMS may have $12 copay if test provided independent of office visit)					
Ambulance Services	None	$20				
Home Health Services	None	$12				
Family Health Services	None	$12				
Durable Medical Equipment (greater than $100)	None	20% cost-share				
Emergency Services (network and non-network)	None	$30 copayment				
Outpatient Behavioral Health (limitations apply)	None	$25 copayment $17 group visits				
Immunizations (for required overseas travel)	None	Not covered		Not covered		Not covered
Ambulatory Surgery (same day)	None	$25 copayment (applied to facility charges only)	$25 copayment for hospital charges	20% of contracted fee	$25 copayment for hospital charges	*Professional:* 25% of maximum allowable charge *Facility:* 25% of maximum allowable charge OR billed charges, whichever is less
Eye Examinations (limitations apply)	None	Clinical Preventive Service	15% of contracted fee	Not covered	20% of maximum allowable charge	Not covered
Prescription Drugs– Network Pharmacy	$3 copayment for each 30-day supply of **generic** medication $9 copayment for each 30-day supply of **brand name** medication					
Prescription Drugs– National Mail Order Pharmacy	$3 copayment for each 90-day supply of **generic** medication $9 copayment for each 90-day supply of **brand name** medication (Note: if the beneficiary has primary insurance that covers presciption medication, the beneficiary is not eligible for the mail order pharmacy benefit)					
Prescription Drugs– Non-network Pharmacy	$9 or 20% of total cost (whichever is greater) plus deductible					

*No enrollment fee for those who are eligible for Medicare (enrolled in Part B) on the basis of disability or end-stage renal disease

NOTE: TRICARE Prime Remote—benefits are similar to TRICARE Prime program; however, ADSMs have no copayment costs-share or deductible

Program for Persons with Disabilities—no deductible; monthly cost-share varies from $25 to $250, depending on sponsor's rank

Figure 19-4 TRICARE plans: eligibility and benefits. (From Fordney MT: *Insurance handbook for the medical office,* ed 8, St Louis, 2004, Saunders.)

PROCEDURE 19-2

Apply Managed Care Policies and Procedures: Perform Verification of Eligibility and Benefits

CAAHEP COMPETENCY: 3.a.(3)(a)
ABHES COMPETENCY: 3.t

GOAL: *Confirm patient's insurance is in effect and determine what benefit and exclusions are covered.*

EQUIPMENT and SUPPLIES

- Patient record
- Precertification form
- Patient's insurance information
- Telephone and fax machine
- Pen

PROCEDURAL STEPS

1. When a patient calls for an appointment, identify the patient's insurance plan or managed care organization.
   PURPOSE: To prepare for and begin gathering required information to perform both insurance verification and insurance claim completion procedures.

2. At the time of the appointment, obtain and photocopy both sides of the patient's insurance ID card(s).
   PURPOSE: To ensure the correct ID, group, and policy numbers are obtained, as well as the name, address, and phone number of the insurance carrier(s).

3. Complete the patient portion of the Verification of Eligibility and Benefit form, including demographic and insurance information for the patient, and the contact information for the insurance plan. Complete one form for each of the patient's insurances.

PURPOSE: To document the information needed to perform the verification of eligibility and benefits. This form will later be filed in the patient's insurance record.

4. Contact the insurance carrier(s) by phone to a) verify that the patient is eligible for benefits and the insurance is in effect; b) determine the basic benefits, exclusions, or non-covered services of the insurance plan; c) determine if there are deductibles, co-payments or any other out-of-pocket expenses the patient is responsible for paying; d) determine if preauthorization is required for referrals to specialists or for any procedures and/or services.
   PURPOSE: To confirm the insurance is in effect, and to determine what benefits, preauthoritizations, deductibles and/or out-of pocket expenses the patient is responsible for.

5. Obtain the name, title, and phone number of the person contacted.
   PURPOSE: To identify and document the name of the individual providing the benefits and eligibility information, and to have as a reference if additional questions arise.

6. Document the information collected in the patient's medical record and on the Verification of Eligibility and Benefits form.

---

exclusions or non-covered services, and whether pre-authorization is required for referrals to specialists or for any procedures and/or services. Obtain the name, title, and phone number of the person contacted.

- Document the information collected in the patient's medical record and on a Verification of Benefits form.
- Give the patient a letter to read and sign, outlining the plan requirements and possible restrictions or non-covered items.
- When referrals are required, explain the procedure to the patient so it is understood that without the referral, it is the patient's responsibility to pay for the physician's services.
- Collect any copayments or deductibles.

PRECERTIFICATION AND PREAUTHORIZATION

Most insurance companies require precertification or preauthorization, usually within 24 hours, when a patient is going to be hospitalized or undergo certain procedures. In addition, most managed care systems require preauthorization for a patient to be referred to a specialist or even for certain laboratory tests or other procedures. Insurance claims for payment will be denied if proper authorization is not obtained.

It is standard when a new patient makes an appointment to ask what type of insurance the patient has and to collect the patient and insured's personal, employment, and insurance information on a patient registration form. The patient registration form will be discussed further in Chapter 20. If the patient belongs to an HMO, the medical assistant should check that plan contract for precertification or preauthorization requirements. Typically, only HMOs require preauthorization (precertification); however, it is recommended that the need for preauthorization be obtained during the verification of eligibility and benefits for all insurance carriers. The following lists the information that should be obtained and recorded on the preauthorization form (Figure 19-5) before the contact with the insurance carrier is made.

- Patient name, address, phone number and identification number(s)
- Provider name, address, phone number, and provider identification number (PIN)
- Plan name, address, and contact person
- Telephone number (or numbers) of contact person and fax number
- Preliminary diagnosis
- Planned surgery, diagnostic test or reason for referring patient to a specialist

Mary Jo Smith
College Clinic
4567 Broad Avenue, WH
Telephone No.: (555) 486-9002
Fax No.:(555) 487-8976

MANAGED CARE PLAN AUTHORIZATION REQUEST

☐ Health Net   ☐ Met Life
☐ Pacificare   ☐ Travelers
☐ Secure Horizons   ☐ Pru Care
☐ Other

Member/Group No.: 54098XX

**TO BE COMPLETED BY PRIMARY CARE PHYSICIAN
OR OUTSIDE PROVIDER**

Patient Name: Louann Campbell   Date: 7-14-20XX

☐ Male   ☐ Female   Birthdate: 4-7-1952   Home Telephone Number: (555) 450-1666

Address: 2516 Encina Avenue, Woodland Hills, XY 12345-0439

Primary Care Physician: Gerald Practon, MD   Provider ID #: TC 14021

Referring Physician: Gerald Practon, MD   Provider ID #: TC 14021

Referred to: Raymond Skeleton, MD   Office Telephone Number: (555) 486-9002

Address: 4567 Broad Avenue, Woodland Hills, XY 12345

Diagnosis Code: 724.2   Diagnosis Low back pain

Diagnosis Code: 722.10   Diagnosis Sciatica

Treatment Plan: Orthopedic consultation and evaluation of lumbar spine; R/O herniated disc L4-5

Authorization requested for: ☐ Consult Only   ☐ Treatment Only   ☐ Consult/Treatment

☐ Consult/Procedure/Surgery   ☐ Diagnostic Tests

Procedure Code: 99244   Description: New patient consultation

Procedure Code: _____   Description: _____

Place of service: ☒ Office ☐ Outpatient ☐ Inpatient ☐ Other   Number of Visits: 1

Facility: _____   Length of Stay: _____

List of potential future consultants (i.e., anesthetists, surgical assistants or medical/surgical):

Physician's Signature: *Gerald Practon, MD*

TO BE COMPLETED BY PRIMARY CARE PHYSICIAN

PCP Recommendations: See above   PCP Initials: GP

Date eligibility checked: 7-14-20XX   Effective Date: 1-15-20XX

TO BE COMPLETED BY UTILIZATION MANAGEMENT

Authorized: _____ Auth. No. _____ Not Authorized _____

Deferred: _____   Modified: _____

Comments: _____

Figure 19-5 Sample preauthorization (referral) form.

- Name, address, phone number of facility or specialist
- Copayment amount or deductible
- Hospital benefits for inpatient and outpatient surgery
- Participating hospitals, radiology service providers, laboratories, and physicians

Once the information is collected it should be faxed to the insurance company. In case of an emergency, the authorization may be obtained by phone; however, the form should be faxed as soon as possible afterward. The form will be faxed back to the provider from the insurance carrier with the authorization number and other vital information as described in the next section. The **birthday rule** determines the primary insurance for those who are covered by more than one policy.

Obtaining preauthorization for referrals or certain procedures and services is required. Typically, the PCP or "gatekeeper" is responsible for obtaining the authorization. A gatekeeper

PROCEDURE 19-3

Apply Managed Care Policies and Procedures: Perform Preauthorization (Precertification) and/or Referral

CAAHEP COMPETENCY: 3.a.(3)(a)
ABHES COMPETENCY: 3.u

GOAL: *Using the information in the case study, obtain precertification from a patient's HMO for requested services or procedures.*

EQUIPMENT and SUPPLIES

- Patient record
- Precertification form
- Patient's insurance information
- Telephone and fax machine
- Pen

PROCEDURAL STEPS

1. Assemble the necessary documents and equipment.
2. Examine the patient record, and determine the service or procedure for which preauthorization is being requested, including, if applicable, the specialist's name and phone number and the reason for the request.
   PURPOSE: To correctly complete the required form for gaining authorization from the patient's insurance carrier for the specified treatment.
3. Complete the referral form, providing all pertinent information requested.

PURPOSE: To document for the insurance carrier the patient demographic and insurance information, the physician's identification information, and either the diagnosis and planned procedure or treatment, or the name and contact information of the physician to whom the patient is being referred.
4. Proofread the completed form.
   PURPOSE: To ensure the accuracy of the information.
5. Fax the completed form to the patient's insurance carrier.
   PURPOSE: To inform the insurance carrier of the patient's medical condition; to request preauthorization for the requested treatment; to request a verification number; and to confirm the specific number of physical therapy sessions, or to obtain authorization for referral of the patient to a specialist.
6. Place a copy of the returned, completed approval form in the patient's medical record.

---

can be a PCP, a general or family practitioner, an internist, a pediatrician, and in some instances an obstetrician or a gynecologist.

Referral is a term used in managed care when a patient is referred from a PCP to a specialist. When completing a referral form, it is imperative that all necessary information be included (Procedure 19-3). A referral can take from a few minutes to a few days to be reviewed and approved or denied. The three types of referral are as follows:

- A regular referral usually takes 3 to 10 working days for review and approval. This type of referral is used when a patient has not responded to a PCP's treatment and/or medication and the physician believes that the patient must see a specialist to continue treatment.
- An urgent referral will usually take about 24 hours for approval. This type of referral is used when an urgent situation occurs but is not life-threatening.
- A STAT referral can be approved by telephone immediately after faxing it to the utilization review department. A STAT referral is used in an emergency situation as indicated by the physician, such as life-or-death situations, miscarriage, loss of limb, or other conditions of similar magnitude. Usually the physician will refer the patient by telephone and will fax the information with the referral afterward.

A regular referral is the most common and can be inconvenient for the patient. Most managed care plans require contacting the member services department to check the status

of a referral. A cardinal rule is to never tell the patient that the referral has been approved unless you have a hard copy of the authorization. *Authorization* is a term used in managed care for an approved referral. A referral becomes an authorization after it is reviewed by utilization management and/or the medical director and has been approved. When a referral is approved, the PCP's office will receive a copy of the authorization by mail or fax. Always review the authorization thoroughly. The patient will receive a letter with an authorization number and the approved services. The patient must present the authorization to the specialist's office receptionist on the day the services will be provided. An authorization provides the following information to both the referring PCP and the specialist:

1. An authorization code, which may be alphabetic, numeric, or alphanumeric.
2. The date on which it was received by utilization management, the date on which it was approved, and the expiration date.
   a. An authorization is good for 60 days.
   b. If services are provided after the expiration date, the services will be denied. If this happens, you need to contact utilization management or member services, ask for an extension, and answer a few questions. Sometimes it is necessary to involve the patient and/or the specialist's office.
   c. If the authorization expires and services have not been provided, an extension may be requested. Utilization

management will change the expiration date and will fax a copy to the PCP and specialist or will generate a new authorization with a new number.

3. A diagnosis code.

4. The name, address, and telephone number of the contracted specialist where services will be provided. Sometimes the PCP will refer the patient to a specialist but will not receive approval for that specialist and must get approval for another. Always be sure that any specialist to whom the physician refers a patient is contracted with the same managed care plan as the PCP.

5. The comments section is the most critical area of a referral, because this area will designate what services are approved.

   a. It includes the specified number of authorized visits to the specialist.

   b. An authorization may be issued for (1) evaluation only, (2) evaluation and treatment plan, (3) evaluation and biopsy, (4) evaluation and one injection, etc.

   c. When authorization for only an evaluation and/or treatment plan is given, the medical assistant must inform the patient that there will not be any treatment—only an evaluation and/or a treatment plan.

If a referral is denied because of insufficient information or no medical necessity, the PCP's office will be notified. Some medical groups will notify both the PCP and the patient. When the PCP's office provides the utilization management committee with the necessary information, the referral will be reviewed again for approval.

Managed care changes on a day-to-day basis. To compete within this market, some insurance companies have added a benefit that will allow a member or patient to self-refer (meaning an authorization is not required to see a specialist). Many plans for senior citizens now have a **self-referral** and a copayment as well as some other insurance coverage. The procedure for obtaining a self-referral is essentially the same as for a provider of service. An authorization form is completed by the patient or with the assistance of the referred provider and faxed to the insurance company for approval.

CRITICAL THINKING APPLICATION

Many private carriers and managed health plans have precertification or preauthorization requirements. How can Ann explain the rationale of preapproval to inquiring patients?

FEE SCHEDULES

A healthcare practitioner has three commodities to sell—time, judgment, and services. In every case the healthcare practitioner must place an estimate on the value of these services. Fees for medical procedures and services differ from office to office based on the type of practice and the needs of the facility. The physician or physicians establishing the practice normally set the fees for procedures and services. In the past most physicians worked on a fee-for-service basis (e.g., patients were charged

for the provider's service based on each individual service performed).

In recent years **third-party payors** (particularly government and managed healthcare organizations) have greatly influenced what healthcare providers can charge by establishing what is referred to as the *allowable charge*. The allowable charge is the maximum that third-party payors will pay for a particular procedure or service (Procedure 19-4).

When healthcare providers establish a fee schedule, other factors influence what the charge for a particular procedure or service can be; these factors include the relative value scale (RVS) and the RBRVS.

Relative Value Scale

The RVS was pioneered by the California Medical Association in 1956 to help physicians establish rational, relative fees. Other states soon followed suit. Hundreds of the most commonly performed procedures were compiled, given procedure numbers similar to those in the AMA's Current Procedural Terminology (CPT) code list, and assigned a unit value. The assigned unit value represented the value of that procedure in relation to other procedures commonly performed. Although no monetary value was placed on the units, many insurance companies used the RVS to determine benefits by applying a conversion factor to assign a monetary value to the unit value. In 1978 the Federal Trade Commission (FTC) interpreted the California RVS as a fee-setting instrument and prohibited its publication and distribution. The FTC was attempting to make medical practice more competitive by ruling against the setting of fees and by encouraging physicians to advertise.

Resource-Based Relative Value Scale

As discussed earlier in this chapter, CMS developed the first comprehensive RBRVS-based fee schedule, which was adopted by Medicare in 1992. The RBRVS-based fee schedule adjusts fees for differences in resources used to provide each service. The amount of resources required to perform a service is determined through the use of relative value units (RVUs) assigned to the CPT codes developed by the AMA. This system was implemented to standardize payment with an adjustment for overhead costs in different geographic areas. Since Medicare's introduction of RBRVS, most third-party payors have adopted similar approaches in developing their fees.

DEDUCTIBLES AND CO-INSURANCE

Many types of health insurance plans, such as indemnity, managed care, and Medicare, require a deductible and co-insurance amount that the patient must pay out of pocket. These plans typically have an annual deductible amount the patient must pay before the plan pays anything. In addition, members usually must also pay a percentage of each charge, which is called *co-insurance*. Most indemnity plans have an annual "out-of-pocket limit" on the amount members must pay for co-insurance payments. This type of plan takes the major expense out of medical bills and helps keep premium costs down.

PROCEDURE 19-4

Apply Third-Party Guidelines

<u>CAAHEP COMPETENCY:</u> 3.a(3)(b)
<u>ABHES COMPETENCY:</u> 8.c

GOAL: *To ensure that claims are processed quickly and result in the highest allowable reimbursement.*

EQUIPMENT and SUPPLIES

- Managed care contracts
- Managed care handbooks
- Clerical supplies
- Forms from managed care organizations
- Claim forms

PROCEDURAL STEPS

1. Determine the patient's health insurance plan.
   <u>PURPOSE:</u> To bill the correct health insurance plan for services rendered.
2. Review the rules and regulations that govern that particular organization.
   <u>PURPOSE:</u> To be sure that the claim is accurate according to the guidelines in place for the patient's policy.
3. Make certain that a signature is on file for the patient.
   <u>PURPOSE:</u> The signature authorizes the provider to release medical information to the insurance carrier and authorizes the carrier to pay the provider directly.
4. Determine the procedures and services that are to be billed on the claim.
5. Determine if all procedures and services to be billed are covered by the health insurance plan.
   <u>PURPOSE:</u> Procedures and services that are not covered should not be billed on the health insurance claim form; the patient must pay for those services.
6. Make sure that the patient is aware of any procedures that will not be covered by the health insurance plan.
7. Pay close attention to the blocks on the insurance claim form that are designated "for local use.".
   <u>PURPOSE:</u> These blocks are designed to include information particular to certain policies.
8. Determine that all procedures and services that are billed on the claim pertain to one or more of the diagnoses listed.
   <u>PURPOSE:</u> All of the procedures and services must relate to one or more diagnoses to be deemed medically necessary.
9. Submit the claim to the correct address or clearinghouse.

	Column A	Column B
Total charge	$10,000	$20,000
Deductible (paid by Mrs. Jones)	(500)	(500)
5% (Mrs. Jones' portion)	(500)	(500)
Total amount paid by Mrs. Jones	$900	$1000
Total amount paid by insurance	$9000	$19,000

Figure 19-6 Calculation of deductible and co-insurance.

For example, Mrs. Jones' plan has a $500 deductible, after which the insurance company pays 95% of all charges, which leaves Mrs. Jones with a 5% co-insurance expense in addition to the deductible. In addition, she has a $1000 out-of-pocket expense maximum for which she is responsible, which means that once Mrs. Jones has paid $1000 total, the insurance company then pays 100% of any balance remaining. She has incurred a $10,000 charge for a cardiac surgery performed by her physician. Column A in Figure 19-6 shows that Mrs. Jones' total out-of-pocket expense is $1000. She paid the $500 deductible, and 5% of 10,000, or an additional $500. The insurance company then paid the remaining balance of $9000. Column B in Figure 19-6 shows that the cardiac surgery in this instance was $20,000. Mrs. Jones' total out-of-pocket expense remains $1000, therefore, in this instance the insurance company is responsible for payment of the balance of $19,000. Because her maximum out-of-pocket expense according to the plan described is $1000, even though the charges were doubled, she still only pays the $1000 total out-of-pocket expense.

With Medicare and some other plans, a limit is placed on the amount that will be reimbursed for any procedure or service. This limit is called an *allowable amount*. The allowable amount can be all or part of a charge for a service or procedure. For example, for a level I office visit if the provider typically charges $80, the insurance company benefit allowable amount might only be $60. Depending on the contract between the provider and insurance carrier, the provider will either write-off the $20 difference or pass the non-allowed portion of the charge on to the guarantor for payment. The contracts between the physician and provider vary greatly, it is important for the medical assistant to examine the explanation of benefits from the insurance carrier closely, and to be knowledgeable about the contract provisions between the provider of service and all insurance carriers the provider uses.

CRITICAL THINKING APPLICATION

An elderly patient comes to the office complaining that Medicare did not pay her bill in full. "Medicare is supposed to pay 80% of all of my bills and I have already paid my portion," she insists.

- What information does Ann need to get to the bottom of this problem?
- How can she explain situations like this to patients?

PROCEDURE 19-5

Apply Managed Care Policies and Procedures: Perform Deductible, Co-Insurance, and Allowable Amount Calculations

<u>CAAHEP COMPETENCY:</u> 3.a.(3)(a)
<u>ABHES COMPETENCY:</u> 3.t

GOAL: *To calculate the patient's out-of-pocket expense or amount to be billed to a secondary insurance carrier, and to determine what amounts are to be written off and/or passed on to the patient for payment.*

EQUIPMENT and SUPPLIES

- Explanation of benefits (EOB) form (or explanation of Medicare benefits (EOMB) form or remittance advice (RA) form OR Verification of eligibility and benefits form
- Patient accounts receivable ledger
- Calculator
- Pen
- Paper

PROCEDURAL STEPS

1. Assemble the required materials and equipment.
   <u>REMEMBER:</u> Deductibles and co-insurance are generally deducted from the total charge for services rendered; however, depending on the policies and procedures of the provider they can be calculated for each individual charge. Allowable amounts are almost always deducted from an individual charge.

2. Using the EOB, EOMB, and/or the RA and/or the Verification of Eligibility and Benefits form; and the patient accounts receivable ledger:
   - Write down the total charge from the EOB and/or the patient accounts receivable ledger.
   - Subtract the deductible amount from the total charge. If the deductible exceeds the total amount, subtract only that amount of the deductible that equals the total charge, and stop—do not continue with the other steps. Proceed to the other steps only after all of the patient's deductible has been paid.
   <u>PURPOSE:</u> To calculate and record the appropriate amount of deductible that must be met (and paid) by the patient according to the terms of his or her insurance policy.

3. If it is determined that all of the patient's deductible has been met, proceed by then identifying the co-insurance amount that the patient must pay (e.g., 20%).
   - Multiply this amount (e.g., 20%) by the total charge.
   - Subtract the sum from the total charge balance.

<u>PURPOSE:</u> To calculate and record the appropriate amount of co-insurance that must be met (and paid) by the patient according to the terms of his or her insurance policy.

4. Record the deductible and, if applicable, co-insurance amount(s) on separate lines in the patient balance due column of the patient's account receivable ledger. The sum becomes the patient's responsibility, or if the patient has a secondary insurance carrier, the sum can be billed to the secondary insurance carrier.
   <u>PURPOSE:</u> To maintain a current balance and audit trail on the patient accounts receivable ledger and, when appropriate, to submit a statement to the patient for payment and/or submit a claim to a secondary insurance company.
   <u>NOTE:</u> If there is an allowable amount shown on the EOB, EOMB, or RA which is less than the amount of either the total charge or the individual charge for the date of service, proceed to steps 5 and 6. Otherwise, stop here.

5. Subtract the allowable amount of each individual charge from the actual (billed) charge.

6. Record the difference either in the adjustments or patient balance column.
   - If the provider of service writes off the difference either as a courtesy, hardship adjustment, or as part of the contract the provider has with the insurance company, the amount is recorded in the adjustments column.
   - If the patient is responsible for paying the difference between the actual charge and the allowable amount, the amount is recorded in the patient balance column.
   <u>PURPOSE:</u> To adjust and reconcile the patient accounts receivable ledger and deduct the appropriate allowable amounts from the patient ledger; or, pass those amounts on to the patient for payment.

The steps for calculating deductible, co-insurance, and allowable amounts are illustrated in Procedure 19-5. Calculating deductibles, co-insurance, and allowable amounts is relatively simple. The deductible and co-insurance are subtracted from the total charge for the services and procedures. The sum becomes the patient's responsibility, or if the patient has a secondary insurance, it can be billed to the secondary insurance carrier. Deductibles and co-insurance are generally deducted from the total charge for services rendered; however, depending on the policies and procedures of the provider they can be calculated for each individual charge. Allowable amounts are almost always deducted from an individual charge. Using the example in Figure 19-7, if the allowable amount for Mrs. Jones' $10,000 cardiac surgery is $8500, the $1500 difference between the physician's charge and the allowed amount would either be written off or passed on to the patient as an out-of-pocket expense. In Figure 19-7, Column A, a line has been added to show the $8500 allowable amount and that $1500 has been

	Column A	Column B
Total charge	$10,000	$20,000
Deductible (paid by Mrs. Jones)	(500)	(500)
5% (Mrs. Jones' portion)	(500)	(500)
Allowable amount $8500	(1500)	
Allowable amount $8500 with write off		(1500)
Total amount paid by Mrs. Jones	$2500	$1000
Total amount paid by insurance	$7500	$17,500

Figure 19-7 Calculation of allowable amount.

billed to the patient. In Column B, the amount has been written off, or absorbed as a cost, by the provider. Notice, too, that the insurance carrier pays $1500 less for the cardiac surgery charge in Figure 19-7 than in Figure 19-6.

CRITICAL THINKING APPLICATION

Ann has been working with Max Carter, who is having coronary bypass surgery in one week. Discuss the possible differences in Max's coverage if he has Medicare, Medicaid, or commercial insurance.

UTILIZATION MANAGEMENT

Patient care review by healthcare professionals who do not provide the care is a necessary component of managed care to control costs. A **utilization review** committee reviews individual cases to make certain that medical care services are medically necessary and to study how providers use medical care resources. This committee reviews all physician referrals and cases of emergency department visits and urgent care. After review this department will either approve or deny the referral, so it is important to submit exact documentation and precise statements. The medical assistant should contact this department directly; it should never be left to the patient or covered member to contact this department.

THE *FEDERAL REGISTER*

The *Federal Register* is the official daily publication for rules, proposed rules, and notices of federal agencies and organizations, as well as Executive Orders and other presidential documents. Publications are sponsored by the Office of the *Federal Register* (OFR) and produced by the Government Printing Office (GPO). The system was established to regulate complex social and economic issues after it was decided that agencies and the general public needed a centralized filing and publication system to keep track of rules and regulations.

Medical assistants can use the *Federal Register* for researching rules and regulations governing health insurance and coding. The *Federal Register* website is user-friendly and can be accessed by typing http://fr.cos.com into the computer's browser (such as Internet Explorer or Netscape) address line and pressing Enter. The *Federal Register* search page will be accessed, and from

that point a search can be launched by topic, issue, or agency. Medical assistants may want to take a few minutes to browse this interesting website.

CRITICAL THINKING APPLICATION

■ Ann has obtained precertification and knows the benefits that will be paid toward Max's bill. Discuss how to best explain insurance benefits, exclusions, co-insurance, deductibles, and allowable amounts to Max. Should the medical assistant explain other bills, such as those to the hospital and anesthesiologist?

■ Suppose that Max has two different insurance policies in effect. Discuss the tasks and procedures associated with collecting information about his insurance. How does the medical assistant determine the primary carrier?

CLOSING COMMENTS

Understanding how insurance plans handle reimbursement of benefits is challenging for a patient as well as a medical assistant. However, it is important that patients understand how their insurance works. Many, especially elderly persons, believe that if they have health insurance, all charges for their healthcare will be covered, and they do not always understand the intricacies of deductibles, copayments, medical necessity, and allowable charges.

The responsibilities of a medical assistant include keeping the patient informed and answering questions as they arise. Often medical facilities will provide informational brochures to their patients that explain how health insurance and reimbursement works, giving definitions of some of the more common terms used in the insurance claims process. If patients are well advised and comfortable with insurance facts before treatment begins, the medical experience will go more smoothly, and collection of fees not covered by the carrier will be easier. The medical assistant must use good communication skills, patience, and tact when discussing third-party reimbursement issues with patients.

Throughout their careers, medical assistants must remember that an individual's medical record is personal and private. Conversations between patients and their healthcare providers (and staff) are considered privileged communication. Nearly every day a medical assistant is in a position to read and hear information of a private medical nature, and both the caregiver and the patient expect that this information will not leave the medical office.

Unauthorized release of medical information carries over into the insurance claims processing area. Even though the patient expects the insurance form to be filled out and submitted for payment, this cannot be done without proper written release. This medical release form should be kept in the patient's chart, and it should be updated on a regular basis.

Managed care has often been criticized by the news media. Some types of managed care can create a physician-patient barrier that did not exist during the fee-for-service era. An extra effort in human relations by the medical assistant can help to overcome this barrier and put the patient at ease.

SUMMARY OF SCENARIO

There is still a lot of information on health insurance to digest, but Ann is now much more comfortable with its concepts and no longer feels that understanding the various topics is impossible. Ann understands that there are many different types of insurance carriers, including federal and state programs, commercial carriers, health maintenance organizations, and preferred provider organizations, and that each of these programs offers different benefits, and has different requirements. Ann understands that the best way to remember all of the carriers and benefits offered is to keep an up-to-date manual or computer record that keeps track of addresses, phone numbers, and benefits information for each carrier. In addition, she's learned that failure to verify benefits

and eligibility, or authorization for referrals, treatments, or procedures, can result in a denial of payment for services rendered.

In addition, understanding how to calculate the deductibles, co-insurance, and allowed amounts for procedures and services benefits both the provider and patient. The provider's productivity, income, and losses can be easily tracked, and the patient can be educated as to the exact amounts he or she is responsible for paying.

Now that Ann understands the basics about health insurance, she can look forward to learning the procedure for completing insurance claim forms for various insurance carriers for reimbursement.

SUMMARY of LEARNING OBJECTIVES

1. Define, spell, and pronounce the terms listed in the vocabulary.
   - Spelling and pronouncing medical terms correctly adds credibility to the medical assistant. Knowing the definition of these terms promotes confidence in communication with patients and co-workers.
2. Discuss the purpose of health insurance.
   - Medical assistants should have an understanding of the purpose of health insurance. This will help in the workplace not only by facilitating their knowledge of the subject, but also in helping them educate patients. The trend for insurance policies to encourage preventive medicine can be appreciated.
3. Differentiate among the various types of insurance policies.
   - Insurance policies fall into many different categories and are available in many different forms. The ability to differentiate among the various types of insurance policies gives medical assistants a solid background in what is available on the market, what is included in each policy category, and the function of each. It is also important for medical assistants to understand and appreciate that there are still many people in this country who cannot afford and do not receive high-quality healthcare.
4. Explain the numerous classifications of insurance benefits available.
   - Insurance packages are often tailored to the needs of each individual or group, and the ways to combine benefits are limitless. Health insurance policies normally contain a combination of the different benefits discussed in this chapter (e.g., surgical, basic medical, and major medical).
5. Explain how insurance benefits are determined.
   - Benefits are determined and paid in one of several ways: indemnity schedules, service benefit plans, UCR fees, and relative value studies and scales. Medical assistants should become familiar with each of these methods and understand the ramifications of all.

6. Differentiate among the different types of managed care options.
   - *Managed care* is a broad term used to describe a variety of health plans developed to provide healthcare services at lower costs. When the medical assistant is employed in a medical facility, he or she will undoubtedly be working with many types of managed care plans. Therefore it is important to know the various types (e.g., HMO, IPA, and PPO) and understand how each one functions. Managed care has had both positive and negative effects on modern medicine. The medical assistant should be well informed about the managed care policies most frequently seen in the practice.
7. List and discuss other major third-party payors.
   - Other major third-party payors the medical assistant should become familiar with are BC/BS, Medicaid, Medicare, CHAMPVA, TRICARE, and workers' compensation. Medicare is the largest third-party insurer in the country, making high-quality healthcare affordable for the elderly and select other groups. Medicaid is another government-sponsored healthcare plan for individuals who qualify for these benefits. Workers' compensation covers employees who are injured or who become ill as a result of accidents or adverse conditions in the workplace. Disability programs reimburse individuals for monetary losses incurred as a result of an inability to work for reasons other than those covered under workers' compensation. The medical assistant should be familiar with the major plans that are presented in the practice.
8. Interpret the procedure for verifying insurance benefits.
   - Many problems can be prevented for both the patient and the medical office if the medical assistant develops and follows a procedure for verifying insurance benefits before services are rendered. This procedure includes gathering as much information as possible about the demographics of the patient and his or her insurance coverage. A pragmatic and tactful discussion with all new patients explaining the established

Continued

SUMMARY of LEARNING OBJECTIVES

Continued

policy that the medical office adheres to regarding the insurance claims process and the collection of fees not covered by their policy will pay off in the end.

9. Discuss the different types of fee schedules.
   - It is important for both the medical assistant and patients to realize that fees for medical procedures and services differ from office to office based on the type of practice and the needs of the facility. Until the advent of managed care, most physicians operated on a fee-for-service basis in which the provider would render his or her services and charge accordingly. In recent years, government and managed care organizations have greatly influenced what healthcare providers can charge. Many third-party payors base reimbursements on what is referred to as the allowable charge. Other fee schedule types include the RVS and the RBRVS.

10. Obtain managed care referrals and precertifications.
    - Obtaining precertifications and making referrals is a process that must be done according to the guidelines of the individual insurance companies. If uncertain about the procedure, always

refer to the company's insurance manual or check the process online, if possible.

11. Perform eligibility and verification of benefits procedures.
    - Verification of insurance benefits is done to make certain that the physician will be reimbursed for his or her services performed on the patient. The process for verifying insurance benefits is outlined in Procedure 19-1.

12. Perform a preauthorization procedure.
    - Preauthorization helps the medical assistant to ensure that the physician will be paid for the services provided to the patient. The process for obtaining preauthorization or precertification is outlined in Procedure 19-2.

13. Demonstrate how insurance benefits are determined by calculating deductible and co-insurance payments.
    - Medical assistants should become proficient at calculating the amounts due to the physician, considering deductibles, copayments, and coinsurance amounts. The process for calculating insurance payments is outlined in Procedure 19-3.

CONNECTIONS

Study Guide Connection: Go to Chapter 19 Study Guide. Read the Case Study and Workplace Applications and complete the assignments. Do online research for answers to the questions in the Internet Activities associated with third-party reimbursement.

CD Connection: Go to the Medical Assisting Competency Challenge CD and do the training activities under Health Insurance Activities.

Evolve Connection: For more information related to third-party reimbursement, go to http://evolve.elsevier.com/kinn/ admin and visit related weblinks for Chapter 19. Click on the Medical Assisting Exam Review and do the practice questions to sharpen your test-taking skills. To learn more about office software, do the exercises for the Altapoint demo that is on the CD.

The Health Insurance Claim Form 20

Carline A. Dalgleish
Alexandra Patricia Young

SCENARIO

The school where Machelle Van Cleve receives her medical assistant training offers an optional job-shadowing module. For her assignment she chose a nearby health center, where she observed the administrative responsibilities of the medical assistants employed in this multi-specialty practice. Machelle found that some of the offices were organized and efficient, whereas others lacked a structured routine, especially in the insurance department. Machelle, a detail-oriented person who enjoyed her studies related to billing and coding, heard numerous comments from employees in the administrative area related to the volumes of work in the billing offices. Her office manager explained that the mountainous paperwork was created as a result of managed care requirements, rejected claims needing further research, and inconsistencies in the demands of the various insurance companies. Machelle agreed that keeping up with the requirements and regulations of the many third-party payors and government entitlement programs must be an overwhelming task. She concluded that billing and reimbursement are at the heart of the medical facility, and the correct completion of insurance claim forms is central to the success of the practice. She realized that becoming familiar with the complexities of the insurance claims process would be challenging, but she was convinced that through education, organization, and dedication she could become a valuable employee and an advocate for the patients who needed her assistance in resolving issues related to their claims for reimbursement.

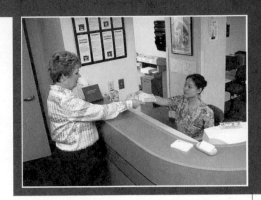

While studying this chapter, think about the following questions:

- What will Machelle find is one of the most important, and basic, tasks that must be done properly before even beginning the insurance claim preparation?
- Why was it important for Machelle to learn the specific insurance billing requirements of different insurance companies and third party payers?

- What has Machelle learned about the importance of auditing claims before they're sent to the insurance carrier for reimbursement?
- What does Machelle know about reimbursement and insurance claims followup?

LEARNING OBJECTIVES

1. Define, spell, and pronounce the terms listed in the vocabulary.
2. Discuss the differences between paper claims and electronic claims.
3. Understand the guidelines for completing the CMS-1500 claim form.
4. Explain how to complete each of the 33 blocks of the CMS-1500 claim form.

5. Differentiate between "clean" and "dirty" claims.
6. Discuss methods of preventing claim rejections.
7. Describe ways of checking the status of claims.
8. Gather information for use on insurance claim forms.
9. Complete a CMS 1500 insurance claim form appropriately for various federal, state and commercial third-party payors.

National Accreditation Competencies and Content

CAAHEP COMPETENCIES

Administrative
3.a.(3)(a). Apply managed care policies and procedures
3.a.(3)(b). Apply third-party guidelines
3.a.(3)(e). Complete insurance claim forms

General
3.c.(2)(a). Identify and respond to issues of confidentiality
3.c.(2)(b). Perform within legal and ethical boundaries
3.c.(2)(d). Document appropriately
3.c.(3)(a). Explain general office policies
3.c.(4)(c). Utilize computer software to maintain office systems

ABHES COMPETENCIES

Professionalism
1.b. Maintain confidentiality at all times
1.d. Be cognizant of ethical boundaries

Administrative Duties
3.d. Apply computer concepts for office procedures
3.t. Apply managed care policies and procedures
3.u. Obtain managed care referrals and pre-certification
3.w. Complete insurance claim forms
3.x. Use physician fee schedule

Legal Concepts
5.a. Determine needs for documentation and reporting
5.b. Document accurately

Instruction
7.a. Orient patients to office policies and procedures

VOCABULARY

assignment of benefits The transfer of the patient's legal right to collect benefits for medical expenses to the provider of those services, authorizing the payment to be sent directly to the provider.

audit A process done prior to claims submission to examine claims for accuracy and completeness. An audit can be performed manually or, if computer billing software is used, electronically.

audit trail The path left by a transaction when it has been completed; often referred to when tracking medical services used by patients or researching claims.

clean claims Insurance claim forms that have been completed correctly (no errors or omissions) and can be processed and paid promptly if they meets the restrictions on covered services and items.

clearinghouse A centralized facility to which insurance claims are transmitted. Clearinghouses separate, check, and redistribute claims electronically to various insurance carriers and may offer additional services to the physician.

direct billing A method of electronic claims submission where computer software allows a provider to submit an insurance claim directly to an insurance carrier for payment.

dirty claims Claims that contain errors or omissions which must be corrected and resubmitted to an insurance carrier in order to obtain reimbursement.

electronic claims Claims that are submitted to insurance processing facilities using a computerized medium, such as direct data entry, direct wire, dial-in telephone digital fax, or personal computer download or upload.

Electronic Data Interchange (EDI) The transfer of data back and forth between two or more entities using an electronic medium.

electronic (or digital) signature A scanned signature or other such mark that is accepted as proof of approval of and/or responsibility for the content of an electronic document.

employer identification number (EIN) The number used by the Internal Revenue Service that identifies a business or individual functioning as a business entity for income tax reporting.

incomplete claim A claim that is missing information and is returned to the provider for correction and resubmission. This is sometimes also called an invalid claim.

Intelligent Character Recognition (ICR) The electronic scanning of printed items as images and use of special software to recognize these images (or characters) as ASCII text for upload into a computer database.

National Provider Identifier (NPI) A lifetime number consisting of 10 digits that Medicare will use to replace the Provider Identification Number (PIN) and the Unique Physician Identification Number (UPIN).

paper claims Hard copies of insurance claims that have been completed and sent by surface mail.

provider Any company, individual, or group that provides medical, diagnostic, or treatment services to a patient.

Provider Identification Numbers (PINs) Numbers assigned to providers by a carrier for use in submission of claims.

rejected claims Claims returned unpaid to the provider for clarification of any question and that must be corrected before resubmission.

Unique Provider Identification Number (UPIN) A number

List continues on next page

List continued from previous page

assigned by fiscal intermediaries to identify providers on claims for services.

universal claim form The form developed by the Health Care Financing Administration (HCFA) (now known as the Centers

for Medicare and Medicaid Services [CMS]) and approved by the AMA for use in submitting all government-sponsored claims. Also known as the CMS-1500 form.

Medical insurance means many things to many people. To some, it is a mound of paperwork. To others, it is a mass of confusion and regulations that seem to constantly change. To a patient with an illness or injury, health insurance helps defray the high costs associated with health care.

The **universal claim form,** originally called the *HCFA-1500,* was first developed in 1988 by the Health Care Financing Administration (HCFA) and approved for use by physicians and **providers** of outpatient services when submitting Medicare Part B claims for reimbursement. A provider is any health care worker who performs any diagnostic assessment or treatment in relation to a patient's illness or injury. In July 2001, HCFA was renamed the Centers for Medicare and Medicaid Services (CMS) and the claim form was renamed the CMS-1500. The form was subsequently adopted by almost all health insurance companies and third-party payors for use in submitting physician claims for reimbursement.

TYPES OF CLAIMS

A medical assistant may submit insurance claims to a third-party payor or an insurance carrier either on **hard copy** (paper) or electronically. Hard copy claims are insurance claims submitted manually, on paper, by surface mail (i.e., the U.S. postal service). **Electronic claims** are insurance claims that are submitted to an insurance carrier via electronic media, such as the internet. Most of today's computer programs generate claims internally from the information that is entered into the database. There are advantages and disadvantages associated with hard-copy or **paper claims** creation. The advantages include minimal start-up costs, because the forms are readily available through many vendors, and the ability to attach documentation explaining unusual circumstances that might affect reimbursement. The cost in time, labor, and postage is higher with paper claim submission, and reimbursement is much slower. Paper claims also require a lot of storage space.

Electronic Claims

Electronic claims are insurance claims that are transmitted over the Internet from the **provider** to the health insurance company. Most claims-processing software is designed to permit electronic claims generation, and with the standardization of the process that was mandated by the Health Insurance Portability and Accountability Act (HIPAA) security and privacy rules, it is far less complicated to send claims electronically. One of

the mandates coming out of HIPAA includes the development of "transaction and code sets" for all insurance-related information sent electronically, including claim form submissions, claims status requests, and remittance (payment) processing. The transaction and code sets for the CMS-1500 electronic claims submission is called the **837P (HIPAA Health Care Claim: Professional).**

Electronic claims can be submitted in several ways. Claims can be transmitted directly to the insurance carrier, also known as **direct billing,** or to a claims **clearinghouse,** which then submits the claims to the insurance carrier. Direct billing occurs when an insurance carrier allows a provider to submit insurance claims directly to the carrier electronically. Most major insurance carriers, including Medicare and Medicaid, provide small computer programs that assist providers in the transmission of the claims. A clearinghouse is a vendor which, for a small fee per claim, provides a service which allows a provider to submit all of the insurance claims generated by the provider to the clearinghouse using special software. The clearinghouse then audits and sorts the claims, and sends them in batches electronically to each of the different insurance carriers. A clearinghouse charges the healthcare provider a small fee for the service of receiving claim transmissions, checking and preparing the claims for processing, consolidating claims so that one transmission can be sent to each carrier, and submitting claims in correct data format to the applicable insurance payor. Clearinghouses typically also provide the following additional services:

- Audit claims to make sure all required fields are completed and data are correct
- Report the number of claims submitted and the number of errors and their specifics
- Forward claims to insurance carriers that accept electronic claims (Medicare, Medicaid, Blue Cross/Blue Shield, and others) or to another clearinghouse that may hold the contracts with specific payors
- Keep provider offices updated as new carriers are added to the database
- Generate informative statistical reports

Typically, with electronic claims processing, payments are received in less than half the time required for turnaround of paper claims. Very soon after claims are transmitted, tracking reports will be sent from the clearinghouse that describe which claims were received, audited, and forwarded to the insurance carrier. These tracking reports also provide information regarding **rejected claims** and those needing additional information.

HIPAA 837 Health Care Claim: Professional (837P) Overview

In Chapter 16 information about HIPAA was introduced that discussed the privacy and security of patient information. As part of HIPAA, standards were developed to protect patient health information being transmitted electronically. These standards, known also as *Transaction and Code Sets,* mandate the format of insurance claims, remittance information, claims attachments, and claims status submitted electronically. The insurance claim form for physician and provider services is called the *HIPAA 837 Health Care Claim: Professional,* or *837P.* This standard contains the format and establishes the data contents of the Health Care Claim Transaction Set (837) for use within the context of an **Electronic Data Interchange (EDI)**—data that are transmitted electronically via the Internet. This transaction set can be used to submit healthcare claim billing information, encounter information, or both from providers of healthcare services to payors, either directly or via intermediary billers and claims clearinghouses.

After 2003 all insurance claims submitted electronically, whether the claim was submitted directly to the payor or a clearinghouse, must be submitted using the 837P standard, in order to comply with the HIPAA mandates. Any provider, payor, employer, or other entity found not using these standards can be removed from participation in federal programs such as Medicaid, Medicare, and TRICARE and could also face stiff civil and/or criminal fines and imprisonment. All vendors, providers, clearinghouses, employers, and health insurance carriers that transmit protected health information electronically must have updated software that conforms to the HIPAA standards, including but not limited to the 837P. These software upgrades will be transparent to the medical assistant entering data into the computer for insurance claims processing—in other words, the format, screens, steps, and processes for entering data into the computer for the purpose of generating insurance claim forms, whether on paper to be mailed, or to be transmitted electronically, should look and feel the same as before the transaction and code sets were implemented.

For more information about the Transaction and Code Sets for the HIPAA 837 Health Care Claim: Professional, and the standards for other electronically submitted data, such as the Claims Payment and Remittance Advice (835), Healthcare Claims Status (276/277), Coordination of Benefits (837), and Referral Certification and Authorization (278), log on to the CMS website

Advantages and Disadvantages: Electronic vs. Paper Billing

Electronic Claims

Advantages

- Cost savings from shorter preparation time
- Cost savings in postage
- Quicker payment turnaround time
- Generation of claim status reports
- New HIPAA rules make claims submission, attachments, and claims status follow-up quicker and easier

Disadvantages

- Computer hardware/software glitches and/or power outages can delay preparation or transmission
- Creating electronic attachments can be problematic
- Initial start-up is expensive

Paper Claims

Advantages

- Minimal start-up costs
- Can attach documentation explaining unusual circumstances

Disadvantages

- The cost in time, labor, and postage is higher
- Reimbursement is much slower
- Require much more storage space

Electronic claims processing reduces payment turnaround time by shortening the payment cycle and can reduce average error rates to less than 1% or 2%. Some insurance companies even waive the attachment requirements for many procedures when claims are submitted electronically.

CRITICAL THINKING APPLICATION

Machelle is interested in learning more about filing claims electronically. In the medical facility where she is doing her externship, she has asked to work with Mrs. Leonard, who performs this procedure in the office. How can working closely with Mrs. Leonard benefit Machelle with regard to this subject?

National Provider Identifier

In the past, each insurance carrier, including government programs, assigned an identifier to each provider of service. Now, also as part of HIPAA, all allied healthcare providers of service will be assigned one individual **National Provider Identifier (NPI)** that the provider can use regardless which insurance carrier is being billed for reimbursement. The NPI is a uniform, national identification number providers will use in lieu of the many provider identification numbers currently used. The NPI, which should be issued in 2007, will replace Medicare's **Unique Provider Identification Number (UPIN)** and almost all other federal, state, and private insurance carriers' **Physician Identification Numbers (PINs).** When following the steps for preparing a health insurance claim form, use the UPIN and PIN numbers where indicated, unless and until the provider's NPI has been issued. At that time, use the NPI in lieu of any references to a UPIN or PIN. This NPI does not replace the Social Security number (SSN), employer identification number (EIN), or federal tax identification number (TIN) used by a provider of service. The SSN, EIN, and TIN are used for income and tax purposes and for reporting to the Internal Revenue Service.

DATA GATHERING GUIDELINES

When the first appointment is made for a patient, it is routine to ask the patient for all pertinent insurance information. Much of this information is on the patient information form that is completed when the patient comes to the medical office for the initial visit and is inserted into the medical chart as well as entered into the computer's patient database. This information should always be collected from every new patient seen by the provider. Returning or established patients should be asked during each visit whether their insurance information is complete and current. Many offices use a form that allows the patient to provide address and phone updates, as well as new insurance information.

The information required to properly complete an insurance claim form includes a patient registration form, verification of eligibility and benefits, referral and authorization information (when required by the insurance carrier), the patient's medical record and/or encounter form or charge ticket, and a CMS-1500 insurance claim form.

The patient registration form (Figure 20-1) is generally divided into several sections. The first section includes the patient information, including the full name, address, phone number, date of birth, gender, and insurance information.

The information needed to complete an insurance claim form includes patient and guarantor demographic and insurance information, the name, address, and phone number of the insurance company, the diagnostic, treatment, and procedures and services information, and the provider's billing information, including name, address, phone number, place of service, and the tax and provider identification numbers.

A medical assistant can use the following general guidelines for collecting information in preparation for insurance claim preparation. More information about the importance of collecting this information and its use in completing an insurance claim form will be discussed later in this chapter.

- Photocopy the back and front of the patient's insurance card, and place the photocopy in the medical record and/or patient insurance file.
- Obtain the patient's full name, address, phone number, date of birth, gender, and employer or, if a student, school information.
- If a patient has more than one insurance policy, it is important to get the name, address, group, and policy number for each company.
- Record the name of the subscriber or guarantor if it is someone other than the patient, and obtain the guarantor's address, date of birth, employer information, and the guarantors relationship to the patient (i.e., spouse, parent, self, or other)
- Signatures to authorize insurance billing, supplying of information to insurance companies, and acceptance of assignments of benefits (if appropriate) should be obtained from all new patients.

Verification of Eligibility and Benefits

Once this information has been collected, the next step is to verify the patient's eligibility and benefits. This is done, usually by phone, by calling the insurance carrier(s) for the patient and confirming that the patient is covered by the insurance, and to obtain a general overview of the benefits available for the patient from the insurance policy. Figure 20-2 is an example of a basic form to use as a guide when completing the eligibility and benefits verification.

THE CMS-1500 HEALTH INSURANCE CLAIM FORM

The CMS-1500 Health Insurance Claim Form (Figure 20-3) is used for most health payors for claims submitted by physicians and suppliers. In the 1960s, there were a number of different claim forms used by third-party payors, but no standardized form for physicians to use in reporting health care services. In the 1980s, the American Medical Association and the Centers for Medicare and Medicaid Services (then known as the Health Care Financing Administration or HCFA) formed a group called the Uniform Claim Form Task Force. The group was charged with creating a standardized claim form and promoting its use among the insurance entities.

In the mid 1990s, the Uniform Claim Form Task Force was replaced by the National Uniform Claim Committee (NUCC). The goal of NUCC was to develop a standardized data set for use in an electronic environment, but still be applicable to and consistent with evolving paper claim form standards.

The CMS-1500 claim form has been revised slightly to accommodate the National Provider Identifier (NPI) and current identifiers until the NPI is fully implemented. An instruction manual is available on the NUCC website for completion of the claim form. The date of the new form is 08-05, replacing the old CMS-1500 form, dated 12-90. Physicians can use either form during the time period between October 1, 2006 and March 31, 2007. On April 1, 2007, the CMS-1500 (12-90 version) will be discontinued and all claims must be submitted on the CMS-1500 (08-05 version). NUCC will provide a data set crosswalk between the 837P and the CMS-1500. The data set is currently being revised to reflect the changes in the CMS-1500 and updated information will be available on the NUCC website when available.

Each item number, or box, in the guidelines below contains the box title, instructions, description, field specifications, and an example. Examples are only for completion of the information required in the box and are not indicative of billing methods. Punctuation is noted in the instructions for each box.

Insurance cards copied   ☒
Date: Jan. 20, 20XX

**Patient Registration
Information**

Account #: __84516__
Insurance #: H-550-64-5172-02
Co-Payment : $ OV $10 ER $50

Please PRINT AND complete ALL sections below!

Is your condition the result of a work injury? YES (NO) An auto accident? YES (NO)
Date of injury: _____

PATIENT'S PERSONAL INFORMATION Marital status ☐ Single ☒ Married ☐ Divorced ☐ Widowed
Sex: ☐ Male ☒ Female
Name: _____FUHR_____ _____LINDA_____ __L.__
       last name   first name   initial
Street Address: __3070 Tipper Street__ (Apt # 4) City: _Oxnard_ State: _CA_ Zip: _93030_
Home phone:(555)276-0101 __ Work phone:(555)372-1151 __ Social Security # _550-XX-5172_
Date of Birth: 11 /05 /65 __ Driver's License: (State & Number) G0075012
Employer/Name of School Electronic Data Systems   ☒ Full Time ☐ Part Time
Spouse's Name: __FUHR__ __GERALD__ __T.__ Spouse's Work phone: (555)921-0075
              last name   first name   initial
How do you wish to be addressed?____LINDA____ Social Security # _____545-XX-2771_____

PATIENT'S/ RESPONSIBLE PARTY INFORMATION
Responsible party: __GERALD T. FUHR__ Date of Birth: _06-15-64_
Relationship to patient: ☐ Self ☒ Spouse ☐ Other   Social Security # _545-XX-2771_
Responsible party's home phone:(555) 276-0101 __ Work phone:(555)921-0075
  Address: _____3070 Tipper Street_____ (Apt # 4) City: _Oxnard_ State: _CA_ Zip: _93030_
Employer's Name: _General Electric_ Phone number: (555) 485-0121
  Address: _____317 East Main_____ City: _Oxnard_ State: _CA_ Zip: _93030_
Your occupation: _Technician_
Spouse's Employer's Name: _Electronic Data Systems_ Spouse's Work phone: (555)372-1151
  Address: _2700 West 5th Street_ City: _Oxnard_ State: _CA_ Zip: _93030_

PATIENT'S INSURANCE INFORMATION Please present insurance cards to receptionist.
PRIMARY insurance company's name: __ABC Insurance Company__
Insurance address: _P.O. Box 12340_ City: _Fresno_ State: _CA_ Zip: _93765_
Name of insured: _Linda L. Fuhr_ Date of Birth:_11/05/65_ Relationship to insured: ☒ Self ☐ Spouse
                                                                                    ☐ Other ☐ Child
Insurance ID number: _H-550-XX-5172-02_ Group number: _17098-020-00004_
SECONDARY insurance company's name: _None_
Insurance address: _____ City: _____ State: ___ Zip: _____
Name of insured: _____ Date of Birth: _____ Relationship to insured: ☐ Self ☐ Spouse
                                                                                  ☐ Other ☐ Child
Insurance ID number: _____ Group number:_____
Check if appropriate: ☐ Medigap policy ☐ Retiree coverage

PATIENT'S REFERRAL INFORMATION   (Please circle one)
Referred by: _Margaret Taylor (Mrs. W. T.)_ If referred by a friend, may we thank her or him? (Yes) No
Name(s) of other physician(s) who care for you: _Jason Smythe, MD_

EMERGENCY CONTACT
Name of person not living with you:_Hannah Gildea_ Relationship: _Aunt_
Address: __4621 Lucretia Avenue__ City: _Oxnard_ State: _CA_ Zip: _93030_
Phone number (home):(555) 274-0132 __ Phone number (work):(__)_____

Assignment of Benefits • Financial Agreement

I hereby give lifetime authorization for payment of insurance benefits be made directly to Gerald Practon, MD,
and any assisting physicians, for services rendered. I understand that I am financially responsible for all charges
whether or not they are covered by insurance. In the event of default, I agree to pay all costs of collection, and
reasonable attorney's fees. I hereby authorize this healthcare provider to release all information necessary to
secure the payment of benefits.
I further agree that a photocopy of this agreement shall be as valid as the original.
Date: _Jan 20, 20XX_ Your signature:_Linda L Fuhr_
Method of payment: ☐ Cash ☒ Check ☐ Credit Card

Figure 20-1 Patient registration form. (Courtesy
Bibbero Systems, Inc., Petaluma, Calif.)

ASSIGNMENT OF INSURANCE BENEFITS

I, the undersigned, represent that I have insurance coverage with and do hereby authorize
_____ to pay and assign directly to _____
        (NAME OF COMPANY)   (NAME OF DOCTOR)
all surgical and/or medical benefits, if any, otherwise payable to me for services as described on the
attached forms hereof, but not to exceed the charges for those services. I understand that I am
financially responsible for all charges whether or not paid by said insurance. I hereby authorize said
assignee to release all information necessary to secure the payment of said benefits.

Date _____ Signed _____

Figure 20-2 Insurance Eligibility/
Preauthorization form.

1500

HEALTH INSURANCE CLAIM FORM

APPROVED BY NATIONAL UNIFORM CLAIM COMMITTEE 08/05

| | PICA | | | | | | | | PICA | | |

1. MEDICARE (Medicare #) **MEDICAID** (Medicaid #) **TRICARE CHAMPUS** (Sponsor's SSN) **CHAMPVA** (Member ID#) **GROUP HEALTH PLAN** (SSN or ID) **FECA BLK LUNG** (SSN) **OTHER** (ID) **1a. INSURED'S I.D. NUMBER** (For Program in Item 1)

2. PATIENT'S NAME (Last Name, First Name, Middle Initial)

3. PATIENT'S BIRTH DATE MM | DD | YY **SEX** M F

4. INSURED'S NAME (Last Name, First Name, Middle Initial)

5. PATIENT'S ADDRESS (No., Street)

6. PATIENT RELATIONSHIP TO INSURED Self Spouse Child Other

7. INSURED'S ADDRESS (No., Street)

CITY   STATE

8. PATIENT STATUS Single Married Other

Employed Full-Time Student Part-Time Student

CITY   STATE

ZIP CODE   TELEPHONE (Include Area Code) ( )

ZIP CODE   TELEPHONE (Include Area Code) ( )

9. OTHER INSURED'S NAME (Last Name, First Name, Middle Initial)

10. IS PATIENT'S CONDITION RELATED TO:

11. INSURED'S POLICY GROUP OR FECA NUMBER

a. OTHER INSURED'S POLICY OR GROUP NUMBER

a. EMPLOYMENT? (Current or Previous) YES NO

a. INSURED'S DATE OF BIRTH MM | DD | YY **SEX** M F

b. OTHER INSURED'S DATE OF BIRTH MM | DD | YY **SEX** M F

b. AUTO ACCIDENT? PLACE (State) YES NO

b. EMPLOYER'S NAME OR SCHOOL NAME

c. EMPLOYER'S NAME OR SCHOOL NAME

c. OTHER ACCIDENT? YES NO

c. INSURANCE PLAN NAME OR PROGRAM NAME

d. INSURANCE PLAN NAME OR PROGRAM NAME

10d. RESERVED FOR LOCAL USE

d. IS THERE ANOTHER HEALTH BENEFIT PLAN? YES NO If yes, return to and complete item 9 a-d.

READ BACK OF FORM BEFORE COMPLETING & SIGNING THIS FORM.
12. PATIENT'S OR AUTHORIZED PERSON'S SIGNATURE I authorize the release of any medical or other information necessary to process this claim. I also request payment of government benefits either to myself or to the party who accepts assignment below.

SIGNED _____ DATE _____

13. INSURED'S OR AUTHORIZED PERSON'S SIGNATURE I authorize payment of medical benefits to the undersigned physician or supplier for services described below.

SIGNED _____

14. DATE OF CURRENT: MM | DD | YY ILLNESS (First symptom) OR INJURY (Accident) OR PREGNANCY(LMP)

15. IF PATIENT HAS HAD SAME OR SIMILAR ILLNESS. GIVE FIRST DATE MM | DD | YY

16. DATES PATIENT UNABLE TO WORK IN CURRENT OCCUPATION MM | DD | YY FROM TO MM | DD | YY

17. NAME OF REFERRING PROVIDER OR OTHER SOURCE

17a.
17b. NPI

18. HOSPITALIZATION DATES RELATED TO CURRENT SERVICES MM | DD | YY FROM TO MM | DD | YY

19. RESERVED FOR LOCAL USE

20. OUTSIDE LAB? YES NO $ CHARGES

21. DIAGNOSIS OR NATURE OF ILLNESS OR INJURY (Relate Items 1, 2, 3 or 4 to Item 24E by Line)

1. |___|.|___| 3. |___|.|___|

2. |___|.|___| 4. |___|.|___|

22. MEDICAID RESUBMISSION CODE ORIGINAL REF. NO.

23. PRIOR AUTHORIZATION NUMBER

24. A. DATE(S) OF SERVICE					B. PLACE OF SERVICE	C. EMG	D. PROCEDURES, SERVICES, OR SUPPLIES (Explain Unusual Circumstances)		E. DIAGNOSIS POINTER	F. $ CHARGES	G. DAYS OR UNITS	H. EPSDT Family Plan	I. ID. QUAL.	J. RENDERING PROVIDER ID. #
From MM DD YY			To MM DD YY				CPT/HCPCS	MODIFIER						
1													NPI	
2													NPI	
3													NPI	
4													NPI	
5													NPI	
6													NPI	

25. FEDERAL TAX I.D. NUMBER SSN EIN

26. PATIENT'S ACCOUNT NO.

27. ACCEPT ASSIGNMENT? (For govt. claims, see back) YES NO

28. TOTAL CHARGE $

29. AMOUNT PAID $

30. BALANCE DUE $

31. SIGNATURE OF PHYSICIAN OR SUPPLIER INCLUDING DEGREES OR CREDENTIALS (I certify that the statements on the reverse apply to this bill and are made a part thereof.)

SIGNED _____ DATE _____

32. SERVICE FACILITY LOCATION INFORMATION

a. NPI   b.

33. BILLING PROVIDER INFO & PH # ( )

a. NPI   b.

NUCC Instruction Manual available at: www.nucc.org

APPROVED OMB-0938-0999 FORM CMS-1500 (08/05)

CARRIER

PATIENT AND INSURED INFORMATION

PHYSICIAN OR SUPPLIER INFORMATION

Figure 20-3 CMS-1500 Insurance Claim form.

Completing the CMS-1500 (08-05)

The CMS-1500 Claim Form is divided into three sections. The first contains the address of the insurance carrier and is located at the top of the form (Figure 20-4). The second section contains information about the patient and insured person, and contains Boxes 1 through 13. The third section contains Boxes 14 through 33 and details physician or supplier information. The following text provides a brief description of each of the blocks on the form. Procedure 20-1 outlines detailed instructions on how to complete each block.

CARRIER BLOCK The name and address of the payor is entered in this block. The payor is the carrier, health plan, third-party administrator, or other payor who will handle the claim. Use the format shown in Figure 20-4.

Suggestions for Claims Submission Planning

Medical assistants might consider the following items when creating a work-friendly routine for completing insurance claims:

- If possible, set aside a definite time for completing insurance claims.
- Have a central location for all insurance forms.
- Have readily available the necessary manuals, code books, and other references needed.
- Create a master list of codes most often used by the practice, including fourth and fifth digits, if appropriate. The list should be updated annually and should never be considered a replacement for the coding manuals.
- Make it a practice to complete the forms as soon as possible after service is rendered, usually at the end of the day.
- Complete the forms by type of insurance category (e.g., all Blue Cross, all Medicare).
- Transmit claims electronically whenever possible.

Patient/Insured Section—Blocks 1 to 8 (Figure 20-5)

Block 1 **Type of Insurance.** This block indicates the type of insurance that the patient has. The "other" block is used when the insurance type is HMO, commercial insurance, automobile accidents, liability, or workers compensation. This information directs the claim to the correct payor and may establish primary liability. EXAMPLE: If the claim is primary for Medicare, check the Medicare box. If Medicare is secondary, check the "Other" box.

Block 1a **Insured's ID Number.** The ID number identifies the patient to the payer. The patient may not be the insured, but the ID number should identify that the patient is covered for benefits.

Block 2 **Patient's Name.** The name of the patient is the person who received treatment or supplies.

Block 3 **Patient's Birth Date and Sex.** The patient's birth date and sex help to identify the patient and distinguishe patients with similar names.

Block 4 **Insured's Name.** The insured's name identifies the person who owns the policy. For employee-sponsored plans, the insured would be the employee.

Block 5 **Patient's Address.** The patient's address and telephone number are entered here. Use the patient's permanent address; do not use a temporary or school address.

Block 6 **Patient Relationship to Insured.** "Self" indicates that the patient is the insured. "Spouse" indicates that the patient is married to the insured. "Child" means that the patient is the insured's minor

Figure 20-4 CMS-1500 insurance claim form: carrier information.

Figure 20-5 CMS-1500 insurance claim form: patient and insured information, blocks 1 to 8.

PROCEDURE 20-1

Complete an Insurance Claim Form

<u>CAAHEP COMPETENCY:</u> 3.a.(3)(e)
<u>ABHES COMPETENCY:</u> 3.x

GOAL: *Accurately complete a CMS-1500 (formerly HCFA-1500) claim form.*

EQUIPMENT and SUPPLIES

- Patient registration form
- Photocopy of patient's insurance ID card
- Encounter form
- Patient record
- Patient's ledger
- CMS-1500 form
- Typewriter or computer

PROCEDURAL STEPS

Carrier Section

Enter the name and address of the payer to whom this claim is being sent in the following format:
1st Line: Name of carrier
2nd Line: First line of address
3rd Line: Second line of address, If needed
4th Line: City, State, and Zip code

Patient/Insured Section

Block 1   Place an "X" in the appropriate box to indicate the type of healthcare coverage that applies to this claim. Mark only one box. <u>NOTE</u>: One (1) character may be entered in any box within the field. Only one box can be marked.

Block 1a   Enter the insured's ID number as shown on the health insurance ID card for the specific payor that this claim addresses. <u>NOTE</u>: A total of twenty-nine (29) characters may be entered in this block.

Block 2   The patient's full last name, first name, and middle initial should be entered into Block 2. Suffixes should be entered after the last name. Do not include titles or professional suffixes. Use commas to separate each name. Do not use periods. Use a hyphen for hyphenated names. <u>NOTE</u>: A total of twenty-eight (28) characters may be entered in this block.

Block 3   Use an 8-digit birth date (MM/DD/YYYY). Enter an "X" in the correct box to indicate the sex of the patient. Only one box can be marked. Leave blank if the gender is for some reason unknown. <u>NOTE</u>: Two (2) characters may be entered for month and date, and four (4) characters may be entered for the year. One (1) character may be entered in the box denoting sex.

Block 4   Enter the insured's full last name, first name, and middle initial. Suffixes should be entered after the last name. Do not include titles or professional suffixes. Use commas to separate each name. Do not use periods. Use a hyphen for hyphenated names. <u>NOTE</u>: Twenty-nine (29) characters may be entered in this box.

Block 5   Enter the patient's mailing address and phone number. The first line is for the number and street, the second line is for the city and state, while the third line is for the zip code and phone number. Do not use punctuation in the address, other than a hyphen in a nine digit zip code. Do not use a hyphen in the phone number. <u>NOTE</u>: Twenty-eight (28) characters are allowed for the street address, twenty-four (24) characters are allowed for the city, and three (3) for the state. Twelve (12) characters are allowed for the zip code, three (3) for the area code, and ten (10) for the phone number.

Block 6   Place an "X" in the correct box that indicates the relationship of the patient to the insured. Mark only one box. <u>NOTE</u>: One (1) character may be entered in any box. Only one box should be marked.

Block 7   Enter the insured's address in this block. The first line is for the number and street, the second line is for the city and state, while the third line is for the zip code and phone number. Do not use punctuation in the address, other than a hyphen in a nine digit zip code. Do not use a hyphen in the phone number. <u>NOTE</u>: Twenty-nine (29) characters are allowed for the street address, twenty-three (23) characters are allowed for the city, and four (4) for the state. Twelve (12) characters are allowed for the zip code, three (3) for the area code, and ten (10) for the phone number.

Block 8   Place an "X" in the appropriate box indicating marital status and employment status. Mark only one box on each line. <u>NOTE</u>: Only one (1) character may be marked in the boxes and only one box per line should be marked.

Block 9   Complete blocks 9 and 9 a-d only if block 11d is marked. Use this block when other group health coverage exists. Enter the last name, first name, and middle initial of the other insured if it is different from block 2. Suffixes should be entered after the last name. Do not include titles or professional suffixes. Use commas to separate each name. Do not use periods. Use a hyphen for hyphenated names. <u>NOTE</u>: Twenty-eight (28) characters may be entered in this block.

Block 9a   Enter the group number or policy of the other insured. <u>NOTE</u>: Twenty-eight (28) characters can be entered in this field.

Block 9b   Use an 8-digit birth date (MM/DD/YYYY). Enter an "X" in the correct box to indicate the sex of the other insured. Only one box can be marked. Leave blank if the gender is for some reason unknown. <u>NOTE</u>: Two (2) characters may be entered for month and date, and four (4)

Continued

PROCEDURE 20-1—*cont'd*

Block 9c   Enter the name of the other insured's employer or school. NOTE: Twenty-eight (28) characters may be entered in this field.

Block 9d   Enter the other insured's insurance plan or program name. NOTE: Twenty-eight (28) characters may be entered in this field.

Block 10a-c   Enter an "X" in the correct box to indicate whether one or more of the services described in block 24 are for a condition or injury that occurred on the job or as a result of an automobile or other accident. Only one box on each line can be marked. Place the state postal code in the blank next to auto accident if the "yes" box is marked in that line. NOTE: One (1) character may be entered per line in either box, and two (2) characters may be entered in the place/state field.

Block 10d   Refer to the most recent instructions from the applicable public or private payor regarding the use of this field. NOTE: Nineteen (19) characters may be entered in this field.

Block 11   The policy, group, or FECA number should be entered as it appears on the health care identification card. If block 4 was completed, then this block must be completed. NOTE: Twenty-nine (29) characters may be entered in this field.

Block 11a   Enter an 8-digit date of birth, in the MM/DD/YYYY format. Place an "X" in the box that indicates the sex of the patient. NOTE: Two characters are allowed in the month and day spaces, and four in the year space. One entry is allowed in the block to indicate sex.

Block 11b   Enter the name of the insured's employer or school. NOTE: Twenty-nine (29) characters are allowed in this block.

Block 11c   The insurance plan or program name should be placed in this block. Some payors prefer an identification number of the primary insurer instead of a name in this block. NOTE: Twenty-nine (29) characters are allowed in this field.

Block 11d   Mark the appropriate box. If there is another health plan, blocks 9 and 9a-d must be completed. NOTE: One (1) character may be entered in either box.

Block 12   Enter either "signature on file," "SOF," or an actual legal signature. When using a legal signature, enter the date signed in 6-digit format (MMDDYY) or 8-digit format (MMDDYYYY). NOTE: Use the space available to enter the signature and date.

Block 13   Enter either "signature on file," "SOF," or an actual legal signature. When using a legal signature, enter the date signed in 6-digit format (MMDDYY) or 8-digit format (MMDDYYYY). NOTE: Use the space available to enter the signature.

Block 14   Enter the 6-digit (MMDDYY) or 8-digit (MMDDYYYY) date of the first time the present illness, injury, or pregnancy began. In the case of pregnancy, use the date of the last menstrual period (LMP). NOTE: Two (2) characters may be entered under MM and DD, and four (4) characters may be entered under the YYYY.

Block 15   Enter the first date that the patient experienced the same or a similar illness in either 6-digit (MMDDYY) or 8-digit (MMDDYYYY) format. Do not indicate previous pregnancies. Leave blank if unknown. NOTE: Two (2) characters may be entered under MM and DD, and four (4) characters may be entered under the YYYY.

Block 16   If the patient is employed and is unable to work in the current occupation, use the 6-digit (MMDDYY) or 8-digit (MMDDYYYY) date in the "from" and "to" spaces that explain the time period that the patient was unable to work in his or her current occupation. NOTE: Two (2) characters may be entered under MM and DD, and four (4) characters may be entered under the YYYY.

Block 17   Enter the name (first name, middle initial, last name) and credentials of the professional who referred or ordered the service(s) or supply(ies) on the claim. Do not use period or commas within the name. A hyphen can be used for hyphenated names. NOTE: Twenty-six (26) characters may be entered in this field.

Block 17a   The other ID number is the referring provider, ordering provider, or other source and is reported in 17a in the shaded area. The qualifier indicating what the number represents is reported in the qualifier field to the immediate right of 17a. The NUCC defines the qualifiers (see Table 20-1), since they are the same as those used in the electronic 837P. NOTE: Two (2) characters may be entered in the qualifier field and seventeen (17) characters may be entered in the other ID# field.

Block 17b   Enter the NPI number of the referring provider, ordering provider, or other source in block 17b. NOTE: This field allows for the entry of a ten (10) digit NPI number.

Block 18   Enter the date that the patient was in the hospital, beginning with the admission date and ending with the discharge date in 6-digit (MMDDYY) or 8-digit (MMDDYYYY) format. If the patient is not yet discharged, leave the discharge date blank. This block is used only when the hospitalization is related to the current illness or injury. NOTE: This field allows for the entry of the following in each of the date fields: Two (2) characters may be entered under MM and DD, and four (4) characters may be entered under the YYYY.

Block 19   Please refer to the most current instructions from the applicable public or private payor regarding the use of this field. Some payors ask for certain identifiers in this field. If identifiers are reported in this field, enter the appropriate qualifiers describing the identifier. Do not

Continued

PROCEDURE 20-1—*cont'd*

enter a space, hyphen, or other separator between the qualifier code and the number. Refer to Table 20-1 for the qualifiers, which are the same as those used on the 837P. <u>NOTE</u>: Eighty-three (83) characters are allowed in this field.

Block 20   Use this field when billing for purchased services. Enter an "X" in "yes" if the reported services were performed by an entity other than the billing provider. Then enter the purchase price of those services. A "yes" mark indicates that an entity other than the one billing for the services performed the purchased services. A "no" mark indicates that no purchased services are included on the claim. When "yes" is marked, Block 32 must be completed. When billing for multiple purchased services, each service should be submitted on a separate claim form. Only one box can be marked. When entering the charge amount, enter the amount in the field to the left of the vertical line. Enter the number right justified to the left of the vertical line. Do not use commas or a decimal point when reporting amounts. Negative dollar amounts are not allowed. Dollar signs should not be entered. Use "00" for the cents if the amount is a whole number. Leave the righthand field blank. <u>NOTE</u>: One (1) character may be entered in either box in the Outside Lab area and eight (8) characters to the left of the vertical line and in the charges area.

Block 21   Enter the patient's diagnosis/condition. List up to four ICD-9-CM diagnosis codes. Relate lines 1, 2, 3, and 4 to the lines of service in 24E by line number. Use the highest level of specificity. Do not provide narrative descriptions in this field. When entering the number include a space (accommodated by the period) between the two sets of numbers. If entering a code with more than three beginning digits, (e.g., E codes), enter the fourth digit on top of the period. <u>NOTE</u>: The field allows for the entry of three (3) characters prior to the period, one (1) character above or on the period, and four (4) characters after the period in each of the four line areas.

Block 22   List the original reference number for resubmitted claims. Please refer to the most current instructions from the applicable public or private payor regarding the use of this field. <u>NOTE</u>: This field allows for the entry of eleven (11) characters in the code area and eighteen (18) characters in the original reference number area.

Block 23   Enter any of the following: prior authorization number, referral number, mammography precertification number, or Clinical Laboratory Improvement Amendments number, as assigned by the payor for the current service. Do not enter hyphens or spaces within the number. <u>NOTE</u>: Twenty-nine (29) characters are allowed in this field.

Block 24   The six service lines in block 24 have been divided horizontally to accommodate submission of both the NPI and to accommodate the submission of supplemental information to support the billed service. The top area of the six service lines is shaded and is the location for reporting supplemental information. It is NOT intended to allow billing for twelve items. <u>NOTE</u>: The shaded area of lines 1 through 6 allow for the entry of sixty-one (61) characters from the beginning of 24A to the end of 24G.

Block 24A   Enter the dates of service, both from and to. If there is one date of service only, enter that date under "from" and leave the "to" blank or re-enter the date placed in "from." <u>NOTE</u>: Two (2) characters are allowed for each section of month, day, and year.

Block 24B   Enter the appropriate 2-digit code from the Place of Service code list for each item used or service performed. <u>NOTE</u>: Two (2) characters are allowed in the unshaded area.

Block 24C   Determine if the services provided were an emergency. If required, place a "Y" for "yes" and an "N" for "no" in the bottom, unshaded section of the field. The definition of emergency would be either defined by federal or state regulations or programs, payor contracts, or as defined in the electronic 837P implementation guide. <u>NOTE</u>: Two (2) characters may be entered in the unshaded area.

Block 24D   Enter the CPT or HCPCS code(s) and modifiers (if applicable) from the appropriate code set in effect on the date of service. This field accommodates the entry of up to four 2-digit modifiers. The procedure code must be shown without a narrative description. <u>NOTE</u>: Six (6) characters may be entered in the unshaded area of the CPT/HCPCS field and four sets of two (2) characters in the modifier area.

Block 24E   In 24E, enter the diagnosis code reference number (pointer) as shown in Block 21 to relate the date of service and the procedures performed to the primary diagnosis. When multiple services are performed, the primary reference number for each service should be listed first, other applicable services show follow. The reference numbers should be 1, 2, 3, or 4, or multiple numbers as explained. ICD-9-CM diagnosis codes should be entered in Block 21 only. Do NOT enter them in 24E. Enter the numbers justified to the left. Do not use commas between the numbers. <u>NOTE</u>: Four (4) characters may be entered in the unshaded area.

Block 24F   Enter the charge for the listed service or procedure. Enter the number right justified in the dollar area of the field. Do not use commas when reporting dollar amounts. Negative dollar amounts are not allowed. Dollar signs should not be entered. Enter 00 in the cents column area if the amount is a whole number. <u>NOTE</u>: Six (6) characters may be entered to the left of the vertical line and two (2)

Continued

characters to the right of the vertical line in the unshaded area.

Block 24G Enter the number of days or units. This is usually used for multiple visits, units of supplies, anesthesia units or minutes, or oxygen volume. If only one service is performed, enter "1." Enter numbers right justified in the field. No leading zeros are required. If reporting a fraction of a unit, use the decimal point. Refer to Table 20-3 for a description of qualifiers. <u>NOTE</u>: This field allows for the entry of three (3) characters in the unshaded area.

Block 24H If the claim is Early & Periodic Screening, Diagnosis, and Treatment related, enter "Y" for "yes" or "N" for "no" in the unshaded area of the field. If the claim is family planning, enter "Y," or leave blank if "N" is in the unshaded area of the field. <u>NOTE</u>: One (1) character is allowed in this field.

Block 24I Enter in the shaded area of 24I the qualifier identifying if the number is a non-NPI. The Other ID# of the rendering provider is reported in 24J in the shaded area. The NUCC qualifiers are defined in Table 20-1, which are used in the 837P. <u>NOTE</u>: This field allows for entering two (2) characters in the shaded area.

Block 24J The individual rendering the service is reported in 24J. Enter the non-NPI ID number in the shaded area of the field. Enter the NPI number in the unshaded area of the field. <u>NOTE</u>: Eleven (11) characters can be entered in the shaded area and ten (10) characters for the NPI number are allowed in the unshaded area.

Block 25 Enter the federal tax ID number or social security number. Place an "X" in the appropriate box to show which was provided. Do not enter hyphens with numbers. Enter numbers left justified in the field. <u>NOTE</u>: Fifteen (15) characters may be entered for the federal tax ID number or social security number and one (1) character for the description of which number is being provided.

Block 26 Enter the patient account number, if desired. <u>NOTE</u>: This field allows for fourteen (14) characters.

Block 27 Enter an "X" in the correct box. Only one box can be marked. <u>NOTE</u>: One (1) character is allowed per box.

Block 28 Enter the total charges for the services in 24F. <u>NOTE</u>: Seven (7) characters may be entered to the left of the vertical line and two (2) characters may be entered to the right of the vertical line.

Block 29 Enter the total amount that was paid toward this claim by the patient or guarantor. <u>NOTE</u>: Six (6) characters may be entered to the left of the vertical line and two (2) characters may be entered to the right of the vertical line.

Block 30 Enter the total amount due. This information does not exist in the 837P. <u>NOTE</u>: Six (6) characters may be entered to the left of the vertical line and two (2) characters may be entered to the right of the vertical line.

Block 31 Enter the legal signature of the practitioner or supplier, "signature on file," or "SOF." Enter a 6-digit (MMDDYY) date or 8-digit (MMDDYYYY) date reflecting the day that the claim was signed.

Block 32 Enter the name, address, city, state, and zip code of the location where the services were rendered. Enter the name and address in the following format:
> 1st line: Name
> 2nd line: Address
> 3rd line: City, State, and Zip code

<u>NOTE</u>: Seventy-eight (78) characters may be used in this block.

Block 32a Enter the NPI number of the service facility location in 32a. <u>NOTE</u>: Ten (10) characters may be entered in this space.

Block 32b Enter the 2-digit qualifier identifying the non-NPI number followed by the ID number. Do not enter a space, hyphen, or other separator between the qualifier and number. Refer to Table 20-1 for qualifiers. <u>NOTE</u>: Fourteen (14) characters may be entered in 32b.

Block 33 Enter the provider's or supplier's billing name, address, and use the following format:
> 1st line: Name
> 2nd line: Address
> 3rd line: City, State, and Zip Code

Block 33 identifies the provider that is requesting to be paid and should always be entered. <u>NOTE</u>: Three (3) characters are available for area code, nine (9) for phone number, and eighty-seven (87) for billing provider information.

Block 33a Enter the NPI number of the billing provider. <u>NOTE</u>: Ten (10) characters are allowed.

Block 33b Enter the two digit qualifier as shown in Table 20-1. <u>NOTE</u>: Thirty-three (33) characters may be entered in this space.

Final Steps

1. Review the claim for accuracy and completeness.
   <u>PURPOSE:</u> To double-check that no blocks or fields are inaccurate or missing required information.
2. Run or prepare an insurance claims log for all claims completed. For paper claims, make copy of claim and place in tickler file.
   <u>PURPOSE:</u> To provide an audit trail of claims submitted.
3. For paper claims:
   a. Paperclip any attachments to be sent with the claim.
   b. Group all claims going to the same carrier and mail together in one large envelope.
   c. Address the envelope, weigh the contents, attach postage, and mail.
4. For claims to be submitted electronically, follow the computer software instructions for the software being used.
   <u>PURPOSE:</u> To submit all claims electronically or by surface mail to the appropriate insurance carrier.

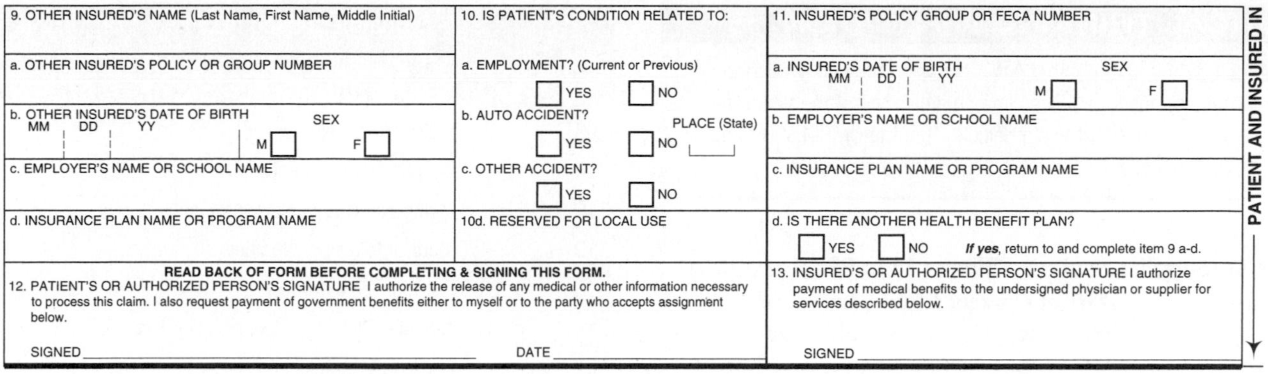

9. OTHER INSURED'S NAME (Last Name, First Name, Middle Initial)	10. IS PATIENT'S CONDITION RELATED TO:	11. INSURED'S POLICY GROUP OR FECA NUMBER
a. OTHER INSURED'S POLICY OR GROUP NUMBER	a. EMPLOYMENT? (Current or Previous) YES NO	a. INSURED'S DATE OF BIRTH MM DD YY SEX M F
b. OTHER INSURED'S DATE OF BIRTH MM DD YY SEX M F	b. AUTO ACCIDENT? PLACE (State) YES NO	b. EMPLOYER'S NAME OR SCHOOL NAME
c. EMPLOYER'S NAME OR SCHOOL NAME	c. OTHER ACCIDENT? YES NO	c. INSURANCE PLAN NAME OR PROGRAM NAME
d. INSURANCE PLAN NAME OR PROGRAM NAME	10d. RESERVED FOR LOCAL USE	d. IS THERE ANOTHER HEALTH BENEFIT PLAN? YES NO *If yes*, return to and complete item 9 a-d.

READ BACK OF FORM BEFORE COMPLETING & SIGNING THIS FORM.

12. PATIENT'S OR AUTHORIZED PERSON'S SIGNATURE I authorize the release of any medical or other information necessary to process this claim. I also request payment of government benefits either to myself or to the party who accepts assignment below.

SIGNED ____ DATE ____

13. INSURED'S OR AUTHORIZED PERSON'S SIGNATURE I authorize payment of medical benefits to the undersigned physician or supplier for services described below.

SIGNED ____

Figure 20-6 CMS-1500 Insurance Claim form: patient and insured information, blocks 9 to 13.

dependent. "Other" could mean that the patient is an employee, ward, or other dependent as defined by the insured's plan.

Block 7 **Insured's Address.** The insured's address and telephone number are entered here. Use the insured's permanent address, which may be different from the patient's address in block 5.

Block 8 **Patient Status.** These boxes are important in determining liability and for coordinating benefits. Mark the employment box if the patient has a job. Full- or part-time student would be marked depending on the school's definition of full- and part-time status.

Patient/Insured Section—Blocks 9 to 13 (Figure 20-6)

Block 9 **Other Insured's Name.** The other insured's name indicates that there is a holder of another policy that may cover the patient.

Block 9a **Other Insured's Policy or Group Number.** The other insured's group number or policy number identifies coverage for the insured as indicated in block 9.

Block 9b **Other Insured's Date of Birth and Sex.** The other insured's birth date and sex help to identify the birth date and gender of the insured as indicated in block 9.

Block 9c **Employer's Name or School Name.** This block identifies the other insured's employer or school name as indicated in block 9.

Block 9d **Insurance Plan or Program Name.** The insurance plan name or program name identifies the name of the plan or program of the other insured as indicated in block 9.

Blocks 10a to 10c **Is Patient's Condition Related to.** This block indicates whether the patient's condition is the result of an employment injury or illness, auto accident, or other accident.

Block 10d **Reserved for Local Use.** Some third-party payors require that this boxed be used. Refer to the applicable third-party payor instructions.

Block 11 **Insured's Policy, Group, or FECA Number.** The policy, group, or FECA number is the alphanumeric identifier for the insurance plan coverage. Workers' compensation claims use the carrier's alphanumeric identifier. FECA numbers are the 9-digit alphanumeric identifier assigned to the patient claiming a work-related condition under the Federal Employees Compensation Act.

Block 11a **Insured's Date of Birth, Sex.** This information applies to the person identified in block 1a.

Block 11b **Insured's Employer's Name or School Name.** This refers to the name of the employer or school attended by the insured as indicated in Box 1a.

Block 11c **Insurance Plan Name or Program Name.** The insurance plan name or program name refers to the name of the plan or program of the insured as indicated in Block 1a.

Block 11d **Is There another Health Benefit Plan.** This block indicates whether the patient has insurance coverage other than that indicated in Block 1.

Block 12 **Patient's or Authorized Person's Signature.** The signature is an authorization for the release of any medical or other information necessary to process or adjudicate the claim.

Block 13 **Insured or Authorized Person's Signature.** The insured's or authorized person's signature indicates that there is a signature on file authorizing payment of medical benefits.

CRITICAL THINKING APPLICATION

It is office policy to request that patients assign benefits when the patient does not pay for services immediately. One of the patients, Mr. Jones, seems hesitant to sign block 13 of the CMS-1500 form. How should Machelle explain the office policy to Mr. Jones?

TABLE 20-1 Qualifiers Used in Blocks 17a, 19, 24I, 32b, and 33b

QUALIFIER	DESCRIPTION
0B	State License Number
1B	Blue Shield Provider Number
1C	Medicare Provider Number
1D	Medicaid Provider Number
1G	Provider UPIN Number
1H	TRICARE CHAMPUS Identification Number
E1	Employer's Identification Number
G2	Provider Commercial Number
LU	Location Number
N5	Provider Plan Network Identification Number
SY	Social Security Number (cannot be used for Medicare)
X5	State Industrial Accident Provider Number
ZZ	Provider Taxonomy

Physician/Supplier Section—Blocks 14 to 23 (Figure 20-7)

Block 14   **Date of Current Illness, Injury, or Pregnancy.** The date should be the first date of the onset of the illness, the date the injury happened, or the LMP in case of pregnancy.

Block 15   **Same or Similar Illness.** A patient having had same or similar illnesses would indicate that the patient had a previously related condition.

Block 16   **Dates Patient Unable to Work in Current Occupation.** This section refers to the time span that the patient was unable to work in his or her current occupation.

Block 17   **Name of Referring Provider or Other Source.** The name of the referring provider, ordering provider, or other source that referred or ordered the service or supply on the claim.

Block 17a   **Other ID.** The non-NPI number of the referring provider, ordering provider, or other source refers to the payor assigned unique identifier number of the professional. The qualifier indicating what the number represents is reported in the qualifier field to the immediate right of 17a. Table 20-1 shows the two-character qualifiers used in this block.

Block 17b   **NPI Number.** The NPI number refers to the HIPAA National Provider Identifier Number.

Block 18   **Hospitalization Dates Related to Current Services.** The hospitalization dates related to current services would refer to an inpatient stay and indicates the admission and discharge dates associated with the service on the claim.

Block 19   **Reserved for Local Use.** Some payors ask for certain identifiers in this field. Refer to the applicable third-party payor instructions. (See Table 20-1 for a list of the identifiers used in this block.)

Block 20   **Outside Lab and Charges.** This field refers to services that have been rendered by an independent provider as indicated in Block 32 and the related costs.

Block 21   **Diagnosis or Nature of Illness or Injury.** The diagnosis or nature of illness or injury refers to the signs, symptoms, complaint, or condition of the patient relating to the services on the claim. It should be coded to the highest level of specificity.

Block 22   **Medicaid Resubmission.** Medicaid resubmission means the code and original reference number assigned by the destination payor or receiver to indicate a previously submitted claim or encounter.

Block 23   **Prior Authorization Number.** The prior authorization number refers to the

14. DATE OF CURRENT: ◄ ILLNESS (First symptom) OR INJURY (Accident) OR PREGNANCY(LMP) MM DD YY	15. IF PATIENT HAS HAD SAME OR SIMILAR ILLNESS. GIVE FIRST DATE MM DD YY	16. DATES PATIENT UNABLE TO WORK IN CURRENT OCCUPATION MM DD YY FROM MM DD YY TO
17. NAME OF REFERRING PROVIDER OR OTHER SOURCE	17a. 17b. NPI	18. HOSPITALIZATION DATES RELATED TO CURRENT SERVICES MM DD YY FROM MM DD YY TO
19. RESERVED FOR LOCAL USE		20. OUTSIDE LAB? YES NO $ CHARGES
21. DIAGNOSIS OR NATURE OF ILLNESS OR INJURY (Relate Items 1, 2, 3 or 4 to Item 24E by Line) 1. 2. 3. 4.		22. MEDICAID RESUBMISSION CODE ORIGINAL REF. NO. 23. PRIOR AUTHORIZATION NUMBER

Figure 20-7 CMS-1500 Insurance Claim form: physician or supplier information, blocks 14 to 23.

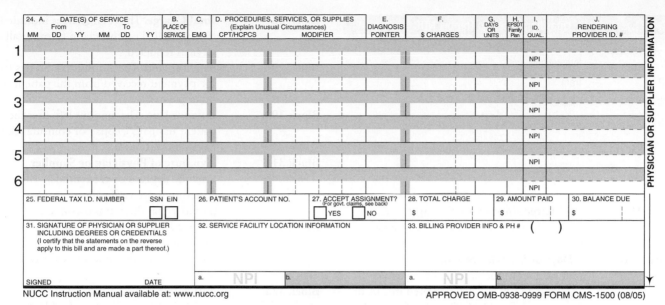

Figure 20-8 CMS-1500 Insurance Claim form: physician or supplier information, blocks 24 to 33.

TABLE 20-2	Place of Service Codes		
CODE	**DESCRIPTION**	**CODE**	**DESCRIPTION**
11	Doctor's office	51	Inpatient psychiatry facility
12	Patient's home	52	Psychiatric facility-partial hospitalization
21	Inpatient hospital	53	Community mental health care (outpatient, twenty-four-hours-a-day services, admission screening, consultation, and educational services)
22	Outpatient hospital		
23	Emergency department—hospital		
24	Ambulatory surgical center	54	Intermediate care facility/mentally retarded
25	Birthing center	55	Residential substance abuse treatment facility
26	Military treatment facility/uniformed service treatment facility	56	Psychiatric residential treatment center
31	Skilled nursing facility (swing bed visits)	60	Mass immunization center
32	Nursing facility (intermediate/long-term care facilities)	61	Comprehensive inpatient rehabilitation facility
33	Custodial care facility (domiciliary or rest home services)	62	Comprehensive outpatient rehabilitation facility
34	Hospice (domiciliary or rest home services)	65	End-stage renal disease treatment facility
35	Adult living care facilities (residential care facility)	71	State or local public health clinic
41	Ambulance-land	72	Rural health clinic
42	Ambulance-air or water	81	Independent laboratory
50	Federally qualified health center	99	Other unlisted facility

payor-assigned number authorizing the service(s).

Physician/Supplier Section—Blocks 24 to 33 (Figure 20-8)

Block 24A   **Date(s) of Service (lines 1-6).** Date(s) of service indicate the actual month, day, and year that the service was provided.

Block 24B   **Place of Service (lines 1-6).** This section identifies where the services were provided. Table 20-2 shows the two-digit place of service codes.

Block 24C   **EMG (lines 1-6).** This field is used to indicate whether or not the services provided involved an emergency.

Block 24D   **Procedures, Services, or Supplies (lines 1-6).** The procedures, services, or supplies refer to a listing of identifying codes for reporting medical services and procedures.

Block 24E   **Diagnosis Pointer (lines 1-6).** The diagnosis pointer refers to the line number from Block 21 that relates to the reason the services were performed.

TABLE 20-3 Qualifiers Used to Report NDC Units	
QUALIFIER	DESCRIPTION
F2	International unit
GR	fram
ML	milliliter
UN	unit

Block 24F **$ Charges (lines 1-6).** $ charges refers to the total billed amount for each service line.

Block 24G **Days or Units (lines 1-6).** Days or units refer to the number of days that correspond to the dates entered in 24A or units as defined in CPT or HCPCS coding manual(s). Table 20-3 shows the qualifiers to be used in this block.

Block 24H **EPSDT/Family Plan (lines 1-6).** The EPSDT/Family Plan identifies certain services covered under state plans.

Block 24I **Rendering Provider ID Qualifier (lines 1-6).** The Rendering Provider is the person or company who rendered or supervised the care. If the provider does not have an NPI number, enter the appropriate qualifier and identifying number in the shaded area. There will always be providers who do not have an NPI and will need to report non-NPI identifiers on their claim forms. The qualifiers will indicate the non-NPI number being reported. See Table 20-1 for the two-character qualifiers used in this block.

Block 24J **Rendering Provider ID Number (lines 1-6).** The individual performing/rendering the service is reported in 24J and the qualifier indicating if the number is a non-NPI goes into 24I. The non-NPI ID number of the rendering provider refers to the payor assigned unique identifier of the professional.

Block 25 **Federal Tax ID Number.** The federal tax ID number refers to the unique identifier assigned by a federal or state agency.

Block 26 **Patient's Account Number.** The patient's account number is that which is assigned by the provider and leads to the patient's financial information.

Block 27 **Accept Assignment.** The accept assignment indicates that the provider agrees to accept assignment under the terms of the Medicare program.

Block 28 **Total Charge.** The total charges indicate the amount billed on this claim form for all services rendered.

Block 29 **Amount Paid.** The amount paid refers to the payment received from the patient or other payors.

Block 30 **Balance Due.** The amount left after the patient has paid a copay or coinsurance is placed in this block.

Block 31 **Signature of Physician or Supplier (include degrees or credentials).** The signature is the verification from the provider that the claim is correct.

Block 32 **Service Facility Location Information.** The name, address, city, state, and ZIP code identify the site where services were rendered.

Block 32a **NPI Number.** The NPI number refers to the HIPAA National Provider Identifier Number of the service facility.

Block 32b The non-NPI number of the service facility refers to the payor-assigned unique identifier of the facility. The qualifier for the non–NPI number is entered here (see Table 20-1 for the two-character qualifiers used in this block.).

Block 33 **Billing Provider Info and Phone Number.** This block refers to the address and phone number of the provider that wishes to be paid on this claim.

Block 33a **NPI Number.** The NPI number of the billing provider is entered here. The NPI number refers to the HIPAA National Provider Identifier Number.

Box 33b **Other ID Number.** The non–NPI number of the billing provider refers to the payor-assigned unique identifier of the professional. The two-character qualifier of the non–NPI number is also entered here (see Table 20-1).

PREVENTING CLAIM REJECTION

It is important for the medical assistant to understand and comply with the guidelines specific to completion of a CMS-1500 form for each third-party payor and insurance company to prevent delays in reimbursement—or worse, denial of payment. The guidelines for Medicare, Medicaid, TRICARE, and worker's compensation can be found online at any of the fiscal intermediaries—e.g., Medicare billing guidelines are on the CMS website. Most computer software billing systems have built-in "claim scrubbers" that help in the process, and if claims are sent electronically through a clearinghouse, claims auditing is done before the clearinghouse submits the claim to the third-party payor. Claims without significant errors of any type are called **clean claims.** Claims with incorrect, missing, or insufficient data are called **dirty claims.**

Guidelines for Claims Review Before Submission

- Proofread the form carefully for accuracy and completeness.
- Make certain any necessary attachments are included with the completed form.
- Follow office policies and guidelines for claim review and signatures.
- Forward the original claim to the proper insurance carrier either by mail or electronically.
- If creating a paper claim, make a copy of the completed and signed claim form for the office records.
- Enter the appropriate information in the insurance log, and record the insurance submission information on the patient's ledger.
- The patient's and/or insured's name, address, and ID, group, and/or policy number should be identical to the information printed on the insurance card.
- Patient's birth date and sex should correspond with the medical record.
- The word "NONE" should appear in block 11 if Medicare is the primary payor.
- The referring, consulting, or ordering provider's name and identification number should be entered in blocks 17 and 17a, if applicable.
- Accept assignment should be checked "yes" if the physician is a participating provider (PAR).
- Be sure the diagnosis is not missing or incomplete.
- The diagnosis must be coded accurately and must correspond with the treatment.
- The patient must have authorized the release of information, and block 12 should contain a handwritten signature, the words "Signature on File," or the acronym SOF.
- The patient section (blocks 1-13) should be completed accurately according to the guidelines of the insurance carrier.
- Fees for each charge must be listed individually.
- All required fields of the diagnosis and procedure section of the claim form (blocks 14-24K) should be accurate and completed according to the guidelines of the third-party payor or insurance company.
- The physician signature must be on the form in an accepted manner.
- The federal **Employer Identification Number (EIN)** or Social Security number (SSN) should be double-checked to identify potential number transposition.
- The physician's correct billing or provider identification number corresponding to the insurance carrier being billed should be entered in block 24k and again to the right of "PIN #" in block 33, when required

Intelligent Character Recognition

Only claims which are completed on hard copy (paper) and submitted via surface mail such as the postal service are affected by the **Intelligent Character Recognition (ICR)** system and the guidelines given below. ICR is a system used to scan documents and capture claims information directly from the CMS-1500 form. Medicare, Medicaid, TRICARE (formerly CHAMPUS), and many other insurance carriers have adopted the ICR system.

The ICR system replaces the more antiquated optical character recognition (OCR) process, which had been in use until the early twenty-first century. The ICR scanners transfer the information on claim forms to their carrier's computer memories using a red bulb scanner, which causes the red preprinted portion of the CMS-1500 form to disappear or "drop out," and "transfers" to the computer only those characters printed in black ink. The resulting image allows for "clean" recognition of the data inserted without the characters being obstructed by the lines and text of the form. The benefits of ICR scanning include greater efficiency in processing claims, improved accuracy, more control over the data input, and reduced data entry cost for the insurance carrier.

There are rules for completing the CMS-1500 form in order for the insurance carriers to scan the claims; these rules include the following:

- Entries should be clear and sharp; carbon copies are not acceptable.
- A proportionally spaced 12-point font such as Courier works best.
- All uppercase letters should be used.
- All punctuation should be omitted.
- The MM DD CCYY format (with a space between each set of digits) should be used for all birth dates.
- All entries should be kept within their respective boxes. Xs must fall completely within the designated box.
- For the following, a blank space should be substituted:
  - Dollar signs and decimal points in charges and ICD codes
  - Dashes preceding procedure code modifiers
  - Parentheses around telephone area codes
  - Hyphens in Social Security numbers
- Titles and other designations, such as Sr., Jr., II, or III, should be omitted unless they appear on the identification (ID) card.
- When the charge is expressed in whole dollars, two zeros should be used in the "cents" column.
- If a typewriter is used, do not use lift-off tape, correction tape, or correction fluid.
- Because photocopies of claims cannot be scanned, all resubmissions must be prepared using the original (red print) claim form.
- No handwritten data (other than signatures) may be included on the forms.
- Nothing should be stapled to the form.
- The name and address of the insurance company should be inserted in the proper area in the top margin of the claim form.

Denied or Rejected Claims

The two main reasons for denial of payment are technical errors and insurance policy coverage issues. Technical errors include incorrect or incomplete information or typographic or mathematic errors. A common reason for insurance coverage rejections is that a procedure listed on the claim is not a covered service or is involved with a preexisting condition. The reason for a claim denial or reduction in reimbursement is listed on

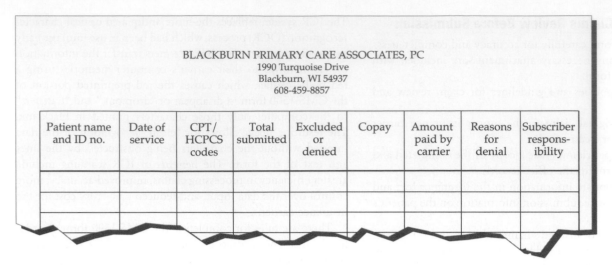

Figure 20-9 Example of explanation of benefits form. (From Hunt SA: *Saunders fundamentals of medical assisting*, Philadelphia, 2002, Saunders.)

the explanation of benefits (EOB) of commercial carriers, the remittance advice (RA) for commercial carriers and on Medicaid claims, and the explanation of Medicare benefits (EOMB) on Medicare claims. The EOMB, EOB and RA are hard copy or electronic forms that list the amount paid by the insurance company, as well as information about any non-covered services, denied claims (and the reason), deductible and/or co-insurance amounts, and other information about the claim or claims submitted. Figure 20-9 is an example of an insurance carrier benefits explanation.

A complete, accurate claim is called a **clean claim.** Claims returned unpaid by the third-party payor can be called "dingy," (also known as "incomplete,") or "rejected."

- **Dingy claims.** An inaccurate or incomplete insurance claim returned for more information or correction.
- *Rejected claims.* A claim for which payment has been denied for any reason (e.g., non-covered service, pre-existing condition, or ineligibility) is called an incomplete claim.

At times, a denied claim may involve policy issues beyond the control of the medical assistant. When this happens, he or she should contact the patient and discuss the problem. Normally, it is the patient's responsibility to resolve disputes regarding payment with the payor. The insurance policy is a contract between the company and the insured. However, the provider and those involved with the billing process in the medical facility should have a good understanding of the guidelines and requirements for the types of claims and various insurers handled most often in the facility.

CRITICAL THINKING APPLICATION

In her externship at the women's health center, Machelle sees a file containing a number of rejected claims. On closer examination she notices that similar errors in certain blocks are repeatedly the cause for rejection. Discuss common errors on the CMS-1500 claim form and what can be done to prevent these mistakes and/or omissions.

CHECKING CLAIM STATUS

It is often necessary to send a **"tracer"** to an insurance company to determine the status of a delinquent insurance claim. The accepted practice is to submit the tracer a day or two after the usual turnaround time of the payor, generally 30 to 60 days. A tracer is typically a form letter asking the insurance company about the status of an unpaid insurance claim. An example of a tracer letter is shown in Figure 20-10.

A duplicate copy of all submitted claims should be retained either in paper form or in the computer billing software. A structured routine for following up on claims unpaid within a specific time frame should be created to prevent overlooking a claim that should be filed or that has not been paid. The Insurance Claim Register (Figure 20-11), tickler files, and reports from the insurance database all help to keep track of paid and pending claims. If using software to file claims, an insurance pending report and an insurance aging report (among others) can be generated. The insurance aging report can be sorted by age of the claim, typically 30, 60, 90, and 120 days (or more), and by the payor, such as Medicare, Medicaid, and so on. Any of these methods suggested is useful in the follow-up of claims that have yet to be paid.

If claims are being submitted electronically either directly or through a clearinghouse, the medical assistant might allow 10 business days for claim turnaround time before expecting reimbursement. For paper claims, allow an additional week or two to allow for necessary manual processing and mailing time. Time between when a claim is submitted and when it is paid varies from payor to payor; however, an experienced medical assistant will soon become familiar with individual payment patterns of third-party payors and their claim turnaround times. Most states have laws that require payment within 45 days for clean claims.

Audit Trails

Electronic transactions leave behind a path or trail as they are processed, and this trail can be tracked or audited to provide a

INSURANCE CLAIM TRACER

INSURANCE COMPANY NAME _____ DATE _____

ADDRESS: _____

PATIENT NAME _____ INSURED: _____

POLICY/CERTIFICATE NUMBER _____ GROUP NAME/NUMBER _____

EMPLOYER NAME AND ADDRESS: _____

DATE OF INITIAL CLAIM SUBMISSION _____ AMOUNT: _____

An inordinate amount of time has passed since submission of our original claim as described above. We have not received a request for additional information and still await payment of this assigned claim. Please review the attached duplicate and process for payment within seven (7) days.

If there is any difficulty with this claim, please check one of these below and return this letter to our office.

Claim pending because: _____
Payment of claim in process: _____
Payment made on claim: Date: _____ To whom: _____
Claim denied: (Reason) _____
Patient notified: Yes _____ No _____
Remarks: _____

Thank you for your assistance in this important matter. Please contact _____ in our office if you have any questions regarding this claim.

Office of: _____ M.D.

Address: _____
_____ TELEPHONE NUMBER: _____

Figure 20-10 Example of an insurance claim tracer. (From Fordney MT: *Insurance handbook for the medical office,* ed 9, St Louis, 2006, Saunders.)

INSURANCE CLAIMS REGISTER   Page No._____

Figure 20-11 Insurance claims register.

Patient's Name Group/Policy No.	Name of Insurance Company	Claim Submitted		Follow-Up		Claim Paid		Difference
		Date	Amount	Date	Date	Date	Amt	
Jones, Bob	BC/BS	1-7-03	319.37			2/28/03	294.82	24.55
Carson, David	BC	1-8-03	268.08	2-10-03	3-10-03			
Linden, Jan	Medicaid	1-9-03	146.15	2-10-03				
Paul, Emma	Medicare	1-10-03	96.28	2-10-03				
Cortez, Jose	Unicare	1-10-03	647.09	2-10-03				
Dimico, Joe	Tricare	2-1-03	134.78	3-10-03				
Coldman, Billy	Aetna	2-4-03	607.67	3-10-03				
Fritz, Renee	Travelers	2-10-03	564.55	3-10-03				
Wong, Chang	Prudential	2-15-03	1515.79					
Billings, Harry	Allstate	2-21-03	121.21					
Green, James	BC	2-24-03	124.99					

record. This record, called an **audit trail** (Figure 20-12), can be used to verify that information was processed correctly or to locate the source of an error. If an office uses a computerized accounting program and submits claims electronically, the task of keeping track of claims is simple, because the software is capable of printing out an "insurance aging report" by date, by patient name, or by carrier name. If paper claims are used, however, the medical assistant should establish a follow-up procedure for tracking insurance claims. This can be accomplished by using an insurance claims register or log. This document can be developed and updated with little effort using a spreadsheet computer program, such as Microsoft Excel if the provider's office is computerized. If a physician financial management and billing software is used by the provider, an audit trail report can be generated automatically from the software program.

Blackburn Primary Care Associates
Patient Aging

NAME	CURRENT 0 - 30	PAST 31 - 60	PAST 61 - 90	PAST 91 - 120	PAST over 120	Total Balance
Mary Smith Last Payment on 08/08/xx	$120.00					$120.00
John Payne Last Payment on 07/06/xx		$250.00				$250.00
Jack Desmonde Last Payment on 05/25/xx			$500.00			$500.00
Jill Jayne Last Payment on 04/02/xx		$80.00		$100.00		$180.00
Report Aging Totals Percent of Total Aging	$120.00 11.4%	$330.00 31.4%	$330.00 47.6%	$100.00 9.5%		$1,050.00 100.0%

Figure 20-12 Sample accounts aging record. (From Hunt SA: *Saunders fundamentals of medical assisting,* Philadelphia, 2002, Saunders.)

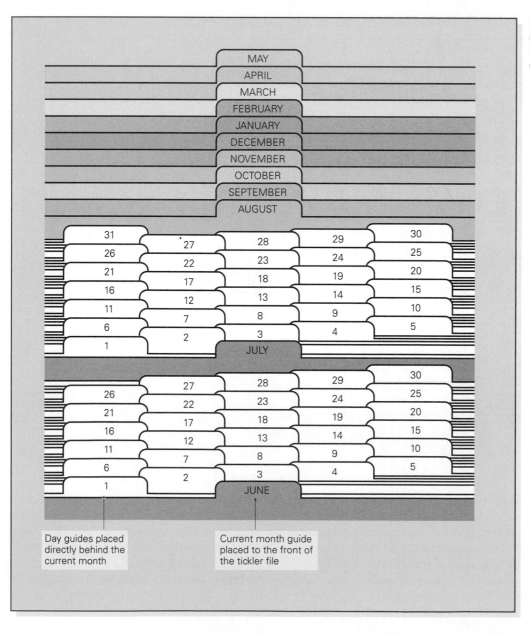

Figure 20-13 Example of an insurance claims tickler file. (From Fordney MT: *Insurance handbook for the medical office,* ed 9, St Louis, 2006, Saunders.)

Another method of tracking claims is a tickler file (Figure 20-13), also called a *suspense* or *follow-up file*. With this method, a copy of each insurance claim is filed chronologically, and the file is checked periodically for unprocessed (delinquent) claims. When the claim is paid, the copy is removed, and the information is posted on the patient's ledger card.

Delinquent claims remaining in the file after the normal contract time limits are pulled, then traced. If the claim has been denied, a letter may be sent to the insurance carrier's appeals department with a copy to the patient.

Claim Status

Obtaining timely and correct payment from third-party payors is a concern for many medical practices. Lost claims, delayed claims, and dirty claims result in healthcare providers waiting months for payment of professional services rendered. Most providers would agree that claim-processing payment issues are at the heart of most provider-payor conflicts.

Rejected Claims

A rejected claim is one that has missing or incorrect information. Rejected claims subsequently require investigation, need further clarification, and/or possibly require answers to or documentation regarding specific questions.

Denied Claims

Claims can be denied as the result of a technical error but are usually not paid because the medical service submitted is not covered under the policy, is an ineligible service, or must be applied to the deductible in accordance with the policy.

CLOSING COMMENTS

Patient Education

The medical assistant should be able to explain confusing technical issues to patients in simple, understandable terms. Patients, especially elderly ones, quickly become confused and frustrated over insurance issues—especially Medicare rules and regulations, which change nearly every year. The medical assistant should attempt to keep patients fully informed of changes in insurance guidelines and patiently explain why some procedures and services are paid for and others are not.

Legal and Ethical Issues

The practice of medicine and the responsibilities of the medical assistant are greatly affected by the legislative process. It is extremely important to stay current on the laws that affect medicine, federal and state insurance programs, such as Medicare, Medicaid, workers' compensation, and TRICARE, and the completion of the CMS-1500 claim form.

The Health Insurance Portability and Accountability Act of 1996 (HIPAA), developed by CMS, is responsible for the implementation of various acts that protect individuals' health insurance and privacy standards. Medical assistants should familiarize themselves with this important insurance act.

Because of the emphasis on compliance in medical practices today, every medical office must create and implement a plan to identify potential compliance problems and correct them before a liability risk is incurred. It is mandated that all providers avoid fraud and abuse charges by following the regulations and guidelines provided by governmental entities and third-party payors.

SUMMARY OF SCENARIO

Machelle feels that she now has a better understanding of the insurance claims process. Before becoming a medical assisting student, she did not give much thought to what went on behind the scenes when she visited a medical office for her own personal healthcare. She now understands why all of the information is collected at the time of her visits to the doctor, including the patient registration form listing her demographic and insurance information – Machelle has learned that the gathering of accurate data and verification of eligibility and benefits are some of the most important tasks performed, before she even begins to complete an insurance claim form. This information and the procedure to verify eligibility and benefits greatly reduce the chance of insurance claim denials or requests for additional information. No matter where she works and whether or not the office is computerized, organization, communication, dedication, and attention to detail head the list of requirements for becoming successful.

Machelle has asked for her instructor's help in developing a reference manual for the various third-party payors common to her area which will help her understand the requirements of the insurance carriers when submitting an insurance claim form. This too will greatly reduce the number of claims that are returned for more information which will delay reimbursement for services rendered. She is looking forward to more hands-on experience in the medical office where she is doing her externship so she can gain as much knowledge as possible in every facet of medical assisting. She is also establishing positive relationships with the staff at her externship site. She feels the knowledge and expertise they share with her will do much to round out her education in the medical field in preparation for her career.

SUMMARY of LEARNING OBJECTIVES

1. Define, spell, and pronounce the terms listed in the vocabulary.
   - Spelling and pronouncing medical terms correctly adds credibility to the medical assistant. Knowing the definition of these terms promotes confidence in communication with patients and co-workers.
2. Discuss the differences between paper claims and electronic claims.
   - Insurance claims can be submitted in two forms: paper and electronic. Both have advantages and disadvantages; however, electronic claims normally have fewer errors and historically are paid faster.
3. Understand the guidelines for completing the CMS-1500 claim form.
   - The insurance claim cycle begins when the patient first makes an appointment. The medical assistant should follow an established list of guidelines for CMS-1500 form completion, including obtaining a signed authorization to release information and assign benefits, if applicable.
4. Explain how to complete each of the 33 blocks of the CMS-1500 claim form.
   - There are 33 blocks in the CMS-1500 claim form, and, except for a few blocks that ask for standard information, completion requirements vary from payor to payor. The medical assistant should familiarize himself or herself with each major payor's unique requirements in order to maximize reimbursement.

5. Differentiate between "clean" and "dirty" claims.
   - Clean claims are those that can be processed and paid quickly; dirty claims contain errors and/or omissions that often result in rejection, thus greatly slowing the reimbursement process.
6. Discuss methods of preventing claim rejections.
   - Claim rejection and delay cost the medical facility time and money. Proven methods of preventing claim rejections should be established and adhered to.
7. Describe ways of checking the status of claims.
   - It is important to track claims once they are submitted. An insurance claim register, or log, can be created and used as one method of tracking claims. A routine should be established for claims follow-up.
8. Gather information for use on insurance claim forms.
   - The medical assistant who completes claim forms must have accurate, complete information to work with.
9. Complete a CMS-1500 insurance claim form appropriately for various federal, state, and commercial third-party payors.
   - Accuracy in completing insurance claim forms is mandatory. The process for completing claim forms appropriately is outlined in Procedure 20-1.

CONNECTIONS

 Study Guide Connection: Go to Chapter 20 Study Guide. Read the Case Study and Workplace Applications and complete the assignments. Do online research for answers to the questions in the Internet Activities associated with the health insurance claim form.

 CD Connection: Go to the Medical Assisting Competency Challenge CD and do the training activities under Health Insurance Activities.

 Evolve Connection: For more information related to the health insurance claim form, go to http://evolve.elsevier.com/kinn/admin and visit related weblinks for Chapter 20. Click on the Medical Assisting Exam Review and do the practice questions to sharpen your test-taking skills. To learn more about office software, do the exercises for the Altapoint demo that is on the CD.

Professional Fees, Billing, and Collecting

21

SCENARIO

Myra Morrison has worked for Dr. Jerry Wallace, an endocrinologist, for 3 years. She began as a receptionist, but she always had a knack for mathematics. Dr. Wallace was confident enough in her abilities to place her in charge of the accounting functions for the practice. When patients are ready to leave, Myra totals their bill and enters the charges and payments into the computerized ledger system. She also schedules their return appointments. Myra has learned quite a bit about medical insurance as well, so she can answer the patients' questions about their coverage and the benefits or exclusions of their insurance policies. In many instances, she was able to decipher a confusing insurance claim and explain the reimbursement to the patient. Myra has a great attitude about assisting patients with insurance questions and does not hesitate to call the insurance company to ask questions on behalf of the patient. She provides the patients with exceptional customer service.

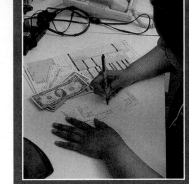

Myra knows that care must be taken when dealing with numeric transactions. Her handwriting is clear and legible, and she writes numbers the same way each time to avoid confusion and errors. She is able to use a manual pegboard but prefers the computer programs that do most of the work for her. Myra has some basic accounting background, so she can find errors easily and correct them. She even enjoys balancing the accounts on a daily basis to be sure all transactions were entered correctly.

Myra provides a valuable service to the patients who visit Dr. Wallace. She can always be counted on to follow up on any detail that needs attention. When patients call her for assistance, she takes no more than 24 hours to respond with the answers to their questions. She is a great patient advocate in the office. Some patients even tease her by asking her to balance their checkbooks! Myra is also willing to help any staff member with other duties whenever necessary. She is an enthusiastic team player who puts the patients first.

While studying this chapter, think about the following questions:

- Why do the provider's usual fees influence the amount of reimbursement received from third-party payors?
- Why is professional courtesy used less frequently than in the past?
- How does the medical assistant effectively explain fees to patients?
- Why might some providers still use a manual pegboard accounting system?

LEARNING OBJECTIVES

1. Define, spell, and pronounce the terms listed in the vocabulary.
2. List three values that are considered in determining professional fees.
3. Distinguish among the terms *usual*, *customary*, and *reasonable*.
4. Discuss the value of estimates for patient treatment.
5. Explain the concept of professional courtesy.
6. Name the ways by which payment for medical services is accomplished.
7. Explain why itemizing statements is important.
8. Discuss why patients fail to pay accounts.
9. Explain how to handle a "skip."
10. Briefly explain some of the guidelines of telephone collecting.
11. Explain professional fees to patients.
12. Effectively use a pegboard system.
13. Establish credit arrangements for patient payment.
14. Prepare accurate monthly statements.
15. Evaluate patient accounts for necessary collection procedures.
16. Perform accounts receivables procedures.
17. Post adjustments to patient accounts.
18. Process a credit balance on a patient account.
19. Process refunds and send overpayments to patients, when appropriate.
20. Post non-sufficient fund checks to patient accounts.
21. Post payments to accounts that have been turned over to a collection agency.
22. Age accounts receivable.

National Accreditation Competencies and Content

CAAHEP COMPETENCIES

Administrative

3.a.(2)(b). Post entries on a day sheet
3.a.(2)(c). Perform accounts receivable procedures
3.a.(2)(d). Perform billing and collection procedures
3.a.(2)(e). Post adjustments
3.a.(2)(f). Process a credit balance
3.a.(2)(g). Process refunds
3.a.(2)(h). Post non-sufficient fund (NSF) checks
3.a.(2)(i). Post collection agency payments

General

3.c.(3)(a). Explain general office policies

ABHES COMPETENCIES

Administrative Duties

3.k. Post entries on a day sheet
3.l. Perform billing and collection procedures
3.o. Post adjustments
3.p. Process credit balance
3.q. Process refunds
3.r. Post NSF checks
3.s. Post collection agency payments
3.x. Use physician fee schedule

Instruction

7.d. Orient patients to office policies and procedures

Financial Management

8.a. Use manual and computerized bookkeeping systems
8.e. Maintain records for accounting and banking purposes

VOCABULARY

account A statement of transactions during a fiscal period and the resulting balance.

account balance The amount owed on an account.

accounts receivable ledger A record of the charges and payments posted on an account.

credit An entry on an account constituting an addition to a revenue, net worth, or liability account; the balance in a person's favor in an account.

debit An entry on an account constituting an addition to an expense or asset account or a deduction from a revenue, a net worth, or a liability account.

debit cards Cards that looks like credit cards and by which money may be withdrawn or the cost of purchases paid directly from the holder's bank account without the payment of interest.

disbursements (dis-buhr'-smunts) Funds paid out.

fee profile A compilation or average of physician fees over a given period of time.

fee schedule A compilation of preestablished fee allowances for given services or procedures.

fiscal agent An organization under contract to the government as well as some private plans to act as financial representatives in handling insurance claims from providers of health care; also referred to as *fiscal intermediary.*

guarantor (gar-uhn-tor') A person who makes or gives a guarantee of payment for a bill.

instigate (in'-stuh-gat) To goad or urge forward; to provoke.

medically indigent Able to take care of ordinary living expenses but not able to afford medical care.

payables Balances due to a creditor on an account.

pegboard system Also called the *write-it-once system;* a method of tracking patient accounts that allows the figures to be proved accurate through mathematic formulas.

posting Transferring or carrying from a book of original entry to a ledger; entering figures in an accounting system.

premium The consideration paid for a contract of insurance.

preponderance (pri-pahn'-duh-rents) A superiority or excess in number or quantity; a majority.

professional courtesy Reduction or absence of fees to professional associates.

receipts (ri-sets') Amounts paid on patient accounts.

receivables Total monies received on accounts.

third-party payor Someone other than the patient, spouse, or parent who is responsible for paying all or part of the patient's medical costs.

transaction (tran-zak'-shun) An exchange or transfer of goods, services, or funds.

The practice of medicine is a business as well as a profession, and the details of conducting the business aspects are often the responsibility of the medical assistant. Although service to the patient is the primary concern of the medical profession, a physician must charge and collect a fee for such services to continue providing medical care. The physician is one of many contributors in determining the amount of the fees. The medical assistant usually has the responsibility of informing the patient about financial matters, collecting the payment, and in some cases making arrangements for deferred payment.

WHY PATIENTS DO NOT PAY

Most patients truly want to pay the bills that they owe. However, there may be times that the patient experiences difficulties in meeting his or her obligations. The patient may have lost a job or insurance coverage. An emergency could arise that depletes finances. When patients are in a position in which they must choose between paying their medical bills or having electricity, the physician is often forced to wait for reimbursement for the services rendered. Although a few patients will absolutely refuse to pay for medical care they have received, most are honest and willing to pay but may need help with a payment plan. Terms can be arranged for collecting payment in full when both the office and the patient cooperate with each other. The medical assistant should attempt to work out a plan that the patient can abide by, and the patient should be expected to make promised payments.

HOW FEES ARE DETERMINED

Setting fees is no simple matter. The physician has three commodities to sell—time, judgment, and services. Yet the value of these commodities is never exactly the same to any two individuals. Medical care has little value except to the patient, and the value may not be consistent with his or her ability to pay. In every case the physician must place an estimate on the value of the services. Such an arrangement is known as *fee for service*. This value may then be modified by other considerations.

Impact of Managed Care

An important consideration in today's atmosphere of managed care is the **preponderance** of patients who are enrolled in health maintenance organization (HMO) insurance contracts. Under managed care the physician agrees to accept predetermined fees for specific procedures and services instead of the fee-for-service arrangement described in the preceding paragraph. The patient may be subject to a copayment that is determined by the insurance contract and is collected at the time of service. A base capitation plan pays the provider a set amount for each patient enrolled that is meant to cover all of the person's healthcare expenses. Usually, capitation plans cover a group of individuals.

Prevailing Rate in the Community

One of the bases for determining charges on the fee-for-service basis is the economic level of the community. Different communities have different living scales, and this situation is reflected in medical fees as well. Consequently, the prevailing rate in the community—the average composite fee—must be taken into consideration by each physician. Strangely enough, fees that are too low drive patients away just as quickly as fees that are too high, because the average person tends to judge worth of a product on its cost—low cost translates as low value.

Usual, Customary, and Reasonable Fees

Most insurance plans base their payments on what has become known as a *usual, customary, and reasonable* (UCR) fee for a given procedure.

- Usual—The physician's usual fee for a given service is the fee that an individual physician most frequently charges for the service.
- Customary—The customary fee is a range of the usual fees charged for the same service by physicians with similar training and experience practicing in the same geographic and socioeconomic area. There is now a growing tendency for fees to be determined by national trends rather than by local custom.
- Reasonable—The term *reasonable* usually applies to a service or procedure that is exceptionally difficult or complicated, requiring extraordinary time or effort on the part of the physician.

To illustrate, let us suppose that Dr. Wallace usually charges patients $100 for a first office visit. The usual fees charged for a first visit by other physicians in the same community with similar training and experience range from $75 to $125. Dr. Wallace's fee of $100 is within the customary range and would therefore be paid by an insurance plan that pays on a usual and customary basis. If, on the other hand, the range of usual fees in the community is from $60 to $85, the insurance plan would allow only the maximum within the range, or $85, to Dr. Wallace.

UCR rates were developed many years ago when indemnity plans were the most common type of health insurance coverage. However, because the majority of insurance plans today are some type of managed care, the UCR rates now are based on the prevailing managed care rate of payment in a region.

CRITICAL THINKING APPLICATION

Myra realizes that many of Dr. Wallace's patients are confused about insurance policies and are easily frustrated when payments are not as high as the patient thinks they should be. How can Myra help patients understand their policies better?

Fee Setting by Third-Party Payors

The physician does not act alone in determining fees. A **third-party payor** may provide the physician with a schedule of predetermined fees that it will approve for payment. Some require preapproval of the fee before service is rendered. A third-party payor may require precertification before it will pay for a specific service. Government programs such as Medicare and Medicaid have strict guidelines regarding reimbursement for fees and the raising of fees.

Physician's Fee Profile

The **fiscal agent,** or fiscal intermediary, for government-sponsored insurance programs as well as some private plans keeps a continuous record of the usual charges submitted for specific services by each physician. When these fees have been compiled and averaged over a given period, usually a year, the physician's **fee profile** is established. This fee profile is then used in determining the amount of third-party liability for services under the program. One of the objections voiced by physicians is the lag between the time of a private fee increase and the time it is reflected in payments by an insurance carrier. It may be as long as 2 to 3 years.

Insurance Allowance

In some individual cases the physician may not wish to charge the patient more than what will be allowed by the patient's insurance. This is often a **professional courtesy** extended to other healthcare professionals. The full fee should be quoted to the patient and charged to the **account,** with the understanding that after the insurance allowance has been received, the balance may be discounted. If a smaller fee is quoted and charged, the following problems may arise:

- The lower fee will alter the physician's fee profile.
- If it becomes necessary to bring suit for payment of the fee, only the reduced fee can be recovered.
- If the insurance allowance is paid on the basis of a certain percentage of the physician's fee and a lower fee is charged, the insurance allowance will be correspondingly lower.
- If the physician does this with many patients, the insurance company may take the position that the reduced fee is the physician's usual fee and base its payments accordingly. It may even be considered fraudulent in some instances.

EXPLAINING COSTS TO PATIENTS

It is natural for the patient, particularly one new to the practice, to wonder, "How much is this going to cost?" However, some patients may be reluctant to voice this concern. Do not wait for the patient to ask about the fees. It is the responsibility of the physician or the medical assistant to approach the subject if the patient does not do so (Procedure 21-1). Be prepared to discuss costs with any patient who is interested, and ask all patients if they have questions about the fees. A good way to open the discussion would be to ask the following:

"Mr. Willardson, do you have any questions about the costs of your operation? If you do, I'll be glad to review them."

In this preliminary discussion of fees the physician or medical assistant must not sidestep the issue by saying, "Don't worry

---

PROCEDURE 21-1

Explain General Office Policies: Explain Professional Fees

CAAHEP COMPETENCY: 3.c.(3)(a)
ABHES COMPETENCY: 7.d

GOAL: *To explain the physician's fees so that the patient understands his or her obligations and rights for privacy.*

EQUIPMENT and SUPPLIES

- Patient's statement
- Copy of physician's fee schedule
- Quiet, private area where the patient feels free to ask questions

PROCEDURAL STEPS

1. Determine that the patient has the correct bill.
   PURPOSE: To make certain that the bill belongs to this patient and that the insurance numbers, the address, and the telephone number are correct.
2. Examine the bill for possible errors.
   PURPOSE: To demonstrate that the patient's concerns are important and that you are willing to make any necessary adjustments.
3. Refer to the fee schedule for services rendered.
   PURPOSE: To explain how physicians determine their fees. If an error has occurred, correct it immediately with a sincere apology.

4. Explain itemized billing:
   - Date of each service
   - Type of service rendered
   - Fee.
   PURPOSE: To make certain that the patient realizes the number and extent of the services rendered.
5. Display a professional attitude toward the patient.
   PURPOSE: To reassure the patient that you have a thorough understanding of the fee schedule and show willingness to answer questions politely and completely.
6. Determine whether the patient has specific concerns that may hinder payment.
   PURPOSE: To provide an opportunity for making special arrangements if needed.
7. Make appropriate arrangements for a discussion between the physician and patient if further explanation is necessary for resolution of the problem.

about the bill; let's just get you well first." The patient may later complain about the bill because he or she misunderstood the complexity of the service.

Even in cases in which the physician quotes a fee, the medical assistant often has the responsibility of explaining the physician's fees to the patient. The medical assistant must know how fees are determined and why charges vary, as well as have a thorough knowledge of the physician's practice and policies, to handle perplexing situations involving fees.

As the medical assistant's understanding of the practice increases, he or she can build respect for the physician's services by educating patients that money spent for medical care is an excellent investment in the future. It is a rare patient who understands the intricate procedures involved in diagnosis and treatment, especially when third-party payors are involved. Be patient and understanding when questions arise in this area.

CRITICAL THINKING APPLICATION

Mr. Reynolds, one of Dr. Wallace's long-standing patients, continually complains about his insurance policies and the small payments made on his medical claims. He frequents the office at least twice a month for checkups and goes into a long speech about the problems with his insurance each time he stops to pay his bill at Myra's desk. He will continue complaining even when other patients come to pay their bills. How can Myra tactfully handle Mr. Reynolds and stop his complaints?

Advance Discussion of Fees

Advance fee discussions help the patient plan ahead for medical expenditures (Figure 21-1). Most patients want to meet their financial obligations but rightly insist on an accurate estimate of those obligations before they contract for purchase of goods

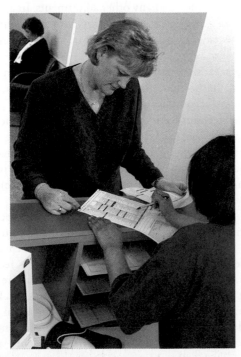

FIGURE 21-1 Taking a short amount of time to explain fees will often result in prompt payment for services.

or services. When a physician frankly discusses fees in advance with patients, even to the point of describing how a fee is established, misconceptions and complaints about overcharging and fee discrepancies are usually eliminated.

Explanation of Additional Costs

Explanations of medical costs should extend beyond the physician's own charges. For example, if a patient is to undergo surgery, the physician should also explain the costs of the operation, the anesthesiologist's and radiologist's charges, the laboratory fees, and the approximate hospital bill. The importance of calling in another physician for consultation should be explained to patients when consultation becomes necessary. It should be made clear, in advance, that there will be a separate bill submitted by the consulting physician. Patients do not always understand that the consultation is for the benefit of the patient, not the physician.

Estimates of Costs

Some physicians give patients an estimate of medical expenses before hospitalization. A few medical societies cooperatively develop estimate sheets or forms with local hospitals. Individual physicians occasionally work up their own estimate forms when a patient is embarking on long-term treatment. The physician should, however, emphasize that it is an estimate only and that the actual cost may vary somewhat.

Estimate slips should be prepared in duplicate so that the patient may have a copy while the original is retained in the patient's file. Using duplicate estimate slips may help in the following ways:

- It may help to avoid forgetting that a fee was quoted.
- It may help eliminate the possibility of later misquoting the fee.
- It may help simplify collection by preventing misunderstanding and confusion over charges.

Guarantor's Ultimate Responsibility: The Bill

Patients must understand that the **guarantor** is the person ultimately responsible for the entire bill. The insurance policy is a contract between the policy holder and the insurance company or between a group of people (such as an employer) and a managed care organization. The actual physician is not a party to that contract. Therefore it is not the responsibility of the physician or staff to pursue insurance payment for the benefit of the patient. However, it is in the best interest of the staff to actively assist the patient if problems occur in securing payment for several reasons.

First, the staff is almost always more knowledgeable about the insurance business than the patient. Many patients have never even read their insurance policies and have no idea what is or is not covered. Some patients expect the insurance to pay all costs simply because they are paying a high **premium.** The medical assistant may need to educate these patients about their policies and offer advice regarding how the patients can effectively work with the insurance company to get answers to questions and make certain that they are receiving all of the benefits to which they are entitled.

Second, it is in the best interest of the staff to assist the patient in collecting from the insurance company so that the physician will be compensated for services rendered. Helping the patient in this area will usually result in the bill for care being paid. Another reason to actively assist the patient is that the medical assistant will gain knowledge about the insurance industry. The more experience the medical assistant has in working with third-party payors, the more helpful he or she can be to the patients of the clinic. It is a good idea to keep a notebook with specific information about each type of policy that the office handles. This reference notebook will provide excellent guidance and suggestions for the medical assistant when working with a particular payor.

Always be sure to secure guarantors in writing. Most patient information sheets have a section that refers to the guarantor. There may be a statement that the guarantor signs indicating an agreement to pay the costs of medical care. States have varying statutes that deal with guarantors, so be sure that the office policies reflect compliance with those laws. It is especially important to secure a written agreement to pay for services when the care will be long term or when a costly treatment or surgical procedure must be done.

CRITICAL THINKING APPLICATION

- Madeline Amos has a 12-year-old diabetic son, Eric, who is Dr. Wallace's patient. Ms. Amos is divorced from her son's father, but the father is required to keep a medical insurance policy on the son. Myra knows that Ms. Amos has had numerous problems with the father. On a visit to the office, it is discovered that the insurance policy on the son has been cancelled. How does Myra explain this to Ms. Amos?
- What steps, if any, can be taken to assist Ms. Amos in paying her son's account?

ENCOUNTER FORMS

Encounter forms are the slips that are attached to charts while the patient is in the office; they are used for billing purposes. The encounter form provides information about the patient, such as the name, account number, and previous balance. Current charges and payments for the visit are added after the physician sees the patient. The physician can indicate on the encounter form when the patient should return to the clinic (Figure 21-2). The medical assistant then schedules an appointment and can even use the patient's copy of the encounter form to note the next appointment date and time.

The encounter form normally consists of three parts, with a white top sheet, a yellow sheet, and a pink sheet. The colors can vary, but usually the white copy is kept as a permanent record by the office, and the yellow and pink copies are given to the patient. The yellow copy is used by the patient for insurance billing (if not done by the office), and the pink copy is a receipt for the patient.

Encounter forms are sometimes designed to work with a **pegboard system** or may be available in continuous forms that can be placed in the printer for computer use. Encounter forms have been known by many aliases throughout the years; these include *superbills*, *charge slips*, and *multipurpose billing forms*.

PATIENT ACCOUNT TRANSACTIONS

A business **transaction** is the occurrence of an event or of a condition that must be recorded. For example, when a service is performed for which a charge is made, when a debtor makes a payment on account, when a piece of equipment is purchased, or when the monthly rent is paid, a business transaction has been completed.

Each of these examples is a transaction that must be recorded within the accounting system. The medical assistant will very likely encounter various other business transactions as he or she becomes more familiar with the individual needs of the employer's practice.

A patient's financial record is called an *account*. All of the patients' accounts together constitute the **accounts receivable ledger.** Account cards vary in design, but all will have at least three columns for entering figures. In the manual system these columns are as follows:

- **Debit** column—It is on the left, is used for entering charges, and is sometimes called the *charge column*.
- **Credit** column—It is to the right, is sometimes headed *Paid*, and is used for entering payments received.
- Balance column—It is on the far right and is used for recording the difference between the debit and the credit columns.

An adjustment column is available in some systems and is used for entering professional discounts, write-offs, disallowances by insurance companies, and any other adjustments. In a computer system, when a patient is called up by name or identification number, the patient's balance will appear. This is the individual patient's ledger.

Posting means the transfer of information from one record to another. Transactions are posted from the journal to the ledger; this is accomplished in one writing on the pegboard system. The **account balance** is normally a debit balance, which means that the charges exceed the payments on the account. A debit balance is entered by simply writing the correct figure in the balance column. A credit balance exists when payments exceed charges (e.g., when a patient pays in advance). This is common in obstetric practices.

Discounts are also credit entries and are entered in the adjustment column; if there is no adjustment column, the discount is entered in the debit column and enclosed in parentheses. When the entry is made this way, it is recognized as a subtraction from the charges. When columns are totaled, any figure in red or in parentheses is always subtracted. **Receipts** are cash and checks taken in payment for professional services. **Receivables** are charges for which payment has not been received—amounts that are owing. **Disbursements** are cash amounts paid out. **Payables** are amounts owed to others but not yet paid.

LIC. # 999999
S.S. # 111-22-3333
UPIN # A12365

JANE A. SMITH, M.D.
Reproductive Endocrinology
123 FIRST AVENUE
ANYTOWN, N.Y. 22222

TELEPHONE: (212) 555-4444
FAX: (212) 555-4545

PATIENT'S LAST NAME	FIRST	INITIAL	BIRTHDATE / /	SEX ✔FEMALE	TODAY'S DATE / /
ADDRESS	CITY	STATE	ZIP	RELATION TO SUBSCRIBER	REFERRING PHYSICIAN
SUBSCRIBER OR POLICYHOLDER				INSURANCE CARRIER	
ADDRESS	CITY	STATE	ZIP	INS. ID	COVERAGE CODE	GROUP

OTHER HEALTH COVERAGE? ☐ NO ☐ YES IDENTIFY

DISABILITY RELATED TO: ☐ IND. ☐ ACCIDENT ☐ PREGNANCY ☐ OTHER

DATE SYMPTOMS APPEARED, INCEPTION OF PREGNANCY, OR ACCIDENT OCCURRED: / /

ASSIGNMENT & RELEASE: I hereby assign my insurance benefits to be paid directly to the undersigned physician. I am financially responsible for non-covered services. I also authorize the physician to release any information required to process this claim.
SIGNED: (Patient, or Parent, if Minor)   DATE: / /

PATIENT INFORMATION

✔ DESCRIPTION	CODE	FEE
OFFICE VISIT		
New Patient		
Consultation	99204	
Comprehensive	99205	
OFFICE VISIT		
Established Patient		
Limited	99211	
Intermediate	99212	
Extended	99213	
Comprehensive	99214	
Comprehensive	99215	
SURGERY		
D & C	58120	
Pregnancy Termination	59840	
Laparoscopy	56305	
Hysteroscopy	56351	
Laporotomy	49000	
Myomectomy	58140	
Hysterectomy	58150	

✔ DESCRIPTION	CODE	FEE
OFFICE PROCEDURES		
Sperm Wash	58323	
Cauterization of Cervix	57510	
Cervical Biopsy	57500	
Endocervical Curettage	57505	
Endometrial Biopsy	58100	
Office Endometrial Curettage	58102	
Post Coital Test	89300	
Artificial Insemination	58310	
Pelvic Sonogram	76856	
Vulvar Biopsy	56600	
Bilateral Mammogram	76091	
Unilateral Mammogram	76090	
Breast Ultrasound	76645	
Abdominal Ultrasound	76700	
Polypectomy	57500	

✔ DESCRIPTION	CODE	FEE
LABORATORY - IN OFFICE		
Pregnancy Test	85160	
Urinalysis	81002	
Stool Occult Blood	82270	
Lyme Titer	86317	
Estradiol	82670	
Chemistry	80019	
CBC, pit., Diff.	85024	
T3 Uptake	84479	
T4	84435	
TSH	84443	
ESR	85650	
Pregnancy Test	84702	
FSH	83000	
Prolactin	84146	

DIAGNOSIS: ICD-9
☐ Abortion, Incomplete 634.71
☐ Abortion, Spontaneous 634.90
☐ Alopecia 704.09
☐ Amenorrhea 626.0
☐ Anemia 285.9
☐ Anovulation 628.0
☐ Atrophic Vaginitis 627.3
☐ Breast Cyst 610.1
☐ Breast Mass 611.72
☐ Breast Pain 611.71
☐ Cervical Polyp 622.7
☐ Cervicitis 616.0
☐ Condyloma 091.3
☐ Cyclic Adrenal Hyperplasia .255.2
☐ Cystocele 618.0
☐ Cystitis 595.9

☐ Diabetes Mellitus 250.0
☐ Dysmenorrhea 625.3
☐ Dyspareunia 625.0
☐ Dysuria 788.1
☐ Ectopic Pregnancy 633.9
☐ Edema 782.3
☐ Endometrial Hyperplasia . . .621.3
☐ Endometriosis 617.0
☐ Fatigue 780.7
☐ Fibrocystic Breast Disease .610.1
☐ Galactorrhea 676.6
☐ Headache 784.0
☐ Hemorrhoids 455.6
☐ Herpes 054.1
☐ Hypercholesterolemia 272.0
☐ Hyperprolactinemia 253.1
☐ Hypertension 401.9

☐ Hyperthyroidism 242.9
☐ Hypothyroidism 244.9
☐ Infertility 628.9
☐ Luteal Phase Insufficiency .628.8
☐ Menometrorrhagia 626.2
☐ Menopausal Syndrome 627.2
☐ Menorrhagia 626.2
☐ Monilial Vaginitis 112.1
☐ Obesity 278.0
☐ Osteoarthritis 715.9
☐ Osteopenia 733.9
☐ Osteoporosis 733.0
☐ Ovarian Cyst 620.2
☐ Ovarian Insufficiency 256.3
☐ Pelvic Pain 625.9
☐ Polycystic Ovary Syndrome 256.4
☐ Postmenopausal Bleeding .627.1

☐ Pregnancy V22.2
☐ Pregnancy Termination . . .V72.4
☐ Premature Ovarian Failure .256.3
☐ Premenopausal Menorrhagia .627.0
☐ Prolactinoma 253
☐ Prolapsed Uterus 618.1
☐ Rectocele 569.1
☐ Thyroiditis 245.2
☐ Trichomonas 131.0
☐ Urinary Tract Infection 599.0
☐ Uterine Fibroids 218.9
☐ Vasomotor Instability 780.2
☐ Vaginitis 616.1
☐ Vulvitis 616.1

DIAGNOSIS: (IF NOT CHECKED ABOVE)   ADDITIONAL INFORMATION: DOCTOR'S SIGNATURE

SERVICES PERFORMED AT: ☐ OFFICE   ☐ University Hospital ☐ Day Surgery / University Hosp.
345 Second Avenue   678 Third Avenue
Anytown, N.Y. 23333 Anytown, N.Y. 23444

ACCEPT ASSIGNMENT? ☐ YES ☐ NO

TOTAL TODAY'S FEE	
PREVIOUS BALANCE	
AMT. REC'D. TODAY	
NEW BALANCE	

REFERRING PHYSICIAN:

INSTRUCTIONS TO PATIENT FOR FILING INSURANCE CLAIMS:
1. COMPLETE UPPER PORTION OF THIS FORM; SIGN AND DATE.
2. MAIL THIS FORM DIRECTLY TO YOUR INSURANCE COMPANY. YOU MAY ATTACH YOUR OWN INSURANCE COMPANY'S FORM IF YOU WISH, ALTHOUGH IT IS NOT NECESSARY.
PLEASE REMEMBER THAT PAYMENT IS YOUR OBLIGATION, REGARDLESS OF INSURANCE OR OTHER THIRD PARTY INVOLVEMENT.

INSUR-A-BILL ® BIBBERO SYSTEMS, INC. • PETALUMA, CA • © 5/95 (SB M-N)   (REV. 9/96)

FIGURE 21-2 An encounter form. The encounter form is used by the physician and staff to document what was done to the patient during an office visit and to indicate when the physician wishes the patient to return. The copies of the form may be used to bill third-party payors. (Courtesy Bibbero Systems, Inc., Petaluma, Calif. 94954, (800) 242-2376, www.bibbero.com.)

Manual Posting

All charges and payments for professional services are posted to the ledger daily. The ledger then becomes a reliable source of information for answering all inquiries from patients about their accounts.

A separate account card or page is prepared for each patient at the time of the first visit or service. The heading of the account should include all information pertinent to collecting the account, such as the following:

- Name and address of person responsible for payment (the guarantor)

- Insurance identification
- Social Security number
- Home and business telephone numbers
- Name of employer
- Any special instructions for billing

Billing statements to the patient and the patient's insurance carrier are prepared from the ledger.

Computer Posting

The patient's name, date, diagnosis, and procedures are posted when the patient leaves the office. The database will retrieve the correct charges and post the charges on the computerized patient record and the accounts receivable ledger.

WRITE-IT-ONCE, OR PEGBOARD, SYSTEM

The initial cost of materials for the pegboard system is slightly more than that for other accounting systems but is still moderate. The system is simple to operate, and training is included in most medical assisting programs.

The system gets its name from the lightweight aluminum or Masonite board with a row of pegs along the side or top that holds the forms in place. The accounting forms are perforated for alignment on the pegs. All of the forms used in any system must be compatible so that they may be aligned perfectly on the board. The pegboard system generates all the necessary financial records for each transaction with one writing, as follows:

- Encounter form
- Receipt
- Ledger card
- Journal entry

It may also include a statement and bank deposit slip.

The system provides current accounts receivable totals and a daily record of bank deposits and cash on hand, in addition to the record of income and expenses. The need for separate posting to patient accounts is eliminated, and the chance for error is decreased.

Using the Pegboard System

The pegboard system provides positive control over cash, collections, and receivables and ensures that every cent is accounted for and properly entered. It provides a record of every patient, every charge, and every payment, plus a daily recap of earnings—a running record of receivables and an audited summary of cash. The system requires a minimum of time. One writing allows a medical assistant to do the following:

- Enter a transaction on the day sheet
- Give the patient a receipt for payment
- Bring the patient's account up to date
- Provide a current statement of account for the patient
- Give the patient a notation of the next appointment

All of these features communicate the money message to patients effectively and courteously and generate good financial records.

Gathering Required Materials

The pegboard may be of inexpensive Masonite construction with pegs down the left side, or it may be a more sophisticated aluminum sliding board that allows flexible positioning of materials. The basic pegboard forms follow:

- Day sheet (Figure 21-3)
- Patient ledger
- Encounter form

All of the forms must be compatible and are available from medical office supply companies. They may be customized to the practice, incorporating the usual services and procedure codes of the practice.

Preparing the Board

At the beginning of each day, place a new day sheet on the accounting board. Some systems have a sheet of clean carbon attached to the day sheet, others use special carbon with holes for the pegs, and some use NCR (no carbon required) paper. The carbon goes on top of the day sheet. Over the carbon, place the encounter form. The receipt has a carbonized writing line that should align with the first open writing line on the day sheet. If the slips are shingled, lay the entire bank of receipts over the pegs, with the top one aligned as mentioned. The remainder will be automatically in place. Receipts should be used in numeric order.

Pulling the Ledger Cards

If a great many patients are to be seen in a day, pull the ledger cards for all scheduled patients in the morning to save time (Figure 21-4). Keep the cards in the order in which the patients are scheduled to be seen.

Entering and Posting Transactions

As each patient arrives, insert the patient's ledger card under the first receipt, aligning the first available writing line of the card with the carbonized strip on the receipt. Enter the receipt number and date, the account balance in the space labeled *previous balance,* and the patient's name. The information recorded on the receipt is automatically posted to the ledger and the day sheet (Figure 21-5). The charge slip is then detached and clipped to the patient chart to be routed to the physician, who now has an opportunity to see how much the patient owes and can discuss the account in privacy, if desired.

After the service has been performed, the physician enters the service on the encounter form and asks the patient or the nurse to return it to the medical assistant. The assistant then has an opportunity to ask the patient whether this is to be a charge or cash transaction before completing the posting. Again, insert the ledger card under the proper receipt, checking the number that was previously entered to make sure the correct card is being used. Record the service by procedure code, post the charge from the **fee schedule,** enter any payment made, and write in the current balance (Procedure 21-2, p. 409). If there is no balance, place a zero or a straight line in the balance column. If another appointment is required, enter the date and time at the bottom of the receipt.

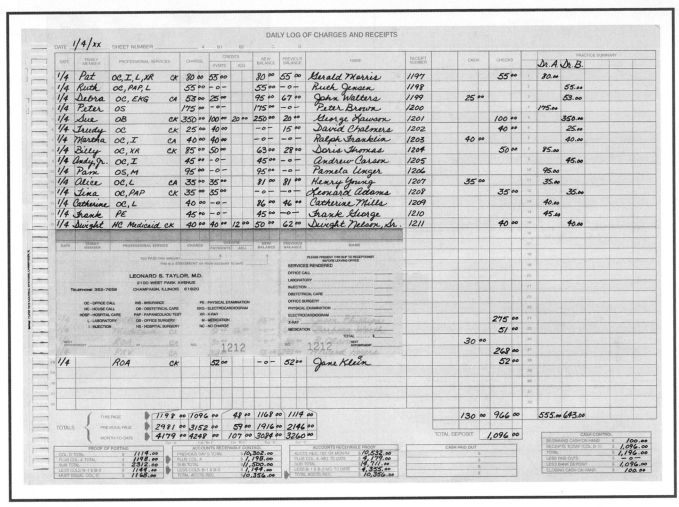

FIGURE 21-3 Sample day sheet for use with a pegboard bookkeeping system. The pegboard system allows the user to write bookkeeping entries once, prepare deposit slips, and perform business analysis functions. (Courtesy Colwell Systems, Inc., Champaign, Ill.)

The transaction has now been posted to the journal and the ledger, and if payment was made by the patient, a receipt has been generated. The service receipt is given to the patient; no other receipt is necessary. The ledger card is ready for refiling.

File the encounter forms in numeric order for any internal audit. At the end of the month, the total of the encounter forms should equal the total of the charges recorded on the day sheets for the month (Figure 21-6, p. 410).

Recording Other Payments and Charges

Payments will be received in the mail and may be brought in by patients some time after a service was performed. These payments are entered on the day sheet and the ledger card in the same manner as previously explained. Payments by mail do not require a receipt.

The physician may have daily charges for visits to patients in a hospital or convalescent facility. Enter these charges on the day sheet and ledger card only. Surgery fees are usually recorded as one entry that includes the surgery and aftercare.

Summarizing Accounting Transactions

At the end of the day, all columns must be totaled and proved. Although all bookkeeping is done in ink, it is a good idea to write the totals in pencil until they have been proved. If an error is discovered, correct the entry in which it occurred. Do not attempt to erase or write over the incorrect entry. Simply draw one line through it and make a new entry on the first open writing line. Remember to reinsert the ledger card for these corrections. Also, if the entry included a receipt for the patient, make a new receipt and notify the patient of the correction.

STATEMENT

LEONARD S. TAYLOR, M.D.
2100 WEST PARK AVENUE
CHAMPAIGN, ILLINOIS 61820

TELEPHONE 351-5400

| DATE | FAMILY MEMBER | PROFESSIONAL SERVICE | CHARGE | CREDITS | | BALANCE |
				PAYMENTS	ADJ.	
		BALANCE FORWARD ◇				
5/13/00		Office consult 99203	60 –	60 –		Ø

Form 1825   PAY LAST AMOUNT IN THIS COLUMN

OC - OFFICE CALL	INS - INSURANCE	PE - PHYSICAL EXAMINATION
HC - HOUSE CALL	OB - OBSTETRICAL CARE	EKG - ELECTROCARDIOGRAM
HOSP - HOSPITAL CARE	PAP - PAPANICOLAOU TEST	XR - X-RAY
L - LABORATORY	OS - OFFICE SURGERY	M - MEDICATION
I - INJECTION	HS - HOSPITAL SURGERY	NC - NO CHARGE

FIGURE 21-4 Patient ledger card. A ledger card showing the charge and payment for an office consultation. (Courtesy Colwell Systems, Inc., Champaign, Ill.)

SPECIAL BOOKKEEPING ENTRIES

The following special entries are necessary occasionally and may be used with a pegboard or any other accounting system:

- Adjustments
- Credit balances
- Refunds
- Insufficient funds checks

Adjustments

At times, it is necessary to enter a credit adjustment. These could be for professional discounts, insurance disallowances, account write-offs, or payments that come to the office after the account has been placed for collection (Procedure 21-3, p. 411). If a patient or guarantor files for bankruptcy, the charge will usually have to be adjusted off the books.

If the system has an adjustment column, enter adjustments there. Otherwise, because the adjustment is actually a subtraction from the charge, enter it in the charge column with the figure enclosed in parentheses or circled and with an explanation of the entry in the description column. When the column of figures is totaled, the circled figure is subtracted rather than added. The learner has a tendency to ignore the circled figures. This is incorrect—they must be subtracted.

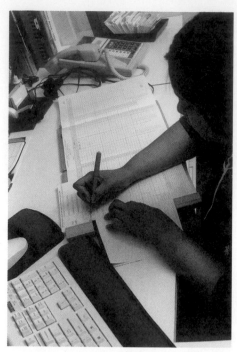

FIGURE 21-5 The pegboard system saves time by allowing several entries to be made at one time.

Credit Balances

A credit balance occurs when a patient has paid in advance or there has been an overpayment or duplicate payment (Procedure 21-4, p. 411). For example, an overpayment occurs if the patient made a partial payment and later the insurance allowance was more than the remaining balance. The difference between the total amount of money received and the amount owed must be entered in the balance column and enclosed within parentheses or circled. This indicates a credit balance. Some credit balances are created when an error has been made in posting.

The credit balance is money owed to the patient. If the patient has paid in advance or wishes to leave the overpayment in the account in anticipation of future charges, care must be taken in figuring the balance on future transactions. Whereas normally a charge increases the balance, it will decrease a credit balance.

Refunds

If a patient wishes to have an overpayment refunded, write a check for the amount due and enter the transaction on the day sheet. In most cases, the refund will result in a patient balance of zero (Procedure 21-5, p. 412).

PROCEDURE 21-2

Post Entries on a Daysheet

CAAHEP COMPETENCY: 3.a.(2)(b)
ABHES COMPETENCY: 3.k

GOAL: *To post 1 day's charges and payments and compute the daily bookkeeping cycle using a pegboard.*

EQUIPMENT and SUPPLIES

- Pegboard
- Calculator
- Pen
- Day sheet
- Receipts
- Ledger cards
- Balances from previous day

PROCEDURAL STEPS

1. Prepare the board.
   - Place a new day sheet on the board.
   - Place a bank of receipts over the pegs, aligning the top receipt with the first open writing line on the day sheet.
2. Carry forward balances from the previous day.
   <u>PURPOSE:</u> To keep all totals current.
3. Pull ledger cards for patient being seen that day.
4. Insert the ledger card under the first receipt, aligning the first available writing line of the card with the carbonized strip on the receipt.
   <u>PURPOSE:</u> To ensure that one writing will correctly post the entry to receipt, ledger, and day sheet.
5. Enter the patient's name, the date, the receipt number, and any existing balance from the ledger card.
6. Detach the charge slip from the receipt and clip it to the patient's chart.

<u>PURPOSE:</u> The physician will indicate the service performed on the charge slip and return it to you.

7. Accept the returned charge slip at the end of the visit.
8. Enter the appropriate fee from the fee schedule.
9. Locate the receipt on the board with a number matching the charge slip.
   <u>PURPOSE:</u> To make certain it is the correct receipt.
10. Reinsert the patient's ledger card under the receipt.
11. Write the service code number and fee on the receipt.
12. Accept the patient's payment, and record the amount of payment and the new balance.
    <u>PURPOSE:</u> To bring the patient's account up to date and provide a current statement for the patient.
13. Give the completed receipt to the patient.
14. Follow your agency's procedure for refilling the ledger card.
15. Repeat Steps 4 to 14 for each service of the day.
16. Total all columns of the day sheet at the end of the day.
    <u>PURPOSE:</u> To determine total amount of the charges, receipts, and resulting balances for the day.
17. Write preliminary totals in pencil.
    <u>PURPOSE:</u> To facilitate any necessary changes.
18. Complete proof of totals and enter totals in ink.
19. Enter figures for accounts receivable control.
    <u>PURPOSE:</u> To complete daily accounting cycle.

Insufficient Funds Checks

Sometimes, a patient sends in a check without having sufficient funds to cover it; this check is later deposited to the physician's account. The bank will return the check to you marked NSF ("nonsufficient funds"). Two accounting functions must be performed. First, deduct the amount from the practice's checking account balance. Then add the amount back into the patient's account balance by entering the amount in the paid column in parentheses and increasing the balance by the same amount. Write a brief explanation of the transaction in the description column (Procedure 21-6, p. 412).

Balancing the Accounts Receivable and Accounts Receivable Control

The accounts receivable control is a daily summary of what remains unpaid on the accounts. Most offices also complete an end-of-day summary. These are integral parts of the office accounting system and are discussed in Chapter 23.

PAYING FOR MEDICAL SERVICES AND TREATMENT

The payment for medical services is accomplished in the following four ways:
- Payment at the time of service
- Internal billing when extension of credit is necessary
- Internal insurance or other third-party billing
- Outside billing and collection assistance

Payment at the Time of Service

A large percentage of patients will have some type of health insurance for at least major items. Every practice in which there are patient visits should encourage time-of-service collection. It is especially important to collect co-payments and payment for office visits not covered by insurance. If patients get into the habit of paying their current charges before they leave the office, there are no further billing and bookkeeping expenses. If patients are informed when making an appointment that payment is expected at the time of service, they are not surprised

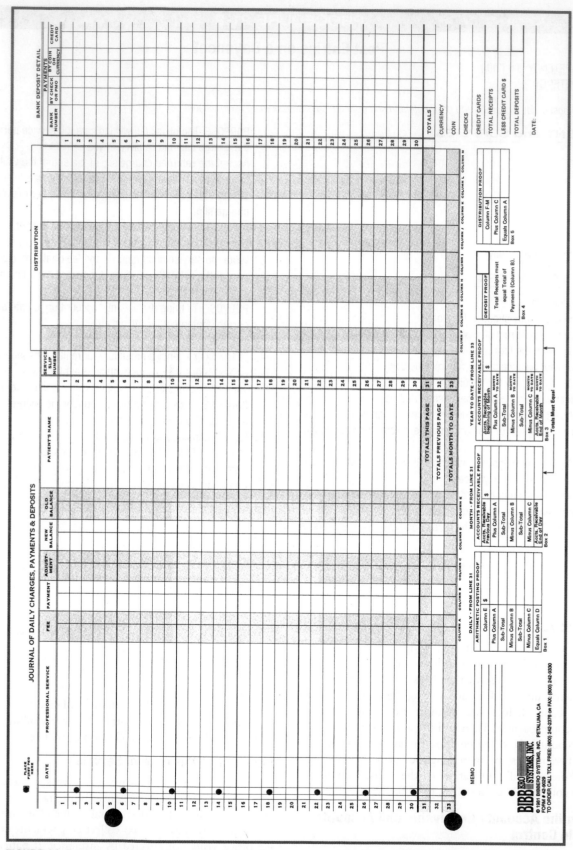

FIGURE 21-6 Sample day sheet used to log patient charges and receipts. (Courtesy Bibbero Systems, Inc., Petaluma, CA 94954, (800) 242-2376, www.bibbero.com.)

PROCEDURE 21-3

Post Adjustments

CAAHEP COMPETENCY: 3.a(2)(e)
ABHES COMPETENCY: 3.o

GOAL: *To process adjustments to patient accounts accurately.*

EQUIPMENT and SUPPLIES

- Patient ledgers
- Office policy manual
- Explanation of benefits and remittance advice
- Bookkeeping system
- Clerical supplies
- Payments
- Calculator

PROCEDURAL STEPS

1. Open checks that arrive in the mail as payment on patient accounts.
2. Paper-clip the check to the explanation of benefits or remittance advice.
   PURPOSE: To keep the check with the EOB as payments are posted.
3. Post the payment to the patient's account.
4. Determine if an adjustment is necessary on the patient account.
   PURPOSE: Adjustments may be necessary in cases of disallowed charges, noncovered services, and so on.
5. Review the office policy manual to ascertain the correct procedure to follow regarding adjustments to patient accounts.
   PURPOSE: To make certain that office policies are followed and are consistent with regard to patient accounts and adjustments.
6. Make sure that the ledger card is aligned with the day sheet correctly.
7. Write the adjustment amount in the adjustment column of the ledger card.
8. Check the math to make certain the adjustment was posted correctly.

PROCEDURE 21-4

Process a Credit Balance

CAAHEP COMPETENCY: 3.a(2)(f)
ABHES COMPETENCY: 3.p

GOAL: *To return overpayments to patients in a timely manner.*

EQUIPMENT and SUPPLIES

- Patient ledgers
- Office policy manual
- Explanation of benefits and remittance advice
- Bookkeeping system
- Clerical supplies
- Payments
- Calculator

PROCEDURAL STEPS

1. Review the office policy manual to determine the guidelines for credit balances.
   PURPOSE: To make certain that office policy is followed.
2. Review the payment received and the explanation of benefits or remittance advice.
3. Post the payment to the patient's account.
4. Determine if an overpayment has been made.
5. Review the account to determine if more insurance is expected on the account.
   PURPOSE: Some credit balances need not be made if more activity exists on the account; only refund amounts that remain after the complete bill has been paid.
6. Adjust the credit balance off of the patient's account.
   PURPOSE: To refund the credit balance if it is due to the patient.

when asked for payment at the end of the visit. Use a phrase, such as the following:

> "Your charge for today is $25.00. Will that be cash, check, or credit card?"

Many patients are hesitant to ask about charges and are unsure whether to offer to pay or to wait until asked. Make it easier for the patients by offering to accept their payments, because most people are prepared to pay small bills on a cash basis. If a patient requests to be billed, the medical assistant may say:

> "Our normal procedure is to pay at the time of service unless other arrangements are made in advance."

PROCEDURE 21-5

Process Refunds

CAAHEP COMPETENCY: 3.a(2)(g)
ABHES COMPETENCY: 3.q

GOAL: *To process patient refunds in a timely manner.*

EQUIPMENT and SUPPLIES

- Patient ledgers
- Office policy manual
- Explanation of benefits and remittance advice
- Bookkeeping system
- Clerical supplies
- Payments
- Calculator

PROCEDURAL STEPS

1. Determine the amount of the refund to be processed.
   PURPOSE: To make certain that the patient receives a refund in the correct amount.
2. Write a check for the amount of the refund.

PURPOSE: Always use a check to pay refunds so that the patient's name is on the back of the check as endorsement, proving that the patient received the refund.

3. Give the check to the physician for a signature.
   PURPOSE: Most physicians prefer to sign their own checks.
4. Determine the correct mailing address for the patient.
   PURPOSE: To make certain that the patient has not reported a change of address.
5. Make a copy of the check, and place it in the patient medical record.
   PURPOSE: The copy will show that a check was mailed to the patient.
6. Mail the refund check to the patient.

PROCEDURE 21-6

Post Nonsufficient Fund Checks

CAAHEP COMPETENCY: 3.a(2)(h)
ABHES COMPETENCY: 3.r

GOAL: *To correctly note that a patient's check was returned because of insufficient funds.*

EQUIPMENT and SUPPLIES

- Patient ledgers
- Office policy manual
- Bookkeeping system
- Clerical supplies
- Calculator

PROCEDURAL STEPS

1. Pull the ledger card that corresponds with the patient who wrote the check.
   PURPOSE: To post charges to the correct patient account.
2. Determine the amount to be added back to the account as a result of the returned check.

PURPOSE: The physician's bank usually charges a fee for all checks that are returned by the bank because of insufficient funds.

3. Post the total amount onto the patient's ledger card.
   PURPOSE: To account for the original check amount plus the fee for the returned check.
4. Send a certified letter to the patient notifying him or her of the returned check and demanding fast payment.
   PURPOSE: Many states require that certified mail be used when notifying patients about insufficient funds checks.
5. Note this collection activity in the patient medical record.

Many offices accept credit cards for the convenience of their patients. **Debit cards** are now widely accepted for payment as well. Computers have made the electronic transfer of funds easy and convenient.

The medical assistant must believe that the physician and the facility have a right to charge for the services provided. Do not be embarrassed to ask for payment for the value of the service. When tact and good judgment are used in billing and collecting, patients appreciate the service they receive and the help the medical assistant provides. Give individual attention and personal consideration to each patient, and be courteous, showing a sincere desire to help the patient who has financial problems.

Billing after Extension of Credit

In some types of practice, particularly those involving large fees for surgery or long-term care, it becomes necessary to extend credit and establish a regular system of billing. This requires informing the patient of what the charges will be, what professional services these charges cover, and what the credit policy of the office is (Procedure 21-7).

Many practices do not have a true credit policy; thus each account continues to be evaluated individually. It is almost impossible to judge accounts objectively and equitably under such circumstances.

The physician and the staff should think through their situation, decide what they expect of patients with respect to payments, and how they will inform the patient. Although there will always be exceptions to any rule, there must be a rule, which should be in writing and conveyed to the patient at the outset of the relationship.

Some medical practices prepare an information booklet that includes the payment policy. New patients are given a copy of the booklet. Any patient who needs special consideration can be counseled by the medical assistant. The medical assistant who has the guidance and support of an established credit policy can perform with confidence when handling patient accounts. The credit policy must be fair and must address the following issues:

- Time when payment is due from patients
- Payment at the time of service
- Times when or if assignment of insurance benefits is accepted
- Completion of insurance forms by the office staff (or not)
- Billing procedures
- Collection protocol
- Length of time an account will be carried without payment
- Telephone collection protocol
- Use of a collection agency

Installment Buying of Medical Services

Because installment buying is so much a part of our economic system today, the physician's office must be prepared to help patients budget for their medical care. Patients expect to use their credit resources and appreciate business-like assistance in establishing a payment plan. The medical profession has too long suffered a poor collection record because of its fear

---

PROCEDURE 21-7

Explain General Office Policies: Make Credit Arrangements with a Patient

CAAHEP COMPETENCY: 3.c.(3)(a)
ABHES COMPETENCY: 7.d

GOAL: *To assist the patient in paying for services by making mutually beneficial credit arrangements according to established office policy.*

EQUIPMENT and SUPPLIES

- Patient's ledger
- Calendar
- Truth in Lending form
- Assignment of benefits form
- Patient's insurance form
- Private area for interview

PROCEDURAL STEPS

1. Answer all questions about credit thoroughly and kindly.
2. Inform the patient of the office policy regarding credit:
   - Payment at the time of first visit
   - Payment by bank card
   - Credit application

   PURPOSE: To ensure complete understanding of mutual responsibilities.
3. Have the patient complete the credit application.
   PURPOSE: To comply with office practices on the extension of credit.

4. Check the completed credit application.
   PURPOSE: To confirm that all the necessary information is included.
5. Discuss with the patient the possible arrangements and ask the patient to decide which of those arrangements is most suitable.
   PURPOSE: To ensure better compliance, which can be expected when the patient makes the choice.
6. Prepare the Truth in Lending form and have the patient sign it if the agreement requires more than four installments.
   PURPOSE: To comply with Regulation Z.
7. Have the patient execute an assignment of insurance benefits.
   PURPOSE: To comply with credit policy.
8. Make a copy of the patient's insurance card, and have the patient sign a consent for release of the information to the insurance company.
   PURPOSE: To ensure that a claim can be processed because consent for the release of information is necessary on most insurance forms.
9. Keep credit information confidential.

of appearing too commercial. The physician should be ready to arrange credit when medical bills will be high or when a patient for some reason is unable to pay at the time of service. In general, fees for routine office calls and small medical bills should be kept on a pay-as-you-go basis.

In recent years companies have begun to offer credit or loans specifically for medical procedures. This is very popular for cosmetic surgeries. Offices that offer these types of procedures may wish to investigate these alternative financing services.

Truth in Lending Act

Regulation Z of the Truth in Lending Act, which is enforced by the Federal Trade Commission, requires that when a bilateral agreement exists between physician and patient for the physician to accept payment in more than four installments, the physician is required to provide disclosure of information regarding finance charges (Figure 21-7). Even if there are no finance charges involved, the form must be completed stating this fact. The physician retains a copy of the form, and the original is given to the patient. Specific wording is required in the disclosure. Have the patient sign the agreement in your presence, because you must have proof of signing. The disclosure statement must be kept on file for 2 years. Although the disclosure statement is designed as protection for the debtor, it can be a good collection tool for the creditor.

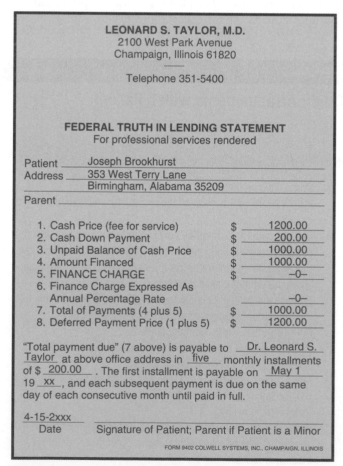

LEONARD S. TAYLOR, M.D.
2100 West Park Avenue
Champaign, Illinois 61820

Telephone 351-5400

FEDERAL TRUTH IN LENDING STATEMENT
For professional services rendered

Patient _____ Joseph Brookhurst
Address _____ 353 West Terry Lane
_____ Birmingham, Alabama 35209
Parent _____

1. Cash Price (fee for service)	$	1200.00
2. Cash Down Payment	$	200.00
3. Unpaid Balance of Cash Price	$	1000.00
4. Amount Financed	$	1000.00
5. FINANCE CHARGE	$	–0–
6. Finance Charge Expressed As Annual Percentage Rate		–0–
7. Total of Payments (4 plus 5)	$	1000.00
8. Deferred Payment Price (1 plus 5)	$	1200.00

"Total payment due" (7 above) is payable to _Dr. Leonard S. Taylor_ at above office address in _five_ monthly installments of $ _200.00_ . The first installment is payable on _May 1_ 19 _xx_ , and each subsequent payment is due on the same day of each consecutive month until paid in full.

4-15-2xxx
Date   Signature of Patient; Parent if Patient is a Minor

FORM 9402 COLWELL SYSTEMS, INC., CHAMPAIGN, ILLINOIS

FIGURE 21-7 Disclosure statement. An example of a document for compliance with the Federal Truth in Lending Act. (Courtesy Colwell Systems, Inc., Champaign, Ill.)

It is recognized that physicians generally permit their patients to pay in installments, and as long as no specific agreement has been made for payment to the physician to be made in more than four installments and no finance charge is assessed, the account is not subject to the regulation. If the patient chooses to pay in installments instead of the full amount, this is considered a unilateral action. The physician, in accepting such payments, probably would not be subject to the provisions of the regulation. The physician's office, however, must be certain to bill for the full balance each time. If the statement is for only a partial payment, it then becomes a bilateral agreement and as such is subject to Regulation Z.

Helping patients budget their medical expenses is a rather new aspect of the business side of medical practice. However, it is a real service to patients and demonstrates that the physician and the office staff are sincerely anxious to help patients pay their own way. It may also prevent many collection problems.

Confidentiality

Obtaining Credit Information

Credit information is confidential. It should be guarded as carefully as a confidential medical history and should be disclosed to no one. When asking for credit information from patients in the office, do so in a private area where others cannot overhear the conversation. A desk or table away from the reception area where a patient can sit in total privacy and complete a credit application is a great asset. Credit information is personal—it should be kept that way.

Credit Bureaus

Some physicians join a credit bureau, particularly in large cities where it is more difficult to gauge informally the patients' ability to pay. Credit bureaus gather credit information from many sources, pool it, and make it available to dues-paying bureau members. If the office receives a request for credit information about a patient, it is permissible to furnish it because the debtor, by giving the physician's name as a reference, has given implied consent; otherwise, the credit bureau would not have contacted the office. According to the Fair Credit Practices Act Amendments of 1975, only the following information can be given:

- When the account was opened
- How much the patient now owes
- What the highest amount of the account is at any time

You should avoid any reference to the following:

- Character
- Paying habits
- Credit rating

Billing Insurance or Other Third Parties

Insurance billing in the medical office is a courtesy to patients. Often, patients do not understand the policies and appreciate the assistance given by the medical office. Information on completing insurance forms and diagnostic and procedure coding is found in Chapters 17 through 20.

Independent Billing and Collection Services

Many healthcare facilities find it advantageous to refer their billing and collections to an independent billing service. The information related to services and fees is sent to the billing service on a daily or weekly basis. The servicing agent then handles all billing and collections, as well as any telephone inquiries. This system frees the regular office staff for more patient-oriented duties. An added advantage is that a person who is not connected with the patient care on a personal basis handles any dispute that may arise.

INTERNAL BILLING BY THE ACCOUNT MANAGER

Billing Methods

In a practice with only a moderate number of accounts, the medical assistant handles the preparation and mailing of statements. This may be accomplished by using the following:

- A computer-generated statement
- An encounter form
- A typewritten statement
- A photocopied statement

The appearance of the statement carries a visual impact just as a letter does, so the statement heads should be carefully chosen and the typing clean and accurate. Statement heads are usually imprinted with the same information as the physician's letterhead. They should be of good quality and large enough to allow itemization of charges. Envelopes should be imprinted with Address Correction Requested under the return address to maintain up-to-date mailing lists. A self-addressed return envelope included with the statement encourages prompt payment. This is mainly for the convenience of patients who do not always have stationery available for sending a return payment or who are less likely to return a payment immediately if they must address an envelope.

Computer-Generated Statement

Patient accounts are generated and stored in the computer, and a statement can be produced whenever needed. The statement can show the service rendered on each date, the charge for each service, the date on which a claim was submitted to the insurance company, the date of payment, and the balance due from the patient. The computer may also be programmed to print messages on the statement, such as "Balance now 30 days past due" or various other messages.

Encounter Form as a Bill

There are variations in style, but encounter forms are usually personalized for the practice. The form has space for all the elements required in submitting medical insurance claims, such as the following:

- Name and address of the patient
- Name of the insurance carrier
- Insurance identification number
- Brief description of each service by code number
- Fee for each service
- Place and date of service

- Diagnosis
- Physician's name and address
- Physician's signature

The encounter form can be used as a charge slip for office treatments if the physician checks the services performed at the completion of the visit and asks the patient to hand it to the medical assistant when leaving. Either the physician or the medical assistant may write in the amount of the fee. If a payment is made, it can be so indicated. Instructions to the patient for filing insurance claims are on the bottom left.

Statements

Statements must be correct and must include the patient's name and address as well as the balance owed. If statements are photocopied or microfilmed, special care must be taken that the ledger card is correct because it will be duplicated in the billing process.

Typewritten Statements

The use of continuous-form billing statements is a timesaver. The statements are printed in a roll with perforated edges for separation. The roll is fed into the typewriter for the first statement and remains until the last statement is typed, eliminating the time and energy necessary for inserting and removing each statement form from the typewriter. These statements are rarely used in this age of computers.

Photocopied Statements

Coordinated ledger cards and copy paper are used in preparing photocopied statements. A perfect statement is ready for mailing in minimal time. Extra care must be used in posting the ledgers. A black pen should be used in making entries on the ledger card, because other ink colors do not reproduce well. Writing must be clear and legible. No personal notes should be made on the ledger cards unless there is something you wish conveyed to the patient. (It is possible to buy pencils with nonreproducible lead if you believe this is necessary for making collection entries.) Usually, a window envelope is used for mailing, which means that the name and address on the ledger must be neat, correct, and positioned correctly for the envelope window.

Internal Billing Procedures

Itemizing the First Statement

If the medical fee has been explained in advance, the monthly statement is merely a confirmation of what is owed, and there should be no misunderstanding. However, it is good business practice and a courtesy to the patient to itemize the charges. This is essential if the statement is to be used for billing the patient's insurance. Patients are entitled to an understanding of the physician's statement for medical services.

Itemizing statements is not difficult, and computerized statements usually automatically itemize the first statement. The simplest method is merely to allow space on the original statement, below the "For Professional Services" line, in which to list the separate charges for office visits, hospital calls, or treatments or tests performed in the medical facility (Procedure 21-8).

PROCEDURE 21-8

Perform Accounts Receivable Procedures

CAAHEP COMPETENCY: 3.a(2)(c)
ABHES COMPETENCY: 8.e

GOAL: *To collect amounts due to the physician or medical facility.*

EQUIPMENT and SUPPLIES

- Patient ledgers
- Office policy manual
- Telephone
- Letterhead and envelopes
- Clerical supplies

PROCEDURAL STEPS

1. Determine the billing cycle for the medical facility according to the office policy manual.
   PURPOSE: The billing cycle specifies which groups of accounts are billed at different times of the month.

2. Determine amounts due to the physician and who owes these amounts.
   PURPOSE: To specify which accounts need to be billed.

3. Group accounts together when necessary.
   PURPOSE: Some physicians prefer to separate regular billings from past-due billings.

4. Print bills using the computer system, or make copies of ledger cards.

5. Mail bills to patients.

6. Post payments to patient accounts as they arrive at the office.
   PURPOSE: To credit the patients' accounts with payments that they submit to the medical facility.

Many physicians have devised their own itemized encounter forms, which are given to the patient when payment is made at the time of service or later mailed in a combination statement-reply envelope. The use of such charge slips simplifies the itemization procedure, because filling out the slips is usually just a matter of checking the procedures listed. Although the itemization of bills may seem tedious, the medical assistant will spend less time in explaining services provided, clearing up misunderstandings with patients, and following up on delinquent accounts by itemizing.

CRITICAL THINKING APPLICATION

Mrs. Deaton is frustrated because she claims she was never sent an itemized statement and now refuses to pay her account. Myra believes that this is a delay tactic, because she specifically recalls sending an itemized statement to the patient. How can this situation be remedied?

Time and Frequency of Billing

A regular system of mailing statements should be put into operation. Most people expect to receive statements from their creditors, and they plan their budgets around first-of-the-month bills received. Punctuality in billing encourages prompt payment.

Statements should be sent at least once each month. Some offices send bills immediately after treatment; others bill all patients on the same day each month. Mailing statements twice a month (e.g., half of the accounts on the tenth and the remaining half on the twenty-fifth) is also a common practice.

Once-a-Month Billing

If a monthly pattern is followed, bills should leave the office in time to reach the patient no later than the last day of each month and preferably before the twenty-fifth of the month. Planning ahead for the preparation of statements can lighten the burden of once-a-month billing (Procedure 21-9). The statement can be prepared at the time of service, postdated, and mailed at the end of the month.

Cycle Billing

Many physicians prefer to use the cycle billing system, which calls for the billing of certain portions of the accounts receivable at given times during the month instead of the preparation of all statements at the end of each month. Cycle billing is used in large businesses such as department stores, banks, and utility companies. Its many advantages include avoiding once-a-month peak workloads and stabilizing the cash flow. In a small office in which billing is done only once a month, the unexpected illness or absence of the medical assistant for any emergency can leave the physician in a financial bind if the statements do not go out.

The accounts are separated into fairly equal divisions, with the number of divisions depending on how many times billing will be done during a month. For example, if the office expects to bill twice per month, divide the accounts into two equal groups; for weekly billing, divide into four groups; and for daily billing, divide into 20 groups.

Small alphabetic groups can be combined to keep the divisions nearly equal in the number of statements to prepare on each billing day. If the files are color-coded, the medical assistant may wish to use the same alphabetic breakdown in billing. Regardless of constant changes in the individual accounts, the mailing dates for accounts in each section remain the same. A schedule for processing and mailing is therefore established, and the workload is apportioned throughout the entire month.

Cycle billing allows the medical assistant to continue all routine duties each day, handling the statements on a day-to-day

PROCEDURE 21-9

Perform Billing Procedures

<u>CAAHEP COMPETENCY:</u> 3.a(2)(d)
<u>ABHES COMPETENCY:</u> 3.l

GOAL: *To bill insurance companies for patient procedures and services and obtain the maximum legal reimbursement.*

EQUIPMENT and SUPPLIES

- Patient ledgers
- Accounting system
- Calculator
- Claim forms
- Encounter forms
- Clerical supplies

PROCEDURAL STEPS

1. Read the medical record or encounter form to determine the procedures and services that are to be billed.
   <u>PURPOSE:</u> To make certain that all procedures and services performed by the provider are billed so that he or she can receive the correct reimbursement.
2. Determine the diagnosis code for each diagnosis noted by the provider.
   <u>PURPOSE:</u> To use the proper code to note each diagnosis.
3. Determine the procedure codes for all procedures noted by the provider.
   <u>PURPOSE:</u> To use the proper code to note each procedure.
4. Complete the insurance claim form, following the directions provided for each block.
5. Determine the amount of money that the provider is billing for on this claim.
   <u>PURPOSE:</u> To bill for the correct amount in reimbursement.
6. Complete the claim form according to the directions for each block.
7. Determine the address where the claim forms should be mailed.
   <u>PURPOSE:</u> To eliminate unnecessary delays in the carrier's receipt of the claim form.
8. Mail the claim form.
9. Note the date that the claim should receive follow-up to make certain it is paid.

or weekly schedule rather than in one intensive period at the end of the month. This means that whole days need not be sacrificed from other duties to get statements in the mail. When the billing is spaced throughout the month, more time and consideration can be given to each statement, the itemization of bills is less burdensome, and the likelihood of error is decreased.

Patients generally accept the cycle billing system quickly, often with enthusiasm. However, if your office decides to change from a once-a-month billing system to a cycle billing system, patients should be notified in advance, and the new plan should be explained to them. To explain the new system to established patients, enclose a notice in each statement for 2 months before the transfer, describing the plan and indicating the future dates on which each patient will receive the bill.

Before a physician adopts the cycle billing system, particularly in a small community, several factors should be taken into consideration, such as the following:

- What is the general income level of the community, and how and when does the average patient get paid?
- Do local companies pay employees at various times during the month, or are most paychecks handed out at the beginning of the month?
- Would cycle billing benefit patients as well as the overall operation of the office?

Billing Third-Party Payors

Collection problems may arise if the medical assistant fails to get the necessary insurance information, particularly Medicare and Medicaid information. In some instances, if the insurance forms are not completed correctly the claim may be denied because of minor infractions such as failing to name the responsible party or omitting Social Security information, the policy number, or the group number.

Time limits must also be observed in billing third-party payors. In cases of Medicare patients with a terminal illness, it may be best to accept assignment of benefits. If the physician does not take assignment, he or she may receive nothing because the family is not obligated to pay, and Medicare will not pay after a certain time or if the claim has not been correctly filed.

Billing Minors

Minors cannot be held responsible for payment of a bill unless they are emancipated. Bills for minors must be addressed to a parent or legal guardian. If a bill is addressed to a minor, the parent or parents could take the attitude that they are not responsible because they never received the bill.

If the parents are separated or divorced, the parent who brings the child in for treatment is responsible for payment. Whatever financial agreement exists between the parents is strictly their personal business and should not concern the medical office. The responsible parent should be so informed from the beginning.

If a minor appears in the office and requests treatment and you can ascertain that the person is legally emancipated, the minor is responsible for the bill. It may be wise to make a determination either with the business manager or with the physician as to whether your office wishes to treat this emancipated minor.

CARE FOR THOSE WHO CANNOT PAY

The medical profession has traditionally accepted the responsibility of providing medical care for individuals unable to pay for these services. In spite of the increased scope of government-sponsored care for the **medically indigent,** physicians still donate thousands of dollars' worth of such medical services each year.

In many instances medical care of the indigent is available through social service agencies. The medical assistant should learn about any local organizations and agencies that can aid the patient in obtaining the necessary assistance. The physician can provide only medical services. Other agencies must provide hospitalization, for example, or arrange for paying the costs of special therapy, rehabilitation, or medications. Unfortunately, there is still another segment of the population that consists of uninsured employees who are not eligible for public assistance, are not covered under a group policy, and cannot afford the high premiums for private medical insurance. Special attention must be given to helping these people arrange to pay their medical bills.

If a physician accepts a case for which a fee will not be paid, complete records must still be kept on the patient. The only deviation in procedure is that the financial record indicates no charge (n/c) in the debit column.

Fees in Hardship Cases

Sometimes a physician is faced with the problem of deciding whether to reduce or cancel a fee in a hardship case. Before adjusting or canceling a fee, the physician or the medical assistant should engage in a frank discussion of the patient's financial situation. Find out whether the patient is entitled to an insurance settlement of some kind. For instance, if the patient's injuries are the result of a car accident, there may be insurance through the automobile policy. Circumstances may qualify the patient for local or state public assistance, such as crime victim assistance. If so, the assistant may direct the patient to the appropriate agency.

If the circumstances of hardship are known before the services are rendered, a thorough discussion of what the fee will be and how it will be paid should take place at that time. The physician may suggest that a medically indigent patient seek care at a county hospital with public assistance. A physician should be free to choose his or her form of charity and should not feel obligated to substantially reduce or cancel a fee when the circumstances are known in advance.

After the physician and patient have agreed on a fee, special circumstances may arise that create a hardship. If the physician then agrees to reduce the fee, the patient should be told that the reduction will be effective only after the adjusted amount is paid in full. For instance, if a fee of $500 is reduced to $350, the full amount of the $500 charge should appear on the ledger, and when $350 has been received the remainder can be written off as an adjustment.

PITFALLS OF FEE ADJUSTMENTS

When a physician begins to reduce his or her fees, problems can arise. Patients may begin to expect that fees will be reduced in all circumstances. Patients may even doubt the competency of a physician who habitually reduces fees.

Great care should be taken in reducing the fee for care of a patient who dies. The physician's sympathy is with the family in such instances, but the physician's generosity in reducing a fee could be misinterpreted and result in a suit for malpractice. The family may suspect that the fee was reduced because the physician knows he or she made an error.

If the physician agrees to settle for a reduced fee in a situation in which the patient is disputing the fee, care should be taken to make certain the negotiations are without prejudice. By taking this precaution, the physician protects the right to collect the original sum should the patient refuse to pay the lowered fee. The offer of a discount therefore should be made in writing, with the insertion of the words "without prejudice" and a definite time limit for making payment stated. Prepare two copies of the agreement and have the signatures witnessed. Keep the original for the physician and give a copy to the patient.

A fee should never be reduced on the basis of a poor result or as a means of obtaining payment to avoid the use of a collection agency. A reduction for these reasons degrades the physician and the practice of medicine.

PROFESSIONAL COURTESY

Traditionally, physicians do not charge professional colleagues or their immediate dependents for medical care. Although the concept of professional courtesy is often attributed to Hippocrates, the foundations of professional courtesy today are derived from Thomas Percival's Code of 1803.

In some cases, giving professional courtesy represents the loss of a large amount of potential income. If there is a substantial outlay in the cost of materials, the professional colleague will probably wish to reimburse the physician for the materials used. Most physicians today subscribe to a health insurance plan. If the care they receive is covered by insurance, it is entirely ethical for the attending physician to accept the insurance benefits in payment for services.

If the services are frequent enough to involve a significant portion of the physician's professional time or if they extend over a long time, the physician may wish to charge on an adjusted basis. When professional courtesy has been offered and the recipient still insists on paying, the physician need not hesitate on ethical grounds to accept a fee for service.

Professional courtesy is often extended beyond fellow physicians and their dependents. Most physicians treat their own medical assistants, and often their families, without charge and grant discounts to nurses and medical assistants not in their direct employ. Student externs should never expect to be treated while serving in an externship capacity. Professional courtesy is sometimes extended to others in the healthcare field (e.g., pharmacists and dentists).

COLLECTION TECHNIQUES

Sometimes, it becomes necessary to aggressively attempt to collect the balances that patients owe the physician (Procedures 21-10 and 21-11). Persuasive collection procedures include telephone calls, collection reminders and letters, and personal interviews.

Telephone Collection Calls

A telephone call at the right time, in the right manner, will be more successful than notes, a statement, or a collection letter. The personal contact of a telephone call will bring in more money than if a call is not made. In the absence of time to make calls, the collection letter is the next best avenue. If collections are a serious problem, it may pay to hire an extra person to do the telephoning. Written notification is a must before making a final demand for payment indicating that legal or collection proceedings will be started. There are no hard and fast rules for pursuing collections by telephone. Each case should be handled individually on the basis of the experience with the person involved.

Collection Letters or Reminders

Some consultants believe that a printed collection letter or reminder enclosed with a statement is more effective than a personal letter. Their attitude is that a patient may be embarrassed by a personal letter and feel that he or she has been singled out for attention. An impersonal printed message will probably encourage the debtor to send a payment. The printed form is a time saver and is recommended if a lack of time is contributing to poor collection follow-up. Standard printed forms are readily available, and the medical assistant can also design original forms.

Letters that are friendly requests for an explanation of why payment has not been made are still effective in many cases. These letters should indicate that the physician is sincerely interested in the patient and wishes to help straighten out the financial obligations. The patient should be invited to visit the office to explain the reasons for nonpayment so that, if possible, special arrangements can be worked out. To give the patient an opportunity to save face, these letters can suggest that the patient may have overlooked previous statements.

PROCEDURE 21-10

Perform Collection Procedures

CAAHEP COMPETENCY: 3.a(2)(d)
ABHES COMPETENCY: 3.l

GOAL: *To collect the maximum amount of funds on each account.*

EQUIPMENT and SUPPLIES

- Patient ledger
- Office policy manual
- Clerical supplies
- Scripts for telephone collections
- Letters for collection efforts
- Telephone
- Letterhead and envelopes
- Copies of claim forms previously filed

PROCEDURAL STEPS

1. Be familiar with office policy regarding turning accounts over to collections.
   PURPOSE: To make certain that policy is followed when accounts are turned over to collection agencies.
2. Review the patient ledger to determine if it needs collection activity.
   PURPOSE: Some accounts may be past due, but patients have made arrangements to pay them; in this case, collection activities should not commence.
3. Determine the type of collection activity the account needs.
   PURPOSE: The account that is only slightly past due does not need a harsh collection letter; determine the best approach for each particular account.
4. Begin collection efforts with telephone calls or postcards.
   PURPOSE: Many patients only need a small reminder that their account is past due.
5. Progress to more stringent collection efforts if the patient does not pay the account as promised.
6. Once all collection efforts have been exhausted, report the account to the physician for further disposition.
   PURPOSE: The physician should decide which accounts are given to collection agencies and which are simply written off as bad debts.
7. Document the final collection activity on the ledger and/or in the patient medical record.

PROCEDURE 21-11

Perform Accounts Receivable Procedures: Age Accounts Receivables

CAAHEP COMPETENCY: 3.a.(2)(c)
ABHES COMPETENCY: 3.l

GOAL: *To determine the age of accounts and decide what collection activity is needed.*

EQUIPMENT and SUPPLIES

- Patient ledger cards with a balance due
- Pen
- Computer
- Calculator

PROCEDURAL STEPS

1. Prompt the computer to compile a report on the age of accounts receivable. Many programs will have this as an easily accessed report option.
   PURPOSE: To determine which accounts have a balance due.

2. Divide the accounts into categories as listed below:
   - 0-30 days old
   - 30-60 days old
   - 60-90 days old
   - 90-120 days old
   - Over 120 days old
   PURPOSE: To determine how old the various accounts are and place the accounts into categories as to when the last payment was made.

3. If the computer program does not perform this function, manually pull all ledger cards that have a balance due and divide them into the categories listed above.

4. Examine the accounts to see which are awaiting an insurance payment. Action need not be taken if an insurance payment is expected and is not long overdue. Return those ledgers to the ledger tray.
   PURPOSE: To avoid collection activity on accounts for which a payment is expected.

5. Follow the office procedure for collections on the accounts left. Collection reminder stickers may be placed on the statements sent to the patient, or a collection letter may be sent. Be sure that the stickers are inside the envelope, not on the outside.
   PURPOSE: To prompt the patient to make a payment by pointing out the age of the account.

6. Call patients whose accounts are over 90 days old. Attempt to make payment arrangements with the patient.
   PURPOSE: To attempt to collect from the patient or determine why the patient has not yet paid the account.

7. Send a collection letter to patients whose accounts are over 120 days old, if indicated, to encourage the patient to pay the bill. If it is the office policy, mention that the account is in danger of being sent to a collection agency.
   PURPOSE: To reach patients who are not available by telephone.

8. Add the total accounts receivable for each category and arrive at a figure outstanding for each. The physician may wish to have a report weekly or monthly on these figures.
   PURPOSE: To have a current accounting of the amounts owed to the physician, and to double-check the amount outstanding according to the pegboard system or software system.

9. Note in the chart and/or on the ledger any arrangements made with patients regarding payment of the accounts. Send a follow-up letter to remind the patients of their payment agreements.
   PURPOSE: To document arrangements made and remind the patients of their obligation and promise to pay.

On receipt of such a letter, most patients make some effort to explain their failure to make payment. If a patient really is having financial difficulties, the physician may be able to get public assistance for him or her. If it is a temporary financial embarrassment, the physician and the patient may together be able to work out a satisfactory installment plan for payment.

The medical assistant often is given a free hand in designing collection patterns and composing collection letters. Many medical assistants compose a series of collection letters, using model letters that they have found to be effective (Figure 21-8). Such a series usually includes at least five letters in varying degrees of forcefulness.

Sometimes even the person with poor paying habits will pay the bill if treated with respect and consideration. The medical assistant should never go beyond the authority granted by the physician in pursuing collections. If there are questions about special collection problems, always check with the physician

before proceeding. This is particularly important with patients whom you do not know personally (e.g., patients whom the physician has seen in the hospital or at home and patients with no credit history). It is difficult to say whether the effects of pressing collections too hard (which can result in loss of patient good will) are more detrimental than the effects of not pursuing collections diligently enough (which can result in loss of revenue). The physician and the medical assistant together should agree on general collection policies as outlined earlier in this chapter, then the policies should be followed. In all cases in which an account is to be assigned to a collection agency, be certain that the physician is aware of it.

Signing Collection Letters

In most medical offices, the medical assistant signs collection letters with the identification "Assistant to Dr. Brown" or "Financial Secretary" below the typewritten signature. Some

1. Your account has always been paid promptly in the past, so this must be an oversight. Please accept this note as a friendly reminder of your account due in the amount of $ _____ .

2. Since your care in this office in March, we have had no word from you in regard to how you are feeling or your account due. If it is impossible for you to pay the full amount of $ _____ at this time, please call this office before June 15 so that satisfactory arrangements can be worked out.

3. Medical bills are payable at the time of service unless special credit arrangements are made. Please send your check in full or call this office before June 30.

4. If you have some question about your statement, we will be happy to answer it for you. If not, may we have a payment before the end of this month?

5. Unless some definite arrangement is made to reduce your balance of $ _____ , we can no longer carry your account on our books. Delinquent accounts are turned over to our collection agency on the 25th of the month.

6. **When a payment plan has been established, it can be reinforced by recognizing the first remittance with a letter of acknowledgment:**

   Thank you for the recent payment of $ _____ on your account. We are glad to cooperate with you in this arrangement for clearing your account. We will look for your next check at about the same time next month, and your final payment the following month.

7. **When a payment schedule has been arranged by a telephone call, it can be confirmed by letter.**

   As agreed upon in our telephone conversation today, we will expect you to mail a payment of $50 on February 10; $50 on March 10; and the balance on April 10. If some emergency should prevent your making one of these payments on time, please notify us immediately by telephone.

DO'S AND DON'TS

DO:

1. Individualize letters to suit the situation.

2. Design your early letters as mere reminders of debt.

3. Always imply that the patient has good intentions to pay, until lack of response over a period of time proves otherwise.

4. Send letters with a firmer tone only after you have sent one or two friendly reminders.

DON'T

1. Use the same collection letter for a patient with good paying habits as for one who is known to neglect financial obligations.

2. Place an overdue notice of any kind on a postcard or on the outside of an envelope. This is an **invasion of privacy.**

FIGURE 21-8 Suggestions for composing collection letters. Brief collection letters that ask patients to explain the lack of payment are often effective.

physicians may wish to personally sign these communications, but generally the medical assistant who handles the accounts also signs the collection letters.

Personal Interviews

Personal interviews with patients can sometimes be more effective than a whole series of collection letters. By talking to a patient face to face, the medical assistant can come to an understanding of the problem more quickly, and an agreement about future payment plans can be reached.

Occasionally a patient may undergo a long course of treatment and yet make no attempt to pay anything on account. Perhaps such a patient is only waiting for the physician or the medical assistant to suggest that a payment be made. When there is advance knowledge that the patient will require extensive treatment, the matter of payment should be discussed early in the course of treatment, the credit policy explained, and some agreement reached as to a payment plan.

Because medical services are far more intangible than any commercial service, collection efforts must not be delayed too long. Any responsible, sincere patient will call or write the physician's office after receiving a second statement and explain the delay in payment or ask for a payment plan.

If it becomes necessary to refer the account to a collector, a good agency should have a 35% to 40% recovery rate with an account that is assigned within 4 or 5 months. This may drop to 25% if the account is held only a few more months. If recovery by the agency is greater than 40%, it may indicate that the collection effort by the medical assistant needs to be intensified.

The value of medical accounts diminishes in direct proportion to the length of time that has elapsed since service was rendered.

General Rules to Follow in Telephone Collections

What to Do

- Call the patient when it can be done with privacy.
- Call between 8 am and 9 pm.
- Determine the identity of the person with whom you are speaking. If you ask, "Is this Mrs. Noble?" and she answers, "Yes," it could be the patient's mother-in-law or daughter-in-law, who is also "Mrs. Noble." Use the person's full name.
- Be dignified and respectful. One can be friendly and formal at the same time.
- Ask the patient if it is a convenient time to talk. Unless you have the attention of the called party, there is little to be gained by continuing. If told that it is an inopportune time, ask for a specific time to call back, or get a promise that the patient will call the office at a specified time.
- After a brief greeting, state the purpose of the call. Make no apology for calling, but state the reason in a friendly, businesslike way. The physician expects payment and the medical assistant is interested in helping the patient meet the financial obligation. Open the call with a phrase such as, "This is Alice, Dr. Wallace's financial secretary. I'm calling about your account." A well-placed pause at this point in the call sometimes gets an immediate response from the debtor in regard to the nonpayment.
- Assume a positive attitude. For example, convey the impression that the patient intended to pay and it is only a matter of working out some suitable arrangements.

- Keep the conversation brief and to the point, and avoid threats of any kind.
- Try to get a definite commitment—payment of a certain amount by a certain date.
- Follow up on promises. This is best accomplished by a tickler file or a note on the calendar. If the payment does not arrive by the promised date, remind the patient with another call. If the medical assistant fails to do this, the whole effort has been wasted.

What Not to Do

- Do not call between 9 PM and 8 AM. To do so may be considered harassment.
- Do not make repeated telephone calls.
- Do not call the debtor's place of work if the employer prohibits personal calls.
- If a call is placed to the debtor at work and the person cannot take the call, leave a message asking the debtor to "call Mrs. Black at 727-9238" without revealing the nature of the call; that is, do not state that the call is from "Dr. Wallace's office" or "Dr. Jones's medical assistant."
- Do not show hostility. An angry patient is a poor-paying patient. Insulted patients often do not pay at all.

Do not fight the law of diminishing returns. All collection activity is costly. Know when to stop and call on the services of a professional agency.

Special Collection Situations

Tracing "Skips"

When a statement is returned marked "Moved—no forwarding address," you may consider this account as a "skip." This generally is accepted as an indication that the patient is attempting to avoid liability for debts. Some so-called skips are innocent errors. The person may have been careless in not leaving a forwarding address, or the mistake may have occurred in the physician's office; the wrong name or address may have been placed on the statement. However, immediate action should be taken in regard to returned statements. Do not wait until the next billing time to attempt to trace the debtor.

The tracing of skips is a challenge to any medical assistant. A certified letter can be sent; by paying additional fees, you can ask the Postal Service to obtain a receipt including the address where the letter was delivered. The certified letter may be sent in a plain envelope so that the patient will not refuse to accept the letter because of the return address.

If all attempts fail, turn the account over to a collection agency without delay. Do not keep a skip account too long, because the trail may become so cold as time elapses that even collection experts will be unable to follow it.

Claims Against Estates

A bill owed by a deceased patient may be handled a little differently than regular bills. Courtesy dictates that a bill not be sent during the initial period of bereavement, but do not delay more than 30 days. The person responsible for settling the affairs of the estate will be assembling outstanding accounts and will expect to receive the medical bills along with all others. Address the statement using the following format:

Estate of (name of patient)
c/o (spouse or next of kin, if known)
Patient's last known address

Do not address the statement to a relative unless you have a signed agreement that that person will be responsible. If for some reason the statement cannot be addressed as just suggested (e.g., if the patient was in a convalescent home and there is no name of a relative), seek information from the county seat in the county in which the estate is being settled.

A will is generally filed within 30 days of a death. A request to the Probate Department of the Superior Court, County Recorder's Office, will usually provide the name of the executor or administrator. The time limits for filing an estate claim are determined by the state in which the decedent resided.

After the name of the administrator or executor of the estate has been obtained, a duplicate itemized statement of the account should be sent to that person by certified mail, return receipt requested. If no response is received in 10 days, contact the executor or the county clerk where the estate is being settled and obtain forms for filing a claim against the estate. (Some states do not have special claim forms but will accept simple itemized statements.) This claim against the estate must be made within a certain length of time, varying from 2 to 36 months, depending on the state in which it is filed.

The executor of the estate will either accept or reject the claim and if it is accepted, will send an acknowledgment of the debt. Payment is often delayed because of the legal complications in settling an estate, but if the claim has been accepted, you will receive your money in due time. If the claim is rejected and there is full justification for claiming the bill, file a claim against the executor within a limited time, according to state laws. The time limit in such cases starts with the date on the letter of rejection that was sent in response to the original claim.

Because states have different time limits and statutes in regard to such matters, it is advisable for the medical assistant to contact the physician's attorney or the local court for the exact procedure to follow.

Bankruptcy

Bankruptcy laws were passed to secure equal distribution of the assets of an individual among the individual's creditors. Bankruptcy laws are federal and are applicable in all states. When notified that a patient has declared bankruptcy, do not send statements or make any attempt to collect on the account from the patient.

Chapter VII bankruptcy is usually a "no asset" situation. Because the physician's fee is an unsecured debt, there is little

---

purpose in pursuing collection. Chapter XIII is known as *wage-earner bankruptcy*. Under Chapter XIII, the patient-debtor pays a fixed amount (agreed on by the court) to the trustee in bankruptcy. This is then passed on to the creditors. During this period, none of the creditors can attach the debtor's wages or otherwise attempt to collect the debt. It is sometimes beneficial to file a claim under Chapter XIII because small payments will be made by the debtor under the supervision of the court over a period of 3 years.

USING OUTSIDE COLLECTION ASSISTANCE

When everything possible has been done internally to follow up on an outstanding account and the office has not received payment, the question arises as to what step to take next, as follows:

- Should the facility sue for the payment?
- Should the account be sent to a collection agency?
- Should the account be written off as a bad debt?

Before forcing an account, first consider the time element: Has the patient been given a fair chance to pay this bill? Have statements been sent regularly, and has a systematic method of following the account been used? Ask if there might be a misunderstanding about the fee charged. Was the first statement fully itemized? A large unexplained bill may frighten a patient into making no payments at all because the whole balance looks too large.

If the correct registration forms to secure advance credit information were used, the medical assistant should know the financial abilities of the patient to pay. However, illness may have caused a loss of salary and resulted in temporary inability to pay. Try to thoroughly analyze the situation.

Could the patient have been dissatisfied with the care received? For some unknown reason, a patient may feel that he or she was not treated correctly. Perhaps the patient expected a complete cure too soon. Only an explanation of the condition, prognosis, and care can enlighten such patients, and this is best handled by the physician. If payment of a bill is pressed too hard and the patient is dissatisfied for some reason, a malpractice suit may be filed by the patient to seek retribution against the physician. The court can approve a period longer than 3 years in special cases, but cannot approve a period longer than 5 years.

Collecting Through the Court System

Making the Decision to Sue

Will a physician lose more good will by suing for a bill than by writing it off as a loss? One management official has related that, strangely enough, when a physician-client sued two patients for large amounts, the patients lost the cases, paid up, and were back in the office for treatment very shortly! However, most physicians believe it is unwise to resort to the court to collect medical bills unless there are extraordinary circumstances.

An account must be considered a 100% loss to the physician before legal proceedings are started. Remember to never threaten to **instigate** legal proceedings unless prepared to carry out the

---

Suggestions for Tracing Skips

- Examine the patient's original office registration card.
- Call the telephone number listed on the card. Occasionally a patient may move without leaving a forwarding address but will transfer the old telephone number. The new telephone number may be given when you call the old number.
- If you are unable to contact the individual by telephone, make a few discreet calls to the references listed on the registration card to get leads.
- Check the Internet to secure the names and telephone numbers of neighbors or the landlord, and contact these people to secure information about the debtor's whereabouts.
- Do not inform a third party that the person owes you money. Simply state that you are trying to locate or verify the location of the individual.
- Check the debtor's place of employment for information. If the person is a specialist in his or her field of work, the local union or similar organizations may be contacted. Although they may not give you the person's current address, they will relay the message that you are seeking to contact him or her. Often people will be stirred into paying a bill if they think that their employer may learn of their payment failure.
- Do not communicate with a third party more than once. This is specifically forbidden by law (Public Law 95-109, Sec. 804) unless the third party requests the collector to do so.

threat, and have the physician's consent to such a warning being issued. If the physician decides in favor of a lawsuit, investigate thoroughly before taking action. Litigation to collect a bill is generally in order when the following occur:

- The patient can afford to pay without hardship.
- The physician can produce office records that support the bill.
- The physician can justify the amount of the bill by comparing it with fee practices in the community.
- The patient's general condition after treatment is satisfactory.
- The persuasive powers of an ethical collection agency have been exhausted, and the agency advises suing.
- The patient can be given ample warning of the physician's intention to sue.
- The defendant (whether a patient or a parent or legal guardian) is legally liable for the services rendered to the patient.
- The statute of limitations has ruled out any possible malpractice action.
- The physician is not indignant or in a negative frame of mind.

Small Claims Court

Many medical practices find the small claims court a satisfactory and inexpensive way to collect delinquent accounts. The law places a limit on the amount of debt for which relief may be sought in the small claims court. Because this varies from state to state (from $300 to $5000) and in some instances even within a state, this limit should be checked locally before seeking recovery in this manner.

Parties to small claims actions cannot be represented by an attorney at the trial but may send another person to court in their behalf to produce records supporting the claim. Physicians often send their bookkeeper or medical assistant with records of unpaid accounts to show the judge.

If the court awards a judgment for the amount owed, the plaintiff in small claims court may also recover the costs of the suit. For a very small investment in time and money, the physician who uses this method has done the following:

- Saved the time of a regular court action
- Had no attorney's fee to pay
- Not sacrificed the commission charged by a collection agency

After being awarded a judgment, the medical assistant must still collect the money. The only person in a small claims action who has the right of appeal is the defendant. An appeal by the defendant may have the judgment set aside. The plaintiff cannot file an appeal in a small claims action; the decision of the court is final.

The necessary papers for filing action and full instructions on the course to follow may be obtained from the clerk of the small claims court. The medical assistant who has never appeared in the court would probably be wise to attend once as a spectator to preview the procedure and feel more at ease when appearing for the physician.

A collection agency to which an account may have been assigned may not file or handle a small claims action. It must either sue in the regular municipal or justice court or attempt to collect the debt in some other manner.

Using a Collection Agency

The medical assistant should try every means possible to collect accounts before they become delinquent. As soon as the account is determined uncollectible through the office (i.e., the patient has failed to respond to the final letter or has failed to fulfill a second promise on payment), send the account to the collector without delay. Skips should be assigned immediately.

Even though collection by an agency will mean sacrificing from 40% to 60% of the amount owed, further delay will only reduce the chances of recovery by the professional collector. If the agency finds that the case deserves special consideration, it will seek the physician's advice before proceeding further.

CRITICAL THINKING APPLICATION

- Myra has had several complaints about the collection agency used by the office. Patients have called to report that the collectors are threatening and unprofessional. How should Myra approach the collection agency about these complaints?
- The office manager refuses to take these patients seriously, saying that because they owe the money, the collection agency's job is to collect the account in whatever way necessary. Myra does not agree with her philosophy. What should she do?

Selecting a Collection Agency

A number of agencies are either owned and operated as an integral part of the county medical society or are operated separately from the medical society but supervised by the medical profession. These bureaus provide specialized medical collection services.

Another type of collection agency is a division of the local credit association, recognized by the National Retail Credit Association. If the local credit association does not maintain a collection department, it will be able to recommend a reputable one. A nationally recognized credit association has considerable responsibility and a high standard to maintain. These factors serve as monitors to its reliability.

The most common type of collection agency throughout the United States is the privately owned and operated agency. Many of these work with the local professional societies and strive to adhere to a high ethical standard. Because a few bureaus are unethical and unscrupulous in their tactics, care should be taken to be sure that the one chosen is reliable and ethical. For the sake of comparison, many healthcare facilities use two or three agencies.

Responsibilities to the Collection Agency

When a reputable agency is selected, the medical assistant must be prepared to provide the agency with all the necessary data to enable it to begin prompt collection procedures on overdue accounts. The agency should receive the following:

PROCEDURE 21-12

Post Collection Agency Payments

<u>CAAHEP COMPETENCY:</u> 3.a(2)(i)
<u>ABHES COMPETENCY:</u> 3.s

GOAL: *To post payments received on an account after it has been turned over to a collection agency.*

EQUIPMENT and SUPPLIES

- Patient ledgers
- Office policy manual
- Bookkeeping system
- Clerical supplies
- Calculator

PROCEDURAL STEPS

1. Determine that a payment has been received on an account that is now being serviced by a collection agency.

2. Notify the collection agency that the payment has been made. <u>PURPOSE:</u> The collection agency is entitled to a portion of money collected when a payment is sent to the medical office.

3. Send a notice to the patient, if necessary, to explain that the payment has been forwarded to the collection agency for credit.

4. Instruct patients to forward additional payments straight to the collection agency.

- Full name of the debtor
- Name of the spouse
- Last known address
- Full amount of the debt
- Date of the last entry on account (debit or credit)
- Occupation of the debtor
- Business address
- Any other pertinent data

After an account has been released to a collection agency, the office makes no further collection attempts. Once the agency has begun its work, the following guidelines and procedures should be adhered to:

- Send no more statements.
- Mark the patient's ledger or stamp it so that everyone will know it is now in the hands of the collector.
- Refer the patient to the collection agency if he or she contacts the office in regard to the account.
- Promptly report any payments made directly to your office (a percentage of this payment is due the agency).
- Call the agency if any information is obtained that will be of value in tracing or collecting the account.
- Do not push the agency with frequent calls. The representatives of the agency will report regularly and will keep the office posted on collection progress.

Collection Agency Payments

If a patient sends a payment after the account has been turned over to a collection agency, the amount will need to be adjusted on the patient ledger. The collection agency will be due a percentage of the payment (Procedure 21-12).

CLOSING COMMENTS

Billing and collecting are critical duties in the medical office, and a responsible medical assistant is a great asset in this important area. Always maintain a positive attitude with the patients and guarantors. Remember that those who are ill or facing challenges are not always at their best and may not respond in a positive way to calls regarding their accounts. Make every attempt to work with each patient to develop a workable plan to clear his or her account.

Most patients are unaware of the actual coverage they have through their insurance policies. The medical assistant should encourage patients to read the entire policy so that they become familiar with its limitations and exclusions. Tell patients that when calling the company with questions, they should always write down the date, time, and name of the person with whom they spoke. Using email is helpful, because a record of the correspondence can be easily saved or printed. It is well worth the effort to make sure that patients have a general understanding of their health insurance coverage.

Often, patients do not dispute or question the company when a claim is rejected or not paid in the expected amount. Encourage them to call the company and question rejections if they do not understand why the claim was denied. Patients are paying for coverage and they should receive all of the benefits to which they are entitled.

Patients appreciate receiving an office policy brochure or booklet that informs them about payment and credit options. The patient can use the printed booklet as a reference whenever questions arise, and its regular use by most patients will reduce the number of calls made to the office. Encourage patients to use the booklet. Helpful phone numbers or extensions, as well as instructions as to whom the patient should call for answers to questions at the medical facility, should be included.

A patient who has filed for bankruptcy cannot be contacted or billed further. A threat to take collection action must be fulfilled or the creditor is in violation of the federal Fair Debt Collection Practices Act. Never say that the physician intends to take action if he or she does not plan to follow through.

The Federal Equal Credit Opportunity Act of 1977 bars discrimination in all areas of credit. If the physician agrees to extend credit to one credit-worthy patient, then the same arrangement must be offered to any other patient who requests it, as long as the patient is also credit worthy.

Because laws vary greatly from state to state, the medical assistant should review the statutes pertaining to billing and

collecting in the area in which he or she lives. Develop a good understanding of what is required of the small business, such as a physician's office, in collecting fees and billing for amounts due. Remember that laws change often, and constantly update policies to reflect current statutes.

SUMMARY OF SCENARIO

Myra is a well-respected member of Dr. Wallace's office team. Her friendly attitude and flexibility attract patients, and she enjoys the interaction with them. She knows that there are only a few patients for whom she cannot work out some type of payment arrangements. She is professional in her dealings with those whom she contacts about outstanding accounts.

Dr. Wallace has noticed that more and more patients pay their accounts, and he attributes this to the care that Myra shows when working with them. She is never hesitant to ask for payment from patients but is sensitive to their needs and struggles at the same time. She urges her patients to cooperate and make a good attempt to pay their accounts, and in return, Myra arranges a payment schedule that the patient can meet.

Although she was initially nervous about explaining fees to patients and asking for payments, she has become more comfortable in doing this aspect of her job, since she understands the business aspect of the practice. The physician is operating the practice to make a profit and support his family, and the practice is a source of support for the employees' families as well. Patients understand that physicians must charge for their services, and have become used to copayments and coinsurance amounts. Many times, these fees are collected in advance before the patient sees Dr. Wallace. This practice saves time on checkout and most patients feel that the copay is a small cost compared to the entire fee that physicians charge to manage their care in one office visit.

Myra has noticed that the usual, customary, and reasonable fees that Dr. Wallace charges his patients directly affect the

reimbursements that are paid by various insurance and managed care companies. She has handled several claims in which the payor questioned the fee when it fell outside of the UCR ranges. Dr. Wallace commented that he uses professional courtesy much less frequently than in the past because of the many rules and regulations placed on providers by managed care companies. He still offers the occasional patient a professional discount when it does not violate the managed care contract that he holds with the insurer or managed care company.

Myra's flexibility as an employee has paid off for Dr. Wallace several times. During a week-long period when the computer bookkeeping system was malfunctioning, Myra was able to retrieve information from her backup disks and use a pegboard system until the system was repaired. Her preparation allowed the office to continue operations without skipping a beat. Most patients did not even notice that the computer was not in use for the week.

Many physicians still use the manual pegboard system out of habit and because it is a reliable method of keeping up with patient accounts. Some simply trust manual, written records more than computerized systems. Since this is a matter of personal choice, either system will work in the physician's office.

Myra has been able to fill in for other employees because of the versatility she gained from her medical assistant training. She has scheduled appointments and even assisted Dr. Wallace with minor office surgery. Myra feels that performing other duties is a nice change periodically, and she keeps her skills sharp. She has proved herself to be a valuable and efficient employee.

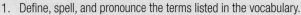

SUMMARY of LEARNING OBJECTIVES

1. Define, spell, and pronounce the terms listed in the vocabulary.
   - Spelling and pronouncing medical terms correctly adds credibility to the medical assistant. Knowing the definition of these terms promotes confidence in communication with patients and co-workers.
2. List three values that are considered in determining professional fees.
   - Medical services are valuable to the patient who receives them. The physician sets fees based on three commodities. The physician offers the patient his time and makes the most

accurate judgments possible about the patient's medical condition. The services provided to the patient also figure into the fees that are set for various procedures.
3. Distinguish among the terms usual, customary, and reasonable.
   - Many third-party payors use the UCR method of determining fees for procedures. The usual fee is what the physician normally charges for a given service. The customary fee is the range of fees charged by physicians who have similar experience in the same geographic area. Services or procedures that are exceptionally complicated and that require

Continued

SUMMARY of LEARNING OBJECTIVES
Continued

extra time deserve a reasonable fee and may be higher than the usual fee.

4. Discuss the value of estimates for patient treatment.
   - Providing estimates for medical care helps patients plan their finances when an illness or injury occurs. When estimates are provided, the possibility of later misquoting the fee is avoided. The office staff should keep a copy of the estimate in the patient's chart, which will help to avoid misunderstandings and confusion over charges.

5. Explain the concept of professional courtesy.
   - Some physicians choose to extend professional courtesy to other physicians, medical professionals, and medical staff employees. This means that the physician either discounts or eliminates the charges for all or part of the services provided. The decision to offer professional courtesy should remain with the physician.

6. Name the ways by which payment for medical services is accomplished.
   - Payment for medical services is accomplished in several ways. Most physicians prefer that payment be received at the time of service. When the extension of credit is offered, internal billing is necessary. Some offices contract with external billing services. Often, patients have some type of insurance or managed care policy that pays at least a portion of the bill. When patients fail to meet their obligations, outside collection services may be used.

7. Explain why itemizing statements is important.
   - The first statement should always be itemized. This provides the patient and the guarantor with a record of each procedure and each charge. Insurance companies require itemized bills to reimburse the charges.

8. Discuss why patients fail to pay accounts.
   - Rarely do patients not wish to meet their bill-paying obligations. Some do not have the money to pay for medical services, and if they do not have health insurance, it could be even more difficult to obtain medical care. The financial problem that the patient faces may be temporary, or it may be a long-standing situation. Only a few patients are actually unwilling to pay, so the medical assistant should work with the patient to develop a payment plan that the patient can meet.

9. Explain how to handle a "skip."
   - Immediate action should be taken when the office classifies a patient as a "skip." Search the patient chart for all possible telephone numbers, and call those that the patient has given. Do not reveal that the patient owes money. If it is necessary to leave a message, do not indicate that the call is from a physician's office. The employer may be called if the patient has not given specific permission not to call the place of business. Never communicate with a third party more than once unless invited to call back. A certified letter may be sent, and when address corrections are requested, the new address

is often obtainable. Unless the skip is found quickly, the account is generally turned over to a collection agency.

10. Briefly explain some of the guidelines of telephone collecting.
    - When making collection calls to patients or guarantors, be sure to call within accepted calling hours, which are 8 am to 9 pm. Be sure to correctly identify the person speaking, and always be respectful and courteous. State the purpose of the call, and keep the conversation businesslike and professional. Keep a positive attitude, and convey to the patient that the call is to help devise a way that his or her obligations to the physician can be met. Never threaten the patient, and make every effort to get a commitment as to when payment can be expected. Most important, follow up on collection calls to ensure that patients send in the payment as promised.

11. Explain professional fees to patients.
    - The medical assistant will periodically be required to explain the physician's professional fees to patients. The process for explaining fees to patients is outlined in Procedure 21-1.

12. Effectively use a pegboard system.
    - The pegboard system is effective in allowing the physician to know his or her accounts receivable on a daily basis. The process for posting entries on a daysheet is outlined in Procedure 21-2.

13. Establish credit arrangements for patient payment.
    - From time to time, the medical assistant will be required to make credit arrangements with patients who are unable to pay their accounts in full at the time of service. The process for making credit arrangements with patients is outlined in Procedure 21-7.

14. Prepare accurate monthly statements.
    - Billing statements sent in cycles through the month allow the physician to receive a constant flow of income. The process for preparing billing statements is outlined in Procedure 21-9.

15. Evaluate patient accounts for necessary collection procedures.
    - Some accounts will require collection activities. The process for performing collection procedures is outlined in Procedure 21-10.

16. Perform accounts receivables procedures.
    - The medical assistant may be required to work with receivables in the business office of the practice. The process for performing accounts receivable procedures is outlined in Procedure 21-8.

17. Post adjustments to patient accounts.
    - Various adjustments will be made to patient accounts in situations such as adjusting the allowable charge or writing off bad debt accounts. The process for posting adjustments is outlined in Procedure 21-3.

18. Process a credit balance on a patient account.
    - When an overpayment is made on a patient's account, the patient will receive funds back from the practice. The process for a credit balance is outlined in Procedure 21-4.

SUMMARY of LEARNING OBJECTIVES
Continued

19. Process refunds and send overpayments to patients, when appropriate.
    - Once a credit balance has been discovered, the patient will be due a refund. The process for refunds is outlined in Procedure 21-5.
20. Post non-sufficient fund checks to patient accounts.
    - When a patient writes a check that is returned to the practice for non-sufficient funds, the check must be added back to the patient's ledger account. The process for posting non-sufficient fund checks is outlined in Procedure 21-6.
21. Post payments to accounts that have been turned over to a collection agency.

- Once an account has been turned over to a collection agency, the physician should no notify the collection agency that a payment has been made. The process for posting collection agency payments is outlined in Procedure 21-12.
22. Age accounts receivable.
    - The medical assistant must periodically evaluate patient accounts to determine their age and decide what action needs to be taken on the account. The process for aging accounts receivables is outlined in Procedure 21-11.

CONNECTIONS

 Study Guide Connection: Go to Chapter 21 Study Guide. Read the Case Study and Workplace Applications and complete the assignments. Do online research for answers to the questions in the Internet Activities associated with professional fees, billing, and collecting.

 CD Connection: Go to the Medical Assisting Competency Challenge CD and do the training activities under Financial Management.

Evolve Connection: For more information related to professional fees, billing, and collecting, go to http://evolve.elsevier.com/kinn/admin and visit related weblinks for Chapter 21. Click on the Medical Assisting Exam Review and do the practice questions to sharpen your test-taking skills. To learn more about office software, do the exercises for the Altapoint demo that is on the CD.

Banking Services and Procedures 22

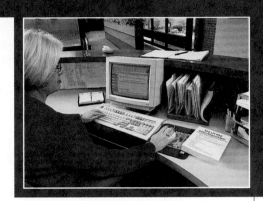

SCENARIO

Laura Anderson likes working with figures and has always been interested in bookkeeping. In high school she took all the bookkeeping and accounting courses that were offered, and during the summer months she helped out in the accounting department of the family business. In addition to her schooling and on-the-job experience, Laura wants to learn all she can about the financial transactions common to a medical practice. She is especially interested in electronic banking and all of the possibilities that it has to offer. Once her career in medical assisting is launched, Laura hopes to specialize in helping medical offices set up and run electronic banking systems.

Although Laura has had considerable bookkeeping experience, she realizes that she still has a lot to learn about the daily financial duties in a medical office, including accounts payable, working with the business checkbook, making deposits, reconciling bank statements, and many other banking responsibilities.

Taking on the bookkeeping functions of a medical office involves not only responsibilities to the physician and employer, but also to patients and the vendors from whom the medical office purchases supplies. Laura realizes that to perform well in her upcoming career as a medical assistant, she must learn all she can about the topics pertinent to her special interest areas and stay current with the rapidly changing world of finance.

While studying this chapter, think about the following questions:

- How has banking changed over the years?
- How safe is Internet banking?

- How can an office manager know that an employee can be trusted with banking procedures?
- Why is it a good idea to make daily deposits?

LEARNING OBJECTIVES

1. Define, spell, and pronounce the terms listed in the vocabulary.
2. Explain how the Internet has changed traditional banking practices.
3. State the four requirements of a negotiable instrument.
4. Discuss the advantages of using checks.
5. Identify the three most common types of bank accounts.
6. Explain how you would handle mistakes made in preparing a check.
7. List and discuss eight precautions to observe in accepting checks.

8. Name and compare the four kinds of endorsements.
9. Discuss the actions necessary when a deposited check is returned.
10. Correctly write checks for bill payment.
11. Prepare a bank deposit and appropriate office documents.
12. Accurately reconcile a bank statement with the office checking account.

National Accreditation Competencies and Content

CAAHEP COMPETENCIES

Administrative
3.a.(2)(a). Prepare a bank deposit

General
3.c.(4)(c). Utilize computer software to maintain office systems

ABHES COMPETENCIES

Administrative Duties
3.i. Prepare a bank statement and deposit record
3.j. Reconcile a bank statement
3.m. Prepare a check

Financial Management
8.e. Maintain records for accounting and banking purposes

VOCABULARY

clearinghouses Networks of banks that exchange checks with one another.

disbursements Money (funds) paid out.

drawee Bank or facility on which a check is drawn or written.

drawer Person who writes a check.

e-banking Electronic banking via computer modem or over the Internet.

endorser Person who signs his or her name on the back of a check for the purpose of transferring title to another person.

holder Person presenting a check for payment.

m-banking Banking through the use of wireless devices, such as cellular phones and wireless Internet services.

maker In reference to a check, any individual, corporation, or legal party who signs a check or any type of negotiable instrument.

negotiable Legally transferable to another party.

payee Person named on a draft or check as the recipient of the amount shown.

payor Person who writes a check in favor of the payee.

power of attorney A legal statement in which a person authorizes another person to act as his or her attorney or agent. The authority may be limited to the handling of specific procedures. The person authorized to act as the agent is known as the *attorney in fact*.

principal A capital sum of money due as a debt or used as a fund for which interest is either charged or paid.

reconciliation The process of proving that a bank statement and checkbook balance are in agreement.

Uniform Commercial Code (UCC) A unified set of rules covering many business transactions; it has been adopted in all 50 states, the District of Columbia, and most U.S. territories. It regulates the fields of sales of goods; commercial paper, such as checks; secured transactions in personal property; and particular aspects of banking, letters of credit, warehouse receipts, bills of lading, and investment securities.

Financial transactions in the professional office nearly always involve banking services and the use of checks. Therefore a medical assistant must understand the responsibilities involved in accepting payments, endorsing and depositing checks, writing checks, and regularly reconciling bank statements. Payments received in the medical office should be deposited as soon as possible—ideally, on the same day. The medical assistant may very well be in charge of these financial responsibilities; therefore he or she must understand each transaction and what its function is.

BANKING IN TODAY'S BUSINESS WORLD

With the advent of the Internet, banking as we once knew it has changed. People once had to fight traffic and wait in line at crowded banks; today they can sit in the comfort of their own homes and do their banking on the computer at any time of day. It is now possible to conduct such electronic banking transactions as buying and selling shares, paying bills, and transferring funds between accounts. In addition, customers have access to information about stock market prices and news and historical analyses of shares, which makes buying or selling decisions easier.

In fact, it is no longer necessary to sit in front of a computer terminal to conduct banking transactions. Instead, customers can sit on a bus or a train or be waiting for a flight and still make their investments or carry out other bank transactions. All of this is possible by just turning on a mobile telephone.

Online Banking

Online banking is a means to perform banking services via the Internet. It is also called *personal computer (PC) banking, home banking, electronic banking, **e-banking**,* or *Internet banking*. There are many facilities to choose from; most of them offer both basic and advanced services. Basic services usually include these:

- Checking account balances
- Transferring funds between accounts
- Paying bills electronically

Some of the advanced services that banks offer include the following:

- Applying for loans
- Downloading account information
- Trading stocks or mutual funds
- Viewing images of transactions (checks and deposits)

Online banking has advantages and disadvantages. One of the most obvious advantages is the ability to bank at one's own convenience in one's own home or office at any time. This can save considerable time and expense, especially if banking must be done daily. Many people find online banking a convenient and comprehensive method for money management. Other advantages include ease of use, portability, and availability.

Disadvantages of e-banking include having to learn the software—it is less versatile than physical banking—and the fact that service options are often more limited. In addition, some experts believe that there may be a slight increase in risk as compared with conventional banking, although this has been debated by e-banking proponents. Forecasts show, however, that in spite of the disadvantages, banking via the Internet is becoming more popular, with an estimated 20% to 25% of homes and businesses using it.

The cost of online banking varies from bank to bank. Some charge a flat rate (from $5 to $10 per month), with varying fees for additional transactions.

Online Loans

Online lending is becoming more common as well. Loans are available for nearly anything consumers want to purchase—from homes and cars to small business loans and student loans for college tuition. Although online lending still has many loopholes, consumers can save time and money by comparison shopping the dozens of lenders available to find a good rate. Application forms can be downloaded for processing to initiate the process quickly, but the complicated loan process—especially for home mortgages—still requires coordination among many parties, and the sensitive financial and personal information needed for loan approval can raise online security concerns. Despite these issues, many people are "surfing the Web" for loans.

Online Convenience

Convenience is probably the number one reason people and businesses use the Internet for their financial services. There is no frenzied drive to the bank during rush hour, waiting in line, or working around the confines of banking hours. Online banking is available 24 hours a day, 7 days a week. In addition to Internet banking services, consumers can also pay bills online, without the delay of mailing. Credit card holders can check their balances and transaction status. Costly fees can be avoided for financial transactions left until the last minute, because online transactions can be accomplished in a matter of seconds. The need to wait and worry if the mail will get it there in time is eliminated.

Customer-Oriented Banking

Americans are becoming more and more mobile. They want to conduct business and take care of personal concerns over cell phones on their way to and from work. In addition, the rapid pace of life requires rapid or "instant" solutions: people are buying take-out food at a record rate; some churches even offer drive-up services. It is no wonder that today's mobile consumers want the ability to conduct their financial transactions on the go, every day, at any time.

Banks no longer consider customers to be merely account numbers; to stay competitive, banks are being forced to look at the total customer picture. Some banks even offer a type of interactive voice response system that operates through speech recognition, allowing customers to conduct business through a combination of talking into the telephone and using the telephone keypad. The call centers of some banks employ live customer service personnel to answer questions and fulfill requests for all types of bank transactions.

Another customer-oriented innovation is mobile banking, or **m-banking**, which is emerging through the wireless technology market. Through the use of wireless devices such as cellular phones and wireless Internet services, customers can conduct a variety of financial transactions, set up alerts and notifications when bills are due, and make electronic transfers to pay these bills.

CRITICAL THINKING APPLICATION

Laura is excited about all of the possibilities available with e-banking and m-banking. Where can Laura learn more about electronic banking and its advantages and disadvantages compared with conventional banking?

CHECKS

A check is a bank draft or order to pay a certain sum of money payable on demand to a specified person or entity. The concept of writing and depositing checks as a method of conducting financial transactions dates back as far as the Roman Empire. Widespread check-writing didn't become popular, however, until the 1500s, when people in Holland began depositing excess cash with Dutch "cashiers," as a safer alternative than keeping money in their homes. These cashiers then paid the debts of the "depositors" on receipt of a written order. The word "check" was coined in England nearly 200 years later, when serial numbers were marked on these written orders of payment as a way to "check" on them. About 90% of all financial transactions in the United States are said to be accomplished by check.

A check is considered to be a **negotiable** instrument. For a check to be negotiable, it must:

- Be written and signed by a **maker**
- Contain a promise or order to pay a sum of money
- Be payable on demand or at a fixed future date
- Be payable to order or bearer

Types of Checks

A medical assistant is probably familiar with the standard personal check, but there are many additional types of checks used in business transactions. He or she should also be familiar with other types of checks, which are discussed next.

Bank Draft

A bank draft is a check drawn by a bank against funds deposited to its account in another bank.

Advantages of Using Checks

Using checks for the transfer of funds has many advantages:

- Checks are both safe and convenient, particularly for making payments by mail.
- Expenditures are quickly calculated.
- Specific payments can be easily located from the check record.
- A stop-payment order can protect the payor from loss resulting from stolen, lost, or incorrectly drawn checks.
- Checks provide a permanent reliable record of disbursements for tax purposes.
- The deposit record provides a summary of receipts.
- Checking accounts protect the money while on deposit.

Cashier's Check

A cashier's check is a bank's own check drawn on itself and signed by the bank cashier or other authorized official. It is also known as an *officer's* or *treasurer's check*. A cashier's check is obtained by paying the bank cashier the amount of the check, in cash or by personal check. Many banks charge a fee for this service. Cashier's checks are often issued to accommodate the savings account customer who does not maintain a checking account.

Certified Check

A certified check is the depositor's own check, on the face of which the bank has placed the word *certified* or *accepted* with the date and a bank official's signature. Because the bank deducts the amount of the check from the depositor's account at the time it certifies the check, the bank can guarantee that the amount is available. A certified check, like a cashier's check, can be used when an ordinary personal check might not be acceptable. If not used, a certified check should be redeposited promptly, so that the funds previously set aside are credited back to the depositor's account.

Limited Check

A check may be limited as to the amount written on it and as to the time during which it may be presented for payment—30, 60, or 90 days. The limited check is often used for payroll or insurance checks.

Money Order

Domestic money orders are sold by banks, some stores, and the United States Postal Service. Money orders are often used for paying bills by mail when an individual does not have a checking account. The maximum face value varies according to the source. International money orders may be purchased for limited amounts, indicated in U.S. dollars, for use in sending money abroad.

Traveler's Check

Traveler's checks are designed for persons traveling where personal checks may not be accepted or for use in situations in which it is inadvisable to carry large amounts of cash. Traveler's checks are usually printed in denominations of $10, $20, $50, and $100, and sometimes $500 and $1000. They require two signatures of the purchaser, one at the time of purchase and the other at the time of use. They are available at banks and some travel agencies. The use of traveler's checks is becoming less common, because major credit cards are widely accepted throughout the world.

Voucher Check

A voucher check has a detachable voucher form. The voucher portion is used to itemize or specify the purpose for which the check is drawn. It is used for the convenience of the **payor** and shows discounts and various other itemizations. This portion of the check is removed before the check is presented for payment and provides a record for the **payee** (Figure 22-1).

THE BANKING SYSTEM

The Federal Reserve

Wanting to provide the nation with a safer, more flexible, and stable monetary and financial system, Congress created the Federal Reserve in 1913 as the central bank of the United States. It consists of a seven-member Board of Governors with headquarters in Washington, DC and 12 Reserve Banks located in major cities throughout the country.

Figure 22-2 shows how the country is divided into the 12 regional Federal Reserve districts. For additional information on the Federal Reserve System and its regional banks, visit its website; the Web address is found at the end of this chapter.

American Bankers Association Number

The American Bankers Association (ABA) number is part of a coding system originated by the ABA. It appears in the upper right area of a printed check. The number is used as a simple way to identify the area where the bank on which the check is written is located and the particular bank within the area. The code number is expressed as a fraction (Figure 22-3), for example:

$$\frac{90\text{-}1822}{1222}$$

In the top part of the fraction, before the hyphen, the numbers 1 to 49 designate cities in which Federal Reserve banks are located or other key cities; the numbers from 50 to 99 refer to states or territories. The part of the number following the hyphen is a number issued to each bank for its own identification purposes. The ABA number is used in preparing deposit slips, to identify each check. The bottom part of the fraction includes the number of the Federal Reserve district in which the bank is located and other identifying information.

HOW CHECKS ARE PROCESSED

When a check is presented for payment, the **drawee** (bank or facility on which the check is drawn or written) pays the specified sum of money written on the face of the check to the **holder** (person presenting the check for payment). Checks received

CARB-OUT

Seattle Optical Company
222 Elm
Seattle, WA 90202
Date _____ 093   78-31 / 5467

Pay to the
Order of _____ | $ _____

_____ **Dollars**

United Trust Company
P.O. Box 327
Anytown, U.S.A.

Sample-VOID

Memo _____

⑈ 1 2 3 4 0 0 0 5 ⑆ 0 8 5 ⑆ 0 3 8 2 9 4 8 3 9 ⑈

DETACH AND RETAIN THIS STATEMENT
Seattle Optical Company   THE ATTACHED CHECK IS IN PAYMENT OF ITEMS DESCRIBED BELOW
Seattle, WA 90202   IF NOT CORRECT PLEASE NOTIFY US PROMPTLY. NO RECEIPT DESIRED

DATE	INVOICE NO.	AMOUNT	DISC.	NET	DATE	INVOICE NO.	AMOUNT	DISC.	NET

FIGURE 22-1 Page from a bank order book showing a sample voucher check.

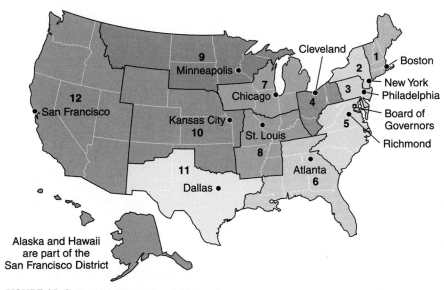

FIGURE 22-2 The 12 federal reserve districts.

by the bank are turned over daily to a regional clearinghouse, which cancels each one by stamping, mechanically punching, or embossing them. The identifying code numbers, printed on the face of the check with magnetic ink, enables this "clearing" process to be accomplished quickly and efficiently. Checks due from and to all banks outside of a specific region are settled by means of computerized entries. The cancelled check is then either kept by the financial institution or returned to the **drawer** (person who wrote the check). Many banks no longer provide cancelled checks on a regular basis with the advent of Internet banking services and most sophisticated computer systems. If the drawer needs proof of payment, a copy of the check can be requested from the bank if the checks are not returned in the monthly bank statement.

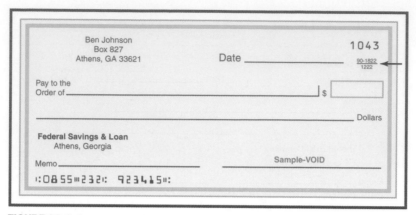

FIGURE 22-3 Sample check. The arrow indicates the American Bankers Association number.

Clearinghouses

As the use of checks increased, the system became confusing because so many different banks were involved. At first, messengers were used for collection; however, this involved a lot of traveling and carrying a lot of cash. Then, in a London coffee shop a solution came about when two bank messengers discussing the shortcomings of the system realized they both had checks for each other. They decided to exchange them and save some time and effort. This practice evolved into a system of check **clearinghouses**–networks of banks that exchange checks with one another–that is still in use. Today banks in the United States can present checks to the Federal Reserve System or private clearinghouses for regional and national check collection.

Magnetic Ink Character Recognition

Characters and numbers printed in magnetic ink are found at the bottom of checks. They represent a common machine language, readable by machines as well as by humans. When a check is deposited, the amount of the check can also be printed in magnetic ink below the signature. Magnetic ink character recognition (MICR) identification facilitates processing through a high-speed machine that reads the characters, sorts the checks, and does the bookkeeping.

BANK ACCOUNTS

Common Types of Accounts

Checking Accounts

By placing an amount of money on deposit in a bank, a depositor can set up a checking account. Simply stated, a checking account is a bank account against which checks can be written. Many variations in checking accounts have been developed over the years. Instead of a straight, non–interest-bearing account, one might have an insured money market checking account, which bears interest at the daily money market rate if a certain minimum balance is maintained. Most banks, however, do not offer interest-bearing checking accounts for businesses.

A physician often requires three different checking accounts:

- An account for personal and family expenses
- A separate checking account for office expenses

- A high-yield interest-bearing account for funds reserved for paying insurance premiums, property taxes, and other seasonal expenses

A medical assistant's use will probably be limited to the office checking account.

Savings Accounts

Money that is not needed for current expenses can be deposited into a savings account. In most cases, savings accounts earn interest on the amounts deposited–that is, the bank pays the depositor a certain percentage monthly or quarterly for the use of the money in the savings account. An ordinary savings account draws interest at the lowest prevailing rate and has no minimum balance requirement and no check-writing privileges.

Interest

Interest is a charge (or payment) in exchange for the use of money. It is usually figured as a percentage of the **principal.** Simple interest is computed annually; compound interest is figured on the principal as well as any previous interest that has been added to the original sum of money and can be computed using a variety of time increments–daily, monthly, quarterly, and so on. Certain checking accounts draw a small amount of interest–1% or 2% on the average daily balance. Savings accounts usually pay a higher rate of interest than checking accounts–2% to 3%. However, these rates fluctuate with the financial market.

Money Market Savings Account

An insured money market savings account requires a minimum balance, anywhere from $500 to $5000; draws interest at money market rates (which is usually a higher percentage rate than drawn by a regular savings account); and allows the writing of a specified number of checks (frequently three) per month. There may be a minimum fee charged for each transaction. Such checks are usually written for transfer of funds to a checking account. Some businesses transfer excess funds from the business checking account to a money market account over the weekend or over an extended holiday period to draw interest on the funds (Figure 22-4).

014143759	R		1	12/20/02
Account Number	Type	Items	Page No.	Statement Date

Statement of Account   14700 CT

001

Current Balance	Previous Statement Date	Previous Balance
2896.34	11/21/02	2886.59

ANSWERS TO YOUR BANKING QUESTIONS 24 HOURS A DAY,
7 DAYS A WEEK.   CALL ANSWERLINE TODAY

**** SUPER INSURED MONEY MARKET ACCOUNT ****

YOUR OPENING BALANCE OF: 2,886.59

NO   DEPOSITS LISTED TOTALING: .00

- OTHER CREDITS -

12-20 SUPER INSURED MONEY MKT. INT. PAID   9.75

1   CREDITS LISTED TOTALING: 9.75

NO   CHECKS LISTED TOTALING: .00

NO   DEBITS LISTED TOTALING: .00

EQUALS YOUR ENDING BALANCE OF: 2,896.34

DAILY ACCOUNT BALANCES

DATE	BALANCE	DATE	BALANCE	DATE	BALANCE
12-20	2896.34				

- - - - - - - - - - - - - - - - - - SUPER INSURED MONEY MARKET STATEMENT - - - - - - - - - - - - - - - - -

DATE	COLLECTED BALANCE	INTEREST RATES	DATE	COLLECTED BALANCE	INTEREST RATES
11-22	2,886.59	04.40	11-25	2,886.59	04.40
11-26	2,886.59	04.40	11-27	2,886.59	04.40
12-02	2,886.59	04.40	12-03	2,886.59	04.40
12-04	2,886.59	04.15	12-05	2,886.59	04.15
12-06	2,886.59	04.15	12-09	2,886.59	04.15
12-10	2,886.59	04.15	12-11	2,886.59	04.15
12-12	2,886.59	04.15	12-13	2,886.59	04.15
12-16	2,886.59	04.15	12-17	2,886.59	04.15
12-18	2,886.59	04.15	12-19	2,886.59	04.15
12-20	2,886.59	04.15			04.15

FIGURE 22-4 Example of a money market account statement. This type of check-writing has limited privileges.

Individual Retirement Accounts

Individual Retirement Accounts (IRAs) are a type of individual savings plan that are allowed special tax treatment at the federal and sometimes the state level. This tax-favored status is what distinguishes an IRA from an ordinary savings account; however, you must follow specific rules to get the tax savings. IRA rules are stricter than those for ordinary savings accounts.

Several different types of IRAs are available, such as traditional, Roth, and Education. IRAs are often used as a way to prepare for retirement for several reasons:

- Savings grows tax-deferred.
- Tax deductions are realized for contributions (for traditional IRAs).
- Interest earned may not be taxed at withdrawal (for Roth IRAs).

IRAs come in all shapes and sizes. It is important to study and know the rules of each one before deciding which is best for an individual's needs.

CRITICAL THINKING APPLICATION

One of Laura's co-workers wants to open an account at her local bank. She knows Laura has more experience in this field than she, so she asks for her advice. How might Laura advise her on this?

The Business Account

A business bank account is used for business or company operations and managing cash related to day-to-day business functions. A wide variety is available for businesses today, including checking, savings, and money market accounts, as well as other types of financial elements. When setting up a business account, careful consideration should be given to each of these elements to determine which account best meets the particular needs of a business.

What to Look for in a Business Account

Most businesses want "the most bang for their buck." In other words, they want to have the most services possible for the least amount of money—just as individuals do with personal accounts. Some of the service components available for business accounts include the following:

- Business checking with interest, accruing interest with either checking or savings accounts
- Free checks and deposits, with a maintained minimum balance (which varies from bank to bank)
- Overdraft protection, accomplished by linking the account to a savings account or to a bank-issued credit or debit card
- Online banking

Perks for Businesses

Many financial institutions are offering perquisites ("perks") for businesses opening accounts at their facility by offering special features. These may include the following:

- Business Express: A computerized cash management system that allows access to account information by telephone.
- "Sweep" account: An account in which excess funds over a minimum balance are "swept" into a higher yielding interest-bearing investment account. Then, when the balance in the account drops below the minimum, funds are "swept" back into it automatically.
- Business checking with "special features": A customized bank account designed for businesses with low to moderate transaction volumes and limited cash balances. This service helps business owners manage their day-to-day business and/or personal finances.

- Cash management account: Combines a checking account with a money market fund and a brokerage account. All cash activities are summarized on one monthly statement. This is ideal for business owners who do not have time for managing their money and/or investments.
- Other special features: Automatic bill paying, payroll preparation, and timed business deposits.

Business Checks

The checkbook most widely used in the professional office is a ledger-type book with three checks per page and a perforated stub at the left end of the check (Figure 22-5).

Checks may be bound in a soft cover or punched for a ring binder. The checks and matching stubs are numbered in sequence and preprinted with the depositor's name and account number, along with any additional information, such as address and telephone number. Check quantities of 100 to 300 are usually ordered at one time, and the cost is charged against the account. Numbered deposit slips in separately bound books are also supplied to the depositor.

Computer-Generated Checks. Instead of ordering checks to be printed by the bank, personalized checks can be ordered from printing houses to fit your computer's financial software program (e.g., Quicken). Checks can be prepared on the computer in much the same manner as using a typewriter. The checks may have one or more copies that serve as the record of checks written.

One-Write Check Writing. A one-write system of writing checks can save time and minimize errors in medical office **disbursements.** The office with a pegboard bookkeeping system may wish to include one-write check writing. By using a combination check-writing system, such as the one illustrated in Figure 22-6, one check and one record of checks drawn handle both bill paying and payroll check writing.

When the check is written, a permanent record is created through the carbonized line of the check onto the record of checks drawn and the employee's payroll record, including a record of all deductions. Space is provided for the payee's address, so that the check can be mailed in a window envelope. This not only saves time but also ensures that the check will go to the right address. Suppliers of basic pegboard systems can also provide a check-writing system such as the one described.

BILL PAYING AND CHECK WRITING

Establishing a Bill-Paying System

A systematic plan should be established for the writing of checks and the paying of bills. Some offices have incorporated an online bill-paying system and pay bills as soon as they are received. For those using manual systems, check writing usually is done on a specific day or days of each month. An exception sometimes arises when it is possible to realize a good discount if payment of a bill is made within a specified time, such as 10 days. Such discounts are usually indicated at the bottom of invoices or billing statements.

When a check is written in payment of a statement or invoice, it is good practice to write on the invoice the number

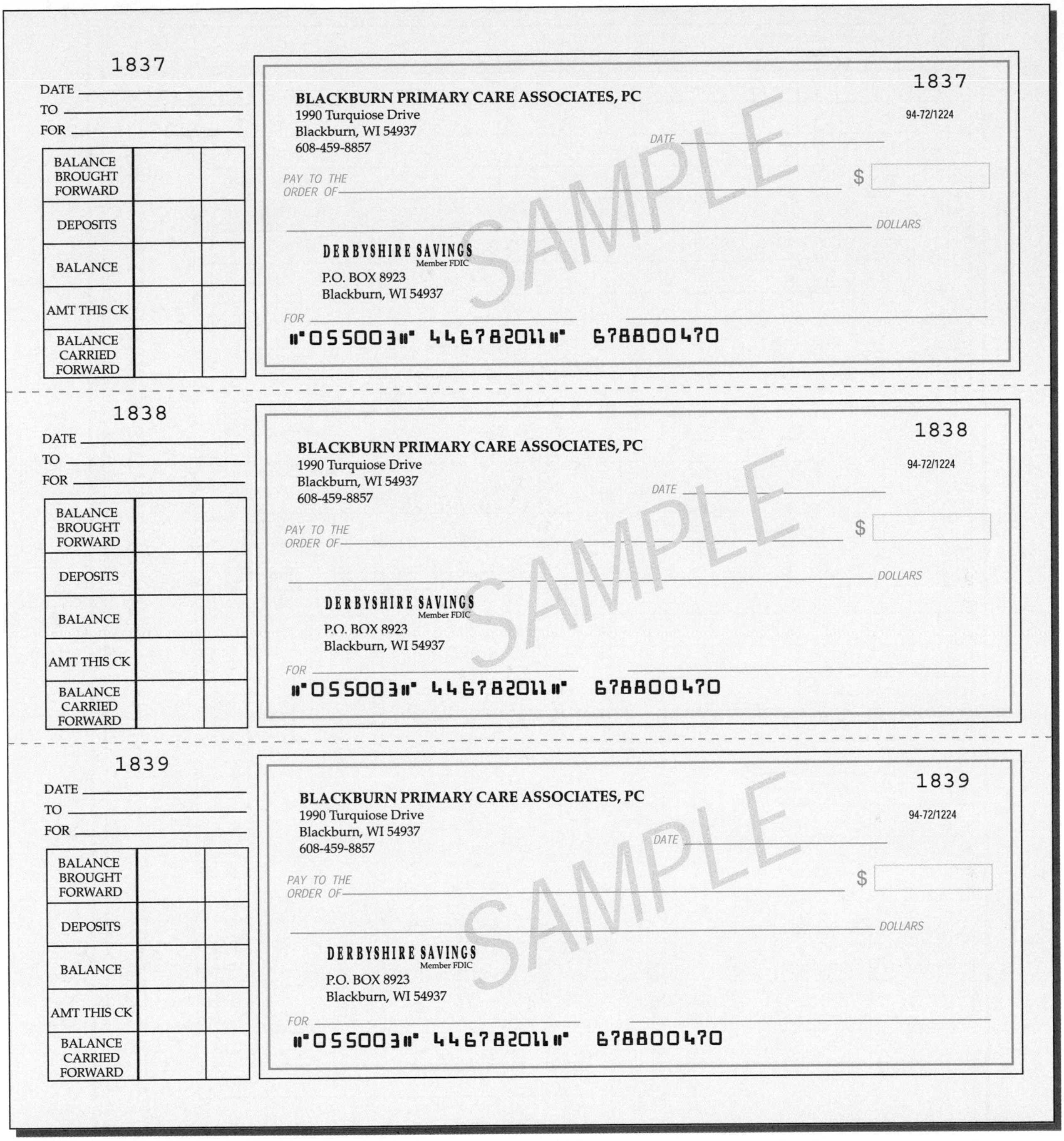
1837
DATE
TO
FOR
BALANCE BROUGHT FORWARD
DEPOSITS
BALANCE
AMT THIS CK
BALANCE CARRIED FORWARD

BLACKBURN PRIMARY CARE ASSOCIATES, PC
1990 Turquiose Drive
Blackburn, WI 54937
608-459-8857
1837
94-72/1224
DATE
PAY TO THE ORDER OF $
DOLLARS
DERBYSHIRE SAVINGS
Member FDIC
P.O. BOX 8923
Blackburn, WI 54937
FOR
⑈055003⑈ 446782011⑈ 678800470
SAMPLE

1838
DATE
TO
FOR
BALANCE BROUGHT FORWARD
DEPOSITS
BALANCE
AMT THIS CK
BALANCE CARRIED FORWARD

BLACKBURN PRIMARY CARE ASSOCIATES, PC
1990 Turquiose Drive
Blackburn, WI 54937
608-459-8857
1838
94-72/1224
DATE
PAY TO THE ORDER OF $
DOLLARS
DERBYSHIRE SAVINGS
Member FDIC
P.O. BOX 8923
Blackburn, WI 54937
FOR
⑈055003⑈ 446782011⑈ 678800470
SAMPLE

1839
DATE
TO
FOR
BALANCE BROUGHT FORWARD
DEPOSITS
BALANCE
AMT THIS CK
BALANCE CARRIED FORWARD

BLACKBURN PRIMARY CARE ASSOCIATES, PC
1990 Turquiose Drive
Blackburn, WI 54937
608-459-8857
1839
94-72/1224
DATE
PAY TO THE ORDER OF $
DOLLARS
DERBYSHIRE SAVINGS
Member FDIC
P.O. BOX 8923
Blackburn, WI 54937
FOR
⑈055003⑈ 446782011⑈ 678800470
SAMPLE

FIGURE 22-5 Example of business checks with stubs. (From Hunt SA: *Fundamentals of medical assisting*, Philadelphia, 2002, Saunders.)

of the check and the date it was paid. Then if any question arises about whether or when the bill was paid, you can readily locate the check stub. The handling and writing of checks must be done with extreme care (Procedure 22-1).

Designated Times

Rather than haphazardly paying bills as they are received in the office, the medical assistant should establish a routine for paying bills at designated times, such as on the fifteenth and thirtieth days of each month. Most vendors allow a 30-day cycle to elapse before adding on interest or late fees.

One method of handling accounts payable is to create a chronologic "tickler file" with dividers for each pay cycle (e.g., the tenth of the month, the twentieth, and the thirtieth). Behind each of the dividers, the invoices can be arranged alphabetically, if desired. When the date arrives, the medical assistant can pull all of the bills from that section and prepare the checks.

Paying Bills to Maximize Money

In establishing the procedure for accounts payable, a medical assistant should keep in mind that most vendors allow 30 days to pay. When each invoice is received, check the "terms," which

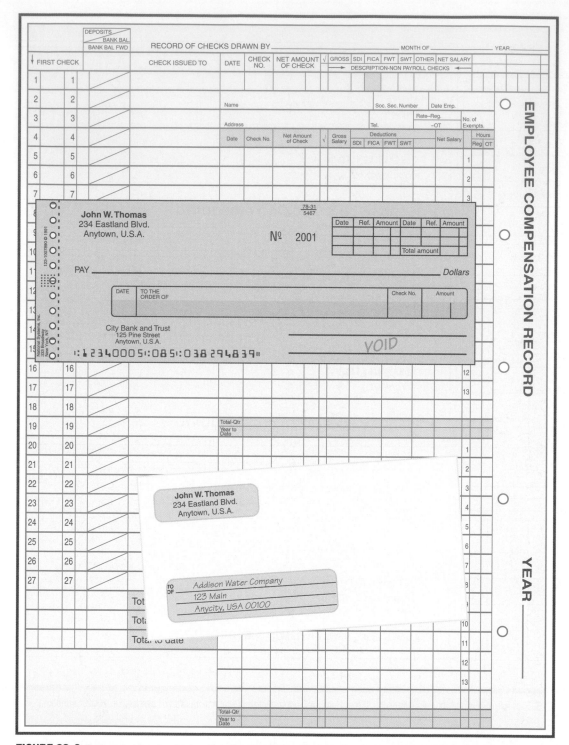

FIGURE 22-6 Pegboard system for check writing. (Courtesy Bibbero Systems, Inc., Petaluma, Calif. 94954, (800) 242-2376, www.bibbero.com.)

are usually located at the top of the document. A few vendors offer a discount (normally 1% to 2%) if bills are paid within a shorter period of time. If the terms say "Net 30," this means the total amount of the bill is due within 30 days. Remember to allow a certain number of days (2 to 5, depending on where payment is to be sent) for mailing. If the business checking account is an interest-bearing one, do not pay bills before their due date. In this way the funds in the account will continue to draw interest until it is time to write the check.

Also, if the practice has a weekly service, such as a laundry or cleaning service that bills several times a month, accumulate the invoices and issue only one check per month. Checks are costly, and some banks charge businesses a fee for each transaction.

PROCEDURE 22-1

Write Checks in Payment of Bills

ABHES COMPETENCY: 3.m

GOAL: *To correctly write checks for payment of bills.*

EQUIPMENT and SUPPLIES

- Checkbook
- Bills to be paid

PROCEDURAL STEPS

1. Locate the first bill to be paid. Before writing the check, fill out the stub or the place designated for recording expenditures. Include the date, name of payee, amount of check, the new balance to be carried forward, and usually, the purpose of the check.
   PURPOSE: To prevent the possibility of delivering or mailing a check without entering the information in the checkbook.
2. Complete both the check and the stub with pen or typewriter.
   PURPOSE: To avoid danger of alteration for any reason.
3. Date the check the day it is written (do not postdate).
4. Write the name of the payee after the printed words, "Pay to the Order of _____," with the necessary information following. Do not use abbreviations unless so instructed.
5. Leave no space before the name, and follow it with three dashes if space remains.
6. Omit personal titles from the names of payees.
7. If a payee is receiving a check as an officer of an organization, the name of the office should follow the name. Example: "John F. Jones, Treasurer."
8. Start writing at the extreme left of each space. Leave no blank spaces. Keep the cents notation close to the dollars figure to prevent alteration.
9. Verify that the amount of the check is recorded correctly on the stub, in the box for the dollar ($) amount, and on the line where the amount is written in words.
10. If a check is written for an amount less than 1 dollar, the figures by the $ sign may be circled or enclosed in parentheses ($0.65) to emphasize the amount.

Automatic Withdrawals and Deductions

Some routine bills that occur monthly or on a regular billing cycle, such as insurance premiums, rent payments, and utility bills, can be set up to be paid automatically through prior arrangements with the bank.

Online Bill-Paying

An online bill-paying account can be established with a bank or other business entity. The bank then pays bills by automatically debiting the customer's account and crediting the merchant's account. More banks are offering this service; however, not all vendors accept electronic transfers in payment of bills. If a business decides to take advantage of online bill-paying, the options should be researched carefully, with consideration of the advantages and disadvantages involved.

Writing Checks

Instructions

Writing checks is a routine and basically simple function; however, certain guidelines should be followed to prevent potential problems. Figure 22-7 illustrates several correct methods to use when writing checks.

Figure 22-8 shows the correct method for writing a check for an amount less than a dollar *(top)*. The check on the bottom illustrates an incorrect method of check writing. Note the incomplete name and space for altering (e.g., $6.00 could easily be changed to $26.00 or more, and 00 could be made into 88). When writing in the numeric amount of a check, begin as far to the left in the block as possible. When inserting the written amount of the check, again start as far to the left as possible, allowing no space for added or altered words. Writing checks for less than a dollar is not recommended.

Checkbook Stubs

The check stub (the part that remains in the book after the check has been written and removed) is the depositor's own record of checks written—date, amount, payee, and purpose (Figure 22-9). It is important that the stub be completed before the check is written.

This prevents the possibility of writing a check and neglecting to complete the stub. If the stub is not completed and the check is sent out, you will have no record of the payee and the amount taken from the account until the cancelled check is returned at a later date. Consequently, the account cannot balance nor can one determine the amount on hand until the bank returns those cancelled checks. It is possible to get this information from the bank after the check has been cashed. There may be a charge for this service.

Signing Checks

After all checks have been written, place them along with the invoices or other verifying information on the physician's desk for signature. In some practices, the medical assistant who is in charge of the financial matters is also allowed to sign the checks. This is accomplished by filing a **power of attorney** at the depositor's bank. The power of attorney may limit the check-signing authorization to a certain amount or to a limited time period.

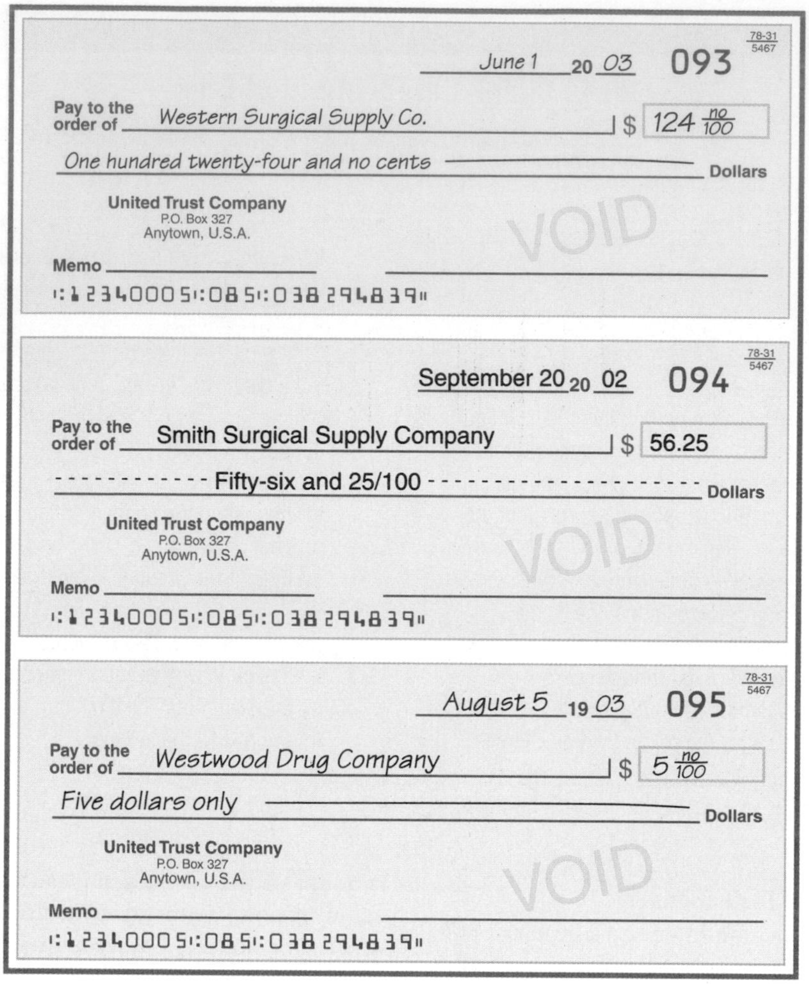

FIGURE 22-7 Correct methods of writing checks.

Handling Corrections

Do not cross out, erase, or change any part of a check. Checks are printed on sensitized paper so that erasures are easily noticeable, and the bank has the right to refuse to pay on any check that has been altered. (See Figures 22-7 and 22-8 for examples of correct and incorrect check writing.) If a mistake is made, write the word "VOID" on the stub and the check, but do not throw out or destroy the check. It should be filed with the canceled checks so that it is available for auditing purposes.

Writing Cash Checks

A cash check is made payable to Cash or Bearer. Such checks are completely negotiable. Because these checks are easily cashed without positive identification, it is poor policy to write cash checks unless they are to be cashed at the time they are written. Some bank personnel may require that the person receiving the cash endorse the check. Many experts in the banking business advise their customers not to endorse a check written for cash or petty cash; often if there is a problem the person who endorses the check is liable. A medical assistant should never endorse a check written for cash or petty cash, as he or she is not a party in the transaction.

Mailing Checks

When checks are sent through the mail, the check should not be visible through the envelope. Either place the check within a letter or fold it into a plain sheet of paper. Checks may be folded at the right end to conceal the amount of money written. Make certain the envelopes are sealed before mailing, and the medical assistant should personally mail all checks as soon as possible after writing.

Special Problems with Checks

Special problems may arise when a check is written on non-existent funds or when a payor wishes, for a legitimate reason, to prevent the payee from cashing a check.

Overdraws or Overdrafts

When a depositor draws a check for more than the amount on deposit in the account, the account becomes overdrawn. In most states it is illegal to issue a check for more than the amount on deposit in the bank. Should this happen through error or oversight, the bank may refuse to honor the check and will return it to the bank that presented it for payment. Such a check is said to "bounce."

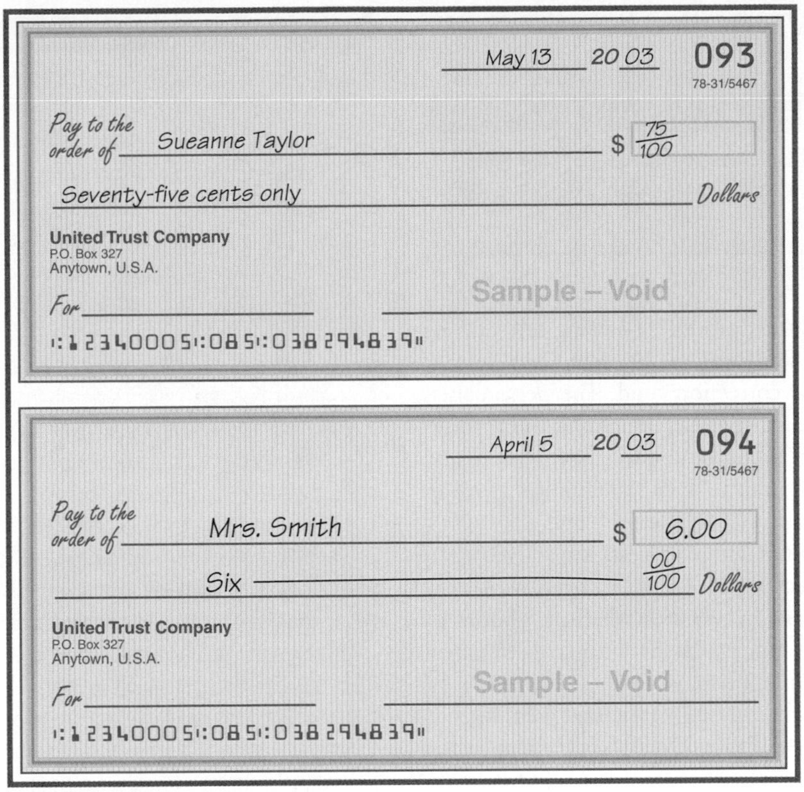

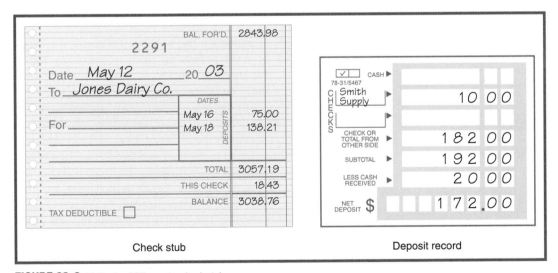

FIGURE 22-8 *Top,* Correct method of writing a check. *Bottom,* Incorrect method of writing a check, with incomplete name and space for altering (e.g., 6.00 could be made into 26.00 or more, and 00 could be made into 88).

FIGURE 22-9 Methods of filling out a check stub.

If a check is written by an established depositor, the bank may honor the check and notify the depositor that the account is overdrawn. If the bank thus pays or covers the check, it issues an overdraft on the depositor's account. Considerable fees (from $10 to $30) are normally charged when an overdraft occurs. Some accounts allow automatic withdrawals from savings accounts to cover overdrafts without additional charges.

Stop-Payments

A depositor or check writer who wishes to rescind the check has the right to request that the bank stop payment on it. Stop-payment orders should be used only in emergencies. Reasons for stop-payment requests include the following:

- Loss of a check
- Disagreement about a purchase
- Disagreement about a payment

As with overdrafts, most banks charge a fee for stop-payment orders.

Check Washing

Check washing is the fraudulent process of erasing or "washing out" the ink on a check with common household chemicals, such as bleach, benzene, or correction fluid. The person then rewrites the check to himself or herself, increasing the amount payable by hundreds or even thousands of dollars. It is estimated that check-washing fraud amounts to over $800 million a year in this country, and it is increasing at an alarming rate.

The National Check Fraud Center suggests the following to minimize the chance of check fraud:

- Ask your bank to advise your office when new books of checks are ready, then either pick them up or use a parcel delivery service to deliver them.
- Make sure cancelled checks are in a secured area, such as a bank lock box or a wall safe. Don't throw them in the trash.
- Check bank statements immediately after receiving them. If check fraud is not reported within 30 days of receipt of a monthly statement, the bank does not have to reimburse the loss (**Uniform Commercial Code [UCC]** Code 4-406).
- Print a return address on an envelope. A signature can be traced, duplicated, or forged.
- Don't discard credit card records or bills with trash.

For more information on how to avoid check fraud or what to do when fraud occurs, log onto the National Check Fraud Center's website, listed at the end of this chapter.

ACCEPTING CHECKS

Precautions in Accepting Checks

A medical assistant is presented with checks for payment of physician's services on a daily basis. In most cases these are personal checks.

Acknowledging Payment in Full

If payment in full is to be recognized with regard to a given check, the statement "Payment in Full to Date" must appear on the back of the check, above the endorsement, not on the face of the check. Canceled checks are a receipt for the maker of the check, not for the payee.

Guidelines for Accepting Checks

- Scan the check carefully for the correct date, amount, and signature.
- Do not accept a check with corrections on it.
- If you do not know the person presenting a personal check, ask for identification and compare signatures.
- Accept an out-of-town check, government check, or payroll check only if you are well acquainted with the person presenting it and it does not exceed the amount of the payment.
- Acceptance of a third-party check is generally unwise. A third-party check is one made out to your patient by a party unknown to you. A check from the patient's health insurance carrier is an exception.
- When accepting a postal money order for payment, make certain it has only one endorsement. Postal money orders with more than two endorsements will not be honored.
- Do not accept a check marked "Payment in Full" unless it does pay the account in full up to and including the date on which it is received. If a check so marked is less than the amount due, you will be unable to collect the balance on the account once you have accepted and deposited such a check. It is illegal for you to scratch out the words "Payment in Full."
- Accepting checks written for more than the amount due and returning cash for the difference between the amount of the check and the amount owed is poor policy. If the check is not honored by the bank, your office will suffer the loss not only of the amount of the check but also of the amount returned in cash.

Returned Checks

Occasionally the bank may return a deposited check because of some irregularity, such as a missing signature or missing endorsement. More often, it is because the payor has insufficient funds on deposit to cover the check.

If a check is stamped "NSF," indicating insufficient funds, do not delay in contacting the person who gave the check. If unable to contact the maker of a bad check, waste no time in tracking down all leads, such as referrals, numbers obtained from credit cards, driver's license, and so forth. Bad checks may be reported to several places. Credit associations are often a great help when such problems arise. Turn the account over to a qualified collection agency if you do not succeed in collecting on the account yourself within a short time.

If a check is returned to your office marked "No Account" and it is a check that had been deposited promptly, the office has obviously been swindled. This check should be given to the police, the local Better Business Bureau, or a collection agency.

Charging Fees

To cover their overhead costs, most banks currently charge both the payor and payee a fee of $15 to $30 dollars for a check that has been returned because of "insufficient funds." It is customary for the medical assistant to notify the person responsible for writing the check that it has been returned. Often the individual will have a plausible excuse and simply requests that the check be "run through again." If this is the case, it is a wise practice to first call the bank and ask if there are sufficient funds to do this, thereby avoiding additional time delay and fees. Some offices add these charges to the patient's account in an attempt to recoup the expense.

Collecting Returned Checks

There are several options available for collecting returned checks. As mentioned previously, the medical assistant might want to make an initial collection attempt by either telephoning or writing a letter to the patient. Many NSF problems can be cleared up quickly and easily using courtesy and tact, assuming that the situation was simply a mistake or oversight. If this method proves unsuccessful, the office might consider registering with a company that specializes in collecting bad checks. This can be done online or physically, using a local collection agency.

Legal Options

After all reasonable options for collecting NSF checks have been exhausted, a medical assistant may employ a collection method using the court system. Small claims court is a special court in which disputes are resolved inexpensively and quickly; it is a commonly used method that avoids costly attorney fees. Filing fees are in the $20 to $30 range, and there is usually a charge for having the papers served. There are restrictions, however. The amount for which the plaintiff (individual or company initiating the suit) can sue in a small claims lawsuit is limited to $5000. Other limitations vary from state to state. Contact the local Clerk of the District Court for the necessary forms and instructions in completing a small claims suit. For more information on filing small claims, refer to the government legal department's website.

> ### CRITICAL THINKING APPLICATION
>
> When opening the mail, Laura notices a form from the bank with a check attached. It is a check from Elliott Benson, a new patient seen in the office the previous week, being returned for insufficient funds. How should Laura handle this problem?

It is important that the medical assistant learn how to become "proactive" rather than "reactive" when it comes to problem patients. He or she should discuss fees with the patient on the first visit and gather all the financial and insurance information necessary to make a judgment as to whether the patient is able and willing to pay. An experienced medical assistant can often sense a "red flag" during this initial information-gathering process. If this happens, requesting payment in advance might be wise. This practice should not be abused, however, and the medical assistant should follow the established office policy or discuss the matter with the office manager or physician when necessary.

ENDORSEMENTS

An endorsement is a signature plus any other writing on the back of a check by which the **endorser** transfers all rights in the check to another party. Endorsements are made in ink, with either pen or rubber stamp, on the back of the check across the left (or perforated) end.

Why an Endorsement Is Necessary

The Uniform Negotiable Instrument Act, applicable in all states, explains the need for an endorsement as follows:

> An instrument is negotiated when it is transferred from one person to another in such a manner as to pass title to another party. If payable to bearer, it is negotiated by delivery. If payable to order, it is negotiated by the endorsement of the holder completed by delivery.

The name of the last endorser of the check shows who last received the money. If a check is cashed for someone who did not endorse it and is returned for some reason, the bank will charge the check to the last endorser, not to the last person receiving the money. For this reason, it is not wise to cash a check made payable to another party without having the endorsement of the person who delivered the check to you for cashing.

Types of Endorsements

There are four principal kinds of endorsements. Blank and restrictive endorsements are the ones most commonly used.

Blank Endorsement

The payee signs only his or her name. This makes the check payable to the bearer. It is the simplest and most common type of endorsement on personal checks but should be used only when the check is to be cashed or deposited immediately.

Restrictive Endorsement

This specifies the purpose of the endorsement. A restrictive endorsement is used in preparing checks for deposit to the physician's checking account. An example is shown in Figure 22-10.

Special Endorsement

This endorsement includes words specifying the person to whom the endorser makes the check payable. For instance, a check naming Helen Barker as the payee may be endorsed to the physician by writing on the back of the check as follows:

Pay to the order of
Theodore F. Wilson, M.D.
Helen Barker

The check is still negotiable but requires Dr. Wilson's signature or endorsement.

> Pay to the Order of
> Midwest National Bank
> Main Branch
> For Deposit Only
> CARLOS MACAULEY
> 301-012697

FIGURE 22-10 Example of a restrictive endorsement.

Qualified Endorsement

The effect of the endorsement is qualified by disclaiming or destroying any future liability of the endorser. Usually the words "without recourse" are written above by an attorney who accepts a check on behalf of a client but who has no personal claim in the transaction.

Methods of Endorsement

Stamp

As checks from patients and other sources arrive, they should be recorded on the ledger and immediately stamped with the restrictive endorsement "For Deposit Only." This is a safeguard against lost or stolen checks.

Any endorsement should agree exactly with the name on the face of the check. If the name of the payee is misspelled, it is usually necessary for the payee to endorse the check the way the name is spelled on the face, followed by the correctly spelled signature. UCC, Section 3-203, states:

Where an instrument is made payable to a person under a misspelled name or one other than his own, he may endorse in that name or his own or both; but signature in both names may be required by a person paying or giving value for the instrument.

Most banks accept routine stamp endorsement that is restricted to deposit only, if the customer is well known and maintains an established account.

Signature

Some insurance checks or drafts require a personal signature endorsement; a stamped endorsement is not acceptable. This will be stated on the back of the check. In such cases, ask the payee to endorse the check, then stamp immediately below the signature the restrictive endorsement "For Deposit Only."

MAKING DEPOSITS

The financial duties of a medical assistant include depositing checks and reconciling the bank statements with the checkbook. Checks should be deposited promptly, for these reasons:

- A stop-payment order may be placed.
- The check may be lost, misplaced, or stolen.
- Delay may cause the check to be returned because of insufficient funds.
- The check may have a restricted time for cashing.
- It is a courtesy to the payor.

Preparing the Deposit

Deposit slips are itemized memoranda of cash or other funds that a depositor presents to the bank with the money to be credited to the account. All deposits must be accompanied by a deposit slip. A carbon or photocopy of the deposit slip should be kept on file (Procedure 22-2).

There are several types of deposit slips, sometimes called *deposit tickets*. The commercial slip is used for the office checking account. The deposit slips are printed with the number of the account in magnetic ink characters to correspond with the checks. Preprinted deposit slips are ordered along with the checks.

Some write-it-once accounting systems include a deposit slip that the bank will accept as the itemization if it is attached to the customer's numbered deposit slip. The deposit slip should be prepared before you go to the bank, with the money organized and ready to present to the bank teller.

PROCEDURE 22-2

Prepare a Bank Deposit

CAAHEP COMPETENCY: 3.a.(2)(a)
ABHES COMPETENCY: 3.i

GOAL: *To prepare a bank deposit for the day's receipts and complete appropriate office records related to the deposit.*

EQUIPMENT and SUPPLIES

- Currency
- Checks for deposit
- Deposit slip
- Endorsement stamp (optional)
- Typewriter
- Envelope

PROCEDURAL STEPS

1. Organize currency.
   PURPOSE: To arrange currency in the best order for speedy and accurate presentation to the teller.
2. Total the currency, and record the amount on the deposit slip.
3. Place restrictive endorsements on the checks, using an endorsement stamp or the typewriter.

PURPOSE: To transfer the title and protect checks from loss or theft.

4. List each check separately on the deposit slip, with the ABA number and the amount.
5. Total the amount of currency and checks, and enter on the deposit slip.
6. Enter the amount of the deposit in the checkbook.
   PURPOSE: To record the current balance in the account.
7. Prepare a copy of the deposit slip for the office record, including the names of the payors.
   PURPOSE: For verification of checks deposited, if necessary.
8. Place the currency, checks, and deposit slip in an envelope for transporting to the bank.

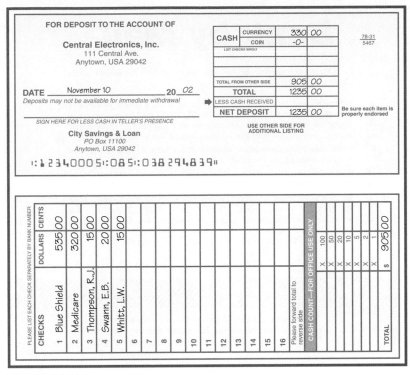

FIGURE 22-11 Front and back of a deposit slip.

Payment on patient accounts is generally made by check, but some payments are made in currency (paper money). Each type of fund is recorded separately on the deposit slip. The currency is usually listed first. Organize the currency so that all of the bills are facing in the same direction—for example, with the black-ink (portrait) side up. Place the largest-denomination bills on top.

Some banks prefer that checks be recorded individually by the ABA number; others use just the maker's name. If the checks are arranged alphabetically by the names of the patient accounts, with these names included on your office copy of the deposit slip, you will have a ready reference of checks deposited should a question arise regarding a patient's payment. Follow the following procedure for preparing a deposit slip (Figure 22-11):

1. List all checks on the back of the deposit slip.
2. Transfer the total to the front of the slip.
3. Enter the amount of the total deposit on the deposit slip stub.

Money orders, either postal, express, or others, are identified by "PO Money Order" or "Express MO." Remember that money orders cannot have more than two endorsements.

The deposit slip should be carefully totaled, and the total entered in the checkbook. Any torn bills should be mended with transparent tape. Clip the currency together, and clip the checks in a separate packet. Then place the entire amount in a heavy envelope for taking to the bank. Deposit the currency and checks daily if possible.

Deposits by Mail

Depositing by mail saves time and is easily accomplished if the deposit consists of checks only. Banks usually supply their customers with special mailing deposit slips and envelopes on request (Figure 22-12). Although the majority of banking that is not done in person is performed on the internet, some offices do still use mail services for banking procedures, especially if the physician has accounts at banks in other cities or states.

Some mailing deposit slips have an attached portion that the bank will stamp and return to the customer as a receipt. Others may provide the customer with a receipt card that is sent along with the deposit each time for the bank's notation. The mailer shown in Figure 22-12 has a peel-off receipt for the depositor's records. Mailed deposits are prepared in the same manner as are regular deposits, but certain precautions should be observed.

Direct Deposits

Direct deposit is a plan in which payments are transferred, usually electronically, by a paying agency directly into the account of a recipient. Direct deposits are commonly used for paying salaries; paychecks are credited to employees' accounts—checking, savings, or any other type of account—at any financial institution.

Precautions for Deposits Made by Mail

- Do not send cash or currency by mail. If this is absolutely necessary, then send it by registered mail.
- Use only a restrictive endorsement; use a deposit stamp or write the notation "For Deposit Only to the account of _____ ."
- If you have not obtained mailing deposit slips or your bank does not provide them, make duplicate slips and mail them with your deposit. Ask the bank to stamp one copy and return it to you as a receipt.

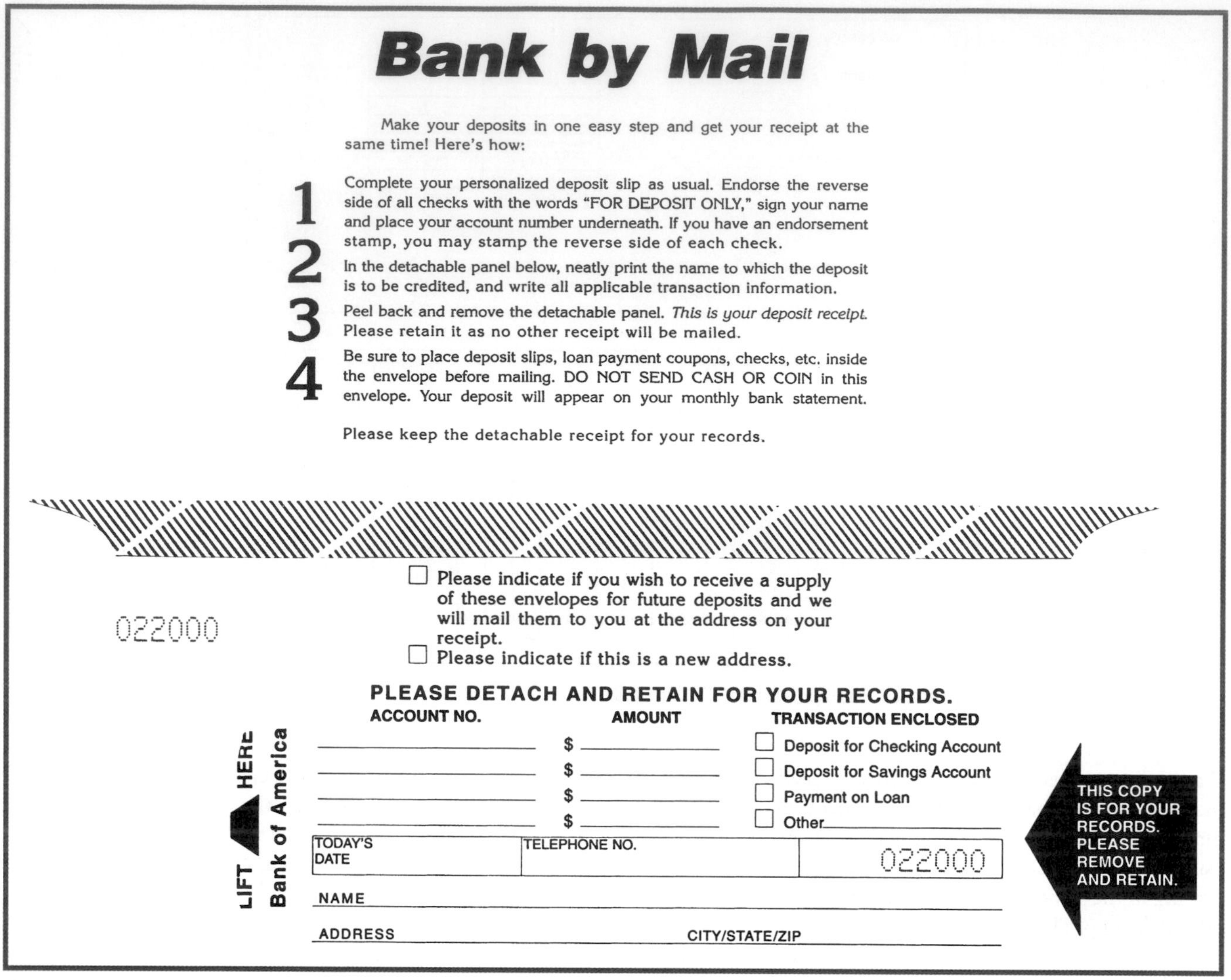

Bank by Mail

Make your deposits in one easy step and get your receipt at the same time! Here's how:

1 Complete your personalized deposit slip as usual. Endorse the reverse side of all checks with the words "FOR DEPOSIT ONLY," sign your name and place your account number underneath. If you have an endorsement stamp, you may stamp the reverse side of each check.

2 In the detachable panel below, neatly print the name to which the deposit is to be credited, and write all applicable transaction information.

3 Peel back and remove the detachable panel. *This is your deposit receipt.* Please retain it as no other receipt will be mailed.

4 Be sure to place deposit slips, loan payment coupons, checks, etc. inside the envelope before mailing. DO NOT SEND CASH OR COIN in this envelope. Your deposit will appear on your monthly bank statement.

Please keep the detachable receipt for your records.

022000

☐ Please indicate if you wish to receive a supply of these envelopes for future deposits and we will mail them to you at the address on your receipt.
☐ Please indicate if this is a new address.

PLEASE DETACH AND RETAIN FOR YOUR RECORDS.

ACCOUNT NO.	AMOUNT	TRANSACTION ENCLOSED
	$	☐ Deposit for Checking Account
	$	☐ Deposit for Savings Account
	$	☐ Payment on Loan
	$	☐ Other_____

TODAY'S DATE	TELEPHONE NO.	022000

NAME

ADDRESS _____ CITY/STATE/ZIP

LIFT ▲ HERE   Bank of America

THIS COPY IS FOR YOUR RECORDS. PLEASE REMOVE AND RETAIN.

FIGURE 22-12 Example of a bank-by-mail deposit envelope. (Courtesy Valley Bank of Nevada, Las Vegas, Nev.)

Other Methods of Deposit

Advances in computer technology have allowed financial institutions to offer other methods of deposit to consumers and business customers. Some automated teller machines (ATMs) will accept deposits, and there are checking accounts available that allow the customer to conduct the majority of banking services using the computer and ATMs. These types of accounts may limit the amount of times the customer can use teller services without a fee.

Online banking allows customers to view their accounts, make transfers, order checks, pay bills, and perform numerous other transactions simply by logging onto the bank website and accessing the account with a password. Online banking is also an excellent way to research the checks that have cleared the bank and compute accurate bank balances.

BANK STATEMENTS AND RECONCILIATION

A statement is periodically sent by the bank to the customer; it shows the status of the customer's account on a given date. This statement indicates the following:

- Beginning balance
- Deposits received
- Checks paid
- Bank charges
- Ending balance

Mailed Statements

Bank statements, similar to the one illustrated in Figure 22-13, are prepared at regular intervals (usually once a month) and are usually mailed to the bank's customers. These statements may or may not include the accompanying cancelled checks, depending on bank policy and account type. The back of each page of the statement usually includes a reconciliation page so that the customer can determine what checks have still not cleared the bank, what deposits are not yet shown on the statement, and the accurate account balance.

Online Statements

Online statements, or e-statements, are an electronic version of a paper bank statement. Financial establishments that offer online banking services in an attempt to make banking easier

0821-402054

#821

Hihuuhlhlulunhlululuhuullllluuhuuhhlululull

N
2

CALL (888) 555-2932
24 HOURS/DAY, 7 DAYS/WEEK
FOR ASSISTANCE WITH
YOUR ACCOUNT.

PAGE 1 OF 2   THIS STATEMENT COVERS: 6/22/02 THROUGH 7/22/02

INTEREST CHECKING 0821-402054	**SUMMARY**				
	PREVIOUS BALANCE	252.10		MINIMUM BALANCE	142.55
	DEPOSITS	68.74 +		AVERAGE BALANCE	220.00
	INTEREST EARNED	.18 +		ANNUAL PERCENTAGE	
	WITHDRAWALS	109.55 −		YIELD EARNED	.96 %
	CUSTOMER SERVICE CALLS	.00 −			
	INTERLINK/PURCHASE FEE	.00 −		INTEREST EARNED 1994	2.23
	MONTHLY CHECKING FEE				
	AND OTHER CHARGES	.00 −			
	▶ NEW BALANCE	**211.47**			

USE YOUR EXPRESS CARD TO MAKE UNLIMITED PURCHASES AT RETAILERS DISPLAYING
THE INTERLINK SYMBOL. (A $1 MONTHLY FEE MAY APPLY.)

TRY IT TODAY AT ARCO . . . MOBIL . . . LUCKY . . . RALPHS . . . SAFEWAY & MORE!

CHECKS AND WITHDRAWALS	CHECK	DATE PAID	AMOUNT	CHECK	DATE PAID	AMOUNT
	202	7/05	15.05	203	7/15	94.50

DEPOSITS					DATE POSTED	AMOUNT
	CUSTOMER DEPOSIT				7/22	68.74
	INTEREST PAYMENT THIS PERIOD				7/22	.18

BALANCE INFORMATION	DATE	BALANCE	DATE	BALANCE	DATE	BALANCE
	6/22	252.10	7/05	237.05	7/15	142.55
					7/22	211.47

24 HOUR CUSTOMER SERVICE

EACH ACCOUNT COMES WITH 3 COMPLIMENTARY CALLS PER STATEMENT PERIOD.

CALLS TO 24 HOUR CUSTOMER SERVICE THIS STATEMENT PERIOD: 0

INTEREST INFORMATION	FROM	THROUGH	INTEREST RATE	ANNUAL PERCENTAGE YIELD (APY)
	6/22	7/22	1.00%	1.01%

INTEREST RATE/APY AS OF 7/22/02 IF YOUR BALANCE IS

$ 0 - 4,999 . . . . .1.00%	1.01%
$ 5,000 - 9,999 . . . . .1.00%	1.01%
$ 10,000 AND OVER. 1.00%	1.01%

CALL 1-800-555-2932 IN CALIFORNIA ANYTIME FOR CURRENT RATES.

MEMBER FDIC

STATEMENT

FIGURE 22-13 Example of a regular checking account statement.

for their customers claim that e-statements are a user-friendly way of viewing account balances and checking financial images online.

With e-statements, there is no need to continue receiving paper statements. The benefits include the following:

- Receiving statements quickly and easily
- Being able to save statements in an electronic file for examination and printing at the customer's convenience
- Keeping fees low by minimizing unnecessary paper and mailing costs

Various banks offer different options, and fees vary. If the medical assistant has been authorized to set up an online banking account with the financial institution used by the medical facility, he or she should visit the bank to discuss the details of what is involved.

Reconciling the Bank Statement

The bank statement balance and the customer's checkbook balance usually differ, except in a relatively inactive account. The two balances must be reconciled. The reconciliation discloses any errors that may exist in the checkbook or, on rare occasions, in the bank statement (Figure 22-14).

The bank statement may include an entry for service charges that must be deducted from the checkbook balance. In all types of accounts, the bank may charge a fee for services. Usually in the case of an individual account, it is a flat fee; in a business account, the fee is based on services rendered. If the average or minimum balance is maintained at an established level, the bank may forego a service charge.

Most banks ask to be notified within a reasonable amount of time (e.g., 10 days) of any error found in the statement. The bank statement should be reconciled as soon as it is received. You will usually find a form to follow in carrying out this procedure on the back of the bank statement.

The **reconciliation** procedure may be put in a formula, as shown below.

If the two corrected balances agree, you may stop there. If they do not agree, subtract the lesser figure from the greater figure; the difference will usually give you a clue to the error (Procedure 22-3).

Bank Statement Reconciliation Formula	
Bank statement balance	$ _____
Less outstanding checks	$ _____
Plus deposits not shown	$ _____
Corrected bank statement balance	$ _____
Checkbook balance	$ _____
Less any bank charges	$ _____
Corrected checkbook balance	$ _____

SIGNATURE CARDS

When an account is first opened at a banking facility, the depositor will be required to affix his or her handwritten signature to a card, which is then kept on file at the bank. If

Questions to Ask in Searching for a Possible Error
• Is your arithmetic correct?
• Did you forget to include one of the outstanding checks?
• Did you fail to record a deposit or did you record one twice?

a check comes through, and some suspicion arises that the depositor's signature has been forged, the bank personnel compare the signature on the check with the original one on the signature card.

In a business situation, as in a medical office, the physician often delegates the responsibility of paying bills to the medical assistant or other office staff members. In this case, any staff member who has been authorized to sign the medical facility's checks must go to the bank and add his or her handwritten signature to the signature card. Only the people whose names appear on the signature card are authorized to sign checks, and it is the bank's responsibility to verify any questionable signatures.

BONDING

To protect their business establishments from embezzlement or other financial loss caused by employees who handle large sums of money, physicians often purchase fidelity bonds. Fidelity bonds reimburse the physician for any monetary loss caused by employees. The three types of bonding methods are as follows:

- Position-schedule bonding, which covers a specific position rather than an individual, such as bookkeeper or receptionist
- Blanket-position bonding, which covers all employees
- Personal bonding, which covers specific individuals

For individuals to be bonded, a personal background investigation is normally necessary.

CLOSING COMMENTS

Patient Education

Medical assistants might want to encourage patients to pay for professional services rendered with a personal check because of the numerous benefits checks offer. If a patient attempts to pay for services with a third-party check (other than an insurance reimbursement), the medical assistant should tactfully explain why this is not a wise practice. In addition, if a patient makes a mistake when writing a check, it is the responsibility of the medical assistant to point it out and request a new one, as corrections on the face of a check often render the check useless.

When a patient's check is returned from the bank marked "insufficient funds," the medical assistant should immediately call the patient and explain the problem, requesting that he or she correct the matter as soon as possible. It is important to remember, however, that most overdrafts are simply the result of mathematic errors or a delay in deposited funds being available

THIS WORKSHEET IS PROVIDED TO HELP YOU BALANCE YOUR ACCOUNT

1. Go through your register and mark each check, withdrawal, Express ATM transaction, payment, deposit or other credit listed on this statement. Be sure that your register shows any interest paid into your account, and any service charges, automatic payments, or Express Transfers withdrawn from your account during this statement period.

2. Using the chart below, list any outstanding checks, Express ATM withdrawals, payments or any other withdrawals (including any from previous months) that are listed in your register but are not shown on this statement.

3. Balance your account by filling in the spaces below.

ITEMS OUTSTANDING		
NUMBER	**AMOUNT**	
TOTAL	$	

ENTER

The NEW BALANCE shown on this statement _ _ _ _ _ _ _ _ _ _ _ _ _ _ _ _ _ _ _ $_____

ADD

Any deposits listed in your register $_____
or transfers into your account $_____
which are not shown on this $_____
statement.   +$_____

TOTAL _ _ _ _ _ _ _ _ +$_____

CALCULATE THE SUBTOTAL _ _ _ _ _ _ _ _ _ _ $_____

SUBTRACT

The total outstanding checks and withdrawals from the chart at left _ _ _ _ _ _ _ _ _ −$_____

CALCULATE THE ENDING BALANCE

This amount should be the same as the current balance shown in your check register _ _ _ _ _ _ _ _ _ _ _ _ _ _ _ _ $_____

IF YOU SUSPECT ERRORS OR HAVE QUESTIONS ABOUT ELECTRONIC TRANSFERS

If you believe there is an error on your statement or Express ATM receipt, or if you need more information about a transaction listed on this statement or an Express ATM receipt, please contact us immediately. We are available 24 hours a day, seven days a week to assist you. Please call the telephone number printed on the front of this statement. Or, you may write to us at United Trust Company, P.O. Box 327, Anytown, USA.

1) Tell us your name and account number or Express card number.

2) As clearly as you can, describe the error or the transfer you are unsure about, and explain why you believe there is an error or why you need more information.

3) Tell us the dollar amount of the suspected error.

You must report the suspected error to us no later than 60 days after we sent you the first statement on which the problem appeared. We will investigate your question and will correct any error promptly. If our investigation takes longer than 10 business days (or 20 days in the case of electronic purchases), we will temporarily credit your account for the amount you believe is in error, so that you may have use of the money until the investigation is completed.

FIGURE 22-14 Reverse side of a bank statement to be used for reconciling a checking account.

PROCEDURE 22-3

Reconcile a Bank Statement

ABHES COMPETENCY: 3.j

GOAL: *To reconcile a bank statement for a checking account.*

EQUIPMENT and SUPPLIES

- Ending balance of previous statement
- Current bank statement
- Canceled checks for current month
- Checkbook stubs
- Calculator
- Pen

PROCEDURAL STEPS

1. Compare the opening balance of the new statement with the closing balance of the previous statement.
   PURPOSE: To determine that the balances are in agreement.
2. Compare the canceled checks with the items on the statement.
   PURPOSE: To verify that they are your checks and that they are listed in the right amount.
3. Arrange the canceled checks in numeric order, and compare with the checkbook stubs.
4. Place a checkmark on each stub for which a canceled check has been returned.
   PURPOSE: To locate any outstanding checks.

5. List and total the outstanding checks.
6. Verify that all previous outstanding checks have cleared.
7. Subtract the total of the outstanding checks from the bank statement balance.
   NOTE: Do not include any certified checks as outstanding because their amount has already been deducted from the account.
8. Add to the total in step 7 any deposits made but not included in the bank statement.
   PURPOSE: To correct the credits in the bank statement balance.
9. Total any bank charges that appear on the bank statement, and subtract them from the checkbook balance. Such charges may include service charges, automatic withdrawals or payments, and NSF checks.
   PURPOSE: To correct the checkbook balance.
10. If the checkbook balance and the statement balance do not agree, match the bank statement entries with the checkbook entries.

---

for withdrawal. So the medical assistant should be patient and courteous when discussing NSF issues with patients. Patients need to know, however, that overdrafts are costly not only to them, but also to the medical facility.

Legal and Ethical Issues

If a mistake is made in preparing a check, do not destroy this check. Rather, write "VOID" across the face of the check, make a note on the check stub, and file the check with the cancelled checks for auditing purposes.

A stop-payment order may be placed with the bank in an emergency, such as when a check is lost or a disagreement occurs with regard to a purchase or payment.

Do not accept a check made payable to another party without having the endorsement of the person who gives the check to you. If the check is returned by the bank for any reason, the check will be charged to the last endorser, not the last person to receive the money.

SUMMARY OF SCENARIO

Laura has gained considerable knowledge through her experiences and work with the various aspects of the banking world. The goals she set for completing the assignments and competencies were accomplished in the time frame allowed by the instructor. She is comfortable now that she can readily apply this knowledge to whatever medical facility she works in.

Laura spent extra time outside of class exploring online banking and bill paying on the Internet and found a wealth of information available. Laura now plans to visit several banks in her area to see what kind of e-banking services they offer.

The versatility of the medical assistant's role and the variety of the opportunities available reinforce to Laura that she has made the right career choice.

SUMMARY of LEARNING OBJECTIVES

1. Define, spell, and pronounce the terms listed in the vocabulary.
   - Spelling and pronouncing medical terms correctly adds credibility to the medical assistant. Knowing the definition of these terms promotes confidence in communication with patients and co-workers.

2. Explain how the Internet has changed traditional banking practices.
   - The Internet has changed conventional banking as we know it, and it offers expansive opportunities without leaving home. As with everything, however, e-banking has both advantages and disadvantages, and these should be thoroughly researched before an online account is opened.

3. State the four requirements of a negotiable instrument.
   - For an instrument (e.g., a check) to be "negotiable," it must meet certain criteria: (1) be written and signed by a maker, (2) contain a promise or order to pay a sum of money, (3) be payable on demand or at a fixed future date, and (4) be payable to order or bearer.

4. Discuss the advantages of using checks.
   - There are many advantages to using checks. These advantages include safety and convenience, quick calculation of expenditures, and a permanent record for tax purposes.

5. Identify the three most common types of bank accounts.
   - The three most common types of bank accounts are checking accounts, savings accounts, and money market savings accounts. Each one is slightly different, and each has its special uses.

6. Explain how you would handle mistakes made in preparing a check.
   - Normally, when a mistake is made on a check, it should be marked "VOID" and a new check should be written. Some banks will accept minor errors if the maker initials the error. Erasures are not allowed, nor is the use of correction fluid.

7. List and discuss eight precautions to observe in accepting checks.
   - Scan the check carefully for the correct date, amount, and signature.
   - Do not accept a check with corrections on it.
   - If you do not know the person presenting a personal check, ask for identification and compare signatures.
   - Accept an out-of-town check, government check, or payroll check only if you are well acquainted with the person presenting it and it does not exceed the amount of the payment.
   - Acceptance of a third-party check is generally unwise. A third-party check is one made out to your patient by a party unknown to you. A check from the patient's health insurance carrier is an exception.
   - When accepting a postal money order for payment, make certain it has only one endorsement. Postal money orders with more than two endorsements will not be honored.
   - Do not accept a check marked "Payment in Full" unless it does pay the account in full up to and including the date on which it is received. If a check so marked is less than the amount due, you will be unable to collect the balance on the account once you have accepted and deposited such a check. It is illegal for you to scratch out the words "Payment in Full."
   - Accepting checks written for more than the amount due and returning cash for the difference between the amount of the check and the amount owed is poor policy. If the check is not honored by the bank, your office will suffer the loss not only of the amount of the check but also of the amount returned in cash.

8. Name and compare the four kinds of endorsements.
   - The four kinds of endorsements are (1) blank endorsement, in which the payee simply signs his or her name on the back of the check; (2) restrictive endorsement, which specifies which bank and what specific account the funds are to be deposited in; (3) special endorsement, which names a specific person on the back of the check as payee; and (4) qualified endorsement, which disclaims future liability. This type of endorsement is used when the person who accepts the check has no personal claim in the transaction.

9. Discuss the actions necessary when a deposited check is returned.
   - When a deposited check is returned, the maker should be contacted immediately, informed of the situation, and asked to remedy the situation either by immediately depositing funds in his or her account to cover the check or by paying the bill by alternative means—cash or money order.

10. Correctly write checks for bill payment.
    - The medical assistant may be required to write checks on the practice account to pay bills. The process for writing a check is outlined in Procedure 22-1.

11. Prepare a bank deposit and appropriate office documents.
    - Bank deposits should be made on a daily basis. The process for preparing a bank deposit is outlined in Procedure 22-2.

12. Accurately reconcile a bank statement with the office checking account.
    - Bank statements should be reconciled as soon as they arrive at the physician's office or should be printed from the bank's website for reconciliation. The process for reconciling a bank statement is outlined in Procedure 22-3.

CONNECTIONS

Study Guide Connection: Go to Chapter 22 Study Guide. Read the Case Study and Workplace Applications and complete the assignments. Do online research for answers to the questions in the Internet Activities associated with banking services and procedures.

CD Connection: Go to the Medical Assisting Competency Challenge CD and do the training activities under Financial Management.

Evolve Connection: For more information related to banking services and procedures, go to http://evolve.elsevier.com/kinn/admin and visit related weblinks for Chapter 22. Click on the Medical Assisting Exam Review and do the practice questions to sharpen your test-taking skills. To learn more about office software, do the exercises for the Altapoint demo that is on the CD.

23

Management of Practice Finances

Brenda Newman is the office manager for Dr. Susan Wilkins, a neurologist who is beginning her second year of practice. Dr. Wilkins is financially savvy and takes care with the money she has invested in her business. She encourages her employees to plan for the future and offers them a retirement plan as well as opportunities for investing in mutual funds through payroll deduction. Her accountant, Grant Schmidt, assists Dr. Wilkins with the financial aspects of her practice and is always willing to counsel the employees of the clinic about finances.

Mr. Schmidt has taught Brenda several methods of keeping track of the practice finances. Brenda is interested in learning more about general accounting rules and bookkeeping. She is able to perform computerized accounting duties and is also able to use a pegboard system. She is able to work with patients when they need to make payment arrangements and has an excellent collection ratio.

Dr. Wilkins is cost conscious and does not order random supplies and equipment. Instead, she and Brenda plan the inventory for a 6-month period and have needed to order supplies only every 6 months. By ordering in precise amounts, Dr. Wilkins saves money and uses the extra funds for staff development events and seminars. Each month, the budget is reviewed to ensure that the office is on track with expenses.

The team effort among Dr. Wilkins, Brenda, and Mr. Schmidt results in a balanced budget for the clinic, and subsequently the staff is able to enjoy more benefits and perks.

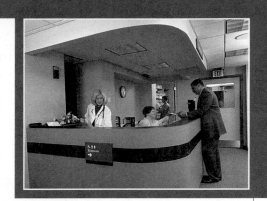

While studying this chapter, think about the following questions:

- Why is a constant flow of income preferable to a once-a-month influx for a physician's office?
- Why should the person entering numbers on a manual system make all numerals exactly alike all the time?
- From a legal standpoint, why is positive identification required before hiring individuals to work in the physician's office?
- How do practice finances affect the income of the medical assistant?

LEARNING OBJECTIVES

1. Define, spell, and pronounce the terms listed in the vocabulary.
2. List the four items that all financial records should show at any given time.
3. Distinguish between accounts payable and accounts receivable.
4. List and explain the three most common bookkeeping systems found in physicians' offices today.
5. Explain the importance of a trial balance.
6. State the types of employment records required by the IRS.
7. Discuss the basis for the withholding amounts that are taken from employees' earnings.
8. Name the five common periodic accounting reports.
9. Explain the purpose of the W-4 form.
10. Explain the requirements of the Federal Insurance Contributions Act.
11. Discuss the importance of setting a budget each fiscal year.
12. Maintain a petty cash fund.
13. Accurately process an employee payroll.

National Accreditation Competencies and Content

CAAHEP COMPETENCIES

Administrative
3.a.(2)(c). Perform accounts receivable procedures

General
3.c.(4)(a). Perform an inventory of supplies and equipment
3.c.(4)(c). Utilize computer software to maintain office systems

ABHES COMPETENCIES

Administrative Duties
3.j. Reconcile a bank statement
3.l. Perform billing and collection procedures
3.m. Prepare a check
3.n. Establish and maintain a petty cash fund

Office Management
6.c. Inventory equipment and supplies
6.d. Evaluate and recommend equipment and supplies for practice

Financial Management
8.a. Use manual and computerized bookkeeping systems
8.d. Manage accounts payable and receivable
8.e. Maintain records for accounting and banking purposes
8.f. Process employee payroll

VOCABULARY

accounts payable Debts incurred and not yet paid.

accounts receivable Amounts owed to the physician.

accounts receivable trial balance A method of determining that the journal and the ledger are in balance.

accrual basis of accounting Method of accounting in which income is recorded when earned and expenses are recorded when incurred.

assets The entire property of a person, association, corporation, or estate applicable or subject to the payment of debts.

balance sheet A financial statement for a specific date that shows the total assets, liabilities, and capital of the business.

bookkeeping The recording of business and accounting transactions.

cash basis of accounting Method of accounting in which income is recorded when received and expenses are recorded when paid.

cash flow statement A financial summary for a specific period that shows the beginning balance on hand, the receipts and disbursements during the period, and the balance on hand at the end of the period.

disbursements journal A summary of accounts paid out.

equities The money value of a property or of an interest in a property in excess of claims or liens against it.

fiscal year An accounting period of 12 months.

in balance State in which the total ending balances of patient ledgers equals total of accounts receivable.

invoice A paper describing a purchase and the amount due.

liabilities Things that are owed; debts.

packing slip An itemized list of objects in a package.

petty cash fund A fund maintained to pay small unpredictable cash expenditures.

statement A request for payment.

statement of income and expense A summary of all income and expenses for a given period.

trial balance A method of checking the accuracy of accounts.

A physician's business records are the key to good management practice. The medical assistant who can keep accurate financial records and who will conduct the administrative side of the practice in a businesslike fashion is genuinely needed and appreciated.

Financial records that are complete, correct, and current are essential for the following:

- Prompt billing and collection procedures
- Professional financial planning
- Accurate reporting of income to federal and state agencies

WHAT IS ACCOUNTING?

Accounting is a system of recording, classifying, and summarizing financial transactions. **Bookkeeping** is mainly the recording part of the accounting process. The bookkeeping must be done daily and is the responsibility of the administrative medical assistant in a small practice and of the office manager or financial manager in a larger practice.

Accounting Bases

There are two general bases, or methods, for accounting: the cash basis and the accrual basis. Most physicians use the **cash**

basis of accounting, which means that charges for services are entered as income when payment is received, and expenses are recorded when they are paid. Merchants, on the other hand, generally use an **accrual basis of accounting.** Income is considered earned when services have been performed or goods have been sold, even though payment may not have been received. Expenses are recognized and recorded when incurred, even though they have not been paid.

Financial Summaries

The financial records of any business should at all times show the following:
- How much was earned in a given period
- How much was collected
- How much is owed
- The distribution of expenses incurred

From the daily entries, the accountant can prepare monthly and annual summaries that provide a basis for comparing any given period with another similar period. Periodic analyses of the financial records can result in improved business practices, better management of time, curtailment or elimination of unprofitable services, and better budgeting of expenses. With the appropriate software these analyses can be accomplished using the computer. The medical assistant may notice notations of AP/AR, which stand for **accounts payable** and **accounts receivable.**

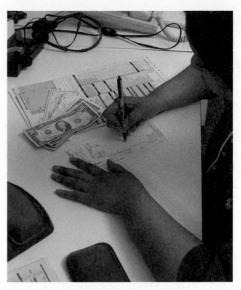

FIGURE 23-1 Accurate records reflect competency in the medical office. The medical assistant should use a calculator when adding figures and should be careful not to transpose numbers.

CRITICAL THINKING APPLICATION

- Brenda has noticed several errors on encounter forms lately. These errors seem to be a result of not using a calculator when adding the charges once the patient checks out. Brenda has approached the person who assists the patients in this area but has not seen any improvement in the errors. How might she convince the employee to follow precautions in adding charges?
- How might Mr. Schmidt educate the staff about the importance of accurate financial records?

The Cardinal Rules of Bookkeeping

There are many rules that apply to bookkeeping that the medical assistant must learn. First, use good penmanship so that the records are clearly legible, even years later. Use the same pen style and type of ink consistently. Keep columns of figures straight, and write well-formed figures (a careless 9 may look like a 7; an open 0 may resemble a 6). Carry decimal points correctly.

Enter all charges and receipts immediately in the daily record or journal. Write a receipt in duplicate for any currency received (Figure 23-1). Writing receipts for checks is optional, but a consistent pattern should be followed. Post all charges and receipts to the patient ledger daily. Checks should be endorsed for deposit as soon as received. Verify that the total of the deposit plus the amount on hand equals the total to be accounted for in the daily journal. The **petty cash fund** should be used to pay for small unpredictable expenses. Pay all other expenses by check. A cancelled check is the best proof of payment. Bills should be

paid before their due dates, after checking them for accuracy. Place date of payment and number of check on paid bills.

Do not erase, write over, or blot out figures. If an error is made, a straight line should be drawn through the incorrect figure, and the correct figure written above it. Bookkeeping procedures are not complicated, but they do require concentration to avoid errors. There is no such thing as almost correct financial records. The books either balance or they do not balance. The bookkeeping is either right or wrong. This is not the place to be creative or take shortcuts.

The medical assistant should set aside a certain time each day for bookkeeping tasks, if possible. Do not attempt to work on financial records when busy attending patients or when other distractions are present.

Kinds of Financial Records

Daily Journal

The daily journal day sheet is the chronologic record of the practice—the financial diary. All information regarding services rendered, charges, and receipts is first recorded in the daily journal. It is important that every transaction be recorded.

In addition to professional services rendered in and out of the office, there may be income from other sources, such as rentals, royalties, interest, and so forth. Usually a special place is provided in the journal for such income. Any income that is not practice related should be recorded separately from patient receipts.

Checkbook

Receipts are usually deposited in the checking account, and a record of the deposit is entered in the journal and on the check stub. A copy of each deposit slip should be kept with the financial records. Bills are usually paid by check or via online bill-paying services, and a record of the payment is entered on the check stub and in the disbursements section of the general journal.

Disbursements Journal

Manual Posting. In simplified accounting systems, the **disbursements journal** usually consists of a section at the bottom of each day sheet and a check register page at the end of each month, plus monthly and annual summaries. It must show the following:

- Every amount paid out
- Date and check number
- Purpose of payment

Computer Posting. Use the cash or check payments screen. Enter payment information and the computer can print the check, or enter information after the check has been manually prepared.

Petty Cash Records

A petty cash fund and voucher system should be established to take care of minor unpredictable expenditures such as postage due, parking fees, small contributions, emergency supplies, and miscellaneous small items. In the average facility $25 to $50 is sufficient for the petty cash fund. If a larger sum is available, there is a tendency to pay too many bills out of petty cash instead of writing a check.

When the check for this fund is exchanged at the bank for small bills and coins, the money is placed in a cashbox or drawer that can be locked or kept in the safe at night. One person only should be in charge of the petty cash fund. This person must be able to account for the full amount of the fund at any time.

Payroll Records

The payroll record is an auxiliary disbursement record. A separate page or card for each employee, as well as a summary record, should be kept. This procedure is discussed in more detail later in this chapter.

COMPARISON OF COMMON BOOKKEEPING SYSTEMS

Success in bookkeeping requires a thorough understanding of the system and what it is expected to accomplish. Many variations in bookkeeping systems exist, from simple to complex, no one of which can meet the needs of every physician. The basic principles are the same for all; only the system of recording varies. The three most common systems found in the professional office are as follows:

- Single-entry
- Double-entry
- Pegboard or write-it-once

An overview of the three systems is presented here. More detailed instruction for the pegboard system, the most widely used manual system in medical practices, is found in Chapter 21.

Single-Entry System

Single-entry bookkeeping is inexpensive, is simple to use, and requires very little training. It is the oldest and simplest of bookkeeping systems and includes at least three basic records:

- A general journal, also called a daily log, daybook, day sheet, daily journal, or charge journal
- A cash payment journal, which in its simplest form is a checkbook
- An accounts receivable ledger, which is a record of the amounts owed by all the patients. The accounts receivable ledger may be a bound book, a loose-leaf binder, a card file, or loose pages in a ledger tray

There may also be auxiliary records for petty cash and payroll records.

The records of charges and receipts are usually entered into a bound journal with a page for each day of the year, monthly summary pages, and an annual summary. Daily pages have columns for entering each transaction that show the patient's name, the service performed and the charge, any payments received, and the totals for charges and receipts. The daily totals are entered on the monthly summary, and the monthly totals are carried forward to the annual summary.

The same bound book may also have space for recording cash payments, or the checkbook may be the only cash payment journal. Monthly and annual summaries would be done from the checkbook.

The accounts receivable ledger usually consists of an account card for each patient, on which are entered the charges and payments from the general journal. The patients' statements are prepared from these cards. In a single-entry system, each entry is made separately.

Although the single-entry system may satisfy the requirements for reporting to government agencies, it does have some drawbacks:

- Errors are not easily detected.
- There are no built-in controls.
- Periodic analyses are inadequate for financial planning.

The single-entry system was at one time widely used in healthcare facilities but has been largely replaced by more complete accounting systems.

Double-Entry System

Double-entry bookkeeping is also inexpensive but requires a trained and experienced bookkeeper or the regular services of an accountant. The transactions may be recorded manually or by computer. In addition to the basic journals used in a single-entry system, there may be numerous subsidiary journals. The system is based on the following accounting equation:

Assets = Liabilities + Proprietorship (Capital)

Every transaction requires an entry on each side of the accounting equation, and the two sides must always be **in balance.** For this reason the system is called *double-entry bookkeeping.* It is the most complete of the three systems. An understanding of the basics of double-entry bookkeeping will help to clarify the principles of all systems.

Assets are the properties owned by a business, such as bank accounts, accounts receivable, buildings, equipment, and furniture. The rights to these assets are called **equities.** The equity of the owner is called *capital, proprietorship,* or *owner's equity.* The equities of the creditors to whom money is owed are called **liabilities.** The owner's equity or capital is what remains of the value of the assets after the creditor's equities or liabilities have been subtracted.

For example, if the physician purchased equipment for $1000, paid $250 down, and gave a promissory note for $750, the accounting equation would be as follows:

Assets		$1000 =	Liabilities	$750
			+	
			Capital	250
		$1000		$1000

The total value of the asset is $1000. The owner's equity is $250, and the creditor's equity is $750. The accounting terms *capital, proprietorship, owner's equity,* and *net worth* are used interchangeably.

Few medical assistants are trained in accounting. If a double-entry system is used, a practice management consultant or the accountant who does most of the actual bookwork and reports usually sets it up. The medical assistant in this instance generally maintains only the daily journal, from which the accountant takes the figures once a month.

The double-entry system provides a more comprehensive picture of the practice and its effect on the physician's net worth. Errors show up readily, and there are many built-in accuracy controls; however, because of the time and skill required, it is not frequently used in the small practice.

Pegboard or Write-It-Once System

The pegboard is the most commonly used manual method of accounting in the physician's office. It is discussed at length in Chapter 21.

CRITICAL THINKING APPLICATION

Mr. Schmidt has taught Brenda all three types of accounting systems. Which seems to be the easiest system to use in the medical office? What is the basis for this choice?

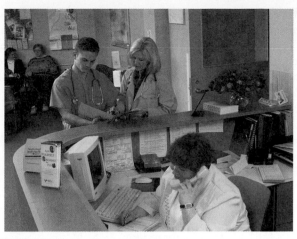

FIGURE 23-2 Ask the physician when unsure about financial information. When an unfamiliar statement arrives, check with the physician to be sure it should be paid.

END-OF-DAY SUMMARIZING

Most computer accounting systems will perform end-of-the-day summarizing automatically. If the office uses the pegboard system, the bottom of the day sheet has three sections to be completed that will show that the accounts have balanced for the day.

The first section is the proof of posting section, which deals with the transactions that occurred that day on the day sheet. The second section is month-to-date accounts receivable proof, and the day's totals being added to the month-to-date totals should balance to the penny. The last section is the year-to-date accounts receivable proof, which adds the accounts, including the day's totals, to the year-to-date total.

Most systems also have a deposit ticket, which can be double-checked when adding the cash receipts and the checks. This is handy when preparing the day's deposit.

The totals at the bottom of the second and third sections must be identical. When the end-of-the-day summarizing does not balance, the medical assistant should first check the addition of each column, both horizontally and vertically. This will result in finding most errors (Figure 23-2). Be sure that the instructions are followed to the letter. To avoid frustrating mistakes, it is best to use a calculator, even when adding small numbers.

TRIAL BALANCE OF ACCOUNTS RECEIVABLE

A **trial balance** should be done once per month after all posting has been completed and before preparing the monthly statements. The purpose of a trial balance is to disclose any discrepancies between the journal and the ledger. It does not prove the accuracy of the accounts. For example, if a charge or payment was posted to the wrong account, or if the wrong amount was entered in the journal then posted to the ledger, the totals would still "balance," but the accounts would not be accurate.

To begin, pull all the account cards that have a balance, enter each balance on the calculator, and total the figures. This should equal the accounts receivable balance figure on the control.

If there is no daily control, total all of the charges, all of the payments, and all of the adjustments for the month, then do the computation illustrated as follows. The end-of-the-month accounts receivable figure must agree with the figure arrived at by adding all the account card balances. The accounts are then said to be *in balance*. If the two totals do not agree, the error must be located.

Example of Balancing End-of-Month Accounts Receivable

Accounts receivable at first of month	$ _____
Plus total charges for month	$ _____
Subtotal	$ _____
Less total payments for month	$ _____
Subtotal	$ _____
Less total adjustments for month	$ _____
Accounts receivable at end of month	$ _____

Locating and Preventing Errors

After checking the tape and verifying that no error in calculation has been made, the first step in locating an error in the trial balance is to find the difference between the two totals. Then search the daily journal pages and the account cards for an entry for the identical amount. Check each one found, and verify that it was posted correctly. Of course, more than one error may add up to this amount.

If only one error has been made and the amount of the error is divisible by 9, a figure may have been transposed. For example, if the difference is $81 (a number divisible by 9), the person who posted to the account may have written $209 instead of $290. If the amount of the error is divisible by 2, the amount may have been posted to the wrong column, reversing a debit and a credit.

A common error is made by entering the wrong amount in the previous balance column or in figuring the new balance. This kind of error will show up on the pegboard daily proof but could easily go undetected in the single-entry system. Carrying forward the wrong amount results in another common error total from one day to the next (e.g., carrying forward the beginning accounts receivable total rather than the ending accounts receivable total). There is always a chance of sliding a number, which means writing the first digit in the wrong column, such as writing 400 for 40 or 60 instead of 600.

Many bookkeepers avoid errors in the cents column by using a line (−) instead of writing two zeros when only even dollars are involved. For example, instead of writing $12.00, the bookkeeper will write $12.−. This eliminates the possibility of misreading zeros as other numbers. It also speeds the adding process when columns must be totaled.

If the medical assistant is unable to locate any numeric error, then an account card may have been lost or overlooked or transferred as paid in full.

CRITICAL THINKING APPLICATION

- What should Brenda do if she has repeatedly reviewed records in search of an error and is still unable to find it?
- To whom should this be reported?

ACCOUNTS PAYABLE PROCEDURES

Invoices and Statements

When an item is not paid for at the time of purchase, the vendor usually includes a **packing slip** with delivery of the merchandise. A packing slip describes the items enclosed. The vendor may also enclose an **invoice.** An invoice describes the items and shows the amount due. Always check to verify that the items listed on the packing slip and invoice are included in the delivery.

Invoices should be placed in a special folder until paid. The facility may be making more than one purchase from the same vendor during the month. Some vendors request that payment be made from the invoice; others expect to send a **statement** later. A statement is a request for payment.

Paying for Purchases

At the time of payment, compare the statement with the invoice to verify accuracy, fasten the statement and invoice together, write the date and check number on the statement, and place it in the paid file.

CRITICAL THINKING APPLICATION

- Brenda does not recall ordering a certain item from the office supply company. However, it was included in her last shipment and listed on the packing list. How can she recount whether the item was ordered?
- How would Brenda correct this problem if the item was in fact not ordered?

Recording Disbursements

Both the pegboard and the single-entry bookkeeping systems provide pages for recording disbursements. This is sometimes called a *check register.* On these pages disbursements are distributed to specific expense accounts such as the following:

- Auto expense
- Dues and meetings
- Equipment
- Insurance
- Medical supplies
- Office expenses
- Printing, postage, and stationery
- Rent and maintenance
- Salaries
- Taxes and licenses
- Travel and entertainment
- Utilities
- Miscellaneous
- Personal withdrawals

Each check should be entered on the disbursement page, showing the date, the name of the company to which the check was written, the number and amount of the check, and the payment allocated to one or more of the expense accounts. It is important to separate personal expenditures from business expenses. Business expenses are tax deductible and are

PROCEDURE 23-1

Account for Petty Cash

<u>ABHES COMPETENCIES:</u> 3.m, 3.n

GOAL: *To establish a petty cash fund, maintain an accurate record of expenditures for 1 month, and replenish the fund as necessary.*

EQUIPMENT and SUPPLIES

- Form for petty cash fund
- Pad of vouchers
- Disbursement journal
- Two checks
- List of petty cash expenditures

PROCEDURAL STEPS

1. Determine the amount needed in the petty cash fund.
2. Write a check in the determined amount.
   <u>PURPOSE:</u> To establish a fund.
3. Record the beginning balance in the petty cash fund.
4. Post the amount to Miscellaneous on the disbursement record.
   <u>PURPOSE:</u> To account for the original amount in the fund.
5. Prepare a petty cash voucher for each amount withdrawn from the fund.
   <u>PURPOSE:</u> The vouchers will be used for internal audit.

6. Record each voucher in the petty cash record, and enter the new balance.
   <u>PURPOSE:</u> To record current balance and determine the need for replenishing the fund.
7. Write a check to replenish the fund as necessary.
   <u>NOTE:</u> The total of the vouchers plus the fund balance must equal the beginning amount.
8. Total the expense columns, and post to the appropriate accounts in the disbursement record.
   <u>PURPOSE:</u> To record expenditures in the correct expense category.
9. Record the amount added to the fund.
10. Record the new balance in the petty cash fund.

---

considered in determining net income from the practice, but personal expenditures are not. Although personal expenses are not deductible in determining net income from the practice, some qualify as personal deductions in computing personal income tax, so a careful accounting should be kept. Deductible expenses would include property taxes, interest paid out, contributions, and so on.

Accounting for Petty Cash

The petty cash fund is a revolving fund (Procedure 23-1). It does not change in amount except to increase or decrease the established fund. To establish the petty cash fund, a check is written payable to Cash or Petty Cash and entered in the disbursements journal under Miscellaneous. This is the only time that the petty cash check is charged to Miscellaneous.

Each time the fund is replenished, the amount of the check is spread among the various accounts for which the money was used. This is determined from a record of expenditures. The headings of the columns should correspond to headings in the disbursements journal to which they will be posted.

A pad of petty cash vouchers is kept in or near the cash box. For every disbursement from the fund, the petty cashier should either have a receipt or prepare a voucher. The total of the petty cash vouchers and receipts plus the amount of cash in the box must always equal the original amount of the fund.

At the end of the month, or sooner if the fund is depleted, a check is written to Cash for replenishing the fund, but instead of being charged to Miscellaneous as previously, the amount of the check is divided among the various accounts affected.

Avoid the habit of borrowing from the petty cash fund. This admonition applies to the physician as well as to the medical assistant. If the physician requests cash from the fund, request a personal check or an office check in exchange for cash from the fund. It is also poor policy to use the petty cash fund for making change. In facilities where patients frequently pay with currency, a separate change fund should be kept.

PERIODIC SUMMARIES

Financial summaries are compiled on monthly and annual bases. They may be prepared either by the medical assistant manually or on the computer or by the accountant. Common summary reports include the following:

- **Statement of income and expense**
- **Cash flow statement**
- Trial balance
- **Accounts receivable trial balance** and aging analysis
- **Balance sheet**

The statement of income and expense is also known as the *profit and loss statement* and covers a specific period. It lists all the income received and all expenses paid during the period. The total income is called *gross income* or *earnings*. The income after deduction of all expenses is the *net income*.

A cash flow statement starts with the amount of cash on hand at the beginning of the month (or for any specified period). It then lists the cash income and the cash disbursement made throughout the period and concludes with a statement of the amount of cash remaining on hand at the end of the period.

A trial balance is necessary to determine that the books are in balance. All of the columns on the disbursements journal must be totaled at the end of the month. The combined totals of all the expense columns must be equal to the total of the checks written. If the figures do not balance, it is necessary to recheck every entry until an error is found.

The accounts receivable trial balance is done before the monthly statements are sent out. First, record the total of the accounts receivable ledger at the end of the previous month; then add the charges for the current month and subtract the adjustments and the payments received. The remainder should equal the total of the accounts receivable ledger at the end of the current month.

The balance sheet, also known as a *statement of financial condition*, shows the financial picture of the practice on a specific date. Often, it is done only on an annual basis. The balance sheet is set up using the following accounting equation:

$$\text{Assets} = \text{Liabilities} + \text{Proprietorship}$$

The title of the statement had its origin in the equality of the elements—the balance between the sum of the assets and the sum of the liabilities and proprietorship.

At the end of the accounting year, it is very simple to combine the monthly reports to compile the annual summaries. The annual summaries simplify the reporting of income for tax returns.

PAYROLL RECORDS

Handling payroll records, whether for one employee or dozens of employees, involves frequent reporting activities (Procedure 23-2). Government regulations require the withholding of taxes from employees and payment of certain taxes due from both employees and employers. To comply with government regulations, complete records must be kept for every employee. All records of employment taxes must be kept for at least 4 years. These should be available for review by the Internal Revenue Service (IRS). Such records include the following:

- Social Security number of the employee
- Number of withholding allowances claimed
- Amount of gross salary
- All deductions for Social Security and Medicare taxes; federal, state, and city or other subdivision withholding taxes; state disability insurance; and state unemployment tax, where applicable

CRITICAL THINKING APPLICATION

- On Friday Brenda hired a new employee, who reported to work on Monday. The new employee states that she cannot produce her Social Security card. Can Brenda allow the individual to work?
- Investigate the procedures for verifying a Social Security number.

PROCEDURE 23-2

Process an Employee Payroll

ABHES COMPETENCY: 8.f

GOAL: *To process payroll and compensate employees, making deductions accurately.*

EQUIPMENT and SUPPLIES

- Checkbook
- Computer and payroll software, if applicable
- Pen
- Tax withholding tables
- Federal Employers Tax Guide

PROCEDURAL STEPS

1. Be sure that all information and paperwork have been collected from the employees, including a copy of the Social Security card, a W-4 form, and an I-9 form.
   PURPOSE: To make certain that the employee is eligible to work in the United States and to determine what withholding amounts should be deducted from paychecks.

2. Review the time cards for all employees. Determine if any employees need counseling because of late arrivals or habitual absences.
   PURPOSE: To address problem issues immediately and help to correct habits that can lead to employee termination.

3. Figure the salary or hourly wages that are due the employee for the period worked.
   PURPOSE: To ascertain the amount owed to the employee.

4. Figure the deductions that must be taken from the paycheck. These usually include but are not limited to the following:
   - Federal, state, and local taxes
   - Social Security withholdings
   - Medicare withholdings
   - Other deductions, such as insurance, savings, and so on
   - Donations to organizations, such as the United Way.
   PURPOSE: To comply with federal, state, and local laws and deduct amounts for insurance, savings plans, and so on.

5. Write the check for the balance due the employee. Most software can print the checks and explanations of deductions.

6. Have employees sign for their paychecks, if that is the policy of the office.

Payroll Reporting Forms

Each employee and each employer must have a tax identification number. The Social Security number is the employee's tax identification number. Any person who does not have a Social Security number should apply for one, using Form SS-5, available from any Social Security Administration office.

The employer applies for a number for federal tax accounting purposes using Form SS-4, available at Social Security Administration offices. In states that require employer reports, a state employer number must also be obtained.

Before the end of the first pay period, the employee should complete an Employee's Withholding Allowance Certificate (Form W-4) showing the number of withholding allowances claimed (Figure 23-3). Otherwise, the employer must indicate withholding on the basis of a single person with no exemptions.

The employee should complete a new form when changes occur in marital status or in the number of allowances claimed. Each employee is entitled to one personal allowance and one for each qualified dependent. The employee may elect to take fewer or no allowances, in which case the tax withheld will be greater and a refund may be due when the employee's annual tax report is filed (Figure 23-4). If an employee claims more than 10 withholding allowances or an exemption from withholding and his or her wages would normally be more than $200 per week, the employer is required to send copies of these W-4 forms to the IRS.

A supply of all the necessary forms for filing federal returns, preprinted with the employer's name, will be furnished to an employer who has applied for an employer identification number. Extra forms may be obtained from the IRS office.

CRITICAL THINKING APPLICATION

- Mr. Schmidt has explained to Brenda that the more withholding deductions an employee claims, the less tax is taken from the paycheck. If Brenda's new employee wishes to claim seven deductions and she has only three children and is single, could she do so legally?
- Why or why not?
- Why might it be risky to claim all of the deductions to which a person is legally entitled?

Income Tax Withholding

Employers are required by law to withhold certain amounts from employees' earnings. These amounts must be reported and forwarded to the IRS to be applied toward payment of income tax. The amount to be withheld is based on the following:

- Total earnings of the employee
- Number of withholding allowances claimed
- Marital status of the employee
- Length of the pay period involved

The Federal Employer's Tax Guide includes tables to be used in determining the amount to be withheld. There is one table for single persons and unmarried heads of households and one for married persons. The tables cover monthly, semimonthly, biweekly, weekly, and daily or miscellaneous periods.

Employers Income Tax

The physician who is practicing as an individual is not subject to withholding tax but is expected to make an estimated tax payment four times a year. The accountant prepares four copies of Form 1040-S, Declaration of Estimated Tax for Individuals, for the ensuing year when the annual income tax return is prepared. The first form and the quarterly estimated tax for the next year are filed at the same time as the tax return. The remaining three forms, with the estimated tax due, must be filed on June 15, September 15, and January 15. It may be the business manager's responsibility to see that these returns are filed when due. The employer also contributes to Social Security and Medicare in the form of a self-employment tax.

Social Security, Medicare, and Income Tax Withholding

The Federal Insurance Contributions Act (FICA) provides for a federal system of old age, survivors, disability, and hospital insurance. The tax rate is reviewed frequently and is subject to change by Congress. As of 2001, the wage base for Social Security tax is $84,900 and the tax rate is 6.2% each for employers and employees. All wages are subject to the Medicare tax at a rate of 1.45% each for both employees and employers.

Quarterly Returns

Each quarter of the year, all employers who are subject to income tax withholding (including withholding on sick pay and supplemental unemployment benefits) of Social Security and Medicare taxes must file an Employer's Quarterly Federal Tax Return on or before the last day of the first month after the end of the quarter (Figure 23-5). Due dates for this return and full payment of the tax are April 30, July 31, October 31, and January 31. If deposits equaling full payment of taxes due have been made, the due date for the return is extended 10 days.

Annual Returns

The employer is required to furnish two copies of Form W-2, the Wage and Tax Statement, to each employee from whom income tax or Social Security tax has been withheld or from whom income tax would have been withheld if the employee had claimed no more than one withholding allowance. The forms should be given to employees by January 31. If employment ends before December 31, the employer may give the W-2 form to the terminated employee any time after employment ends. If the employee asks for Form W-2, the employer should give the employee the completed copies within 30 days of the request or the final wage payment, whichever is later.

Employers must file Form W-3, the Transmittal of Income and Tax Statement, annually to transmit wage and income tax withheld statements (Form W-2) to the Social Security Administration. These forms are processed by the Social Security Administration, which then furnishes the IRS with the income tax data that it needs from those forms. Form W-3 and its attachments must be filed separately from Form 941 on or before the last day of February after the calendar year for which the W-2 forms are prepared.

Form W-4 (2002)

Purpose. Complete Form W-4 so your employer can withhold the correct Federal income tax from your pay. Because your tax situation may change, you may want to refigure your withholding each year.

Exemption from withholding. If you are exempt, complete only lines 1, 2, 3, 4, and 7 and sign the form to validate it. Your exemption for 2002 expires February 16, 2003. See **Pub. 505,** Tax Withholding and Estimated Tax.

Note: *You cannot claim exemption from withholding if (a) your income exceeds $750 and includes more than $250 of unearned income (e.g., interest and dividends) and (b) another person can claim you as a dependent on their tax return.*

Basic instructions. If you are not exempt, complete the **Personal Allowances Worksheet** below. The worksheets on page 2 adjust your withholding allowances based on itemized deductions, certain credits, adjustments to income, or two-earner/two-job situations. Complete all worksheets that apply. **However, you may claim fewer (or zero) allowances.**

Head of household. Generally, you may claim head of household filing status on your tax return only if you are unmarried and pay more than 50% of the costs of keeping up a home for yourself and your dependent(s) or other qualifying individuals. See line **E** below.

Tax credits. You can take projected tax credits into account in figuring your allowable number of withholding allowances. Credits for child or dependent care expenses and the child tax credit may be claimed using the **Personal Allowances Worksheet** below. See **Pub. 919,** How Do I Adjust My Tax Withholding? for information on converting your other credits into withholding allowances.

Nonwage income. If you have a large amount of nonwage income, such as interest or dividends, consider making estimated tax payments using **Form 1040-ES,** Estimated Tax for Individuals. Otherwise, you may owe additional tax.

Two earners/two jobs. If you have a working spouse or more than one job, figure the total number of allowances you are entitled to claim on all jobs using worksheets from only one Form W-4. Your withholding usually will be most accurate when all allowances are claimed on the Form W-4 for the highest paying job and zero allowances are claimed on the others.

Nonresident alien. If you are a nonresident alien, see the **Instructions for Form 8233** before completing this Form W-4.

Check your withholding. After your Form W-4 takes effect, use Pub. 919 to see how the dollar amount you are having withheld compares to your projected total tax for 2002. See Pub. 919, especially if you used the **Two-Earner/Two-Job Worksheet** on page 2 and your earnings exceed $125,000 (Single) or $175,000 (Married).

Recent name change? If your name on line 1 differs from that shown on your social security card, call 1-800-772-1213 for a new social security card.

Personal Allowances Worksheet (Keep for your records.)

A   Enter "1" for **yourself** if no one else can claim you as a dependent . . . . **A** _____

B   Enter "1" if:
- You are single and have only one job; or
- You are married, have only one job, and your spouse does not work; or
- Your wages from a second job or your spouse's wages (or the total of both) are $1,000 or less.

. . **B** _____

C   Enter "1" for your **spouse.** But, you may choose to enter "-0-" if you are married and have either a working spouse or more than one job. (Entering "-0-" may help you avoid having too little tax withheld.) . . . . **C** _____

D   Enter number of **dependents** (other than your spouse or yourself) you will claim on your tax return . . . . . . **D** _____

E   Enter "1" if you will file as **head of household** on your tax return (see conditions under **Head of household** above) . **E** _____

F   Enter "1" if you have at least $1,500 of **child or dependent care expenses** for which you plan to claim a credit . . **F** _____

(**Note:** *Do not include child support payments. See Pub. 503, Child and Dependent Care Expenses, for details.*)

G   **Child Tax Credit** (including additional child tax credit):
- If your total income will be between $15,000 and $42,000 ($20,000 and $65,000 if married), enter "1" for each eligible child plus **1 additional** if you have three to five eligible children or **2 additional** if you have six or more eligible children.
- If your total income will be between $42,000 and $80,000 ($65,000 and $115,000 if married), enter "1" if you have one or two eligible children, "2" if you have three eligible children, "3" if you have four eligible children, or "4" if you have five or more eligible children. **G** _____

H   Add lines A through G and enter total here. **Note:** *This may be different from the number of exemptions you claim on your tax return.* ▶ **H** _____

For accuracy, complete all worksheets that apply.
- If you plan to **itemize or claim adjustments to income** and want to reduce your withholding, see the **Deductions and Adjustments Worksheet** on page 2.
- If you have **more than one job** or are **married and you and your spouse both work** and the combined earnings from all jobs exceed $35,000, see the **Two-Earner/Two-Job Worksheet** on page 2 to avoid having too little tax withheld.
- If **neither** of the above situations applies, **stop here** and enter the number from line H on line 5 of Form W-4 below.

- **Cut here and give Form W-4 to your employer. Keep the top part for your records.** - - - - - - - - - - - - - - -

Form **W-4**

Department of the Treasury
Internal Revenue Service

Employee's Withholding Allowance Certificate

▶ **For Privacy Act and Paperwork Reduction Act Notice, see page 2.**

OMB No. 1545-0010

2002

1 Type or print your first name and middle initial	Last name		**2** Your social security number

Home address (number and street or rural route)	**3** ☐ Single ☐ Married ☐ Married, but withhold at higher Single rate.
City or town, state, and ZIP code	**Note:** *If married, but legally separated, or spouse is a nonresident alien, check the "Single" box.*

4 If your last name differs from that on your social security card, check here. You must call 1-800-772-1213 for a new card. ▶ ☐

5   Total number of allowances you are claiming (from line **H** above **or** from the applicable worksheet on page 2)   **5** _____

6   Additional amount, if any, you want withheld from each paycheck . . . .   **6** $ _____

7   I claim exemption from withholding for 2002, and I certify that I meet **both** of the following conditions for exemption:
- Last year I had a right to a refund of **all** Federal income tax withheld because I had **no** tax liability **and**
- This year I expect a refund of **all** Federal income tax withheld because I expect to have **no** tax liability.

If you meet both conditions, write "Exempt" here . . . . ▶   **7**

Under penalties of perjury, I certify that I am entitled to the number of withholding allowances claimed on this certificate, or I am entitled to claim exempt status.

Employee's signature
(Form is not valid
unless you sign it.) ▶   Date ▶

8 Employer's name and address (Employer: Complete lines 8 and 10 only if sending to the IRS.)	**9** Office code (optional)	**10** Employer identification number

Cat. No. 10220Q

FIGURE 23-3 IRS Form W-4: Employee's Withholding Allowance Certificate.

Form W-4 (2002)   Page **2**

Deductions and Adjustments Worksheet

Note: *Use this worksheet only if you plan to itemize deductions, claim certain credits, or claim adjustments to income on your 2002 tax return.*

1 Enter an estimate of your 2002 itemized deductions. These include qualifying home mortgage interest, charitable contributions, state and local taxes, medical expenses in excess of 7.5% of your income, and miscellaneous deductions. (For 2002, you may have to reduce your itemized deductions if your income is over $137,300 ($68,650 if married filing separately). See **Worksheet 3** in Pub. 919 for details.) . . .   **1** $ _____

2 Enter:
{ $7,850 if married filing jointly or qualifying widow(er)
  $6,900 if head of household
  $4,700 if single
  $3,925 if married filing separately }   . . . .   **2** $ _____

3 **Subtract** line 2 from line 1. If line 2 is greater than line 1, enter "-0-" . . . .   **3** $ _____

4 Enter an estimate of your 2002 adjustments to income, including alimony, deductible IRA contributions, and student loan interest   **4** $ _____

5 **Add** lines 3 and 4 and enter the total. Include any amount for credits from **Worksheet 7** in Pub. 919. .   **5** $ _____

6 Enter an estimate of your 2002 nonwage income (such as dividends or interest) . . . .   **6** $ _____

7 **Subtract** line 6 from line 5. Enter the result, but not less than "-0-" . . . .   **7** $ _____

8 **Divide** the amount on line 7 by $3,000 and enter the result here. Drop any fraction . . . . . .   **8** _____

9 Enter the number from the **Personal Allowances Worksheet,** line H, page 1 . . . .   **9** _____

10 **Add** lines 8 and 9 and enter the total here. If you plan to use the **Two-Earner/Two-Job Worksheet,** also enter this total on line 1 below. Otherwise, **stop here** and enter this total on Form W-4, line 5, page 1 .   **10** _____

Two-Earner/Two-Job Worksheet

Note: *Use this worksheet only if the instructions under line H on page 1 direct you here.*

1 Enter the number from line H, page 1 (or from line 10 above if you used the **Deductions and Adjustments Worksheet**)   **1** _____

2 Find the number in **Table 1** below that applies to the **lowest** paying job and enter it here . . . . .   **2** _____

3 If line 1 is **more than or equal to** line 2, subtract line 2 from line 1. Enter the result here (if zero, enter "-0-") and on Form W-4, line 5, page 1. **Do not** use the rest of this worksheet . . . .   **3** _____

Note: *If line 1 is **less than** line 2, enter "-0-" on Form W-4, line 5, page 1. Complete lines 4–9 below to calculate the additional withholding amount necessary to avoid a year end tax bill.*

4 Enter the number from line 2 of this worksheet . . . .   **4** _____

5 Enter the number from line 1 of this worksheet . . . .   **5** _____

6 **Subtract** line 5 from line 4 . . . .   **6** _____

7 Find the amount in **Table 2** below that applies to the **highest** paying job and enter it here . . . . .   **7** $ _____

8 **Multiply** line 7 by line 6 and enter the result here. This is the additional annual withholding needed . .   **8** $ _____

9 Divide line 8 by the number of pay periods remaining in 2002. For example, divide by 26 if you are paid every two weeks and you complete this form in December 2001. Enter the result here and on Form W-4, line 6, page 1. This is the additional amount to be withheld from each paycheck . . . .   **9** $ _____

Table 1: Two-Earner/Two-Job Worksheet

Married Filing Jointly				All Others			
If wages from **LOWEST** paying job are—	Enter on line 2 above	If wages from **LOWEST** paying job are—	Enter on line 2 above	If wages from **LOWEST** paying job are—	Enter on line 2 above	If wages from **LOWEST** paying job are—	Enter on line 2 above
$0 - $4,000	0	44,001 - 50,000	8	$0 - $6,000	0	75,001 - 95,000	8
4,001 - 9,000	1	50,001 - 55,000	9	6,001 - 11,000	1	95,001 - 110,000	9
9,001 - 15,000	2	55,001 - 65,000	10	11,001 - 17,000	2	110,001 and over	10
15,001 - 20,000	3	65,001 - 80,000	11	17,001 - 23,000	3		
20,001 - 25,000	4	80,001 - 95,000	12	23,001 - 28,000	4		
25,001 - 32,000	5	95,001 - 110,000	13	28,001 - 38,000	5		
32,001 - 38,000	6	110,001 - 125,000	14	38,001 - 55,000	6		
38,001 - 44,000	7	125,001 and over	15	55,001 - 75,000	7		

Table 2: Two-Earner/Two-Job Worksheet

Married Filing Jointly		All Others	
If wages from **HIGHEST** paying job are—	Enter on line 7 above	If wages from **HIGHEST** paying job are—	Enter on line 7 above
$0 - $50,000	$450	$0 - $30,000	$450
50,001 - 100,000	800	30,001 - 70,000	800
100,001 - 150,000	900	70,001 - 140,000	900
150,001 - 270,000	1,050	140,001 - 300,000	1,050
270,001 and over	1,150	300,001 and over	1,150

FIGURE 23-3, cont'd For legend see previous page.

SINGLE Persons—WEEKLY Payroll Period
(For Wages Paid in 2002)

If the wages are—		And the number of withholding allowances claimed is—										
At least	But less than	0	1	2	3	4	5	6	7	8	9	10
		The amount of income tax to be withheld is—										
$0	$55	$0	$0	$0	$0	$0	$0	$0	$0	$0	$0	$0
55	60	1	0	0	0	0	0	0	0	0	0	0
60	65	1	0	0	0	0	0	0	0	0	0	0
65	70	2	0	0	0	0	0	0	0	0	0	0
70	75	2	0	0	0	0	0	0	0	0	0	0
75	80	3	0	0	0	0	0	0	0	0	0	0
80	85	3	0	0	0	0	0	0	0	0	0	0
85	90	4	0	0	0	0	0	0	0	0	0	0
90	95	4	0	0	0	0	0	0	0	0	0	0
95	100	5	0	0	0	0	0	0	0	0	0	0
100	105	5	0	0	0	0	0	0	0	0	0	0
105	110	6	0	0	0	0	0	0	0	0	0	0
110	115	6	0	0	0	0	0	0	0	0	0	0
115	120	7	1	0	0	0	0	0	0	0	0	0
120	125	7	1	0	0	0	0	0	0	0	0	0
125	130	8	2	0	0	0	0	0	0	0	0	0
130	135	8	2	0	0	0	0	0	0	0	0	0
135	140	9	3	0	0	0	0	0	0	0	0	0
140	145	9	3	0	0	0	0	0	0	0	0	0
145	150	10	4	0	0	0	0	0	0	0	0	0
150	155	10	4	0	0	0	0	0	0	0	0	0
155	160	11	5	0	0	0	0	0	0	0	0	0
160	165	11	5	0	0	0	0	0	0	0	0	0
165	170	12	6	0	0	0	0	0	0	0	0	0
170	175	13	6	1	0	0	0	0	0	0	0	0
175	180	13	7	1	0	0	0	0	0	0	0	0
180	185	14	7	2	0	0	0	0	0	0	0	0
185	190	15	8	2	0	0	0	0	0	0	0	0
190	195	16	8	3	0	0	0	0	0	0	0	0
195	200	16	9	3	0	0	0	0	0	0	0	0
200	210	17	10	4	0	0	0	0	0	0	0	0
210	220	19	11	5	0	0	0	0	0	0	0	0
220	230	20	12	6	0	0	0	0	0	0	0	0
230	240	22	13	7	1	0	0	0	0	0	0	0
240	250	23	15	8	2	0	0	0	0	0	0	0
250	260	25	16	9	3	0	0	0	0	0	0	0
260	270	26	18	10	4	0	0	0	0	0	0	0
270	280	28	19	11	5	0	0	0	0	0	0	0
280	290	29	21	12	6	0	0	0	0	0	0	0
290	300	31	22	14	7	1	0	0	0	0	0	0
300	310	32	24	15	8	2	0	0	0	0	0	0
310	320	34	25	17	9	3	0	0	0	0	0	0
320	330	35	27	18	10	4	0	0	0	0	0	0
330	340	37	28	20	11	5	0	0	0	0	0	0
340	350	38	30	21	12	6	1	0	0	0	0	0
350	360	40	31	23	14	7	2	0	0	0	0	0
360	370	41	33	24	15	8	3	0	0	0	0	0
370	380	43	34	26	17	9	4	0	0	0	0	0
380	390	44	36	27	18	10	5	0	0	0	0	0
390	400	46	37	29	20	11	6	0	0	0	0	0
400	410	47	39	30	21	13	7	1	0	0	0	0
410	420	49	40	32	23	14	8	2	0	0	0	0
420	430	50	42	33	24	16	9	3	0	0	0	0
430	440	52	43	35	26	17	10	4	0	0	0	0
440	450	53	45	36	27	19	11	5	0	0	0	0
450	460	55	46	38	29	20	12	6	0	0	0	0
460	470	56	48	39	30	22	13	7	1	0	0	0
470	480	58	49	41	32	23	15	8	2	0	0	0
480	490	59	51	42	33	25	16	9	3	0	0	0
490	500	61	52	44	35	26	18	10	4	0	0	0
500	510	62	54	45	36	28	19	11	5	0	0	0
510	520	64	55	47	38	29	21	12	6	0	0	0
520	530	65	57	48	39	31	22	14	7	1	0	0
530	540	67	58	50	41	32	24	15	8	2	0	0
540	550	68	60	51	42	34	25	17	9	3	0	0
550	560	70	61	53	44	35	27	18	10	4	0	0
560	570	71	63	54	45	37	28	20	11	5	0	0
570	580	74	64	56	47	38	30	21	12	6	0	0
580	590	76	66	57	48	40	31	23	14	7	1	0
590	600	79	67	59	50	41	33	24	15	8	2	0

FIGURE 23-4 Pages from the 2002 Withholding Tax Table.

MARRIED Persons—MONTHLY Payroll Period
(For Wages Paid in 2002)

If the wages are—		And the number of withholding allowances claimed is—										
At least	But less than	0	1	2	3	4	5	6	7	8	9	10
		The amount of income tax to be withheld is—										
$0	$540	$0	$0	$0	$0	$0	$0	$0	$0	$0	$0	$0
540	560	1	0	0	0	0	0	0	0	0	0	0
560	580	3	0	0	0	0	0	0	0	0	0	0
580	600	5	0	0	0	0	0	0	0	0	0	0
600	640	8	0	0	0	0	0	0	0	0	0	0
640	680	12	0	0	0	0	0	0	0	0	0	0
680	720	16	0	0	0	0	0	0	0	0	0	0
720	760	20	0	0	0	0	0	0	0	0	0	0
760	800	24	0	0	0	0	0	0	0	0	0	0
800	840	28	3	0	0	0	0	0	0	0	0	0
840	880	32	7	0	0	0	0	0	0	0	0	0
880	920	36	11	0	0	0	0	0	0	0	0	0
920	960	40	15	0	0	0	0	0	0	0	0	0
960	1,000	44	19	0	0	0	0	0	0	0	0	0
1,000	1,040	48	23	0	0	0	0	0	0	0	0	0
1,040	1,080	52	27	2	0	0	0	0	0	0	0	0
1,080	1,120	56	31	6	0	0	0	0	0	0	0	0
1,120	1,160	60	35	10	0	0	0	0	0	0	0	0
1,160	1,200	64	39	14	0	0	0	0	0	0	0	0
1,200	1,240	68	43	18	0	0	0	0	0	0	0	0
1,240	1,280	72	47	22	0	0	0	0	0	0	0	0
1,280	1,320	76	51	26	1	0	0	0	0	0	0	0
1,320	1,360	80	55	30	5	0	0	0	0	0	0	0
1,360	1,400	84	59	34	9	0	0	0	0	0	0	0
1,400	1,440	88	63	38	13	0	0	0	0	0	0	0
1,440	1,480	92	67	42	17	0	0	0	0	0	0	0
1,480	1,520	96	71	46	21	0	0	0	0	0	0	0
1,520	1,560	100	75	50	25	0	0	0	0	0	0	0
1,560	1,600	106	79	54	29	4	0	0	0	0	0	0
1,600	1,640	112	83	58	33	8	0	0	0	0	0	0
1,640	1,680	118	87	62	37	12	0	0	0	0	0	0
1,680	1,720	124	91	66	41	16	0	0	0	0	0	0
1,720	1,760	130	95	70	45	20	0	0	0	0	0	0
1,760	1,800	136	99	74	49	24	0	0	0	0	0	0
1,800	1,840	142	105	78	53	28	3	0	0	0	0	0
1,840	1,880	148	111	82	57	32	7	0	0	0	0	0
1,880	1,920	154	117	86	61	36	11	0	0	0	0	0
1,920	1,960	160	123	90	65	40	15	0	0	0	0	0
1,960	2,000	166	129	94	69	44	19	0	0	0	0	0
2,000	2,040	172	135	98	73	48	23	0	0	0	0	0
2,040	2,080	178	141	103	77	52	27	2	0	0	0	0
2,080	2,120	184	147	109	81	56	31	6	0	0	0	0
2,120	2,160	190	153	115	85	60	35	10	0	0	0	0
2,160	2,200	196	159	121	89	64	39	14	0	0	0	0
2,200	2,240	202	165	127	93	68	43	18	0	0	0	0
2,240	2,280	208	171	133	97	72	47	22	0	0	0	0
2,280	2,320	214	177	139	102	76	51	26	1	0	0	0
2,320	2,360	220	183	145	108	80	55	30	5	0	0	0
2,360	2,400	226	189	151	114	84	59	34	9	0	0	0
2,400	2,440	232	195	157	120	88	63	38	13	0	0	0
2,440	2,480	238	201	163	126	92	67	42	17	0	0	0
2,480	2,520	244	207	169	132	96	71	46	21	0	0	0
2,520	2,560	250	213	175	138	100	75	50	25	0	0	0
2,560	2,600	256	219	181	144	106	79	54	29	4	0	0
2,600	2,640	262	225	187	150	112	83	58	33	8	0	0
2,640	2,680	268	231	193	156	118	87	62	37	12	0	0
2,680	2,720	274	237	199	162	124	91	66	41	16	0	0
2,720	2,760	280	243	205	168	130	95	70	45	20	0	0
2,760	2,800	286	249	211	174	136	99	74	49	24	0	0
2,800	2,840	292	255	217	180	142	105	78	53	28	3	0
2,840	2,880	298	261	223	186	148	111	82	57	32	7	0
2,880	2,920	304	267	229	192	154	117	86	61	36	11	0
2,920	2,960	310	273	235	198	160	123	90	65	40	15	0
2,960	3,000	316	279	241	204	166	129	94	69	44	19	0
3,000	3,040	322	285	247	210	172	135	98	73	48	23	0
3,040	3,080	328	291	253	216	178	141	103	77	52	27	2
3,080	3,120	334	297	259	222	184	147	109	81	56	31	6
3,120	3,160	340	303	265	228	190	153	115	85	60	35	10
3,160	3,200	346	309	271	234	196	159	121	89	64	39	14
3,200	3,240	352	315	277	240	202	165	127	93	68	43	18

FIGURE 23-4, cont'd For legend see previous page.

Form **941**
(Rev. January 2002)
Department of the Treasury
Internal Revenue Service (99)

Employer's Quarterly Federal Tax Return

▶ See separate instructions revised January 2002 for information on completing this return.

Please type or print.

Enter state code for state in which deposits were made **only** if different from state in address to the right ▶ (see page 2 of instructions).

Name (as distinguished from trade name)

Trade name, if any

Address (number and street)

Date quarter ended

Employer identification number

City, state, and ZIP code

OMB No. 1545-0029

T	
FF	
FD	
FP	
I	
T	

If address is different from prior return, check here ▶

IRS Use

1	1	1	1	1	1	1	1	1	1	2	3	3	3	3	3	3	3	3	4	4	4	5	5	5

6	7	8	8	8	8	8	8	9	9	9	9	9	10	10	10	10	10	10	10	10	10

If you do not have to file returns in the future, check here ▶ ☐   and enter date final wages paid ▶

If you are a seasonal employer, see **Seasonal employers** on page 1 of the instructions and check here ▶

1	Number of employees in the pay period that includes March 12th . ▶	**1**			
2	Total wages and tips, plus other compensation		**2**	
3	Total income tax withheld from wages, tips, and sick pay		**3**	
4	Adjustment of withheld income tax for preceding quarters of calendar year		**4**	
5	Adjusted total of income tax withheld (line 3 as adjusted by line 4—see instructions)		**5**	
6	Taxable social security wages	**6a**	× 12.4% (.124) =	**6b**	
	Taxable social security tips	**6c**	× 12.4% (.124) =	**6d**	
7	Taxable Medicare wages and tips . . .	**7a**	× 2.9% (.029) =	**7b**	
8	Total social security and Medicare taxes (add lines 6b, 6d, and 7b). Check here if wages are not subject to social security and/or Medicare tax . . . . ▶ ☐		**8**	
9	Adjustment of social security and Medicare taxes (see instructions for required explanation) Sick Pay $ _____ ± Fractions of Cents $ _____ ± Other $ _____ =		**9**	
10	Adjusted total of social security and Medicare taxes (line 8 as adjusted by line 9—see instructions)		**10**	
11	**Total taxes** (add lines 5 and 10)		**11**	
12	Advance earned income credit (EIC) payments made to employees		**12**	
13	Net taxes (subtract line 12 from line 11). **If $2,500 or more, this must equal line 17, column (d) below (or line D of Schedule B (Form 941))**		**13**	
14	Total deposits for quarter, including overpayment applied from a prior quarter		**14**	
15	**Balance due** (subtract line 14 from line 13). See instructions		**15**	

16   **Overpayment.** If line 14 is more than line 13, enter excess here ▶ $ _____
and check if to be: ☐ Applied to next return   **or**   ☐ Refunded.

● **All filers:** If line 13 is less than $2,500, you need not complete line 17 or Schedule B (Form 941).

● **Semiweekly schedule depositors:** Complete Schedule B (Form 941) and check here . . . . ▶ ☐

● **Monthly schedule depositors:** Complete line 17, columns (a) through (d), and check here. . . . . ▶ ☐

17	**Monthly Summary of Federal Tax Liability.** Do not complete if you were a semiweekly schedule depositor.			
	(a) First month liability	**(b)** Second month liability	**(c)** Third month liability	**(d)** Total liability for quarter

Third Party Designee

Do you want to allow another person to discuss this return with the IRS (see separate instructions)?   ☐ **Yes.** Complete the following.   ☐ **No**

Designee's name ▶

Phone no. ▶ (   )

Personal identification number (PIN) ▶

Sign Here

Under penalties of perjury, I declare that I have examined this return, including accompanying schedules and statements, and to the best of my knowledge and belief, it is true, correct, and complete.

Signature ▶

Print Your Name and Title ▶

Date ▶

For Privacy Act and Paperwork Reduction Act Notice, see back of Payment Voucher.   Cat. No. 17001Z   Form **941** (Rev. 1-2002)

FIGURE 23-5 IRS Form 941: Employer's Quarterly Federal Tax Return.

Form 941
Payment Voucher

Purpose of Form

Complete Form 941-V if you are making a payment with **Form 941,** Employer's Quarterly Federal Tax Return. We will use the completed voucher to credit your payment more promptly and accurately, and to improve our service to you.

If you have your return prepared by a third party and make a payment with that return, please provide this payment voucher to the return preparer.

Making Payments With Form 941

Make payments with Form 941 only if:

1. Your net taxes for the quarter (line 13 on Form 941) are less than $2,500 and you are paying in full with a timely filed return or

2. You are a monthly schedule depositor making a payment in accordance with the **accuracy of deposits** rule. (See section 11 of **Circular E,** Employer's Tax Guide, for details.) This amount may be $2,500 or more.

Otherwise, you must deposit the amount at an authorized financial institution or by electronic funds transfer. (See section 11 of Circular E for deposit instructions.) Do not use the Form 941-V payment voucher to make Federal tax deposits.

Caution: *If you pay amounts with Form 941 that should have been deposited, you may be subject to a penalty. See Circular E.*

Specific Instructions

Box 1—Employer identification number (EIN). If you do not have an EIN, apply for one on **Form SS-4,** Application for Employer Identification Number, and write "Applied for" and the date you applied in this entry space.

Box 2—Amount paid. Enter the amount paid with Form 941.

Box 3—Tax period. Darken the capsule identifying the quarter for which the payment is made. Darken only one capsule.

Box 4—Name and address. Enter your name and address as shown on Form 941.

● Make your check or money order payable to the United States Treasury. Be sure to enter your EIN, "Form 941," and the tax period on your check or money order. Do not send cash. Please do not staple this voucher or your payment to the return or to each other.

● Detach the completed voucher and send it with your payment and Form 941 to the address provided on the back of Form 941.

▼ _ _ _ **Detach Here and Mail With Your Payment** _ _ ▼ _ _ _ _ Form **941-V** (2002)

Form **941-V** | **Payment Voucher** | OMB No. 1545-0029
Department of the Treasury Internal Revenue Service (99) | ► **Do not staple or attach this voucher to your payment.** | 2002

1 Enter your employer identification number	2 **Enter the amount of the payment**	Dollars	Cents

3 Tax period		4 Enter your business name (individual name if sole proprietor)
⊘ 1st Quarter	⊘ 3rd Quarter	Enter your address
⊘ 2nd Quarter	⊘ 4th Quarter	Enter your city, state, and ZIP code

FIGURE 23-5, cont'd For legend see previous page.

Form 940

Department of the Treasury
Internal Revenue Service (99)

Employer's Annual Federal Unemployment (FUTA) Tax Return

▶ **See separate Instructions for Form 940 for information on completing this form.**

OMB No. 1545-0028

2001

T	
FF	
FD	
FP	
I	
T	

You must complete this section. ▶

Name (as distinguished from trade name)

Calendar year

Trade name, if any

Address and ZIP code

Employer identification number

A Are you required to pay unemployment contributions to only one state? (If "No," skip questions B and C.) . ☐ Yes ☐ No

B Did you pay all state unemployment contributions by January 31, 2002? ((1) If you deposited your total FUTA tax when due, check "Yes" if you paid all state unemployment contributions by February 11, 2002. (2) If a 0% experience rate is granted, check "Yes." (3) If "No," skip question C.) . . . . ☐ Yes ☐ No

C Were all wages that were taxable for FUTA tax also taxable for your state's unemployment tax? . . . . . ☐ Yes ☐ No

If you answered "No" to any of these questions, you must file Form 940. If you answered "Yes" to all the questions, you may file Form 940-EZ, which is a simplified version of Form 940. (Successor employers see **Special credit for successor employers** on page 3 of the instructions.) You can get Form 940-EZ by calling 1-800-TAX-FORM (1-800-829-3676) or from the IRS Web Site at **www.irs.gov.**

If you will not have to file returns in the future, check here (see **Who Must File** in separate instructions), **and complete and sign the return** . . . . ▶ ☐

If this is an Amended Return, check here. . . . . ▶ ☐

Part I	**Computation of Taxable Wages**

1 Total payments (including payments shown on lines 2 and 3) during the calendar year for services of employees **1**

2 Exempt payments. (Explain all exempt payments, attaching additional sheets if necessary.) ▶ -------------------------------- -- **2**

3 Payments of more than $7,000 for services. Enter only amounts over the first $7,000 paid to each employee. (See separate instructions.) Do not include any exempt payments from line 2. The $7,000 amount is the Federal wage base. Your state wage base may be different. **Do not use your state wage limitation**. **3**

4 Add lines 2 and 3 . . . . **4**

5 **Total taxable wages** (subtract line 4 from line 1) . . . . ▶ **5**

Be sure to complete both sides of this form, and sign in the space provided on the back.

For Privacy Act and Paperwork Reduction Act Notice, see separate instructions. ▼ **DETACH HERE** ▼ Cat. No. 11234O Form **940** (2001)

Form 940-V

Department of the Treasury
Internal Revenue Service

Form 940 Payment Voucher

Use this voucher only when making a payment with your return.

OMB No. 1545-0028

2001

Complete boxes 1, 2, and 3. Do not send cash, and do not staple your payment to this voucher. Make your check or money order payable to the **"United States Treasury."** Be sure to enter your employer identification number, "Form 940," and "2001" on your payment.

1 Enter your employer identification number.

2 **Enter the amount of your payment.** ▶ | Dollars | Cents |

3 Enter your business name (individual name for sole proprietors).

Enter your address.

Enter your city, state, and ZIP code.

FIGURE 23-6 Employer's Annual Federal Unemployment Tax (FUTA) Return.

Form 940 (2001) Page **2**

Part II   **Tax Due or Refund**

1	Gross FUTA tax. Multiply the wages from Part I, line 5, by .062	**1**
2	Maximum credit. Multiply the wages from Part I, line 5, by .054 . . | **2**	
3	Computation of tentative credit (**Note:** *All taxpayers must complete the applicable columns.*)	

(a) Name of state	(b) State reporting number(s) as shown on employer's state contribution returns	(c) Taxable payroll (as defined in state act)	(d) State experience rate period		(e) State experience rate	(f) Contributions if rate had been 5.4% (col. (c) x .054)	(g) Contributions payable at experience rate (col. (c) x col. (e))	(h) Additional credit (col. (f) minus col.(g)) If 0 or less, enter -0-.	(i) Contributions paid to state by 940 due date
			From	To					

3a   Totals . . . ▶

3b   **Total tentative credit** (add line 3a, columns (h) and (i) only—for late payments, also see the instructions for Part II, line 6) . . . . ▶   **3b**

4

5

6	**Credit:** Enter the smaller of the amount from Part II, line 2 or line 3b; or the amount from the worksheet in the Part II, line 6 instructions	**6**
7	**Total FUTA tax** (subtract line 6 from line 1). If the result is over $100, also complete Part III . .	**7**
8	Total FUTA tax deposited for the year, including any overpayment applied from a prior year . .	**8**
9	**Balance due** (subtract line 8 from line 7). Pay to the **"United States Treasury."** If you owe more than $100, see **Depositing FUTA Tax** on page 3 of the separate instructions . . . . . . ▶	**9**
10	**Overpayment** (subtract line 7 from line 8). Check if it is to be: ☐ **Applied to next return** or ☐ **Refunded** . . . . ▶	**10**

Part III   **Record of Quarterly Federal Unemployment Tax Liability** (Do not include state liability.) **Complete only if line 7 is over $100.** See page 6 of the separate instructions.

Quarter	First (Jan. 1–Mar. 31)	Second (Apr. 1–June 30)	Third (July 1–Sept. 30)	Fourth (Oct. 1–Dec. 31)	Total for year
Liability for quarter					

Third Party Designee   Do you want to allow another person to discuss this return with the IRS (see instructions page 4)? ☐ **Yes.** Complete the following. ☐ **No**

Designee's name ▶   Phone no. ▶ ( )   Personal identification number (PIN) ▶

Under penalties of perjury, I declare that I have examined this return, including accompanying schedules and statements, and, to the best of my knowledge and belief, it is true, correct, and complete, and that no part of any payment made to a state unemployment fund claimed as a credit was, or is to be, deducted from the payments to employees.

Signature ▶   Title (Owner, etc.) ▶   Date ▶

✹

Form **940** (2001)

FIGURE 23-6, cont'd For legend see previous page.

Federal Unemployment Tax

Employers also contribute under the Federal Unemployment Tax Act (FUTA). Generally, credit can be taken against the FUTA tax for amounts paid into a state unemployment fund up to a certain percentage. Employers are responsible for paying the FUTA tax; it must not be deducted from employees' wages. For 1998 the FUTA tax was 6.2% of the first $7000 in wages paid to each employee during the calendar year.

For deposit purposes, the FUTA tax is figured quarterly, and any amount due must be paid by the last day of the first month after the quarter ends. The formula for determining the amount due is set forth in the Federal Employer's Tax Guide.

An annual FUTA return must be filed on Form 940 on or before January 31 following the close of the calendar year for which the tax is due (Figure 23-6). Any tax still due is payable with the return. Form 940 may be filed on or before February 10 following the close of the year, if all required deposits were made on time and if full payment of the tax due is deposited on or before January 31.

State Unemployment Taxes

All of the states and the District of Columbia have unemployment compensation laws. In most states, the tax is imposed only on the employer, but a few states require employers to withhold a percentage of wages for unemployment compensation benefits. An employer may be subject to federal unemployment tax and not subject to state unemployment tax. In some states, for instance, the employer with fewer than four employees is not subject to the state unemployment tax. The regulations for a specific state should be checked.

State Disability Insurance

Some states require that employees be covered by disability or sick-pay insurance. The employer may be required to withhold

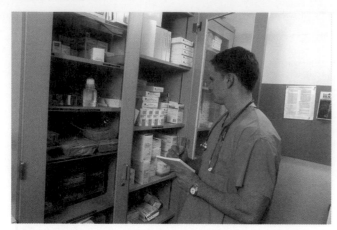

FIGURE 23-7 Inventory supplies and equipment before developing the annual budget. Once a good inventory has been completed, more accurate projections can be made for the expenses for the coming year.

a certain amount from the employee's salary to pay for this insurance.

BUDGETS

Growing businesses must develop budgets that help to plan finances over a certain period. Medical offices should compile a new budget before the beginning of each **fiscal year.** The best way to begin a budget is to look at the expenses from the previous year (Figure 23-7). These expenses should be divided into categories, then a total should be derived for each category. Each month should represent approximately $^1/_{12}$ of the total budget, not including large capital expenses.

Within the individual categories, examine expenses for those that could be eliminated or those that were underbudgeted. For example, if $3345 was spent on office supplies and the budget was $3000, either more money needs to be allotted for this category or cuts in spending are necessary. If $3345 was spent and the budget was $4000, the excess may be placed in another category for the next year.

CRITICAL THINKING APPLICATION

- Brenda has developed a preliminary budget. She realizes that several pieces of equipment need to be replaced in the coming year. However, Dr. Wilkins has expressed that she does not wish to make any capital purchases. How might Brenda approach Dr. Wilkins about the needed equipment?
- How might leasing equipment benefit the office? How can Brenda determine if this would be more or less expensive than purchasing the equipment?

By monitoring expenses on a monthly basis, the physician can see if the facility is over budget, under budget, or right on target. Categories in which overspending has occurred can be reconciled by taking funds from another category (for instance, category B) and adding them to the overspent category (category A). However, the amount taken must be subtracted from category B and added to category A. Those subtracted

funds are no longer available in category B. Specific notes should be kept when categories are overspent, so that an adjustment may be made for the next fiscal year.

The following categories should be considered for the physician's operating budget:

- Insurance
- Rent
- Depreciation
- Loan payments
- Advertising and promotions
- Legal and accounting
- Miscellaneous expenses
- Supplies
- Salaries and wages
- Utilities
- Dues, subscriptions, and fees
- Taxes
- Repairs and maintenance
- Medical equipment
- Administrative equipment
- Medication and pharmacy expenses

The physician should investigate whether leasing equipment might be a better option for the facility. Some leasing programs are very progressive and provide service contracts at no additional cost. Because depreciation costs are high, leasing might be the best answer to a new equipment need.

Insurance

Insurance coverage is one of the physician's major expenses. Almost every physician carries some type of malpractice insurance for protection against the cost of legal liabilities. Property and fire insurance are mandatory, and most physicians carry workers' compensation insurance to cover employee injuries and accidents. The medical assistant may be asked to shop for the best insurance rates at the time of renewals.

CLOSING COMMENTS

The physician will come to rely heavily on the person who manages the finances of the office. It is important that this individual keep information confidential. The entire staff must be conscious of the costs involved in operating a medical office and should adhere to their respective budgets as closely as possible. By being conservative, the physician may be willing to spend more money on pay increases and benefits to reward his or her employees.

There may be times when patients do not fully understand the costs involved in providing high-quality medical care. The medical assistant may need to educate the patient about the basic costs involved with the procedures that are performed in the office. Patients do not need a lengthy explanation but may be set more at ease in knowing that the physician does not set his or her fees arbitrarily. The physician's office is a small business, like thousands of other small businesses, and should be able to pay its overhead and expenses.

The keeping of the financial records is a position of great trust and responsibility. Some physicians require the person placed in charge of the office finances to be bonded. This means that the facility has done a security check on an individual and the person was found worthy to be placed in a position of responsibility. A bond is issued by an entity on behalf of a second party, guaranteeing that the second party will fulfill an obligation or series of obligations to a third party. In the event that the obligations are not met, the third party will recover its losses via the bond.

Records must be accurate and completed on a daily basis. Daily journals should be kept indefinitely in support of tax returns.

SUMMARY OF SCENARIO

Brenda has learned much about the financial management of a physician's office. She is never hesitant to call the practice accountant, Mr. Schmidt, whenever a question arises. As she gains more experience, she comes to understand the budgeting process, cost management, and the various methods of accounting practice.

There are many things that can affect the finances of a medical practice. However, the physician who is fairly conservative about spending and careful with investments should remain a stable part of the community's healthcare professionals. Dr. Wilkins lives by this philosophy and encourages her employees to manage money wisely, too. This attitude among all the staff members promotes a sense of teamwork and cooperation for the benefit of all.

SUMMARY of LEARNING OBJECTIVES

1. Define, spell, and pronounce the terms listed in the vocabulary.
   - Spelling and pronouncing medical terms correctly adds credibility to the medical assistant. Knowing the definition of these terms promotes confidence in communication with patients and co-workers.
2. List the four items that all financial records should show at any given time.
   - The financial records of any business should at all times show how much was earned in a given period, how much was collected, how much is owed, and the distribution of expenses incurred.
3. Distinguish between accounts payable and accounts receivable.
   - *Accounts payable* refers to the amounts of money owed by a business and not yet paid, whereas *accounts receivable* refers to amounts owed to the business that are not yet paid.
4. List and explain the three most common bookkeeping systems found in physicians' offices today.
   - The three most common bookkeeping systems in use today are the single-entry system, double-entry system, and pegboard system. The single-entry method is the oldest accounting method and uses a general journal, a cash payment journal, and an accounts receivable ledger. Payroll records and petty cash records may also be included. The double-entry system, which is more difficult to use than the single-entry system, requires an entry on each side of the accounting equation, and each side must always balance. The pegboard system requires a moderate initial investment to implement but allows the user to perform several accounting functions at one time. It is often called the *write-it-once system*.

5. Explain the importance of a trial balance.
   - A trial balance will reflect discrepancies between the journal and the ledger. It does not reveal errors in the individual accounts but will show errors in the overall balances of accounts.
6. State the types of employment records required by the IRS.
   - The IRS requires that several employment records be kept for at least 4 years. These records include the Social Security number of the employee; the number of withholding allowances claimed; the amount of gross salary; all deductions for Social Security and Medicare taxes; federal, state, and city or other subdivision withholding taxes; state disability insurance; and state unemployment tax.
7. Discuss the basis for the withholding amounts that are taken from employees' earnings.
   - Several deductions are taken from the employee's wages as required by law. These deductions are based on the total earnings of the employee, the number of withholding allowances claimed, the marital status of the employee, and the length of the pay period involved.
8. Name the five common periodic accounting reports.
   - Five common reports are used for accounting in the small business office: the statement of income and expense, the cash flow statement, the trial balance, the accounts receivable trial balance, and the balance sheet.
9. Explain the purpose of the W-4 form.
   - The Employee's Withholding Allowance Certificate, or Form W-4, specifies the number of withholding allowances that the employee is claiming. The more allowances that are

Continued

SUMMARY of LEARNING OBJECTIVES
Continued

claimed, the less money that is taken from the employee's paycheck.

10. Explain the requirements of the Federal Insurance Contributions Act.
    - FICA requires that a certain amount of money be deducted from an employee's wages and designated for Medicare and Social Security programs. The current percentages are 1.45% for the Medicare contribution and 6.2% for Social Security. Both the employer and the employee contribute these amounts.

11. Discuss the importance of setting a budget each fiscal year.
    - The physician's office must set a budget each fiscal year to prepare for all of the expenses that will be involved in running the office. Without a well-planned budget, the physician cannot control expenses. The expenditures from the past year should be evaluated when the new budget is planned, with particular attention paid to the expense categories that exceeded expected amounts.

12. Maintain a petty cash fund.
    - Most offices pay for small, incidental expenses with petty cash. The process for maintaining a petty cash fund is outlined in Procedure 23-1.

13. Accurately process an employee payroll.
    - Employee payroll is an essential function related to practice finances. The process for employee payrolls is outlined in Procedure 23-2.

CONNECTIONS

Study Guide Connection: Go to Chapter 23 Study Guide. Read the Case Study and Workplace Applications and complete the assignments. Do online research for answers to the questions in the Internet Activities associated with management of practice finances.

CD Connection: Go to the Medical Assisting Competency Challenge CD and do the training activities under Financial Management.

Evolve Connection: For more information related to management of practice finances, go to http://evolve.elsevier.com/kinn/admin and visit related weblinks for Chapter 23. Click on the Medical Assisting Exam Review and do the practice questions to sharpen your test-taking skills. To learn more about office software, do the exercises for the Altapoint demo that is on the CD.

Medical Practice Management and Human Resources

24

SCENARIO

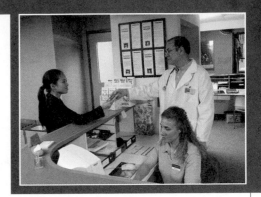

Katherine Martinson is the office manager for Dr. Michael Collins, a family practitioner in a group practice located in a metropolitan area. The office usually carries a full schedule of patients each day. Katherine has been instrumental in the seamless operation of the facility. Before joining Dr. Collins, Katherine worked for a physician in the same group of doctors, Dr. Grant Bradley, who retired last year. She worked as an administrative medical assistant for 6 years before that. Her strength and ability to motivate employees led Dr. Collins to approach her about becoming his office manager once Dr. Bradley retired.

Katherine is a consummate professional but knows the importance of treating each employee as an individual. At weekly staff meetings the employees offer input on the various procedures followed in the office. Katherine regularly consults with the staff members and always asks for input as to how the office can function more effectively. She then implements many of the staff members' suggestions in the day-to-day activities of the office. She knows that employees need to feel a part of the team, and by trying the procedures others suggest she validates them as an asset to the facility.

When a position is open, Katherine is careful about whom she hires, always checking at least three references per applicant and verifying each previous place of employment. She trains each employee on every aspect of the job and keeps checklists that reflect the employee has been given instruction on certain skills.

Katherine makes sure that each person has the tools needed to do his or her job. She also explains overhead costs to employees and helps them to understand what is involved with the daily operation of the practice. With this information the employees are more conservative about use of supplies and care of equipment. Major changes are presented to the entire staff, and although Dr. Collins makes the final decision, he and Katherine seek the input of the employees, too. The cooperative attitude between management and the employees of the office provides a good atmosphere for teamwork, and Katherine and the physician are pleased with the results.

While studying this chapter, think about the following questions:

- How friendly should office managers become with the staff members?
- Why is it important to check references when hiring a new staff member?

- How should negative employee evaluations be handled?
- Why could the patient information folder be considered a management tool?

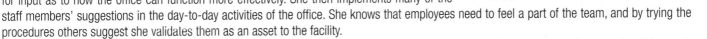

LEARNING OBJECTIVES

1. Define, spell, and pronounce the terms listed in the vocabulary.
2. Explain the importance of management in the medical office.
3. Discuss the desirable qualities of a medical office manager.
4. List and discuss the three types of leaders.
5. Discuss several types of power and whether power is a positive or negative entity.
6. Identify several ways in which employees are motivated.
7. Explain the difference between intrinsic and extrinsic motivation.
8. List several ways to prevent burnout.
9. Discuss what to look for when reviewing resumes and applications.

10. Explain why the telephone voice of an applicant is important.
11. Identify the follow-up activities the office manager should perform after an interview.
12. Explain the importance of mentors for new employees in the medical office.
13. List the various types of staff meetings.
14. Successfully arrange a group meeting.
15. Interview a job candidate for a position at the facility.
16. Conduct a performance review for an employee.

National Accreditation Competencies and Content

CAAHEP COMPETENCIES

General

3.c.(1)(b). Recognize and respond to verbal communications

3.c.(1)(c). Recognize and respond to nonverbal communications

3.c.(2)(b). Perform within legal and ethical boundaries

3.c.(2)(d). Document appropriately

3.c.(4)(c). Utilize computer software to maintain office systems

ABHES COMPETENCIES

Professionalism

1.d. Be cognizant of ethical boundaries

Communication

2.f. Interview effectively

2.k. [Use] principles of verbal and nonverbal communication

Administrative Duties

3.a. Perform basic secretarial skills

3.d. Apply computer concepts for office procedures

Legal Concepts

5.a. Determine needs for documentation and reporting

5.b. Document accurately

Office Management

6.e. Maintain liability coverage

6.f. Exercise efficient time management

Instruction

7.d. Orient and train personnel

VOCABULARY

affable Being pleasant and at ease in talking to others; characterized by ease and friendliness.

agenda (ah-jen'-duh) A list or outline of things to be considered or done.

ancillary (an'-suh-ler-e) Subordinate; auxiliary.

appraisal An expert judgment of the value or merit of; judgment as to quality.

blatant Completely obvious, conspicuous, or obtrusive, especially in a crass or offensive manner; brazen.

burnout Exhaustion of physical or emotional strength or motivation, usually as a result of prolonged stress or frustration.

chain of command A series of executive positions in order of authority.

circumvention To manage to get around, especially by ingenuity or stratagem.

cohesive Sticking together tightly; exhibiting or producing cohesion.

disparaging (dis-pahr'-uh-jing) Slighting; having a negative or degrading tone.

embezzlement Stealing from an employer; to appropriate goods, services, or funds for personal use without permission.

extrinsic (eks-trin'-zik) External to a thing, its essential nature, or its original character.

impenetrable Incapable of being penetrated or pierced; not capable of being damaged or harmed.

incentives Things that incite or spur to action; rewards or reasons for performing a task.

insubordination Disobedience to authority.

intrinsic Originating with or resulting from causes within a body, organ, or part.

mentors Trusted counselors or guides.

meticulous (meh-tiku'-luhs) Marked by extreme or excessive care in the consideration or treatment of details.

micromanage To manage with great or excessive control or attention to details.

morale The mental and emotional condition, such as enthusiasm, confidence, or loyalty, of an individual or group with regard to the function or tasks at hand.

motivation The process of inciting a person to some action or behavior.

reprimands Criticisms for a fault; severe or formal reproofs.

retention The act of keeping in possession or use; keeping in one's pay or service.

subordinate Submissive to or controlled by authority; placed in or occupying a lower class, rank, or position.

targeted Directed or used toward a target; directed toward a specific desire or position.

The management of a professional medical office can greatly influence the success of the operation. Good management will allow the physician to see and treat his or her patients in a functional environment with the confidence that the business side of the facility is operating as it should be. A well-managed office is not something that just happens. Great effort and teamwork are necessary to ensure that the day-to-day activities are carried out efficiently and that the many details needing attention are handled expeditiously.

WHO'S IN CHARGE?

If the office has only one medical assistant, that person must be able to assume many management responsibilities with cooperation from the physician. When there are two medical assistants, one administrative and one clinical, it is often the administrative medical assistant who is expected to assume management duties. In an office with a larger staff, a line of authority must be established.

A facility with three or more employees should designate one person as supervisor or office manager. This individual should have management skills and the ability to deal with personnel matters (Table 24-1). Other employees answer to the office manager, and the office manager answers to the physician or physicians. A **chain of command** allows the office staff to consult with the physician regarding administrative or clinical problems, complaints, or grievances; however, it prompts employees to allow those individuals whom the physician has placed in charge to have the first opportunity to solve problems. It also allows the physician to check on the operation of the office, disseminate information on policy changes, and correct errors or grievances by dealing with one person instead of all employees.

A medical assisting career is challenging and offers great opportunities for advancement. The recently graduated medical assistant, whose first position may have been as a receptionist, can be given more responsibilities and may eventually become the office manager of a large staff. Executive-level personnel work in one of the most critical areas in healthcare.

Management problems can often be avoided by carefully defining the areas of authority and responsibility of each employee. Many physicians say that friction among workers is their most common personnel problem. The importance of the chain of command cannot be overemphasized, and the physician must not undermine the office manager's authority by **circumvention.** When employees know what is expected of them, they can plan both their daily and long-term work more effectively.

Duties of the Medical Office Manager

The duties carried out by medical office managers vary from place to place and practice to practice. Some physicians take on a much more active role in office management than others. The best management plan for the physician is to hire an office manager who is trustworthy and reliable, then allow him or her to run the business aspects of the office. This frees the physician to concentrate on taking care of patients (Figure 24-1).

Some of the tasks performed by the medical office manager include the following:
- Preparing and updating policy and procedure manuals
- Developing job descriptions
- Recruiting new employees
- Performing orientation and training
- Conducting performance and salary reviews
- Dismissing employees
- Planning staff meetings
- Maintaining staff harmony
- Establishing work-flow guidelines
- Ensuring compliance with all federal and state regulations
- Improving office efficiency
- Supervising the purchase and care of equipment
- Educating patients
- Eliminating time-wasting tasks for the physician
- Marketing the practice
- Performing customer service

TABLE 24-1 Qualities of an Effective Manager
• Uses good judgment
• Has good health
• Has the ability to organize
• Is willing to learn
• Possesses original ideas
• Has leadership ability
• Is fair with all employees
• Is flexible
• Has a sense of fairness
• Cares about employees
• Remains calm during crises
• Is open to constructive criticism
• Has good communication skills
• Uses good listening skills
• Is approachable

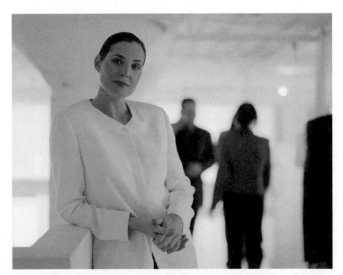

FIGURE 24-1 The office manager ensures that the medical facility runs smoothly so that the physician can concentrate on patient care.

Office management can best be accomplished by developing a thorough office policy and procedure manual. This is discussed later in the chapter.

The Power of Influence

Managers have a great deal of influence over the people they supervise. A successful manager must be interested in people and enjoy working with them on a daily basis. It is said that if one helps others get what they want in life, the individual usually gets what he or she wants as well. An effective manager discovers the **motivation** behind employees' drives to be a part of the profession in which they are employed, then helps them achieve their individual goals. In turn, most employees are enthusiastic about working toward the facility's goals as productive team members.

Successful managers know that their employees should be encouraged to perform at optimal levels, and they are confident enough in their own skills to give credit to those employees who develop ideas and concepts for the team. These managers know how to let their employees help them "look good." A manager with a group of outstanding employees usually is looked on as an effective leader.

CRITICAL THINKING APPLICATION

- When Katherine first began as Dr. Collins's office manager, she found several supportive employees, but a few were concerned about their new boss. How can a new manager help employees be at ease during the first few weeks?
- Katherine scheduled a time with each employee and asked the three things he or she liked best about the office and three things he or she liked the least. How does this help her to manage the office effectively?

The Manager as a Leader

Leaders nurture other people. They take the time to discover what makes people tick, then give them opportunities that will help them rise to new levels of responsibility. Leaders have a strong belief in people, and they express confidence in their abilities, seeing them as successes rather than failures. Often this belief exists before people prove themselves, and that provides motivation for them to reach their potential.

Perhaps most important, leaders listen to their people. Few things are more frustrating than an employee attempting to talk to a manager who is working on some project or typing on the computer. Listening involves eye contact and questions to ensure that the employee is understood. Being willing to take the time to listen is a step toward success as a manager.

Instead of sitting across from employees at a desk, try sitting beside them in the chairs that are usually placed in front of a desk. When discussing issues with employees, this simple change in position places the office manager on an equal plane with the employee and implies more of a team effort. At times this positioning would be inappropriate, such as during discussions about disciplinary matters. Still, when attempting to get an employee to cooperate or come over to the office manager's

way of thinking, position can play a large role in placing people "on the same page."

Types of Leaders

There are three basic types of leaders today, including the charismatic leader, the transactional leader, and the transformational leader. Each has positive qualities, and all can be successful in business.

Charismatic leaders have a special way of inspiring an unswerving allegiance and devotion from their followers. They encourage people to overcome great obstacles and buy into their vision for the organization or business. They also tend to trust people in **subordinate** positions and earn trust in return.

Transactional leaders are structured and organized. They ensure that their subordinates understand their duties and roles. These leaders are fair and provide rewards when they have been earned. The transactional leader is hardworking, a planner, and strict about budgets and time frames.

Transformational leaders are innovative and able to bring about change in an organization. These leaders are relationship builders. They stress shared values and strive to create a common ground among team members. Transformational leaders are the most effective when an organization is experiencing change and reorganization.

Styles of Management

Some managers are democratic and willing to listen to employees. These managers are fair-minded and ask the opinions of the staff when making decisions. In contrast, the autocratic manager is more of a dictator, making demands and insisting tasks be done in a certain way—his or her way. The laissez-faire manager is easygoing and does not make a lot of demands on employees. This is a "go with the flow" manager who lets employees work on their own and does not **micromanage.**

Leading During Transitions and Change

Change is a part of the life of every person and every business. Most people are initially hesitant to face change, and many people try to avoid it completely. However, a business cannot experience growth without change. The manager who is able to lead subordinates through periods of change will be a valuable asset to the organization. Employees will need guidance on maintaining focus on the tasks at hand. The manager should remain visible to the employees during times of change and communicate frequently with status reports and updates on policies and procedures.

The book *Who Moved My Cheese?* by Spencer Johnson, MD, is one of the most innovative stories in recent years. Any manager or employee experiencing a time of change should study this simple, short book. The opening quotes A. J. Cronin, saying:

"Life is no straight and easy corridor along which we travel free and unhampered, but a maze of passages, through which we must seek our way, lost and confused, now and again checked in a blind alley. But always, if we have faith, a door will open for us, not perhaps

one that we ourselves would ever have thought of, but one that will ultimately prove good for us."

Who Moved My Cheese? stresses several points about change that the good manager should remember, including the following:

- Change happens
- Anticipate change
- Monitor change
- Adapt to change quickly
- Move with the change
- Enjoy change
- Be ready to change again quickly, and enjoy it again

The simplicity of this advice does not diminish its truth. Change will happen in any person's job and personal life. Those who learn to adapt quickly and move forward will be the ones who do not become casualties of change.

The Role of Power

Power is the ability to influence employees so that they carry out their directives. Leaders use many types of power.

Coercive power is manipulative, and the leader often makes threats or uses fear to accomplish goals. The fear of losing a job is one manipulation of power.

Granting rewards is a more positive use of power. When the leader is able to give employees some type of reward for a job well done, most strive to reach their goals.

Expert power is a factor when the leader is knowledgeable about a subject. Employees respect leaders who know their job and how things should be done. Most people look up to a person who has a high degree of knowledge about a given subject. When working for someone who knows nothing about procedures or the services offered, employees frequently are frustrated.

Legitimate power is that of position or status. It does not really matter who the President of the United States is—the office itself carries the weight of power. Therefore the individual who serves as President holds legitimate power.

Referent power is granted from subordinates to those who lead by example. It is a power based on the admiration of the leader. **Mentors,** parents, and teachers are often the objects of referent power.

CRITICAL THINKING APPLICATION

- Katherine is a respected office manager in the facility where she works, but several other managers are not as well liked. What makes a good office manager?
- Everyone has worked for at least one supervisor whom they did not like. What traits make a poor office manager?

Abuse of Power and Authority

Unfortunately, many managers have the capacity to abuse the power they have. A manager who puts up barriers and erects emotional walls with the employees will have difficulty forming a **cohesive** team. Some managers use other people as tools to get what they want, whereas others stick to their own level or stature, relating only to the inner circle of decision makers in the facility.

When there are no checks and balances in an organization, it is easy to abuse power. It is difficult to work with a manager who cannot look inside himself or herself and see mistakes. Some managers stress rules and conformity, leaving no gray areas where subordinates are concerned. Some show a false humility and pretend to care, but most employees can see right through this half-effort at a relationship. Others only hire "yes" people, who agree with everything that the manager says. All of these are abuses of power and indications of a poor manager.

The Power of Motivation

What motivates a person to reach a goal?

- A challenge
- Money
- Praise
- Satisfaction
- Freedom
- Fear
- Family
- Insecurity
- Competition
- Fulfillment
- Integrity
- Honor
- Reputation
- Responsibility
- Prestige
- Needs
- Love

All of the motivators listed above could prompt an employee to action. There are two general types of motivation. **Intrinsic** motivation is internal or originates within someone. Intrinsic motivation is long term and can be focused toward a lifelong goal. **Extrinsic** motivation is external and more material in nature. Generally, extrinsic motivation is more short-lived and less satisfying than intrinsic motivation.

CRITICAL THINKING APPLICATION

- Katherine knows that employees have different reasons and motivations for working. Some must work to help support their families, and others work simply because of a love for their field. How can Katherine discover her employees' motivations for working?
- How does this knowledge benefit the office manager?
- Can this knowledge help Katherine achieve her goals?

CREATING A TEAM ATMOSPHERE

Teamwork is critical in the medical profession. In the physician's office the manager must promote an atmosphere in which the employees are willing to work together toward common goals. Low **morale** may exist in the office because of recent changes in policies or procedures, changes in staff or management,

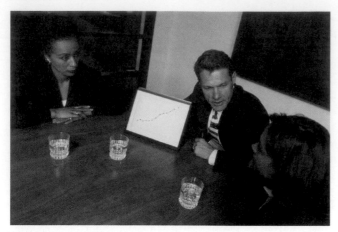

FIGURE 24-2 Communication is vital when building a team. Employees appreciate good communication with management. Sharing good and bad news openly with employees leads to fewer rumors and nervous workers.

Five Essential Elements for Teamwork

- Mutual accountability: Each person on the team holds the others accountable for the success of the organization.
- Common purpose and performance goals: Short-term and intermediate goals must relate to the long-term goals of the group.
- Small size: Most successful teams have a small number of members, and fewer than 10 is optimum.
- Common approach: All of the team members must learn to work together toward the goal.
- Complementary skills: A variety of talents, skills, and abilities is needed for a successful team.

From Katzenbach JR, Smith DK: *Wisdom of teams: creating the high-performance organization*, Boston, 1992, Harvard Business School Publishing.

terminations of recent employees, lack of business, or any number of other reasons. The wise manager will take steps to constantly improve employee morale, including scheduling frequent meetings and keeping the employees abreast of changes and developments that affect them (Figure 24-2). Employees like to be kept "in the loop." Some managers attempt to shield employees from negative information, but this practice can cause rumors to circulate and make morale even worse.

Managers can improve morale by scheduling activities that involve the families of employees and making an obvious effort to include employees in various events. One of the most effective ways to improve employee morale is to communicate. Regular staff meetings are critical for good communication and smooth operation of the medical facility.

Use of Incentives and Employee Recognition

The staff of the physician's office should feel satisfaction with the working conditions and atmosphere in the facility. The office manager plays a part in ensuring that this happens.

Incentives give the employees reason to perform over and above the level expected of them. For instance, if the staff meets or exceeds a goal that has been set, the physician may elect to provide tickets to a sports or entertainment event for the entire staff. A paid day off is always a great incentive for accomplishing a goal. Some physicians have an incentive program that is related to collections for a given period. These ideas provide a goal for the employees to work toward and an opportunity to expand their efforts as a team.

Recognition is a strong method for improving employee morale and encouraging outstanding performance. Certificates for peak performance are a great way to motivate employees. For instance, the office manager may decide to award a certificate each month to the employee who provides the best customer service. Patients could even be involved by allowing them to nominate employees for this honor. When an award is at stake, most employees will enjoy participating and striving to accomplish the goals that have been set.

CRITICAL THINKING APPLICATION

- One of Katherine's employees, Jewel, is very sensitive about performing perfectly on the job. She is an excellent employee, but she does have a few weaknesses. However, she has received a lot of recognition for the good things she has done at work. Katherine still feels that she needs to discuss the areas where Jewel is performing weakly with her but knows that it will upset her. How might Katherine deal with this sticky situation?
- How can Katherine reassure Jewel that she is pleased with her overall performance?

Problem Employees

Occasionally, problem employees disrupt the efficiency of the physician's office. Counseling these employees to find the source of their difficulties is the first step toward resolution. Many employees can be redirected to become productive staff members with a little patience and understanding on the part of the manager. However, some employees have negative attitudes that seem **impenetrable.**

The manager must never hesitate to counsel the employee who is not performing at the expected level, and this includes employees with attitude problems. Establish a set regimen of counseling. Many offices allow one verbal warning before written **reprimands** go into the employee files. If the manager does not make a habit of writing formal reprimands, there may be insufficient documentation of problems with the employee once the manager is ready to terminate him or her. Even small offenses, such as being tardy, should at least be noted in the employee's file. The manager should never be in a position that the termination of an employee cannot be justified by written documents.

Preventing Burnout

Burnout is defined as exhaustion of physical or emotional strength or motivation, usually as a result of prolonged stress or frustration. Medical professionals are particularly susceptible to burnout because of the intensity of their jobs. Even small decisions could affect the life of a patient. Therefore the office

TABLE 24-2 Tips for Preventing Burnout

- Ask for help
- Devote specific times to self-introspection or meditation
- Understand what can be changed and what cannot be changed
- Get some exercise
- Organize and prioritize tasks
- List tasks that are displeasing, and delegate them to others, if possible
- Understand personal limitations
- Take short vacations at least twice a year
- Identify goals, and try to perform only tasks that lead to reaching them
- Consider options, including changing jobs
- Personalize work space with pictures and comforting items
- Get a good understanding of a position and the stress involved before accepting it

manager should take measures to help employees avoid burnout (Table 24-2).

Some of the causes of burnout include a stressful, disorganized home or work environment; poor human relations skills; a feeling of being out of control of one's life; excessive expectations from supervisors or family members; long work hours or time away from family and friends; and not being able to relax either at home or in the work environment.

Keeping the Management Relationship Professional

When people work together for an extended period, they often become **affable,** and sometimes relationships develop into close friendships. This is a normal occurrence, but the office manager must be careful about becoming too close to his or her employees. When the relationship is friendly, it is sometimes difficult to reprimand an employee when needed. Some employees will take advantage of a good relationship with the office manager and may begin to arrive late or call in sick more than usual. A healthy respect for each other must be maintained. The manager can have a good rapport with employees without becoming overly friendly, and this is the best policy. Some facilities have strict rules about fraternization with subordinates outside of the work facility. It is advisable to keep the relationship on a professional level at all times.

CRITICAL THINKING APPLICATION

- The clinical medical assistants usually celebrate payday by going to eat after work every other Friday. After about 6 months on the job, they invited Katherine to join them. Should she go with the employees? Why or why not?
- Most offices plan parties for Christmas or at other times during the year. Are these good for employee morale, or should they be avoided?

SELECTING THE RIGHT STAFF MEMBERS

The most important asset to any medical facility is the staff that cares for the patients. From the doctor to the receptionist,

all play a vital role in the well-being of those who visit the office. Selecting staff members who can be molded into a cohesive team is not an easy task. Care should be taken to choose employees who have the necessary skills and the right personality for the office. Never try to select employees who are all alike. A variety of personality types works better than several similar personalities.

Understanding the Needs of the Office

The office manager should discuss with the physician the type of employee needed when an opening arises. Ask what qualities he or she desires in the person who occupies that particular position and what tasks the person will be responsible for. Once the need has been established and the duties confirmed, the office manager can begin the recruiting process.

One of the most effective methods of finding new employees is through word of mouth. Ask other office managers, physicians, or medical professionals if they are aware of a person looking for employment who has the skills needed in the office. It is a good idea to keep a file of resumes that can be accessed when an opening exists in the office. Often the physician or office manager may know of a person working in another area of the clinic or perhaps in a nearby hospital who may be interested in a job change. Be careful in approaching a person who is already employed. There is no harm in asking if a person is interested, but if the reply is negative, do not pursue the issue further.

Employment agencies can be used to find staff members, but they may charge a fee for their services. The office manager may wish to contact a local medical assistant school to secure an extern. If the extern proves to be an asset to the office, then he or she may be offered the permanent position. Newspaper ads are another option for finding employees, but many resumes may be submitted from people who are not qualified, especially when the economy is not at its best. When creating an ad for the newspaper, list the basic requirements for the position. Briefly describe the office and location and the personality type being sought. Some offices list a few of the benefits offered to attract applicants and may disclose a salary range as well.

Reviewing Resumes and Applications

Once several resumes or applications have been submitted, the office manager should set aside quiet time to review the documents. Place them into one of three stacks—stack one should contain resumes of individuals who will be called for an interview, stack two those of possible candidates but not the strongest, and stack three those of applicants who will not be called.

During this preliminary review process, look for several items. First, be sure the documents are neatly prepared and completely legible (Figure 24-3). The person hired will probably write in the patient charts, so this is a good opportunity to ensure that his or her handwriting can be read clearly. Second, look for gaps between positions. Be sure that any lengthy time of unemployment is explained. The application should be filled out completely, and no notations of "see resume" should be included. The application provides important information,

APPLICATION FOR POSITION / Medical or Dental Office
AN EQUAL OPPORTUNITY EMPLOYER

(In answering questions, use extra blank sheet if necessary)

No employee, applicant, or candidate for promotion, training or other advantage shall be discriminated against (or given preference) because of race, color, religion, sex, age, physical handicap, veteran status, or national origin.

PLEASE READ CAREFULLY AND WRITE OR PRINT ANSWERS TO ALL QUESTIONS. DO NOT TYPE.

Date of Application

A. PERSONAL INFORMATION

Name - Last   First   Middle   Social Security No.   Area Code/Phone No. ( )

Present Address: - Street   (Apt #)   City   State   Zip   How Long At This Address?:

Previous Address: - Street   City   State   Zip   Person to notify in case of Emergency or Accident - Name:

From: To: Address: Telephone:

B. EMPLOYMENT INFORMATION

For What Position Are You Applying?:   ☐ Full-Time ☐ Part-Time ☐ Either   Date Available For Employment?:   Wage/Salary Expectations:

List Hrs./Days You Prefer To Work   List Any Hrs./Days You Are Not Available: (Except for times required for religious practices or observances)   Can You Work Overtime, If Necessary? ☐ Yes ☐ No

Are You Employed Now?: ☐ Yes ☐ No   If So, May We Inquire Of Your Present Employer?: ☐ No ☐ Yes, If Yes:

Name Of Employer: Phone Number: ( )

Have You Ever Been Bonded? ☐ Yes ☐ No   If Required For Position, Are You Bondable? ☐ Yes ☐ No ☐ Uncertain   Have You Applied For A Position With This Office Before? ☐ No ☐ Yes   If Yes, When?:

Referred By / Or Where Did You Learn Of This Job?:

Can You, Upon Employment, Submit Verification Of Your Legal Right To Work In The United States?: ☐ Yes ☐ No
Submit Proof That You Meet Legal Age Requirement For Employment? ☐ Yes ☐ No   Language(s) Applicant Speaks or Writes (If Use Of A Language Other Than English is Relevant To The Job For Which The Applicant Is Applying):

C. EDUCATIONAL HISTORY

Name & Address Of Schools Attended (Include Current)	Dates From	Thru	Highest Grade/Level Completed	Diploma/Degree(s) Obtained/Areas of Study
High School				
College				Degree/Major
Post Graduate				Degree/Major
Other				Course/Diploma/License/Certificate

Specific Training, Education, Or Experiences Which Will Assist You In The Job For Which You Have Applied.

Future Educational Plans

D. SPECIAL SKILLS

CHECK BELOW THE KINDS OF WORK YOU HAVE DONE:

		☐ MEDICAL INSURANCE FORMS	☐ RECEPTIONIST
☐ BLOOD COUNTS	☐ DENTAL ASSISTANT	☐ MEDICAL TERMINOLOGY	☐ TELEPHONES
☐ BOOKKEEPING	☐ DENTAL HYGIENIST	☐ MEDICAL TRANSCRIPTION	☐ TYPING
☐ COLLECTIONS	☐ FILING	☐ NURSING	☐ STENOGRAPHY
☐ COMPOSING LETTERS	☐ INJECTIONS	☐ PHLEBOTOMY (Draw Blood)	☐ URINALYSIS
☐ COMPUTER INPUT	☐ INSTRUMENT STERILIZATION	☐ POSTING	☐ X-RAY
OFFICE EQUIPMENT USED: ☐ COMPUTER	☐ DICTATING EQUIPMENT	☐ WORD PROCESSOR	☐ OTHER:

Other Kinds Of Tasks Performed Or Skills That May Be Applicable To Position: Typing Speed   Shorthand Speed

(PLEASE COMPLETE OTHER SIDE)

FIGURE 24-3 Application for employment. Candidates for jobs in the medical office should complete applications accurately, leaving no blanks or unanswered questions. (Courtesy Bibbero Systems, Inc., Petaluma, Calif. 94954, (800) 242-2376, www.bibbero.com.)

E. EMPLOYMENT RECORD

LIST MOST RECENT EMPLOYMENT FIRST   May We Contact Your Previous Employer(s) For A Reference? ☐ Yes ☐ No

1) Employer   Work Performed. Be Specific:

Address   Street   City   State   Zip Code

Phone Number   (   )

Type of Business   Dates   Mo. Yr.   Mo. Yr.
                                 From   To

Your Position   Hourly Rate/Salary
                                 Starting   Final

Supervisor's Name

Reason For Leaving

2) Employer   Worked Performed. Be Specific:

Address   Street   City   State   Zip Code

Phone Number   (   )

Type of Business   Dates   Mo. Yr.   Mo. Yr.
                                 From   To

Your Position   Hourly Rate/Salary
                                 Starting   Final

Supervisor's Name

Reason For Leaving

3) Employer   Worked Performed. Be Specific:

Address   Street   City   State   Zip Code

Phone Number   (   )

Type of Business   Dates   Mo. Yr.   Mo. Yr.
                                 From   To

Your Position   Hourly Rate/Salary
                                 Starting   Final

Supervisor's Name

Reason For Leaving

F. REFERENCES — FRIENDS / ACQUAINTANCES NON-RELATED

(1) _____
     Name   Address   Telephone Number   (☐ Work ☐ Home)   Occupation   Years Acquainted

(1) _____
     Name   Address   Telephone Number   (☐ Work ☐ Home)   Occupation   Years Acquainted

Please Feel Free To Add Any Information Which You Feel Will Help Us Consider You For Employment

READ THE FOLLOWING CAREFULLY, THEN SIGN AND DATE THE APPLICATION

"I certify that all answers given by me on this application are true, correct and complete to the best of my knowledge. I acknowledge notice that the information contained in this application is subject to check. I agree that, if hired, my continued employment may be contingent upon the accuracy of that information. If employed, I further agree to comply with Company/Office rules and regulations."

Signature: _____   Date: _____

FIGURE 24-3, *cont'd*

and an applicant who does not fill it out in its entirety might be classified as lazy and prone to taking shortcuts. Watch for inconsistencies or oversights, including information that seems incomplete. Also look for resumes that are **targeted** toward the job opening available in the clinic. Targeted resumes are written specifically for a certain position. With today's computer capabilities, job seekers can target their resumes for each job applied for, and this strategy tells the manager that the applicant has enough interest in the job to demonstrate that he or she meets the requirements.

Once the entire stack of documents has been reviewed and separated, return to the stack of potential interviews. Careful judgment and objectivity must be used in the search for an employee who is suitable for the practice. Before interviewing any applicant, the manager needs to know several details:

- What personal qualities and abilities must the applicant have?
- What responsibilities are involved with the position?
- What is the salary range that the physician is willing to offer?
- How soon will the position be open?

Once these facts are clear, the manager should review the final resumes and applications with the following questions in mind:

- Do the applicant's appearance and personal grooming meet the standards set forth in the policy manual?
- Has the applicant been employed previously? What duties were performed?
- If previously employed, how long was the applicant in the last position? Why did the applicant leave?
- What are the applicant's skills? Do these meet the requirements for the position as set forth in the office procedure manual?
- Does the applicant seem to accept and enjoy responsibility?
- What is the applicant's formal education? Is he or she registered or certified? If not, is the applicant interested in taking the examination?
- Is the applicant a member of a professional organization? Does he or she attend meetings?

Arranging the Personal Interview

If the applicant sent a letter asking for an interview, note whether the letter was correctly typed and included essential contact information, and whether he or she also provided an attractive resume. Amazingly, many resumes do not include a contact telephone number! Many managers schedule interviews by email, but there are advantages to speaking to applicants directly. By telephoning the applicant, the manager will have an opportunity to judge his or her telephone voice. The manager may wish to prescreen applicants with the telephone call, asking several questions about the person's education and experience. Because the employee probably will speak with patients on the telephone, clarity of speech will be important. Those who perform well during the prescreening should be scheduled for an interview.

Set a time for the personal interview when the applicant can be given undivided attention. An applicant who is being considered for employment should have an opportunity to see the office when there is a fairly normal amount of activity. The prospective employee who is interviewed in a peaceful, quiet office on the physician's day out may not be prepared for the activity on a normal working day.

Before interviewing any applicant, be thoroughly familiar with the federal, state, and local fair employment practice laws affecting hiring practices. Both men and women receive protection from on-the-job discrimination, sexual harassment, mandatory lie detector tests, and unfair discharge. Title VII of the Civil Rights Act of 1964, as amended by the Equal Employment Opportunity Act of 1972, prohibits inquiries into an applicant's race, color, sex, religion, and national origin. Inquiries regarding medical history, arrest records, or previous drug use are also illegal. Most states have laws designed to protect the rights of job applicants, and these laws may impose additional restrictions.

If an application has not been submitted, have the applicant complete it at the time of the interview. The application form can serve as a check of the applicant's penmanship and thoroughness as well as become a permanent record if the individual is hired. Tell the candidate if the form should be completed in the applicant's own handwriting, and be sure to state this on the instructions. Check to see if the applicant was **meticulous** about following instructions and filling in all the blanks. This provides the manager with an indication of the individual's capacity for following directions.

The Interview

The manager's first priority is to make certain that the applicant feels at ease (Figure 24-4). Shake his or her hand and ask a few social questions before starting the interview (Procedure 24-1). In general, use good manners and see that the person to be interviewed is comfortable. Most people feel some butterflies in the stomach when interviewing, but the manager will get a better idea of the person's capabilities if he or she is relaxed and able to discuss strengths and background openly with the manager.

Begin with a few open-ended questions that cannot be answered with a simple "yes" or "no," such as "What were your duties during your last position?" When interviewing a recent graduate who does not have experience, ask questions such as, "What subject did you perform well in at school?" When speaking with the candidate, make a mental note of whether he or she displays essential personal qualities, such as the ability to converse easily, the capacity to listen, and a bright smile. The applicant should be interested enough in the position to ask

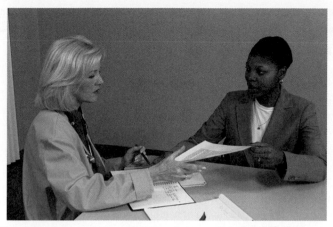

FIGURE 24-4 Put the applicant at ease. Job applicants perform at their peak when relaxed and calm.

Intelligent Questions for Late in the Interview

Interviewers expect candidates to ask intelligent questions concerning the organization and the nature of the work. Always indicate an interest in the position by asking questions. The medical assistant should ask a minimum of two intelligent questions at the end of the interview. Unless a few questions are asked by an interviewee, the interviewer may assume that he or she is not interested in the position. One cautionary note: never allow the first question asked to be about money or benefits. Ask other questions first, and end with a question about money or benefits if that information was not covered in the interview. This way, the interview can progress naturally into a negotiation stage, if the interviewer is ready to move in that direction.

Consider asking some of these questions if they have not been answered earlier in the interview:

- What are the duties and responsibilities of the job?
- How does this position relate to the other positions within the organization?
- How long has this position been a part of the organization, and how long has it been vacant?
- Could you describe the ideal person that you would like to place in this position?
- How have others succeeded or failed in this position in the past?
- With whom would I work?
- What would I be expected to accomplish in the first year?
- How will I be evaluated?
- Are promotions and raises tied to performance evaluations?
- Based on your experience, what type of problems would someone new in this position likely encounter?
- I'm interested in your career with this organization. When did you start? What do you enjoy about your job?
- How can I advance if I am hired at this company?
- What is particularly unique about this organization?
- What does the future look like for this organization?
- What is the salary range for this position? What benefits would I be eligible for, if I am hired?

intelligent questions and appear interested in the office and the physician's specialty.

Avoid inquiries that involve the applicant's privacy. The questions should be related to the available position and the applicant's ability to do the job. An interview is a two-way exchange of information between the applicant and the interviewer. If the applicant appears to be one who will receive serious consideration, explain what will be expected as an employee. Office policies regarding appearance, working hours, overtime, time off, and vacations may be discussed at this stage. Salary and other fringe benefits should be discussed once the manager is ready to offer the job. If the manager fails to mention these items, the applicant may be hesitant to inquire.

Some employers request a credit check before offering employment, especially if the individual will be handling practice finances. It can safely be assumed that one who is unable to handle personal financial affairs will be a poor risk in handling office finances.

Review the job description for the position being filled. The person being interviewed must understand the required duties and responsibilities of the job. Ask if the applicant has any questions, and close the interview on a positive note. Let the candidate know when a decision will be made and what further contact the office will initiate.

During the hiring proceedings, the manager may wish to invite the prospective employee to lunch with the staff or for coffee in the more relaxed atmosphere of the employee lounge. This presents an opportunity to discover whether the applicant's personality will mesh with the atmosphere of the office. Employees appreciate being asked their opinion on those who are potential team members.

An extensive list of interview questions can be found in Chapter 57.

Follow-Up Activities

When the interview is over, immediately take a few moments to rate the applicant while the interview is fresh in the memory. Jot down some notes so that the applicant will be remembered easily when the final decisions are being made as to who will be hired. Do not trust the impressions to memory, especially if several applicants have been interviewed. Never write harmful personal statements; instead, be objective and fair. Should the potential employee ever have cause to bring the physician to court for discrimination in hiring practices, there should be no **disparaging** information written down that would reflect in a negative way on the physician or office manager.

Always carefully check all references and follow through on any leads for information. Use the telephone in checking references, because people are sometimes less than candid in a letter; furthermore, letter writing is time consuming and a reply may never be sent. If the email address for a reference is provided, this is an excellent way to check a reference, and the printed version may be added to the applicant's file.

Prepare a checklist before placing the call. When speaking with the person called, be sure to "listen between the lines." Note the tone of the replies to the questions. Do not ask

PROCEDURE 24-1

Interview a Job Candidate

<u>ABHES COMPETENCY:</u> 2.f

GOAL: *To evaluate job candidates fairly and choose the best person to fill an available position in the medical facility.*

EQUIPMENT and SUPPLIES

- Candidate's completed job application
- Candidate's resume
- Private area in the medical office
- Clerical supplies

PROCEDURAL STEPS

1. Review the job requirements that the candidate will be required to perform.
   PURPOSE: To properly evaluate candidates, one must determine the tasks that the new employee will be expected to perform.

2. Match each job application with the corresponding resume.

3. Separate strong candidates from moderate candidates and poor candidates.
   PURPOSE: To screen the best candidates and invite them to interview for the position.

4. Review each resume and job application again, and determine which candidates should be brought to the office for an interview.

5. Call each candidate and schedule an appointment for an interview.

6. Evaluate the applicant's speaking voice while making the appointment or the interview.
   PURPOSE: To determine the candidate's professionalism and ability to speak clearly and with clarity on the telephone.

7. Select several interview questions in advance to ask all of the applicants.
   PURPOSE: To avoid having to think of questions during the actual interview.

8. Note whether the applicant arrives on time for the interview.
   PURPOSE: If the candidate does not arrive on time for the interview, he or she may be a habitually late employee.

9. Introduce yourself to the applicant, and proceed to a private area to conduct the interview.

10. Make the applicant feel as much at ease as possible.
    PURPOSE: Most individuals are a little nervous during job interviews, and if helped to relax they will be able to present their qualifications and skills confidently.

11. Ask the applicant the chosen questions.

12. Evaluate the answers and make notations about the candidate that are not demeaning or unprofessional.
    PURPOSE: Demeaning comments in an employee file may eventually be seen if there is a subsequent lawsuit, and this can reflect poorly on the person who made the comments.

13. Ask the candidate if he or she has any questions.
    PURPOSE: Evaluate the types of questions that the employee asks; determine whether they are intelligent questions and if they indicate a true interest in the position.

14. Offer strong candidates a brief tour of the facility.

15. Provide a date that a hiring decision will be made, and suggest that the candidate call the facility that day, if desired.

16. Evaluate all applicants fairly according to their experience and training.

17. Select the best three candidates, and call them for a second interview, if desired.

18. Discuss the final hiring decisions with the physician or others with influence.
    PURPOSE: Some physicians want to make the final hiring decisions.

19. Make the final hiring decision.

20. Call the candidate to come to the office to discuss the position.

21. Negotiate salary and benefits.

22. Offer the position.

23. If the offer is declined, call the next candidate to the office to discuss the position until a satisfactory candidate accepts and agrees to a start date.

---

questions that might incriminate the person answering them. The following questions are effective as an introduction:

- When did (the applicant) work for you?
- For how long?
- What were the duties and responsibilities?
- Did the employee assume responsibility well?

Some employers will provide information only on the date of hire, job title, and date of termination of the employment. Respect the company's policy and do not press for further information.

CRITICAL THINKING APPLICATION

- While checking Carol's references, Katherine speaks to her last employer, who makes the statement, "she is not eligible for rehire." The former employer placed strong emphasis on the word "not." All of Carol's other references were glowing. Should Katherine decide not to hire Carol on the basis of this employer's comment?
- How might Katherine find out more about the situation with the last employer?

Any person who is granted an interview should send a thank-you letter to the person who interviewed him or her. Watch the mail to see if any of the applicants perform this important follow-up task.

A second interview may be granted when the field is narrowed to two or three candidates. The physician may wish to participate in these interviews. Some offices conduct a group interview with several staff members present. Remember that these interviews become more and more stressful for the candidate, and the manager should expect some nervousness. Do not "count off" in the interview for mild nervousness.

Making the Selection

When a decision has been reached to hire someone, it is best to bring the successful candidate back into the office to offer the position and negotiate the final details. The office manager may wish to wait until the first-choice candidate has actually accepted the offer before notifying anyone else that the job has been filled. Don't expect the potential employee to answer the offer on the spot. Twenty-four hours is a reasonable time to consider the offer.

Remember to notify all others who have interviewed for the position that it has been filled so that they can continue their job search. They may have hesitated to accept other interviews, and it is unfair to keep individuals who are seeking employment hoping for a telephone call from the physician's office. Good etiquette requires dropping them a note or calling to say that the position is filled. Although this is a rare practice in today's busy clinics, all of the applicants who interviewed were surely the manager's best candidates and professional individuals. Therefore, they deserve a brief call and a wish for success in their job search. Thank the individual for applying, and offer to keep his or her application on file, if the candidate was especially impressive.

ORIENTATION AND TRAINING—CRITICAL FACTORS FOR SUCCESSFUL EMPLOYEES

Recruitment does not end with the hiring. Orientation and training will help new employees to understand what is expected and to develop to their full potential (Figure 24-5). One of the most critical errors in bringing new staff members aboard is not providing them with a fair orientation and training period. The office manager should develop a checklist of the paperwork needed for newly hired staff and all of the information that should be covered with the new employee at the onset of the job.

Some managers assign a mentor to assist the new employee during the initial probationary period. This is a guide whom the new staff member can approach with questions and concerns (Figure 24-6). Using this type of "buddy" system is a good practice, because the new person does not feel isolated and alone during the first few weeks on the job.

Acquaint the new employee with such aspects of the office as the following:

- Staff members and their names
- Physical environment and layout of the office

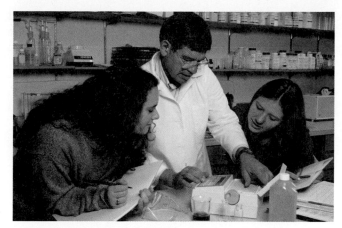

FIGURE 24-5 Training the employee well contributes greatly toward his or her success.

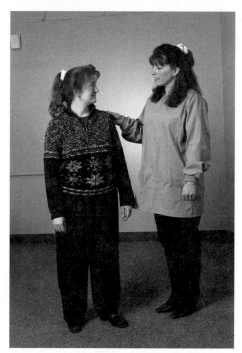

FIGURE 24-6 Mentors are valuable to the new employee. A mentor provides assistance to new employees who are learning their duties and growing accustomed to the medical office.

- Nature of the practice and specialty
- Types of patients seen in the office
- Office policies
- Long-range expectations

All new employees should be required to read the office policy and procedure manual. It is advisable for the manager to require the employee to sign a statement verifying that the manuals were read.

Be sure that all federal and state regulations are met where new employees are concerned. Occupational Safety and Health Administration (OSHA) training must be provided to employees at risk for exposures before they begin any duties. Health Insurance Portability and Accountability Act (HIPAA) training is also required. Certain documents that verify the employee's right to work in the United States must be examined also. It is wise to insist on a fully completed personnel file before allowing the employee to work even 1 hour. Documents that prove worker eligibility are especially important to obtain.

CRITICAL THINKING APPLICATION

Katherine is bringing in a new employee who must begin work on the following Monday, because the staff has been short one person for approximately 2 weeks. However, Katherine will be going on vacation the same day. How can she ensure that the new employee is trained properly?

Job Descriptions

The job description is a tool designed to inform employees about the duties they are expected to perform. Well-written job descriptions list the essential functions of the job and reveal the chain of command that the employee should follow when questions or concerns arise. These documents provide a good guideline for employees so that they will understand exactly what is expected of them and what they are responsible for at work.

The job description should include a statement that says the employee must perform any additional duties as assigned by the supervisor. With this statement in place, the employee cannot say "that is not my job." All employees should be willing to pull together and assist with any tasks, but this statement gives added weight to assignments that are not specified in the written job description.

An effective manager understands the phrase "inspect what you expect." When duties are assigned, the manager should ensure that the tasks were completed correctly and in a timely manner. New employees should be monitored to make certain that their delegated tasks are getting done and getting done right. Without inspection, the manager cannot know that the new employee is meeting expectations. Once employees have earned a degree of trust, inspecting their work is not as necessary as in the beginning. Many managers practice a skill called "management by walking around." By strolling through the areas where subordinates work, managers can observe and hear about issues that might be brewing, while at the same time improve morale by offering encouragement and praise.

Staff Development Training

Continuous training and staff development are vital aspects of any medical office. Constant advancements and technologic changes take place, and employees must be kept up to date on those changes. Meetings should be held at least quarterly to ensure that the staff is using the latest techniques and current regulations when dealing with issues that confront the medical facility.

Delegation of Duties

Delegating duties to subordinates allows managers to concentrate on the most critical aspects of their own jobs. Delegation also provides an opportunity for the employees to grow and learn new skills. Some managers are hesitant to assign duties to employees because they feel the tasks are too important not to be completed by the manager. This hesitation suggests either a refusal to release control or mistrust of the employees. However, this type of manager will soon be overrun with tasks and unable to complete them. Managers should place trust in employees who have earned it and allow them to prove their abilities.

Discover the strengths of individual employees, then assign them tasks that will allow them to use those strengths. If a medical assistant was hired to do administrative duties but is good with phlebotomy, encourage and allow the employee to assist with venipunctures whenever needed.

USING PERFORMANCE EVALUATIONS EFFECTIVELY

A new employee should be granted a probationary period. A period of 60 to 90 days has been traditional, but many employers believe that 2 weeks is sufficient to determine whether the employee will be able to learn and adapt to the position.

Set a definite date for a performance review covering the probationary period at the time of employment. This review should not be squeezed in between patient visits or be given a token few minutes at the end of a day. There should be ample time to relax and talk. At this time, tell the new employee how well expectations have been met and whether there are any deficiencies. Then give the employee an opportunity to ask questions. Sometimes an employee fails to perform because he or she was never told what was expected. Although the probationary period does not always allow time to fully train an individual for a specific position, it is fair to assume that the potential for being a satisfactory employee can be judged at this time. Now is the time to talk out any problems and make suggestions for improvement. Sometimes the employee is released after an unsuccessful probationary period.

The performance **appraisal** includes a judgment of both the quality and quantity of work, personal appearance, attitudes and team spirit, dependability, self-discipline, motivation, attendance, punctuality, and any other qualities essential to satisfactory performance of the job in question (Figure 24-7). The supervisor is responsible for ongoing performance appraisals of all employees, complimenting whenever possible and appropriate and offering helpful criticism when necessary. A formal performance appraisal at the end of the probationary period and at regular 6-month intervals thereafter, with a report to the physician employer, is helpful in the employee's salary review (Procedure 24-2, p. 489).

When negative information is to be relayed to the employee during a performance appraisal, sandwich the negative comment between two positive ones whenever possible. For instance, tell the employee:

"Jewel, you are a pro at greeting patients and making them feel at home. I would like to see you improve your time management skills, however, because I feel you are spending too much time with each individual patient. I must confess that they feel a part of the clinic family. Just watch the time and keep making them feel so welcome!"

PERFORMANCE EVALUATION AND DEVELOPMENT PLAN
(OFFICE AND CLERICAL)

NAME: _____   DATE OF EVALUATION: _____

DATE OF HIRE: _____   DEPARTMENT: _____

JOB TITLE: _____   SUPERVISOR: _____

DATE APPOINTED THIS JOB: _____   MANAGER: _____

LAST REVIEW DATE: _____   LAST REVIEW RATING: _____

NEXT REVIEW DATE: _____   CURRENT REVIEW RATING: _____

PURPOSE

The purpose of this evaluation is to:

1. SET GOALS WITHIN SCOPE OF PRESENT JOB.
2. COMMUNICATE OPENLY ABOUT PERFORMANCE.
3. EVALUATE PAST PERFORMANCE.
4. DISCUSS FUTURE DEVELOPMENT PLANS FOR GROWTH.

INSTRUCTIONS

1. Supervisor to review form prior to completion. If specific items are not applicable they should be left blank.

2. Supervisor and employee to review job description prior to review.

3. In "COMMENTS" section supervisor may indicate which factors should be more heavily weighted in this particular evaluation.

4. Comments should be specific and job-related. All appropriate evaluation factors should be commented on to some degree.

I. POSITION OBJECTIVES AND MAJOR RESPONSIBILITIES. Summarize specific responsibilities of the job.

_____
_____
_____

II. ACCOMPLISHMENTS AND/OR IMPROVEMENTS. What specific accomplishments and/or improvements has employee made since last review with respect to set goals?

_____
_____
_____

PLEASE CONSIDER THE EMPLOYEE'S DEMONSTRATED PERFORMANCE AND MARK THE CIRCLE WHICH MOST CLOSELY DESCRIBES THAT PERFORMANCE.

4 - Performance consistently far exceeds expectations and requirements.
3 - Performance consistently exceeds normal expectations and job requirements.
2 - Performance consistently meets expectations and job requirements
1 - Performance usually meets expectations and minimum job requirements.
0 - Performance does not meet job requirements.

— CONTINUED, NEXT PAGE —

FORM # 72-119 © 1987 BIBBERO SYSTEMS, INC. PETALUMA, CA

TO REORDER CALL TOLL FREE:
800-BIBBERO /(800 242-2376) OR
FAX: (800) 242-9330 MFG IN U.S.A.

FIGURE 24-7 Performance evaluation and development plan. Performance evaluations should be considered tools that will help employees reach their personal goals and the goals of the organization. (Courtesy Bibbero Systems, Inc., Petaluma, Calif. 94954, (800) 242-2376, www.bibbero.com.)

7. <u>DEPENDABILITY:</u> CONSIDER ATTENDANCE, PUNCTUALITY, IDLE TIME AND RELIANCE WHICH CAN BE PLACED ON EMPLOYEE TO PERSEVERE AND CARRY THROUGH TO COMPLETION ALL ASSIGNED TASKS

    ○ 0   ○ 1   ○ 2   ○ 3   ○ 4

_____

_____

_____

8. <u>COMPLIANCE WITH COMPANY POLICIES:</u> DOES THE EMPLOYEE COMPLY WITH RULES AND REGULATIONS WHICH APPLY TO SAFETY, FAIR EMPLOYMENT PRACTICES AND GENERAL ADMINISTRATIVE PROCEDURE.

    ○ 0   ○ 1   ○ 2   ○ 3   ○ 4

_____

_____

_____

9. SPECIFIC PERFORMANCE	1	2	3	4	COMMENTS
A. Ability to handle scheduling:					
B. Willingness to work OT when necessary:					
C. Handling of calls and follow-up:					
D. Maintenance of equipment:					
E. Ability to handle patient complaints:					
F. Tact in dealing with patients:					
G. Speed (in specific technical procedures):					
H. Secretarial accuracy:					
I. Professional terminology:					
J. Assisting procedures:					
K. Laboratory techniques:					
L. X-ray techniques:					
M. Physical therapy:					
N. Collections:					
O. Medical Insurance:					
P. Bookkeeping:					

10. PERSONAL	1	2	3	4	COMMENTS
A. Grooming:					
B. Professional conduct:					
C. Energy, enthusiasm:					
D. Ability to handle stress:					

ADDITIONAL COMMENTS: _____

_____

_____

_____

_____

_____

FIGURE 24-7, *cont'd*

PROCEDURE 24-2

Conduct a Performance Review

ABHES COMPETENCY: 7.d.

GOAL: *To evaluate job performance fairly and determine the strengths and weaknesses of employees.*

EQUIPMENT and SUPPLIES

- Employee's file
- Past evaluations of employee
- Notes and/or reports regarding employee behavior
- Private area in the medical office
- Clerical supplies

PROCEDURAL STEPS

1. Set an appointment with the employee to conduct the review.

2. Allow the employee to complete a self-evaluation of his or her own work.
   PURPOSE: To gain insight into how the employee sees his or her own work performance and allow input as to how the employee feels that he or she has performed during the evaluation period.

3. Review the self-evaluation, then document additional information about the employee and his or her performance.

4. Share the information with any other supervisor or the physician, if dictated by office policy or if additional input is necessary.
   PURPOSE: The physician may have additional input that needs to be documented and discussed during the review.

5. Complete the final written review, and proofread it for accuracy and completeness.

6. Discuss the review with the employee during the evaluation appointment.
   PURPOSE: Discussion should promote an understanding of what is expected by the employer.

7. Progress through the interview, and explain the results of the evaluation to the employee.

8. Allow the employee to respond to any of the points raised during the evaluation, but do not allow an argumentative attitude.
   PURPOSE: o gain insight into the employee's reasons for any poor performance without becoming belligerent.

9. Allow the employee to respond in writing to the evaluation for a limited time, such as 5 days.
   PURPOSE: To give the employee a chance to insert his or her input into the performance report.

10. Ask the employee to sign the evaluation to document that it was reviewed with him or her. (The employee does not have to agree with the evaluation to sign it.)

11. Give a copy of the evaluation to the employee.

12. File the evaluation in the employee's file.

Managers also may use the "feel, felt, found" approach when talking with employees about their performance. Consider the following example:

> *"Jewel, I feel the same way you do about the patients taking up a lot of our time. I know there are some that want to talk with us for hours, and I have felt the pressure of wanting to make them feel comfortable but having so much to do, too. I have found that if I explain that I have a meeting or another patient to assist, they are very understanding and not offended. Perhaps you can try that approach, too."*

Peer Evaluations

Some innovative companies use peer evaluations of employees to get a different view of the work performed by a worker. Asking co-workers to assist in the evaluation process can promote teamwork and cooperation. The rare employee will offer a poor evaluation because of a personal problem with another staff member, but for the most part employees will provide fair, unbiased evaluations, knowing that they will also be evaluated when it is their turn.

Evaluations called *360-degree evaluations* are excellent tools for evaluating any employees, including managers. Such evaluations usually consist of a questionnaire that is given to those who work closely with the employee, and they provide input regarding the performance of the person being evaluated.

Poor Evaluations Made Easier

No supervisor enjoys giving an evaluation that is not a positive one. It is difficult to know where to begin when the employee has not performed as expected or hoped. Perhaps the best way to open the conversation is to say,

> *"Rebecca, your review today is not going to be a positive one. It seems that we do not have a meeting of the minds about your duties and our expectations of you. Let's talk about your performance and discuss whether this position is a good match for you."*

The manager should have good documentation of the problems that led to the poor evaluation. If so, these can be reviewed with the employee with specific times, dates, and descriptions of incidents. If the manager does not document these issues, the conversation can become an argument and grow quite heated. Firm dates and times leave little room for argument and place the manager on the offensive.

The employee may be apprehensive or even defensive at this point, but the phrasing will certainly get his or her attention, and the discussion should produce either the motivation to improve or the clarity that termination is in order.

Terminating Employees

The necessity for dismissing an employee is unpleasant at best, but if the ground rules are decided on in advance, written into the policy manual, and explained to all employees, the problem is partially solved. The policies must be applied equally and impartially to all. The final decision for dismissal probably will be made by the physician but may be based on the recommendation of the office manager or supervisor. The person who does the hiring should do the firing.

The probationary employee who does not prove satisfactory should be dismissed at the end of the probationary period, with tact and a full explanation of the reasons for dismissal. In all fairness, an individual should be told why the employment is being ended and not be given weak excuses or untruths that do not help to correct deficiencies. If the manager is not straightforward in giving the reason for dismissal, the employee will not have the opportunity to grow and improve his or her performance.

An employee who has been in service for some time and is offering unsatisfactory performance should be warned and given an explanation of the specific improvements expected (Figure 24-8). If a second chance does not produce improvement in performance or attitude, then dismissal must follow. It should be done privately, with tact and consideration.

Most practice consultants believe that firing should come close to the end of the day, after all other employees have left, and that the break should be clean and immediate. If the office policy provides for 2 weeks' notice, the physician may wish to offer 2 weeks' pay unless the circumstances that led to the dismissal were extremely **blatant.** A dismissed employee should never be allowed to train or influence a replacement.

The exit meeting should be planned just as carefully as the employment interview. Be honest with the employee. Discuss the employee's assets as well as liabilities, and give the reasons for the termination. There is no need to dwell on the employee's deficiencies. These should have been thoroughly discussed at the warning interview, and the employee need only be told that the necessary improvements have not been made. Do listen to the employee's feedback, unless it becomes abusive. This may reveal some important administrative problems that need correction.

After dismissing an employee, do not leave that person in the office unattended. Request and get the office keys and any other equipment in the employee's possession before the dismissed employee leaves the building. Most states have strict payday laws that will not allow holding the final paycheck for any reason. Do not offer to give the employee a good reference unless it can be done sincerely.

Certain breaches of conduct, such as **embezzlement, insubordination,** and violation of patient confidentiality, are grounds for immediate dismissal without warning.

Occasionally an employee voluntarily terminates a job without giving a valid reason. The physician or office manager may wish to follow up with a letter to the former employee to determine whether a problem prompted the resignation.

Fair Salaries and Raises

Medical office managers should recruit employees who will remain with the office for a long period of time. There are always situations when a part-time worker returns to college, or someone working during the summer months goes back to school. However, good employee **retention** is a goal to work toward.

For good employees to be kept, they must be paid a fair salary and will expect regular raises if they are performing as expected. The office manager can find information about salary comparisons on the Internet. Check the job duties and descriptions found on the web, and see if the salary that the medical facility is offering is comparable to other salaries for similar jobs in the area.

Merit raises are increases based on an employee's commendable performance. Cost-of-living increases are given when earned, usually after specific periods or annually, and are based on national statistics and trends. An employee who is being promoted may be awarded a salary increase, also. When the office pays a fair salary for the work being done, the physician will retain happy employees.

STAFF MEETINGS

There must be some formal mechanism for keeping the office manager and other key employees current on the daily business affairs of the practice. One of the most common complaints from office personnel is that of being unable to discuss problems with the physician. The solution to this problem may be to hold regular staff meetings, which may be scheduled as frequently as weekly but should be held no less often than quarterly (Figure 24-9). Some of the best ideas on improvement come from the office staff, and expressing ideas should be encouraged.

The simplest technique is to set aside a specific time for regular meetings at an hour when the most people can attend

TERMINATION / REHIRE EVALUATION FORM

Employee Name_____   Social Security No. _____

Department _____   Title _____

Termination Date _____

Reason for Termination: _____Resigned _____Laid Off_____Retired

Evaluation of Job Performance	Excellent	Very Good	Average	Poor	Unacceptable
Quality (accuracy, etc.)	☐	☐	☐	☐	☐
Quantity (productivity, consistency, etc.)	☐	☐	☐	☐	☐
Knowledge of Duties	☐	☐	☐	☐	☐
Reliability (absenteeism)	☐	☐	☐	☐	☐
Punctuality	☐	☐	☐	☐	☐
Ability to Cooperate with Co-workers	☐	☐	☐	☐	☐
Relationship with Patients	☐	☐	☐	☐	☐
Overall Attitude (willingness and commitment)	☐	☐	☐	☐	☐
Initiative	☐	☐	☐	☐	☐
Judgment	☐	☐	☐	☐	☐

Recommendation for Rehiring: _____

_____

_____

Comments:_____

_____

_____

_____

_____

_____

_____

_____ Date _____

Supervisor's Signature

FORM # 72-123   PERSONNEL RECORDS ORGANIZING SYSTEMS • © 1987 BIBBERO SYSTEMS, INC. • PETALUMA, CA.
TO REORDER CALL TOLL FREE: (800) BIBBERO (800-242-2376) OR FAX (800) 242-9330   Mғɢ ɪɴ U.S.A.

FIGURE 24-8 Termination form. Document the reasons for terminating employees, and be sure that there is supporting documentation showing warnings and previous counseling efforts. (Courtesy Bibbero Systems, Inc., Petaluma, Calif. 94954, (800) 242-2376, www.bibbero.com.)

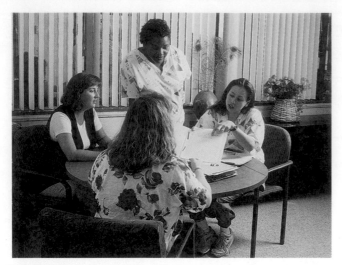

FIGURE 24-9 Periodic staff meetings are important tools for improving communication and resolving problems.

with the least disruption (Procedure 24-3). The meetings need not be long or overly formal, but to be effective they must be planned and organized. There must be a leader, and a secretary should be appointed to take notes. The effectiveness of the leader, a person who can balance firmness with fairness, is an important aspect of the meeting. This is usually either the physician or the office manager or supervisor. All members of the staff should be encouraged to submit ideas for discussion.

Draw up a simple **agenda** listing the issues to be discussed, and prepare any supporting data needed for the meeting. There are many kinds of staff meetings. They may be purely informational, problem-solving, or brainstorming meetings. They may be work sessions for updating manuals, training seminars, or whatever is necessary to that individual practice. Or, meetings may be scheduled to discuss new ideas and any changes in office procedures. Some meetings are held simply to resolve specific problems. The staff meeting must not be allowed to deteriorate into a gripe session. Individual complaints should be handled privately.

The meeting must have a set agenda, with time for topics that need discussion on a regular basis as well as time to handle any current problems. The agenda might be similar to that of any business meeting:

1. Reading of the last meeting's minutes
2. Discussion of any unfinished business
3. Discussion of any problems in the clinical area
4. Discussion of any problems in the administrative area
5. Discussion of any problems in common areas
6. Adjournment

Some physicians like to combine the staff meeting with a breakfast or lunch. The time or place is not important as long as it is neutral and meets the needs of the practice. Meetings should be conducted regularly, democratically, and without interruption. There must be follow-up to the items discussed; otherwise, the only result will be frustration and a reluctance to discuss problems at future meetings.

SEEING THE WHOLE PICTURE

The office manager must keep a bird's-eye view on the office operations. He or she must look at the whole picture when difficulties arise. Remember, there are always two sides to every story, and there is usually truth intermingled with falsity. Do not form the habit of taking every word that an employee says as being 100% accurate. This is not meant to suggest that all employees are not truthful, but to encourage the office manager to look at all sides before making critical decisions.

See issues from the employees' point of view. Try to understand their perspective when dealing with everyday situations in the medical facility. Do not become closed-minded as a manager, unable to grasp what the employees see as important.

OTHER OFFICE MANAGER RESPONSIBILITIES

Patient Information Folder

Only a very small percentage of practices have a booklet that explains the information basic to the operational and service aspects of the practice. Yet, the physician and staff can easily compile a patient information folder cooperatively during a staff meeting. Experience has shown that if such a folder is given to every new patient, the number of incoming telephone calls can be reduced by an average of 20% to 30%. It also can reduce misunderstandings and forgotten instructions. The folder must of necessity be tailored to the specific practice.

The patient information folder should be an introduction to the practice and, if possible, mailed to a new patient before the first visit. A supply also may be left with referring physicians' offices to be given to patients coming to your office. It should be designed to fit easily into a No. 10 business envelope.

The cover should show the name of the practice, its location, and the practice logo, if there is one. Consider using a photo of the medical building for easy identification by the new patient, and a map to the office.

A statement of philosophy frequently is included in the introduction, followed by a description of the practice, such as in the example below:

"The doctors and staff would like to welcome you to our office. We work as a team with the goal of providing prompt and thorough care for your problems. We are always working to improve our care and service in any way possible. Our practice is limited exclusively to the musculoskeletal system and its disorders. Therefore it is important for each patient to have a primary care physician such as a pediatrician, family physician, or internist to oversee the primary medical care for the entire patient. Our role is most effective as a consultant to your primary care physician."

Describe the office policy regarding appointments and cancellations, telephone calls, and the function of the answering service. If a separate business telephone line is available, be sure to include this information, as in the following example:

"This office has two receptionists available to answer telephone calls during regular office hours. The office is very busy, and occasionally you will be asked to hold for a brief period. Please be patient with this. If you wish to speak to a doctor, your call usually will be returned during the next available break period or

PROCEDURE 24-3

Arrange a Group Meeting

ABHES COMPETENCY: 3.a

GOAL: *To plan and execute a productive meeting that will result in achieved goals.*

EQUIPMENT and SUPPLIES

- Meeting room
- Agenda
- Visual aids and equipment
- Handouts
- Stopwatch or clock
- Computer or word processor
- Paper
- List of items for the agenda

PROCEDURAL STEPS

1. Determine the purpose of the meeting, and draft a list of the items to be discussed. Include the desired results of the meeting.
   PURPOSE: To keep the focus on the issues at hand and make the meeting a productive one.
2. Determine where the meeting will be held, the time and date of the meeting, and the individuals who should attend.
   PURPOSE: To have the demographic information about the meeting on hand before posting a notice. Only necessary staff members should attend, so that those not directly involved in the issues to be discussed can continue their regular duties.
3. Send a memo, email, or letter at least 10 days in advance, if possible, to the individuals who should attend the meeting. Send a copy to any supervisors who should be kept informed about the issues to be raised in the meeting.
   PURPOSE: To allow for rescheduling if the key personnel cannot attend on the originally planned time and date. To keep managers informed of important details in areas for which they are ultimately responsible.
4. Be sure that the notice includes the following information:
   - Date
   - Time
   - Place
   - Directions, if not in a common meeting room or if away from the office
   - Speakers and/or meeting topics
   - Cost and registration information, if applicable
   - List of items individuals should bring to the meeting
   PURPOSE: To fully inform those who should attend the meeting of the demographic information and their responsibilities.
5. Finalize the list of items to discuss, and place them in priority order.
   PURPOSE: To keep the focus of the meeting on the issues at hand and to avoid discussion of nonrelated items. To make certain that the time spent in the meeting is productive for all involved.
6. Delegate any tasks that others can accomplish, and follow up to be sure that they fulfill their duties before the meeting.
   PURPOSE: To ensure that all needed information and items are available for the meeting.
7. Assign a staff member the task of taking notes and keeping time during the meeting.
   PURPOSE: To have notes as to what happened so that a permanent record of what was discussed and the decisions that were made can be written after the meeting.
8. Make a list of all items that need to be taken to the meeting, including equipment such as microphones, projectors, screens, computers, disks containing presentations, and so on.
   PURPOSE: To be fully prepared and have all needed items in place during the meeting.
9. Compile the final agenda for the meeting.
10. On the meeting day, transport all items needed to the meeting room. Begin and end the meeting on time. Stay on track, and follow the agenda.
    PURPOSE: Following the plan and being considerate of the time that staff members devote to meetings will promote a positive attitude for meetings and will encourage group participation.
11. Follow up whenever necessary on items discussed in the meetings. Distribute a synopsis of the meeting to all of the individuals who attended, and keep a copy in a binder or folder.
    PURPOSE: To have a permanent record of the meeting and the items discussed and decided.

---

at the end of the office day. We receive many calls during the day, and it is unfair to the patients who have scheduled appointments to continually interrupt the doctor for telephone calls. Therefore the receptionist usually will take a message, and your call will be returned as soon as possible. Please inform the receptionist if your problem is urgent and she will let the doctor know this."

Describe any **ancillary** or laboratory services provided, how test results are reported, and your policy on prescription renewals. Patients need to know the provisions for emergency procedures: What hospitals does the practice use regularly?

What is the night and weekend coverage? Hospitalization procedures and postoperative care and follow-up may also be included:

"One of the doctors in the group is always on call for emergency situations. You may reach him by calling our office telephone number (714) 555-2323, and the answering service will put you in touch with the doctor on call at that time. Our doctors are on staff at St. Joseph Hospital (714) 555-3333 and, for children, Children's Hospital of Orange County (714) 555-4444. In case of emergency, call 911."

List all physicians in the practice; state their educational backgrounds, training, and board certifications; and define their specialties. List the names of key clinical and administrative staff members, such as registered nurses and nurse practitioners, medical assistants, the office manager, and the business manager. Provide the practice address, a map of how to get there, and information about the parking facilities.

Do not just stack these folders in the reception room for patients to pick up. Have the receptionist write the patient's name on the folder, hand it to the patient when he or she registers for the first appointment, and suggest that the patient keep it for future reference.

Financial Policy Folder

A separate small folder covering the financial policies of the office can eliminate many questions and possible misunderstandings. Tailor the financial policy folder to the specific practice. Keep it small enough to fit into the billing envelope, and send it out with the first monthly statement. If the practice sends out a welcome package before the patient's first visit, include the financial policy folder. Otherwise, present one at the first visit.

Spell out policies regarding billing and collection procedures, and make it clear that patients are responsible for the uninsured portion of the fees. If payment is expected at the time of service, put this in the folder. Keep the language simple and straightforward so that the message is clear:

"We ask that our services be paid for at the time they are rendered. You will be provided with an encounter form so that you may bill your insurance company and be reimbursed for services paid at the time of your visit. Simply attach the encounter form to your insurance form and mail it to the insurance company. The appropriate diagnoses and charges will be on the encounter form. There is usually a greater charge for the initial visit, because this involves more time than follow-up visits. If you are sent to an outside office for laboratory testing or special x-ray procedures, you will be billed separately by that office. We will be available to help if special circumstances arise involving difficulty with forms or receiving reimbursement. We will bill your insurance if you have a special situation such as surgery, prepaid health plans, Medicaid, CCS, or Senior Savers. We will complete disability papers as promptly as possible. However, you must obtain the necessary forms from your employer or the disability office."

The financial policy folder should also clearly state that the ultimate responsibility for payment lies with the patient.

Patient Instruction Sheets

In most medical offices there are patient procedures that occur over and over again. Instead of attempting to instruct a patient orally each time, why not develop clearly stated instruction sheets that can be reviewed with the patient, then give the patient the written instructions to take home? The following are suggestions for patient instruction sheets:

- Preparation for x-ray procedure or laboratory tests
- Preoperative and postoperative instructions
- Diet sheets
- Performing an enema
- Dressing a wound

- Taking medications
- Using a cane, crutches, walker, or wheelchair
- Care of casts
- Exercise therapy

Moving a Practice

The thought of moving into a shiny new spacious office can be exciting. However, unless the move is planned in advance, moving day and the weeks that follow can be a nightmare.

Planning the New Quarters

Do some careful measuring to see how the furniture and equipment that will be moved will fit into the new quarters. If possible, draw the rooms to scale and show where each item is to be placed by the mover. Include the location of available electrical outlets in the floor plan. If new furniture, carpets, or equipment is needed, try to have them in place before moving day. Do not expect to have the new carpet installed the day of the move.

Establishing a Moving Date

Decide what day the move will take place and whether the office will close for 1 day or several. Select a mover, and confirm the date. Patients must be notified of the move. As soon as the moving date is established, post a notice in the office and draw the patients' attention to it. Send announcement cards to the active patients. Many physicians place a notice in the local newspapers.

Notifying Utilities and Mailers

At least 60 days in advance of the move, start a change-of-address notification campaign. Notify publishers of journals and suppliers of catalogs. Cards for changes of address are available from the post office. Six weeks' notice generally is required on subscriptions, and postage due on forwarded journals can be very expensive. Notify the telephone company and utility companies well in advance so that there will be no break in service. File a change of address card with the local post office. Order stationery and business cards with the new address.

Packing

The moving company will supply packing cartons. Have each employee be responsible for packing and labeling the items from his or her own work area. Tag each carton with a number, and keep a master list of what is in each numbered carton. This will help in finding items that are needed. Also, if a carton should be lost or mislaid, a record of what was in it will be available. If time allows, just before moving is a good time to cull material from the files and discard old journals, supply catalogs, and any obsolete supplies or equipment.

Moving Day Strategy

Prepare a written outline of the moving day strategy, indicating each person's responsibility, and give each member of the office staff a copy. It may be wise to work in shifts to avoid confusion, but have one person stationed at the new address to direct the movers when they arrive.

Follow-up

After the move, be sure to mention the new address when patients call for appointments. This often is neglected, especially after a few months have passed, and is very upsetting to the patient who tries to check in at the former address.

Closing a Practice

A medical practice may be closed because of retirement, death, a change in geographic location, or a change in profession. If the closing is unexpected, as in the case of sudden death of the physician, much of the burden falls on the staff. If the closing is voluntary and planned for, the physician may wish to consult an attorney or the local medical society for guidelines. The following information is useful in either event.

Advance Notice to Patients

The physician who anticipates retirement can begin cutting back the practice months in advance. Patients can be notified as they come in that the practice will be closing on a specified date and asked to begin arrangements for care from another physician. The physician also can ask that patients pay at the time of service, to minimize accounts receivable at the time of retirement.

Avoiding Abandonment Charge

To avoid a charge of abandonment the physician should notify active patients by letter that the practice is being discontinued. The letter should be sent out at least 3 months in advance, if possible. If a patient has been discharged or has not been given care by the physician for at least 6 years, there is no obligation to send the notice.

Public Announcement

About 1 month after the physician begins telling patients of the closing, an announcement should be placed in a local newspaper, giving the closing date of the office, explaining any arrangements made for continuing care, and thanking patients for their support over the years.

Other Notices

Hospital affiliations should be informed early, particularly if the physician will be leaving the community. If the office space is being rented, be sure to notify the landlord in observance of the rental contract if there is one. Insurance carriers must be advised of the change. The state medical licensure board should be contacted. If the practice is incorporated, an attorney should be consulted about dissolving the corporation.

Patient Transfer and Patient Records

If another physician is taking over the practice, tell the patients about the new physician. However, be sure to explain that a patient's records will be transferred to the physician of his or her choice and that the request for transfer of records must be in writing. For convenience, the physician can have a form available that needs only the patient's signature.

Although the records belong to the physician, they can be transferred legally to another physician only with the consent of the patient. Any records not transferred should be stored, either in bulk or on microfilm or disk, until the statutes of limitations for malpractice and abandonment have run out.

Financial Concerns When a Practice Closes

Income tax returns and supporting documents should be kept for at least 3 years after the tax return was filed. Appoint someone to take care of any remaining outstanding accounts receivable.

Disposition of Controlled Substances

Check with the Drug Enforcement Administration (DEA) for current regulations on disposal of controlled substances and the physician's certificate of registration. Do not simply toss them out. The certificate will have to be sent to the DEA for cancellation, then it will be returned. It may be necessary to produce an inventory of all controlled substances on hand when the practice is terminated, along with duplicate copies of the official order forms that were used to obtain them. Return any unused forms to the DEA. Do not use leftover prescription blanks for note pads. Burn or shred them to prevent misuse.

Professional Liability Insurance

The physician who is discontinuing active medical practice can safely drop the professional liability insurance. However, do not destroy any of the previous policies. Most professional liability claims are covered by the policy that was in effect at the time the alleged act of negligence took place. The suit may be filed many years later, and it is important that the old policy be available.

Furnishings and Equipment

Unfortunately, used office furniture and equipment do not bring much in the marketplace. If another physician is taking over the practice, the value of the furnishings and equipment can be negotiated. Many physicians donate their libraries to the local hospital and declare the gift as an income tax deduction. This is an item to check with the accountant.

A physician may reward loyal employees with severance pay. On average, this equals at least 1 month's salary plus prorated compensation for any unused vacation time. A letter of reference usually is offered.

Many details must be taken care of in closing a medical practice. Contact the local medical society for further guidance.

CLOSING COMMENTS

Successful office managers care about their employees and the vision for the office. They must be strong promoters of the office mission statement. The areas of authority and responsibility must be clearly defined to avoid management problems. A solid office policy and procedure manual will assist the office manager in running an efficient office.

Leadership is an important quality for any manager, and the medical office manager is no exception. The manager should develop good leadership skills, be fair and open-minded, and treat employees and patients as he or she would want to be treated. These actions will help to ensure a pleasant, productive working environment.

Educate patients about the policies and procedures in the office by providing patient information folders or brochures. When these documents are prepared and given to the patients formally, the patient is better informed and fewer calls will come to the office.

Office managers must stay abreast of current employment laws and regulations for all of the different agencies that govern the medical office. Joining an office manager's association will help the manager keep the office up to date and in compliance. Periodic checks on the websites of various organizations, such as OSHA, will help the manager to stay aware of the most recent changes in policies and rules.

Documentation is a critical aspect of the office manager's duties. The manager should keep detailed notes on the performance of employees and always discuss poor performance with employees. Never allow bad habits to go unmentioned. To the extent that it is possible, treat employees in a similar fashion and extend fairness to all.

SUMMARY OF SCENARIO

 Katherine has made an impact on all of the staff members at Dr. Collins's office. She treats her employees well and is fair regarding office policies and procedures. Her subordinates appreciate her flexibility and professionalism as she deals with the many issues surrounding the operation of a medical office. Katherine treats the employees as team members, never speaking to them as if she were superior to them. She shares vital information with the staff so that they feel a part of the whole team and believes that even some negative information should be related to the staff so that everyone is aware of the challenges the office faces. She makes good hiring decisions and firmly believes in a good orientation and training program. Dr. Collins has placed a great deal of trust in Katherine, and she has performed well, proving to be reliable in her position as office manager.

Katherine knows that she should display a friendly attitude toward her staff members when appropriate to do so. She is kind and considerate and treats the staff as individuals. She does not fraternize with them, but is open to having lunch with the staff at various times and participates in all casual office activities. She maintains a healthy distance so that she can be an effective manager, but she listens to those who are experiencing difficulty and is compassionate about helping whenever possible.

Katherine knows that she must be diligent in checking references so that she brings reliable, qualified individuals on board as staff members. Unless she receives acceptable references, she will not hire a medical assistant to become a part of her team. Once she hires someone, she conducts a thorough training program and takes special care to share the experience and skills of the new staff member with the rest of the team.

When Katherine must give a negative employee evaluation, she states that fact at the beginning of their meeting. Although she is compassionate, she is able to point out a staff member's shortcomings in a detailed, fair way. She is usually willing to give an employee time to improve, but if he or she fails to perform, Katherine does not hesitate to end the employment.

Katherine uses patient information folders as management tools. She has instructed her staff to fully explain the folders to patients and tell them about the information contained within them. Because the staff takes the time to review the folders with patients, calls to the office have been reduced and the staff feels that patients are much more informed. They understand office policies much better, and the staff finds that they repeat basic information much less frequently. Katherine heads a cooperative team that functions well together every day, making the office efficient and the work environment a pleasant one of which to be a part.

SUMMARY of LEARNING OBJECTIVES

1. Define, spell, and pronounce the terms listed in the vocabulary.
   - Spelling and pronouncing medical terms correctly adds credibility to the medical assistant. Knowing the definition of these terms promotes confidence in communication with patients and co-workers.
2. Explain the importance of management in the medical office.
   - Management is an important aspect of running a professional medical office. The physician counts on the office manager to run the business aspects of the office so that he or she can focus efforts on good patient care. A high degree of trust is placed with the office manager.

3. Discuss the desirable qualities of a medical office manager.
   - A good office manager is fair and flexible. Good communications skills are necessary, as well as attention to details. The manager should care about the employees and have a sense of fairness. The ability to remain calm in a crisis is important, as is the use of good judgment and ability to organize tasks.
4. List and discuss the three types of leaders.
   - Charismatic leaders inspire allegiance and dedication and encourage individuals to overcome great obstacles. The transactional leader is structured and organized, hardworking,

Continued

SUMMARY of LEARNING OBJECTIVES
Continued

and a planner. The transformational leader is excellent during times of transition and is effective at building relationships.

5. Discuss several types of power and whether power is a positive or negative entity.
   - Power can be both a positive and a negative entity. Power should not be used in a manipulative or coercive manner. Expert power is based on a high degree of knowledge about a certain subject. Using rewards is one form of invoking power, and legitimate power is that of position or status. Referent power is granted from subordinates to those who lead by example.

6. Identify several ways in which employees are motivated.
   - Employees are motivated by various factors, including money, praise, insecurity, honor, prestige, needs, love, fear, satisfaction, and many others. The effective manager attempts to discover what motivates employees to do a good job.

7. Explain the difference between intrinsic and extrinsic motivation.
   - Intrinsic motivation comes from within the employee. Extrinsic motivation has an outside source.

8. List several ways to prevent burnout.
   - Asking for help, first and foremost, can prevent burnout. Managers often take on too many duties and do not delegate as much as they should. Exercise and rest help prevent burnout, as well as understanding one's personal limitations. Focused goals are important and help keep the manager working toward the most critical tasks.

9. Discuss what to look for when reviewing resumes and applications.
   - Resumes and applications should be reviewed for accuracy and completeness. Gaps in employment dates should be explained fully, and the office manager should verify any references given. Documents should be legible, and the information contained should be consistent and without oversights.

10. Explain why the telephone voice of an applicant is important.
    - The telephone voice of an applicant is important because most employees have occasion to answer the telephone while at work. The employee's voice should be clear and easily understandable. Good grammar skills must be used to reflect a professional image.

11. Identify the follow-up activities the office manager should perform after an interview.
    - After interviewing a prospective candidate, the office manager should verify the facts on the resume and application and check several references. A comparison should be made between the candidates and the top two or three chosen for a possible second interview. It is wise to involve other staff members when choosing new employees for the office.

12. Explain the importance of mentors for new employees in the medical office.
    - Mentors assist new employees by offering information regarding policies and procedures. The mentor can be a helpful advocate that the new employee can approach when questions arise about any aspect of the medical office.

13. List the various types of staff meetings.
    - Staff meetings may be held to relay information, solve a problem, or brainstorm ideas. Some meetings are designed as work sessions, whereas others may be scheduled to discuss new policies or changes in procedures.

14. Successfully arrange a group meeting.
    - Meetings will be held on at least a monthly basis in most physician offices. The process for arranging a group meeting is outlined in Procedure 24-3.

15. Interview a job candidate for a position at the facility.
    - By making job candidates comfortable during job interviews, the manager will be able to evaluate the candidate as he or she is expressing the skills that will be pertinent to the position. The process for interviewing a job candidate is outlined in Procedure 24-1.

16. Conduct a performance review for an employee.
    - Performance reviews can be productive, positive experiences, or can lead to termination of employment. The process for conducting a performance review is outlined in Procedure 24-2.

CONNECTIONS

Study Guide Connection: Go to Chapter 24 Study Guide. Read the Case Study and Workplace Applications and complete the assignments. Do online research for answers to the questions in the Internet Activities associated with medical practice management and human resources.

CD Connection: Go to the Medical Assisting Competency Challenge CD and do the training activities under General Office Duties.

Evolve Connection: For more information related to medical practice management and human resources, go to http://evolve.elsevier.com/kinn/admin and visit related weblinks for Chapter 24. Click on the Medical Assisting Exam Review and do the practice questions to sharpen your test-taking skills. To learn more about office software, do the exercises for the Altapoint demo that is on the CD.

Medical Practice Marketing and Customer Service

25

Monica Ray is a medical assistant who is also pursuing a bachelor's degree in marketing. She has worked for Drs. Julie and Robert Todd for 2 years, and based on her interest in marketing the physicians have agreed to allow her to develop some new strategies for their obstetrics and gynecology office.

Monica is highly computer literate and can design Web pages. She plans to incorporate several ideas that she saw on other physicians' websites, including a method of online scheduling. She is quite creative and is excited about the challenge of providing such a service to the patients of the clinic.

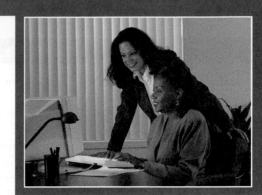

Monica knows that planning is involved in any project, such as the facility's Internet presence. She plans to speak to every employee of the office to get input regarding the design and content of the site. Patients will be able to provide her with additional suggestions as to what features they would like to see.

This new development for the office is just one way that Monica hopes to incorporate more formal customer service techniques. She plans to share the information she is learning in the classroom with the physicians and staff at the clinic. Monica and the doctors are fortunate that the staff is enthusiastic and eager to try new methods of customer service. The physicians will set specific goals with the help of the employees and devise a reward system for reaching them. An exciting few months are ahead for this innovative group of medical professionals!

While studying this chapter, think about the following questions:

- How important is an Internet presence to today's medical office?
- Why has *customer service* become a buzzword in the medical industry?

- How do presentation skills enhance the medical assistant's career?
- Which is more important—the internal or the external customer?

LEARNING OBJECTIVES

1. Define, spell, and pronounce the terms listed in the vocabulary.
2. List the three steps to be followed when preparing to implement a medical marketing strategy.
3. Explain the term *target market*.
4. Discuss how suggestion boxes might help the medical facility to make improvements.
5. List and discuss the "four P's" of marketing.
6. Explain the five steps for developing a plan in marketing.

7. Discuss how community involvement can make a difference in marketing efforts.
8. State the difference between advertising and public relations.
9. Determine ways to promote a new practice.
10. Discuss responses that help the medical assistant identify with the patient.
11. Explain the concept of the internal customer.
12. Design a presentation for a marketing event.
13. Prepare a presentation using PowerPoint.

VOCABULARY

marketing The process or technique of promoting, selling, and distributing a product or service.

objectives Something toward which effort is directed; aims, goals, or ends of action.

outreach The process of using marketing and education strategies to reach and involve diverse audiences through the use of key messages and effective programs.

prosthetic (prohs-thet′-ik) The surgical or dental specialty concerned with the design, construction, and fitting of prostheses, which are artificial devices that replace missing parts of the body.

tangible (tan′-juh-buhl) Capable of being appraised at an actual or approximate value; capable of being precisely identified or realized by the mind.

target market A specific group of individuals toward whom the marketing plan is focused.

Each medical office needs a mission statement that defines the reason for the existence of the office. The physician's philosophy of medicine and reasons for pursing medicine as a career greatly influence the mission statement. With this statement in place, the staff develops goals that will assist them in meeting the mission. The goals can be met through a **marketing** and **outreach** plan for the practice and by providing excellent customer service to patients and visitors of the facility.

DEVELOPING MARKETING STRATEGIES

If a business is to grow, marketing strategies are critical. A marketing strategy is designed to promote the services offered by the organization and encourage new business. Three steps are generally followed when preparing to implement or change medical marketing strategies:

- Evaluate what is being done now to increase patient flow.
- Decide what **objectives** are important and how meeting these objectives will be measured.
- Develop a plan with various means of marketing the practice and a specific methodology for implementing each phase.

CRITICAL THINKING APPLICATION

- Monica knows that the office has never attempted any formal marketing in the past. Because no one at her office is familiar with this task, who might she contact for advice and assistance?
- Even though her fellow staff members are not familiar with marketing, could they provide workable ideas?
- What are some ideas for marketing a medical practice?

Knowing the Target Market

During the strategic phase of developing a marketing plan, the physician and office manager must identify the **target market** for the services provided by the clinic. The target market is the group or groups of individuals that the office wishes to reach. Reaching the target market means that the specific groups are made aware of the clinic and what it has to offer. With managed care restrictions and regulations, competition for patients has become keen among physicians, and a facility that does not pursue growth runs a great risk of not surviving.

Several questions must be answered when discussing the target market. Consider the following:

- What specific outcomes do we hope to accomplish?
- What are the needs and desires of our target market?
- What are the characteristics of a typical member of the target market?
- How can the target market be reached in the most cost-effective ways?

Staff meetings are excellent times to brainstorm about reaching target markets. The staff can relate the needs of the patients who are active at the medical office. If patients have made suggestions, they should be discussed and weighed with regard to which most would benefit the patient population of the facility (Figure 25-1).

CRITICAL THINKING APPLICATION

- What community resources could Monica seek as she is determining the target market of the practice?
- What information does she need to begin her search?

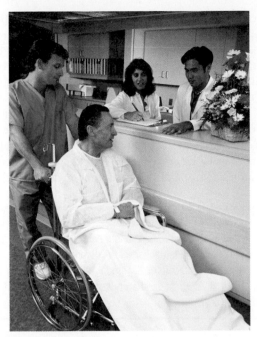

FIGURE 25-1 Friendly staff members are the best marketing tools. A smile is an excellent way to make patients feel welcome in the medical facility.

Suggestion boxes are a great way to solicit patient input. Ask patients for ideas about how the clinic could operate in a smoother fashion and what additional services they would like to see introduced at the facility. Provide and frequently check the suggestion box. If the patient leaves his or her name on the suggestion form, it is a good customer service tactic to reward the patient for the suggestion. Mail the patient a coupon for a free lunch at a local restaurant or a free car wash at a local detailing shop. Involving other businesses in marketing efforts helps both attract new customers.

The "Four P's"

The "four P's" of marketing include product, placement, price, and promotion. A physician's office offers medical services as a product. Some offices have **tangible** retail products that they also offer, such as vitamins, skin-sensitive cosmetics, or **prosthetic** devices. Placement involves the actual location of the medical office. The office may be located in an urban area close to large neighborhoods of young professionals or in a rural area with a few people living several miles apart. Placement can greatly influence the traffic to the facility. Placement can refer also to the setup of the office, the specific suite in a shopping strip where the office is located, or even the placement of retail objects on a shelf.

Price is simply the amount of money charged for goods and services provided. Promotion refers to the methods used to get the product or services to the consumers, or patients in the case of the medical office.

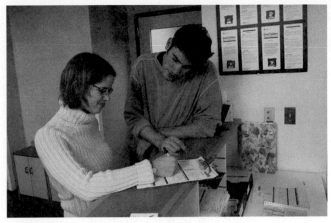

FIGURE 25-2 Offer services that are important in the geographic area of the office. College students may need to see a physician for minor illnesses, and they will appreciate offices that provide short office visits for a reasonable fee.

Deciding What Services to Offer

Once the physician and office manager have identified the target market, decisions can be made regarding what services should be offered to the patients. For instance, suppose the office is situated in a neighborhood of young families. There is a strong possibility that both parents work outside the home, so evening hours would be beneficial to these patients. The physician may decide to extend office hours to 8:00 PM twice a week and to open from 9:00 AM to noon on Saturdays. If there are several schools in the area, particularly junior high and high schools, the physician may wish to offer a special price on sports physicals during the fall. Schools often require physicals, and if the physician offers them at a reasonable price, the entire family may decide to seek medical care from the physician.

If the office is located in a college town, the physician may wish to offer a special student rate for short office visits (Figure 25-2). If a number of senior citizens live in the area, a senior citizen discount might be appropriate. Input from patients and staff members will be valuable in deciding what services to offer in the medical facility.

Developing a Plan

The facility may use several specific planning steps for events, marketing strategies, and any number of other ideas that the physician would like to implement. They are as follows:

• Assessment
• Research
• Planning
• Execution
• Evaluation

Assessment is the phase of planning in which the problem or goals are reviewed. This is another excellent time for brainstorming. Research allows the physician or office manager to investigate the needs of the target market, then decide what the medical office can do to meet those needs. Planning the concept follows, and once a firm plan is in place it is executed or carried out. Afterward, the participants evaluate what went well and what problems occurred so that future efforts will be even more successful.

PROMOTING THE PRACTICE

The physician and office manager should constantly watch for ways to promote the medical practice and keep its name in the public eye. Some of these methods are free of charge, and others will need detailed budgeting and planning. By becoming a member of various civic organizations, such as the Chamber of Commerce, the practice will receive notice of upcoming events and should plan to participate in them on a regular basis. The more that the public sees the physician in the community, the more likely this will affect the growth of the practice.

Tapping into Free Resources

Many good promotional activities are relatively free to the physician. One of the most popular and beneficial to the physician is a professional website. If the physician or an office staff member has sufficient knowledge for website construction, then there is little or no cost to the doctor if one of the free website services is used. Businesses that host websites on the Internet offer very reasonable costs, starting at around $25 per month.

Some newspapers offer an advice column wherein different types of professionals give general medical advice to those who write in with questions. Physicians volunteer to answer these questions in print, and in return the office address, the office telephone number, and often the physicians' pictures are featured. This is an excellent way to generate patient calls and inform the public about the specialties and types of cases the physician handles.

CRITICAL THINKING APPLICATION

- Monica knows there are many opportunities and free resources in her area. Where should she begin to look?
- How might Monica's clinic partner with other businesses and services to provide excellent care to patients and to help one another at the same time?

Community Involvement

Getting involved in the local community is another way to promote a medical practice. Some physicians sponsor Little League football teams, baseball teams, or bowling leagues. Some entire staffs participate in charity events and marathons, wearing T-shirts with the clinic name printed on the back.

The physician or staff may have specific charities that they support on an annual basis, or they may participate in United Way activities, which distribute funds to many different types of worthy organizations through payroll deductions and other gifts. Some medical facilities have volunteer programs in which employees receive recognition for participation in various activities. A good example includes blood donations. Many blood centers offer pins and recognition certificates for the number of pints of blood that volunteers donate. The office staff may set a goal to reach a certain number of donated pints in a year, and as recognition certificates are collected the staff may wish to display them in a prominent place in the office. This is

an indication to patients that the staff is concerned about the community and is volunteer-minded. From a public relations standpoint this is valuable to the medical office, because patients tend to expect medical professionals to be volunteer oriented.

Health fairs are a great avenue for promoting the services offered by the clinic, resulting in name recognition and increasing public visibility. Some health fairs are huge, highly publicized events, whereas others are small, often held at a local shopping mall or grocery store. All of these events could be worthy projects for the physician and the medical office.

CRITICAL THINKING APPLICATION

- What community organizations might help Monica in her efforts to make the office an integral part of the community?
- What resources and community organizations are available in your area that would be good avenues for practice marketing and community service?

Advertising Plans and Agencies

Most physician offices do not use advertising agencies to promote their practices, but on occasion an agency might be useful (Figure 25-3). If a very special event is scheduled that needs extensive planning, then a public relations firm or advertising agency might be consulted. Unfortunately, the cost of these groups is usually high and beyond the reach of sole practitioners or small group practices. However, the investment may be well spent when an event is critical and attendance is important to its success.

There is a difference between advertising and public relations. Advertising could be defined as "creating or changing attitudes, beliefs, and perceptions by influencing people with purchased broadcast time, print space, or other forms of written and visual media." Broadcast time could take the form of television commercials, radio broadcasts, or audiovisual aids. Print could be in a newspaper, magazine, or trade journal, and written and visual media may be a flier, brochure, or billboard. Public relations offerings are influential as well, using news broadcasts, radio reports, and magazine or newspaper articles to reach people. Most public relations efforts are free, but it is often difficult to get others interested enough in the activities the medical office is planning to warrant coverage.

Communication as a Marketing Tool

Many medical offices use communications tools to market the practice and improve customer service. Sending a monthly newsletter through mail or electronically provides health information and news about upcoming events. The newsletter can be very personalized for the office and might even include news about patients and the medical staff, as long as permission is obtained.

Sending birthday cards is an excellent public relations tool. Some offices sign the greetings at staff meetings, and they are placed in a tickler file for the proper mailing date. Sending holiday greetings is another method of wishing patients well.

FINDING A GOOD ADVERTISING AGENCY

1. *Define your objective in hiring an ad agency.* What do you want to achieve? What should be different after the agency goes to work for you? What kind of working relationship do you prefer?
2. *Check out sources.* Consider work you have seen or heard that has impressed you. Call friends and colleagues you trust and get their recommendations. Attend professional or trade association meetings, and talk to members who have used agencies before. Seek out their opinions, and note whose names come up often (both pro and con). Watch for articles about ad agencies in area papers, trade magazines, and related publications, such as chamber of commerce newsletters.
3. *Once you have a list of candidates, screen them by telephone.* Ask about their backgrounds, projects they have worked on, the results they have had, their fees, and anything else important to you. Then set up interviews with the three or four firms that impressed you the most.
4. *Interview the finalists.* Find out the following:
   - *Do they have experience working with your industry?* What is their track record when working with companies like yours? Do they understand your business and the nuances of what you do? If not, are they willing to research the information they need?
   - *Is there chemistry?* You can tell if there is a good "fit" with an ad agency. A good agency will express interest in getting to know you as an individual and learning more about your company. They will be good listeners and quick learners. They will make good suggestions and react quickly to your questions and opinions. They should demonstrate the ability to anticipate what is best for your business and be prepared to disagree with you if they feel you are on the wrong track.
   - *Do they show originality and creativity?* Based on the agency's previous work, do you feel these people understand how best to "sell" your product or service? If you operate a home healthcare agency, for example, you probably do not want an ad campaign that features technology over tenderness. Sensing your clientele, the agency should know enough about you to put together the appropriate message.
   - *Are they reliable and budget conscious?* No amount of chemistry and creativity can make up for a missed deadline or an estimate that is way off. Be sure the agency has not only the creative skills needed but also the time and commitment to devote to your needs. Whether you are the biggest or smallest client in their stable, you should be able to count on consistent attention to detail. Their staff should be available to answer your questions and be accountable for delays and expenses.

FIGURE 25-3 Selecting an advertising or public relations agency. (From Anderson L: *Star makers.* Entrepreneur Magazine, April 1997.)

Automated call distribution is becoming a popular means of communicating with large numbers of people. A computer dials multiple numbers at the same time and plays a recorded message, which can be the actual physician reading a message. Although many people block such calls to their homes and an equal number hang up, the success rate for automatic call distribution is actually quite good.

Many individuals listen and respond to the calls, especially if they come from someone they know and the information is important. For instance, if a medical clinic were planning to move to another part of the city, a program could be initiated to notify all patients with telephone numbers that the office will be moving after a certain date. The message could include the address of the new location, and even prompt patients to "press 1" if they need to schedule an appointment. The same principle could be applied to news about an upcoming health fair, a special seminar about a certain illness, or even an article that will be in the Sunday paper about the clinic.

Promoting a New Practice

Most physicians who open a new practice place an ad in local newspapers to announce the event. Usually a picture of the physician is included, and a map to the exact location may be available on the ad. Some physicians purchase clinics from others who are moving or retiring, but many will open a freestanding clinic in a new building, and the word about the new facility must be spread for the business to be a success.

Providing business cards for all employees is a good way to increase public knowledge about the facility. Some offices offer incentives for patient referrals from the staff or other patients, but the physician must ensure that there are no state statutes or ethical standards that prohibit this. The incentive could be a simple coffee cup with the clinic's logo on it or a book about a healthcare issue. Recognition is the important factor where referrals are concerned. A thank-you card is the minimal acceptable "thanks" for patient referrals.

Some physicians hold an open house when the new facility opens. Often, those individuals who assisted with the business from its inception will attend the open house to lend support to the owners. Bankers, attorneys, accountants, and other physicians will often show their support by attending the open house. Pictures from this event should be placed on the facility's website or in the monthly newsletter.

Developing and Giving Presentations

Today's medical assistant should be comfortable when speaking in front of individuals and groups. By developing additional skills the medical assistant increases his or her value to the physician. Developing and giving presentations is not difficult, although one of the most prevalent fears in the United States is the fear of speaking in public (Procedures 25-1 and 25-2).

There are many different types of speeches, but remember that all public speaking is persuasive. The speaker is attempting to get the audience to do something—whether to buy a new product or convince people to vote. The speaker always has a purpose and must be credible to convince listeners to act. Credibility underlies all persuasion. When the speaker is proficient at persuasion, the audience's questions are answered, their concerns addressed, and their needs fulfilled, while at the same time the speaker's goals are met. If the speaker does a good job, the audience will feel satisfied after hearing a persuasive speech. Persuasion should be nonadversarial and gentle so that the audience feels comfortable in making a decision.

Jerry Weissman, in his book *Presenting to Win: The Art of Telling Your Story*, calls persuasion "audience advocacy"—by that, he means the ability to view the self, a company, a story, or a presentation through the eyes of the audience. Answer the question, "'What's in it for me?" which the audience is constantly thinking. To motivate the audience, the speaker must do the following:

- Know the audience
- Research the audience to know their needs, what they care about, and what they want to know
- Link all presentation information to the audience's needs
- Know the purpose of the presentation
- Rehearse the presentation repeatedly

When designing the content of the presentation, keep the audience in mind, and nail down the most important points that must be conveyed to them.

Overcoming Anxiety

Because the fear of public speaking is so common, the speaker must develop ways to overcome the fear and make a successful presentation. Find the actions that promote relaxation, and practice them before giving a speech. Look for a sympathetic face in the audience, and speak directly to that person. Never begin a presentation with an apology of any type such as, "I didn't have much time to prepare" or "I'm not very good at presentations." This undermines the authority of the speaker. Greeting as many of the guests as possible before the presentation helps to develop a rapport and may reduce anxiety. In addition, the guests feel welcome and special because the speaker took the time to make introductions.

During the Presentation

Make certain that the audience can hear everything that is being said. The presentation cannot be effective if it cannot be heard. Make all movements purposeful; if a hand gesture is used, make it then relax the arms. Do not wander around the room. If moving from place to place, go to a spot then stop. Constant movement distracts from the message of the presentation.

Most individuals speak faster when making a presentation, so slow down the pace just a little. Speak so that all the people in the back of the room can hear, but not so loudly that the people in the front rows have to cover their ears. Possibly most important, remember to relax. The physical reactions felt before speaking, such as an increase in pulse rate and a rush of adrenaline, are natural. Do not allow negative thoughts to enter the mind. Instead, deal with fear by knowing the topic and being confident about the message.

Building a Practice Website

Four basic steps are involved in building a website for the medical practice. These steps include the following:

- Define the objectives of the website.
- Design the pages.
- Locate a Web server to which the pages can be uploaded.
- Upload the pages to the server.

Defining Objectives

When defining objectives, important decisions about specific goals must be considered. The physician and staff should discuss who the audience for the website will be and what will be included on the site. Most websites designed for physician offices and clinics are informational, developed mostly for patient and public use. Once the objectives are clearly defined, specific content can be written to place on the website.

Preparing a Presentation

Answer these important questions when preparing a presentation:

- Who is the audience?
- What are the key points?
- When is the presentation?
- How long is the presentation?
- What will the physical surroundings be?
- Why should the audience listen?
- How will the presentation be done?

PROCEDURE 25-1

Design a Presentation

ABHES COMPETENCY: 2.j

GOAL: *To gain skill in designing presentations that can be used for a variety of projects in the medical facility.*

EQUIPMENT and SUPPLIES

- Information about presentation subject
- Software, such as PowerPoint, if needed
- Computer access
- Peripheral computer equipment, if needed

PROCEDURAL STEPS

1. Determine the goals of the presentation.
   PURPOSE: The goals and purpose of the presentation must be determined before beginning so that the presenter is sure to reach those goals.
2. Write an outline of the entire presentation.
   PURPOSE: The outline helps the presenter prepare so that no important points are left out of the presentation.
3. Build the presentation using software, such as PowerPoint, highlighting the major points of the presentation.
4. Evaluate the audience, and adjust the presentation to appeal to that audience.
   PURPOSE: The presenter must know the audience to ensure a successful presentation.
5. Rehearse the presentation several times in front of a mirror.
   PURPOSE: Rehearsing in front of a mirror builds confidence.
6. Make a list of all equipment and materials to take to the presentation.
   PURPOSE: A list will help the presenter to remember all items that need to be taken to the presentation.
7. Arrive for the presentation between 15 to 30 minutes early, depending on the preparation and setup required.
   PURPOSE: Arriving early gives the presenter the opportunity to set up the presentation before the audience arrives.
8. Deliver the presentation within the prescribed time period.
9. Ask the audience if they have any questions about the information in the presentation.
   PURPOSE: A question-and-answer period allows the presenter to interact with the audience.
10. Thank the audience, and remove all equipment and supplies when appropriate.
11. Send a thank-you note to the organization for allowing the presentation, if appropriate.

Designing Presentation Content

Remember these points when designing a presentation:
- Use bulleted points consistently
- Use white space between bullets
- Align text systematically in one area of a slide, and place graphics on the other side
- Make certain that visuals deal with the subject of the presentation and are necessary
- Time the transition between slides
- Make bulleted points appear in a systematic way so that readers see text as the speaker is talking and not before or after the points are mentioned
- If a physical process is demonstrated, use visuals to enhance the demonstration
- Choose the most readable font
- Use hyperlinks effectively
- Use midrange colors for backgrounds
- Rehearse the narration
- Use titles for charts and illustrations
- Organize content well

Designing Pages

Once the objectives are clear, begin developing ideas about what the site will look like on the computer screen. Color choices, animation, and fonts will enhance the look that is being created and make a strong statement about the medical facility. The menus should be designed so that viewers can navigate easily through the site. Most users appreciate a means to go back to the page previously viewed and grow frustrated with sites that have an excessive number of pop-up boxes. Consistency is important, so it is a good idea to keep the same design theme on each page of the website.

The most important part of the website is the text. It has been said that every word in a book must add to the story, and this is a good way to look at the text in a website. Avoid repetition, and remain clear about what is being communicated on the site. Headings and titles help to clarify the theme of each page. Use a spellchecker before uploading the message and making it available for public viewing.

Photographs, graphics, music, and video can add fun to the website, but be careful not to overdo them. Graphics are often large files that take time to download. Most people will not wait more than about 10 seconds for a Web page to load

PROCEDURE 25-2

Prepare a Presentation Using PowerPoint

ABHES COMPETENCY: 2.j

GOAL: *To enhance presentations using PowerPoint as a visual aid.*

EQUIPMENT and SUPPLIES

- Information about presentation subject
- Software, such as PowerPoint, if needed
- Computer access
- Peripheral computer equipment, if needed

PROCEDURAL STEPS

1. Open the PowerPoint program.
2. Have the outline of the presentation available.
3. Click on the "new slide" icon in the program.
4. Create the title slide using the slide layout section on the right side of the screen.
5. Create additional slides using the slide layout section, or design the slides manually.
6. Limit the number of words on the slides so that a concise message results.
   PURPOSE: Too many words on one slide makes the message difficult to understand.
7. Make certain that the font is as large as possible on the slide, beginning with a size 18 font and increasing from there.
   PURPOSE: The font on a presentation must be easy to read from the back of the room.
8. Do not use more than three font types per slide.
   PURPOSE: More than three font types makes the presentation difficult to read.
9. Avoid using more than three text-only slides in a row.
   PURPOSE: Use clip art, photographs, graphs, and other items to enhance the presentation.
10. Insert photos or clip art into the presentation by clicking on "insert," then clicking on "picture," then choosing "clip art" or "from file."
11. Format the background of each slide, or of all slides, by clicking on "format," then "background," then choose a color or fill effects.
    PURPOSE: A consistent background makes the presentation look more professional.
12. Click on "slide show," and adjust the slide transitions so that the slides appear and disappear as desired and are timed correctly.
13. Click on "custom animation" to change the entrance and exit of the slides to the effect that is desired.
14. Save the presentation frequently while working on it.
    PURPOSE: Saving the presentation frequently ensures the user that the work will not be lost.
15. Click on "view" in the task bar, then on "slide sorter," which will allow moving the slides around in the presentation.
16. To run the show continuously, click on "slide show," then on "set up show," then click the box labeled "loop continuously until escape" in the "show options" box.
    PURPOSE: Running the show continuously is helpful for situations in which the presentation can be watched while people are passing through an exhibit hall, and so on.
17. Make certain the presentation has been saved.
18. Practice giving the presentation several times to smooth all transitions and to be familiar with the content.
    PURPOSE: The more the presentation is practiced, the more comfortable the presenter will be.
19. Anticipate questions that the audience may ask, and have answers prepared.
    PURPOSE: Anticipating questions will help the presenter to better prepare for the presentation and ensure that the presenter knows the material.
20. Offer other visual aids, such as handouts, if appropriate, when giving the presentation.
    PURPOSE: Visual aids will help the audience to remember the presentation and may prompt them to take any action that the presenter wishes them to take.

---

before clicking elsewhere. When designing Web page graphics, remember that smaller is better. Graphics can be found by searching for "index of GIF files" or "GIF library." Once an appropriate file is found, it should be copied onto the hard drive by "right-clicking" the graphic and selecting "save picture as." Music can be found by searching for "mid" or "midi." The search can even specify a certain singer, song, or composer. Always respect any copyrights that are designated on any file used. Many websites offer these files for free.

For a more professional-looking website, consider purchasing Web development software, such as Macromedia's Dreamweaver or Microsoft's FrontPage. These feature-rich products are fairly inexpensive and can help the medical assistant create very attractive, easy-to-maintain websites. Most products integrate tutorial and "help" features that explain how to use them.

Hyperlinks are words or graphics on a Web page that, when clicked, take the viewer to another page or another website. To add a hyperlink, simply highlight the text field or graphic, select the hyperlink icon, and specify the destination address (uniform resource locator [URL]). Always specify the full URL.

The main page should always be assigned the file name "index.htm" or "default.htm." Other pages on the website can be assigned any name; however, keep the names short, and avoid using special characters.

Locating a Web Server

At this point the design of the website is complete, but the files reside on the computer hard drive, not on the Internet. Now the pages are ready to be uploaded, or published, to a Web server that will allow them to be viewed on the Internet. The Internet service provider (ISP) that the office uses for email and online services may offer free Web space to its customers. If not, a number of companies will provide Web space at no charge, but the user usually will be required to use banners on the site that advertise the ISP or other services. If no banner ads are desired, the medical facility may wish to use a paid provider. Some Web hosting companies provide other services free of charge, like simple Web page editors and email addresses.

Uploading Pages

When using a free Web server, instructions and passwords will be sent to the users that describe how to upload files to the server. The password is necessary so that other people cannot alter the files. Copying the files from the local hard disk to the Web server is a simple process. The hosting site will prompt the user for the name of the directory on the hard drive where the files are stored and for the names of the specific files to be uploaded. To avoid confusion, make certain that the files saved on the server have the same file names that were used on the hard drive.

Once all of the files have been uploaded, test the page on the Web server and make certain that it functions properly and that all files have been uploaded correctly. It is also a good idea to test the page using a different computer to ensure that graphic files are being read from the server and not from the local hard drive.

Evaluating the Website

Include an email address where viewers of the website can interact with the creator with comments. When viewers have this option, problems with the site can be readily identified and corrected. It is also advisable to check the site every few days to make certain that it is functioning properly.

Counters often can be added to the website that will indicate how many people viewed it. This helpful tool will allow the medical facility to track how many people are viewing which pages.

HIGH-QUALITY CUSTOMER SERVICE IN THE MEDICAL PRACTICE

Treating the Patient as a Customer

The best way to increase the number of patients in a medical office is through word of mouth. When patients are satisfied with the treatment they receive, they will refer other patients to the physician. However, if they are dissatisfied, they will tell everyone they know!

Because patients often have a choice about who provides their healthcare services, it is important that the physician's office become the patient's first choice. Some patients have such loyalty to a certain physician that even if their healthcare

coverage would no longer pay for visits, they would continue to see that doctor. This happens because of the attitude of the physician and his or her office staff.

Helpful Attitudes

The physician and staff probably project a helpful attitude in every contact with the patient. They sincerely ask, "How may I help you?" then take steps to assist the patient in whatever way possible. Instead of pointing in the general direction of the radiology department, they take the patient there and introduce him or her to the receptionist. Instead of telling a patient on the telephone, "Ann handles the insurance billing—I'll transfer you to her," say, "One moment, Mrs. Brown, let me see if Ann is at her desk." Then place Mrs. Brown on hold, call Ann, and let her know that she has a call. Then return to Mrs. Brown and tell her that Ann is at her desk, and transfer the call at that time. Be courteous and kind to every patient and visitor to the office. Good customer relations must be one of the primary goals of the medical facility. Patients count on the staff members to be reliable and available to help them to the best of their abilities.

Phrases That Undermine Successful Customer Service

Several phrases could be considered the "deadly sins" of customer service. These phrases should never be used when relating to patients and visitors:

- "I don't know."
- "I don't care."
- "I can't be bothered."
- "Ask someone else."
- "It's not my job."
- "It's not my fault."
- "I didn't do it."
- "I know that."
- "I'm right, you're wrong."

All of these phrases will give the patient or visitor a negative view of both the office and those who work in the facility.

Identifying with Patients

Patients appreciate staff members who can identify with the problems they are facing. This is especially effective when a patient is upset or angry. For example, if a patient comes to the

Customer Service at Nordstrom

- Use your good judgment in all situations
- There will be no additional rules

From the *Nordstrom, Inc., Employee Handbook.* Courtesy Nordstrom, Inc.

office complaining that charges were placed on his account for procedures that were not performed, the medical assistant may respond with a phrase similar to the following:

"Mr. Roberts, I understand that you are upset about these additional charges. I know I would be upset if I were billed for something I didn't receive. Let me help you by doing this...."

Identifying with the patient shows an understanding on the part of the staff member, no matter how upset the patient may be. Always acknowledge and restate the patient's concern. It proves that the medical assistant was listening and is interested in resolving the problem.

Remember, it costs much more to find new customers than to keep existing customers happy. Providing helpful, personal service impresses even the most difficult patient. To patients and visitors to the clinic, whomever they speak to represents the whole company. Perceptions and opinions will likely be formed based on experiences with only one person. Each individual employee must be aware that to the patient, each employee is the healthcare facility.

What Do Patients Expect?

First, patients expect to be treated using the golden rule. They expect their concerns to be met with responsiveness, which means that the medical assistant should have a caring attitude. They also expect that the professionals in the medical office are knowledgeable about their field or specialty. An insurance biller should know more than just the basics of insurance filing. The office manager should have a certain degree of authority to handle problems and complaints. Patients also expect confidentiality and trust from the staff of the medical office. They expect an organized office that runs on schedule, and that if a staff member promises to do something, it is as good as done (Figure 25-4).

Remembering the Internal Customer

Most of us do not have problems figuring out who the external customers are in a medical practice. Patients, their families and friends, and visitors to the office are external customers. But who is the internal customer?

Internal customers are employees and staff members of the facility. Although they work for the business, they also are served by the business. If they are not pleased with the atmosphere of the medical facility, they are sure to look elsewhere for employment. Keeping the internal customer is just as important as keeping the external customer.

CLOSING COMMENTS

Providing good customer service is a commitment that must be made by every employee of the medical facility, every single day. There will be times that the customer is not right, but he or she should be treated with dignity and respect at all times. In addition, the expert customer service provider will have the knack for making the customer think he or she was right all along! The medical office is no exception to the requirements for providing good service to its patients, and doing so will result in an excellent reputation for the clinic, built by those who matter most—the patients.

Endless opportunities for patient education exist through the practice's marketing and public relations efforts. Most physicians agree that a part of the obligation to the medical profession is to educate patients about healthcare issues. The public relations and practice's marketing staffs can work together to provide information to patients of the facility and to the general public.

Many physicians attend health fairs, where brochures and pamphlets can be distributed about conditions such as diabetes, heart disease, hypertension, and other disorders. Screenings for cholesterol and blood pressure checks are good ways to market a practice and gain new patients.

The medical assistant who knows how to build and maintain a simple website can be of great value to the physician. The practice website could provide opportunities for educating patients, as well as special sections for upcoming events, an online newsletter, and appointment setting. The website address should be included on stationery, business cards, and other documents used to promote the facility.

The physician must take care that patients do not use the information in brochures or on the practice website as medical advice or a substitute for the physician's counsel. When attaching links to other websites, be sure they are reputable. The patient may consider information on the practice's website to be an extension of the advice of the physician, so make sure that everything on the website is accurate.

The physician should review carefully all printed information that is used to promote the medical facility. Be sure that no misleading statements are included. A disclaimer should be used to remind patients that the information given in brochures and on websites is only general information. Patients should discuss specific medical issues with the physician.

Todd Family Medical Clinic

Julie Todd, M.D.   Robert Todd, M.D.
3343 Smithson Place
Dallas, Texas 75229

We are interested in the customer service you received today as a patient of our clinic. Please return this form by mail and help us evaluate our service to you!

Date of contact or visit: _____   Day of week: _____

Name of employees with which you made contact (if known):

How was this contact made?   ☐ by phone   ☐ by mail   ☐ in person

This is a (please check appropriate box)   ☐ complaint   ☐ comment

Description of situation:

Has the problem been resolved to your satisfaction, if any?   ☐ yes   ☐ no

If not, how can we resolve the problem?

Please rate the following based on your experience with our staff:

	Excellent	Good	Fair	Poor
Greeting to you by name	☐	☐	☐	☐
Familiarity with your account	☐	☐	☐	☐
Courtesy and willingness to help	☐	☐	☐	☐
Quickness in answering the phone	☐	☐	☐	☐
Time placed on hold	☐	☐	☐	☐
Quickness in locating your chart	☐	☐	☐	☐
All of your questions answered	☐	☐	☐	☐
Phone transfers kept to a minimum	☐	☐	☐	☐

Other suggestions and comments:

Name (optional): _____   Phone Number (optional): _____

FIGURE 25-4 Customer service evaluation form for the medical office. By using this form for patient feedback, the medical office manager can better assess patient expectations.

SUMMARY OF SCENARIO

Monica knows that without growth, many businesses eventually fail. She is confident that with a simple marketing plan, the clinic will experience steady, continuous expansion. She has spoken to all of the office staff members and gained input from both employees and the patients of the clinic. Many offered excellent suggestions that Monica can incorporate into her marketing plan.

One of her first activities was to develop an annual calendar of special events and outreach efforts. A monthly newsletter and the practice website will be the main thrusts of her marketing plan. The newsletter will be available both in print and online. The patients in the office database who have email addresses will receive automatically a computer-generated email message containing a link that will take them directly to the online newsletter. Inside, patients will find health information and details about upcoming events.

Monica also planned one special activity for each month of the year. She scheduled a blood drive, a Christmas toy drive, and mini–health fair. Because both Dr. Julie and Dr. Robert Todd are dedicated to students who wish to pursue medicine, Monica even planned a career day for high school students interested in becoming physicians, inviting representatives from the medical school that the Todds attended. Because this is considered a public service, Monica was able to get press coverage on the local radio station and in the newspaper at no cost.

Monica visited a new restaurant located close to the office that serves heart-healthy dishes, met with the manager, and discussed ways that the two businesses could help each other. They decided to provide a "buy one entrée, get one free" coupon to patients who referred other patients to the clinic. In turn, Dr. Robert Todd agreed to hold his free nutrition seminars at the restaurant. This arrangement has proven to work well for both businesses. Monica obtained this new agreement by making an effective presentation to the restaurant manager. Her skills in putting an interesting, informative presentation together helped her secure the agreement.

An Internet presence is important to businesses that wish to grow in today's society. Consumers often look on the Internet first when planning purchases, shopping, or looking for community resources. Monica plans to track responses to each event promoted on the practice website to determine what efforts were the most effective in promoting the clinic. The website will allow her to count the number of times it is accessed, as well as which pages were the most popular within the website. She will keep the physicians informed and be open to their suggestions throughout the year. Monica is anxious to see results of her marketing efforts and feels confident of success.

The staff members understand that no matter what efforts are used to promote the facility and obtain new patients, it is their responsibility to provide exceptional customer service so that the patients will be happy with their experience. In the medical industry today, customer service has become as important as in the retail world. Patients have choices as to who provides their healthcare, so they must be treated cordially and fairly by medical professionals who truly wish to serve their needs. The success and growth of the facility depends on customer service. Monica knows that there is more than one type of customer in the medical office—the internal customers (employees) are critical to clinic success. She includes other employees in marketing decisions and often asks for their input. The more involved employees feel in company decisions, the more they feel as if they are a part of the community that is created in the individual facility. Monica has helped to create a fun, exciting workplace, and she looks forward to going to work every single day.

SUMMARY of LEARNING OBJECTIVES

1. Define, spell, and pronounce the terms listed in the vocabulary.
   - Spelling and pronouncing medical terms correctly adds credibility to the medical assistant. Knowing the definition of these terms promotes confidence in communication with patients and co-workers.
2. List the three steps to be followed when preparing to implement a medical marketing strategy.
   - When preparing to implement marketing strategies, first evaluate what currently is being done toward the marketing effort. Then decide what the objectives of the marketing plan are and how they will be measured. Finally, develop a specific plan and timeline for implementing each phase.

3. Explain the term *target market*.
   - A target market is a very specific group of people or individuals whom the medical facility wishes to serve. Geography, lifestyle, and personality all are ways to classify individuals into specific target markets. When identifying a target market ask, "Who is our patient?" "What does our patient want?" and "Why is it wanted?" These questions will help the medical facility to design a marketing plan to meet the needs of these individuals.
4. Discuss how suggestion boxes might help the medical facility to make improvements.
   - Suggestions from patients and employees should always be welcomed in the medical office. Often these people see the

Continued

SUMMARY of LEARNING OBJECTIVES
Continued

facility from a different point of view, and their suggestions can enhance the atmosphere and services that are offered.

5. List and discuss the "four P's" of marketing.
   - A marketing plan must always address the "four P's," which are product, placement, price, and promotion. The product in a medical office would include the services and any actual retail items that might be sold. Placement relates to the location of the office and its convenience to the patients, and the placement of retail items in the facility. Price represents the charges for goods and services, and promotion entails the ways in which the services are promoted to the general public and the target market.

6. Explain the five steps for developing a plan in marketing.
   - When developing a marketing plan, the facility should first assess the efforts that have been made in the past, then research the results of those efforts. Next the plan is developed, which should include very specific steps for each aspect of the endeavor. After the plan is executed, the staff must evaluate its effectiveness and determine whether the goals were met. The evaluation is important in planning future marketing strategies.

7. Discuss how community involvement can make a difference in marketing efforts.
   - Involvement in the community is an excellent way to give to the medical profession and to remain in the public eye. These efforts can result in new patients for the facility. The public sees medical professionals as caring and compassionate, so volunteer activities reinforce this attitude and help to meet patient expectations.

8. State the difference between advertising and public relations.
   - Advertising is defined as a medium that attempts to create or change attitudes, beliefs, and perceptions through purchased broadcast time, printed material, or other forms

of communication. Public relations is a similar field but relies more on news broadcasts or reports, magazine or newspaper articles, and radio reports to reach the audience.

9. Determine ways to promote a new practice.
   - The new medical practice can be promoted by placing an announcement in the newspaper about its opening. Some physicians hold an open house, inviting the public to visit the office. A website is an excellent promotional tool and should be listed on business cards and stationery. Community service and volunteer activities that mention the practice will also help to spread the word about the services that are available.

10. Discuss responses that help the medical assistant identify with the patient.
    - Identifying with the patient is an effective customer service tool. The medical assistant should express his or her understanding about the patient's concerns. Then, tell the patient that the situation can be resolved and how it will be resolved. Four magic words in customer service are, "Let me help you."

11. Explain the concept of the internal customer.
    - External customers are those who visit the facility, such as patients. However, staff members and employees are internal customers who wish to derive a sense of satisfaction from working for the medical office. The internal customers are just as important as the external customers.

12. Design a presentation for a marketing event.
    - A sharp, effective presentation will help the medical assistant to or secure permission to hold or promote a marketing event. The process for designing a presentation is outlined in Procedure 25-1.

13. Prepare a presentation using PowerPoint.
    - PowerPoint is a user-friendly program that will produce effective presentations. The process for preparing a presentation using PowerPoint is outlined in Procedure 25-2.

CONNECTIONS

 Study Guide Connection: Go to Chapter 25 Study Guide. Read the Case Study and Workplace Applications and complete the assignments. Do online research for answers to the questions in the Internet Activities associated with medical practice marketing and customer service.

 CD Connection: Go to the Medical Assisting Competency Challenge CD and do the training activities under Communication.

Evolve Connection: For more information related to medical practice marketing and customer service, go to http://evolve.elsevier.com/kinn/admin and visit related weblinks for Chapter 25. Click on the Medical Assisting Exam Review and do the practice questions to sharpen your test-taking skills. To learn more about office software, do the exercises for the Altapoint demo that is on the CD.

Assisting with Medical Emergencies

26

Cheryl Skurka, CMA, has been working for Dr. Peter Bendt for approximately 6 months. During that time a number of patient emergencies have occurred in the office, and even more potentially serious problems have been managed by the telephone screening staff. Cheryl is concerned that she is not prepared to assist with emergencies in the ambulatory care setting. She decides to ask Dr. Bendt for assistance, and he suggests she work with the experienced screening staff to learn how to manage phone calls from patients calling for assistance.

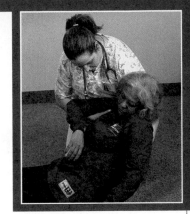

While studying this chapter, think about the following questions:

- What should Cheryl learn about the medical assistant's responsibilities in an emergency situation?
- What are some of the general rules for managing a medical emergency in an ambulatory care setting?
- What types of questions are asked by the phone triage staff if a patient calls with a medical emergency?
- What information from these phone calls should be documented?
- Is it important that Cheryl be able to recognize and be prepared to respond to life-threatening emergencies?

- What are some of the typical patient emergencies that occur in a healthcare facility?
- How should Cheryl instruct a patient to control bleeding from a hemorrhaging wound?
- Are there patient education areas related to common health emergencies that Cheryl should be prepared to share?
- What legal factors should Cheryl be aware of when handling ambulatory care emergencies?

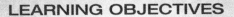

LEARNING OBJECTIVES

1. Define, spell, and pronounce the terms listed in the vocabulary.
2. Describe the medical assistant's responsibilities in an emergency.
3. Identify supplies and equipment for emergency situations.
4. Demonstrate the use of an automated external defibrillator.
5. Summarize the general rules for managing emergencies.
6. Demonstrate screening techniques and documentation guidelines for ambulatory care emergencies.
7. Recognize and respond to life-threatening emergencies in the ambulatory care setting.
8. Perform adult rescue breathing and CPR.

9. Administer oxygen through a nasal cannula to a patient in respiratory distress.
10. Identify and assist a patient with an obstructed airway.
11. Determine appropriate action and documentation procedures for common ambulatory care emergencies.
12. Assist and monitor a patient who has fainted.
13. Control a hemorrhagic wound.
14. Apply patient education concepts to medical emergencies.
15. Discuss legal and ethical concerns regarding medical emergencies.

National Accreditation Competencies and Content

CAAHEP COMPETENCIES

Clinical
3.b.(4)(a). Perform telephone and in-person screening

General
3.c.(1)(d). Demonstrate telephone techniques
3.c.(2)(b). Perform within legal and ethical boundaries
3.c.(2)(d). Document appropriately

ABHES COMPETENCIES

Professionalism
1.d. Be cognizant of ethical boundaries

Communication
2.e. Use proper telephone techniques

Clinical Duties
4.e. Recognize emergencies
4.f. Perform first aid and CPR

Legal Concepts
5.b. Document accurately

VOCABULARY

asystole (ay-sis'-toh-le) The absence of a heartbeat.

bradycardia Slow heart rate; pulse is below 60 beats per minute.

cyanosis (si-an-oh'-sis) Blue color of the mucous membranes and body extremities caused by lack of oxygen.

dyspnea Difficult or painful breathing.

ecchymosis (e-ki-moh'-sis) A hemorrhagic skin discoloration commonly called *bruising*.

emetic (eh-met'-ik) A substance that causes vomiting.

fibrillation Rapid, random, ineffective contractions of the heart.

hematuria (hi-ma-tuhr'-e-uh) Blood in the urine.

idiopathic Pertaining to no known cause of a condition or disease.

mediastinum (meh-de-ast'-uhn-um) Space in the center of the chest under the sternum.

myocardium (my-oh-kar'-de-um) The muscular lining of the heart.

necrosis (neh-kroh'-sis) The death of cells or tissue.

photophobia Visual sensitivity to light.

polydipsia Excessive thirst.

polyuria Excreting large amounts of urine.

thrombolytics Agents that dissolve blood clots.

transient ischemic attack Temporary neurologic symptoms caused by a gradual or partial occlusion of a cerebral blood vessel.

First aid is defined as the immediate care given to a person who has been injured or has suddenly taken ill. Knowledge of first aid and related skills can often mean the difference between life and death, temporary and permanent disability, and rapid recovery and long-term hospitalization. The medical assistant may be responsible for initiating first aid in the office and continuing to administer first aid until the physician or trained medical team arrives. Every medical assistant should successfully complete a course for the professional in cardiopulmonary resuscitation (CPR) and should continue to hold a current CPR card as long as employed (see Procedure 26-2). Basic knowledge of CPR and life-support skills needs to be updated on a regular basis because of changes in procedures as new techniques are developed. For example, both the American Red Cross and the American Heart Association now recommend the inclusion of automated external defibrillator (AED) training for all healthcare workers (see Procedure 26-1). Medical assistants need up-to-date training in current emergency practices and should encourage their local professional chapters to offer workshops on the management of emergencies in the ambulatory care setting.

Medical assistants are not responsible for diagnosing emergencies but are expected to make decisions regarding emergency situations based on their medical knowledge and training. If any doubt exists about how to manage a particular situation or emergency phone call, do not hesitate to refer to the physician, office manager, or a more experienced member of the healthcare team.

The Medical Assistant's Role in Performing Emergency Procedures

- Perform only the emergency procedures in which you are trained.
- If an emergency occurs in the office, notify the physician.
- If a physician cannot be located, contact the local emergency medical services (EMS) team.

MAKING THE FACILITY ACCIDENT-PROOF

Usually it is the medical assistant's responsibility to make the office as accident-proof as possible by keeping cupboard doors and drawers closed, wiping up spills immediately, and picking up dropped objects. All medications should be kept out of sight and away from busy patient areas; dangerous drugs should be kept in locked cupboards. If children are in the office, all sharp objects and potentially toxic substances must be kept out of reach. A medical assistant should never leave a seriously ill patient or a restless, depressed, or unconscious patient unattended.

PLANNING AHEAD

Every healthcare facility should have a standard policy with specific procedures for the management of emergencies on site. When starting a new job, part of the orientation process will be to review the site's policy and procedures manual. Be sure to clarify any questions you have regarding emergency management in that particular facility.

Staff members should discuss possible emergencies that may occur and have an emergency action plan for rapid, systematic intervention. For instance, local industries may present unique problems that call for very specialized care. Plan for these, and ask the physician's advice on what procedures to follow and what supplies to have on hand. If the facility has several employees, each should be assigned specific duties in the event of an emergency. Organization and planning make the difference between systematic care for the patient and complete chaos.

Using Community Emergency Services

Most communities have an emergency medical services (EMS) system. This system includes an efficient communications network, such as the emergency telephone number 911, well-trained rescue personnel, properly equipped ambulances, an emergency facility that is open 24 hours a day to provide advanced life support, and a hospital intensive care unit for the victims.

More than 100 poison control centers in the United States are ready to provide emergency information for treating victims of poisonings. Every healthcare facility is required to post a list of local emergency numbers. This list should be in plain sight and should be known to all office personnel. A good place to post this vital information is next to all of the phones in the facility. Include on the list the local EMS system, poison control center, ambulance and rescue squad, fire department, and police department numbers.

SUPPLIES AND EQUIPMENT FOR EMERGENCIES

Emergency Supplies

Emergency supplies consist of a properly equipped "crash cart" or kit of items needed for a variety of emergencies (Figure 26-1). The contents will vary to some degree according to the type of emergencies each office might expect to encounter. Emergency supplies should be kept in an easily accessible place that is

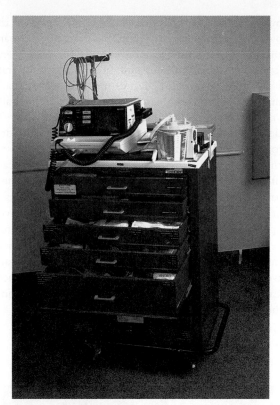

FIGURE 26-1 Office emergency cart with defibrillator. Drawers are marked for easy retrieval of emergency supplies.

known to all personnel in the office, with inventories of supplies completed on a regular basis. Expiration dates of medication and sterile supplies must be checked either weekly or monthly, along with the status of available oxygen tanks and related supplies, and the cart should be replenished with fresh supplies after every use.

Emergency pharmaceutical supplies should include certain basic drugs, such as epinephrine, which has multiple uses in emergency situations. As a vasoconstrictor, it controls hemorrhage, relaxes the bronchioles to relieve acute asthma attacks, and is an emergency heart stimulant used to treat shock. Epinephrine should be in a ready-to-use cartridge syringe and needle unit. These are supplied in 1-ml cartridges.

Additional drugs used are atropine, digoxin (Lanoxin), nitroglycerin (Nitrostat), and lidocaine (Xylocaine). Atropine decreases secretions, increases respiration and heart rate, and is a smooth-muscle relaxant. It is administered in a cardiac emergency for **asystole** or can be used to treat **bradycardia.** Digoxin is a cardiac drug that treats arrhythmias and congestive heart failure (CHF) and is good for emergency use because it has a relatively rapid action. Nitroglycerin is a vasodilator that is given to relieve angina. It acts by dilating the coronary arteries so an increased volume of oxygenated blood can reach the **myocardium.** Lidocaine is used intravenously to treat a cardiac arrhythmia and locally as an anesthetic, and sodium bicarbonate corrects metabolic acidosis that typically occurs after a cardiac arrest.

Emergency medicine supplies should also include an **emetic** such as syrup of ipecac, which causes vomiting soon after swallowing, as well as activated charcoal, an antidote that is swallowed to absorb ingested poisons. Narcan is a narcotic antidote that is administered intravenously for drug overdoses and acts to raise blood pressure and increase respiratory rate. In addition, antihistamines for the treatment of allergic reactions and anaphylaxis need to be available to treat potential allergic responses to medication administered in the facility. These include Benadryl for minor reactions and Solu-Medrol, a corticosteroid, for a severe anaphylactic response.

Other medications that may be found on a crash cart are isoproterenol (e.g., Isuprel, Medihaler-Iso, Norisodrine), an antispasmodic that is used to treat bronchospasms (such as those experienced during an asthma attack) and is also effective as a cardiac stimulant; metaraminol (Aramine) (50%, in a prefilled syringe) for severe shock; phenobarbital, amobarbital sodium (Amytal), and diazepam (Valium) for convulsions and/or sedative effects; furosemide (Lasix) for CHF; and glucagon, primarily used to counteract severe hypoglycemic reactions in diabetic patients taking insulin.

Defibrillators

The medical assistant may be required to assist the healthcare team with defibrillation of emergency patients. Defibrillation is indicated when a patient is in ventricular **fibrillation** (VF). VF is a severe cardiac arrhythmia that is caused by an uncoordinated, rapid firing of the electrical system of the heart, making it impossible for the ventricles to empty. In the absence of ventricular emptying, the patient has no pulse, the blood pressure drops to zero, and the patient could die within 4 minutes unless help is given immediately.

Defibrillators are devices that send an electrical current through the myocardium by means of hand-held paddles or self-adhesive pads applied to the chest. This electrical shock causes momentary asystole, giving the heart's natural pacemaker an opportunity to resume the heart rate at a normal rhythm. The AED has a computerized system that analyzes a cardiac rhythm and delivers voice-prompt instructions on how to operate the device (Figure 26-2 and Procedure 26-1). An AED uses self-

Basic Emergency Supplies

Equipment

- Adhesive tape in 1- and 2-inch widths
- Airways—variety of types and sizes
- Alcohol wipes
- Ambu bag with assorted sizes of facial masks
- Antimicrobial skin ointment
- Bandage scissors
- Cotton balls and cotton swabs
- CPR masks—both adult and pediatric
- Defibrillator
- Elastic bandages in 2- and 3-inch widths
- Filter needles
- Flashlight with batteries
- Gauze pads, 2- × 2- and 4- × 4-inch widths, and roller bandage—both sterile and nonsterile
- Gloves, sterile and nonsterile, in multiple sizes
- Hot and cold packs (instant type)
- Intravenous catheters, tubing, solutions (variety of types including D5W and Ringer's lactate), and tourniquet
- Laryngoscope with blades
- Lubricant
- Personal protective equipment (PPE), including impervious gowns, splash-guards or goggles, and booties
- Portable oxygen tank with regulator, mask, and nasal cannula
- Roller gauze (Ace bandages and gauze dressing) in various sizes
- Sharps container
- Sphygmomanometer—both pediatric and adult regular and large sizes
- Splints—various sizes
- Sterile dressings—miscellaneous sizes, including two abdominal pads
- Steri-Strips or suturing material
- Suction machine and catheters
- Syringes and needles in assorted sizes and gauges
- Tongue blades
- Tubex cartridge system
- Venipuncture supplies and butterfly units

Medications

- Activated charcoal, bottle of 30-50 g
- Amobarbital (Amytal)
- Antihistamine, injectable and oral
- Atropine
- Dextrose
- Diazepam (Valium)
- Digoxin (Lanoxin), injectable
- Diphenhydramine (Benadryl)
- Epinephrine (Adrenalin), injectable
- Furosemide (Lasix)
- Glucagon and/or glucose tablets
- Ipecac syrup
- Isoproterenol (Isuprel), aerosol inhaler and injectable
- Lidocaine (Xylocaine), injectable and spray
- Metaraminol (Aramine)
- Narcan
- Nitroglycerin tablets
- Phenobarbital, injectable
- Sodium bicarbonate, injectable
- Solu-Medrol
- Sterile water and saline for injection

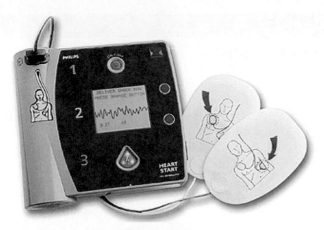

FIGURE 26-2 Fully automated external defibrillator. (From Aehlert B: *Mosby's comprehensive pediatric emergency care*, St Louis, 2005, Mosby.)

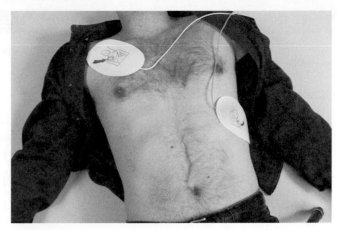

FIGURE 26-3 Connect the adhesive pads to the AED cables, then apply the pads to the patient's chest at the upper-right sternal border and the lower-left ribs over the cardiac apex. (From Chapleau W: *Emergency medical technician: making the difference*, St Louis, 2007, Mosby.)

adhesive pads that record and monitor the cardiac rhythm, and the device instructs the rescuer when to deliver the electrical charge. The apex-anterior position is the most commonly used paddle position, with the anterior (sternum) paddle or pads placed to the right of the upper sternum and the apex one under the patient's left nipple at the left mid-axillary line (Figure 26-3). For defibrillating a female patient, the apex paddle or pad is placed either next to or underneath the left breast.

Automated External Defibrillator Precautions

- Both patient and caregiver should not be in contact with any metal during defibrillation. Do not place the AED pad over jewelry, and remove patient's glasses to avoid injuries.
- A pediatric dose AED system should be used when available for children 1 to 8 years of age. These systems deliver a reduced shock dose for victims up to about 8 years of age or 55 pounds in weight.
- All clothing (including bras) must be removed; pads must be applied directly to the skin. If there is a great deal of hair on the chest, try to push the hair aside before applying the pads, or it may be necessary to shave the areas for complete paddle contact. The machine will prompt you by stating "check electrode" if the connection is poor.
- Make sure the patient is lying on a dry surface and that the chest is dry before applying the paddles, to avoid burns.
- If the patient has an implanted defibrillator or pacemaker it will be obvious from the bulged area under the surface of the skin on the chest. Apply AED pads at least 1 inch away from implants to avoid interference.

GENERAL RULES FOR EMERGENCIES

A medical assistant will face two types of emergencies in the ambulatory care setting: office emergencies and home emergencies. Common office emergencies and their management are discussed later in this chapter. Besides dealing with actual emergency situations on-site, a medical assistant is frequently the first person to interact with patients facing potential emergencies at home. It is estimated that one third of the telephone calls received in a physician's office are for some type

of problem that requires attention. An immediate decision must be made on how to manage that problem—by giving home care advice, scheduling an appointment, or in extreme emergencies notifying EMS personnel. When faced with an emergency, either on the phone or in the facility, the medical assistant should follow some general rules:

- It is most important to stay calm. Reassure the patient, and make him or her as comfortable as possible.
- Assess the situation to determine the nature of the emergency. Decide whether the need is immediate. This decision requires calm judgment and medical knowledge.
- Obtain as much information as possible to determine the appropriate action.
- Immediately refer any concerns to the office supervisor or physician.

Telephone Screening

Each time the phone rings in a healthcare setting there could be a potential life-or-death situation on the other end of the line. One of the most important tasks performed by medical assistants every day is answering the phones and managing patient needs efficiently and appropriately. *Triage* is the process of sorting patients, in this case patient phone calls, according to the patients' need for care. Emergency action principles serve as a guide for managing emergency phone calls in the ambulatory care setting:

- If the patient's situation is life-threatening, activate EMS/911.
  - *Never put the caller with a life-threatening emergency on hold, and always be the last to hang up.*
  - Remain on the line until help arrives and you have talked to EMS personnel.
- Immediately record the name of the caller and that of the patient, location, and phone number in case the connection is lost.
- If you are unsure how to manage the emergency situation, contact the physician.
- If the patient is referred to an emergency department (ED) or emergency room (ER), call the ER to notify them of the

PROCEDURE 26-1

Use an Automated External Defibrillator

<u>ABHES COMPETENCY:</u> 4.f.

GOAL: *To defibrillate adult victims with cardiac arrest. The majority of adult victims in sudden cardiac arrest are in ventricular fibrillation. Survival rates for victims with ventricular fibrillation are as high as 90% when defibrillation occurs within the first minute of collapse. Survival rates for cardiac arrest caused by ventricular fibrillation decrease by 7% to 10% with every minute that defibrillation does not occur.*

EQUIPMENT and SUPPLIES

- Practice automated external defibrillator (AED)
- Approved mannequin

PROCEDURAL STEPS (To be performed on an approved mannequin only)

If the healthcare worker witnesses a cardiac arrest, an AED should be used as soon as it is available. If an arrest is not witnessed, five cycles of CPR should be administered before using an AED. One cycle of CPR consists of 30 compressions and two breaths. When compressions are delivered at a rate of about 100 per minute, five cycles of CPR should take roughly 2 minutes.

1. Place the AED near the victim's left ear. Turn the AED on.
2. Attach electrode pads as pictured on the AED. Place electrodes at the sternum and apex of the heart. Make sure pads have complete contact with the victim's chest and they do not overlap (see Figure 26-3).
3. All rescuers must clear away from the victim. Press the ANALYZE button. The AED will analyze the victim's coronary status, will announce if the victim is going to be shocked, and automatically charges the electrodes (Figure 1*).
4. All rescuers must clear away from the victim. Press the SHOCK button if the machine is not automated. May repeat three analyze-shock cycles.
5. Deliver one shock, leaving the AED attached, and immediately resume CPR, starting with chest compressions.
6. After five cycles (about 2 minutes) of CPR, repeat the AED analysis and deliver another shock if indicated. If a nonshockable

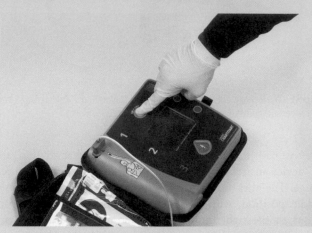

FIGURE 1

rhythm is detected, the AED should instruct the rescuer to resume CPR immediately, beginning with chest compressions.

7. If the machine gives the "no shock indicated" signal, assess the victim. Check the carotid pulse and breathing status and keep the AED attached until emergency medical services arrives. <u>PURPOSE:</u> Continue to monitor breathing and circulation because these can stop at any time. Keep AED pads in place to quickly diagnose ventricular fibrillation if it occurs.

*From Chapleau W: *Emergency medical technician: making the difference,* St Louis, 2007, Mosby.

---

patient's arrival and make a follow-up call to determine the patient's condition.

- Gather as much information as possible about what is wrong with the patient and when the problem started. Obtain details regarding the patient's condition, including:
  - Level of consciousness: Alert, responsive, lethargic, or confused? Did the patient lose consciousness at any time? If so, for how long?
  - Character of respirations (and pulse if the caller is able to determine this): normal, rapid, shallow, or difficult?
  - Is there bleeding? If so, how much, and from where?
  - Is there a suspected head or neck injury? If so, has the patient been moved? Is there a suspected fracture? Where?
  - Does the patient have a history of this problem?
  - Any other symptoms, such as fever, vomiting, diarrhea, or pain?

- Details regarding what has been done for the patient:
  - Medication: What, when? Dose, effectiveness? Current allergies?
- Thoroughly document the information gathered and any actions taken, including notification of EMS, whether the patient was sent to the ER or an appointment was scheduled, all home care recommendations, and whether the physician was notified and when.

Based on the outcome of the telephone interaction, a decision is made about when the practitioner will see the patient (Procedure 26-2). Emergency calls require either activation of EMS or immediate attention as soon as the patient arrives. Urgent calls require a same-day appointment if the patient has an acute condition or is in severe discomfort. This would include a young child with a high fever or a patient complaining of moderate to severe abdominal pain. The new patient will

PROCEDURE 26-2

Perform Telephone Screening and Appropriate Documentation

<u>CAAHEP COMPETENCY:</u> 3.b.(4)(a), 3.c.(1)(d), C.3.c.(2)(d)
<u>ABHES COMPETENCY:</u> 2.e., 5.b.

GOAL: *To asses the direction of emergency care and document information appropriately in the patient record.*

EQUIPMENT and SUPPLIES

- Note pad with pen or pencil
- Patient record
- Facility's emergency procedures manual
- Appointment book or program
- Area emergency numbers

PRACTICE SCENARIO

Cheryl is working with the phone triage staff when they receive a call from the mother of a 5-year-old patient; the mother reports that her son fell and cut his arm. What type of information should Cheryl gather about the injury? What action should be taken? How should the incident be documented?

PROCEDURAL STEPS

1. Stay calm and reassure the caller.
   <u>PURPOSE:</u> To enable gathering of accurate details regarding the patient's condition.

2. Verify the identity of the caller and the injured patient.

3. Immediately record the name of the caller and the patient, location, and phone number.
   <u>PURPOSE:</u> To be able to contact them if the connection is lost.

4. Determine if the patient's condition is life-threatening. Quantify the amount of blood loss, if the patient is alert and responsive, if breathing is normal. Notify EMS if necessary.
   <u>PURPOSE:</u> Immediately notify emergency services if the patient is in danger.

5. If EMS is notified, stay on the line with the caller until EMS personnel arrive at the scene.
   <u>PURPOSE:</u> Never break a phone connection in the case of a life-threatening emergency.

6. If emergency services are not needed, gather details about the injury to determine if the patient can be seen in the office or should be referred to an emergency room (ER). Consider the following questions:
   - Is there a suspected head or neck injury? Has the patient been moved?
   - Is there a possible fracture? If so, where?
   - Are there any other symptoms?
   - Is there anything pertinent in the patient's health history that would complicate the situation?
   - Has the caller administered any first aid? What?

7. Based on information gathered, determine when the patient should be seen in the office if he or she has not been referred to an ER.
   <u>PURPOSE:</u> The majority of emergencies would be scheduled for an immediate office visit. This may require altering the current appointment schedule.

8. At any point in this process, do not hesitate to consult the physician or experienced staff or refer to the facility's emergency procedures manual to determine how to manage the patient's problem.

9. Always allow the caller to hang up first, just in case more information or assistance is needed.

10. Document information gathered, actions taken or recommended, any home care recommendations, and whether the physician was notified.
    <u>PURPOSE:</u> To have a legal record of the management of the emergency and a comprehensive description of the patient's condition and recommended management.

See Appendix D for a charting example.

---

have to be worked into the day's schedule, which may cause a delay in currently scheduled appointments. Patients with other, less urgent problems can be scheduled for appointments within the next 3 to 4 days.

Management of On-Site Emergencies

An emergency can occur at any time to anyone. Always implement Occupational Safety and Health Administration (OSHA) standard precautions when at risk for coming into contact with blood and/or body fluids. When an emergency occurs, it is impossible to determine the level of infection. All body fluids must be considered infectious, and the appropriate

Documentation of an On-Site Emergency

1. Patient's name, address, age, and health insurance information
2. Allergies, current medications, and pertinent health history
3. Name and relationship of any person with the patient
4. Vital signs and chief complaint
5. Sequence of events, beginning with how the problem occurred, any changes in the patient's overall condition, and any observations made regarding the patient's condition
6. Details regarding procedures or techniques performed on the patient

precautions must be employed to prevent cross-contamination. If the situation is life-threatening, notify EMS and stay with the patient until you are relieved by the EMS provider or the physician. It is important to document all details regarding the incident in the patient record.

> ### CRITICAL THINKING APPLICATION
>
> Cheryl is working the front desk when a patient comes into the office limping, saying she fell in the parking lot and hurt her ankle. Role-play the situation with a classmate, and make a list of at least 10 questions Cheryl should ask the patient.

Life-Threatening Emergencies

If a patient in the facility exhibits any signs of nonresponsiveness, the clinician must be brought to the patient immediately. If there is no clinician in the facility, EMS should be activated. Even in situations in which a physician is present, the physician may order you to call 911 for immediate emergency care. Before beginning assessment of the patient, put on gloves, because any emergency situation may necessitate exposure to blood or body fluids.

Nonresponsive Patient

If the patient is nonresponsive, the physician must be notified immediately. The physician may instruct the medical assistant to activate EMS.

If a patient is able to talk to you, then you know that he or she has an open airway. If the patient does not respond to a simple question such as "Are you OK?" then gently shake the shoulder to check responsiveness. If the patient does not respond, then you must assume that the patient is unconscious. Immediately call for help and activate EMS if that is office policy.

Caring for a patient who is nonresponsive first requires assessing the patient's respirations to determine the presence of breathing. Perhaps when the patient collapsed, the tongue went limp and occluded the trachea. Just by changing the individual's position and opening the airway you may provide all the assistance the patient needs to breathe independently.

Position the patient on the back, and apply the head tilt–chin lift movement to open the airway. The tongue is attached to the lower jaw, so moving the jaw forward will automatically open the patient's airway. If there is a suspected head or neck injury, the neck should be manipulated as little as possible, so open the airway with the jaw thrust maneuver. Both of these actions relieve possible obstruction of the trachea by the tongue. Check for breathing by looking for a rise in the chest and either listening or feeling for air exchange (Figure 26-4). Breathing may suddenly cease for a variety of reasons, including shock, disease, and trauma. If no breaths are detected, artificial ventilation must be started immediately, because death may occur within 4 to 6 minutes. There should be barrier devices on hand for artificial respirations (Figure 26-5), which should be used if rescue breaths are required (Procedure 26-3).

After giving the patient two slow breaths, check for signs of normal breathing or movement. If there are still no signs of

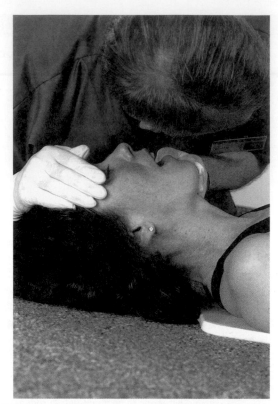

FIGURE 26-4 Checking for breathing in an unconscious patient.

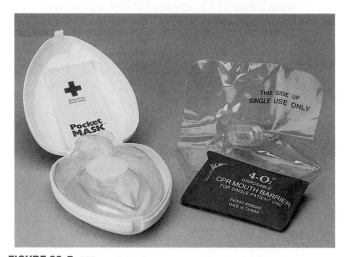

FIGURE 26-5 CPR mouth barriers.

responsiveness, check for cardiac circulation at the carotid pulse in the adult or child or the brachial pulse in the infant (Figure 26-6). Gently feel for the pulse while continuing to assess the patient for possible signs of recovery for 5 to 10 seconds. If the pulse is present, continue ventilating the lungs with slow breaths every 4 to 5 seconds in an adult or every 3 seconds in a child or infant. If the pulse is absent, begin cycles of 30 chest compressions followed by two slow breaths.

When both breathing and pulse stop, the victim has suffered sudden death. There are many causes of sudden death, including heart disease, choking, drowning, poisoning, suffocation, electrocution, and smoke inhalation. CPR must be started immediately in an attempt to revive the patient and

PROCEDURE 26-3

Perform Adult Rescue Breathing and One-Rescuer CPR

<u>ABHES COMPETENCY:</u> 4.f.

GOAL: *To restore a victim's breathing and blood circulation when respiration, pulse, or both stop.*

EQUIPMENT and SUPPLIES

- Disposable gloves
- CPR ventilator mask
- Approved mannequin

PROCEDURAL STEPS (To be performed on an approved mannequin only)

1. Establish unresponsiveness. Tap the victim and ask, "Are you OK?" Wait for victim to respond.
   <u>PURPOSE:</u> To determine whether the victim is conscious.

2. Activate the emergency response system. Put on gloves and get ventilator mask.
   <u>PURPOSE:</u> As soon as it is determined that an adult victim requires emergency care, immediately activate EMS. Most adults with sudden, nontraumatic cardiac arrest are in ventricular fibrillation. The time from collapse to defibrillation is the single most important predictor of survival.

3. Tilt the victim's head by placing one hand on the forehead and applying enough pressure to push the head back and with the fingers of the other hand under the chin, lift up and pull the jaw forward. Look, listen, and feel for signs of breathing. Place your ear over the mouth and listen for breathing. Watch the rising and falling of the chest for evidence of breathing (Figure 1*). If breathing is absent or inadequate, open the open airway and place the ventilator mask over the victim's nose.
   <u>PURPOSE:</u> To open the airway and determine if the victim is breathing.

4. Give two slow breaths (1½ to 2 seconds per breath for an adult and 1 to 2 seconds per breath for an infant or child), holding the ventilator mask tightly against the face while tilting the victim's chin back to keep the airway open (Figure 2*). Remove your mouth from the mouthpiece between breaths to allow time for patient exhalation between breaths.

5. Check the patient's pulse (at the carotid artery for an adult or older child or brachial artery for an infant). If a pulse is present, continue rescue breathing (one breath every 4 to 5 seconds, about 10 to 12 breaths per minute for an adult, or one breath about every 3 seconds, about 12 to 20 breaths per minute, for an infant or child). If no signs of circulation are present, begin cycles of 30 chest compressions (at a rate of about 100 compressions per minute for an adult) followed by two slow breaths.

6. To deliver chest compressions, kneel at the victim's side a couple of inches away from the chest. Move your fingers up the ribs to the point where the sternum and the ribs join in the center of the lower part of the sternum but above the xiphoid process.

7. Place the heel of your hand on the chest over the lower part of the sternum.

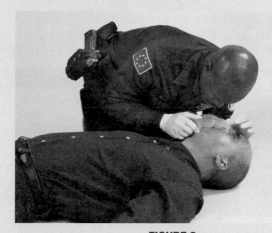

FIGURE 2

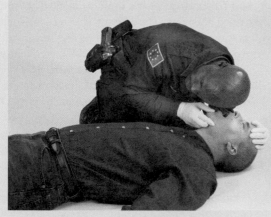

FIGURE 1

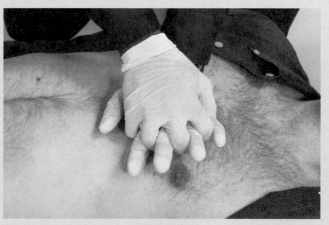

FIGURE 3

Continued

PROCEDURE 26-3—cont'd

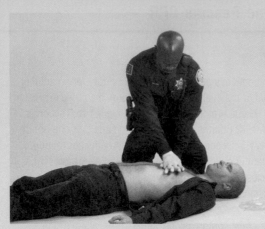

FIGURE 4

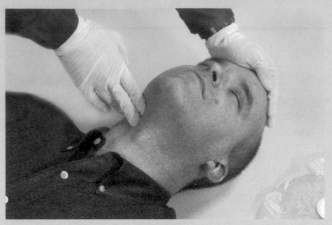

FIGURE 5

8. Place your other hand on top of the first, and either interlace or lift your fingers upward off of the chest (Figure 3*).
   PURPOSE: This position gives you the most control, allowing you to avoid injuring the victim's ribs as you compress the chest.

9. Bring your shoulders directly over the victim's sternum as you compress downward, and keep your elbows locked (Figure 4*).

10. Depress the sternum 1½ to 2 inches in an adult victim. Relax the pressure on the sternum after each compression, but do not remove your hands from the victim's sternum.
    PURPOSE: The depth of compression is needed to circulate blood through the heart. Movement of the hands may cause injury to the victim.

11. After performing 30 compressions (at a rate of about 100 compressions per minute), open the airway and give two slow rescue breaths.

12. After five cycles of compressions and breaths (30:2 ratio, about 2 minutes) recheck breathing and carotid pulse (Figure 5). If there is a pulse but no breathing, continue rescue breathing (one breath every 5 seconds, about 10 to 12 breaths per minute) and reevaluate the victim's breathing and pulse every few minutes. If no signs of circulation are present, continue 30:2 cycles of compressions and ventilations, starting with chest compressions. Continue giving CPR until an AED is available or EMS relieves you.

13. Remove gloves and the ventilator mask valve and dispose in the biohazard container. Disinfect the ventilator mask per manufacturer recommendations. Wash hands.

14. Document the procedure and patient condition.

From Chapleau W: *Emergency medical technician: making the difference,* St Louis, 2007, Mosby.

prevent permanent damage to body organs, especially the brain. After five cycles of compressions and ventilations in the adult patient, recheck the pulse. If no signs of circulation are present, continue CPR until help arrives. If there is a pulse but no breathing, continue rescue breathing and occasionally monitor the pulse until help arrives.

Refer to the American Red Cross *Standard First Aid Manual* or *American Heart Association CPR Manual,* or the organizations' websites for specific procedures and precautions in the management of respiratory and cardiac emergencies. As stated earlier, all healthcare workers must have current CPR Certification for the Professional.

Cardiac Emergencies

Chest pain or angina can be associated with heart and lung disease, as well as a few other conditions. It can be quite serious; a patient with chest pain is treated as a cardiac emergency until a physician has ruled this out. The patient is often sweating and may have a gray, ashen appearance. The lips and fingernails may be blue, which is a sign of **cyanosis** (Figure 26-7). Frequently the patient will clutch the chest in pain. This pain may radiate from the **mediastinum** down the left arm and up the left side of the neck. The pulse may be rapid and weak, and the patient often complains of nausea.

If a patient has any of these signs or symptoms, report this to the clinician immediately. If the physician is not available, activate EMS. Use a wheelchair to move the patient to an examination room. Breathing will be easier if the patient's head is slightly elevated or in Fowler's position. Keep the patient quiet and warm. Loosen all tight clothing. Take vital signs, including both apical and radial pulses. The physician may order oxygen started on the patient to relieve **dyspnea**

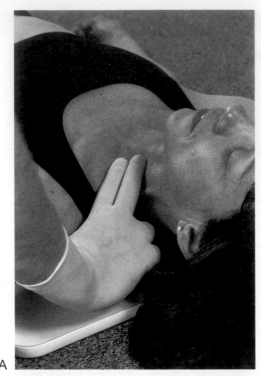

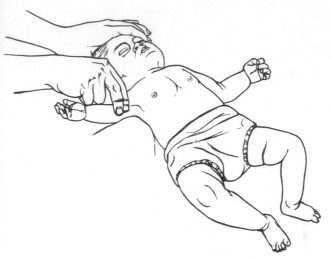

FIGURE 26-6 A, In an adult, check for carotid pulse. **B,** In an infant, check for brachial pulse.

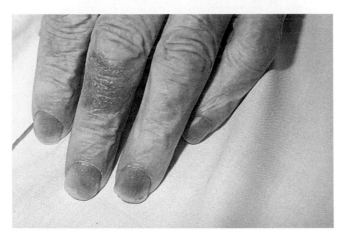

FIGURE 26-7 Cyanosis of nail beds. (From Henry MC, Stapleton ER: *EMT prehospital care*, ed 3, Philadelphia, 2004, Saunders.)

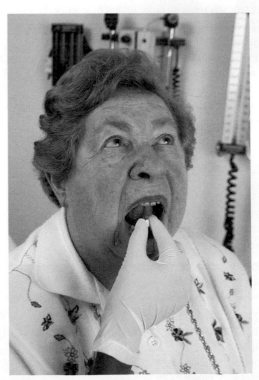

FIGURE 26-8 Nitroglycerin is administered beneath patient's tongue.

(Procedure 26-4). Bring the emergency cart into the room and open the medication drawer so the physician is able to quickly prepare the medications needed. These may include epinephrine (adrenaline), atropine, digitalis, calcium chloride, or morphine.

If the patient is conscious, ask about any medication that he or she has recently taken or is carrying. If the patient has an established heart disorder, the patient may be carrying nitroglycerin tablets. Nitroglycerin tablets are administered sublingually and may be given with the patient's consent (Figure 26-8). If the physician is in the office or is on the way, connect the patient to the electrocardiograph and record a few tracings. If the patient becomes unresponsive before the physician or EMS arrives, it may be necessary to start rescue breathing if there is no evidence of respirations. If chest pain progresses to cardiac arrest and loss of circulation, CPR must be perform until help arrives.

Signs of a Heart Attack

A heart attack, or *myocardial infarction,* is usually caused b blockage of the coronary arteries that decreases the amoun

PROCEDURE 26-4

Administer Oxygen

ABHES COMPETENCY: 4.f.

GOAL: *To provide oxygen for a patient in respiratory distress.*

EQUIPMENT and SUPPLIES

- Portable oxygen tank
- Pressure regulator
- Flow meter
- Nasal cannula with connecting tubing
- Physician order
- Patient chart

PROCEDURAL STEPS

1. Gather equipment and wash hands.
2. Identify the patient and explain the procedure.
   PURPOSE: A nasal cannula is applied with a nasal prong in each nostril and the tab resting above the upper lip. Patients who will be using oxygen at home need to be taught how to open an oxygen tank or to use an oxygen compressor. It is vital that patients and their families understand the dangers of oxygen use in the home. They must avoid open flames and not smoke when oxygen is in use, because it is combustible. The physician will typically write an order for the number of liters of oxygen to be delivered and for home healthcare services to set up the equipment in the patient's home.
3. Check the pressure gauge on the tank to determine the amount of oxygen in the tank.
4. If necessary, open the cylinder on the tank one full counterclockwise turn, then attach the cannula tubing to the flow meter.
5. Adjust the administration of the oxygen according to the physician's order. Usually the flow meter is set at 12 to 15 liters per minute (LPM). Check to make sure oxygen is flowing through the cannula.
6. Insert cannula tips into the nostrils, and adjust the tubing around the back of the patient's ears (Figure 1).
7. Make sure the patient is comfortable and answer any questions.
8. Wash hands.
9. Document the procedure, including the number of liters of oxygen being administered and the patient's condition. Continue to monitor the patient throughout the procedure, and document any changes in condition.

See Appendix D for a charting example.

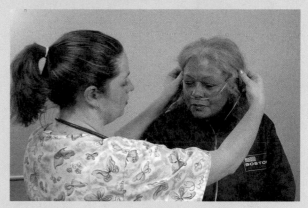

FIGURE 1

Signs and Symptoms of Myocardial Infarction in Women

Women may experience different symptoms than those traditionally associated with a heart attack. These include a combination of the following:

- Back pain or aching and throbbing in the biceps or forearms
- Shortness of breath (SOB)
- Clammy perspiration
- Dizziness (*vertigo*)—unexplained lightheadedness or *syncopal* episodes
- Edema—especially of the ankles and/or lower legs
- Fluttering heartbeat or tachycardia
- Gastric upset
- Feeling of heaviness or fullness in the mediastinum

blood being delivered to the myocardium. The most common signal of a heart attack is an uncomfortable pressure, squeezing, fullness, or pain in the center of the chest. This may spread to the shoulder, neck, jaw, or arms. The pain may not be severe. Other symptoms include sweating *(diaphoresis)*, nausea or indigestion, shortness of breath (SOB), cold and clammy skin, and a feeling of weakness *(general malaise)*. If these signs persist longer than 5 minutes, the patient should activate EMS. However, the vast majority of people will deny that the problem is serious until they require immediate medical attention.

Choking

Choking is usually caused by a foreign object, often a bolus of food, lodged in the upper airway. The victim may clutch the neck between the thumb and index finger (Figure 26-9). This universal distress signal should be viewed as a sign that the

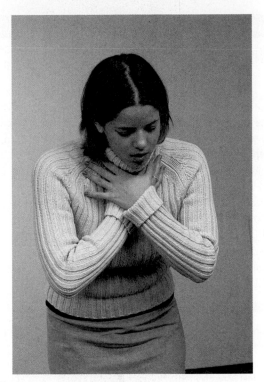

FIGURE 26-9 Universal sign of choking.

need help. If the patient is unable to speak, breathe, or cough, a complete airway obstruction exists and quick action must be taken to clear the airway. With a complete obstruction the patient will eventually lose consciousness from lack of oxygen to the brain. This condition may lead to respiratory and cardiac arrest. If the object is not removed, the victim may die within 4 to 6 minutes. Refer to Procedure 26-5 to learn the steps involved in clearing an obstructed airway on an adult. The procedure for removal of a foreign airway obstruction is exactly the same for a child over the age of 1 year.

To dislodge a foreign object from the airway of an infant up to age 1 year, place the baby face down over your forearm and across your thigh. The head should be lower than the trunk, and you should support the baby's head and neck with one hand. Using the heel of your other hand, deliver five blows to the back, between the infant's shoulder blades (Figure 26-10, *A*). Holding the baby between your arms, turn the infant face up, keeping the head lower than the trunk. Using two fingers, deliver five thrusts to the midsternal area at the infant's nipple line (Figure 26-10, *B*). Examine the infant's mouth, and if the object is visible, pluck it out with your fingertips, but never perform a finger sweep on an infant. A baby's oral cavity is too small for a finger sweep; such an action may only lodge the obstruction farther into the airway. If the obstruction is not visible, administer two rescue breaths by covering both the baby's nose and mouth with your mouth or use a pediatric ventilator mask if available. Repeat the sequence until the foreign body is expelled or help arrives.

It is possible to perform the abdominal thrust maneuver on yourself if you are choking and no one is nearby to help you. Press your fist into your upper abdomen with quick upward thrusts, or lean forward and press the abdomen quickly against a firm object, such as the back of a chair. In the case of a woman

victim needs help. If the victim has good air exchange or only partial airway obstruction and can speak, cough, or breathe, do not interfere but encourage the patient to continue coughing until the object is expelled. Monitor the patient for signs of respiratory distress, such as pallor and cyanosis. If the patient has a pronounced wheeze or a very weak cough, he or she has a partial airway obstruction with poor air exchange and may

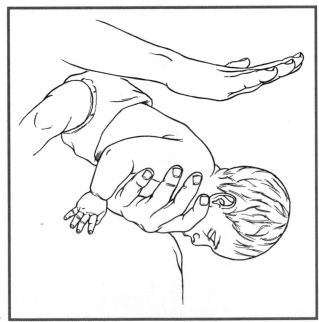

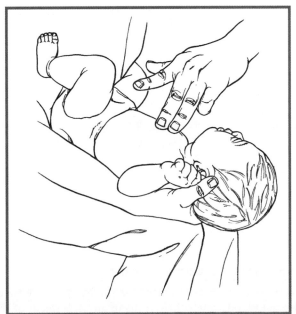

A   B

FIGURE 26-10 A, Back blows are administered to an infant supported on the arm and thigh. **B,** Chest thrusts are administered in the same position as for cardiac compressions. (From Henry MC, Stapleton ER: *EMT prehospital care*, ed 3, Philadelphia, 2004, Saunders.)

PROCEDURE 26-5

Respond to an Adult with an Obstructed Airway

<u>ABHES COMPETENCY:</u> 4.f.

GOAL: *To remove an airway obstruction and restore ventilation.*

EQUIPMENT and SUPPLIES

- Disposable gloves
- Ventilation mask (for unconscious victim)
- Approved mannequin to practice unconscious foreign body airway obstruction (FBAO)

PROCEDURAL STEPS (Unconscious maneuver to be performed on an approved mannequin only)

1. Ask "Are you choking?" If victim indicates yes, ask "Can you speak?" If the victim is unable to speak, tell the victim you are going to help.
   <u>PURPOSE:</u> If the victim is unable to speak, is coughing weakly, and/or is wheezing, there is an obstructed airway with poor air exchange and the obstruction must be removed before respiratory arrest occurs.

2. Stand behind the victim with feet slightly apart.
   <u>PURPOSE:</u> With an obstructed airway, the victim may lose consciousness at any time. The rescuer must be prepared to safely lower the unconscious victim to the floor.

3. Reach around the victim's abdomen and place an index finger into the victim's navel or at the level of the belt buckle. Make a fist of the opposite hand (do not tuck the thumb into the fist) and place the thumb side of the fist against the victim's abdomen above the navel. If the victim is pregnant, place the fist above

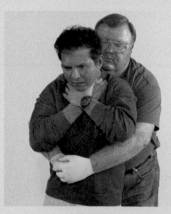

FIGURE 1

the enlarged uterus. If the victim is obese, it may be necessary to place the fist higher in the abdomen. It may be necessary to perform chest thrusts on a victim who is pregnant or obese.
<u>PURPOSE:</u> The fist should be placed in the soft tissue of the abdomen to avoid injury to the sternum or rib cage.

4. Place the opposite hand over the fist, and give abdominal thrusts in a quick inward and upward movement (Figure 1*).
   <u>PURPOSE:</u> Abdominal contents pushing against the diaphragm force trapped air out of the lungs and with it the obstruction.

5. Repeat the abdominal thrusts until the object is expelled or the victim becomes unresponsive.

UNRESPONSIVE ADULT VICTIM

6. Carefully lower the patient to the ground, activate the emergency response system, and apply disposable gloves.

7. Immediately begin CPR with 30 compressions and two breath cycles.
   <u>PURPOSE:</u> Higher airway pressures are maintained with chest compressions rather than abdominal thrusts.

8. Each time the airway is opened to deliver a rescue breath during CPR, look for an object in the victim's mouth and remove it if visible. If no object is found, immediately return to the cycle of 30 chest compressions.

9. A finger sweep should only be used if the rescuer can see the obstruction.

10. Continue cycles of 30 compressions to two rescue breaths until either the obstruction is removed or EMS arrives.

11. If the obstruction is removed, assess the victim for breathing and circulation. If a pulse is present, but the patient is not breathing, begin rescue breathing.

12. Once either the patient is stabilized or EMS has taken over care, remove gloves and the ventilator mask valve and dispose in the biohazard container. Disinfect the ventilator mask per manufacturer recommendations. Wash hands.

13. Document the procedure and patient condition.

*From Chapleau W: *Emergency medical technician: making the difference*, St Louis, 2007, Mosby.
See Appendix D for a charting example.

---

in the late stages of pregnancy, chest compressions should be delivered to prevent possible trauma to the infant.

Cerebrovascular Accident (Stroke)

A cerebrovascular accident (CVA), or stroke, is a disorder of the cerebral blood vessels that results in an impairment of the blood supply to part of the brain. This interruption in normal circulation of blood through the brain leads to some degree of neurologic damage, either temporary or permanent, depending on the severity of the oxygen deprivation to the brain cells.

A minor stroke or **transient ischemic attack** (TIA) usually does not cause unconsciousness, and symptoms depend on the location of the circulatory problem in the brain as well as the amount of brain damage. TIA symptoms are temporary and may include headache, confusion, vertigo, ringing in the ears *(tinnitus)*, temporary paralysis or weakness of one side of the body, transient limb weakness, slurred speech, and vision problems. TIA episodes indicate that the patient is at risk for a major stroke.

Symptoms of a major stroke include unconsciousness, paralysis on one side of the body, difficulty in breathing and swallowing, loss of bladder and bowel control, unequal pupil size, and slurring of speech.

Home recommendations for a patient who has suffered a major stroke should begin with notifying the physician and/or activating EMS. Keep the patient lying down and lightly covered. Maintain an open airway. Position the head so that any secretions will drain from the side of the mouth to prevent choking. If the patient did not fall and no indications of a head or neck injury are present, the patient can be placed in the recovery position, which uses gravity to drain fluids from the mouth and keep the trachea clear. Do not give the patient anything to eat or drink. Vital signs should be measured at regular intervals and recorded for the physician.

The recovery position is used as follows:

1. Place the patient on the left side. If the patient is lying on his or her back, raise the left arm above the head and cross the right leg over the left. Roll the patient toward you while keeping the head and neck in alignment.
2. Place the left arm behind the patient (similar to Sims' position).
3. Bend the right arm, and place the right hand under the side of the face.

Advances made in the early treatment of strokes show great promise in preventing long-term neurologic deficits. However, to prevent permanent brain damage, **thrombolytics** must be administered intravenously within 3 hours of the onset of symptoms. If a patient does not know when symptoms began, for example if he or she woke up with the symptoms, or if the patient cannot accurately tell the physician when the symptoms started, then the time allotted for administration begins from when the patient was last known to be asymptomatic. Intracranial hemorrhage must be ruled out before treatment begins. The earlier the treatment starts, the better the neurologic outcomes. The best possible outcomes are seen in those patients who received thrombolytic therapy within 90 minutes of the onset of symptoms.

CRITICAL THINKING APPLICATION

Thomas Antonio, a 67-year-old patient, calls to report that when he woke up this morning the left side of his face was drooping and he had difficulty seeing out of his left eye. The symptoms went away in about 2 hours, and he is feeling fine now. There are not any openings in the schedule for 2 days. When should Cheryl make Mr. Antonio an appointment? What questions should Cheryl ask Mr. Antonio?

Shock

Shock is a state of collapse resulting from failure of the circulatory system to deliver enough oxygenated blood to the body's vital organs. An injury, hemorrhage, infection, anesthesia, drug overdose, burns, pain, fear, or emotional stress may cause this

Types and Causes of Shock

- Anaphylactic—a severe allergic reaction
- Insulin—overdose of insulin causing severe hypoglycemia
- Psychogenic or mental—excessive fear, joy, anger, or emotional stress
- Hypovolemic or hemorrhagic—excessive loss of blood
- Cardiogenic—myocardial infarction, pulmonary embolism, or severe congestive heart failure
- Neurogenic—dilation of blood vessels resulting from brain or spinal cord injuries
- Septic—systemic infection

physiologic reaction. Shock can be immediate or delayed or mild or severe and is potentially fatal. Many different types of shock may occur, but the signs and symptoms are universal. The most common indicators of shock are a pale, gray, or cyanotic appearance; moist but cool skin; dilated pupils; weak and rapid pulse; marked hypotension; shallow and rapid respirations; lethargy or restlessness; nausea and vomiting; and extreme thirst.

If a patient exhibits signs of shock, maintain an open airway and check for breathing and circulation. Place the patient supine with the legs elevated approximately 1 foot to return the blood from the legs to vital organs. Loosen all tight clothing, and cover the patient with a blanket for warmth. Do not move the patient unnecessarily. Fluids may be given by mouth if the patient is alert. Because shock can develop into a life-threatening situation, it is advisable to administer only basic first aid care and to have the patient transported to the hospital as soon as possible.

COMMON OFFICE EMERGENCIES

The remainder of the chapter highlights typical emergencies seen either in the ambulatory care setting or in telephone triage situations. Table 26-1 summarizes common emergencies, the questions that should be asked, and possible home care advice.

Fainting (Syncope)

Fainting or *syncope* is a common emergency problem. Syncope is usually caused by a transient loss of blood flow to the brain, such as a sudden drop in blood pressure, which results in a temporary loss of consciousness. It can occur without warning, or the patient may appear pale; may feel cold, weak, dizzy, or nauseated; and may have numbness of the extremities before the incident. The greatest danger to the patient is an injury from falling during the attack. Therefore if the patient presents with syncopal symptoms, immediately place the patient in a supine position. Loosen all tight clothing and maintain an open airway. Apply a cold washcloth to the forehead. Measure the patient's pulse, respiration rate, and blood pressure, and report the findings to the physician. Keep the patient in a supine position for at least 10 minutes after consciousness has been regained. A complete patient history helps diagnose the possible

TABLE 26-1 Telephone Triage Approach

EMERGENCY SITUATION	SCREENING QUESTIONS	HOME CARE ADVICE
Syncope	Was the patient injured? Does the patient have a history of heart disease, seizures, or diabetes?	Does not necessarily indicate a serious disease. If injured from a fall, the patient may need to be evaluated and treated. The patient should get up very slowly to prevent a recurrence, take it easy, and drink plenty of fluids. If the patient is to be seen, someone should accompany him or her to the clinician's practice.
Animal bites	What kind of animal (pet or wild)? How severe is the injury? Where are the bites? When did the bite occur?	The health department or police should be notified. Every effort must be made to locate the animal and monitor its health. If the skin is not broken, wash well and observe for signs of infection.
Insect bites and stings	Does the patient have a history of anaphylactic reaction to insect stings? Does the patient have difficulty breathing, have a widespread rash, or have trouble swallowing?	If there is a history of anaphylaxis and the patient has an EpiPen, it should be administered immediately and EMS notified. Activate EMS if the patient is having systemic symptoms. An antihistamine (Benadryl) relieves local pruritus.
Asthma	Does the patient show signs of cyanosis? Has the patient used the prescribed inhalers?	If a patient with asthma is unable to speak in sentences, has poor color, and is struggling to breathe even after inhaler use, he or she should be seen immediately or EMS should be activated.
Burns	Where are the burns located, and what caused them? Are there signs of shock (moist, clammy skin, altered consciousness, rapid breathing and pulse)? Are there signs of infection (foul odor, cloudy drainage) in a burn more than 2 days old?	Activate EMS for burns on the face, hands, feet, or perineum, those caused by electricity or a chemical, or burns associated with inhalation. Activate EMS if there are signs of shock. The patient must receive a tetanus shot if it has been more than 10 years since the last one. Schedule an urgent appointment if signs of infection are reported.
Wounds	Is the bleeding steady or pulsating? How and when did the injury occur? Does the patient have any bleeding disorders or is the patient on anticoagulant drugs? Is the wound open and deep?	Pulsating bleeding usually indicates arterial damage; activate EMS. If the injury was caused by a powerful force, other injuries may exist. For patients taking anticoagulants or with diabetes or anemia, schedule an urgent appointment. A gaping, deep wound requires sutures.
Head injury	Did the patient pass out or have a seizure? Is the patient confused or vomiting? Is there clear drainage from nose or ears?	If the answer is 'yes' to any of these symptoms, EMS should be activated.

causes of the attack, such as history of heart disease or diabetes. Document the details of the episode and how long it took for complete recovery (Procedure 26-6).

If the patient does not recover quickly, the physician may activate EMS for transport to the hospital. Syncope might be a brief episode in the development of a serious underlying illness, such as an abnormal heart rhythm, that may lead to sudden cardiac death.

Poisoning

Poisonings are considered medical emergencies and are the sixth leading cause of accidental pediatric deaths in the United States. Poisoning can occur by oral intake, absorption, inhalation, or injection. Over-the-counter medications such as acetaminophen, detergents and bleach, plants, cough and cold medicines, and vitamins cause the majority of poisoning cases seen in young children. Other typical household poisons include drain cleaners, turpentine, kerosene, furniture polish, and paints (Figure 26-11). Signs and symptoms of poisoning vary greatly and include burns on the hands and mouth, stains on the victim's clothing, open bottles of medicines or chemicals, changes in skin color, nausea or stomach cramps, shallow breathing, convulsions, heavy perspiration, dizziness or drowsiness, and unconsciousness.

What to Ask When a Poisoning Is Reported

- The name, weight, and age of the victim
- The name of the poison taken and any information on the label
- How much was taken
- How long ago the poison was ingested
- Whether vomiting has occurred
- Any pertinent symptoms, such as difficulty breathing or an altered state of consciousness
- Any first aid given

PROCEDURE 26-6

Care for a Patient Who Has Fainted

ABHES COMPETENCY: 4.f.

GOAL: *To provide emergency care for and assessment of a patient who has fainted.*

EQUIPMENT and SUPPLIES

- Patient record
- Sphygmomanometer
- Stethoscope
- Watch with second hand
- Blanket
- Foot stool or box
- Pillows
- Oxygen equipment, if ordered by physician:
    - Portable oxygen tank
    - Pressure regulator
    - Flow meter
    - Nasal cannula with connecting tubing

PROCEDURAL STEPS

1. If warning is given that the patient feels faint, have the patient lower the head to the knees to increase the blood supply to the brain (Figure 1*). If this does not stop the episode, either have the patient lie down on the examination table or lower the patient to the floor. If the patient collapses to the floor when fainting, treat with caution because of possible head or neck injuries.

2. Immediately notify the physician of the patient's condition, and assess the patient for life-threatening emergencies such as respiratory or cardiac arrest. If the patient is breathing and has a pulse, monitor the patient's vital signs.

3. Loosen any tight clothing and keep the patient warm, applying a blanket if needed.

4. If there is no concern about a head or neck injury, elevate the patient's legs above the level of the heart using the footstool with pillow support if available (Figure 2*).
   <u>PURPOSE:</u> Elevating the legs will assist with venous blood return to the heart. This may relieve symptoms of fainting by elevating the blood pressure and increasing blood flow to vital organs.

5. Continue to monitor vital signs, and apply oxygen via nasal cannula if ordered by the physician.

6. If vital signs are unstable or the patient does not respond quickly, activate emergency medical services.
   <u>PURPOSE:</u> Fainting may be a sign of a life-threatening problem.

7. If the patient vomits, roll the patient on his or her side to avoid aspiration of vomitus into the lungs.

8. Once the patient has completely recovered, assist the patient into a sitting position. Do not leave the patient unattended on the examination table.

9. Document the incident, including a description of the episode, patient symptoms, vital signs, length of time, and any complaints. If oxygen was administered, document the number of liters and length of administration.

---

*From Bonewit-West K: *Clinical procedures for medical assistants*, ed 5, Philadelphia, 2000, Saunders.
See Appendix D for a charting example.

FIGURE 1

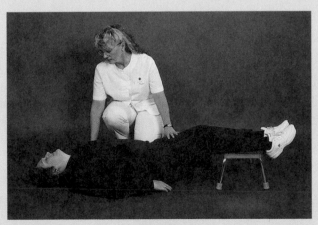

FIGURE 2

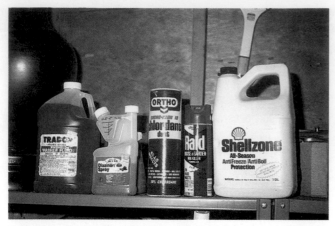

FIGURE 26-11 Hazardous household materials. (From Henry MC, Stapleton ER: *EMT prehospital care*, ed 3, Philadelphia, 2004, Saunders.)

Instruct the caller not to hang up and not to leave the victim unattended. Call the local poison control center, and forward all directions to the caller. Syrup of ipecac, which will cause vomiting within 15 to 20 minutes, should be used only if ordered by the physician or poison control center, because some substances can cause irritation to the tissues when vomited. Do not induce vomiting if the victim is either not alert or having a convulsion because of the risk of aspiration. If syrup of ipecac is recommended, give 2 teaspoons to infants 9 to 12 months old after the child has drunk about 4 oz of warm water. For a child 1 to 4 years old, administer 1 tablespoon after the child has drunk 4 to 8 oz of warm water. If the patient is to be seen by the physician or sent to the hospital, tell the caller to bring the container of poison or sample of vomitus with them so the chemical contents of the substance can be verified.

CRITICAL THINKING APPLICATION

A young mother calls in a panic to report her 18-month-old daughter swallowed at least half a bottle of cough syrup. The child is fussy and very sleepy, and the mother wants to give her ipecac immediately. What should Cheryl do?

Animal Bites

Potential complications from animal bites include rabies, tetanus, and local skin infections. Any animal bite that is extensive or deep should be seen by a physician. Human infection with rabies is rare, but if the bite occurs from a domestic animal, it is recommended that the animal be kept quarantined and under observation for 10 days to monitor for signs of the disease. The animal should not be killed, because a positive rabies identification is almost impossible to make if the animal has been dead for a period of time. If the bite is from a bat, raccoon, or any other wild animal, the animal is assumed to be rabid and the patient must undergo a series of rabies vaccine injections. Local skin infections can be prevented by immediately cleansing the area with antimicrobial soap and water. If the bite (including human) breaks the skin, the patient's tetanus immunization status must be checked and, if needed, a booster or the entire four-dose tetanus series must be administered as indicated.

Insect Bites and Stings

The bite or sting of an insect can be irritating and painful because of the chemical toxin injected from the insect, but it usually is not serious. Typical symptoms—inflammation, itching *(pruritus)*, and edema—are local and confined to the area of the bite. Rarely a severe allergic reaction occurs, which is a potentially dangerous situation that can lead to anaphylaxis. Signs and symptoms of a systemic allergic reaction include a dry cough, feeling of tightening in the throat or chest, swelling or itching around the eyes, widespread hives *(urticaria)*, wheezing, dyspnea, and hypotension. Difficulty in talking is a sign of urticaria or edema in the throat and may indicate the onset of complete airway obstruction. This is a sign of a true emergency. Epinephrine and oxygen should be ready for immediate administration on the physician's orders. Antihistamines may be used, as well as corticosteroids, but the action of these agents is considerably slower than that of epinephrine. If the patient develops acute anaphylactic shock, death may occur within 1 hour unless medical intervention is initiated.

If the stinger is still lodged in the skin, scrape it off with a dull knife, credit card, or fingernail. Be careful not to squeeze the stinger, because that will inject more venom into the skin. Apply an ice bag to the site to relieve pain and slow the absorption of the venom. Calamine lotion or hydrocortisone cream may be applied to relieve itching. If the patient has a history of allergies, especially to insect venom, he or she should have access to an EpiPen injection system and use it immediately after the sting occurs and should be transported to the nearest hospital for immediate care.

Tick Removal

Ticks can cause a number of diseases, including Rocky Mountain spotted fever and Lyme disease. They embed their heads in the skin to obtain blood and should be removed intact by the following method:
1. Do not handle ticks with uncovered fingers; use tweezers to prevent personal contamination.
2. Place the tips of the tweezers as close as possible to the area where the tick has entered the skin.
3. With steady slow motion, pull the tick away from the skin. Try not to squeeze or crush the tick. If the entire tick's body is not removed, make a physician's appointment to evaluate the site.
4. After removal, place the tick directly into a sealable container. Disinfect the area around the bite site using standard procedures.
5. The physician may suggest the tick be brought to the office to be tested for disease.

Asthma Attacks

Asthma is a condition characterized by expiratory wheezing, coughing, a feeling of tightness in the chest, and SOB. During an asthma attack two different physiologic responses occur. The lining of the respiratory tract becomes inflamed and edematous and produces mucus, which results in a narrowing of the air passages. At the same time, bronchospasms occur that also constrict the airways. The quality and severity of attacks vary greatly among patients, and treatment must be individualized to minimize or eliminate chronic symptoms. If the patient is prescribed a bronchodilator inhaler, it should be used at the first indication of symptoms. Depending on the severity of the attack, give the patient an appointment for the same day of the call or consult the physician. The physician may recommend the patient go directly to the ER for emergency respiratory care.

Seizures

Seizures may be **idiopathic** or may result from trauma, injury, or metabolic alterations, such as hypoglycemia or hypocalcemia. A *febrile* seizure is transient and occurs with a rapid rise in fever over 101.8° F (38.8° C). Febrile seizures typically occur in children between 6 months and 5 years of age. Many different types of seizures occur, but they all are caused by a disruption in the electrical activity of the brain.

If a patient suffers a grand mal seizure, which involves uncontrolled muscular contractions, the most important factor is protecting the patient from possible injury. Clear everything away from the patient that could cause accidental injury, and observe the patient until the seizure ends. Do not place anything in the patient's mouth, because it may damage the teeth or tongue. Do not hold the patient down, because that may result in muscle injuries or fractures. If the patient remains unconscious after the seizure has subsided, place the patient in the recovery position to maintain an open airway and allow drainage of excess saliva. After the seizure is over, let the patient rest or sleep, but never leave the patient alone. If the physician is not in the office, check the office procedure manual to determine how to manage the situation.

Call 911 for emergency assistance in any of the following situations:

- The patient has not regained consciousness within 10 to 15 minutes.
- The seizure does not stop within a few minutes.
- The patient begins a second seizure immediately after the initial one.
- The patient is pregnant.
- Signs of head trauma are present.
- The patient is a known diabetic.
- The seizure was triggered by a high fever in a child.

Abdominal Pain

Abdominal pain is a symptom caused by many different problems and may range from acute discomfort to life-threatening complications. The clinician should see every patient who reports abdominal pain; the question is how soon the patient should be seen. A patient with acute onset of severe and persistent abdominal pain, especially when this is accompanied by fever, should receive medical attention as soon as possible. Abdominal pain has a variety of causes, including intestinal infections, appendicitis, ectopic pregnancy, inflammation, hemorrhage, obstruction, and tumors.

Triage Guidelines for Assessing Abdominal Pain

- Investigate the presence of shock-related signs and symptoms—diaphoresis; cold, clammy skin; cyanosis or gray pallor; rapid respirations; altered state of consciousness.
- Is the pain severe and constant, or does it come in waves?
- Has the patient had any bloody or tarry stools?
- Is there a fever greater than 101° F?
- Could the patient be pregnant, or has she missed a menstrual period?
- Has the patient experienced continuous vomiting or severe constipation?
- Are there any urinary symptoms such as frequency, **hematuria,** or flank pain?
- Does the patient have chest pain, SOB, or continuous cough?
- Is there a history of serious illness such as diabetes, heart disease, or cancer?

Treatment in the ambulatory care setting depends on the cause of the pain; however, the medical assistant should observe the following general guidelines:

- Keep the patient warm and quiet
- Have an emesis basin available
- Administer nothing by mouth (NPO)
- Do not apply heat to the abdomen unless so instructed by the physician
- Administer analgesics as ordered
- Check and record the patient's vital signs, and follow the physician's orders

Sprains and Strains

Sprains are tears of the ligaments that support a joint, and *strains* are injuries to a muscle and its tendons. Both types of injury may also cause damage to surrounding soft tissue, blood vessels, and nearby nerves. With a sprain the victim develops edema and **ecchymosis** around the injury, and any movement of the joint, especially a twisting one, results in pain. There usually is no swelling or discoloration with a strain and only mild tenderness unless the injured muscle or tendon is used. Tendon strains and ligament sprains take several weeks to heal, whereas muscle tears usually heal in 1 to 2 weeks, because muscle has such a rich blood supply. These injuries are treated by elevating the affected area and applying mild compression and ice. Swelling is reduced if ice is applied within 20 to 30 minutes of the injury. After 24 to 36 hours, alternately applying mild heat and ice is usually indicated. The patient may be advised to immobilize the part.

Fractures

A fracture is a break or crack in a bone and can result from trauma or disease. Fractures are very painful and affect the patient's ability to freely move the injured part. When a patient with a fracture is brought into the office, the medical assistant should make the patient as comfortable as possible. Place the patient in a position that does not place strain on the area. Notify the physician immediately, and proceed according to the orders given. Emergency treatment for fractures includes preventing movement of the injured part through splinting, elevation of the affected extremity, application of ice, and control of any bleeding. If a patient with an open fracture is seen in an ambulatory care setting, he or she should be transported to the ER.

Burns

Burns are among the most frequent causes of injuries in the United States. Burn injuries can result from flame, heat, scalds, electricity, chemicals, or radiation. The skin surface may be reddened, blistered, or charred. The depth and extent of burns are the major determinants in classifying the severity of the burn. The extent of the pain is directly proportional to the extent of the surface area burned, as well as the depth and nature of the burn.

To triage a burn injury, it is necessary to understand what caused the burn, its location and approximate size, the depth of the burn, and whether any additional injuries also occurred. The percentage of the body surface area burned can be estimated using the Rule of Nines (Figure 26-12). This is an assessment tool that helps caregivers make a quick calculation of the amount of burnt tissue. With the Rule of Nines, the body is divided into areas approximately equal to 9% of the total body surface area. When a burn victim is assessed, the affected regions are combined to estimate the total percentage of burned tissue. Partial-thickness burns over 15% of the total body surface

and full-thickness burns of less than 2% can be treated in the ambulatory care setting if the patient can be seen immediately. Patients with larger body surface area involvement or other complications should be immediately transported to a hospital, preferably one with a burn unit.

Lacerations

Lacerations are a common presentation in a primary care physician's office. A lacerated wound displays a jagged or irregular tearing of the tissues. The severity depends on the mechanism, site, and extent of the injury and the presence of foreign bodies or contamination in the wound. The injury that caused the laceration may also have caused damage to blood vessels, nerves, bones, joints, and organs within the body cavities.

When the patient arrives at the facility, apply gloves and notify the physician immediately. Have the patient lie down. Cover the injured area with a sterile dressing; use a dressing that is thick enough to absorb the bleeding (Procedure 26-7). Reassure the patient and explain your actions as much as possible. Ask the patient when he or she last received a tetanus inoculation, and record the date in the patient's record. If it has been more than 10 years, the physician will probably want a booster injection given.

Wounds that are not bleeding severely and that do not involve deep tissue damage should be cleansed with antimicrobial soap and water to remove bacteria and other foreign matter. If the laceration is extremely dirty, the physician may want the area irrigated with a sterile normal saline solution.

A butterfly closure strip may be used over small lacerations to hold the edges together. If the wound is superficial and has straight edges, it may be closed with a microporous tape (such as Steri-Strips), which eliminate the discomfort of suturing and suture removal. Other wound closure devices include Dermabond fluid, which forms a strong, flexible closure that is similar in strength to nylon suture material. It is very useful for the closure of simple lacerations in children and provides an antimicrobial and waterproof coating to the wound site that will last for several days even with repeated washing.

After the clinician has completed the wound closure, the medical assistant typically applies a sterile dressing to the site. The dressing will vary in size and thickness according to the wound.

Figure 26-13 shows a patient handout from an ER on potential danger signs as well as instructions for follow-up care. Patient education forms should be printed in different languages for non–English-speaking patients.

Nosebleeds (Epistaxis)

A nosebleed, or *epistaxis*, is a hemorrhage that usually results from the rupture of small vessels within the nose. Nosebleeds can be caused by injury, disease, hypertension, strenuous activity, high altitudes, exposure to cold, overuse of anticoagulant medications such as aspirin, or nasal recreational drug use. Bleeding from the anterior nostril area is usually venous while that in the posterior region is usually arterial and more difficult

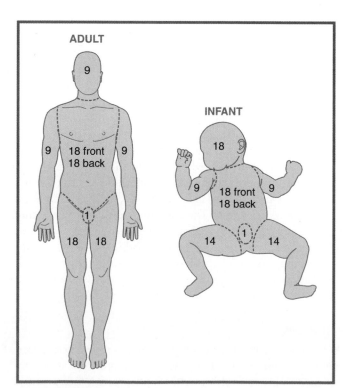

FIGURE 26-12 Rule of Nines classification of burns.

PROCEDURE 26-7

Control Bleeding

ABHES COMPETENCY: 4.f.

GOAL: *To stop hemorrhaging from an open wound.*

EQUIPMENT and SUPPLIES

- Gloves, sterile if available
- Appropriate personal protective equipment (PPE) according to OSHA guidelines including:
  - Impermeable gown
  - Goggles or face shield
  - Impermeable mask
  - Impermeable foot covers if indicated
- Sterile dressings
- Bandaging material
- Biohazard waste container
- Patient record

PROCEDURAL STEPS

1. Wash hands, and apply appropriate personal protective equipment.
   PURPOSE: To meet OSHA standard precautions.
2. Assemble equipment and supplies.
3. Apply several layers of sterile dressing material directly to the wound, and exert pressure.
   PURPOSE: Direct pressure to the wound will slow down or stop bleeding. Sterile supplies are needed to prevent wound infection.
4. Wrap the wound with bandage material. Add more dressing and bandaging material if bleeding continues.
5. If bleeding persists and the wound is located on an extremity, elevate the extremity above the level of the heart. Notify the physician immediately if bleeding cannot be controlled.
6. If bleeding still continues, maintain direct pressure and elevation; also apply pressure to the appropriate artery. If bleeding is in the arm, apply pressure to the brachial artery by squeezing the inner aspect of the mid-upper arm. If bleeding is in the leg, apply pressure to the femoral artery on the affected side by pushing with the heel of the hand into the femoral crease at the groin. If bleeding cannot be controlled, it may be necessary to activate the emergency medical system.
7. Once the bleeding is controlled and the patient is stabilized, dispose of contaminated materials into the biohazard waste container.
8. Disinfect the area, remove gloves, and dispose into biohazard waste.
9. Wash hands.
10. Document the incident, including the details of the wound, when and how it occurred, patient symptoms, vital signs, physician treatment, and the patient's current condition.

---

to stop. Treatment of epistaxis varies according to the amount of bleeding and the presence of other conditions or the use of anticoagulant medications.

If the bleeding is mild to moderate and from one side of the nose, the patient should sit up, lean slightly forward, and apply direct pressure to the affected nostril by pinching the nose. Continue constant pressure for 10 to 15 minutes to allow clotting to take place. Repeat if bleeding cannot be controlled, insert a clean pad of gauze into the nostril, and notify the physician. If the physician is not available, proceed with standard EMS protocols. Bleeding that is bilateral and continuous or in a patient with a bleeding disorder or on anticoagulant therapy should be considered a medical emergency.

Head Injuries

The severity of a head injury can vary greatly. The history of the injury–details about what it is and how it happened–is crucial for determining appropriate management. With a head injury, the patient may appear normal; may experience dizziness, severe headache, mental confusion, or memory loss; or may even be unconscious. The loss of consciousness may be brief or prolonged; it may appear immediately or may be delayed. The victim may experience vomiting; loss of bladder and bowel control; and bleeding from the nose, mouth, or ears. The pupils of the eyes may be unequal and nonreactive to light.

All head injuries must be considered serious. Notify the physician or contact EMS immediately. If there is evidence of neck injury, stabilize the neck and do not attempt to move the victim. Do not administer anything by mouth. Keep the patient warm and quiet. Watch the pupils of the eyes, and record any changes. Measure vital signs and record the extent and duration of any unconsciousness. If the patient is at home or is sent home after physician assessment, he or she should be watched closely for 24 hours after the injury for any change in mental status.

Foreign Bodies in the Eye

The eye is a delicate organ whose unique structure demands special handling. This kind of emergency is most uncomfortable, and it is often extremely difficult to keep the patient from rubbing the eye. Tell the patient not to touch the eye in any way. The physician may order ophthalmic topical anesthetic drops to relieve the patient's pain. The patient should be placed in a darkened room to wait for the physician, because **photophobia** is common with eye irritations. If a contusion and swelling are present, cold, wet compresses will help. Ask the patient to close both eyes and cover them with eye pads until the physician arrives. The physician may order an eye irrigation to remove the object. Unless the foreign object is clearly visible, do not attempt to search for it or to remove it.

LACERATIONS

What you need to know . . .

It is important to prevent infection and to allow your cut to heal. Call your doctor or return to him or her immediately if any of the "danger signs" occur.

Return for recheck in _____ days
Return for suture removal in _____ days

Danger signs to watch for . . .

1. Increasing pain, swelling, redness, and warmth in the injured area.
2. Pus in or around the cut.
3. Fever greater than 100°F (38°C).
4. Blood soaking through the dressing.

If any of these signs occur, contact your doctor or return to the Emergency Department.

What to do at home . . .

1. Take all medicines exactly as directed.
2. Raise the injured area above your heart level for 1 to 2 days.
3. Keep the wound and bandage clean and dry. For cuts on the face, a bandage is often not necessary. All finger dressings must be changed within 24 hours.
4. Remove the bandage/dressing in 24 hours.
5. After 24 hours, you may shower or bathe. Begin cleaning the wound with clear water twice each day to remove crusting and scabbing. Then apply ointment (Polysporin).
6. Prevent sunburn. Use a sunscreen for 6 months (e.g., Pre-Sun or Eclipse).
7. If you have a private doctor or are a member of an HMO (e.g., Kaiser), you should call for an appointment for your recheck and suture removal. If you can't get an appointment, you are welcome to return here to complete your care.

Please remember . . .

1. The exam and treatment you have just received are not intended to provide complete medical care. You need to call your doctor to schedule a follow-up visit.

2. The X-rays or ECG taken today will be reviewed by a specialist. If there is any change in your diagnosis, we will contact you.

FIGURE 26-13 Educational materials about lacerations for home care of a wound.

Heat and Cold Injuries

Exposure to extremes in temperature can cause minor to severe injuries. Heat injuries occur most often on hot, humid days and result in cramps, heat exhaustion, or heat stroke. Heat-related muscle cramps may be the first sign of *heat exhaustion,* which is a serious heat-related condition. Patients with heat exhaustion appear flushed and report headaches, nausea, vertigo, and weakness. *Heat stroke,* the most dangerous form of heat-related injury, results in a shutdown of body systems. Patients with heat stroke have red, hot, dry skin; altered levels of consciousness; tachycardia; and rapid, shallow breathing. This is a true medical emergency. If heat-related problems are recognized in the early stages and adequately treated, the patient does not usually develop heat stroke. Management of heat-related illnesses includes getting the person out of the heat; loosening clothing or removing perspiration-soaked clothing; and giving the person cool drinks if he or she is alert. An effective way to lower the victim's temperature is to apply cool, wet cloths and to fan the moist skin so heat is released from the body by evaporation.

There are two types of cold-related injuries: frostbite and hypothermia. *Frostbite,* which is the actual freezing of tissue, occurs when the skin temperature falls to a range of 14° to 25° F. Prolonged exposure of the skin to cold causes damage similar to a burn. The tissue may appear gray or white, be swollen, have clear blisters, or, in full-thickness frostbite, show signs of tissue **necrosis,** including blackened areas and severe deformity. The more advanced the frostbite, the more serious the tissue damage, and the more likely the body part will be lost. There is no feeling in tissue that is frozen, but as thawing occurs, the patient reports itching, tingling, and burning pain. Mild frostbite can be managed by applying constant warmth to the affected areas either by immersing the area in warm water (no warmer than 105° F) or wrapping it in warm, dry clothing. Friction should never be used, because this would increase tissue damage. If blisters have formed or if there is evidence of full-thickness frostbite, the patient should be transported to the nearest ER.

Hypothermia is a medical emergency that may result in death unless the patient receives immediate assistance. Systemic hypothermia occurs when the core body temperature, preferably taken with an Ototemp (tympanic thermometer), is less than 95° F. Signs and symptoms of hypothermia include shivering, numbness, apathy, and loss of consciousness. If hypothermia is suspected, activate EMS and care for any life-threatening conditions until help arrives. Remove the victim's wet clothing and wrap the victim in blankets while moving him or her to a warm place. If the victim is alert, give warm liquids and apply heating pads (using a barrier to avoid burns) to help slowly warm the core body temperature.

Dehydration

A person dehydrates when he or she excretes more water than is taken in. Dehydration can be a very serious health emergency, leading to convulsions, coma, and even death. Infants, young children, and older adult patients are at greatest risk for developing serious complications from dehydration. Severe dehydration may be caused by excessive heat loss, vomiting, diarrhea, or lack of fluid intake. Symptoms include vertigo; dark yellow urine or no urine output for 8 to 10 hours; extreme thirst; lethargy or confusion; and abdominal or muscle cramps. If the patient exhibits any of these symptoms and is not able to retain fluids, schedule an urgent appointment or recommend the patient be taken to the ER. Replacing lost fluids is vital, so the patient should be encouraged to drink water, tea, sports drinks, fruit juice, or Pedialyte.

Diabetic Emergencies

Diabetes mellitus is caused by either a malfunction in the production of insulin in the pancreas or an inability of the cells to use insulin. Insulin is required on the cellular level so that glucose can be used for energy. Two different diabetic emergencies are caused by either *hyperglycemia* (high blood glucose levels) or *hypoglycemia* (low blood glucose levels).

Insulin shock is caused by severe hypoglycemia, because the diabetic patient has taken too much insulin, has not eaten enough food, or has exercised an unusual amount. Signs and symptoms have a rapid onset and include tachycardia, profuse sweating (diaphoresis), headache, irritability, vertigo, fatigue, hunger, seizures, and coma. It is important to provide glucose immediately, preferably in the form of glucose tablets, because they have a known concentrated quantity of glucose.

Diabetic coma results from severe hyperglycemia, which develops because the body is not producing enough insulin; the patient ate too much food or is very stressed; or the patient has an infection. Symptoms of impending diabetic coma develop more slowly than those of insulin shock; these include general malaise, dry mouth, **polyuria, polydipsia,** nausea, vomiting, SOB, and acetone- or "fruity"-smelling breath. If the patient or caregiver calling for an appointment reports these symptoms, notify the physician immediately, because the patient would typically be admitted to the hospital.

In an emergency situation, if a patient who has been diagnosed with diabetes mellitus exhibits signs and symptoms of a diabetic emergency, the patient should be given glucose. If the problem is caused by insulin shock (hypoglycemia), the patient will improve quickly after receiving glucose; if it is caused by diabetic coma (hyperglycemia), a small amount of added glucose will not affect the patient's condition, and he or she will need to be transported to the hospital regardless.

CLOSING COMMENTS

Patient Education

Emergencies can occur anywhere. Patients need to learn how to handle emergency situations both by the example of healthcare workers and through instruction. The medical assistant must remain calm, triage the situation, call for help, and be prepared to administer appropriate first aid intervention. Brochures regarding home safety can be used to help educate patients about methods for avoiding accidents in the home.

All patients, even children, should understand how to contact EMS. This is especially important for families with members who have chronic diseases that are potentially life-threatening, such as heart conditions, severe allergic reactions, diabetes, and asthma. Patients should be encouraged to post emergency numbers, such as for the local EMS, poison control center, and their primary care physician, next to the telephone. Families with young children need to "childproof" their homes, being especially careful to keep potentially poisonous substances stored where children cannot get into them. "Mr. Yuk" stickers placed on poisonous containers can be an excellent educational tool for young children.

Remember to keep your American Red Cross and American Heart Association certifications current. Take advantage of community workshops to maintain and extend your skills. Post a list of community safety workshops in an area where it can be seen by patients, and encourage them to attend. Your participation in emergency care workshops and your encouragement to have others participate may help to save lives.

Legal and Ethical Issues

The medical assistant works in the healthcare environment as the physician's agent. Although you are responsible for your own actions, the physician is legally responsible for the care you administer to patients while working in the healthcare facility. You are responsible for knowing the limitations placed on medical assistants in your state and for strictly adhering to your employer's emergency care policies and procedures. Medical assistants are not qualified to diagnose a patient problem but are responsible for acting appropriately in a medical emergency. In addition to legal responsibilities, you have an ethical responsibility to your patients to provide the highest standard of care. Always act in the best interest of the patient, and never hesitate to ask the physician and/or office manager for immediate assistance when faced with a medical emergency.

Most states have enacted Good Samaritan laws to encourage healthcare professionals to provide medical assistance at the scene of an accident without fear of being sued for negligence. These statutes vary greatly, but all have the intent of protecting the caregiver. A physician or other healthcare professional is not legally obligated to give emergency care at the site of an accident, regardless of the ethical and moral considerations. Legal liability is limited to gross neglect of the victim or willfully causing further injury to the victim. As a caregiver, you are required to act as a reasonable person and cannot be held liable for personal injury resulting from an act of omission. Good Samaritan statutes provide for the evaluation of the caregiver's judgment but are only in effect at the site of an emergency, not at your place of employment.

If you have never been trained in CPR, you cannot be expected to perform the procedure at the emergency site. However, in many states a healthcare provider with CPR training and skills who is present at the scene can be declared negligent if cardiac arrest occurs and he or she does not administer CPR to the victim.

If the victim is conscious or if a member of his or her immediate family is present, obtain verbal consent to perform emergency care. Consent is implied if the patient is unconscious and no family member is present.

Many types of emergencies can be handled in the physician's office. In an emergency situation, decisions that must be made quickly can determine whether the patient lives. A medical assistant must be prepared to act calmly and efficiently in all emergency situations.

SUMMARY OF SCENARIO

Cheryl has learned through her work with the triage team and involvement with emergencies in the office how important it is to gather complete information about emergency situations as well as to act calmly and knowledgeably when managing patient problems. She knows she must maintain her certification in CPR for the Professional and continue to participate in workshops on emergency care to be prepared for the wide variety of patient problems seen in the ambulatory care setting. Working with the screening staff has also reinforced the need to document all interactions on the telephone as well as information gathered during patient visits. Cheryl recognizes that medical assistants in the office must follow the facility's policy and procedure manual for handling emergencies, plan ahead and complete her designated duties if an emergency occurs, use community emergency services as needed, and keep emergency supplies and equipment well stocked and ready for any potential emergency situation. She recognizes that understanding first aid practices for common patient emergencies allows her to assist patients either through instruction by phone or by performing specific skills when emergencies occur in the facility. Cheryl has investigated her legal standing as a medical assistant in her home state and recognizes her responsibilities when a patient either calls or shows up at the office with a medical emergency. She will continue to refer to the more experienced screening staff or Dr. Bendt when she has questions, but she now feels more confident in managing emergency situations at work.

SUMMARY of LEARNING OBJECTIVES

1. Define, spell, and pronounce the terms listed in the vocabulary.
   - Spelling and pronouncing medical terms correctly adds credibility to the medical assistant. Knowing the definition of these terms promotes confidence in communication with patients and co-workers.
2. Describe the medical assistant's responsibilities in an emergency.
   - A medical assistant should be familiar with the healthcare facility's policy and procedures on the management of emergencies and must maintain certification in CPR. Perform only the procedures in which you are trained, always notify the physician or activate EMS if the physician is unavailable. The medical assistant must make sure the facility is accident-proof to prevent patient injuries on site, participate in planning for emergency situations, and post emergency telephone numbers for reference during an emergency.
3. Identify supplies and equipment for emergency situations.

- A physician's office must have a centrally located crash cart or emergency bag for all emergency supplies, equipment, and medication. This material must be consistently inventoried and maintained. The chapter provides a detailed list of materials that should be readily available for an on-site emergency, including a defibrillator if indicated by the physician's practice.
4. Demonstrate the use of an automated external defibrillator.
   - Procedure 26-1 describes the use of an AED.
5. Summarize the general rules for managing emergencies.
   - Managing emergencies requires a calm, efficient approach to the situation. Assess the nature of the emergency and determine whether EMS should be activated or whether the patient requires an immediate or urgent appointment. Gather as many details as possible about the situation, and refer to the physician when in doubt.

Continued

SUMMARY of LEARNING OBJECTIVES
Continued

6. Demonstrate screening techniques and documentation guidelines for ambulatory care emergencies.
   - Telephone screening is one of a medical assistant's most important tasks. Emergency action principles should be used to determine the level of a patient's emergency. These include determining whether the situation is life-threatening and obtaining the patient's contact information as well as all pertinent information regarding the injury and patient signs and symptoms. This information must be shared with the physician, and all details must be documented in the patient's chart.

7. Recognize and respond to life-threatening emergencies in the ambulatory care setting.
   - Life-threatening emergencies require immediate assessment, referral to the physician, and, if the physician is not present, activation of EMS. While waiting for assistance, determine the presence of breathing and circulation. Administer rescue breaths or CPR if indicated. Depending on the patient's signs and symptoms, monitor the patient for signs of a heart attack; administer the Heimlich maneuver if there is an obstructed airway; evaluate for signs of a CVA; and assess for shock. Ask for assistance when indicated, and perform appropriate skills based on the patient's presenting condition.

8. Perform adult rescue breathing and CPR.
   - Procedure 26-3 describes how to perform adult rescue breathing and CPR.

9. Administer oxygen through a nasal cannula to a patient in respiratory distress.
   - Procedure 26-4 describes how to administer oxygen with a nasal cannula.

10. Identify and assist a patient with an obstructed airway.
    - Procedure 26-5 demonstrates how to respond to and assist an adult with an obstructed airway. Infants with an obstructed airway should receive alternating back blows and chest thrusts with attempted rescue breaths until the item is dislodged or help arrives.

11. Determine appropriate action and documentation procedures for common ambulatory care emergencies.
    - Always follow standard precautions when caring for a patient with a medical emergency. Documentation of emergency treatment should include information about the patient; vital signs; allergies, current medications, and pertinent health history; the patient's chief complaint; the sequence of events, including any changes in the patient's condition since the incident; and any physician's orders and procedures performed.

12. Assist and monitor a patient who has fainted.
    - Procedure 26-6 demonstrates the steps for caring for a patient who has fainted.

13. Control a hemorrhagic wound.
    - Procedure 26-7 describes how to control wound hemorrhage.

14. Apply patient education concepts to medical emergencies.
    - Patients should know how to contact emergency personnel, and families with young children should have poison control telephone numbers posted. Educating patients about how to care for minor emergencies at home is an important part of telephone triage in the ambulatory care setting. Encouraging patients to participate in community safety workshops and to become CPR certified may help them to avoid emergencies as well as save lives.

15. Discuss legal and ethical concerns regarding medical emergencies.
    - Good Samaritan laws vary from state to state but are designed to protect any individual, whether a healthcare professional or layperson, from liability if he or she provides assistance at the site of an emergency. The law does not require a medically trained person to act, but if emergency care is given in a reasonable and responsible manner, the healthcare worker is protected from being sued for negligence. This protection, however, does not extend to the workplace.

CONNECTIONS

Study Guide Connection: Go to Chapter 26 Study Guide. Read the Case Study and Workplace Applications and complete the assignments. Do online research for answers to the questions in the Internet Activities associated with assisting with medical emergencies.

CD Connection: Go to the Medical Assisting Competency Challenge CD and do the training activities under Patient Care. For a better understanding of cardiopulmonary function when assisting with medical emergencies, view the animation for normal cardiopulmonary physiology.

Evolve Connection: For more information related to assisting with medical emergencies, go to http://evolve.elsevier.com/kinn/admin and visit related weblinks for Chapter 26. Click on the Medical Assisting Exam Review and do the practice questions to sharpen your test-taking skills.

Career Development and Life Skills

27

SCENARIO

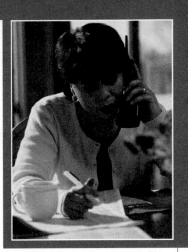

Lisa Walker is 1 month away from graduating from her medical assisting program. She has been an excellent student and is looking forward to beginning her career in the medical field. Lisa wants to begin her job search now to minimize the time during which she is not employed after her externship ends.

Lisa has participated in several volunteer activities while she has been attending school. She plans to list these experiences on her resume. She met many office managers and physicians while doing volunteer work, and she will be contacting those people in hopes of obtaining more job leads.

Lisa began saving for interview clothing when she first began school. She is on a strict budget, but she found several outfits appropriate for interviews at secondhand clothing shops and discount stores. Her best-looking suit cost only $25!

Not a person afraid to interview, Lisa looks forward to sharing her skills and experience with potential employers. She looks on each interview as a practice session for the next one, and this helps her to relax more and present a true picture of herself to the office manager. She has a great smile and projects a natural friendliness and positive attitude.

Lisa has given much thought to what she wants from her first job as a medical assistant. She knows that she may not start at a high salary, but she also realizes that there are benefits and perquisites ("perks") to working in a physician's office. She plans to commit to working for 2 years on her first job, gaining experience before looking for her next job at a higher salary and with additional benefits.

Lisa is excited about her future as a medical assistant. She is ready to put the training she received to work with actual patients. She plans to perform exceptionally well at her externship site and to go above and beyond her designated duties to impress the staff in that facility, who will become references for her first paid position. Lisa is dedicated to becoming the best medical assistant possible and becoming indispensable to her employer.

While studying this chapter, think about the following questions:

- How can the medical assistant prepare for his or her first job throughout the duration of training?
- What is meant by "writing your resume every day"?

- How can the medical assistant organize the job search?
- How can the new medical assistant employee make a positive, lasting impression on co-workers and supervisors?

LEARNING OBJECTIVES

1. Define, spell, and pronounce the terms listed in the vocabulary.
2. Discuss the reasons that job search training is important to a medical assistant.
3. List three expectations that employers have of employees.
4. Understand the three types of employee skill strengths.
5. Explain the two best job search methods.
6. Describe some of the errors that should be avoided on a resume.
7. Explain the importance of having demographic information about former jobs before appearing for an interview.
8. List the four phases of the interview process.

9. Discuss the importance of the probationary period for a new employee.
10. List some mistakes that should be avoided by a new employee.
11. Explain why a performance appraisal's ratings are usually not perfect.
12. Prepare a resume.
13. Organize a job search.
14. Complete a job application.
15. Interview for a job.
16. Negotiate a salary.

National Accreditation Competencies and Content

CAAHEP COMPETENCIES

General
3.a.(1)(a). Schedule and manage appointments
3.c.(1)(a). Respond to and initiate written communications
3.c.(1)(b). Recognize and respond to verbal communications
3.c.(1)(c). Recognize and respond to nonverbal communications

ABHES COMPETENCIES

Professionalism
1.a. Project a positive attitude
1.g. Evidence a responsible attitude
1.i. Conduct work within scope of education, training, and ability

Communication
2.e. User proper telephone techniques
2.f. Interview effectively
2.j. Use correct grammar, spelling, and formatting techniques in written works
2.o. Fundamental writing skills
2.q. Allied health professions and credentialing

VOCABULARY

appraisals Expert judgments of the value or merit of; also, evaluations of work performance.

counteroffer Return offer made by one who has rejected an offer or job.

defaults Fails to pay financial debts, such as a student loan.

deferment Postponement, especially of a student loan.

genuineness Expressing sincerity and honest feeling.

intolerable Not tolerable or bearable.

mock Simulated; intended for imitation or practice.

networking Exchange of information or services among individuals, groups, or institutions; also, meeting and getting to know individuals in the same or similar career fields and sharing information about available opportunities.

pertinent (pur′-tuh-nent) Having a clear, decisive relevance to the matter at hand.

proofread To read and mark corrections.

ramifications Consequence; outgrowth; something produced by a cause or necessarily following from a set of conditions.

rectify (rek′-tuh-fy) To correct by removing errors.

subtle Ingenious; artful; delicate.

succinct (suhk-sinkt′) Marked by compact, precise expression without wasted words.

synopsis Condensed statement or outline.

vocation The work in which a person is regularly employed.

Each day that a person exists is a small portion of a whole—in this case, the person's entire lifetime. The events that happen during a day, no matter how small, shape the future. In the same way, the events that happen in the life of a medical assistant play a role in shaping his or her career. Every day, he or she "writes a resume"–through actions that will reveal strengths, highlight skills, and summarize accomplishments–that builds on the medical assistant's **vocation.** Each duty performed becomes a part of the medical assistant's sum of experience and is important in the overall growth of the individual. Each action taken can have an impact on the future for the medical assistant. If the actions are professional, accurate, and performed to his or her utmost ability, the resume that the medical assistant is writing through these actions will be one that will lead to greater opportunities. If the medical assistant performs poorly, the resume will be one that will not reflect trustworthiness and dependability. The small decisions that are made every day are those that greatly affect the overall impressions that the medical assistant makes in the workplace.

Approximately 85% of persons seeking employment have never had any type of formal training in the job search process. A newly graduated medical assistant should take advantage of job search training for three reasons:

- The training will decrease the amount of time spent searching for a job.
- The training will increase the chances of receiving better wages through negotiations.
- The training will help to eliminate the fears of looking for work and interviewing.

WHAT DOES THE EMPLOYER WANT?

Employers have three basic desires when they are interviewing individuals for a job:

- They want a person who has a neat appearance and looks as if he or she fits the job (Figure 27-1).
- They want an individual who is dependable and can prove that he or she has been a reliable team member in other job positions.
- They want a person with the skills to do the job.

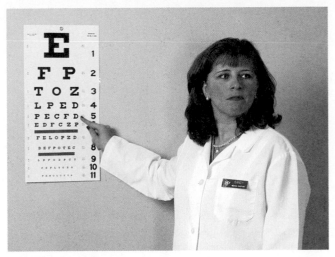

Figure 27-1 A professional appearance is mandatory in the medical office.

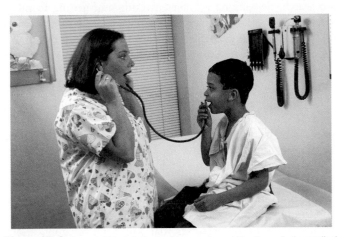

Figure 27-2 A great attitude is the best personal asset. Employers in the medical profession want medical assistants who will exhibit a positive attitude with the patients.

From the beginning of the job search process, a medical assistant's attitude is the most critical part of his or her potential success in getting a job (Figure 27-2). A good attitude is not a trait that can be developed overnight. For this reason a medical assistant must have a positive outlook in all situations, so the **genuineness** of his or her demeanor will be clear during job interviews.

CRITICAL THINKING APPLICATION

Lisa knows that attitude is of primary importance on a job. How can she prove to a potential employer in an interview that she has a good attitude? What exactly constitutes a good attitude? A bad attitude? What does it take to change an attitude from bad to good?

ASSESSING STRENGTHS

Before promoting himself or herself as a potential employee, a medical assistant must first determine the strengths that make him or her a valuable team member. There are three types of skill strengths: job skills, self-management skills, and transferable skills.

Job skills are the abilities that the medical assistant needs to perform the job. This includes such skills as performing venipuncture, billing insurance, answering the telephone, scheduling appointments, giving injections, and handling other tasks.

Self-management skills relate to the medical assistant's personality and character traits. They include such attributes as honesty, integrity, and enthusiasm.

Transferable skills can be taken from one job to another. For instance, if the medical assistant has the ability to communicate effectively, this skill can be used on every job. Leadership is a transferable skill, as are the ability to follow directions and the ability to manage people.

CRITICAL THINKING APPLICATION

Lisa expects potential employers to ask her what her strengths are. She has determined six specific strengths that she can prove with examples from past positions or her externship. What six strengths can you prove? Give examples of each of these strengths.

DEVELOPING CAREER OBJECTIVES

Each medical assistant has a reason for entering the healthcare field. This basic desire should influence decisions concerning his or her career choices. Because medical assisting is such a versatile profession, a medical assistant will have numerous options after graduation.

It is wise to take some time to think about what the medical assistant wants from his or her career. While he or she is attending school and subsequently completing an externship, ideas may surface about what specialty to enter.

When developing career objectives, the medical assistant should start by asking several questions:
- Where am I today?
- Where will I be in 5 years?
- Where will I be in 10 years?
- What additional skills do I need to get where I want to go?

Write down the questions and answers, and go into specific detail. Set realistic goals, and develop a plan as to how and when they will be reached. It is helpful to put a list of goals in a prominent place at home, where they will be seen every day. Some people use the front of the refrigerator, and some post the goals on the mirror in the area where they get dressed every day. Write goals in a visible place to keep them in mind even on the more difficult days, when they seem far from sight.

CRITICAL THINKING APPLICATION

Lisa knows that goals are important when attempting to achieve in life. She has five goals written regarding her job search and her first position as a medical assistant. What are some goals that are realistic regarding the job search? What realistic goals could be developed with regard to the first position as a medical assistant?

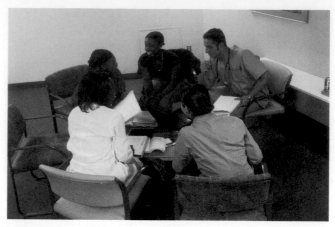

Figure 27-3 Enjoyment of the job is paramount. Medical assistants should enjoy their job and give compassionate, friendly care to all patients.

Figure 27-4 Stay in touch with classmates. Classmates are excellent networking contacts and may be able to provide job leads.

KNOWING PERSONAL NEEDS

A medical assistant must evaluate all of the needs that he or she requires in a work situation. Most people have a minimum salary that they require, as well as certain benefits. For example, if the medical assistant is a single mother, she may require a moderate salary and insist on health insurance benefits. We also have intrinsic needs, which are those internal desires that are important to us personally.

A helpful activity is to write a **synopsis** of a typical day on an ideal medical assisting job. Imagine the type of office, the job title, the daily duties, and the salary and benefits that would be a part of the ideal job (Figure 27-3). This will help to develop a focus and a goal to work toward as the medical assistant's career develops.

FINDING A JOB

Many people have misconceptions about the job market that exists today. Graduation from a medical assisting program does not guarantee that the student will obtain employment. Completion of the program will give the medical assistant the job skills needed to work, but a good attitude and positive outlook are essential for success in the job search.

Some job seekers assume that potential employers will not interact with students until they graduate. However, prospecting before graduation is a smart idea, and there are **subtle** ways of introducing oneself to a facility without bluntly asking for employment. Many also think that they must have work experience to be hired, but employers are more interested in attitude and teachability than a long resume full of experience. In fact, many physicians like hiring students fresh from school so that they can teach them how they want procedures done.

The Two Best Job Search Methods

Although there are many ways to find employment, two methods have proved to be the best and most effective. These are **networking** and direct contact with employers.

Networking is the exchange of information or services among individuals, groups, or institutions. When related to a job search, networking involves meeting and getting to know individuals in the same or similar career fields and sharing information about available opportunities. A medical assistant should begin to form a network of friends, business associates, co-workers, and acquaintances early in training, and he or she should stay in contact with these people throughout the job search effort (Figure 27-4).

How does one network? One way is by joining professional medical assisting organizations. The members that attend regular meetings often know about job leads in the area. The medical assistant should also tell his or her personal physician(s) about being in school and the approximate time of graduation. Friends and family members can be on the lookout for potential opportunities and may help by asking their personal physicians if they are aware of positions that will open for applications soon. Always keep a few resumes on hand—the opportunity to network could come at any time.

Networking is not limited to job searching, and many organizations are formed to develop networks of individuals or groups that assist one another and refer clients to one another. However, these groups are useful to the person who is looking for employment, and by attending meetings and get-togethers held for networking purposes, the medical assistant may happen onto the ideal job he or she has been looking for.

CRITICAL THINKING APPLICATION

Lisa knows that networking is a great way to secure employment. She is making a list of people with whom she can share her resume or inform that she is now ready to seek employment as a medical assistant. How many people can you think of who are good prospects for networking?

Direct contact with employers is also an effective method of job searching. Medical assistants often know of specific clinics or facilities that they would like to investigate as job possibilities. Compile a list of these places, and learn as much about them as possible. If the facility has a website, read it thoroughly. Ask for brochures about the employer. Some have an annual report that lists details about the organization. All of this information will help the medical assistant get a good basic idea of why the facility exists and what it does for the community.

Contact with employers does not necessarily begin only after the student has graduated. Students can begin networking and contacting employers from the very start of their enrollment at school. The student may wish to keep a file of potential employers. Make a list of facilities that are good prospects for employment, then begin researching them. Call to find out who supervises medical assistants in the facility. In a physician's office, this is usually the office manager. Then call the office manager and ask to make an appointment to learn about the facility. Even the busiest people are usually willing to help a student investigate healthcare facilities in the area.

Do not express to the office manager that the objective of the appointment is a job offer. The goal at this point is to learn about the facility, what it offers the community, and what roles the medical assistants in the facility perform. Suggest that the appointment be set at his or her convenience. Then treat the appointment like an actual job interview, dressing appropriately and arriving on time. Have a list of questions about the facility prepared in advance, and do not take too much of the office manager's time. Take notes about what the office manager says about the facility so that they can be referred to on graduation, during the actual job search.

After the appointment with the office manager, ask for a business card and always send a thank-you note or letter. Do not fail to remember this critical point! This helps the office manager to remember the name of the medical assistant and is a pleasant addition to the daily mail. Everyone enjoys being recognized for his or her efforts, and the office manager will appreciate the thank-you note.

Toward the time that he or she is to graduate, the medical assistant may wish to perform an externship at one of the facilities visited early in training. Check with school regulations to determine whether this is possible. Then the office manager can be approached about allowing the student to extern in the office. Be sure to follow school guidelines when investigating these possibilities. Some schools allow students to secure their own externship sites, but this must be discussed with the externship supervisor at school. Performing an externship at a medical facility is usually the first practical experience the student will have in the medical field and can be used as a reference in building a resume.

After the externship is completed, the medical assistant may wish to send a resume to all of the office managers met through the direct contact efforts made earlier in his or her training. A professional resume with a cover letter that refers to the earlier meeting will prompt the office manager to remember the student. Ask in the cover letter whether any opportunities exist in the facility. Express to the office manager that the facility and staff were impressive on the first meeting and that it would be an exciting place to begin a career. In the letter, request that if the office manager does not have any positions available at that time, the resume be kept on file or be passed along to an acquaintance who is looking for an additional staff member.

The Internet and the Job Search

The Internet opens a whole new world of opportunity when it comes to job searching. The medical assistant can find a gargantuan amount of information about writing resumes, interviewing, and follow-up methods, but perhaps most important, the Internet can provide information about who is hiring right now.

Many databases provide information about job openings. Monster, Yahoo! Jobs, and the Online Career Center are a few examples. The search can be targeted to specific geographic areas, certain career fields, or even specific job titles. Conduct a search in a selected state (or metropolitan area), then look for jobs in the medical profession, then narrow the field even more by asking for information on jobs specifically for medical assistants.

The medical assistant can also express interest in a job by perusing the company website then contacting the employer directly on the "contact us" page. Anyone looking at the website should be able to find an email address to use for gathering additional information. Express that the school encourages seeking quality businesses as potential employers, and ask for information that could be presented to a class. Most employers are happy to get the word out about their company and may give all kinds of pamphlets and "freebies" to share with a class. By sending a thank-you note and staying in touch with the company, the medical assistant creates a new lead for the job search.

Just remember, the information available to one medical assistant on the Internet is also available to every other medical assistant. The Internet is great for researching positions and companies, but networking and direct contact are still the most successful ways to obtain a job. The medical assistant's "whole package"—meaning the resume, application, interview, follow-up, attitude, appearance, and job skills—all combine to make an impression on the employer. Will that impression be favorable enough to result in a job offer?

Traditional Job Search Methods

The more traditional job search methods may be effective but are usually not as successful as networking and contacting employers directly.

Newspaper Ads

Newspaper ads normally produce a huge number of applicants and resumes for the employer. A resume or application will have to stand out in the crowd to be noticed when it arrives at the facility. Some applicants use clear envelopes, which draw attention to the resume quickly in a stack of mail.

Employment Agencies

Employment agencies usually charge a fee for their services. Even when the employer pays the fee, the medical assistant may be offered a lower wage to compensate for the fee. These agencies can be useful, however. In salary negotiation the agency will know the salary range the employer is willing to pay. This means that medical assistants can command a salary within that range and not be short-changed by asking for a salary that is much lower than the employer was willing to pay.

Professional Societies

Joining local chapters of medical assistant organizations helps the student in many ways. Not only will valuable information be exchanged at the meetings, but the medical assistant may also hear of positions that are becoming available in various medical facilities. This is a form of networking.

Volunteering

By volunteering in medical offices or facilities, the medical assistant will meet other professionals who may be able to provide job leads. Volunteer activities should be added to the resume, because these valuable experiences can often be used in the physician's office as well. It does not matter that the position was not a paid job; experience counts, whether paid or not.

Mailing Resumes

Mailing a large number of resumes is not a very effective method of job search. Out of 100 resumes sent, one or two potential employers may respond with a request for an interview. It is much more effective to network first, then follow up with a good cover letter and resume. Resumes can be used when contacting employers directly, and this approach allows the medical assistant to meet at least one employee of the facility when the document is delivered. Be sure to ask for a business card and write down the name of the person to whom the resume was delivered. For impressive facilities, send a note of thanks to the person who accepted the resume, asking to be considered for future positions.

Cold Calling

Cold calling is contacting employers by phone and prospecting for available positions. If the medical assistant asks, "Are you hiring?" at the beginning of the conversation, he or she should expect a negative answer and has just wasted the call. This is all but useless in the job search effort. However, an assistant who calls for information about the clinic and schedules an appointment with the office manager may have more success. Never attempt to get a job over the phone. Even when interested employers call and ask questions, attempt to set up an interview to discuss your qualifications in person.

Performing Well on Externships

Performing well on externships may be one of the best ways to secure a job. If an opening exists, the medical assistant extern is already oriented to the practice and may be the perfect fit for the job. Perform duties assigned on the externship as if they were final examinations at school. Even when the office does not have a position available at that time, there may be one soon, or the office manager or physician may know of an office that has an opening. Do the best job possible, and there may be an employment offer waiting at the conclusion of the externship. Be ready to learn from the moment the externship begins until the moment it ends.

ORGANIZING THE JOB SEARCH

Seeking a job is a full-time job. The new medical assistant must put forth effort, have stamina, and be persistent. Do not expect to get a job with the first practice that offers an interview. By keeping track of opportunities found, one will be more likely to obtain employment in a short time after graduation (Procedure 27-1).

A job lead is any information that could lead to a position, either now or in the future. Some of the most promising job leads for the newly graduated medical assistant come from the externship experience. Be friendly and meet as many people as possible while completing this part of training. Ask for business cards, and stay in contact with the medical professionals met at the externship site and nearby hospitals. Be willing to shake hands and make introductions at all times so that the circle of promising contacts for job leads continues to expand.

The medical assistant would be wise to keep a record of all job leads (Figure 27-5). The name and address of the facility, contact name, and phone numbers are all important items of information. Keep track of where the lead was obtained so that if it is provided by an individual, that person can be thanked properly, especially if the lead results in a job offer. These records are an excellent starting place when making calls to set up job interviews. Remember, the placement office at school is a resource for job leads but should not be the only source used for obtaining leads. Each medical assistant graduate must take personal responsibility for finding and following up on job opportunities.

The job lead is not the only information that should be recorded during job search efforts. Keep a record of arrangements when an interview is secured, including information such as the following:

- Day, date, and time of the interview
- Directions to the interview site
- Name of the person to interview with
- Items to bring to the interview
- Information about the company or facility

As soon as the interview is over, the medical assistant should record information about the interview itself. After several interviews, it may be difficult to remember which opportunity offered what salary, which had medical benefits, and which was closest to home. By keeping accurate records, the medical assistant can follow up in whatever way is appropriate and send a note or letter of appreciation to the person who conducted the interview (Figure 27-6).

DEVELOPING A RESUME

A resume is a fact sheet that summarizes an applicant's qualifications, education, and experience. A medical assistant must

PROCEDURE 27-1

Organize a Job Search

ABHES COMPETENCY: 6.f

GOAL: *To devote adequate time to and organize the job search in an efficient way so that proper follow-up can be conducted.*

EQUIPMENT and SUPPLIES

- Record of a Job Lead form
- Record of an Interview form
- Copies of resume
- List of interview questions
- Contact information for former employers and references
- Map of geographic area or printout from Internet mapping program
- Internet access
- Computer
- Job search weblinks
- Local newspapers
- Contact information for friends and family

PROCEDURAL STEPS

1. Format the resume as an accurate, up-to-date document.
   PURPOSE: If the resume is kept on a computer, it can be easily updated and targeted for various job opportunities.
2. Make copies of the record of job lead form and record of interview form.
3. Research job search websites and newspapers for job leads.
4. Network and contact employers directly to obtain job leads.
   PURPOSE: Networking and direct employer contact are the best two methods of job searching.
5. Gather information on job leads, and complete a record of Job Lead form for each one.
   PURPOSE: Employers are impressed when the person being

interviewed is familiar with the company; much information can be found on the company's website.

6. Prepare a targeted copy of the resume for each job lead.
   PURPOSE: Targeted resumes are designed to highlight the candidate's skills for a particular job, and the resume can be tailored for each specific company easily on a computer.
7. Take the resume to the facility and ask to complete an application, or….
8. Email the resume to the facility according to directions listed in the job advertisement.
9. Document all activity on each job lead.
   PURPOSE: The job search should be an organized process.
10. Schedule interviews for as many facilities as possible.
    PURPOSE: The more interviews, the better prepared the candidate will be.
11. Keep a record of job details on the record of the interview form for later reference.
    PURPOSE: Keeping a record of the details about each job possibility helps to keep them organized and is useful in comparing job offers.
12. Send thank-you notes to all professionals who grant an interview when the appointment is over.
    PURPOSE: Never fail to send a thank-you note, because this gesture may be the deciding factor in securing the job.
13. Compare opportunities when making a choice between offered positions.

---

determine what to include in the resume, remembering that he or she is "selling" himself or herself to an employer (Procedure 27-2). The resume should be developed before cover letters are written or job applications are completed so that strengths can be identified and highlighted on all job search documents.

There are many types of resumes. Three of the most common include the chronologic resume, the functional resume, and the targeted resume. A chronologic resume highlights the medical assistant's abilities in a logical order, such as most recent jobs back to the beginning of the individual's career (Figure 27-7, p. 549). A functional resume highlights specific skill sets, emphasizing the most important abilities or the most valuable experiences that the medical assistant has performed (Figure 27-8, p. 549). A targeted resume is perhaps the most effective: it emphasizes the skills that relate specifically to the job for which the medical assistant is applying (Figure 27-9, p. 550).

A medical assistant should target the resume toward the specific job that he or she is applying for. This means that the job requirements should be compared with the skills on the resume, and those skills should be highlighted in the document

using action words (Figure 27-10, p. 550). Of course, to do this effectively the medical assistant must actually know the job requirements. One can assume that clinical and administrative duties will be similar from place to place, but the ad for the position may provide further information about the scope of duties for the position. A medical assistant should read these carefully and emphasize that those are a part of his or her skill set on the resume.

Compose the resume and save it on the computer hard drive, a CD, or other storage device. Keep a copy on a flash drive so that the information is readily available if needed when away from the primary computer. Then as each job opportunity presents itself the resume can be modified to fit the job. For instance, if the resume lists back-office skills first and the job is for an administrative position, the administrative skills should be moved to the top to draw more attention to them. This is easy to accomplish when the resume is on a computer, because the medical assistant can cut and paste where necessary to make changes and save several versions of the resume. Then an original can be printed on high-quality paper for every job for which he or she applies.

Record of a Job Lead

Job Title _____ Medical Office/Facility Name _____

Phone Number_____Fax Number _____

Contact Name _____ Contact Title _____

Contact Phone Number/Extension _____

Physician(s) _____Office Manager _____

Office/Facility Address _____

City _____ State _____ Zip _____

Referred By _____ Phone Number _____

Date First Contacted _____ Person Spoken To _____

Information Submitted:

☐ Cover Letter ☐ Resume ☐ References

Date Sent _____ Date Sent _____ Date Sent _____

First Interview Scheduled: Day/Date _____ Time _____

Interviewer Name _____ Phone _____

Second Interview Scheduled: Day/Date _____ Time _____

Interviewer Name _____ Phone _____

Travel Directions _____

_____

_____

Office/Facility Information _____

_____

Basic Job Duties _____

_____

Miscellaneous Information _____

_____

_____

_____

(staple a business card to this form from the office/facility – use back for additional information)

Figure 27-5 Record of a job lead.

Record of an Interview

Job Title _____ Medical Office/Facility Name _____

Phone Number_____Fax Number _____

Contact Name _____ Contact Title _____

Contact Phone Number/Extension _____

Physician(s) _____Office Manager _____

Office/Facility Address _____

City _____ State _____ Zip _____

Interviewer Name _____ Phone _____

Travel Directions _____

_____

_____

Office/Facility Information _____

_____

Basic Job Duties _____

_____

Benefits/Salary Discussed _____

_____

Hours/Days to Work _____

General Impression of Office and Personnel _____

Questions as a result of interview _____

_____

Self-Evaluation of Interview Performance _____

_____

Thank-you sent ❏ yes ❏ no Date _____ Job Offer ❏ yes ❏ no (use back for notes)

Other Follow-up _____

_____

_____

(staple a business card to this form from the office/facility – use back for additional information)

Figure 27-6 Record of an interview.

PROCEDURE 27-2

Prepare a Resume

<u>ABHES COMPETENCY</u>: 2.j

GOAL: *To write an effective resume for use as a tool in gaining employment.*

EQUIPMENT and SUPPLIES

- Scratch paper
- Pen or pencil
- Former job descriptions, if available
- List of addresses of former employers and schools and names of supervisors
- Computer or word processor
- Quality stationery and envelopes

PROCEDURAL STEPS

1. Perform a self-evaluation by making notes about your strengths as a medical assistant. Consider job skills, self-management skills, and transferable skills.
   <u>PURPOSE:</u> To determine the strongest aspects of your abilities so that they can be highlighted on the resume.

2. Explore formatting, and decide on a professional resume appearance that best highlights your skills and experience. Use the templates available in word processing software, or design your own.
   <u>PURPOSE:</u> To construct an attractive document.

3. Place your name, address, and two telephone numbers where you can be contacted at the top of the resume.
   <u>PURPOSE:</u> To make certain that potential employers have a means of contact.

4. Write a job objective that specifies your employment goals.
   <u>PURPOSE:</u> To give the prospective employer an idea of what you are looking for in a medical assisting position.

5. Provide details about your educational experience. List degrees and/or certifications obtained.

6. Provide details about your work experience. Include all contact information and names of supervisors. Do not include salary expectations or reasons for leaving former jobs.
   <u>PURPOSE:</u> No negative information should be put on the resume. Salaries should be discussed; if a certain salary is listed on the resume, it may limit the amount that the facility will offer the medical assistant.

7. Prepare a cover letter and a list of references. Send the references with the resume only when requested.

8. Type the resume carefully, and make certain that there are no errors on the document.
   <u>PURPOSE:</u> Resumes submitted with errors are often discarded without consideration.

9. Proofread the resume. Allow another person to read it as well and look for missed errors.
   <u>PURPOSE:</u> To make certain that the resume is error free.

10. Print the resume on high-quality paper. Review the resume again for errors and to assure that it looks attractive on the printed page.

11. Target each resume to a specific person or position. Do not send generic resumes to each prospective employer.
    <u>PURPOSE:</u> Targeted resumes get better results during the job search.

12. For all resumes that are distributed, follow up with a phone call to arrange an interview.
    <u>PURPOSE:</u> A resume sent without follow-up is usually ineffective.

A resume is an important job search tool, but it should never be expected to get the medical assistant a job on its own merit. It is but one of many tools that should be used when looking for employment. Developing a professional resume takes some time and effort, and it will prove to be a good investment. Give the document some thought, and follow generally accepted guidelines for its construction.

CRITICAL THINKING APPLICATION

Lisa has drafted her resume and given a copy to her placement director. She has recommended that Lisa remove the mention of her volunteer experience, because it was not in the medical field. Should Lisa do this? Why or why not?

Critical Resume Errors

The first error that should be avoided on a resume is just that—any error. There should be no errors at all on a resume;

many employers will automatically disqualify a job candidate if one is found.

One medical assistant who was having a difficult time finding a job consulted her placement director at school. The director suggested that she come in for a **mock** interview. About halfway through the interview, the placement director realized the problem. The medical assistant had worked for 2 years at a local grocery store and had misspelled the name of the store on the resume. From an employer's point of view, a person who cannot spell the name of a facility in which she worked for a length of time, even though she cashed a paycheck with the company name on it, might well make critical errors in charting or in other aspects of her duties. Within a week after this error was corrected, the medical assistant found a job.

Never list salary expectations on the resume. If the medical assistant lists a salary of $25,000 on the last job held, the future employer might not offer more than $26,000 to $27,000, realizing that this is a step up from the last salary. However, if

Ruby Dunham
9362 Caesar Creek Road
Mytown, OH 45458
(937) 555-1899
rdunham@comcast.net

Education

• 1998: A.S. in Medical Assisting, Community College, Mytown, OH

Experience:

1995–present: Medical Transcriptionist, Community Hospital,
Mytown, OH

• Transcribe 55 wpm
• Specialist in medical terminology
• Excellent attendance record
• Detail oriented
• Increased personal productivity each quarter

1990–1995: Secretary, State University School of Medicine,
Mytown, OH

• Coordinated schedules of four full-time professors
• Maintained office supply and assistant budget
• Created final examination scheduling guidelines for department
• Developed excellent written communication skills
• Familiar with a variety of office machines

1986–1990: Shift Manager, Burger World, Mytown, OH

• Managed 10 employees, including hiring, training, evaluating,
  and firing
• Developed excellent oral communication skills and team player
  concept
• Improved inventory supply techniques, reducing losses by 10%
• Maintained cleanliness standards highest in chain
• Developed customer-focused service goals for store

Figure 27-7 Chronologic resume.

Max Bryan
1234 Rolling View Court
Mytown, OH 45431
(937) 555-3137
maxbryan@yahoo.com

OBJECTIVE

• An entry level position in medical assisting, with the opportunity to
  utilize and refine skills and training

EDUCATION

• 1998: A.S. in Medical Assisting, Community College, Mytown, OH
  Dean's list senior year, cumulative GPA 3.5

STRENGTHS

• Possess excellent interpersonal and communication skills
• Demonstrate consistent positive attitude and high energy
• Caring and compassionate
• Responsible, self-motivated, precise in work
• Experienced in customer-focused service

ACCOMPLISHMENTS

• Tutored students in medical assisting and 12-lead EKG courses
  Received excellent evaluations and positive results
• Certified Medical Assistant, active member of local AAMA
• Experienced in MS Office programs
• Consistent "excellent" ratings in clinical externships

COMMUNITY ACTIVITIES

• 1995–present: Organized, recruited, and trained 20 others for church
  hand bell choir, direct weekly practices and monthly performances
• 1996–present: Teach community CPR twice yearly to high school
  students
• Vice-President Student Government, Community College, Mytown,
  OH. Recruited members, organized fund-raisers, campaigned
  successfully for policy changes

EMPLOYMENT

• 1996–present: Tutor, Community College, Mytown, OH
• Waiter, Scott's Place, Mytown, OH

Figure 27-8 Functional resume.

they had been willing to pay $32,000, the medical assistant has lost an opportunity for much higher wages.

Avoid using "I" or other personal pronouns on the resume. If abbreviations are used on the resume, be sure to spell them out for clarity the first time they are used, if they are not well-known abbreviations. Never include personal information, such as height, weight, age, marital status, number of children, or any other information that is not **pertinent** to the job requirements.

Do not list dates along the left-hand side of the paper. This is distracting and draws attention away from the points that should be emphasized. A resume must be visually appealing and easy to read. The medical assistant should make good use of spacing, margins, indention, capitalization, and underlining to ensure an attractive document. **Proofread** the document several times to be sure there are no errors. It is helpful to have someone else proofread it, because many times the writer of a document misses errors when proofreading.

Never include a photograph with the resume. Photographs can be a discriminatory factor in the hiring process, and the medical assistant should be wary of any employer who requests a photograph with the resume.

One of the most senseless errors common to resumes is not having the appropriate contact information, such as an address

and telephone number. Two phone numbers are suggested, such as a cell phone number and a home phone number, so that there is a better chance of reaching the candidate when it is time to schedule an interview. Place an email address on the front page so that potential employers can make contact quickly. If an interview time becomes available late in the day, having access to job candidates by email may make a difference in who is scheduled and who ultimately gets the job.

The Argument about Length

Professionals disagree about the acceptable length of a resume. One page may be considered the ideal length, but a person with 20 years' experience in the job market will never get all of his or her skills on one page. A medical assistant without previous work experience may easily fit the resume on one page.

Recent trends indicate that a good rule of thumb is to allow one page for every 6 years of experience. If a person has a 20-

Roscoe Patterson
3472 Vienna Woods Lane
Mytown, OH 45449
(937) 555-8874
rpatt@aol.com

Job Target:

• A long-term medical assistant position in a busy and
varied medical office

Education:

• 1992: BA in Art History, State University, Mytown, OH
• 1998: AS in Medical Assisting, Community College, Mytown, OH

Capabilities:

• Excellent interpersonal skills and caring attitude
• Detail oriented, with strong analytical and problem-solving abilities
• Utilize solid organizational and time-management abilities in
coordinating multiple projects
• Self-starter, take initiative to ensure jobs get done properly and
efficiently
• Upbeat, personable, and highly energetic
• Ability to communicate in Spanish and American Sign Language

Accomplishments/Achievements:

• Campaigned for and raised consistent 15% annual increase in
contributions and grants, allowing expansion of exhibits and needed
renovations to art museum
• Maintained museum budget with 100% accountability
• Organized annual "Art Ball" for 100 contributors under budget
• Museum employee of the year 1995
• Certificates in CPR and EKG; Certified Nursing Assistant; will sit for
CMA exam this November

Work History:

• 1998–present: Certified Nursing Assistant, Friendly Nursing Home,
Mytown, OH
• 1992–1998: Assistant to the Curator, Mytown Museum of Art,
Mytown, OH

Figure 27-9 Targeted resume.

USEFUL ACTION WORDS

Accelerated	Manage
Actively	Motivated
Adapted	Organized
Administered	Originate
Analyze	Participated
Approve	Perform
Completed	Pinpointed
Conceived conduct	Plan
Control	Proficient
Coordinate	Program
Created	Proposed
Delegate	Proved
Demonstrate	Provide
Develop	Recommended
Direct	Reduced
Effect	Reinforced
Eliminated	Reorganized
Established	Responsibilities
Evaluate	Revamped
Expanded	Review
Expedite	Revise
Founded	Schedule
Generated	Significantly
Implemented	Simplify
Improved	Solve
Increased	Strategy
Influence	Streamline
Interpret	Structure
Launched	Successfully
Lead	Supervise
Lecture	Support
Maintain	Teach

Figure 27-10 Use action words when describing skills on the resume.

year career, the resume would be approximately three pages long. This is a general guideline; the document should be as **succinct** as possible while clearly communicating the strengths and background of the applicant. Make certain that contact information such as name, phone number, and an email address are provided on each subsequent page of the resume. The pages should also be numbered if there is more than one.

The Purpose of a Resume

The purpose of a resume is not to get the medical assistant a job, although this is a commonly held belief. The purpose of the cover letter is to get the employer to look at the resume. The purpose of the resume is to get the applicant an interview. The purpose of the interview, of course, is to get the job. Remember this, and use the resume as a tool, along with other strategies for job searching.

The medical assistant should be the person to write the resume, or at the very least should have a hand in its composition. Professional resume services may be helpful, but the person who

knows the most about the experience and education gained is the medical assistant.

CRITICAL THINKING APPLICATION

Lisa has been asked by a potential employer to email her resume. She has used an unusual font on her cover letter and the top of the resume. What concerns should Lisa have about emailing the document? How can Lisa make certain that her document arrives in a readable format when sending it electronically?

THE COVER LETTER

When sending a resume, always include a cover letter (Figure 27-11). This is the introduction to the resume and the person sending the document. A cover letter should always be sent to an individual, not to the facility or "to whom it may concern." A simple phone call will usually reveal the name of the person to whom the resume should be sent. Ask for the name of the office manager, or if this information is not obtained, address it specifically to the physician.

Brutis Walter
2345 Morrow Court
Mytown, OH 45310
(937) 555-7426

May 23, 1998

Andrea Foreman, CMA
Office Manager
Family Health, Inc.
123 Timberleaf Drive
Mytown, OH 45432

Ms. Foreman:

I will be graduating from Community College with an A.S. in Medical Assisting on June 9 and am interested in an entry-level medical assistant position in your office. I will consider part-time or temporary work to gain experience in a diverse office such as yours.

My training includes hands-on experience in pediatrics, cardiology, internal medicine, obstetrics, and geriatrics. My administrative training would allow me to fill in wherever needed in the office. I am highly motivated and have supported myself and paid my own way through college. I understand responsibility and am a true team player. Belinda Mallet, RN, a fellow church member, told me the office will be short-staffed this summer owing to vacations and a maternity leave. I believe I could help your office run smoothly this summer, and beyond.

I look forward to hearing from you. I am available Tuesday and Thursday afternoons and Friday mornings until graduation. I will call you next Tuesday to set up an appointment for an interview. Thank you for your consideration.

Very truly yours,

Brutis Walter

Figure 27-11 Basic cover letter.

The purpose of the cover letter is to gain attention. Many potential employers will schedule an interview with an individual based strictly on the content of the cover letter. Some are general letters that provide basic information without targeting the requirements of one specific job. An executive briefing, as described by Martin Yate in his book *Cover Letters That Knock 'Em Dead*, is a variation on the traditional cover letter. It provides a comprehensive picture of a thorough professional, plus a personalized, fast, and easy-to-read synopsis that details exactly how the applicant meets the major job requirements. This type of cover letter is extremely effective, but the applicant must have some idea of the job requirements in advance. To produce a dynamic executive briefing, the medical assistant should choose the most important qualifications listed on the ad for the job, then explain how he or she fits those qualifications (Figure 27-12).

Remember, not all direct supervisors will be the first recipient of the resume, so the impression formed by the cover letter may make the difference in getting to the next step in the hiring process. Make it easy for screeners to find the strengths that match the job description. The cover letter should be brief and interesting. Use the same paper stock weight and color as

EXECUTIVE BRIEFING

Allison Aubrey, R.M.A.
3040 Wood Branch Drive
Austin, Texas 78716
512-434-9902

James Richardson, M.D.
Family Practice Clinic
5508 Lamar Blvd.
Austin, Texas 78752

Dear Dr. Richardson:

Although my attached resume will provide you with a general outline of my work history, my problem-solving abilities, and some of my achievements, it may take longer than a few moments to peruse. For your convenience, I have listed your specified requirements for the medical assistant position at the Lakewood office below, and the skills I have developed that match those specifications. I hope this briefing will allow you to quickly determine my eligibility for the position and will prompt you to contact me for an interview.

Your Requirements:	My Skills:
1. Two years' experience as a medical assistant.	1. Three years' experience as a registered medical assistant.
2. Ability to work with a larger supervisory team in planning, budgeting, and policy formulating.	2. Experience as employee council president, intricately involved in planning and budgeting.
3. Familiarity with HIPAA regulations.	3. Trained in HIPAA compliance and received three certificates for continuing education related to HIPAA compliance.
4. Ability to work with others as a team.	4. Awarded "Employee of the Quarter" honors twice during past year, and nominated for "Employee of the Year" by my coworkers.

I know that my experience and abilities will be of benefit to your organization. I look forward to discussing my qualifications and your requirements in person. I am confident that we can develop an exceptional working relationship and that I am the right individual for your organization. I will telephone you on Monday to arrange an interview to take place at your convenience.

Sincerely yours,

Allison Aubrey, R.M.A.

Figure 27-12 Executive briefing.

the resume. Be sure to include contact information, such as an address and at least two phone numbers, even if these are on the attached resume. The supervisor may separate the two documents, so there must be a method of contact on each one. Never start a cover letter with the sentence, "I saw your ad in the newspaper" or a similar phrase. Be creative with the opening line, and try to capture the attention of the reader.

A cover letter should be one to three paragraphs long. The final section should include a call to action that will prompt an interview. If the document concludes with a request for a meeting, the medical assistant should state when he or she will call for a time and date.

JOB APPLICATIONS

Many facilities require a job application along with a resume (Figure 27-13). Arrive 15 minutes before the scheduled interview to allow time to fill out an application (Procedure 27-3).

Job applications can be considered a legal document if the person is hired. Therefore they should be neat and filled out correctly and completely. Always read the application before filling it out, so that directions make sense and information is not placed in the wrong area of the form. Carry a planner or address book to the interview so that former employers' and supervisors' names, addresses, and phone numbers are handy. The medical assistant should not be in a position that he or she must ask for a phone book to get an address. Have all of this information ready for when it is needed.

Applications often ask for a date that the medical assistant is available for work. Be careful with this question. If the applicant currently has a job, yet writes that he or she is "immediately available," it may indicate that the applicant intends to quit without notice. On the other hand, the current employer may be aware that the person is seeking other employment and may have granted him or her permission to quit immediately once a new job is found.

Be careful on the sections that ask the reason for leaving former positions. Think about the answers that are listed in those spaces, and try to put the information in as positive a light as possible. Ask the advice of the placement counselor if unsure what to say in these sections.

If there are sections available for listing special skills and qualifications, fill them out fully. Describe cardiopulmonary resuscitation (CPR) and first aid certifications and any professional organizations joined. If references are requested, list the name, title, employer, and a means of contact. Be sure to get permission before using someone as a reference.

One of the most common mistakes on the job application is writing "see resume." This is an indication of laziness and must be avoided. Even if the same information is found on the resume, the application must still be completed in its entirety. In addition, most job applications include a disclaimer that states that if a false or incomplete statement is made on the application, the individual can be dismissed from any position for which he or she was hired.

THE JOB INTERVIEW

A medical assistant may interview with the office manager, the physician, or both. It is possible that other staff members may be brought in for a portion of the interview. This is especially true in offices that have a cohesive team of employees.

The interview is usually the most stressful of the job search steps. Some individuals dread job interviews and become extremely nervous at the prospect of interviewing. Others are

---

PROCEDURE 27-3

Complete a Job Application

ABHES COMPETENCY: 2.j

GOAL: *To complete an accurate, detailed job application legibly in order to secure a job offer.*

EQUIPMENT and SUPPLIES

- Record of a Job Lead form
- Record of an Interview form
- Copies of resume
- Contact information for former employers and references
- Contact information for friends and family

PROCEDURAL STEPS

1. Read the entire job application before completing any portion of the document.
   PURPOSE: Reading through the entire application helps to avoid mistakes while filling out the document.
2. Gather any information that may be necessary to answer all questions on the application.
   PURPOSE: The candidate should have all information available for completing a job application.
3. Begin to complete the application legibly.
   PURPOSE: The interviewer will evaluation the candidate's handwriting to make certain that it would be legible on medical records.

4. Answer each question on the document, or write "not applicable."
5. Do not leave any space blank.
   PURPOSE: Leaving a space blank on the application may suggest that the candidate did not wish to answer a certain question or accidentally overlooked it. By writing "not applicable" on such questions, the candidate demonstrates competence and attention to detail.
6. Do not write "see resume" anywhere on the document.
   PURPOSE: Many supervisors view this practice as laziness. Always completely fill out the job application, and do not leave blank spaces.
7. Be completely honest about every fact written on the document.
8. Sign the document and date it.
9. Proofread the document and make certain that no information conflicts with the resume.
   PURPOSE: Proofreading will help the candidate to catch any errors before submitting the application.
10. Submit the application.

APPLICATION FOR POSITION / Medical or Dental Office
AN EQUAL OPPORTUNITY EMPLOYER

(In answering questions, use extra blank sheet if necessary)

No employee, applicant, or candidate for promotion, training or other advantage shall be discriminated against (or given preference) because of race, color, religion, sex, age, physical handicap, veteran status, or national origin.

PLEASE READ CAREFULLY AND WRITE OR PRINT ANSWERS TO ALL QUESTIONS. DO NOT TYPE.

Date of Application

A. PERSONAL INFORMATION

Name - Last   First   Middle   Social Security No.   Area Code/Phone No. (   )

Present Address: - Street   (Apt #)   City   State   Zip   How Long At This Address?:

Previous Address: - Street   City   State   Zip   Person to notify in case of Emergency or Accident - Name:

From: To: Address: Telephone:

B. EMPLOYMENT INFORMATION

For What Position Are You Applying?:   ☐ Full-Time ☐ Part-Time ☐ Either   Date Available For Employment?:   Wage/Salary Expectations:

List Hrs./Days You Prefer To Work   List Any Hrs./Days You Are Not Available: (Except for times required for religious practices or observances)   Can You Work Overtime, If Necessary? ☐ Yes ☐ No

Are You Employed Now?: ☐ Yes ☐ No   If So, May We Inquire Of Your Present Employer?: ☐ No ☐ Yes, If Yes:

Name Of Employer: Phone Number: (   )

Have You Ever Been Bonded? ☐ Yes ☐ No   If Required For Position, Are You Bondable? ☐ Yes ☐ No ☐ Uncertain   Have You Applied For A Position With This Office Before? ☐ No ☐ Yes   If Yes, When?:

Referred By / Or Where Did You Learn Of This Job?:

Can You, Upon Employment, Submit Verification Of Your Legal Right To Work In The United States?: ☐ Yes ☐ No
Submit Proof That You Meet Legal Age Requirement For Employment? ☐ Yes ☐ No   Language(s) Applicant Speaks or Writes (If Use Of A Language Other Than English Is Relevant To The Job For Which The Applicant Is Applying:

C. EDUCATIONAL HISTORY

Name & Address Of Schools Attended (Include Current)	Dates From	Dates Thru	Highest Grade/Level Completed	Diploma/Degree(s) Obtained/Areas of Study
High School				
College				Degree/Major
Post Graduate				Degree/Major
Other				Course/Diploma/License/Certificate

Specific Training, Education, Or Experiences Which Will Assist You In The Job For Which You Have Applied.

Future Educational Plans

D. SPECIAL SKILLS

CHECK BELOW THE KINDS OF WORK YOU HAVE DONE:

☐ MEDICAL INSURANCE FORMS   ☐ RECEPTIONIST

☐ BLOOD COUNTS	☐ DENTAL ASSISTANT	☐ MEDICAL TERMINOLOGY	☐ TELEPHONES
☐ BOOKKEEPING	☐ DENTAL HYGIENIST	☐ MEDICAL TRANSCRIPTION	☐ TYPING
☐ COLLECTIONS	☐ FILING	☐ NURSING	☐ STENOGRAPHY
☐ COMPOSING LETTERS	☐ INJECTIONS	☐ PHLEBOTOMY (Draw Blood)	☐ URINALYSIS
☐ COMPUTER INPUT	☐ INSTRUMENT STERILIZATION	☐ POSTING	☐ X-RAY
OFFICE EQUIPMENT USED: ☐ COMPUTER	☐ DICTATING EQUIPMENT	☐ WORD PROCESSOR	☐ OTHER:

Other Kinds Of Tasks Performed Or Skills That May Be Applicable To Position: Typing Speed   Shorthand Speed

(PLEASE COMPLETE OTHER SIDE)

Figure 27-13 Application for employment. (Courtesy Bibbero Systems, Petaluma Calif. 94654, (800) 242-2376, www.bibbero.com.)

E. EMPLOYMENT RECORD

LIST MOST RECENT EMPLOYMENT FIRST

May We Contact Your Previous Employer(s) For A Reference? ☐ Yes ☐ No

1) Employer

Work Performed. Be Specific:

Address   Street   City   State   Zip Code

Phone Number ( )

Type of Business

Dates   Mo. Yr.   Mo. Yr.
From   To

Your Position

Hourly Rate/Salary
Starting   Final

Supervisor's Name

Reason For Leaving

2) Employer

Worked Performed. Be Specific:

Address   Street   City   State   Zip Code

Phone Number ( )

Type of Business

Dates   Mo. Yr.   Mo. Yr.
From   To

Your Position

Hourly Rate/Salary
Starting   Final

Supervisor's Name

Reason For Leaving

3) Employer

Worked Performed. Be Specific:

Address   Street   City   State   Zip Code

Phone Number ( )

Type of Business

Dates   Mo. Yr.   Mo. Yr.
From   To

Your Position

Hourly Rate/Salary
Starting   Final

Supervisor's Name

Reason For Leaving

F. REFERENCES — FRIENDS / ACQUAINTANCES NON-RELATED

(1) _____

Name   Address   Telephone Number   (☐ Work ☐ Home)   Occupation   Years Acquainted

(1) _____

Name   Address   Telephone Number   (☐ Work ☐ Home)   Occupation   Years Acquainted

Please Feel Free To Add Any Information Which You Feel Will Help Us Consider You For Employment

READ THE FOLLOWING CAREFULLY, THEN SIGN AND DATE THE APPLICATION

"I certify that all answers given by me on this application are true, correct and complete to the best of my knowledge. I acknowledge notice that the information contained in this application is subject to check. I agree that, if hired, my continued employment may be contingent upon the accuracy of that information. If employed, I further agree to comply with Company/Office rules and regulations."

Signature: _____   Date: _____

Figure 27-13, _cont'd_ For legend see previous page.

very comfortable and consider the interview as much for their own purposes as for the employer's.

There are four phases to interviews. These are the preparation, the interview itself, the follow-up, and the negotiation.

Preparation for the Interview

When preparing for an interview, the medical assistant should learn everything possible about the employer. Look on the Internet for information about the facility. Practice answering potential interview questions. Prepare an outfit to wear to interviews. It is wise to drive to the interview site on a day preceding the interview date if the location is unfamiliar to avoid getting lost on the day of the important event. The better prepared the medical assistant is, the more comfortable he or she will be while interviewing.

The critical part of the interview is the medical assistant's ability to present himself or herself as the best candidate for the job. By preparing to answer interview questions before the interview, the medical assistant will be much more prepared. Although no one can guess exactly what questions will be asked, some standard interview questions are very common (Figure 27-14).

Review these questions thoroughly, answer them in writing, then study them before the interview. Then when the medical assistant is asked, "What are your three greatest strengths?" he or she can confidently answer, "I am professional, reliable, and honest."

When preparing on the day of the interview, be conservative with wardrobe choices. For women a skirt and blouse or business suit is appropriate. For men a business suit is the best choice. Depending on the office situation, one may be given very specific instructions on wardrobe. Some office managers or physicians will even tell the potential employee to arrive in jeans. Is this a test? The physician may be curious as to whether the medical assistant can follow directions and actually wear jeans. Obtain a hint about clothing by visiting the office before the interview, even if it is just to ask for directions. This way, the potential employee can see what the office staff members are wearing. Similar wardrobe should be sufficient for an interview. If the staff wears scrubs, then wear neatly pressed scrubs with clean shoes, avoiding the slouchy scrubs one might find in a hospital surgical suite. Conservative business suits should always be acceptable in an interview.

Be sure clothing is fresh and wrinkle free and shoes are shined. It is a good idea to carry a planner or other method of taking notes during the interview. This makes a good impression and indicates interest in the job. Always arrive 15 minutes early for the interview. Do not use heavy perfumes or colognes, do not chew gum, and avoid excessive jewelry. Never take anyone along on a job interview, especially children, even if they are older.

Pay particular attention to other aspects of appearance (Figure 27-15). Be sure that the hair is clean and styled attractively, teeth are clean, and breath is fresh. Nails are also important and should be clean and well groomed, because the medical assistant will want to give the interviewer a firm handshake. Expect to be a little nervous. Any interview can be a stressful situation. The

better prepared the medical assistant is, the more of a success the interview will be.

The Interview

During the actual interview, maintain good eye contact. Many supervisors refuse to hire people who seem uncomfortable with making strong eye contact. Never take control of the interview. Allow the supervisor to ask questions at his or her own pace. Do not fidget in the chair, and observe the interviewer's body language for clues as to how interested he or she might be. Do not volunteer any negative information, be honest, and do not exaggerate experience or lengths of employment. Never speak negatively about former employers.

Remember that the interview is centered on the medical assistant, so freely discuss the skills and attributes that will be brought to the job. The better prepared the medical assistant is, the smoother the interview will be. Be able to prove the skills claimed, and explain how they meet the needs of the company or facility. Avoid a "know-it-all" attitude, which indicates overconfidence and reluctance in taking direction. Always express an interest in the employer and its projects as opposed to what the employer can do for the employee. Ask intelligent questions at the end of the interview if given the opportunity. Never let your first question be, "How much will I be paid?" Money, although important, cannot seem to be your primary concern.

Before the interview ends, the medical assistant should ask when a decision will be made and if it would be acceptable to call to follow up (Procedure 27-4, p. 558).

CRITICAL THINKING APPLICATION

Lisa is enjoying a good interview when the supervisor, a man, asks her if she is married. When Lisa replies that she is not, he asks if she has a steady boyfriend. What might the supervisor's motive be with this line of questioning? How should Lisa respond? Are these questions inappropriate, or do they serve a purpose?

Follow-Up after the Interview

Follow-up is critical after an interview. Always send a written thank-you note or letter to the person who conducted the interview. Many employers wait to see who sends a thank-you letter before making the final hiring decision. Limit follow-up calls to no more than one or two a week. Most employers will give an indication of when the hiring decision will be made. The company should notify all those who interviewed once a decision has been made, unless specific protocols were set during the interview about follow-up. For instance, if the office manager says that a decision will be made on Friday, and the final three candidates will be called for a second interview, then the medical assistant knows if a call is not received to continue the job search. Although not all companies provide this type of notification, it is considered professional etiquette to tell the candidates who interviewed for the job if they are no longer under consideration. Never place all hope on one job—continue to prospect until an offer is made and accepted. In addition, always be on the watch for the next job opportunity.

TOP 100 INTERVIEW QUESTIONS

1. Tell me about yourself.
2. Why do you want to work for this company?
3. Why should I hire you?
4. How do you work under pressure?
5. What type of job or salary do you expect to make in 5 years?
6. How do you handle criticism?
7. What do you think your co-workers think about you?
8. What is your opinion of the company you last worked for?
9. Describe your last supervisor.
10. What is your view of management?
11. What would you like to change about yourself and how would you do it?
12. What is your best asset?
13. What adjectives would you use to describe yourself?
14. What aspects of your life are you most happy with?
15. How would you describe the perfect job?
16. Why did you leave your last job?
17. Why did you choose this type of profession?
18. What salary do you expect?
19. What are your strongest and weakest personal qualities?
20. What motivates you?
21. What have you learned from some of your previous jobs?
22. What personal characteristics are necessary for success in your chosen field?
23. What do you know about this facility and our competitors?
24. What were your major courses of study in school?
25. Do you plan to continue your education?
26. Did school meet your expectations or were you disappointed?
27. How did you pay for your education?
28. Sell this pen to me.
29. To what extent do your grades reflect how much you have learned?
30. Do you feel your education was worthwhile?
31. What were the major responsibilities of your last job?
32. What has been your most rewarding experience at work?
33. What was your single most important accomplishment for the company on your last job?
34. What was the toughest problem you have ever solved and how did you do it?
35. How do you see yourself fitting in with our company?
36. What skills did you learn on your last job that can be used here?
37. What would you do if you were fired in two years?
38. What kinds of additional education do you think you need to meet your career goals?
39. How long do you plan to stay with our company?
40. What immediate contribution could you make if you came to work for us today?
41. Do you feel that you have received good general training?
42. If you were starting school all over again, what courses would you take?
43. How much money do you hope to earn in 5 years? 10 years?
44. Do you think that your extracurricular activities were worth the time spent?
45. Are you interested in making money or do you have other reasons for entering this career field?
46. Do you prefer working with others or by yourself?
47. Can you take instructions or criticism without being upset?
48. Tell me a story.
49. What do you know about the opportunities in the field in which you are trained?

50. How long do you expect to work?
51. Have you ever had any difficulty in getting along with a co-worker, classmate, or instructor?
52. Which of your school years was most difficult?
53. Do you like routine work?
54. Define cooperation.
55. Will you fight to get ahead?
56. Do you have an analytical mind?
57. Are you willing to go where the company sends you?
58. What job in this company would you choose if you could?
59. Do you think that employers should consider grades?
60. What have you done that shows initiative and willingness to work?
61. What benefits did you receive from your last employer?
62. What has been your most important accomplishment during your school years?
63. Have you ever helped to reduce operating costs, and how?
64. Have you ever developed or helped develop any programs, and how did you do this?
65. What do you think determines a person's progress in a company?
66. What would you do if a personal problem interfered with your work?
67. What would you do if you became bored with your job?
68. What would you do if you had a personality clash with a supervisor?
69. How will you be getting to work each day?
70. Do you have reliable transportation?
71. How do you feel about working with someone who is HIV positive?
72. What person has most influenced your life?
73. What is the last book you read?
74. Who do you most admire?
75. Who is your favorite relative?
76. What will previous supervisors say about you?
77. What makes a good supervisor?
78. Why would you be successful in this job?
79. Why have you held so many jobs?
80. Can you explain this gap in your employment history?
81. Have you ever been fired from a position?
82. Do you have adequate child care arrangements that will allow you to be at work when scheduled?
83. What is your philosophy of life?
84. How many other positions are you considering?
85. Why were your grades in school so low?
86. Are you a member of any professional organizations?
87. How old were you when you began to support yourself?
88. Do you participate in continuing education activities or seminars?
89. Have you had the hepatitis B injection series?
90. Where did you perform your externship?
91. How many days of school did you miss?
92. Why did you decide to attend the college/school you attended?
93. What kind of boss do you prefer?
94. How do you usually spend your weekends?
95. Why types of people seem to rub you the wrong way?
96. What planning procedures do you use?
97. What frustrates you about your current job?
98. What is unique about you?
99. What have you done that indicates you are qualified for this job?
100. Do you have any questions?

Figure 27-14 Top 100 interview questions.

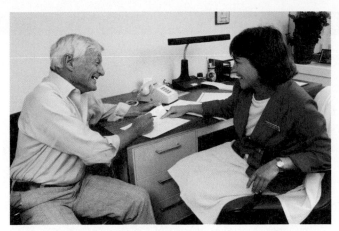

Figure 27-15 Present a professional appearance during the job interview, and be sure to smile often.

Reasons People Do Not Get Hired

Below is a ranked list of reasons that interviewers do not hire job candidates. The list is compiled from the results of a nationwide survey of 153 companies performed by North Central Technical Institute.

1. Poor personal appearance
2. Lack of interest or enthusiasm
3. Overemphasis on money
4. Poor voice, diction, grammar
5. Lack of planning
6. No purpose or goals
7. Condemnation of past employers
8. Poor eye contact
9. Limp, fishy handshake
10. Late to interview
11. Lack of tact
12. Lack of maturity
13. Lack of courtesy
14. Asking no questions
15. Overbearing "know-it-all"
16. Lack of confidence and poise
17. Failure to participate in activities
18. Making excuses, evading unfavorable factors on record
19. Indecisiveness
20. Just shopping around
21. No interest in company
22. Sloppy application form
23. Wanting a job for a short time
24. Unwillingness to relocate
25. Cynical attitude
26. Low moral standards
27. Laziness
28. Intolerance or strong prejudices
29. No sense of humor
30. Narrow interests
31. Inability to take criticism
32. No appreciation for the value of experience
33. Radical ideas
34. Too aggressive during interview

Negotiation

The negotiation stage of job acceptance can be as stressful as the actual interviews. A medical assistant should know the lowest salary he or she can afford, then should ask for a little more than that figure. Bracket salary requests: instead of asking for $12.00 per hour, ask for a salary in the "mid to high twenties." Let the employer mention a figure first, or a range of salary. Usually the person who mentions a salary range first has the disadvantage. If the medical assistant requests $12.00 per hour and the facility was willing to pay $15.00 per hour, the medical assistant will probably get $12.00.

Never say "no" to a job offer on the spot. Request at least 24 hours to consider the offer (Procedure 27-5). A medical assistant should not let the salary amount be the main factor in the decision to accept a position. Consider whether the position carries any authority, the benefits, the hours, the distance from home, and the potential for advancement before accepting or rejecting a job offer. Reasons exist for accepting a job other than the salary; remember the value of experience.

YOU GOT THE JOB!

Once the job offer has been made and accepted, a start date will be determined (Figure 27-16). Before the first day, use the computer to map several ways to get to work. Because you may be unsure of traffic flow, leave home extra early the first day so that arrival on time is guaranteed.

Most employees are placed on a 30- to 90-day probationary period, during which employment may be terminated if the employee's performance is not satisfactory. It is also an opportunity for the employer and employee to learn about each other. The medical assistant will interact with other co-workers, with patients, and with providers. A new medical assistant should volunteer to help others and efficiently complete the duties assigned. Use the probationary period as a testing ground, carefully observing ways in which the office might run in a smoother manner. However, do not make numerous suggestions for change during this period. Discover why certain methods are used, and make an effort to fit in with the rest of the team before suggesting that the routine of the office be changed. Remember, the people at the office may have been employed for substantially longer periods and may resent suggestions from a new staff member. Learn the office's rhythms, procedures, and culture first, and demonstrate a team-oriented attitude.

Common Early Mistakes

Some medical assistants make mistakes early on a new job. Never be disruptive to the office by gossiping or complaining. A medical assistant must realize that there may be different ways of performing procedures and that the way he or she was taught in school is probably not the only correct way. Be open to learning new ideas, concepts, and procedures. Although some mistakes are to be expected, be certain that once a mistake is pointed out, it is corrected. Do not make the same mistakes over and over.

Supervisors may or may not work very closely with the medical assistants. Some will be expected to carry out orders

PROCEDURE 27-4

Recognize and Respond to Verbal Communications: Interview for a Job

CAAHEP COMPETENCIES: 3.c.(1)(b), 3.c.(1)(c)
ABHES COMPETENCY: 2.f

GOAL: *To project a professional appearance during a job interview and be able to express the reasons that the medical assistant is the best candidate for the position.*

EQUIPMENT and SUPPLIES

- Record of a Job Lead form
- Record of an Interview form
- Job application
- Copies of resume
- Contact information for former employers and references
- Contact information for friends and family
- Sample interview questions

PROCEDURAL STEPS

1. Prepare for the interview by studying sample interview questions and researching basic information about the facility.
   PURPOSE: Employers are impressed by candidates who have researched the company and know some details about its operation.

2. Know all of the information that is contained on the resume so that it can be discussed confidently during the interview.

3. Prepare clothing that reflects a professional image for the facility in which the medical assistant is hoping to gain employment.
   PURPOSE: Most medical facilities prefer conservative dress.

4. Gather all materials that might be needed during the interview, such as copies of resumes, contact information, and copies of earned certificates.
   PURPOSE: All information must be handy and prepared in advance of the interview.

5. Arrive for the interview at least 15 minutes early.
   PURPOSE: Arrive early in case there are papers to complete in advance of the interview.

6. Stand and shake hands with the interviewer when he or she appears.
   PURPOSE: A confident, firm handshake is a positive gesture.

7. Listen intently to the interviewer as the position is described, and be ready to explain how you fit the requirements for the position.
   PURPOSE: The interviewer will evaluate how well the candidate listens and answers the questions asked.

8. Answer all interview questions confidently, smiling when appropriate, and displaying a positive attitude.

9. Ask intelligent questions after the interviewer finishes.
   PURPOSE: The questions asked at the end of an interview should indicate an interest in the position and should not focus on how the candidate would benefit from the job, but rather on what the candidate can do for the company.

10. Determine a day and time when the next contact will be made.

11. Express interest in the position.
    PURPOSE: Employers expect some type of confirmation that the candidate is interested in the job.

12. Send a thank-you note or letter to the interviewer within 24 hours of the interview.
    PURPOSE: A thank-you note is impressive and reinforces the candidate's interest in the position.

13. Follow-up as appropriate on the interview.

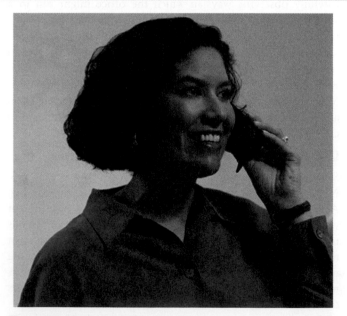

Figure 27-16 Congratulations, you're hired! The first job after school is an exciting experience for a medical assistant.

on their own. Do not make too much supervision necessary or force the office manager to constantly check the work that is done. Finish all assigned duties in a timely manner, and avoid procrastination. When problems arise, communicate them openly with the supervisor and attempt to find a quick resolution. Last, limit absences and tardy days to a minimum and miss work only when absolutely necessary—especially during the probationary period.

How to Be a Good Employee

There are several ways in which a medical assistant can be a better employee. First and foremost, arrive for the scheduled shift on time and do not leave early. Even the best medical assistant cannot benefit an office when he or she does not come to work. Be honest and demonstrate trustworthiness and professionalism. Get along with co-workers in the facility. A medical assistant should be able to resolve simple problems with others easily without involving the supervisor. Reflect a friendly attitude toward others, even if they are difficult to get along with. Arrive every single day ready to learn. The medical

PROCEDURE 27-5

Recognize and Respond to Verbal Communications: Negotiate a Salary

CAAHEP COMPETENCIES: 3.c.(1)(b), 3.c.(1)(c)
ABHES COMPETENCY: 2.i

GOAL: *To develop negotiation skills that will help the medical assistant obtain the salary and benefits that will sustain his or her family.*

EQUIPMENT and SUPPLIES

- Record of a Job Lead form
- Record of an Interview form
- Information about job offers received
- Contact name at medical facility

PROCEDURAL STEPS

1. Study the job offer at hand.
2. Determine if the offer is sufficient as it stands.
3. Make a list of what additional salary requirements and/or benefits are needed at a minimum.
   PURPOSE: Know the minimum salary and benefits that you can accept when evaluating a job offer.
4. Arrive at the second or subsequent interview appointment to discuss the job with the hiring supervisor.
5. Thank the supervisor for the offer that has been presented, and express interest in the position.
6. Express the additional salary and/or benefits desired.
   PURPOSE: The candidate should be able to express what he or she needs with regard to salary and benefits.
7. Discuss whether the facility would be willing to increase the offer to match your desires.
8. Express valid reasons that explain why the additional benefits should be offered, based on past performance, experience, or other valid factors.
9. Discuss reasonable compromises regarding the additional salary and/or benefits.
   PURPOSE: The ability to compromise is a valuable employee trait.
10. Ask what level of performance is expected for salary and/or benefits to be increased.
11. Express interest in and promise serious consideration of the position.
12. Determine the next contact time with the supervisor.
13. Weigh the offer and compromises to make a good decision about the job offer.

---

assistant's education does not end on graduation from school. The medical field is one of constant change, and those who work in it must learn and change along with the field.

A medical assistant should constantly be performing assigned duties and not expect frequent breaks in the medical office. Most offices are fast paced, and the supervisor will expect the medical assistant to keep up with the activity. Even when there are slow periods, there is always a counter to clean or filing to do. Be supportive of the leadership in the facility, and ask for more responsibility if necessary. Take initiative to perform duties that are cumbersome or repetitive, and get them done quickly.

It is vital to treat the patients with compassion. Remember that they are not always at their best when ill, so be kind and courteous to them and their families. The patients are the reason that the facility exists. Treat them with great respect and care.

CRITICAL THINKING APPLICATION

On Lisa's second day at the externship site, she clearly sees a co-worker taking and using a controlled drug from the storage area. What should Lisa do? What potential problems will this situation prompt? To whom should Lisa report this incident, if anyone?

Dealing with Supervisors

Supervisors appreciate employees who come to them when there are questions but who are able to handle minor decisions on their own. Never hesitate to approach supervisors when there is an issue at hand that needs their attention. Do not allow a situation to go unaddressed and then say, "I didn't want to bother you with that." It is the responsibility of the office manager to deal with difficult issues, and these should be handled immediately when they arise.

A medical assistant should never attempt to cover up a mistake; admitting the error is a much better approach to solving the problem. When talking with the supervisor, do not hesitate to speak and do not avoid the subject. State the problem clearly, and explain what routes are available to **rectify** the situation. Work with the supervisor to resolve issues and accept the advice given with a positive attitude.

Performance Appraisals

Performance **appraisals** are usually done after the initial probationary period and annually after that. The performance appraisal is designed to inform the employee of his or her strengths and weaknesses on the job, according to the supervisor's point of view. Most of these appraisals offer a scale to rate the employee's performance, such as 1 to 5. Do not expect to receive a perfect appraisal, because employees are seldom perfect in all aspects of their jobs. If the supervisor gives perfect scores to an employee, there is no room for growth or improvement. It is the rare employee who completes all duties without any errors. When asked to sit down with your supervisor for a performance appraisal, go into the meeting open to addressing areas that may need improvement. Ask questions and work with the supervisor to improve in the areas that may need more effort or a different approach.

If the employee strongly disagrees with any area of the performance appraisal, discuss this with the supervisor. There may have been a misunderstanding as to the duties involved. Clarify this, and strive to do better next time.

Asking for a Raise

Most facilities have some type of schedule for pay increases. Some offer a cost of living increase on an annual basis; others use a merit system, offering raises only when earned and deserved based on performance.

There may come a time when the medical assistant feels the need to ask for a raise. Before doing so, a little self-reflection should be performed to determine whether a raise is in order. Has attendance been exemplary? How many times was the medical assistant tardy? Does he or she work well with little supervision? Has he or she performed all the expected duties well and in a timely manner?

Approach the supervisor at a relatively calm part of the day, and ask how a salary raise might be earned in the near future. Do not expect a raise of more than 4% to 5% at any given time. If the supervisor is unable to grant a raise, determine whether the reasons are valid. If they are not, the medical assistant may wish to pursue other employment options. It is always easier to find a job if one already has a job, so do not quit outright unless the work environment is **intolerable.** Begin networking again, and discover the options available.

Leaving a Job Professionally

Always offer at least a 2-week notice when resigning from a job. Give the supervisor a written notice of resignation, and take this to him or her in person. Do not just leave it on a desk or place it in the interoffice mail.

It is a dangerous practice to resign from a job just to attempt to get a salary increase. Once the employer doubts the employee's loyalty, the future is usually not bright for the employee at that facility. Resign only after a final decision has been made. If the medical assistant is resigning to take another position, the current employer may be expected to make a **counteroffer.** However, be wary about accepting counteroffers. What led to looking for a new job in the first place? Has the situation been resolved? Ask these questions before agreeing to stay with the current employer.

LIFE SKILLS

To be successful in the job search, the medical assistant must have the basic entry-level skills needed to perform in the workplace. Even more important, however, he or she must develop certain life skills that are essential to excel in any profession. If these skills are not developed and refined, the medical assistant may find fewer opportunities and advancements available, as well as less impressive salaries and benefits.

The most important life skill one can possess is the willingness to change. Many employees insist on doing things the same way they have always been done, and they resist any changes in policy or procedure. However, a medical assistant who does not welcome and work hard to adjust to change is a failure waiting to happen.

Personal Growth

Personal growth is a comprehensive term that applies to many aspects of a person's mental, physical, and spiritual health. This growth is a result of goals that are set for self-improvement. Without clear goals, people rarely experience personal growth that is initiated from within. There may be growth that is a result of some outside influence, but a conscious effort toward personal growth is an innate decision.

No matter how great the training or how many opportunities are placed in front of a person, fear and doubt can sabotage efforts to improve the self-image, confidence, and future potential of an individual. Personal growth involves such traits as self-control, self-esteem, problem-solving skills, decision-making skills, and stress management.

Self-Control

Self-control is a vital trait in the medical office. Some patients may not be at their best because of their illness, and this may make them less than cordial toward the staff. Remember that this is usually a temporary situation. A medical assistant must exercise self-control and not respond in kind to patients who are disagreeable.

Self-control is important in other areas of the medical office. Never remove drugs from the storage areas without permission, and be careful when dealing with petty cash. A medical assistant must get enough rest during the work week that he or she can care for the patients in an enthusiastic manner.

Self-Esteem

Everyone has certain strengths and weaknesses. Good self-esteem is the result of knowing what those strengths are and overcoming the weaknesses. It is having a positive outlook about the self and others. A person with good self-esteem is motivated, able to express love, and capable of handling criticism. A person's self-esteem will improve if he or she has developed adaptive skills. Especially in the medical profession, one thing that is guaranteed in the workplace is change. Change can be positive or negative; this depends mostly on the way it is viewed by the individual.

A person is not doomed to live with poor self-esteem forever. With a degree of effort and open-mindedness, an individual can work toward better self-esteem, which can make a tremendous difference in the individual's future potential.

Problem-Solving Skills

For individuals to work together, they must have a degree of trust and be willing to make suggestions for the good of the group. The phrase "two heads are better than one" is still true when it comes to problem solving. Employees usually want to play a part in solving the problems in the workplace, and they appreciate knowing that their opinions make a difference. A medical assistant who can listen to the concerns of others and is willing to give and take will be an excellent problem solver.

Decision-Making Skills

People who know how to make good decisions are usually successful. Thinking through a decision requires logic, and it is best to take some time to carefully think of all of the "pros and cons." Unfortunately, a medical assistant may not always have time to consider decisions in a leisurely fashion, especially when dealing with emergencies. A good decision-maker is honest when identifying the real problems and attempts to keep personal feelings isolated from the process.

There are several steps toward making a sound decision. The problem must be specifically defined and evaluated so that the individual understands clearly what needs to happen to resolve the situation at hand. Gather as much information as possible and consider all alternatives. It is sometimes helpful to choose an alternative then consider all of the **ramifications** of making a decision using that alternative. Then, when the best alternative is determined, the decision should be made and put into action. Care should be taken to avoid making a decision simply because it is easy and comfortable, because more problems could arise later as a result of not addressing the true problem in the beginning.

CRITICAL THINKING APPLICATION

Lisa has been on several interviews and likes the prospect of working for three different physicians. If an offer is made at each office, how can Lisa decide which to accept? What will help Lisa make this decision?

Stress Management

The demands of the medical profession make it a stressful environment at times. Stress is not always bad. In fact, some stress is a positive motivator toward a goal. A stressor is a stimulus that prompts a reaction from the body. Positive stress, or eustress, includes exhilarating activities or success, which often leads to higher expectations from the person experiencing the eustress. The opposite is distress, which includes disappointment, failure, or embarrassment. Stress management is a conscious effort toward controlling the stressors and resulting reactions so that the body and mind operate evenly, even when stress is present in an individual's life.

By learning to recognize the signs of stressful overload, a medical assistant can possibly ward off the negative reactions that are so physically and mentally draining to the body. Many people notice a headache or fatigue when overly stressed. Breathing correctly is one way to reduce stress. Often an accelerated breathing pattern that is quick and shallow is a stress indicator. Breathing from the abdomen at a slower pace, inhaling through the nose, and exhaling through the mouth may help reduce tension. Taking time for relaxing activities and getting plenty of exercise are other methods of stress reduction.

Planning a Budget

A newly graduated medical assistant should formulate a simple budget and attempt to live within that budget. It is helpful to track spending with checkbook ledgers, bill stubs, receipts, and daily records for 3 months before developing a firm budget, so that there is a realistic accounting of where money goes when it leaves the checkbook. Use that information to design a spending plan for monthly income that accounts for monthly, quarterly, and annual expenses, as well as special activities.

Even when making only a small salary, building savings is important. A medical assistant should set aside 5% to 10% of the net income in a savings account. The money in savings should not be touched except in emergencies. It is even better to establish an emergency fund, which would ideally hold 3 months' salary. This way, there is enough cash to pay bills for 3 months in case of a sudden job loss or emergency. No one can do this immediately when beginning a new job, but it can be done over a period of time if one is committed to the effort.

Avoid going into debt whenever possible. If credit cards are used, they should be used conservatively and not for impulse purchases. Instead of using credit, set spending goals and save for a purchase or use layaway programs. Make more than the minimum payment on credit cards to avoid excessive interest from accruing on the account. Everyone should work toward being debt free as soon as possible.

Limit housing and utilities to no more than 30% of the net income. Other monthly installment debt should total less than 15% of the net income. Many financial institutions figure a debt ratio when they consider loaning money to an individual. If that debt ratio is too high, the bank may not lend money, even to a person with stellar credit.

Student Loans

Student loans are extremely important and are designed to provide the opportunity to obtain a good education. They must be paid back. If an individual **defaults** on a student loan, he or she becomes ineligible for future student loans until the original loan is paid back, and amounts owed may be deducted from tax refunds involuntarily. There is never a reason to default on a student loan. The medical assistant should contact the company that services the student loan and explain any problems that are keeping him or her from repaying the debt. These companies want to work with students to clear their accounts. Often a **deferment** is available, which allows the student to postpone the payments for a period of time (Figure 27-17). Deferments may be available when the student is unemployed, attending school to continue his or her education, suffering economic hardship, completing a graduate fellowship, completing rehabilitation training, or in other situations. Contact the lender to find out whether a deferment is in order.

The Guideline Budget

Dealing with personal finances can be a stressor. Developing a realistic budget will assist a medical assistant in planning his or her spending. When careful planning is implemented, more can be accomplished with less money if a commitment has been made to staying on budget and resisting the temptation to spend.

Dangerous Habits

Some individuals practice dangerous habits related to finances. For instance, if this month's bills are arriving and last month's

IN-SCHOOL DEFERMENT REQUEST

Federal Family Education Loan Program

OMB No. 1845-0005
Form Approved
Exp. Date 09/30/XXXX

SCH

WARNING: Any person who knowingly makes a false statement or misrepresentation on this form or on any accompanying documents shall be subject to penalties which may include fines, imprisonment or both, under the U.S. Criminal Code and 20 U.S.C. §1097.

SECTION 1: BORROWER IDENTIFICATION

Please enter or correct the following information.

SSN |___|___|___| – |___|___| – |___|___|___|___|

Name _____

Address _____

City, State, Zip _____

Telephone - Home (   ) _____

Telephone - Other (   ) _____

E-mail Address (optional) _____

SECTION 2: DEFERMENT REQUEST

Before answering any questions, carefully read the entire form, including the instructions and other information in Sections 5 and 6.

■ I meet the qualifications for the deferment checked below and request that my loan holder defer repayment of my loan(s):

❑ While I am enrolled at an eligible school as a **FULL-TIME STUDENT** . (For borrowers with a FFEL Program loan.)

❑ While I am enrolled at an eligible school as a **LESS THAN FULL-TIME BUT AT LEAST HALF-TIME STUDENT**. (For borrowers who, on the date they signed the promissory note, did not have an outstanding balance on a FFEL Program loan made **before July 1, 1987**.)

NOTE: *Your promissory note or other loan documents may state that a borrower with an outstanding balance on a FFEL Program loan made **prior to July 1, 1993**, must receive another loan in order to qualify for a half-time student deferment. This requirement was eliminated by the Higher Education Amendments of 1998. **Effective October 1, 1998**, no FFEL Program borrower who is eligible for a deferment based on enrollment as at least a half-time student is required to receive another loan in order to qualify for this deferment.*

SECTION 3: BORROWER UNDERSTANDINGS AND CERTIFICATIONS

■ **I understand that: (1)** I am not required to make payments of loan principal during my deferment. Interest will not be charged on my subsidized loan(s) during my deferment. However, interest will be charged on my unsubsidized loan(s). **(2)** I have the option of making interest payments on my unsubsidized loan(s) during my deferment. **(3)** I may choose to make interest payments by checking the box below. Interest that I do not pay during the deferment period will be capitalized by my loan holder.

❑ I wish to make interest payments on my unsubsidized loan(s) during my deferment.

(4) My deferment will begin on the date the condition that qualifies me for a deferment began, as certified by the authorized official who completes Section 4 of this form. **(5)** My deferment will end on the earlier of the date that I no longer meet the condition that qualifies me for the deferment, or the ending date of that condition as certified by the authorized official. **(6)** If my deferment does not cover all my past due payments, my loan holder may grant me a forbearance for all payments due before the begin date of my deferment or—if the period for which I am eligible for a deferment has ended—a forbearance for all payments due at the time my deferment request is processed. **(7)** If I am eligible for a post-deferment grace period on loans made before October 1, 1981, my loan holder may grant me a forbearance on my other loans for this period so that I can begin repayment of all my loans at the same time. I understand that my loan holder may capitalize the interest that accrues on my other loans during the six-month period and that this will increase the principal balance of my other loans. **(8)** My loan holder may grant me a forbearance on my loans for up to 60 days, if necessary, for the collection and processing of documentation related to my deferment request. Interest that accrues during the forbearance will not be capitalized.

■ **I certify that: (1)** The information I provided in Sections 1 and 2 above is true and correct. **(2)** I will provide additional documentation to my loan holder, as required, to support my deferment status. **(3)** I will notify my loan holder immediately when the condition(s) that qualified me for the deferment ends. **(4)** I have read, understand, and meet the eligibility criteria of the deferment for which I have applied.

Borrower's Signature _____   **Date** _____

SECTION 4: AUTHORIZED OFFICIAL'S CERTIFICATION

NOTE: As an alternative to completing this section, the school may attach its own enrollment certification report listing the required information.

I certify, to the best of my knowledge and belief, that the borrower named above:

(1) is/was enrolled as (check the appropriate box) ❑ a full-time student ❑ at least a half-time student

during the academic period from |___|___| – |___|___| – |___|___|___|___| to |___|___| – |___|___| – |___|___|___|___| and

(2) is reasonably expected to complete his/her program requirements on |___|___| – |___|___| – |___|___|___|___|.

Name of Institution _____   OPE-ID _____

Address _____   City, State, Zip _____

Name/Title of Authorized Officia _____   Telephone (   ) _____

Authorized Official's Signature _____   **Date** _____

Page 1 of 2

Figure 27-17 In-school deferment form. Do not allow yourself to default on your student loans. Contact the financial aid office at your educational institution for assistance and answers to questions about student loans.

SECTION 5: INSTRUCTIONS FOR COMPLETING THE FORM

Type or print using dark ink. Report dates as month-day-year (MM-DD-YYYY). For example, 'January 31, 2002' ='01-31-2002'. An authorized school official must either (A) complete Section 4, or (B) attach the school's own enrollment certification report listing the required information. If you need help completing this form, contact your loan holder.

Return the completed form and any required documentation to the address shown in Section 7.

SECTION 6: DEFINITIONS FOR IN-SCHOOL DEFERMENT REQUEST

- The **Federal Family Education Loan (FFEL) Program** includes Federal Stafford Loans (both subsidized and unsubsidized), Federal Supplemental Loans for Students (SLS), Federal PLUS Loans, and Federal Consolidation Loans.

- A **deferment** is a period during which I am entitled to postpone repayment of the principal balance of my loan(s). The federal government pays the interest that accrues during an eligible deferment for all subsidized Federal Stafford Loans and for Federal Consolidation Loans for which the Consolidation Loan application was received by my loan holder **(1)** on or after January 1, 1993, but before August 10, 1993, **(2)** on or after August 10, 1993, if it includes *only* Federal Stafford Loans that were eligible for federal interest subsidy, or **(3)** on or after November 13, 1997, for that portion of the consolidation loan that paid a subsidized FFEL Loan or a subsidized Federal Direct Loan. I am responsible for the interest that accrues during this period on all other FFEL Program loans.

- **Forbearance** means permitting the temporary cessation of payments, allowing an extension of time for making payments, or temporarily accepting smaller payments than previously scheduled. I am responsible for the interest that accrues on my loan(s) during a forbearance. If I do not pay the interest that accrues, the interest may be capitalized.

- The **holder** of my FFEL Program loan(s) may be a lender, guaranty agency, secondary market, or the U.S. Department of Education.

- **Capitalization** is the addition of unpaid interest to the principal balance of my loan. This will increase the principal and the total cost of my loan.

- An **authorized certifying official** for an In-School Deferment is an authorized official of the school where I am/was enrolled as a full-time or at least half-time student.

SECTION 7: WHERE TO SEND THE COMPLETED DEFERMENT REQUEST

RETURN THE COMPLETED DEFERMENT REQUEST AND ANY REQUIRED DOCUMENTATION TO:
(IF NO ADDRESS IS SHOWN, RETURN TO YOUR LOAN HOLDER)

SECTION 8: IMPORTANT NOTICES

Privacy Act Notice

The Privacy Act of 1974 (5 U.S.C. 552a) requires that the following notice be provided to you:

The authority for collecting the requested information from and about you is §428(b)(2)(A) et seq. of the Higher Education Act of 1965, as amended (20 U.S.C. 1078(b)(2)(A) et seq.) and the authority for collecting and using your Social Security Number (SSN) is §484(a)(4) of the HEA (20 U.S.C. 1091(a)(4)). Participating in the Federal Family Education Loan (FFEL) Program and giving us your SSN are voluntary, but you must provide the requested information, including your SSN, to participate.

The principal purposes for collecting the information on this form, including your SSN, are to verify your identity, to determine your eligibility to receive a loan or a benefit on a loan (such as a deferment, forbearance, discharge, or forgiveness) under the FFEL program, to permit the servicing of your loan(s), and, if it becomes necessary, to locate you and to collect on your loan(s) if your loan(s) become delinquent or in default. We also use your SSN as an account identifier and to permit you to access your account information electronically.

The information in your file may be disclosed to third parties as authorized under routine uses in the appropriate systems of records. The routine uses of this information include its disclosure to federal, state, or local agencies, to other federal agencies under computer matching programs, to agencies that we authorize to assist us in administering our loan programs, to private parties such as relatives, present and former employers, business and personal associates, to credit bureau organizations, to educational institutions, and to contractors in order to verify your identity, to determine your eligibility to receive a loan or a benefit on a loan, to permit the servicing or collection of your loan(s), to counsel you in repayment efforts, to enforce the terms of the loan(s), to investigate possible fraud and to verify compliance with federal student financial aid program regulations, to locate you if you become delinquent in your loan payments or if you default, to provide default rate calculations, to provide financial aid history information, to assist program administrators with tracking refunds and cancellations, or to provide a standardized method for educational institutions efficiently to submit student enrollment status.

In the event of litigation, we may send records to the Department of Justice, a court, adjudicative body, counsel, party, or witness if the disclosure is relevant and necessary to the litigation. If this information, either alone or with other information, indicates a potential violation of law, we may send it to the appropriate authority for action. We may send information to members of Congress if you ask them to help you with federal student aid questions. In circumstances involving employment complaints, grievances, or disciplinary actions, we may disclose relevant records to adjudicate or investigate the issues. If provided for by a collective bargaining agreement, we may disclose records to a labor organization recognized under 5 U.S.C. Chapter 71. Disclosures may also be made to qualified researchers under Privacy Act safeguards.

Paperwork Reduction Notice

According to the Paperwork Reduction Act of 1995, no persons are required to respond to a collection of information unless it displays a currently valid OMB control number. The valid OMB control number for this information collection is 1845-0005. The time required to complete this information collection is estimated to average 0.16 hours (10 minutes) per response, including the time to review instructions, search existing data resources, gather and maintain the data needed, and complete and review the information collection. *If you have any comments concerning the accuracy of the time estimate(s) or suggestions for improving this form, please write to:*

U.S. Department of Education, Washington, DC 20202-4651

If you have any comments or concerns regarding the status of your individual submission of this form, write directly to the address shown in Section 7.

Figure 27-17, *cont'd* For legend see previous page.

Top Ten Ways to Avoid Defaulting on a Student Loan

1. Understand your rights and responsibilities regarding your repayment obligation as well as your repayment options.
2. Borrow for college expenses only. Borrow only the amount you need and only what you can reasonably expect to be able to repay.
3. Keep all records regarding your loan. Make copies of all letters, canceled checks, and any forms you sign.
4. Notify your lender or servicer when you have a change of address, phone number, or name or if you change schools or your enrollment status.
5. Seek help as early as possible if you have any difficulty maintaining your student loan repayment arrangement.
6. If you have any questions, talk to your lender or student loan guarantor about the particular terms of your loan.
7. Keep credit card debt to a minimum or avoid credit card debt completely.
8. Create and maintain a budget that is within your monthly income.
9. Consider making nominal student loan payments while in school. This will reduce the amount you owe after graduation.
10. Make loan payments on time.

Courtesy Texas Guaranteed Student Loan Corporation. Available at: www.tgslc.org.

MONTHLY INCOME	AMOUNT
Net Income	
Spouse Net Income	
Child Support	
Other Income	

MONTHLY EXPENSES	AMOUNT
Rent	
Gas	
Electric	
Home/Renters Insurance	
Water/Sewage	
Trash	
Home Telephone	
Cell Telephone	
Pager	
Cable TV/Satellite	
Internet/DSL	
Child Care	
Lawn Care	
Clothing	
Food - Home	
Food - Work or School	
Food - Eating Out	
Laundry/Dry Cleaning	
Medical Expenses	
Dental Expenses	
Life Insurance	
Medical Insurance	
Dental Insurance	
Eyeglasses	
Prescriptions	
Automobile Payment	
Automobile Insurance	
Repairs	
Gas/Oil	
Furniture	
Beauty/Barber Shop	
Pet Expenses	
Student Loan	
Other Loans	
Credit Cards	
Church/Charities	
Birthdays	
Anniversaries	
Christmas	
Vacation Planning	
Entertainment	

Figure 27-18 The guideline budget.

have not been paid, frustration and depression may result. Some people may even avoid opening letters or bills just so they do not have to deal with seeing the balance due. Writing checks on funds that are not in the checking account is not only unwise—it is also illegal. All states have laws related to insufficient fund checks, and most legislation considers this a form of theft. It is possible to be arrested for writing "hot" checks. People headed for financial disaster also purchase daily items, such as bread and milk, with a credit card. All of these behaviors are signs of financial trouble.

A sample budget outline is shown in Figure 27-18. Take an honest look at each item listed, and determine what amount is spent monthly in each category. Compare these amounts with the monthly income and see if the current budget is positive or negative. Remember that the gross salary is the amount earned before taxes and other deductions. The net salary is the take-home pay. Adjustments may be needed to bring the budget into balance.

CLOSING COMMENTS

The period surrounding graduation will be a celebration, but also a busy time for which much planning is required. Cooperate with the school when securing externship sites, and make an effort to obtain a site that will be of the most benefit to the career desired. Do not take an externship just because it is close to home. Think about the skills that will be offered, and learn as much as possible. Then perform well, so that the staff

and physicians are happy to offer a good reference to potential employers. Strive to attain goals and once they are reached, set additional goals to continue moving forward in life.

Even though the medical assistant educational experience ends, remember that there is constantly something new to learn in the medical profession. Join professional societies, and participate in as many educational seminars and continuing education classes as possible. Remain in a continual state of learning, and be determined to be the best medical assistant you can be.

Steps for Achieving Goals

- Decide what you want
- Write the goal down
- Set the date for accomplishment
- Read the goal three times daily
- Think of the goal often
- See yourself accomplishing the goal
- Develop a plan of action for reaching the goal
- Do not discuss the plan with others who might be discouraging
- Be confident
- Act successful, and you will be!

Always be completely honest when completing a job application and offering information on a resume. Most facilities stipulate that if an individual is not truthful on these documents, his or her employment can be terminated once the deception is discovered. Employers are more interested in honesty and a forthright explanation than in minor problems that affect the job performance.

If a medical assistant has had some brush with the law that requires disclosure on the job application, the best policy is to be honest and deal with the ramifications of telling the truth. Most businesses can verify whether a potential employee has any type of criminal record. A solid explanation of the facts, admission of a past mistake, and excellent, current references will often prompt an employer to have faith and make a positive decision about extending employment.

SUMMARY OF SCENARIO

The end of medical assistant training is a time of great excitement and perhaps a small bit of apprehension. Lisa is prepared to accept the challenges ahead as she readies herself for her future in her new career. She has begun her externship and has been expanding her network of acquaintances in the medical profession for several months. Lisa has met many office managers and a few physicians and has learned a great deal about several area medical facilities. Through her research, she has decided that she would like to work with one of three local physicians who need a medical assistant. One is a pediatrician, another is a well-known neurologist, and the third is a family practitioner just out of medical school. Lisa has gathered information about all of these professionals, and each has invited her for a job interview.

Lisa knows that she will need to be at her best, so she takes care of herself and gets plenty of rest. She has a long list of interview questions and has taken the time to write out answers to the questions in preparation for her interviews. She is careful about her grooming every day that she reports to the externship, because she knows that the physician at her site is her first reference in the medical field. In addition, she knows that she may be called for an interview any day that might be scheduled just after her workday ends. Looking professional prepares her for this each day.

Lisa is comfortable during her interviews because she is well prepared. She has identified her strengths and can share them with a potential employer. She is focused on her objectives and knows what the minimum requirements will be for her to accept a position. She has a healthy self-esteem, and her good decision-making skills will help her to determine which position will be right for her. Her enthusiasm and excitement show in her eyes, and she is dedicated to making a difference in the lives of her patients and co-workers.

SUMMARY of LEARNING OBJECTIVES

1. Define, spell, and pronounce the terms listed in the vocabulary.
   - Spelling and pronouncing medical terms correctly adds credibility to the medical assistant. Knowing the definition of these terms promotes confidence in communication with patients and co-workers.
2. Discuss the reasons that job search training is important to a medical assistant.
   - Because approximately 85% of individuals do not have any formal training in job search skills, taking the time to learn the best methods will place the medical assistant at an advantage. Training decreases the time spent looking for work and increases the benefits and salary offered when using good

negotiating skills. The medical assistant will also be more comfortable during interviews and throughout the job search process.
3. List three expectations that employers have of employees.
   - Employers have three basic expectations of their medical assistant employees. They want an employee with a good appearance, who looks as if he or she fits in the medical profession. A medical assistant should also be dependable and have the skills to do the job for which he or she was hired.
4. Understand the three types of employee skill strengths.
   - There are three types of skill strengths that may be used by employees. Job skills are those used to actually perform

Continued

SUMMARY of LEARNING OBJECTIVES

Continued

a job, such as venipunctures or scheduling appointments. Self-management skills are usually a part of the medical assistant's personality; these include honesty and dependability. Transferable skills are those that can be taken from one job to another or used on any job. Examples include the ability to communicate effectively and lead and manage individuals.

5. Explain the two best job search methods.
   - Networking and contacting employers directly are the two best methods of job searching. Networking involves developing a network of individuals that can assist in finding employment. This group may include co-workers, other students, relatives, or friends who provide leads to potential employers. Contacting employers directly includes taking resumes to specific offices or setting appointments to gain knowledge about the facility, then later using that knowledge during the job search. These two methods are more effective than most traditional means of finding a job.

6. Describe some of the errors that should be avoided on a resume.
   - Any error on a resume should be avoided. Be sure that everything is spelled correctly, but do not rely on the computer's spell-check feature alone. Proofread the document, and have someone else proofread it to catch errors that may have been overlooked. Salary expectations should never be stated on the resume, and a photograph should not be included. Do not include personal information, such as height and weight.

7. Explain the importance of having demographic information about former jobs before appearing for an interview.
   - Demographic information on other employers should be taken to interviews and kept handy when filling out job applications. A medical assistant should never have to ask for a phone book to look up the address of a former employer. This demonstrates a lack of preparation and planning on the part of the potential employee.

8. List the four phases of the interview process.
   - The four phases of the interview process include the preparation, the actual interview, the follow-up, and the negotiation. The preparation includes all efforts made before the actual interview in obtaining information about the company, deciding on the wardrobe, and making sure nails are groomed and shoes are shined. The interview itself is designed to help the employer and potential employee get to know each other and discover whether they are compatible. The follow-up is perhaps the most critical stage, wherein the medical assistant should send a thank-you letter and continue to stay in touch with the facility until the job is filled. The negotiation includes discussion of the salary and benefits that will be offered to the new employee.

9. Discuss the importance of the probationary period for a new employee.
   - The probationary period is a time for the new medical assistant to become oriented to the facility. It also allows the employer to assess whether the medical assistant fits with the team and performs the duties of the job in a satisfactory way. During this time, the medical assistant should demonstrate that he or she is a productive team member with an excellent attitude. There should never be idle time; instead, look for ways to assist others when all duties are completed.

10. List some mistakes that should be avoided by a new employee.
    - A new employee in the medical office should avoid arriving late or being absent, especially during the probationary period. Never participate in office gossip, and make a good attempt to get along with every employee. A medical assistant should not make excessive supervision necessary and should be open to learning new ways of performing procedures. Fit in with the team, and the job will be more rewarding.

11. Explain why a performance appraisal's ratings are usually not perfect.
    - No employee is perfect, so performance appraisals rarely have perfect ratings. Even an employee who is doing an excellent job has room for improvement in some area. Without comments that suggest improvement, the employee may not feel that the position offers growth potential. Constructive comments will help a medical assistant to perform better and take on more responsibility.

12. Prepare a resume.
    - The resume must be accurate and error-free. The process for preparing a resume is outlined in Procedure 27-2.

13. Organize a job search.
    - Time management and organizational skills will help the medical assistant to launch an effective job search. The process for organizing a job search is outlined in Procedure 27-1.

14. Complete a job application.
    - Job applications must be competed accurately and in their entirety. The process for completing a job application is outlined in Procedure 27-3.

15. Interview for a job.
    - The interview is the job search step that most influences hiring decisions. The process for interviewing for a job is outlined in Procedure 27-4.

16. Negotiate a salary.
    - The medical assistant should develop skills in negotiating salary after he or she has determined the minimum amount in both benefits and pay that can be accepted. The process for negotiating a salary is outlined in Procedure 27-5.

CONNECTIONS

 Study Guide Connection: Go to Chapter 27 Study Guide. Read the Case Study and Workplace Applications and complete the assignments. Do online research for answers to the questions in the Internet Activities associated with career development and life skills.

 CD Connection: Go to the Medical Assisting Competency Challenge CD and do the training activities under Communication.

 Evolve Connection: For more information related to career development and life skills, go to http://evolve.elsevier.com/kinn/admin and visit related weblinks for Chapter 27. Click on the Medical Assisting Exam Review and do the practice questions to sharpen your test-taking skills.

Procedure A-1: Obtaining a Medical History

Obtain and Record a Patient History

<u>CAAHEP COMPETENCY:</u> 3.b.(4)c
<u>ABHES COMPETENCY:</u> 4.a

Complete this procedure with another student role playing the patient. To make the experience more realistic, choose a student about whom you know very little. To maintain the privacy of your student partner, he or she does not have to share any confidential information while participating in the role-play.

GOAL: *To obtain an acceptable written background from the patient to help the physician determine the cause and effects of the present illness. This includes the chief complaint (CC), present illness (PI), past history (PH), family history (FH), and social history (SH).*

EQUIPMENT and SUPPLIES

- History form
- Two pens—a red pen for recording patient allergies and a black pen to meet legal documentation guidelines
- A quiet, private area

PROCEDURAL STEPS

1. Greet and identify the patient in a pleasant manner. Introduce yourself and explain your role.
   <u>PURPOSE:</u> To make the patient feel comfortable and at ease.
2. Take the patient to a quiet, private area for the interview, and explain to the patient why the information is needed.
   <u>PURPOSE:</u> A quiet, private area is necessary to protect confidentiality and prevent interruptions. An informed patient is more cooperative and therefore more likely to contribute useful information.
3. Complete the history form by using therapeutic communication techniques. Make sure that all medical terminology is adequately explained. A self-history may have been mailed to the patient before the visit. If so, review the self-history for completeness.
   <u>PURPOSE:</u> Therapeutic communication techniques will assist the medical assistant in gathering complete information; the self-history is designed to save time and to involve the patient in the process.
4. Speak in a pleasant, distinct manner, remembering to maintain eye contact with your patient.
   <u>PURPOSE:</u> Positive nonverbal behaviors create a friendly, caring atmosphere.
5. Record the following statistical information on the patient information form:

- Patient's full name, including middle initial
- Address, including apartment number and ZIP code
- Marital status
- Sex (gender)
- Age and date of birth
- Telephone number for home and work
- Insurance information if not already available
- Employer's name, address, telephone number

6. Record the following medical history on the patient history (PH) form:
   - Chief complaint (CC)
   - Past history
   - Social history
   - Present illness
   - Family history
   <u>PURPOSE:</u> This is information that the physician needs to know to make an accurate assessment and diagnosis. The physician usually completes the review of systems (ROS) during the preexamination interview.
7. Ask about allergies to drugs and any other substances, and record any allergies in red ink on every page of the history form, on the front of the chart, and on each progress note page. Some practices apply allergy alert labels to the front of each chart.
   <u>PURPOSE:</u> The presence of an allergy may alter medication and treatment procedures.
8. Record all information legibly and neatly, and spell words correctly. Print rather than writing in longhand. Do not erase, scribble, or use whiteout. If you make an error, draw a single line through the error, write "error" above it, add the correction, and initial and date the entry.
   <u>PURPOSE:</u> To maintain a medical record that is understandable and defensible in a court of law.

Continued

PROCEDURE A-1—cont'd

9. Thank the patient for cooperating, and direct him or her back to the reception area.
10. Review the record for errors before you pass it to the physician.
11. Use the information on the record to complete the patient's chart. Keep the information confidential.
    PURPOSE: All information concerning the patient must remain in the office. This information may be legally and ethically discussed with only the physician.

DOCUMENTATION PRACTICE: Mr. Bonski is a new patient being seen today for the first time. His CC is dizziness for 2 weeks. He denies having headaches and has no previous Hx of ear infections or hypertension. He doesn't take any prescribed medications but uses Tylenol as needed for a headache. T 97.6, P 88, R 22, BP 172/94. Document pertinent patient findings using the SOAPE method.

S: _____

O: _____

_____

English-Spanish Phrases

Commonly Used Phrases

Are you having pain? Where?
¿Siente usted dolor? ¿Dónde?

What does the pain feel like?
¿Qué tipo de dolor es?

How long have you had problems with this?
¿Desde cuándo tiene este tipo de problemas?

When did it start?
¿Cuándo comenzó?

Does your child have a temperature?
¿Tiene fiebre su hijo?

Have you given your child any medication?
¿Le ha dado alguna medicina a su hijo?

Are you allergic to any medication?
¿Es usted alérgico a algo?

How did your child get hurt?
¿Cómo se lastimó su hijo?

What is your name?
¿Cómo se llama usted?

How old are you?
¿Qué edad tiene?

Do you take any medication regularly?
¿Toma usted alguna medicación con regularidad?

How many times have you been pregnant?
¿Cuántas veces ha estado embarazada?

How many children were born alive?
¿Cuántos niños sanos ha dado usted a luz?

Who is your closest relative?
¿Quién es su familiar más cercano?

Do you speak English?
¿Habla usted inglés?

Can someone come with you the next time who does speak English?
¿Puede acompañarle alguien que hable inglés la próxima vez?

Can you read English?
¿Sabe usted leer en inglés?

Does someone in your family read English?
¿Alguien de su familiar sabe leer en inglés?

My name is... You are...
Yo soy... Usted es...

Please put the gown on.
Por favor, póngase la bata.

Your blood pressure is...
Su presión arterial es de...

Your blood sugar is...
Su nivel de azúcar en la sangre es de...

The doctor recommends a low-fat diet.
El médico recomienda una dieta baja en grasa.

Does this hurt?
¿Le duele esto?

Do you have medical insurance?
¿Tiene usted seguro médico?

Please point to where it hurts.
Por favor, indíqueme dónde le duele.

Where do you work?
¿Dónde trabaja usted?

Have you seen blood in your urine?
¿Ha visto algo de sangre en su orina?

Do you have pain when urinating?
¿Siente algún dolor al orinar?

Please fill out this form.
Por favor, llene este formulario.

Do you have an insurance card?
¿Tiene usted una tarjeta del seguro?

Do you have a telephone? What is the number?
¿Tiene usted teléfono? ¿Cuál es el número?

Please come back to see the doctor on…
Por favor, regrese para ver al médico el…

The doctor wants you to see another doctor.
El médico quiere que la vea otro médico.

Go to the hospital.
Vaya al hospital.

Call the ambulance now.
Pida una ambulancia ahora mismo.

Take your medication as ordered.
Tómese la medicación tal como se le indicó.

These are the side effects of your medication.
Su medicación tiene algunos efectos secundarios.

Thank you.
Gracias.

You are welcome.
De nada.

Please.
Por favor.

Please come this way.
Venga por aquí, por favor.

Please come with me.
Acompáñeme, por favor.

Please wait here to see the doctor.
Por favor, espere aquí para ver al médico.

You may leave now.
Ya puede marcharse.

We need to get a blood sample.
Necesitamos una muestra de su sangre.

We need to get a urine sample.
Necesitamos una muestra de su orina.

You owe "xxx" today.
Hoy debe abonar "xxx."

Who should we call to pick you up?
¿A quién debemos contactar para que lo recojan?

Please go to the laboratory at this address.
Por favor, vaya al laboratorio que está en este lugar.

When did you last eat?
¿Cuándo comió por última vez?

Have you had nausea?
¿Ha tenido náuseas?

Have you vomited?
¿Ha vomitado?

Please sign your name here.
Por favor, firme aquí.

Take this medicine (3) times a day.
Tómese esta medicina (3) veces al día.

This paper allows us to file your insurance.
Este papel nos permite presentarle su caso al seguro.

This paper allows the insurance company to pay the doctor.
Este papel es para que el seguro le pague al médico.

The doctor will see you now.
El médico le puede ver ahora.

Good morning.
Buenos días.

Good afternoon.
Buenas tardes.

Here is information (written) about your illness.
Aquí se incluye información (escrita) sobre su enfermedad.

Please follow these directions.
Por favor, siga estas instrucciones.

It is nice to meet you.
Es un placer conocerle.

Thank you for coming.
Gracias por su visita.

Take care of yourself.
¡Cuídese!

Do you drink alcohol?
¿Toma usted alcohol?

Do you smoke? How much?
¿Fuma? ¿Cuántos cigarrillos al día?

Have you had this problem before?
¿Ha tenido antes este problema?

Days of the week

Los días de la semana

Monday
lunes

Tuesday
martes

Wednesday
miércoles

Thursday
jueves

Friday
viernes

Saturday
sábado

Sunday
domingo

Months of the year

Los meses del año

January
enero

February
febrero

March
marzo

April
abril

May
mayo

June
junio

July
julio

August
agosto

September
septiembre

October
octubre

November
noviembre

December
diciembre

Times

Horas

One o'clock
Es la una

Two o'clock
Son las dos

Three o'clock
Son las tres

Four o'clock
Son las cuatro

Five o'clock
Son las cinco

Six o'clock
Son las seis

Seven o'clock
Son las siete

Eight o'clock
Son las ocho

Nine o'clock
Son las nueva

Ten o'clock
Son las diez

Eleven o'clock
Son las once

Twelve o'clock
Son las doce

Numbers

Números

1
uno

2
dos

3
tres

4
cuatro

5
cinco

6
seis

7
siete

8
ocho

9
nueve

10
diez

11
once

12
doce

13
trece

14
catorce

15
quince

16
dieciséis

17
diecisiete

18
dieciocho

19
diecinueve

20
veinte

21
veintiuno

22
veintidos

23
veintitres

24
veinticuatro

25
veinticinco

26
veintiséis

27
veintisiete

28
veintiocho

29
veintinueve

30
treinta

31
treinta y uno

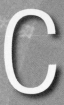

ICD-10-CM and ICD-10-PCS

The tenth revision of Volumes 1, 2, and 3 of the International Classification of Diseases (ICD) brings massive changes. There are now two separate systems: ICD-10-CM for diagnostic coding and ICD-10-PCS for procedural coding.

- ICD-10-CM (International Statistical Classifications of Diseases and Related Health Problems, Tenth Revision, Clinical Modification) is the replacement for Volumes I and II–the diagnoses, signs, symptoms, and health-related codes.
- ICD-10-PCS (International Statistical Classifications of Diseases and Related Health Problems, Tenth Revision, Procedural Coding System) replaces Volume III–the procedures generally performed within a hospital environment.

TENTH REVISION OF ICD

The World Health Organization (WHO) published the tenth revision of the ICD system in 1992 in order to:

- Expand the content, purpose, and scope of system
- Include ambulatory care services
- Increase clinical detail
- Capture risk factors in primary care
- Include emergent diseases
- Group diagnoses for epidemiologic purposes

ICD-10-CM IMPLEMENTATION

The National Center for Health Statistics (NCHS) began testing the clinical modification of ICD-10 in 1997. The American Health Information Management Association (AHIMA), in cooperation with the American Hospital Association (AHA), has begun field testing coding and records management using the ICD-10-CM. Implementation of ICD-10-CM is likely to happen no sooner than October 2007. However, the massive changes to the coding system and the huge impact on all of healthcare in implementing these changes require that planning and training in the new coding system begin now.

BENEFITS OF ICD-10-CM

- Greater specificity
- Added descriptions relevant to ambulatory care and managed care encounters
- Allows for the possibility of expansion

- Extends beyond classification of diseases and injuries to include health-related risk factors
- General terminology and disease classification have been updated to current standards

ICD-10-CM

With the release of Volume 1 of the ICD-10 in 1992 by WHO, the United States requested and was granted permission to develop an adaptation of ICD-10 for use in the United States for government purposes. Currently this clinical modification is underway and is being called *ICD-10-CM*. Other countries have already made or are developing their own modifications of ICD-10 for use within their respective countries. ICD-10-CM will replace ICD-9-CM Volumes 1 and 2 only. Like the ICD-9-CM system, this new coding system is closely related to its ICD counterpart (ICD-10). Therefore it closely follows the changes to ICD-10. It contains significantly more codes than the current ICD-9-CM. It is also alphanumeric and has up to seven digits. Please note that Volume 3 (the inpatient procedures) is not included in ICD-10-CM. A separate coding system, called *ICD-10-PCS* (procedure coding system), has been proposed as a replacement.

COMPARISON OF ICD-10-CM WITH ICD-9-CM

The advantages and benefits of ICD-10-CM are significant in both quality and usefulness of data for various healthcare settings.

- The hierarchic structure is the same for both classification systems, but ICD-10-CM codes are alphanumeric and include all letters except U, which is reserved for new diseases of uncertain etiology.
- ICD-9-CM's V and E codes have been incorporated into the main classification of ICD-10-CM.
- ICD-10-CM codes can be up to seven characters, compared with the maximum of five for ICD-9-CM.
- ICD-10-CM incorporates additional information related to ambulatory care and managed care encounters.
- Conditions that were not uniquely identified in ICD-9-CM have been assigned code numbers in ICD-10-CM.
- In ICD-10-CM, as in ICD-9-CM, some three-character categories are left vacant to allow for code revisions and future additions.
- The ICD-10-CM groups injuries first by site (arm,

shoulder, ankle), then by type (fracture, sprain), rather than just by type, as they are in the ICD-9-CM.

- The Excludes guidelines and notes have been expanded to provide guidance on hierarchy of the chapters and help clarify code assignment.
- Some conditions are listed in more appropriate chapters in the ICD-10-CM.

Some new or expanded features of the ICD-10-CM include the following:

- Combination codes are used for both symptom and diagnosis and for etiology and manifestations.
- Many codes have been expanded to include laterality (identification of a specific side of the body), a feature that was missing from ICD-9-CM.

- Classifications that indicate a patient's trimester are included in the OB chapter. In the section on diabetes, codes are included for types that require insulin therapy and types that do not.
- Codes for postoperative complications have been expanded.
- Codes have been expanded to allow for distinctions between intraoperative complications and postprocedural disorders.

For more information about ICD-10-CM and ICD-10-PCS, contact the National Center for Health Statistics (NCHS) (www.cdc.gov/nchs) or AHIMA (www.ahima.org).

Glossary

abandonment To withdraw protection or support; in medicine, to discontinue medical care without proper notice after accepting a patient.

abstract An outline or summary of the diagnostic statement and/or procedures and services performed. In procedural coding, the outline or summary assists in ensuring that all procedures and services are included in an insurance claim submission, and that nothing was omitted or added to the encounter form or charge ticket; to abstract also means to compile this outline or summary for use in procedural coding.

academic degree A title conferred by a college, university, or professional school on completion of a program of study.

account A statement of transactions during a fiscal period and the resulting balance.

account balance The amount owed on an account.

accounts payable Debts incurred and not yet paid.

accounts receivable Amounts owed to the physician.

accounts receivable ledger A record of the charges and payments posted on an account.

accounts receivable trial balance A method of determining that the journal and the ledger are in balance.

accreditation The process through which an organization is recognized for adherence to a group of standards that meet or exceed expectations of the accrediting agency.

accrual basis of accounting Method of accounting in which income is recorded when earned and expenses are recorded when incurred.

acronyms Abbreviations, such as ECG for electrocardiography.

act The formal action of a legislative body; a decision or determination of a sovereign state, a legislative council, or a court of justice.

adage A saying, often in metaphoric form, that embodies a common observation.

add-on code A code that indicates additional or supplemental procedures carried out in addition to the primary procedure.

advent A coming into being or use.

advocate One who pleads the cause of another; one who defends or maintains a cause or proposal.

affable Being pleasant and at ease in talking to others; characterized by ease and friendliness.

agenda A list or outline of things to be considered or done.

aggressive Forceful or intended to dominate; hostile, injurious, or destructive, especially when referring to a behavior caused by frustration.

allegation A statement by a party to a legal action of what the party undertakes to prove; an assertion made without proof.

allied health fields Occupational disciplines in which professionals involved with the delivery of healthcare or related services assist physicians with the diagnosis, treatment, and care of patients in many different specialty areas.

allocating Apportioning for a specific purpose or to particular persons or things.

allopathic A word used to contrast homeopathic medicine with mainstream medicine; describes medicine supposedly characterized by an effort to counteract the symptoms of a disease by administration of treatments that produce effects that are opposite to the symptoms.

allowed charge (allowable amount) The maximum amount of money that many third-party payors allow for a specific procedure or service.

alphabetic filing Any system that arranges names or topics according to the sequence of the letters in the alphabet.

Alphabetic Index The reference section of the CPT-4 manual that is used to help find a code or code range.

alphanumeric Of or relating to systems made up of combinations of letters and numbers.

alternative medicine A variety of therapeutic or preventative health care practices that are alternatives to mainstream medicine, such as chiropractic, homeopathy, naturopathy, and herbal medicine.

ambiguous Capable of being understood in two or more possible senses or ways; unclear.

ambulatory Able to walk about and not be bedridden.

amenity Something conducive to comfort, convenience, or enjoyment.

amiable Having qualities that make one liked and easy to deal with.

ancillary diagnostic services Services that support patient diagnoses (e.g., laboratory or radiology services).

ancillary Subordinate; auxiliary.

ancillary therapeutic services Services that support patient treatment (specialists or surgery).

"and" In the context of ICD-9-CM, the word *and* should be interpreted as *and/or.*

animate To fill with life; to give spirit and support to expressions.

annotations Notes added by way of comment or explanation.

appeal A legal proceeding by which a case is brought before a higher court for review of the decision of a lower court.

appellate Having the power to review the judgment of another tribunal or body of jurisdiction, such as an appellate court.

application software Computer programs designed to perform specific tasks.

appraisal An expert judgment of the value or merit of; judgment as to quality.

arbitration The hearing and determination of a cause in controversy by a person or persons either chosen by the parties involved or appointed under statutory authority.

arbitrator A neutral person chosen to settle differences between two parties in a controversy.

archaic Of, relating to, or characteristic of an earlier or more primitive time.

archived To have filed or collected records or documents.

artificial intelligence The aspect of computer science that deals with computers taking on the attributes of humans, such as mimicking human thought. One example is expert systems, which are capable of making decisions, such as software that is designed to help a physician diagnose a patient, given a set of symptoms.

ASCII codes Acronym for American Standard Code for Information Interchange; a code representing English characters as numbers, where each is given a number from 0 to 255.

assault An intentional, unlawful attempt of bodily injury to another by force.

assent To agree to something, especially after thoughtful consideration.

assets The entire property of a person, association, corporation, or estate applicable or subject to the payment of debts.

assignment of benefits The transfer of the patient's legal right to collect benefits for medical expenses to the provider of those services, authorizing the payment to be sent directly to the provider.

asystole The absence of a heartbeat.

audit A formal examination of an organization's or individual's accounts or financial situation; a methodic examination and review.

audit trail The path left by a transaction when it has been completed; often referred to when tracking medical services used by patients or researching claims.

augment To make greater, more numerous, larger, or more intense.

authenticated Proved; with regard to medical records, it applies to a signature, initials, or computer keystroke by the maker of the record to verify that the record is correct.

authorization A term used in managed care for an approved referral.

backorder An ordered item that has not been delivered when promised or demanded but will be supplied at a later date.

backup Any type of storage of files to prevent their loss in the event of hard disk failure.

bailiff An officer of some U.S. courts usually serving as a messenger or usher, who keeps order at the request of the judge.

balance sheet A financial statement for a specific date that shows the total assets, liabilities, and capital of the business.

banners Advertisements often found on a Web page that can be animated to attract the user's attention in hopes that he or she will click on the ad, be redirected to the advertiser's home page, and purchase from the site or gain information from the site.

battery An offensive touching or use of force on a person without his or her consent.

beneficence The act of doing or producing good, especially performing acts of charity or kindness.

beneficiary Individual entitled to receive benefits from an insurance policy or program or a governmental entitlement program offering healthcare benefits. Also called a *participant, subscriber, dependent, enrollee,* or *member.*

benefits The amount payable by an insurance company for a monetary loss to an individual insured by that company, under each coverage.

birthday rule Under law, the rule stating that when an individual is covered under two insurance policies, the insurance plan of the policyholder whose birthday comes first in the calendar year (month and day, not year) becomes the primary insurance. This rule applies when there is a question as to whose insurance should be determined as primary, such as for a dependent child, and not used when the individual is the owner of one of the two policies, which would make that the primary policy.

bits The smallest units of information inside the computer, each represented by either the digit "0" or "1"; 8 bits equal 1 byte.

blatant Completely obvious, conspicuous, or obtrusive, especially in a crass or offensive manner; brazen.

bond A durable, formal paper used for documents.

bookkeeping The recording of business and accounting transactions.

bookmarking Marking a document or a specific place within a document for later retrieval; a feature supported by most browsers that allows the user to save the address (or URL) so that the document can be located when it is needed again.

bradycardia Slow heart rate; pulse is below 60 beats per minute.

budget A plan for the coordination of resources and expenditures; the amount of money that is available or required for a particular purpose.

bundled codes Codes designating procedures or services that are grouped together and paid for as one procedure or service.

burnout Exhaustion of physical or emotional strength or motivation, usually as a result of prolonged stress or frustration.

business associates Individuals or organizations that perform or assist a covered entity in the performance of a function or activity that involves the use or disclosure of individually identifiable health information.

byte A unit of data that contains 8 binary digits, or bits.

cache A special high-speed storage that can either be a part of the computer's main memory or can be a separate storage device. One function of a cache is to store websites visited in the computer memory for faster recall the next time the website is requested.

capitation Payment method used by many managed care organizations wherein a fixed amount of money is reimbursed to the provider for patients enrolled during a specific period of time, no matter what services were received or how many visits were made.

caption A heading, title, or subtitle under which records are filed.

cardiac arrhythmias Irregular heartbeats resulting from a malfunction of the electrical system of the heart.

carriers As related to insurance, companies that assume the risk of an insurance policy.

case management The process of assessing and planning patient care, including referral and follow-up, to ensure continuity of care and quality management.

cash basis of accounting Method of accounting in which income is recorded when received and expenses are recorded when paid.

cash flow statement A financial summary for a specific period that shows the beginning balance on hand, the receipts and disbursements during the period, and the balance on hand at the end of the period.

categorically Placed in a specific division of a system of classification.

categories Indented one level below a subsection in the CPT-4 coding manual, usually refers to a specific anatomic site or procedures and/or services.

category I code The primary procedure or service code selected when performing insurance billing or statistical research.

category II codes Special codes that can help providers track revenue and reimbursement.

category III codes Codes for a new or experimental procedure or service.

caustic Marked by sarcasm.

CD burner A device that is capable of "writing" data onto a blank compact disk (CD) or copying data from one CD to a blank CD.

certification The attesting of something as being true, as represented, or as meeting a standard; the result of having been tested, usually by a third party, and awarded a certificate based on proven knowledge.

chain of command A series of executive positions in order of authority.

channels Means of communication or expression; courses or directions of thought.

chapters Broad sections of the ICD-9-CM coding manual grouped by disease or illness, (e.g., Chapter 10 contains diagnostic codes for diseases of the genitourinary system).

characteristics Distinguishing traits, qualities, or properties.

chiropractic A medical discipline that focuses on the nervous system and involves manual adjustment of the vertebral column to affect the nervous system to treat various disorders and to promote patient wellness.

chronologic order Of, relating to, or arranged in or according to the order of time.

circumvent To manage to get around, especially by ingenuity or strategy.

cited Quoted by way of example, authority, or proof or mentioned formally in commendation or praise.

Civilian Health and Medical Program of the Uniformed Services (CHAMPUS) See TRICARE.

Civilian Health and Medical Program of the Veterans Administration (CHAMPVA) A health benefits program run by the Department of Veterans Affairs (VA) that helps eligible beneficiaries pay the cost of specific healthcare services and supplies.

clarity The quality or state of being clear.

clauses Groups of words containing a subject and predicate and functioning as a member of a complex or compound sentence.

clean claims Insurance claim forms that have been completed correctly (no errors or omissions) and can be processed and paid promptly if they meets the restrictions on covered services and items.

clearinghouse A centralized facility to which insurance claims are transmitted. Clearinghouses separate, check, and redistribute claims electronically to various insurance carriers and may offer additional services to the physician.

clinical trials Research studies that test how well new medical treatments or other interventions work in the subjects, usually human beings.

"code also" Used when more than one code is necessary to fully identify a given condition, "code also" or "use additional code" is used.

Code of Federal Regulations (CFR) A coded delineation of the rules and regulations published in the *Federal Register* by the various departments and agencies of the federal government. The CFR is divided into 50 titles that represent broad subject areas, and then chapters that provide specific detail.

coding Converting verbal or written descriptions into numeric and alphanumeric designations.

cohesive Sticking together tightly; exhibiting or producing cohesion.

co-insurance A policy provision frequently found in medical insurance whereby the policyholder and the insurance company share the cost of covered losses in a specified ratio (e.g., 80/20 means 80% is covered by the insurer and 20% by the insured).

collect on delivery (COD) Method of payment used when an article or item is delivered and payment is expected before it is released.

comfort zone A place in the mind where an individual feels safe and confident.

commensurate Corresponding in size, amount, extent, or degree; equal in measure.

commercial insurance Plans that reimburse the insured for expenses resulting from illness or injury according to a specific fee schedule as outlined in the insurance policy and on a fee-for-service basis. Sometimes called *private insurance*.

competent Having adequate abilities or qualities; having the capacity to function or perform in a certain way.

complainant Person making a complaint against a person or organization.

computer A machine that is designed to accept, store, process, and give out information.

concise Expressing much in brief form.

concurrently Occurring at the same time.

condescending Assuming an air of superiority.

congruent Being in agreement, harmony, or correspondence; conforming to the circumstances or requirements of a situation.

connotation An implication; something suggested by a word or thing.

contamination A process by which something is made impure, unclean, or unfit for use by the introduction of unwholesome or undesirable elements.

continuation pages The second and following pages of a letter.

continuing education units (CEUs) Credits for courses, classes, or seminars related to an individual's profession, designed to promote education and to keep the professional up to date on current procedures and trends in his or her field; CEUs are often required for licensing.

continuity of care Continuation of care smoothly from one provider to another, so that the patient receives the most benefit and no interruption in care.

contraindications Factors, such as symptoms or conditions, that make a particular treatment or procedure inadvisable.

contributory negligence Statutes in some states that may prevent a party from recovering some damages if he or she contributed in any way to the injury or condition.

cookies Messages sent to a Web browser from a Web server that identify users and can prepare custom Web pages for them, possibly displaying their name on return to the site.

copayment A sum of money that is paid at the time of medical service; a form of co-insurance.

counteroffer Return offer made by one who has rejected an offer or job.

covered entity An organization that transmits information in an electronic form during a transaction, as defined by HIPAA.

credentialing The act of extending professional or medical privileges to an individual; the process of verifying and evaluating that person's credentials.

credibility The quality or power of inspiring belief.

credit An entry on an account constituting an addition to a revenue, net worth, or liability account; the balance in a person's favor in an account.

critical thinking The constant practice of considering all aspects of a situation when deciding what to believe or what to do.

cross-training Training in more than one area so that a multitude of duties may be performed by one person or so that substitutions of personnel may be made in an emergency or at other necessary times.

cultivate To foster the growth of; to improve by labor, care, or study.

cursor A symbol appearing on the monitor that shows where the next character to be typed will appear.

curt Marked by rude or peremptory shortness.

cyanosis Blue color of the mucous membranes and body extremities caused by lack of oxygen.

cyberspace The nonphysical space of the online world of computer networks in which communication takes place.

damages Loss or harm resulting from injury to person, property, or reputation; compensation in money imposed by law for losses or injuries.

database A collection of related files that serves as a foundation for retrieving information.

debit An entry on an account constituting an addition to an expense or asset account or a deduction from a revenue, a net worth, or a liability account.

debit cards Cards that looks like credit cards and by which money may be withdrawn or the cost of purchases paid directly from the holder's bank account without the payment of interest.

decedent A legal term for a deceased person.

decodes Convert, as in a message, into intelligible form; recognizes and interprets.

deductibles Specific amounts of money a patient must pay out of pocket before the insurance carrier begins paying. Usually this amount ranges from $100 to $500. This deductible amount is met on a yearly or per-incident basis.

defaults Fails to pay financial debts, such as a student loan.

defendant A person required to make answer in a legal action or suit; in criminal cases, the person accused of a crime.

defense mechanisms Psychologic methods of dealing with stressful situations that are encountered in day-to-day living.

deferment Postponement, especially of a student loan.

demeanor Behavior toward others; outward manner.

demographic The statistical characteristics of human populations (as in age or income) used especially to identify markets.

dependents The spouse, children, and sometimes domestic partner or other individuals designated by the insured who are covered under a healthcare plan.

depleted Lessened markedly in quantity, content, power, or value.

detrimental Obviously harmful or damaging.

device driver The program or commands given to a device connected to a computer that enable the device to function. For instance, a printer may come equipped with software that must be loaded onto the computer first, so that the printer will work.

diagnosis The determination of the nature of a disease, injury, or congenital defect.

dictation The act or manner of uttering words to be transcribed.

diction The choice of words especially with regard to clearness, correctness, or effectiveness.

digital subscriber line (DSL) High-speed, sophisticated modulation scheme that operates over existing copper telephone wiring systems; often referred to as "last-mile technologies," because DSL is used for connections from a telephone switching station to a home or office, and not between switching stations.

digital video disk (DVD) An optical disk that holds approximately 28 times more information than a CD; a DVD is most commonly used to hold full-length movies. Compared with a CD, which holds approximately 600 megabytes, a

DVD has the capacity to hold approximately 4.7 gigabytes. Also called a digital versatile disk.

direct billing A method of electronic claims submission where computer software allows a provider to submit an insurance claim directly to an insurance carrier for payment.

direct filing system A filing system in which materials can be located without consulting an intermediary source of reference.

dirty claims Claims that contain errors or omissions which must be corrected and resubmitted to an insurance carrier in order to obtain reimbursement.

disability income insurance Insurance that provides periodic payments to replace income when an insured person is unable to work as a result of illness, injury, or disease.

disbursements Funds paid out.

disbursements journal A summary of accounts paid out.

discrepancies Differences among conflicting facts, claims, or opinions.

discretion The quality of being discrete; having or showing good judgment or conduct, especially in speech.

disk A removable device shaped like a hard plastic square with a magnetic surface capable of storing computer programs; also called *diskettes*, and early versions were called *floppy disks*.

disk drives Devices that load a program or data stored on a disk into the computer.

disparaging Slighting; having a negative or degrading tone.

disparities Fundamentally different and often incongruous elements; elements that are markedly distinct in quality or character.

disposition The tendency of something or someone to act in a certain manner under given circumstances.

disruption An unexpected event that throws a plan into disorder; an interruption that prevents a system or process from continuing as usual or as expected.

dissection Separation into pieces and exposure of parts for scientific examination.

disseminate To disperse throughout.

divulge To make known, as a confidence or secret.

docket A formal record of judicial proceedings; a list of legal cases to be tried.

domestic mail Mail that is sent within the boundaries of the United States and its territories.

downcoding A change in code submitted for reimbursement, usually performed by the insurance company. This change generally occurs because the code submitted does not match in some way to the specifications of the insurance company.

drawee Bank or facility on which a check is drawn or written.

drawer Person who writes a check.

due diligence Also known as *due care;* the effort made by an ordinarily prudent or reasonable party to avoid harm to another party or himself; doing everything possible to prevent something from happening.

due process A fundamental constitutional guarantee that all legal proceedings will be fair; that one will be given notice of the proceedings and given an opportunity to be heard before the government acts to take away life, liberty, or property; a constitutional guarantee that a law will not be unreasonable or arbitrary.

duty Obligatory tasks, conduct, service, or functions that arise from one's position, as in life or in a group.

dyspnea Difficult or painful breathing.

e-banking Electronic banking via computer modem or over the Internet.

e-commerce An abbreviation for electronic commerce; used to describe the sale and purchase of goods and services over the Internet; doing business over the Internet.

e-mail Communications transmitted via computer or computer network.

ecchymosis A hemorrhagic skin discoloration commonly called *bruising*.

effective date The date on which an insurance policy or plan takes effect so that benefits are payable.

electronic (or digital) signature A scanned signature or other such mark that is accepted as proof of approval of and/or responsibility for the content of an electronic document.

electronic claims Claims that are submitted to insurance processing facilities using a computerized medium, such as direct data entry, direct wire, dial-in telephone digital fax, or personal computer download or upload.

electronic data interchange (EDI) The transfer of data back and forth between two or more entities using an electronic medium.

electronic media Means of electronic transmission, including the Internet, private networks, dial-up phone lines, and fax modems; includes information moved from one place to another while stored on an electronic device.

eligibility A term which describes whether a patient's insurance coverage is in effect, and eligible for payment of insurance benefits

emancipated minor A person under legal age who is self-supporting and living apart from parents or guardian; a mature minor considered by the courts to possess a sufficient understanding of self-care and responsibility.

embezzlement Stealing from an employer; to appropriate goods, services, or funds for personal use without permission.

emetic A substance that causes vomiting.

empathy Sensitivity to the individual needs and reactions of patients.

employer identification number (EIN) The number used by the Internal Revenue Service that identifies a business or individual functioning as a business entity for income tax reporting.

encodes Converts from one system of communication to another; converts a message into code.

encounter Any contact between a healthcare provider and a patient that results in treatment or evaluation of the patient's condition; not limited to in-person contact.

encroachments Actions that advance beyond the usual or proper limits.

encrypted Encoded; converted from one system of communication to another.

endorser Person who signs his or her name on the back of a check for the purpose of transferring title to another person.

enunciate To utter articulate sounds; the act of being very distinct in speech.

environment The state of a computer, usually determined by the programs that are running as well as hardware and software characteristics.

eponyms Procedures, services, or diagnoses named after people, such as Mohs' micrographic surgery or Crohn's disease.

equities The money value of a property or of an interest in a property in excess of claims or liens against it.

erroneous Containing or characterized by error or assumption.

established patient (EP) A patient who has been seen by the same physician or same group of physicians over time. An established patient becomes a new patient if not seen by the physician or group in 3 years.

established patients Patients who are returning to the office who have previously been seen by the physician.

etiology The cause of the disorder; a claim may be classified according to etiology.

euthanasia The act or practice of killing or permitting the death of hopelessly sick or injured individuals in a relatively painless way for reasons of mercy.

"excludes" Exclusion terms are always written in italics, and the word "excludes" is often enclosed in a box to draw particular attention to these instructions. Exclusion terms may apply to a chapter, a section, a category, or a subcategory. The applicable code number usually follows the exclusion term.

exclusions Limitations on an insurance contract for which benefits are not payable.

expediency A means of achieving a particular end, as in a situation requiring haste or caution.

expert witnesses People who provide testimony to a court as experts in certain fields or subjects to verify facts presented by one or both sides in a lawsuit, often compensated and used to refute or disprove the claims of one party.

explanation of benefits (EOB) A letter or statement from the insurance carrier describing what was paid, denied, or reduced in payment. It also contains information about amounts applied to the deductible, the patient's co-insurance, and the allowed amounts.

explanation of Medicare benefits (EOMB) The EOMB is the name for an explanation of benefits from Medicare. See explanation of benefits above for the definition.

external noise Sounds or factors outside the brain that interfere with the communication process.

externalization The attribution of an event or occurrence to causes outside the self.

externship or internship A training program that is part of a course of study of an educational institution and is taken in the actual business setting of that field of study; the terms are often interchanged in reference to medical assistant training.

extrinsic External to a thing, its essential nature, or its original character.

fax Abbreviation for facsimile; also, a document sent using a facsimile (fax) machine.

fee for service An established schedule of fees set for services performed by providers and paid by the patient.

fee profile A compilation or average of physician fees over a given period of time.

fee schedule A compilation of preestablished fee allowances for given services or procedures.

feedback The transmission of evaluative or corrective information to the original or controlling source about an action, event, or process.

felony A major crime, such as murder, rape, or burglary; punishable by a more stringent sentence than that given for a misdemeanor.

fermentation An enzymatically controlled transformation of an organic compound.

fervent Exhibiting or marked by great intensity of feeling.

fibrillation Rapid, random, ineffective contractions of the heart.

fidelity Faithfulness to something to which one is bound by pledge or duty.

fine A sum imposed as punishment for an offense; a forfeiture or penalty paid to an injured party or the government in a civil or criminal action.

fiscal agent An organization under contract to the government as well as some private plans to act as financial representatives in handling insurance claims from providers of health care; also referred to as *fiscal intermediary*.

fiscal intermediary An organization that contracts with the government to handle and mediate insurance claims from medical facilities, home health agencies, or providers of medical services or supplies.

fiscal year An accounting period of 12 months during which a company determines earnings and profit; the fiscal year does not necessarily begin in January—instead, the beginning of the fiscal year is determined by the business.

flagged Marked in some way as to remind or remember that specific action needs to be taken.

Flash Animation technology often used on the opening page of a website to draw attention, excite, and impress the user.

flash drive A small portable device that connects into the USB port that can carry 2 to 8 or more gigabytes of information.

flush Directly abutting or immediately adjacent, as set even with an edge of a type page or column; having no indention.

font A design for a set of type characters; a combination of typeface, spacing, pitch, and other qualities. Fonts are named; examples include Times Roman, Arial, and Garamond.

format To magnetically create tracks on a disk where information will be stored, usually done by the manufacturer of the disk.

gametes Mature male or female germ cells, usually possessing a haploid chromosome set and capable of initiating formation of a new diploid individual; a sex cell, whether sperm or ovum.

genome The genetic material of an organism.

genuineness Expressing sincerity and honest feeling.

gigabyte Approximately 1 billion bytes; abbreviated GB.

girth A measure around a body or item.

gleaned Gathered bit by bit (e.g., information or material); picked over in search of relevant material.

government plans Entitlement programs or healthcare plans that are sponsored and/or subsidized by the state or federal government, such as **Medicaid** and **Medicare.**

gradients Changes in response with distance from a stimulus.

grammar The study of the classes of words, their inflections, and their functions and relations in the sentence; a study of what is to be preferred and what avoided in inflection and syntax.

grief Reaction to an unfortunate outcome; a deep distress caused by bereavement, a loss, or a perceived loss.

group policy Insurance written under a policy that covers a number of people under a single master contract issued to their employer or to an association with which they are affiliated.

guarantor The person who is responsible for paying a medical bill.

guardian ad litem Legal representative for a minor.

guidelines Found at the beginning of each of the six sections of the CPT-4. The guidelines define items that are necessary to appropriately interpret and report the procedures and services found in the section.

hard copy The readable paper copy or printout of information.

hardware The physical components of the computer system, such as the CPU, monitor, and printer.

harmonious Marked by accord in sentiment or action; having the parts agreeably related.

HCPCS Health Care Common Procedural Coding System; level II codes created to supplement procedures and services not covered in the CPT-4.

Health Insurance Portability and Accountability Act (HIPAA) The Kassebaum-Kennedy Act, designed to improve portability and continuity of health insurance coverage; to combat waste, fraud, and abuse in health insurance and healthcare delivery; to promote the use of medical savings accounts; to improve access to long-term care services and coverage; to simplify the administration of health insurance; and to serve other purposes.

health insurance Protection in return for periodic premium payments that provides reimbursement of expenses resulting from illness or injury. Includes the following forms of insurance: accident, disability income, medical expense, and accidental death and dismemberment. Also known as *accident and health insurance* or *disability income insurance.*

health maintenance organization (HMO) An organization that provides a wide range of comprehensive healthcare services for a specified group at a fixed periodic payment. HMOs can be sponsored by the government, medical schools, hospitals, employers, labor unions, consumer groups, insurance companies, and hospital-medical plans.

healthcare providers Providers of medical or health services, individually or as organizations, that furnish, bill for, or are paid for services or products.

hematuria Blood in the urine.

holder Person presenting a check for payment.

holistic Related to or concerned with all of the systems of the body, rather than breaking it down into parts.

homeopathy A type of alternative medicine that attempts to stimulate the body to recover itself; a system of therapy based on the concept that disease can be treated with minute doses of drugs thought capable of producing the same symptoms in healthy people as the disease itself.

hospice A concept of care that involves health professionals and volunteers who provide medical, psychologic, and spiritual support to terminally ill patients and their loved ones.

HTML Acronym for HyperText Markup Language, which is the language used to create documents for use on the Internet.

HTTP Acronym for HyperText Transfer Protocol, which defines how messages are formatted and transmitted over the Internet. When a URL is entered into the computer, an HTTP command tells the Web server to retrieve the requested Web page.

hub A common connection point for devices in a network containing multiple ports, often used to connect segments of a LAN.

icons Pictures, often on the desktop of a computer, that represent programs or objects. By clicking on an icon, the user is directed to the program.

idealism The practice of forming ideas or living under the influence of ideas.

idiopathic Pertaining to no known cause of a condition or disease.

immigrant A person who comes to a country to take up permanent residence.

impaired Being in a less-than-perfect or less-than-whole condition; includes having handicaps or functional defects and being under the influence of drugs, alcohol, and/or controlled substances.

impenetrable Incapable of being penetrated or pierced; not capable of being damaged or harmed.

implied consent Presumed consent, such as when a patient offers an arm for a phlebotomy procedure.

in balance State in which the total ending balances of patient ledgers equals total of accounts receivable.

incentives Things that incite or spur to action; rewards or reasons for performing a task.

"includes" This term appearing under a subdivision, such as a category (three-digit code) or two-digit procedure code, indicates that the code and title include these terms. Other terms also classified to that particular code and title are listed in the Alphabetic Indexes.

incomplete claim A claim that is missing information and is returned to the provider for correction and resubmission. This is sometimes also called an invalid claim.

incur To become liable or subject to; to bring down on oneself.

indemnity plans Traditional health insurance plans that pay for all or a share of the cost of covered services, regardless of which physician, hospital, or other licensed healthcare provider is used. Policyholders of indemnity plans and their **dependents** choose when and where to get healthcare services.

indicators An important point or group of statistic values that, when evaluated, indicate the quality of care provided in a healthcare facility.

indicted Charged with a crime by the finding or presentment of a jury according to due process of law.

indigent Totally lacking in something of need.

indirect filing system A filing system in which an intermediary source of reference, such as a card file, must be consulted to locate specific files.

individual policy An insurance policy designed specifically for the use of one person (and his or her dependents), not associated with the amenities of a group policy, namely higher premiums. Often called *personal insurance.*

individually identifiable health information Any part of a patient's health record that is created or received by a covered entity.

infer To derive as a conclusion from facts and premises.

infertile Not fertile or productive; not capable of reproducing.

inflection A change in pitch or loudness of the voice.

informed consent A consent, usually written, which states understanding of what treatment is to be undertaken and of the risks involved, why it should be done, and alternative methods of treatment available (including no treatment) and their attendant risks.

infractions Breaking the law; minor offenses against the rules, usually punishable by fines.

initiative To cause or facilitate the beginning of; to initiate something into happening.

innate Existing in, belonging to, or determined by factors present in an individual since birth.

innocuous Having no effect, adverse or otherwise; harmless.

input Information entered into and used by the computer.

instigate To goad or urge forward; to provoke.

insubordination Disobedience to authority.

insured An individual or organization covered by an insurance policy according to the policy terms, usually the individual or group that pays the premiums. Blue Cross/Blue Shield refers to this person or group as the *subscriber.*

intangibles Qualities that are incapable of being perceived, especially by touch, or incapable of being precisely identified or realized by the mind.

integral Essential; being an indispensable part of a whole.

Intelligent Character Recognition (ICR) The electronic scanning of printed items as images and use of special software to recognize these images (or characters) as ASCII text for upload into a computer database.

interaction A two-way communication; mutual or reciprocal action or influence.

intercom A two-way communication system with a microphone and loudspeaker at each station for localized use.

intermittent Coming and going at intervals; not continuous.

internal noise Factors inside the brain that interfere with the communication process.

International Classification of Diseases, Ninth Revision, Clinical Modification (ICD-9-CM) System for classifying disease to facilitate collection of uniform and comparable health information, for statistical purposes and indexing medical records for data storage and retrieval.

international mail Mail that is sent outside the boundaries of the United States and its territories.

International Statistical Classifications of Diseases and Related Health Problems, Tenth Revision, Clinical Modification (ICD-10-CM) System containing the greatest number of changes in ICD history. To allow more specific reporting of disease and newly recognized conditions, the ICD-10-CMcontains approximately 5500 more codes than ICD-9.

interval Space of time between events.

intolerable Not tolerable or bearable.

intrinsic Belonging to the essential nature or constitution of a thing; indwelling, inward.

introspection An inward, reflective examination of one's own thoughts and feelings.

invariably Consistently; not changing or capable of change.

invasive Involving entry into the living body as by incision or insertion of an instrument.

invoice A paper describing a purchase and the amount due.

jargon The technical terminology or characteristic idiom of a particular group or special activity.

Java A commonly used object-oriented high-level programming language that is well suited for the Internet.

judicial Of or relating to a judgment, the function of judging, the administration of justice, or the judiciary.

jurisdiction A power constitutionally conferred on a judge or magistrate to decide cases according to law and to carry sentence into execution; jurisdiction is original when it is conferred on the court in the first instance, called *original jurisdiction;* or it is appellate when an appeal is given from the judgment of another court.

jurisprudence The science or philosophy of law; a system or body of law or the course of court decisions.

kilobyte Approximately 1024 bytes, abbreviated KB.

language barrier Any type of interference that inhibits the communication process and is related to languages spoken by the people attempting to communicate.

law A binding custom or practice of a community; a rule of conduct or action prescribed or formally recognized as binding or enforceable by a controlling authority.

learning style The way that an individual perceives and processes information to learn new material.

liabilities Things that are owed; debts.

liable Obligated according to law or equity; responsible for an act or circumstance.

libel A written defamatory statement or representation that conveys an unjustly unfavorable impression.

litigious Prone to engage in lawsuits.

mailpiece A piece of mail.

maker In reference to a check, any individual, corporation, or legal party who signs a check or any type of negotiable instrument.

malediction Speaking evil or the calling of a curse.

managed care plans An umbrella term for all healthcare plans that provide healthcare in return for preset monthly payments and coordinated care through a defined network of primary care physicians and hospitals.

manifestation Something that is easily understood or recognized by the mind. *Also* the signs and symptoms of a disease.

marketing The process or technique of promoting, selling, and distributing a product or service.

matrix Something in which a thing originates, develops, takes shape, or is contained; a base on which to build.

m-banking Banking through the use of wireless devices, such as cellular phones and wireless Internet services.

media Term applied to agencies of mass communication, such as newspapers, magazines, and telecommunications.

mediastinum Space in the center of the chest under the sternum.

Medicaid A federal and state sponsored health insurance program for the medically indigent.

medical savings accounts Tax-deferred bank or savings accounts that are combined with a low-premium, high-deductible insurance policy, designed for individuals or families who choose to fund their own healthcare expenses and medical insurance.

medically indigent Able to take care of ordinary living expenses but not able to afford medical care.

Medicare A federally sponsored health insurance program for those over 65 or individuals under 65 but disabled.

Medigap A term sometimes applied to private insurance products that supplement Medicare insurance benefits.

megabyte Approximately 1 million bytes; abbreviated MB.

megahertz The measuring device for microprocessors, abbreviated MHz. A megahertz is 1 million cycles of electromagnetic currency alternation per second and is used as a unit of measure for the clock speed of computer microprocessors. The hertz is a unit of measure named after Heinrich Hertz, a German physicist.

mentors Trusted counselors or guides.

meticulous Marked by extreme or excessive care in the consideration or treatment of details.

microfiche A sheet of microfilm containing rows of microimages of pages of printed matter.

microfilm A film bearing a photographic record on a reduced scale of printed or other graphic matter.

micromanage To manage with great or excessive control or attention to details.

MIDI Acronym for Musical Instrument Digital Interface; a MIDI interface allows computers to record and manipulate sound.

misdemeanor A minor crime, as opposed to a felony, punishable by fine or imprisonment in a city or county jail rather than in a penitentiary.

mock Simulated; intended for imitation or practice.

modem A device that allows information to be transmitted over telephone lines, at speeds measured in bits per second (bps); short for modulator-demodulator. Modem speed is generally listed somewhere on the actual unit.

modifiers Code additions that explain circumstances that alter a provided service, or provide additional clarification or detail about a procedure or service.

monochromatic Having or consisting of one color or hue.

monotone A succession of syllables, words, or sentences in one unvaried key or pitch.

morale The mental and emotional condition, enthusiasm, loyalty, or confidence of an individual or group with regard to the function or tasks at hand.

motivation The process of inciting a person to some action or behavior.

multimedia The presentation of graphics, animation, video, sound, and text on a computer in an integrated way, or all at once. CD-ROMs are efficient multimedia devices.

multitasking Performing multiple tasks at the same time.

municipal courts Courts that sit in some cities and larger towns and that usually have civil and criminal jurisdiction over cases arising within the municipality.

myocardium The muscular lining of the heart.

mysticism The experience of seeming to have direct communication with God or ultimate reality.

national provider identifier (NPI) A lifetime number consisting of 10 digits that Medicare will use to replace the Provider Identification Number (PIN) and the Unique Physician Identification Number (UPIN).

naturopathy An alternative to conventional medicine in which holistic methods are used, as well as herbs and natural supplements, with the belief that the body will heal itself. Naturopathic physicians can currently be licensed in 15 states, Puerto Rico, and the Virgin Islands.

necrosis The death of cells or tissue.

negligence Failure to exercise the care that a prudent person usually exercises; implies inattention to one's duty or business; implies want of due or necessary diligence or care.

negotiable Legally transferable to another party.

networking Exchange of information or services among individuals, groups, or institutions; also, meeting and getting to know individuals in the same or similar career fields and sharing information about available opportunities.

new patient (NP) A patient who has his or her first encounter (visit) with a physician or physician group or who was an established patient with a physician or provider but has not been seen in 3 years.

nonmaleficence Refraining from the act of harming or committing evil.

no-show A person who fails to keep an appointment without giving advance notice.

nosocomial Originating or taking place in a hospital.

notations Notations, also known as instructional notations are found in both the Alphabetic Index and the Tabular Index as instructions or guides in classification assignments, defining category content or the use of subdivision codes.

numeric filing The filing of records, correspondence, or cards by number.

objective information Information that is gathered by watching or observation of a patient.

objectives Something toward which effort is directed; aims, goals, or ends of action.

obliteration Act of making undecipherable or imperceptible by obscuring or wearing away.

Office for Civil Rights (OCR) The division of the federal government that enforces privacy standards.

Office of Inspector General (OIG) Established to protect the integrity of the Department of Health and Human Services

(HHS), the office conducts audits, investigations, and inspections involving the laws that pertain to HHS.

opinions Formal expressions of judgment or advice by an expert; formal expressions of the legal reasons and principles on which a legal decision is based.

optimistic Inclined to put the most favorable construction on actions and events or to anticipate the best possible outcome.

ordinances Authoritative decrees or directions; laws set forth by a governmental authority–specifically, municipal regulations.

osteopathic A type of medicine based on the theory that disturbances in the musculoskeletal system affect other bodily parts, causing many disorders that can be corrected by various manipulative techniques in conjunction with conventional medical, surgical, pharmacologic, and other therapeutic procedures.

other potentially infectious materials (OPIM) Substances or materials other than blood that have the potential to carry infectious pathogens, such as body fluid, urine, semen, and others.

OUTfolder A folder used to provide space for the temporary filing of materials.

OUTguide A heavy guide that is used to replace a folder that has been temporarily moved from the filing space.

output Information that is processed by the computer and transmitted to a monitor, printer, or other device.

outreach The process of using marketing and education strategies to reach and involve diverse audiences through the use of key messages and effective programs.

outsourcing The practice of subcontracting work to an outside company.

packing slip A list of items that are included in a shipment.

pandemic A condition in which the majority of the people in a country, a number of countries, or a geographic area are affected.

paper claims Hard copies of insurance claims that have been completed and sent by surface mail.

paraphrased Restated; applies to restatement of text, passage, or work to convey the meaning in another form.

participating provider (PAR) A physician or other healthcare provider who enters into a contract with a specific insurance company or program, and by doing so agrees to abide by certain rules and regulations set forth by that particular third-party payor.

patient status (PS) The state of a patient as either new or established; appears in the Evaluation and Management section of the CPT-4.

payables Balances due to a creditor on an account.

payee Person named on a draft or check as the recipient of the amount shown.

payor Person who writes a check in favor of the payee.

peer review organization A group of medical reviewers contracted by the Centers for Medicare and Medicaid Services to ensure quality control and medical necessity of services provided by a facility.

pegboard system Also called the *write-it-once system;* a method of tracking patient accounts that allows the figures to be proved accurate through mathematic formulas.

perceiving How an individual looks at information and sees it as real.

perception Capacity for comprehension; an awareness of the elements of the environment.

perjured testimony The voluntary violation of an oath or vow either by swearing to what is untrue or by omission to do what has been promised under oath; false testimony.

perks Extra advantages or benefits from working in a specific job that may or may not be commonplace in that particular profession; a shortened form of *perquisites.*

persona An individual's social facade or front that reflects the role in life the individual is playing; the personality that a person projects in public.

personal health information The patient's own information that pertains to his or her health.

pertinent Having a clear, decisive relevance to the matter at hand.

petty cash fund A fund maintained to pay small unpredictable cash expenditures.

philanthropist An individual who makes an active effort to promote human welfare.

philosopher A person who seeks wisdom or enlightenment; an expounder of a theory in a certain area of experience.

phlebotomy The invasive procedure used to obtain a blood specimen for testing, experimentation, or diagnosis of disease.

phonetic Constituting an alteration of ordinary spelling that better represents the spoken language, that employs only characters of the regular alphabet, and that is used in a context of conventional spelling.

photophobia Visual sensitivity to light.

physical status The physical condition of the patient.

physician office laboratories (POLs) Laboratories owned by a private physician or corporation, such as the laboratory inside a physician's office or a freestanding laboratory.

physiologic noise Physiologic interferences with the communication process.

pitch The property of a sound, especially a musical tone, that is determined by the frequency of the waves producing it; the highness or lowness of sound.

place-of-service (POS) codes Codes that indicate where a procedure or service was performed.

plaintiff The person or group bringing a case or legal action to court.

policyholder A person who pays a premium to an insurance company and in whose name the policy is written in exchange for the insurance protection provided by a policy of insurance.

polydipsia Excessive thirst.

polyuria Excreting large amounts of urine.

portfolio A set of pictures, drawings, documents, or photographs either bound in book form or loose in a folder.

posting Transferring or carrying from a book of original entry to a ledger; entering figures in an accounting system.

postmortem Done, collected, or occurring after death.

power of attorney A legal instrument authorizing one to act as the attorney or agent of the grantor.

preauthorization A process required by some insurance carriers where the provider obtains permission to perform certain procedures or services, or refer a patient to a specialist.

precedence To surpass in rank, dignity, or importance; to be, go, or come ahead or in front of.

precedents A person or thing that serves as a model; something done or said that may serve as an example or rule to authorize or justify a subsequent act of the same kind.

preclude To rule out in advance.

premium The periodic (monthly, quarterly, or annual) payment of a specific sum of money to an insurance company for which the insurer, in return, agrees to provide certain benefits.

preponderance A superiority or excess in number or quantity; a majority.

preponderance of the evidence Evidence that is of greater weight or more convincing than the evidence offered in opposition to it; evidence that as a whole shows that the fact sought to be proven is more probable than not.

prerequisite Something that is necessary to an end or to carry out a function.

pressboard A strong, highly glazed composition board resembling vulcanized fiber; heavy card stock.

prevalent Generally or widely accepted, practiced, or favored.

primary care provider (PCP) A general practice, or non-specialists provider or physician responsible for the care of a patient for some health maintenance organizations. Also called a gatekeeper.

primary diagnosis Initial identification of the condition or complaint that the patient expresses in the outpatient medical setting.

principal A capital sum of money due as a debt or used as a fund for which interest is either charged or paid.

privacy officer A person designated to ensure compliance with privacy standards for a covered entity.

proactive Acting in anticipation of future problems, needs, or changes.

processing How an individual internalizes new information and makes it his or her own.

procrastination Intentionally putting off doing something that should be done.

procurement To get possession of, to obtain by particular care and effort.

professional behaviors Those actions that identify the medical assistant as a member of a healthcare profession, including being dependable, performing respectful patient care, exercising initiative, demonstrating a positive attitude, and using teamwork.

professional courtesy Reduction or absence of fees to professional associates.

professionalism The conduct or qualities characterized by or conforming to the technical or ethical standards of a profession; exhibiting a courteous, conscientious, and generally businesslike manner in the workplace.

proficiency Competency as a result of training or practice.

profit sharing Offer of a part of a company's profits to employees or other designated individuals or groups.

progress notes Notes used in the patient chart to track the progress and condition of the patient.

proofread To read and mark corrections.

prosthetic The surgical or dental specialty concerned with the design, construction, and fitting of prostheses, which are artificial devices that replace missing parts of the body.

protected health information (PHI) Any individually identifiable health information that is transmitted and/or maintained in electronic form.

provider Any company, individual, or group that provides medical, diagnostic, or treatment services to a patient.

Provider Identification Numbers (PINs) Numbers assigned to providers by a carrier for use in submission of claims.

provisional diagnosis A temporary diagnosis made before all test results have been received.

proxemics The study of the nature, degree, and effect of the spatial separation individuals naturally maintain.

prudent Marked by wisdom or judiciousness; shrewd in the management of practical affairs.

public domain The realm embracing property rights that belong to the community at large, are unprotected by copyright or patent, and are subject to use or appropriation by anyone.

putrefaction Decomposition of animal matter that results in a foul smell.

quackery The pretense of curing disease.

quality assurance Activities designed to increase the quality of a product or service through process or system changes that increase efficiency or effectiveness.

quality control An aggregate of activities designed to ensure adequate quality, especially in manufactured products or in the service industries.

queries Requests for information from a database.

ramifications Consequence; outgrowth; something produced by a cause or necessarily following from a set of conditions.

ramifications Consequences produced by a cause or following from a set of conditions.

ream A quantity of paper consisting of, variously, 480, 500, or 516 sheets.

reasonable doubt Doubt based on reason and arising from evidence or lack of evidence; it is not doubt that is imagined or conjured up, but doubt that would cause reasonable persons to hesitate before acting.

receipts Amounts paid on patient accounts.

receivables Total monies received on accounts.

recipient The receiver of some thing or item.

reconciliation The process of proving that a bank statement and checkbook balance are in agreement.

recourse A turning to something or someone for help or protection.

rectify To correct by removing errors.

referral An insurance term used when a primary care provider wants to send a patient to a specialist. Typically, the provider must obtain authorization from the insurance carrier in advance to refer a patient.

reflection The process of considering new information and internalizing it to create new ways of examining information.

rejected claims Claims returned unpaid to the provider for clarification of any question and that must be corrected before resubmission.

relevant Having significant and demonstrable bearing on the matter at hand.

remittance advice (RA) An explanation of benefits which comes from Medicaid. See explanation of benefits above for the definition.

reparations Amends, acts of atonement, or satisfaction given as a result of a wrong or injury.

reprimands Criticisms for a fault; severe or formal reproofs.

reproach An expression of rebuke or disapproval; a cause or occasion of blame, discredit, or disgrace.

requisites Entities considered essential or necessary.

resource-based relative value scale (RBRVS) A fee schedule designed to provide national uniform payment of Medicare benefits after being adjusted to reflect the differences in practice costs across geographic areas.

respondent The person required to make answer in a civil legal action or suit; similar to a defendant in a criminal trial.

retention The act of keeping in possession or use; keeping in one's pay or service.

retention schedule A method or plan for retaining or keeping medical records, and their movement from active, to inactive, to closed filing.

rider A special provision or group of provisions that may be added to a policy to expand or limit the benefits otherwise payable. It may increase or decrease benefits, waive a condition or coverage, or in any other way amend the original contract.

robotics Technology dealing with the design, construction, and operation of robots in automation.

router A device used to connect any number of LANs, which communicate with other routers and determine the best route between any two hosts.

salutation An expression of greeting, goodwill, or courtesy by words or gestures.

sarcasm A sharp and often satirical response or ironic utterance designed to cut or give pain.

scanner Device that reads text or illustrations on a printed page and can translate the information on that page into a form that the computer can understand.

screen Something that shields, protects, or hides; to select or eliminate through a screening process.

search engines Programs that search documents for keywords and return a list of documents containing those words.

section The main divisions of the CPT-4 manual.

"see" A direction given to the coder to look in another place. This term must always be followed and is found in the Alphabetic Index, Volumes 2 and 3.

"see also" A direction given to the coder to look elsewhere if the main term or subterm (or subterms) for that entry are not sufficient for coding the information. If a code number follows, "see also" is enclosed in parentheses. If there is no code number, "see also" is preceded by a dash.

"see category" A direction given to the coder to see a specific category (three-digit code). This must always be followed.

self-insured plan An insurance plan funded by an organization having a large enough employee base that it can afford to fund its own insurance program.

self-referral The act of a patient or insured individual who refers himself or herself to a specialist without requesting the referral from the primary provider, such as a woman seeking an annual gynecologic examination. Managed care guidelines may require the patient to report the self-referral.

sentinel events Unexpected occurrences involving death or serious physical or psychologic injury, or the risk thereof.

sequentially Of, relating to, or arranged in a sequence.

server A computer or device on a network that manages shared network resources.

service benefit plans Plans that provide benefits in the form of certain surgical and medical services rendered, rather than cash. A service benefit plan is not restricted to a fee schedule.

shelf filing A system that uses open shelves rather than cabinets for storing records.

shingling A method of filing whereby one report is laid on top of the older report, resembling the shingles of a roof.

socioeconomic Relating to a combination of social and economic factors.

sociologic Oriented or directed toward social needs and problems.

sound card Device that allows a computer to output sound through speakers that are connected to the main circuitry board, or motherboard.

staff privileges Allowance of a healthcare professional to practice within a specific facility.

standards Models or examples established by authority, custom, or general consent; something set up and established by authority as a rule for the measure of quantity, weight, extent, value, or quality.

STAT Medical abbreviation for immediately; at this moment.

statement A request for payment.

statement of income and expense A summary of all income and expenses for a given period.

stationers Sellers of stationery.

statutes Laws enacted by the legislative branch of a government.

stereotype Something conforming to a fixed or general pattern; a standardized mental picture that is held in common by many and represents an oversimplified opinion, prejudiced attitude, or uncritical judgment.

stipulate To specify as a condition or requirement of an agreement or offer; to make an agreement or covenant to do or forbear from doing something.

stock options Offers of stocks for purchase to a certain group of individuals or certain groups, such as employees of a for-profit hospital.

stressors Stimuli that cause stress.

subcategory Indented one level below a category, usually a procedure or service unique to a specific category.

subjective information Information that is gained by questioning the patient or taken from a form.

subluxations Slight misalignments of the vertebrae or a partial dislocation.

subordinate Submissive to or controlled by authority; placed in or occupying a lower class, rank, or position.

subpoena A writ or document commanding a person to appear in court under a penalty for failure to appear.

subpoena duces tecum A legally binding request to appear in court and provide records or documents that pertain to a particular case.

subsection Indented one level below a section, a subsection usually describes an anatomic site or organ system—e.g., integumentary system or cardiology.

substance number A number based on the weight of a ream of paper containing 500 sheets.

subtle Difficult to understand or perceive; having or marked by keen insight and ability to penetrate deeply and thoroughly.

succinct Marked by compact, precise expression without wasted words.

superfluous Exceeding what is sufficient or necessary.

surrogate A substitute; to put in place of another.

switch In networks, a device that filters information between LAN segments and decreases overall network traffic and increases speed and bandwidth usage efficiency.

synopsis Condensed statement or outline.

system software The operating system and all utility programs that allow the computer to function and perform operations.

tactful Having a keen sense of what to do or say to maintain good relations with others or to avoid offense.

tangible Capable of being appraised at an actual or approximate value; capable of being precisely identified or realized by the mind.

target market A specific group of individuals toward whom the marketing plan is focused.

targeted Directed or used toward a target; directed toward a specific desire or position.

TCP/IP Acronym for Transmission Control Protocol/ Internet Protocol; a suite of communications protocols used to connect users or hosts to the Internet.

tedious Tiresome because of length or dullness

telecommunications The science and technology of communication by transmission of information from one location to another via telephone, television, telegraph, or satellite.

telemedicine The use of telecommunications in the practice of medicine, in which great distances can exist among healthcare professionals, colleagues, patients, and students.

teleradiology The use of telecommunications devices to enhance and improve the results of radiologic procedures.

terabyte Approximately 1 trillion bytes, abbreviated TB.

testimony A solemn declaration usually made orally by a witness under oath in response to interrogation by a lawyer or authorized public official.

thanatology The study of the phenomena of death and of psychologic methods of coping with death.

third-party administrator An organization that processes claims and performs other business-related functions for a health plan.

third-party payor Someone other than the patient, spouse, or parent who is responsible for paying all or part of the patient's medical costs.

thrombolytics Agents that dissolve blood clots.

tickler file A chronologic file used as a reminder that something must be taken care of on a certain date.

transaction An exchange or transfer of goods, services, or funds. *Also* As defined by HIPAA, transmissions of information between two parties to carry out financial or administrative activities related to healthcare.

transcription To make a written copy of, either in longhand or by machine.

transient ischemic attack Temporary neurologic symptoms caused by a gradual or partial occlusion of a cerebral blood vessel.

transposed Altered in sequence; interchanged.

treatises Systematic expositions or arguments in writing including a methodic discussion of the facts and principles involved and the conclusions reached.

triage Process of evaluating the urgency of medical need and prioritizing treatment.

trial balance A method of checking the accuracy of accounts.

TRICARE A government-sponsored program wherein authorized dependents of military personnel receive medical care. This program was originally called *CHAMPUS*.

unbundled codes Codes in which the components of a procedure are separated and reported separately.

Uniform Commercial Code (UCC) A unified set of rules covering many business transactions; it has been adopted in all 50 states, the District of Columbia, and most U.S. territories. It regulates the fields of sales of goods; commercial paper, such as checks; secured transactions in personal property; and particular aspects of banking, letters of credit, warehouse receipts, bills of lading, and investment securities.

unique identifiers Codes used instead of names to protect the confidentiality of the patient in a method of anonymous HIV testing.

unique provider identification number (UPIN) A number assigned by fiscal intermediaries to identify providers on claims for services.

universal claim form The form developed by the Health Care Financing Administration (HCFA) (now known as the Centers for Medicare and Medicaid Services [CMS]) and approved by the AMA for use in submitting all government-sponsored claims. Also known as the CMS-1500 form.

upcoding A deliberate increase in a CPT-4 code, despite the lack of documentation, to the next highest reimbursable code in order to receive higher reimbursements.

URL Acronym for Uniform Resource Locator; specifies the global address of documents or information on the Internet. The URL provides the IP address and the domain name for the Web page, such as microsoft.com.

"use additional code" This term appears only in Volume 1 in those subdivisions in which the user should add further information by means of an additional code to give a more complete picture of the diagnosis. In some cases you will find "if desired" following the term. For the purpose of coding, the "if desired" phrase will not be used. When the term "use additional code...if desired" appears, disregard "if desired" and assign the appropriate additional code.

utilization review A review of individual cases by a committee to make sure that services are medically necessary and to study how providers use medical care resources.

vehemently In a manner marked by forceful energy; intensely emotionally.

veracity A devotion to or conformity with the truth.

verbiage A manner of expressing oneself in words.

verdict The finding or decision of a jury on a matter submitted to it in trial.

versatile Embracing a variety of subjects, fields or skills; having a wide range of abilities.

vested Granted or endowed with a particular authority, right, or property; to have a special interest in.

virtual reality An artificial environment presented to a computer user that feels as if it were a real environment, often involving use of special gloves, earphones, and goggles to enhance the experience.

vocation The work in which a person is regularly employed.

volatile Easily aroused; tending to erupt in violence.

watermark A marking in paper resulting from differences in thickness usually produced by the pressure of a projecting design in the mold or on a processing roll and visible when the paper is held up to the light.

"with" In the context of ICD-9-CM, the terms "with," "with mention of," and "associated with" in a title dictate that both parts of the title be present in the statement of the diagnosis order to assign the particular code.

workers' compensation Insurance against liability imposed on certain employers to pay benefits and furnish care to employees who are injured and to pay benefits to dependents of employees killed in the course of or arising out of their employment.

zip drive A small, portable disk drive that is primarily used for backing up information and archiving computer files. A 100-megabyte Zip disk will hold the equivalent of approximately 70 floppy disks.

Index

Page numbers followed by *t* indicate tables; *f*, figures.